NELSON
ESSENTIALS
OF PEDIATRICS

Second Edition

NELSON

ESSENTIALS
OF PEDIATRICS

Second Edition

Richard E. Behrman, M.D.

Managing Director
Center for the Future of Children
David and Lucile Packard Foundation
Clinical Professor of Pediatrics
Stanford University and University of California, San Francisco
Attending Physician
Lucile Salter Packard Children's Hospital
Stanford, California

Robert M. Kliegman, M.D.

Professor and Chair
Department of Pediatrics
Medical College of Wisconsin
Pediatrician in Chief
Children's Hospital of Wisconsin
Milwaukee, Wisconsin

W. B. SAUNDERS COMPANY
A Division of Harcourt Brace & Company
Philadelphia ■ London ■ Toronto ■ Montreal ■ Sydney ■ Tokyo

W. B. SAUNDERS COMPANY
A Division of Harcourt Brace & Company
The Curtis Center
Independence Square West
Philadelphia, PA 19106

Library of Congress Cataloging-in-Publication Data

Nelson essentials of pediatrics / [edited by] Richard E. Behrman,
    Robert M. Kliegman. – 2nd ed.
        p.   cm.
    Includes bibliographical references and index.
    ISBN 0-7216-3775-2
    1. Pediatrics.   I. Nelson, Waldo E. (Waldo Emerson).
II. Behrman, Richard E.   III. Kliegman, Robert.
IV. Title: Essentials of pediatrics.
    [DNLM: 1. Pediatrics.   WS 100 N425 1994]
RJ45.N418   1994
818.92–dc20
DNLM/DLC   93-24707

International Edition 0-7216-5322-7

NELSON ESSENTIALS OF PEDIATRICS   ISBN 0-7216-3775-2

Last digit is the print number: 9   8   7   6   5   4   3   2

This book is dedicated to those committed to educating the future generations of physicians who will care for children. In a learning process in which "student" and "teacher" are often interchangeable titles, it is hoped that this text will play a catalytic role.

Contributors

HERBERT T. ABELSON, M.D.

Professor and Chairman, Department of Pediatrics, University of Washington School of Medicine; Pediatrician-in-Chief and Director, Department of Medicine, Children's Hospital and Medical Center, Seattle, Washington

Oncology

R. STEPHEN S. AMATO, M.D., Ph.D.

Clinical Professor of Pediatrics, University of Maryland College of Medicine; Lecturer, Pediatrics, Johns Hopkins University; Chairman, Department of Pediatrics, Director, Medical Genetics, Greater Baltimore Medical Center, Baltimore, Maryland

Genetic Disorders

DENNIS D. BLACK, M.D.

Associate Professor of Pediatrics, Pritzker School of Medicine; Associate Professor of Pediatrics, Wyler Children's Hospital, University of Chicago Medical Center, Chicago, Illinois

The Gastrointestinal Tract

STEVEN P. CHERNAUSEK, MD

Associate Professor of Pediatrics, University of Cincinnati School of Medicine, Cincinnati, Ohio. Associate Professor, Children's Hospital Medical Center, Cincinnati, Ohio.

Endocrine Disorders

HOWARD R. FOYE, JR., M.D.

Clinical Associate Professor of Pediatrics, University of Rochester School of Medicine and Dentistry; Associated Attending in Pediatrics, Strong Memorial Hospital, Rochester, New York

Developmental and Behavioral Pediatrics

BRADLEY P. FUHRMAN, M.D.

Professor of Pediatrics, State University of New York at Buffalo; Chief, Pediatric Critical Care, Children's Hospital of Buffalo, Buffalo, New York

The Acutely Ill Child

PAUL C. GILLETTE, M.D.

Professor of Pediatrics and Surgery, Medical University of South Carolina; Director of Pediatric Cardiology; Director, Children's Cardiac Arrhythmia Center, Charleston, South Carolina

The Cardiovascular System

CAROLYN M. KERCSMAR, M.D.

Associate Professor of Pediatrics, Case Western Reserve University, School of Medicine; Director of the Residency Program and the Pediatric Pulmonary Fellowship Program, Cleveland, Ohio
The Respiratory System

BARBARA S. KIRSCHNER, M.D.

Professor of Pediatrics and Medicine, Pritzker School of Medicine, Wyler Children's Hospital, University of Chicago Medical Center, Chicago, Illinois
The Gastrointestinal Tract

ROBERT M. KLIEGMAN, M.D.

Professor and Chair, Department of Pediatrics, Medical College of Wisconsin, Pediatrician in Chief, Children's Hospital of Wisconsin, Milwaukee, Wisconsin
Fetal and Neonatal Medicine

DEBORAH W. KREDICH, M.D.

Associate Clinical Professor of Pediatrics, Duke University School of Medicine, Durham, North Carolina
Rheumatic Disorders of Childhood

RICHARD E. KREIPE, M.D.

Associate Professor of Pediatrics, University of Rochester Medical Center; Acting Chief, Division of Adolescent Medicine, Strong Memorial Hospital, Rochester, New York
Adolescent Medicine

JOHN E. LEWY, M.D.

Professor and Chairman, Department of Pediatrics, Tulane Medical School; Pediatrician-in-Chief, Tulane University Medical Center, New Orleans, Louisiana
Nephrology: Fluids and Electrolytes

ELIZABETH R. McANARNEY, M.D.

Professor and Chairman, Department of Pediatrics, University of Rochester Medical Center; Pediatrician-in-Chief, Strong Memorial Hospital, Rochester, New York
Adolescent Medicine

JOHN F. NICHOLSON, M.D.

Associate Professor of Pediatrics and Pathology, Columbia University College of Physicians and Surgeons; Associate Attending Pediatrician, Director, Clinical Chemistry Service, The Presbyterian Hospital, New York, New York
Inborn Errors of Metabolism

ALICE PRINCE, M.D.

Associate Professor of Pediatrics, Columbia University College of Physicians and Surgeons; Associate Attending Physician, Columbia Presbyterian Medical Center, New York, New York
Infectious Diseases

J. PAUL SCOTT, M.D.

Associate Professor of Pediatrics, The Medical College of Wisconsin; Attending Physician, Children's Hospital of Wisconsin, Milwaukee, Wisconsin
Hematology

MARK A. SPERLING, M.D.

Vira I. Heinz Professor of Pediatrics and Chairman, Department of Pediatrics, University of Pittsburgh, School of Medicine, Pittsburgh, Pennsylvania
Endocrine Disorders

VIRGINIA A. STALLINGS, M.D.

Associate Professor of Pediatrics, University of Pennsylvania, School of Medicine; Chief, Nutrition Section, Children's Hospital of Philadelphia, Philadelphia, Pennsylvania
Pediatric Nutrition and Nutritional Disorders

DENNIS M. STYNE, M.D.

Professor and Chairman, Department of Pediatrics, University of California, Davis, Davis, California
Endocrine Disorders

STEPHEN BRIAN SULKES, M.D.

Associate Professor of Pediatrics, Strong Center for Developmental Disabilities, University of Rochester School of Medicine and Dentistry, Rochester, New York
Developmental and Behavioral Pediatrics

ANDREW M. TERSHAKOVEC, M.D.

Assistant Professor, Department of Pediatrics, University of Pennsylvania School of Medicine; Attending Physician, Division of Gastroenterology and Nutrition, The Children's Hospital of Philadelphia, Philadelphia, Pennsylvania
Pediatric Nutrition and Nutritional Disorders

GEORGE H. THOMPSON, M.D.

Professor of Orthopaedic Surgery and Pediatrics, Director, Pediatric Orthopaedics, Case Western Reserve University; Director, Pediatric Orthopaedics, Rainbow Babies and Children's Hospital, Cleveland, Ohio
Common Orthopaedic Problems in Children

JOHN W. YUNGINGER, M.D.

Professor of Pediatrics, Mayo Medical School; Consultant in Pediatrics and Internal Medicine (Allergy), Mayo Clinic, Rochester, New York
Immunology and Allergy

Preface

The scope of pediatrics has expanded substantially throughout the years that the 14 editions of *Nelson Textbook of Pediatrics* have been published. During this time, progress in biomedical science, technology, and clinical care has advanced our understanding of the normal biology of children and of the pathophysiology and therapy of many diseases of childhood. More recently, advances in biology and genetics have accelerated our basic understanding of genetic disorders and have better enabled us to diagnose and treat diseases that were previously difficult to identify or manage. Consequently, the *Nelson Textbook of Pediatrics* has been expanded in order for it to continue to serve as the major reference text for those who care for children. But this expansion has made it difficult for most medical students to read the entire text during their core pediatric clerkship. In publishing *Nelson Essentials of Pediatrics*, we have focused on essential pediatric problems and have tried to present some overview material to meet the special educational needs of the medical student and the starting house officer.

Nelson Essentials of Pediatrics is primarily intended to introduce important pediatric problems and diseases, representing both the common illnesses of childhood and the less common disorders of special educational importance that exemplify pathophysiologic mechanisms and disease processes. *Nelson Essentials of Pediatrics* is not a "primer" nor is it a synopsis of or a companion to the *Nelson Textbook of Pediatrics*. The term essential does not mean "superficial" or "outlined." Rather, in a readable text with a simplified format and an array of tables and figures, *Nelson Essentials* provides students with sufficient information to improve their understanding of representative pediatric problems and clinical decisions, enabling them to gain a basic understanding of the particular disease process and to develop a clinical approach to a child's problem. In addition, the relatively short text can be digested during the usual length of a core pediatric clerkship.

The contents of this second edition have been updated and it incorporates many helpful suggestions offered by students and faculty who used the first edition. We have organized each chapter in a way that reflects the clinical approach to patients. The student or house officer first should learn to generate a broad differential diagnosis based on the data obtained by taking a history and performing a physical examination; second, to perform an initial analysis of this data, which is facilitated by thinking in terms of the course of the illness (acute or chronic), the organ system involved, and the evidence suggesting that particular pathophysiologic process may be present (e.g., infection or neoplasm); and third, to use this clinical information and its analysis to determine the kind of laboratory data that will further modify and narrow the list of diagnostic possibilities and lead to more specific diagnostic testing.

Besides organizing the chapters to reflect this logical process, we have emphasized both the physiologic and pathophysiologic aspects of pediatric disease, since the understanding of these processes is critical for clinical decision making. Each new contact the student has with a sick child should reinforce their understanding of the pathophysiologic basis of disease.

Presenting the essentials of pediatric medicine does not always permit detailed discussion of the range of variations of each pediatric illness or disease or coverage of all of the less common disorders. To facilitate a student's interests in obtaining additional knowledge, cross references to the relevant sections in the 14th edition of *Nelson Textbook of Pediatrics* are provided as well as selected references to other literature.

The editors wish to express their gratitude and appreciation to the hard working and dedicated authors of the individual chapters. In addition, we thank the many medical students, house staff, and faculty who provided constructive criticism that has improved the final text.

Richard E. Behrman
Robert M. Kliegman

Contents

Developmental and Behavioral Pediatrics

1

Howard R. Foye, Jr.
Stephen B. Sulkes

GROWTH AND DEVELOPMENT

A knowledge of the normal growth and development of children is essential for preventing and detecting disease by recognizing overt deviations from normal patterns. Although the processes of growth and development are not completely separable, it is convenient to refer to "growth" as the increase in the size of the body as a whole or the increase in its separate parts, and to reserve "development" for changes in function, including those influenced by the emotional and social environments. The development of the human organism is a very large, complex topic, but in order to identify and treat underlying disorders, it is important for all who care for children to be familiar with normal patterns of growth and development so that they can recognize abnormal variations.

Every individual's path of growth and development through the life cycle is unique, with a range of complex, interrelated changes occurring from the molecular to the behavioral level. Furthermore, the patterns of development may be very different for individual children within the broad limits that characterize normal development. One goal of pediatrics is to help each child achieve his or her individual potential for growth and development, thus becoming a mature adult. An important means of accomplishing this goal involves periodically monitoring each child for the normal progression of growth and development and screening for abnormalities (Fig. 1–1).

Normal Growth Patterns

Deviations in growth patterns are nonspecific but very important indicators of serious medical disorders. They often provide the first clue that something is wrong, occasionally even when the parents do not suspect a problem. An accurate measurement of height and weight should be obtained at every health supervision visit. In addition, head circumference should be measured at each visit in the first year of life. Serial measurements are much more useful than single measurements because deviations from a particular child's growth pattern can be detected even if the value remains within arbitrarily defined normal limits (e.g., between the 3rd and the 97th percentiles).

Normal growth patterns have spurts and plateaus, so one can expect some shifting on percentile graphs, but large shifts warrant attention. Large discrepancies among height, weight, and head circumference percentiles also deserve attention. For example, when caloric intake is inadequate the weight percentile falls first, then the height, and last the head circumference. A head circumference that is disproportionately large may occur when there is familial megalencephaly, hydrocephalus, or merely "catch-up" growth in a neurologically normal premature infant. Serial measurement of head circumference along with the history (knowing the size of the parents' heads is essential) and the current physical examination would help distinguish among these possibilities.

Whenever possible, growth should be assessed by plotting accurate measurements on growth charts (Figs. 1–2 to 1–14), and comparing them with previous measurements. The most common reasons for deviant measurements are technical (faulty equipment and human errors in measurement or plotting), so the first step in investigating a deviant measurement should be to repeat it. It is also helpful to know some rough rules of thumb, as presented in Table 1–1.

Variability in body proportions occurs from fetal to adult life (Fig. 1–15). In addition, there are individual variations in body forms of normal children (physiques or somatotypes). The **ectomorph** somatotype is characterized by relative linearity, light bone structure, and small mass relative to body length. The **endomorph** has a relatively stocky build, with large amounts of soft tissue, and matures earlier than the ectomorph. The **mesomorph**

1

RECOMMENDATIONS FOR PREVENTIVE PEDIATRIC HEALTH CARE

Committee on Practice and Ambulatory Medicine

Each child and family is unique; therefore these **Recommendations for Preventive Pediatric Health Care** are designed for the care of children who are receiving competent parenting, have no manifestations of any important health problems, and are growing and developing in satisfactory fashion. **Additional visits may become necessary** if circumstances suggest variations from normal. These guidelines represent a consensus by the Committee on Practice and Ambulatory Medicine in consultation with the membership of the American Academy of Pediatrics through the Chapter Presidents. The Committee emphasizes the great importance of **continuity of care** in comprehensive health supervision and the need to avoid **fragmentation of care.**

A **prenatal visit** by the parents for anticipatory guidance and pertinent medical history is strongly recommended.

Health supervision should begin with medical care of the newborn in the hospital.

	INFANCY						EARLY CHILDHOOD					LATE CHILDHOOD					ADOLESCENCE[1]			
AGE[2]	By 1 mo.	2 mos.	4 mos.	6 mos.	9 mos.	12 mos.	15 mos.	18 mos.	24 mos.	3 yrs.	4 yrs.	5 yrs.	6 yrs.	8 yrs.	10 yrs.	12 yrs.	14 yrs.	16 yrs.	18 yrs.	20+ yrs.
HISTORY																				
Initial/Interval	•	•	•	•	•	•	•	•	•	•	•	•	•	•	•	•	•	•	•	•
MEASUREMENTS																				
Height and Weight	•	•	•	•	•	•	•	•	•	•	•	•	•	•	•	•	•	•	•	•
Head Circumference	•	•	•	•	•	•														
Blood Pressure										•	•	•	•	•	•	•	•	•	•	•
SENSORY SCREENING																				
Vision	S	S	S	S	S	S	S	S	S	S	O	O	O	O	S	O	O	S	O	O
Hearing	S	S	S	S	S	S	S	S	S	S	O	O	S[3]	S[3]	S[3]	O	S	S	O	S
DEVEL./BEHAV.[4] ASSESSMENT	•	•	•	•	•	•	•	•	•	•	•	•	•	•	•	•	•	•	•	•
PHYSICAL EXAMINATION[5]	•	•	•	•	•	•	•	•	•	•	•	•	•	•	•	•	•	•	•	•
PROCEDURES[6]																				
Hered./Metabolic[7] Screening	•																			
Immunization[8]		•	•	•			•	•	•			•					•			
Tuberculin Test[9]	←					•→	←		•		→						←		•	→
Hematocrit or Hemoglobin[10]	←				•	→	←		•		→	←		•		→	←		•	→
Urinalysis[11]	←			•		→	←		•		→	←		•		→	←		•	→
ANTICIPATORY[12] GUIDANCE	•	•	•	•	•	•	•	•	•	•	•	•	•	•	•	•	•	•	•	•
INITIAL DENTAL[13] REFERRAL										•										

1. Adolescent related issues (e.g., psychosocial, emotional, substance usage, and reproductive health) may necessitate more frequent health supervision.
2. If a child comes under care for the first time at any point on the schedule, or if any items are not accomplished at the suggested age, the schedule should be brought up to date at the earliest possible time.
3. At these points, history may suffice: if problem suggested, a standard testing method should be employed.
4. By history and appropriate physical examination: if suspicious, by specific objective developmental testing.
5. At each visit, a complete physical examination is essential, with infant totally unclothed, older child undressed and suitably draped.
6. These may be modified, depending upon entry point into schedule and individual need.
7. Metabolic screening (e.g., thyroid, PKU, galactosemia) should be done according to state law.
8. Schedule(s) per Report of Committee on Infectious Disease, *1986 Red Book.*
9. For low risk groups, the Committee on Infectious Diseases recommends the following options: ① no routine testing or ② testing at three times—infancy, preschool, and adolescence. For high risk groups, annual TB skin testing is recommended.
10. Present medical evidence suggests the need for reevaluation of the frequency and timing of hemoglobin or hematocrit tests. One determination is therefore suggested during each time period. Performance of additional tests is left to the individual practice experience.
11. Present medical evidence suggests the need for reevaluation of the frequency and timing of urinalyses. One determination is therefore suggested during each time period. Performance of additional tests is left to the individual practice experience.
12. Appropriate discussion and counselling should be an integral part of each visit for care.
13. Subsequent examinations as prescribed by dentist.

N.B.: **Special chemical, immunologic, and endocrine testing** are usually carried out upon specific indications. Testing other than newborn (e.g., inborn errors of metabolism, sickle disease, lead) are discretionary with the physician.

Key: • =to be performed: S=subjective, by history: O=objective, by a standard testing method.

September 1987

Figure 1–1. Recommendations for preventive pediatric health care. (From Committee on Practice and Ambulatory Medicine, American Academy of Pediatrics. Pediatrics, 81(3), 1988. Copyright American Academy of Pediatrics, 1988.)

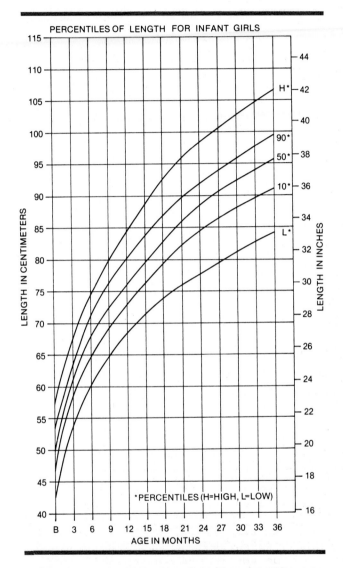

Figure 1–2. Length by age percentiles for girls, ages birth to 36 mo, including highest and lowest values at each age. (From Pomerance HH: Growth Standards in Children. New York, Harper & Row, 1979, p 30.)

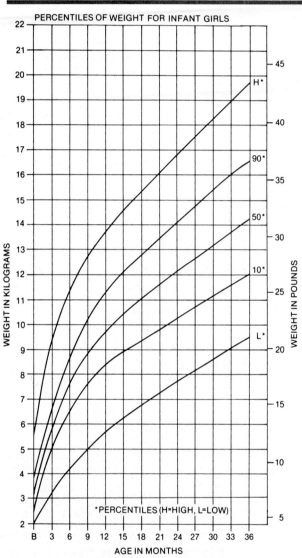

Figure 1–3. Weight by age percentiles for girls, ages birth to 36 mo, including highest and lowest values at each age. (From Pomerance HH: Growth Standards in Children. New York, Harper & Row, 1979, p 26.)

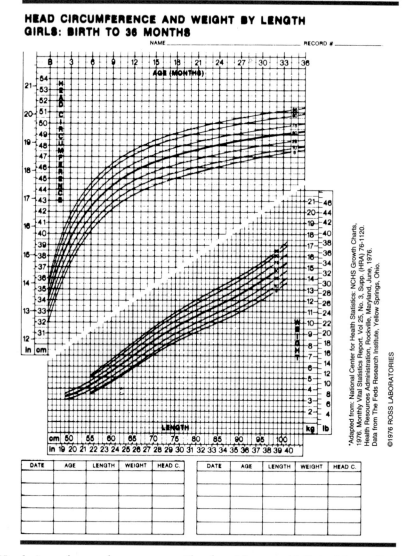

Figure 1–4. *Top,* Head circumference by age percentiles for girls, ages birth to 36 mo. *Bottom,* Weight by length percentiles for girls, ages birth to 36 mo. (From Behrman RE, Vaughn VC [eds]: Nelson Textbook of Pediatrics. 13th ed. Philadelphia, WB Saunders Co., 1992, p 25. Adapted from NCHS Growth Charts by Ross Laboratories.)

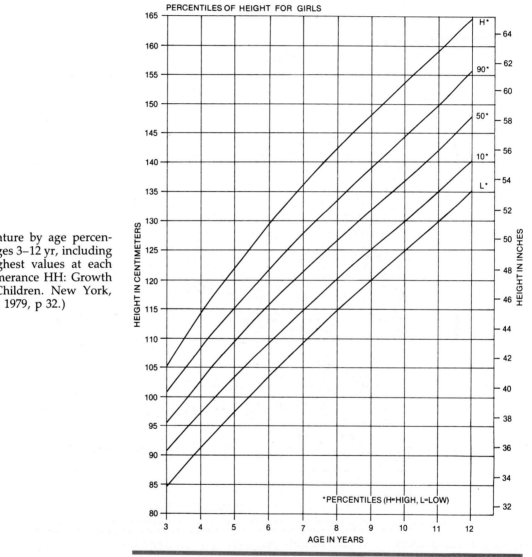

Figure 1–5. Stature by age percentiles for girls, ages 3–12 yr, including lowest and highest values at each age. (From Pomerance HH: Growth Standards in Children. New York, Harper & Row, 1979, p 32.)

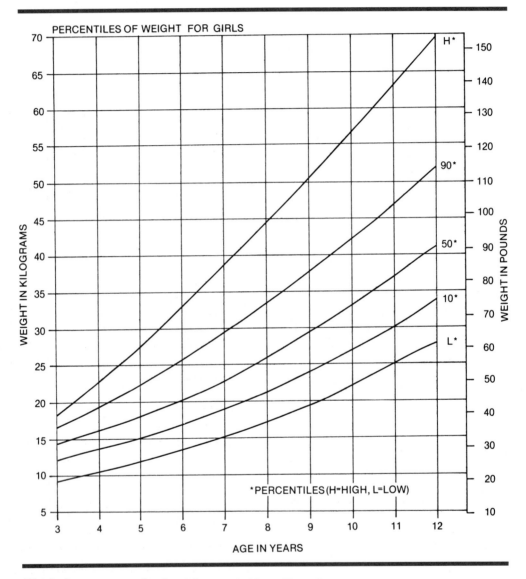

Figure 1–6. Weight by age percentiles for girls, ages 3–12 yr. (From Pomerance HH: Growth Standards in Children. New York, Harper & Row, 1979, p 28.)

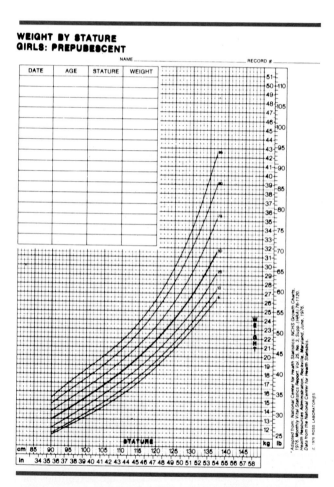

Figure 1–7. Weight by stature percentiles for prepubertal girls. (From Behrman RE, Vaughn VC [eds]: Nelson Textbook of Pediatrics. 13th ed. Philadelphia, WB Saunders Co., 1992, p 25. Adapted from NCHS Growth Charts by Ross Laboratories.)

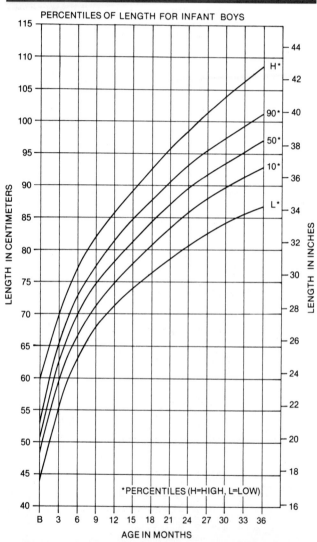

Figure 1–8. Length by age percentiles for boys, ages birth to 36 mo, including highest and lowest values at each age. (From Pomerance HH: Growth Standards in Children. New York, Harper & Row, 1979, p 29.)

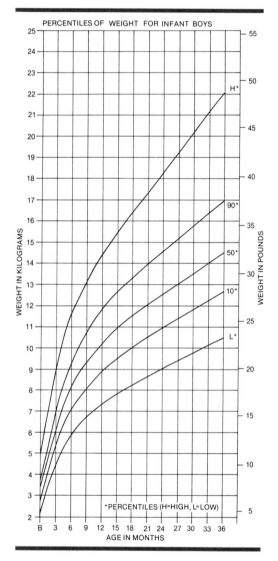

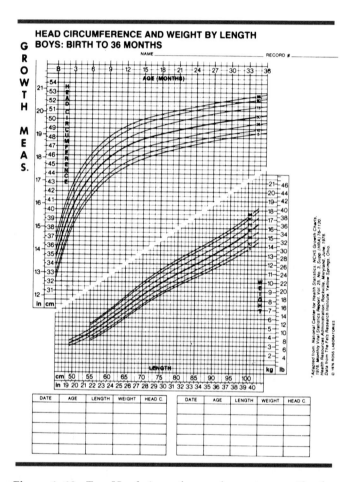

Figure 1–9. Weight by age percentiles for boys, ages birth to 36 mo, including highest and lowest values at each age. (From Pomerance HH: Growth Standards in Children. New York, Harper & Row, 1979, p 25.)

Figure 1–10. *Top,* Head circumference by age percentiles for boys, ages birth to 36 mo. *Bottom,* Weight by length percentiles for boys, ages birth to 36 mo. (From Behrman RE, Vaughn VC [eds]: Nelson Textbook of Pediatrics. 13th ed. Philadelphia, WB Saunders Co., 1992, p 25. Adapted from NCHS Growth Charts by Ross Laboratories.)

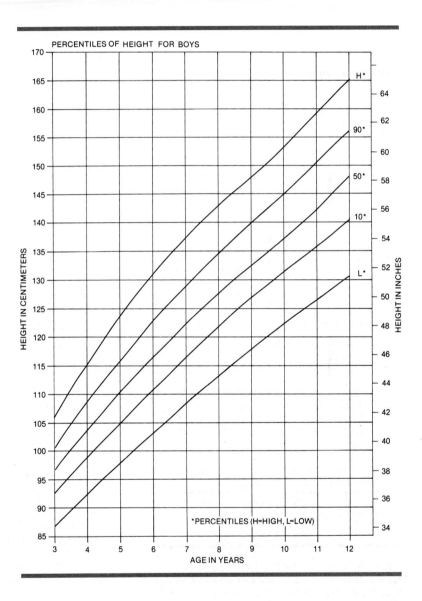

Figure 1–11. Stature by age percentiles for boys, ages 3–12 yr. (From Pomerance HH: Growth Standards in Children. New York, Harper & Row, 1979, p 31.)

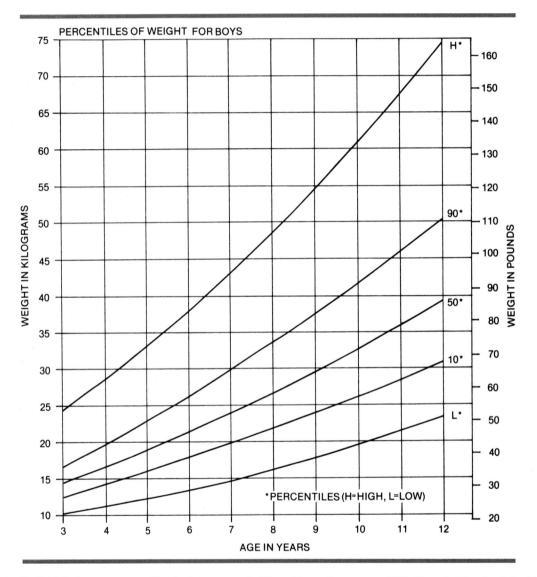

Figure 1–12. Weight by age percentiles for boys, ages 3–12 yr. (From Pomerance HH: Growth Standards in Children. New York, Harper & Row, 1979, p 27.)

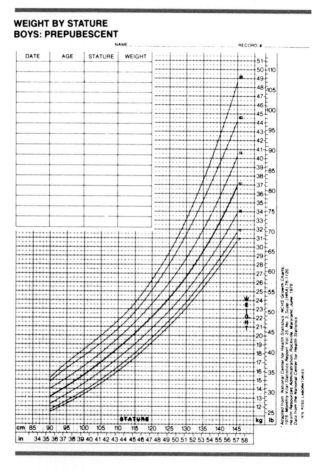

Figure 1–13. Weight by stature percentiles for prepubertal boys. (From Behrman RE, Vaughn VC [eds]: Nelson Textbook of Pediatrics. 13th ed. Philadelphia, WB Saunders Co., 1992, p 25. Adapted from NCHS Growth Charts by Ross Laboratories.)

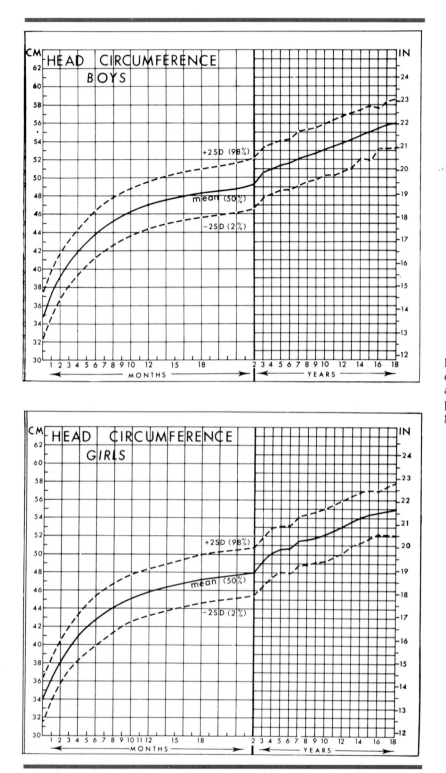

Figure 1–14. Changes in head circumference with age for boys and girls. (From Nellhaus G: Composite international and interracial graphs. Pediatrics 41:106, 1968.)

Table 1–1. Rules of Thumb for Growth

Weight
1. Weight loss in first few days: 5–10% of birth weight
2. Return to birth weight: 7–10 days of age
   Double birth weight: 4–5 mo
   Triple birth weight: 1 yr
   Quadruple birth weight: 2 yr
3. Average weights: 3.5 kg at birth
                      10 kg at 1 yr
                      20 kg at 5 yr
                      30 kg at 10 yr
4. Daily weight gain: 20–30 g for first 3–4 mo
                        15–20 g for rest of the first yr
5. Average annual weight gain: 5 lb between 2 yr and puberty (spurts and plateaus may occur)

Height
1. Average length: 20 in at birth, 30 in at 1 yr
2. At age 3 yr, the average child is 3 ft tall
3. At age 4 yr, the average child is 40 in tall (double birth length)
4. Average annual height increase: 2–3 in between age 4 yr and puberty

Head Circumference (HC)
1. Average HC: 35 cm at birth (13.5 in)
2. HC increases: 1 cm/mo for first yr (2 cm/mo for first 3 mo, then slower)
   10 cm for rest of life

physique lies in between that of the ectomorph and the endomorph and often is relatively muscular. Other differences in body proportions depend on variations in the growth rates of parts of the body or organ systems. Certain growth disturbances result in characteristic changes in the proportional sizes of trunk, extremities, and head.

There are distinctive patterns of proportionate

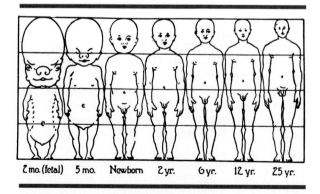

₂ mo. (fetal)   5 mo.   Newborn   2 yr.   6 yr.   12 yr.   25 yr.

Figure 1–15. Changes in body proportions from second fetal month to adulthood. (From Robbins WJ, et al: Growth. New Haven, CT, Yale University Press, 1928, by permission of the publisher.)

growth rates for several body systems that correlate closely with function. Growth of the nervous system is most rapid in the first 2 yr, whereas the growth rate for lymphoid tissue peaks at about 12 yr. Osseous maturation (bone age) is determined from roentgenograms on the basis of (1) the number and size of epiphyseal centers; (2) the size, shape, density, and sharpness of outline of the ends of bones; and (3) the distance separating the epiphyseal center from the zone of provisional calcification. Functional correlations also exist between growing systems. Thus, bone age corresponds more closely to sexual maturity, which is dependent on the growth and development of the endocrine system, than to chronologic age. The heart is relatively large at birth, and a pubertal growth spurt in its size parallels the general growth spurt. Pulse rate and blood pressure vary with age and growth, as do a great many metabolic and nutritional changes.

References

Behrman RE (ed): Nelson Textbook of Pediatrics. 14th ed. Philadelphia, WB Saunders, 1992, Sec. 3.1–3.11.
Knoblock H, Pasamanick B (eds): Gesell and Amatruda's Developmental Diagnosis. 3rd ed. New York, Harper & Row, 1974.
Lowrey GH: Growth and Development of Children. 8th ed. Chicago, Year Book Medical Publishers, 1986.

Developmental Milestones and Theories

The use of developmental milestones to assess development focuses on discrete behaviors that can be observed in the clinical setting or accepted as present by parental report. The approach is based on comparing the patient's behavior with that of many normal children whose behaviors evolve in a uniform sequence and at specific ages. A behavior is the response of the neuromotor system to a specific situation, and the development of this system, like that of other organ systems, is determined largely by genetic endowment. The main influence of the environment on development is its ability to distort the normal pattern.

Norms for discrete behaviors provide a very convenient way to monitor development (see Fig. 1–16 and Assessment section, below), but they provide an incomplete picture. Although a sequence of specific, easily measured behaviors can adequately represent some areas of development (e.g., gross motor, fine motor, language), other areas, particularly social and emotional development, are not adequately assessed by this means. In addition, easily measured developmental milestones are only well established through age 6 yr. Many other types of assessment, including intelligence tests, achievement tests, personality profiles, and neurodevelopmental assessments that expand the developmental milestone approach beyond age 6 yr, are available for all ages, but they generally require time and expertise in administration and/or interpretation that are not available in the primary care medical setting.

Pediatricians therefore need to supplement their screening of developmental milestones with less precise but possibly more important screening of psychosocial issues that are pertinent at each age. The following brief presentation of some developmental theories is intended as an introduction to these important areas. Applications of the theories will be discussed in the sections on assessment, intervention, and topical issues.

PIAGET

Piaget's theory is the major theory of cognitive development. Cognition is defined as the process of knowing in the broadest sense, including perception, memory, judgment, and reasoning. Piaget contends that the development of cognitive ability occurs in a fixed sequence of qualitatively different stages; that is, a child's mind works in different ways in each stage. Table 1–2 presents a brief outline of the major characteristics of each stage. Unrealistic parental expectations often result from lack of understanding about how a child's logic differs from that of an adult. A behavioral problem often can be improved by helping the parent see an episode of problem behavior from the child's perspective.

Piagetian theory also includes the concept of **equilibration,** the mechanism for the formation of knowledge. Equilibration involves two processes that are set in motion when a person is confronted with a new situation that he or she does not fully understand: **assimilation** involves attempts to reshape the new experience to make it fit with accustomed ways of thinking, and **accommodation** involves revisions in the accustomed ways of thinking to fit with the new experience. When the disequilibrium produced by the new experience is resolved by using both processes, a new equilibration is achieved at a higher level of cognitive organization. Disequilibrium, thus, is a necessary stimulus for development. Avoidance of new or unfamiliar experiences will limit the chances for cognitive growth. An important related concept is *cognitive dissonance*, the degree to which a new stimulus differs from familiar stimuli. Novelty attracts children, but if the cognitive dissonance is too great they will be frightened or frustrated and will not achieve a new equilibrium (cognitive growth).

FREUD

Freudian theory contains a number of concepts helpful in understanding child development. The principle of psychic determinism holds that no psychic event happens in a chance or random way but instead is determined by preceding psychic events. "Freudian slips" (e.g., forgetting a meeting that is expected to be stressful) illustrate this principle. At a conscious level these seem to be simple mistakes with no apparent explanation, but the theory contends that unconscious mental processes are responsible for their occurrence. A patient's explanation for a behavior or recounting of an event only taps the conscious level; probing questions may bring more information to the conscious level. The concept of innate sexual and aggressive drives that provide "psychic energy" also is central to Freudian theory. Freud proposed five stages of psychosexual development, with different parts of the body serving as the focus of gratification of the sexual drive at different ages (Table 1–3).

One of Freud's most enduring contributions is his hypothesis about the organization of mental processes into id, ego, and superego. The **id** is the source of the person's impulses and drives and is dominant at birth. The **ego** is the pragmatic, rational part of the mind, consisting of those functions that have to do with the individual's relationship to the environment (sensory perception, motor control, memory, affect, thinking). Initially the ego is the servant of the id, finding ways to achieve gratification of the id impulses. Gradually the ego exerts increasing control over the id in the service of greater long-term gratification and avoidance of discomfort. The **superego,** or "conscience," comprises the moral precepts of an individual's mind and his or her ideal aspirations.

Identification is one of the hypothesized processes by which the ego gains mastery over the id, and is manifested by a child's identifying with people or things that are highly charged with "psychic energy." Identification is apparent in the observation that children behave according to what they see and experience rather than what they are told. Fantasied gratification is another process by which the ego gains mastery over the id. A fantasy (dream or daydream) in which the wishes of the id are represented as fulfilled results in partial gratification of id impulses. The id impulse may be so

Table 1–2. Jean Piaget's Stages of Cognitive Development

Stage	Description	Major Developments
Sensorimotor Birth to 2 yr	Learning occurs through activity, exploration, and manipulation of the environment. Motor and sensory impressions form the foundation of later learning.	Learns to differentiate self from world—beginning sense of self-identity. Formation and integration of schemes—as in learning that sucking on a nipple produces milk or that shaking a rattle produces a noise. Achieves object permanence—that things exist even when not visible. Simple tool use.
Preoperational 2 to 6 or 7 yr	Child capable of symbolic representations of world, as in use of language, play, and deferred imitation. Still not capable of sustained, systematic thought.	Engages in symbolic play—can represent something with something else. Some decline in egocentricity—can take greater account of others' points of view. Develops language and drawing as modes of representing experience.
Concrete Operations 6 or 7 to 11 yr	Child becomes capable of limited logical thought processes, as in seeing relationships and classifying, as long as manipulable, concrete materials are available.	Becomes aware that some aspects of things remain the same despite changes in appearance (conservation). Can mentally reverse a process or action (reversibility). Can focus on more than one aspect of a situation at a time (decentration). Can deduce new relationships from sets of earlier ones (transitivity). Can order things in sequence (seriation). Can group objects on the basis of common features (classification).
Formal Operations 12 yr through adulthood	Can reason logically and abstractly. Can formulate and test hypotheses. Thought no longer depends on concrete reality. Can play with possibilities.	Can deal with abstract ideas. Can manipulate variables in a scientific situation. Can deal with analogies and metaphors. Can reflect on own thinking. Can work out combinations and permutations.

(Adapted from Stone LJ, Church J: Childhood and Adolescence. New York, Random House, 1979, pp 42–43.)

nearly satisfied that it is easy for the ego to control the impulse afterward. This is the idea behind play therapy.

The most important factor in the control of id impulses is anxiety. "Automatic anxiety" develops whenever a child's psyche is overwhelmed by an influx of stimuli too great to be mastered or discharged. These stimuli may be external, but most often they are internal, arising from the id. This type of anxiety is characteristic of infancy because of the immaturity of the ego, but it also is found in adult life in cases of anxiety neurosis. In the course of development, the ego acquires the capacity to produce "signal anxiety" when a potential danger situation arises (i.e., the threat of a traumatic situation), which enables the ego to check or inhibit id impulses. Freud proposed the following sequence of danger situations in early and later childhood that persist unconsciously to some degree throughout life:

Table 1–3. Stage Theories of Socioemotional Development

	Birth–18 mo	18 mo–3 yr	3–6 yr	6–12 yr	Adult
ERIKSON (Psychosocial development)	*Trust vs. Mistrust* Infants learn to trust, or mistrust, that their needs will be met by the world, especially by the mother.	*Autonomy vs. Shame, Doubt* Children learn to exercise will, to make choices, to control themselves, or they become uncertain and doubt that they can do things by themselves.	*Initiative vs. Guilt* Children learn to initiate activities and enjoy their accomplishments, acquiring direction and purpose. If they are not allowed initiative, they feel guilty for their attempts at independence.	*Industry vs. Inferiority* Children develop a sense of industry and curiosity and are eager to learn, or they feel inferior and lose interest in the tasks before them.	*Identity vs. Role Confusion* Adolescents come to see themselves as unique and integrated persons with an ideology, or they become confused about what they want out of life.
FREUD (Psychosexual development)	*Oral Stage* Infants obtain gratification through stimulation of the mouth, as they suck and bite.	*Anal Stage* Children obtain gratification through exercise of the anal musculature during elimination or retention.	*Phallic Stage (Oedipal)* Children develop sexual curiosity and obtain gratification through masturbation. They have sexual fantasies about the parent of the opposite sex and guilt about their fantasies.	*Latency Stage* Children's sexual urges are submerged, they put their energies into acquiring cultural skills.	*Genital Stage* Adolescents have adult heterosexual desires and seek to satisfy them.
PIAGET (see Table 1–2)	*Sensorimotor*	*Preoperational*		*Concrete*	*Formal*

(Adapted from Clarke-Stewart A, Koch JB: Children: Development through Adolescence. New York, John Wiley, 1983, p 11; and Stone LJ, Church J: Childhood & Adolescence. New York, Random House, 1979, pp 42–43.)

1. Loss of the object—separation from a person or thing that is an important source of gratification.
2. Loss of the object's love.
3. Loss of the penis (or analogous genital injury in females).
4. Guilt, or disapproval of the superego.

Defense mechanisms are unconscious ego processes that are focused narrowly on the reduction of anxiety by the control of id impulses. *Repression* occurs when the ego bars from consciousness the unwanted id impulse. Each repression requires a further expenditure of psychic energy. *Suppression* is the conscious equivalent of repression. *Reaction formation* occurs when one of a pair of ambivalent attitudes is made unconscious and kept unconscious by an overemphasis on the other (e.g., love/hate, cruelty/gentleness, and stubbornness/compliance). Reactions to a new sibling may include the use of defense mechanisms like repression (of hostile wishes toward the sibling) and reaction formation (love instead of hate), as well as other ego processes like identification with the mother (imitating caregiving). Other common defense mechanisms include *denial*—the denial of an unpleasant or unwanted piece of external reality (repression involves internal impulses); and *projection*—the attribution of one's own wish or impulse to another person (e.g., the imaginary friend in early childhood). Defense mechanisms are evidence of healthy coping as well as of anxiety. Therefore, in treating anxiety the aim is not to attack the defense mechanism directly, but rather to understand the source of the anxiety that creates the need for the defense mechanism, and to work toward the removal of the source.

According to Freud, the superego is formed as a consequence of identification with the parents' moral demands and prohibitions that arise as part of the resolution of the *Oedipus complex* between the ages of 3 and 6 yr. The Oedipus complex involves an ambivalent attitude toward both parents regardless of the gender of the child (e.g., a wish to eliminate the jealously hated father and take his place in a sensual relationship with the mother). Such wishes arouse fears of retaliation and the loss of love, resulting in the formation of the superego to control the impulses. Subsequently, disapproval by the superego becomes the principal source of anxiety. The consequences of superego functioning may include guilt and unconscious feelings of inferiority but may also include feelings of joy and self-satisfaction.

ERIKSON

Erikson revised and expanded Freud's psychosexual stages into psychosocial stages that span the life cycle. His emphasis is on the development of the ego within a social context rather than on the instinctual drives of the id. Erikson's stages start from a focus on a particular part of the body and then expand to a consideration of the social context of the child's behavior (see Table 1–3). For example, in Freud's oral stage, the major mode of gratification is sucking and feeding. In Erikson's parallel stage, the major psychosocial issue involves the development of "basic trust versus basic mistrust" that the mother will meet the infant's needs. Similarly, in the next stage Erikson goes beyond Freud's narrow focus on bowel control (anal stage) and proposes "autonomy versus shame and doubt" as the central psychosocial issue. Specific behaviors that may serve as the focus of the child's struggle with this psychosocial issue include toilet training but may be generalized to other behaviors that involve control of the body and the environment.

Normal resolution of each psychosocial issue involves the development of a balance between the positive and negative attitudes that characterize the issue, with a ratio favoring the positive. Each issue is never completely resolved but becomes part of the developmental history of the individual, which influences the resolution of each subsequent stage. The sequence of issues proposed by Erikson coincides with the widening circle of societal exposures and demands that are common to all human cultures. Individuals, however, may become fixated at a particular stage, not achieving the balance of attitudes that will permit normal progression to the next stage. More commonly, individuals will **regress** to an earlier stage when a previously attained balance is disrupted by new events and stresses (e.g., birth of a sibling, starting school, illness, separation from loved ones, moves, family turmoil). Puberty and adolescence frequently upset balances achieved in preceding stages and require a reworking of the issues to achieve new balances.

References

Behrman RE (ed): Nelson Textbook of Pediatrics. 14th ed. Philadelphia, WB Saunders, 1992, Sec. 3.13–3.15, 3.19, 3.21.

Brenner C: An Elementary Textbook of Psychoanalysis. Garden City, NY, Doubleday, 1973.

Erikson EH: Childhood and Society. 2nd ed. New York, WW Norton, 1963.

Ginsburg H, Opper S: Piaget's Theory of Intellectual Development. 2nd ed. Englewood Cliffs, NJ, Prentice-Hall, 1979.

Bonding and Attachment

Bonding and attachment are terms that describe the affectional relationships between parents and infants. **Bonding** is a rapid process that occurs immediately or shortly after birth and reflects the feelings of the parents toward the newborn (unidirectional); **attachment** involves reciprocal feelings between parent and infant and develops gradually over the first year. Effective bonding in the postpartum period may enhance the development of attachment. An increased awareness of the importance of bonding has led to significant improvements in routine birthing procedures and postpartum parent-infant contact.

Attachment to a specific, stable mother figure is crucial for a child's normal mental and physical development. Beyond mere feeding and protection, attachment to a primary caregiver also serves to promote exploration of the environment and learning.

Between 9 and 18 mo, children normally become insecure about separation from the primary caregiver. This insecurity coincides with the child's increasing cognitive and motor abilities. The child is beginning to understand simple, immediate, cause-and-effect relationships and thus can anticipate separations (e.g., after Mommy gets her coat), but still has an inadequate appreciation of time and delayed gratification. In addition, the child's new motor skills and attraction to novelty may lead to headlong plunges into new adventures that result in fright or pain followed by frantic efforts to find and cling to the primary caregiver. This often results in dramatic swings from stubborn independence to clinging dependence that can be frustrating and confusing to parents. With a secure attachment, the period of ambivalence may be shorter and less tumultuous.

References

Ainsworth M: The development of infant-mother attachment. In Caldwell BM, Ricciuti HN (eds): Child Development & Social Policy. Review of Child Development Research Series. Vol 3. New York: Russel Sage Foundation, 1973, 1–94.

Behrman RE (ed): Nelson Textbook of Pediatrics. 14th ed. Philadelphia, WB Saunders, 1992, Sec. 3.3, 3.23, 9.6.

Klaus MH, Kennell JH: Parent-Infant Bonding. 2nd ed. St. Louis, CV Mosby, 1982.

Learning Theory

Learning theory postulates that behavior is primarily a product of external environmental determinants and that manipulation of the environmental antecedents and consequences of behavior can be used to modify maladaptive behavior and to increase desirable behavior. **Conditioning** is the process through which behavior is modified by environmental manipulations.

Respondent (classic) conditioning is illustrated by Pavlov's famous experiment in which a dog's salivary response was conditioned to occur at the sound of a bell. The experiment starts with an automatic stimulus–response relationship—food (unconditioned stimulus) stimulating salivation (unconditioned response). Conditioning occurs when another stimulus (bell ringing in Pavlov's experiment) is presented just before or with the unconditioned stimulus (food). After many presentations of the two stimuli together, the bell (conditioned stimulus) alone will elicit the response: salivation (conditioned response). Respondent conditioning has been used to explain **phobic behavior**—a previously unfeared object or stimulus now arouses fear because it is associated with the occurrence of an unconditioned fearful stimulus (e.g., an episode of falling off a diving board leads to a fear of all swimming). Phobias can be treated by desensitization, a process involving training in relaxation techniques, later coupled with gradual exposure to stimuli associated more and more closely with the feared stimulus. The most effective treatment currently available for nocturnal enuresis involves respondent conditioning (see Enuresis).

Operant conditioning modifies behavior by manipulating the antecedents or the consequences of the behavior. The four major methods for operant conditioning are positive reinforcement, negative reinforcement, extinction, and punishment. Many common behavioral problems of children can be helped by these methods.

Positive reinforcement occurs when there is an increase in the frequency of a behavior because it is followed by a favorable event (e.g., the child who eats vegetables more often after he or she receives dessert as a reward). **Negative reinforcement** occurs when there is an increase in the frequency of a behavior because it is followed by the removal or avoidance of an unpleasant event (e.g., a parent's wrath is avoided by staying away from the stove). Reinforcement also may occur unintentionally, increasing the frequency of an undesirable behavior.

Extinction occurs when there is a decrease in the frequency of a previously reinforced behavior because the reinforcement is withheld. This is the principle behind the common advice to ignore behaviors like crying at bedtime or temper tantrums that parents may unwittingly reinforce through attention and comforting. **Punishment** occurs when there is a decrease in the frequency of a behavior because it is followed by an unpleasant consequence.

References

Behrman RE (ed): Nelson Textbook of Pediatrics. 14th ed. Philadelphia, WB Saunders, 1992, Sec. 3.13–3.15.

Hirsh DLO, Russo DC: Behavior management. *In* Levine MD, Carey WB, Crocker AC, Gross RT (eds): Developmental-Behavioral Pediatrics. Philadelphia, WB Saunders, 1983, pp 1068–1099.

Individual Differences

Normal children differ widely in behavior. Failure to appreciate this fact may result in labeling behavior as abnormal or pathologic when the problem may be simply that the behavior does not fit into an expected pattern that is too narrowly defined. Although there are always gray areas between clearly normal and clearly abnormal behavior, in clinical situations the differentiation between abnormal and normal (although perhaps unusual) behavior frequently rests on a judgment of whether the behavior is adaptive. This judgment must be made in the context of the environment in which the individual functions, as well as in the context of the unique physical and mental characteristics of the individual. Alternatively, the physician must avoid explaining away serious problems by attributing them to individual variations in behavior.

There are significant individual differences in the normal development of **temperament** (behavioral style). Thomas and Chess have described three common constellations of temperamental characteristics in a sample of highly educated families.

1. The "easy child" (40%) is characterized by regularity of biologic functions (consistent, predictable times for eating, sleeping, and elimination), positive approach to new stimuli, high adaptability to change, mild or moderate intensity in responses, and a positive mood.
2. The "difficult child" (10%) is characterized by irregularity of biologic functions, negative withdrawal from new stimuli, poor adaptability, intense responses, and a negative mood.
3. The "slow-to-warm-up child" (15%) is characterized by a low activity level, withdrawal from new stimuli, slow adaptability, mild intensity in responses, and somewhat negative mood.

The remaining children had more mixed temperaments. The individual temperament of a child has important implications for parenting and for the advice a pediatrician may give in anticipatory guidance or behavior problem counseling (see Management of Developmental and Behavioral Problems).

References

Behrman RE (ed): Nelson Textbook of Pediatrics. 14th ed. Philadelphia, WB Saunders, 1992, Sec. 3.15.
Thomas A, Chess S: Temperament and Development. New York, Brunner/Mazel, 1977.

Environmental Influences

The important and inseparable contributions of genetic factors (nature) and environmental (nurture) factors are fundamental to the development of each individual and significantly affect the attitudes and advice provided about parenting, education, and governmental policies regarding children. Although we are only beginning to understand the multitude of ways in which the environment can influence development, aspects of the environment clearly play an important role in the etiology and management of many behavioral problems of children.

Reference

Bronfenbrenner U: The Ecology of Human Development. Cambridge, MA, Harvard University Press, 1979.

Adolescence

Early, middle, and late adolescence are characterized by different behavioral and developmental issues (see Table 7–3). The age at which each issue becomes manifest and the importance of the issue will vary widely among individuals, as will the rates of cognitive, psychosexual, psychosocial, or physical development.

During *early adolescence* a young person experiences maximal somatic and sexual growth. Thinking is focused on the present and on the peer group. Identity is focused primarily on the physical changes, and concern is about normality. Exploratory, undifferentiated sexual behavior resulting in physical contact with like-sexed peers is normal during early adolescence, although heterosexual interests can also develop. Strivings for independence are ambivalent.

Middle adolescence can be a most difficult time for both adolescents and the adults who have contact with them. Cognitive processes are more sophisticated. Through formal operational thinking, these adolescents can experiment with ideas, consider things as they might be, develop insight, and reflect on their own feelings and those of others. As they mature cognitively and psychosocially, middle adolescents focus on issues of identity not limited solely to the physical aspects of the body. As middle adolescents socialize with peers, experiment sexually, engage in risk-taking behaviors, and develop employment and interests outside the home, they augment their unique, developing identities. As a result of experimental, risk-taking behaviors, they may experience unwanted pregnancies, drug addiction, or motor vehicle accidents. Middle adolescents' strivings for independence, testing of limits, and need for autonomy are maximal and often distressing to their families, teachers, or other authority figures.

Late adolescence is usually marked by full formal operational thinking, including thoughts about the future (educationally, vocationally, and sexually). Late adolescents are usually more committed to their sexual partners than are middle adolescents. Unresolved separation anxiety from previous developmental stages may emerge at this time as the young person begins to move physically away from the family of origin to college or vocational school, a job, or military service.

References

Behrman RE (ed): Nelson Textbook of Pediatrics. 14th ed. Philadelphia, WB Saunders, 1992, Sec. 3.9.
Sahler OJ, McAnarney ER: The Child from Three to Eighteen. St. Louis, CV Mosby, 1981.

ASSESSMENT

The Primary Care Setting

INITIAL HISTORY AND OBSERVATIONS

Developmental and behavioral problems are more common than any category of problems in pediatrics except acute infections and trauma. Parents often fail to mention these problems because they think the physician is uninterested or cannot help. Therefore, there is a need to screen for their presence in every health supervision visit, particularly in the preschool years when the pediatrician may be the only professional to evaluate the child. The limited time allotted to each health supervision visit will not allow a detailed assessment, but it is essential that a few questions be asked to supplement observations of the child's behavior during the visit. This also will encourage parents to express behavioral and developmental concerns about the child that then can be the focus of anticipatory guidance or early problem solving. Table 1–4 suggests an outline of topics for screening in health supervision visits. The environment in which the child grows and develops is a crucial component of the causes and manifestations of problems, especially behavioral and developmental problems. Furthermore, appropriate approaches to managing these problems depend on the environmental context. Ignorance of the context will result in ineffective and perhaps inappropriate management suggestions from the physician. Table 1–5 lists some of the contextual factors that should be considered in the etiology of a child's behavioral problem.

Building rapport with the parents and the child is a prerequisite for obtaining the often sensitive information that is essential for understanding a behavioral or developmental problem. Rapport usually can be quickly established if the parents sense that the clinician respects them and is genuinely interested in listening to their concerns. Rapport with the child can be developed by engaging him or her in simple conversation or play, providing toys while interviewing the parents, and being

Table 1–4. Topics for Health Supervision Visits

Focus on the Child
Concerns (parent's or child's)
Past problem follow-up
Immunization and screening test update
Routine care (eating, sleeping, elimination, health habits)
Developmental status
Behavioral style and problems

Focus on the Child's Environment
Family
    Caregiving schedule for caregiver who lives at home
    Parent–child and sibling–child interactions
    Extended family role
    Family stresses (work, move, finances, illness, death, marital and other interpersonal relationships)
    Family supports (relatives, friends, groups)

Community
    Caregivers outside the family
    Peer interaction
    School and/or work
    Other activities

Physical environment
    Appropriate stimulation
    Safety

Table 1–5. Context of Behavioral Problems

Child Factors
Health (past and current)
Developmental status
Temperament (e.g., difficult, slow to warm up)
Coping mechanisms

Parental Factors
Misinterpretations of stage-related behaviors
Mismatch of parental expectations and characteristics of child
Parental characteristics (e.g., depression, disinterest, rejection, overprotectiveness)
Coping mechanisms

Environmental Factors
Stress (e.g., marital discord, unemployment, personal loss)
Support (e.g., emotional, material, informational, child care)

Parent–Child Interactions
The common pathway through which the listed factors interact to influence the development of a behavior problem
The key to resolving the behavior problem

sensitive to the fears the child may have. Too often the child is ignored until it is time for the physical examination. Like their parents, children will feel more comfortable if they are greeted by name and involved in pleasant interactions before they are asked sensitive questions or threatened with examinations.

With adolescents, emphasis should be placed on building a doctor–patient relationship with the child that is distinct from the relationship with the parents. This does not mean the parents should be excluded; however, the adolescent should have the opportunity to express concerns to and ask questions of the clinician in confidence. This confidence can be achieved by meeting with the adolescent alone for at least part of each visit. However, confidentiality has limits, and parents must be informed when the clinician has concerns about the health and safety of the child. Often the clinician can convince the child to inform the parents directly of a problem or can reach an agreement with the child about how the parents will be informed.

EXPANDED HISTORY AND OBSERVATIONS

Because the initial health supervision visit is brief, it is best to explore behavioral problems during subsequent visits when more comprehensive information and observations can be obtained, unless the problem is simple and the clinician knows the family well.

Specific interviewing practices will enhance the collection of behavioral information. Responses to open-ended questions often provide clues to underlying, unstated problems and identify the appropriate direction for further, more directed questions. Sensitivity to the way something is said, not just to what is said, provides important clues for content areas to pursue. The interviewer unintentionally may restrict the scope of the discussion by prematurely using directed questions. Histories about developmental and behavioral problems are often vague and confusing, so to reconcile apparent contradictions the interviewer frequently must request clarification (to ascertain the meaning of a word to the patient), more detail, or mere repetition. By summarizing an understanding of the information at frequent intervals and by recapitulating at the close of the visit, the interviewer can ascertain whether he or she and the patient share the same understanding. To build trust and to encourage the patient to talk about difficult issues, the physician must convey respect and empathy for the patient. Empathy is apparent when the physician recognizes the emotions that underlie the patient's responses and communicates this understanding both verbally and nonverbally.

Other techniques for improving the quality of information include the detailed description of a typical day (including parental responses to problem behaviors), and discussion of the physician's observations of the child's behavior and of parent–child and physician–child interactions during the visit. Although the child's behavior during the visit is likely to be unrepresentative of his or her typical behavior, the physician's observations will serve as a springboard for discussion.

A very useful technique is to ask the parents to keep a diary of the occurrence and duration of problem behaviors, as well as the antecedents and parental responses, if possible. This often will reveal a pattern to the behavior that was not previously apparent to the parents. Projective techniques may provide additional useful information (e.g, "What are your happiest, saddest, and maddest moments?" or "If you could have any three wishes, what would they be?"). Third-person techniques (e.g., "Most boys your age are concerned about . . ." or asking about the drinking behavior of friends) may permit a child to talk about an issue that would be too difficult to handle if confronted directly.

If the clinician's impression of the child differs markedly from the parent's description, there may be a crucial parental concern that has not yet been expressed because it may be very difficult for the parent to talk about (e.g., marital problems), or it may be unconscious, or its relevance to the child's behavior may be overlooked by the parent. Alternatively, the physician's observations may be atypical, even with multiple visits. The observations of teachers, relatives, and other regular caregivers may be crucial in sorting out this possibility. The parent also may have a distorted image of the child, rooted in parental psychopathology. A sensitive, supportive, and noncritical approach to the parent may facilitate referral for appropriate therapy.

References

Behrman RE (ed): Nelson Textbook of Pediatrics. 14th ed. Philadelphia, WB Saunders, 1992, Sec. 3.21.

Boyle WE, Hoekelman RA: The pediatrics history. In Hoekelman RA, Blatman S, Friedman SB, et al (eds): Primary Pediatric Care. St. Louis, CV Mosby, 1987, pp 52–62.

SCREENING TESTS

Many clinicians use formal screening tests to detect or better define developmental and/or behavioral problems. The most commonly used tests are described here. As in any screening test, a failed developmental screen implies the need for more conclusive "gold standard" evaluation.

Denver Developmental Screening Test

The Denver Developmental Screening Test (DDST) assesses the development of children from birth to age 6 yr with items in four categories: Personal–Social, Fine Motor–Adaptive, Language, and Gross Motor. Two common criticisms of the DDST include the paucity of language items in the first 2 yr, and questions about its appropriateness for children in some ethnic and social class subgroups. The **Denver II** (see Figs. 1–16 and 1–17) is a substantial revision of the DDST that addresses these criticisms. Language items were added, and all items in the revised test were carefully selected for their reliability and consistency of norms across subgroups. The DDST is very useful as a brief screening instrument but cannot adequately assess the complexities of socioemotional development. In addition, the criteria for passing are set low, which minimizes false positives (labeling normal children as abnormal) but also results in not identifying children with mild but often significant developmental problems. Children with suspect scores therefore must be followed closely.

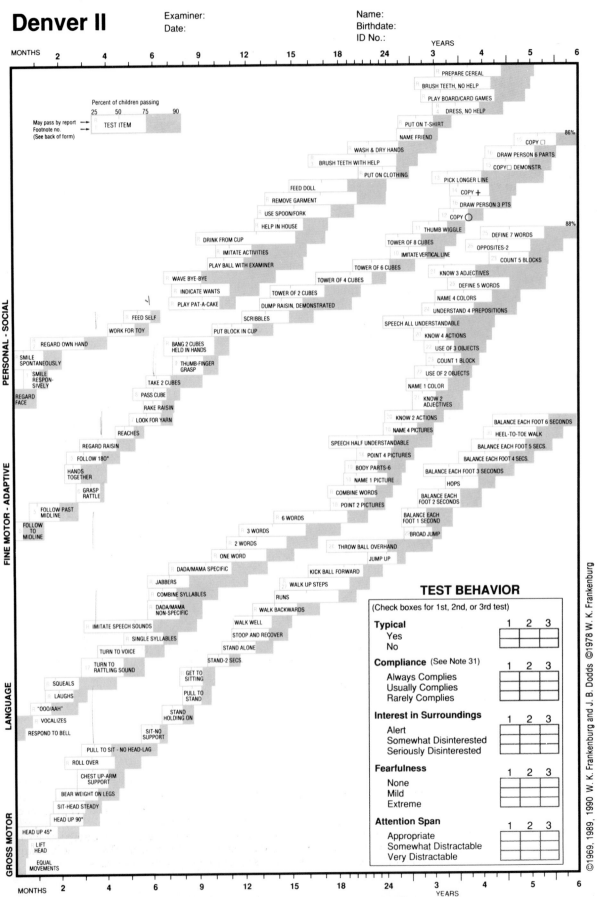

Figure 1–16. Scoring form for Denver Developmental Screening Test (2nd ed.) (Denver II). (From Frankenburg WK, Dodds JB: Denver, CO, Denver Developmental Materials Inc. Copyright 1990 by WK Frankenburg and JB Dodds.)

1. Try to get child to smile by smiling, talking or waving. Do not touch him/her.
2. Child must stare at hand several seconds.
3. Parent may help guide toothbrush and put toothpaste on brush.
4. Child does not have to be able to tie shoes or button/zip in the back.
5. Move yarn slowly in an arc from one side to the other, about 8" above child's face.
6. Pass if child grasps rattle when it is touched to the backs or tips of fingers.
7. Pass if child tries to see where yarn went. Yarn should be dropped quickly from sight from tester's hand without arm movement.
8. Child must transfer cube from hand to hand without help of body, mouth, or table.
9. Pass if child picks up raisin with any part of thumb and finger.
10. Line can vary only 30 degrees or less from tester's line. ∕
11. Make a fist with thumb pointing upward and wiggle only the thumb. Pass if child imitates and does not move any fingers other than the thumb.

12. Pass any enclosed form. Fail continuous round motions.

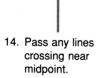

13. Which line is longer? (Not bigger.) Turn paper upside down and repeat. (pass 3 of 3 or 5 of 6)

14. Pass any lines crossing near midpoint.

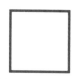

15. Have child copy first. If failed, demonstrate.

When giving items 12, 14, and 15, do not name the forms. Do not demonstrate 12 and 14.

16. When scoring, each pair (2 arms, 2 legs, etc.) counts as one part.
17. Place one cube in cup and shake gently near child's ear, but out of sight. Repeat for other ear.
18. Point to picture and have child name it. (No credit is given for sounds only.)
    If less than 4 pictures are named correctly, have child point to picture as each is named by tester.

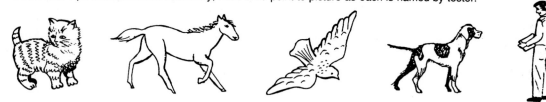

19. Using doll, tell child: Show me the nose, eyes, ears, mouth, hands, feet, tummy, hair. Pass 6 of 8.
20. Using pictures, ask child: Which one flies?... says meow?... talks?... barks?... gallops? Pass 2 of 5, 4 of 5.
21. Ask child: What do you do when you are cold?... tired?... hungry?   Pass 2 of 3, 3 of 3.
22. Ask child: What do you do with a cup? What is a chair used for? What is a pencil used for?
    Action words must be included in answers.
23. Pass if child correctly places and says how many blocks are on paper. (1, 5).
24. Tell child: Put block **on** table; **under** table; **in front of** me, **behind** me. Pass 4 of 4.
    (Do not help child by pointing, moving head or eyes.)
25. Ask child: What is a ball?... lake?... desk?... house?... banana?... curtain?... fence?... ceiling? Pass if defined in terms of use, shape, what it is made of, or general category (such as banana is fruit, not just yellow). Pass 5 of 8, 7 of 8.
26. Ask child: If a horse is big, a mouse is __? If fire is hot, ice is __? If the sun shines during the day, the moon shines during the __? Pass 2 of 3.
27. Child may use wall or rail only, not person. May not crawl.
28. Child must throw ball overhand 3 feet to within arm's reach of tester.
29. Child must perform standing broad jump over width of test sheet (8 1/2 inches).
30. Tell child to walk forward, ∞◁∞◁∞◁➤ heel within 1 inch of toe. Tester may demonstrate.
    Child must walk 4 consecutive steps.
31. In the second year, half of normal children are non-compliant.

OBSERVATIONS:

Figure 1–17. Instructions for DDST (numbers are coded to scoring form [Fig. 1–16]). Abnormal is defined as two or more delays (failure of an item passed by 90% at that age) in two or more categories, or two or more delays in one category with one other category having one delay and an age line that does not intersect one item that is passed. A suspect or questionable score is given if one category has two or more delays or if one or more categories have one delay and in the same category the age line does not pass through one item that is passed. (From Frankenburg WK: Denver Developmental Screening Test [2nd ed.]. Denver, CO, Denver Developmental Materials, Inc.)

An abbreviated DDST has been validated using only 12 items per subject (the three items in each category falling immediately to the left but not touching the age line). This abbreviated test is very helpful in busy clinical settings. A two-stage screening procedure can be used in which every child is given the abbreviated screen and only those with suspect or abnormal scores get a full Denver screen. Another adaptation of the DDST is a parental questionnaire using 97 of the original DDST items (Prescreening Developmental Questionnaire, PDQ). There was a high agreement rate between parent responses and DDST scores in a largely middle-class sample.

Speech and Language Screening

Language screening is important because it correlates best with cognitive development in the early years. Table 1–6 provides some rules of thumb for language development that focus on speech production (expressive language). However, the most dramatic changes in language development in the first years involve the recognition and understanding of speech (receptive language), which is not assessed by these rules and only incompletely assessed by the Denver II. When there is concern about language development, the Early Language Milestone Scales should be used to assess visual, auditory receptive, and auditory expressive communication in the first 36 mo (Fig. 1–18).

Whenever there is a language delay, a hearing deficit must be considered (see Hearing Impairment section). Conditions that have a high risk for an associated hearing deficit are listed in Table 1–7. Early clues that indicate a need for audiologic and speech evaluation are listed in Table 1–8.

Dysfluency ("stuttering") is very common in 3 and 4 yr olds. Unless the dysfluency is severe, is accompanied by tics or unusual posturing, or occurs after age 4 yr, parents should be counseled

Table 1–7. Conditions Considered High Risk for Associated Hearing Deficit

Congenital hearing loss in first cousin or closer relative
Bilirubin of 20 mg/dL or above
Congenital rubella or other nonbacterial intrauterine infection
Defects in the ear, nose, or throat
Birth weight of 1500 g or less
Multiple apneic episodes
Exchange transfusion
Meningitis
5-min APGAR score of 5 or less
Persistent fetal circulation (primary pulmonary hypertension)
Treatment with ototoxic drugs (e.g., aminoglycosides, loop diuretics)

that it is normal and to accept it calmly and patiently. Comments like "relax," "slow down," or "think before you speak" may be counterproductive for a child who already may be too anxious about a behavior over which he or she has little control.

Temperament Questionnaires

The Carey Infant Temperament Questionnaire is widely used to assess temperament in 4 to 8 mo olds. Questionnaires for assessing behavioral style at older ages are also available and can be very helpful in tailoring anticipatory guidance about behavioral issues or management plans for behavioral problems to the individual characteristics of the child.

More Extensive Assessment Instruments

Some pediatricians develop expertise in more extensive assessment instruments, including the Brazelton Neonatal Behavioral Assessment Scale, the Pediatrics Examination of Educational Readi-

Table 1–6. Rules of Thumb for Language Screening

Age (Yr)	Speech Production	Articulation (Amount of Speech Understood by a Stranger)	Following Commands
1	1–3 words		1-step commands
2	2 to 3-word phrases	½	2-step commands
3	Routine use of sentences	¾	
4	Routine use of sentence sequences; conversational give-and-take	Almost all	
5	Complex sentences; extensive use of modifiers, pronouns, and prepositions	Almost all	

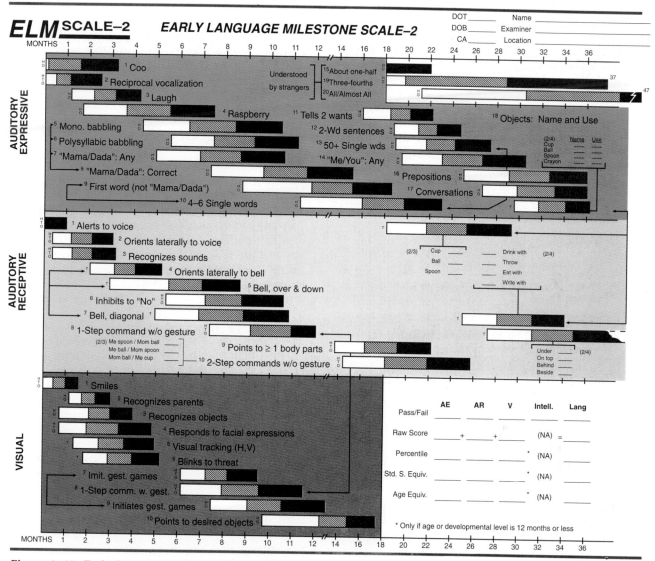

Figure 1–18. Early language milestone scales for auditory and visual development. (Early Language Milestone Scale—2 [ELM Scale—2]: A language screening instrument that covers auditory expressive, auditory receptive, and visual language development from birth to 36 mo, and intelligibility of speech up to 4 yr of age. Austin, TX, PRO-ED, 1987. Copyright 1983, 1993 by James Coplan MD. Reproduced by permission.)

ness, and the Pediatric Early Elementary Examination. These assessments require training for expertise in administration and interpretation.

Team Assessment of Complex Problems

When screening efforts suggest the presence of significant developmental lags, the pediatrician should take responsibility for coordinating the further assessment of the child that is indicated and providing the continuity in the relationship that has developed with the child and family. The physician should become aware of the facilities and programs for assessment and treatment in his or her area. If the child was considered "high risk" because of prematurity or another identified illness that might have long-term developmental impact, a structured follow-up program already may exist to monitor the child's progress. Federal laws mandate that special education programs be provided for all children with developmental disabilities from birth through 21 yr.

MEDICAL ASSESSMENT

The physician's main goals in team assessment are to identify the cause of the developmental dys-

Table 1–8. When a Child with a Communication Disorder Needs Help

0–11 Mo

Before 6 mo, the child does not startle, blink, or change immediate activity in response to sudden loud sounds

Before 6 mo, the child does not attend to the human voice and is not soothed by his or her mother's voice

By 6 mo, the child does not babble strings of consonant + vowel syllables or imitate gurgling or cooing sounds

By 10 mo, the child does not respond to his or her name

At 10 mo, the child's sound-making is limited to shrieks, grunts, or sustained vowel production

12–23 Mo

At 12 mo, the child's babbling or speech is limited to vowel sounds

By 15 mo, the child does not respond to "no," "bye-bye," or "bottle"

By 15 mo, the child will not imitate sounds or words

By 18 mo, the child is not consistently using at least six words with appropriate meaning

By 21 mo, the child does not respond correctly to "Give me - - -," "Sit down," or "Come here" when spoken without gestural cues

By 23 mo, two-word phrases have not emerged that are spoken as single units ("Whatszit," "Thank you," "Allgone")

24–36 Mo

By 24 mo, at least 50% of the child's speech is not understood by familiar listeners

By 24 mo, the child does not point to body parts without gestural cues

By 24 mo, the child is not combining words into phrases ("Go bye-bye," "Go car," "Want cookie")

By 30 mo, the child does not demonstrate understanding of on, in, under, front, and back

By 30 mo, the child is not using short sentences ("Daddy went bye-bye")

By 30 mo, the child has not begun to ask questions, using where, what, why

By 36 mo, the child's speech is not understood by unfamiliar listeners

At any age, the child is consistently dysfluent with repetitions, hesitations, blocks or struggles to say words. Struggle may be accompanied by grimaces, eye blinks, or hand gestures.

(Adapted from Weiss CE, Lillywhite HE: Communication Disorders: A Handbook for Prevention and Early Detection. St. Louis, CV Mosby, 1976.)

function and to identify and interpret other medical conditions that have a developmental impact. The comprehensive history and physical examination should include a careful graphing of growth parameters and an accurate description of dysmorphic features (Chapter 4).

MOTOR ASSESSMENT

Although the traditional neurologic examination provides an excellent basis for evaluating motor function, it should be supplemented by an adaptive functional evaluation. Watching the child at play can aid in such assessment. In addition, standardized tools for evaluating gross and fine motor abilities are utilized by physical and occupational therapists to estimate age-appropriate functional levels.

PSYCHOLOGIC ASSESSMENT

This includes the testing of cognitive ability (Table 1–9) and the evaluation of personality and emotional well-being by a skilled evaluator. IQ and mental age scores, taken in isolation, are only partially descriptive of a person's functional abilities, which are a combination of cognitive, adaptive, and social skills. Tests of achievement are subject to variability based on experience and must be standardized for social factors. Projective and nonprojective tests are useful in understanding the child's emotional status. Although a child should not be labeled as having a problem solely on the basis of a standardized test, such tests do provide important and reasonably objective data for evaluating a child's growth within a particular educational program.

EDUCATIONAL ASSESSMENT

This refers to the evaluation of areas of specific strengths and weaknesses in reading, spelling, written expression, and mathematical skills. Schools routinely screen children with group tests to aid in problem identification and program evaluation. For the child with special needs, this should ultimately lead to individualized testing and the development of an individualized educational plan (IEP) that will enable the child to progress comfortably in school. Diagnostic teaching, in which the child's response to various teaching techniques is assessed, also may be helpful.

Table 1–9. Tests of Cognition

Test	Age Range	Special Features
Infant Scales		
Bayley Scales of Infant Development	2–30 mo	Mental, psychomotor scales, behavior record; weak intelligence predictor
Cattell Infant Intelligence Scale	Birth–30 mo	Used to extend Stanford-Binet downward
Gesell Developmental Schedules	Birth–3 yr	Used by many pediatricians
Ordinal Scales of Infant Psychological Development	Birth–24 mo	Six subscales; based on Piagetian stages; weak in predicting later intelligence
Preschool Scales		
Stanford-Binet Intelligence Scale (4th ed)	2 yr–adult	Four area scores, with subtests and composite IQ score
McCarthy Scales of Children's Abilities	2½–8 yr	6–18 subtests; good at defining learning disabilities; strengths/weaknesses approach
Wechsler Primary and Preschool Test of Intelligence–Revised (WPPSI-R)	3–6½ yr	11 subtests; Verbal, Performance IQs; long administration time; good at defining learning disabilities
Merrill-Palmer Scale of Mental Tests	2–4½ yr	General test for young children
Differential Abilities Scale	2½ yr–adult	Special nonverbal composite; short administration time
School-Age Scales		
Stanford-Binet Intelligence Scale (4th edition)	2 yr–adult	See above
Wechsler Intelligence Scale for Children (3rd ed) (WISC III)	6–16 yr	See comments on WPPSI-R
Leiter International Performance Scale	2 yr–adult	No verbal abilities needed
Wechsler Adult Intelligence Scale–Revised (WAIS-R)	16 yr–adult	See comments on WPPSI-R
Differential Abilities Scale	2½ yr–adult	See above
Adaptive Behavior Scales		
Vineland Adaptive Behavior Scale	Birth–adult	Interview/questionnaire; typical persons + blind, deaf, and retarded
American Association on Mental Retardation (AAMR) Adaptive Behavioral Scale	3 yr–adult	Useful in retardation, other disabilities

SOCIAL ENVIRONMENT ASSESSMENT

Assessment of the environment in which the child is living, working, playing, and growing is also important in understanding the child's development. A home visit by a social worker, community health nurse, or home-based intervention specialist can provide valuable information about the child's social milieu.

References

Behrman RE (ed): Nelson Textbook of Pediatrics. 14th ed. Philadelphia, WB Saunders, 1992, Sec. 3.11–3.15, 3.21, 22.19.

Carey WB: The difficult child. Pediatr Rev 8:39, 1986.

Coplan J: Evaluation of the child with delayed speech or language. Pediatr Ann 14:203, 1985.

Frankenburg WK, Dodds J, Archer P, et al: Denver II: A major revision and restandardization of the Denver Developmental Screening Test. Pediatrics 89:91, 1992.

MANAGEMENT OF DEVELOPMENTAL AND BEHAVIORAL PROBLEMS

Intervention in the Primary Care Setting

After assessment, the clinician must decide whether a problem requires referral for further diagnostic work-up and/or management, or whether management in the primary care setting is appropriate. Some of the counseling roles required in caring for these children are listed in Table 1–10 and discussed below. In this context, the word "patient" refers to the child and/or parent. When a child is young, much of the counseling interaction takes place between the parents and the clinician, but as the child matures direct counseling shifts increasingly toward the child.

The assessment process (particularly that of expanded history and observations) may be therapeutic in itself. By assuming the role of a nonjudgmental, supportive listener, the clinician may create a climate of trust in which the patient feels free to express difficult or even painful thoughts and feelings. Ventilation of these feelings alone may be helpful, but in addition, it may free the patient from a preoccupation with previously unexpressed emotions, allowing the patient to move on to the work of understanding and resolving the problem.

Interview techniques also may facilitate clarification of the problem for the patient as well as the clinician. The patient's ideas about the causes of the problem and descriptions of attempts to deal with it may provide a basis for developing strategies for problem management that are much more likely to be implemented because they emanate in part from the patient. Furthermore, the respect shown by the clinician in endorsing the patient's ideas, when appropriate, can have a positive impact on the patient's self-esteem and sense of competency. The provision of reassurance appropriate to the patient's concern is potentially of great additional benefit but, if given too hastily and nonspecifically, it may suggest a lack of regard for the patient.

The provision of patient education regarding normal and aberrant development and behavior may prevent problems through early detection and anticipatory guidance. Early detection is important because intervention can be started before the problem becomes entrenched and associated problems develop.

Specific parenting advice frequently is provided, because many parents expect and need specific, detailed guidelines from the clinician. Other parents will work out the details if the clinician first provides some general principles and guidelines. When the parents or child play a relatively passive role in the development of the plan, it is particularly important to give them a written copy of the plan to review and to be certain that the details are fully understood. Specific suggestions for changes in the family environment often are very helpful. Perhaps the most frequently helpful suggestion is to arrange for respite and increased emotional support for the primary caregiver, who usually is discouraged and exhausted by the time the clinician hears about the problem. The clinician also may suggest other community services to relieve pressure and to improve the coping ability of the family (e.g., nursery school, tutors, recreational programs, and parent support and education groups).

Most developmental and behavioral problems appear simple when initially presented, and often a small amount of education, reassurance, and a few simple suggestions are sufficient. Follow-up is crucial, however, because complex problems often present as simple problems, and clinicians must be ready to accept failure of their suggestions without attributing the failure to inadequacy in the parents' application of the recommendations. Indications for referral to developmental disability or mental health specialists will vary according to the expertise of the primary care clinician, but children should not be followed for long periods of time in the hope that they will "outgrow" the problem. After referral, the clinician is needed to help coordinate and interpret the evaluations and recommendations.

Table 1–10. Primary Care Counseling Roles

Allow ventilation
Facilitate clarification
Support patient problem solving
Provide specific reassurance
Provide education
Provide specific parenting advice
Suggest environmental interventions
Provide follow-up
Facilitate appropriate referrals
Coordinate care and interpret reports after referrals

Counseling Principles

In order to effect a change in behavior, the change must be learned, not imposed. It is easiest to learn when the lesson is simple, clear, and consistent and presented in an atmosphere free of fear or intimidation. Parents often try to impose behavioral change in an emotionally charged atmosphere. Clinicians often try to "teach" parents with hastily presented advice when the parent is distracted by other concerns. The teacher (parent or clinician) must also remember that patient repetition is the mother of learning.

Apart from management strategies directed specifically at the problem behavior, regular times (at least 15–30 min/day) for *positive parent–child interaction* should be instituted. Frequent, brief, affectionate physical contact over the day may be helpful by providing opportunities for positive reinforcement of desirable child behaviors and for building a sense of competence in the child and the parent.

Guilt is felt by almost all parents when their child has a developmental-behavioral problem. This may be due to the assumption or fear that the problem was caused by inadequacy in their parenting, or they may feel guilty about previous angry responses they have had to the child's behavior (e.g., excessive physical punishment or derogatory comments). The clinician should not unwittingly contribute to parental guilt with insensitive comments that may be construed as criticism by the parents. Guilt may be a serious impediment to problem solving and can be diffused by honestly pointing out how often other parents have similar problems and by empathizing with the difficulties of coping with the problem.

It is usually beneficial to find ways to increase support for the primary caregiver. A mother is better able to nurture a child well when she is well nurtured herself.

The clinician must be careful of using developmental or behavioral labels, even though they may be helpful in diagnosis and management. They can become self-fulfilling prophecies as the people in the child's environment treat the child as "difficult," which becomes part of the child's self-concept.

Interdisciplinary Team Intervention

In many cases, the breadth and quality of services needed to serve appropriately the child who has developmental problems require a team of professionals. This is commonly the case in follow-up programs for infants leaving intensive care nurseries. Although such Early Intervention Programs are now mandated across the United States, the physician may play a key role in guiding the child and family to these services. Once the child reaches school age, the public school system takes increasing responsibility for developmental/educational services, and the physician's role becomes primarily one of consultation on medically related issues.

Educational intervention for the young child begins as a home-based infant stimulation program, often using an early childhood educator, nurse, or occupational, speech, or physical therapist to provide direct stimulation for the child and to train the family to provide the stimulation. As the child matures, a center-based nursery program may be indicated. For the school-age child, special services may range from extra attention given by the classroom teacher to a self-contained special educational classroom. Home-based tutoring or residential programs typically are reserved for only the most behaviorally or cognitively impaired children in this age range.

Psychologic intervention may take several forms. Therapy may be parent or family directed or may become, with the older child, purely child directed. The types of therapy include guidance therapies such as directive advice-giving, counseling the family or child in their own solutions to problems, psychotherapy, behavior management techniques, psychopharmacologic methods, and cognitive therapy.

Motor intervention may be performed by a physical or occupational therapist, or by another professional under his or her direction. Neurodevelopmental therapy (NDT), the most commonly used method, is based on the concept that nervous system development is hierarchical and subject to some plasticity. The focus is on gait training and motor development, including daily living skills and perceptual abilities to assist in the guidance of motor activity, such as eye–hand coordination, spatial relationships, and motor sequencing. A recent trend is to structure sensory experience from the tactile, proprioceptive, and vestibular systems to allow for adaptive motor responses.

Speech and language intervention by the speech therapist is usually part of the overall educational program and is based on the tested language strengths and weaknesses of the child. Children requiring this type of intervention may demonstrate difficulties in reading and other academic areas, as well as develop social and behavioral problems owing to their difficulties in being understood and in understanding others.

Hearing intervention, performed by the audiologist and otolaryngologist, includes monitoring hearing acuity, providing amplification when necessary via hearing aids, and treating ear infections.

Social and environmental intervention generally takes the form of nursing or social work involvement with the family. Frequently the role of case manager, coordinating the services of other disciplines, falls to these specialists.

Medical intervention for the child with a developmental disability involves providing primary care and specific treatment of conditions associated with disability. Curative treatment often is not possible owing to the irreversible nature of many causes of developmental disabilities. Certain general medical problems are found more frequently in the mentally retarded/developmentally disabled population (Table 1–11).

Table 1–11. Recurring Medical Issues in the Developmentally Disabled

Problem	Ask About or Check
Motor	Range of motion examination; scoliosis check; assess mobility; interact with orthopedist, physiatrist, and PT/OT as needed
Other syndrome-specific problems	Ongoing evaluation of other "physical" problems as indicated by known MR/DD etiology
Diet	Dietary history, feeding observation, growth parameter measurement and charting, supplementation as indicated by observations
Sensory impairments	Functional vision and hearing screening; interaction as needed with audiologist, ophthalmologist
Dermatology	Examine ALL skin areas for decubitis ulcers or infection
Dentistry	Examine teeth and gums; confirm access to dental care
Behavioral problems	Aggression, self-injury, pica; sleep problems; psychotropic drug levels and side effects
Advocacy	Educational program, family supports, financial supports
Seizures	Major motor, absence, other suspicious symptoms; monitor anticonvulsant levels and side effects
Infectious diseases	Ear infections, diarrhea, respiratory symptoms, immunizations (especially hepatitis B)
Constipation (GI problems)	Constipation, gastroesophageal reflux, GI bleeding (stool for occult blood)
Sexuality	Sexuality education, hygiene, contraception (when appropriate), ± genetic counseling

GI = gastrointestinal; MR/DD = mental retardation/developmental disability; PT/OT = physical therapist/occupational therapist.

References

Behrman RE (ed): Nelson Textbook of Pediatrics. 14th ed. Philadelphia, WB Saunders, 1992, Sec. 3.55.

Johnston RB, Magrab PR: Developmental Disorders: Assessment, Treatment, and Education. Baltimore, University Park Press, 1976.

Levine MD, Carey WB, Crocker AC (eds): Developmental-Behavioral Pediatrics. 2nd ed. Philadelphia, WB Saunders, 1992, pp 597–674.

Crying

The compelling sound of an infant's cry makes it an effective distress signal and appropriate to the human infant's prolonged dependence on a caregiver. However, cries are discomforting and may be alarming to parents, many of whom find it very difficult to listen to their infant's crying for even short periods of time.

Many reasons for crying are obvious, such as hunger and discomfort due to heat, cold, illness, and lying position. These reasons, however, account for a relatively small percentage of infant crying and usually are recognized quickly and alleviated. In the absence of a discernible reason for the behavior, crying often stops when the infant is held. In most infants, there are frequent episodes of crying with no apparent cause, and holding or other soothing techniques seem ineffective. Infants cry and fuss for a mean of $1\frac{3}{4}$ hr/day at age 2 wk, $2\frac{3}{4}$ hr/day at age 6 wk, and 1 hr/day at 12 wk. Counseling about normal crying may relieve guilt and diminish concerns, but for some the distress caused by the crying cannot be suppressed by logical reasoning. For these parents, respite from exposure to the crying may be necessary to allow them to cope appropriately with their own distress. Without relief, fatigue and tension may result in inappropriate parental responses such as leaving the infant in the house alone or abusing the infant.

Colic

Colic is characterized by periods of unexplained irritability and crying in healthy, well-fed infants. The crying may be intense, and may be brief or last for hours. The episodes typically recur in the late afternoon or evening but may occur at any time. The onset is usually in the first 2–3 wk with resolution by 3 mo, although it sometimes lasts much longer. Colic occurs in 10–20% of infants. Its etiology, although unknown, is probably multifactorial, with infant, parent, and environmental factors playing potentially important roles.

Management begins with sympathetic listening to the parents' frustration and concern, which should not be quickly dismissed with vague reassurance that lots of crying is to be expected. Education about normal crying patterns, specific reassurance about health concerns, suggestions about techniques for consoling the infant, and recommendations for increased support and respite for the primary caregiver often are helpful.

The most effective and appropriate intervention for a crying episode is to pick up and soothe the infant. Greater maternal responsiveness to cries in the first 3 mo is associated with decreased crying and increased use of other forms of communication by the infant later in the first year. For some, however, this is impractical, particularly if the infant must be carried virtually all the time to control crying. Also, when a crying episode does not respond to holding, prolonged attempts to soothe the infant may be counterproductive, serving only to increase parental fatigue and guilt. The interactions may become tense, abrupt, and even hostile, with resulting escalation of the infant's irritability. In order to optimize parental ability to be sensitive and responsive to their infant, parents need to be well rested and to have some time for themselves.

Other techniques that may work include gentle motion (e.g., automatic rockers, stroller or car rides), continuous monotonous noise or music (e.g., mechanical alarm clock, radio), pacifier, or a warm water bottle next to the abdomen. Although only a small percentage of colic cases may be caused by food intolerance, the practice of changing formulas remains popular because it allows time for the colic to resolve on its own. Sedatives may be indicated for a limited time to break the cycle of crying and loss of sleep when the family can no longer cope with the problem; choices include diphenhydramine (1 mg/kg) or chloral hydrate (25 mg/kg) 1 hr before the worst period of crying each day (or before the parents' bedtime) for 1–2 wk. An often effective alternative is to encourage the parents to arrange for a weekend or longer away from the infant.

References

Behrman RE (ed): Nelson Textbook of Pediatrics. 14th ed. Philadelphia, WB Saunders, 1992, Sec. 3.3, 3.30, 3.38, 4.9, 4.13, 20.1.

Mones RL, Asnes RS: The colicky baby: Helping parents cope. Contemp Pediatr April:86–98, 1986.

Discipline

Discipline involves teaching, not merely punishment, to eliminate bad behavior. The ultimate goal is the child's self-control. Overbearing punishment to control a child's behavior will interfere with the learning process and focus on external control at the expense of the development of self-control.

Commonly used and effective techniques to control the undesirable behavior of children include scolding, physical punishment, and threats. However, these techniques have potential adverse side effects on children's sense of security and self-esteem. The effectiveness of scolding diminishes the more it is used, and it should not be allowed to expand from an expression of displeasure about a specific event to derogatory statements about children that may be interpreted as loss of love for them. Scolding also may escalate to the level of psychologic abuse. Frequent mild physical punishment also may become less effective and tempt the parent to escalate the physical punishment, increasing the risk of child abuse. Threats by parents to leave or give up the child are perhaps the most powerful and psychologically damaging ways to control a child's behavior. Children of any age may remain fearful and anxious about loss of the parent long after the threat is made. An alternative common technique is positive reinforcement for desirable behavior. It is a powerful tool for molding a child's behavior, particularly when it is given immediately after the behavior occurs. It fosters self-control and self-esteem.

Parenting involves a dynamic balance between *setting limits* on the one hand and allowing and encouraging freedom of expression and exploration on the other. Children whose behavior is out of control improve when clear limits on their behavior are set and enforced. In general, children find comfort and security in clear limits. However, parents must agree on where the limit will be set and how it will be enforced. Then the limit and the consequence of breaking it must be clearly presented to the child, keeping in mind the cognitive ability of the child. Enforcement of the limit should be consistent and firm. Too many limits will be hard to learn and may thwart the normal development of autonomy. The limit must be reasonable in terms of the child's age and temperament.

The *extinction procedure* is a systematic way to eliminate a frequent, annoying, and relatively harmless behavior by ignoring it. It involves recording the frequency of the behavior in the baseline phase in order to appreciate realistically the magnitude of the problem and to evaluate progress in eliminating it. To determine what reinforces the behavior (and therefore what needs to be consistently eliminated), it is essential to record the consequences of the behavior before any changes are made in the parental response or in other environmental factors. An appropriate behavior is identified to give the child a positive alternative that the parents can reinforce. Parents should be warned that the annoying behavior usually increases in frequency and intensity (may last weeks) before it decreases when the parent ignores it (removes the reinforcement).

The *time-out procedure* is another very useful technique to modify inappropriate behaviors that cannot be ignored. It consists of a short period of isolation that interrupts the behavior. It requires considerable effort by the parents initially. Simple isolation techniques, such as making a child stand in the corner or sending a child to his or her room, may be effective. If they are not, a more systematic procedure may be needed. For example, one very effective protocol for the time-out procedure involves interrupting the child's play when the behavior occurs and having the child sit in a dull, isolated place for a brief period, measured by a portable kitchen timer. This inescapable and unpleasant consequence of the undesired behavior motivates the child to learn to avoid the behavior. If done matter-of-factly and with a minimum of expressed anger by the parent, such a time-out procedure is a potent teaching tool with less chance for adverse side effects than other commonly employed discipline techniques.

References

Behrman RE (ed): Nelson Textbook of Pediatrics. 14th ed. Philadelphia, WB Saunders, 1992, Sec. 3.15, 3.38.
Christophersen ER: Anticipatory guidance on discipline. Pediatr Clin North Am 33:789, 1986.

Enuresis

Enuresis is urinary incontinence at any age when urinary continence is considered normal. Enuresis is primary when the child has never been continent of urine for a prolonged period and secondary when incontinence recurs after a prolonged period of continence (6–12 mo). *Nocturnal enuresis* is the most common type. At least one episode of **bedwetting** per month occurs in 15–30% of 6 yr olds (higher in boys and blacks) and 4–16% of 12 yr olds. The prevalence of bedwetting is so common before age 6 yr that it is not called enuresis. About 20% of bedwetters after age 4 yr, however, have secondary enuresis, which warrants a more careful evaluation. *Daytime enuresis* has a prevalence rate of only about 1% in 6–12 yr olds, with no gender prevalence. Most children are continent of urine during waking hours by age 3–4 yr.

An organic *etiology* is present in less than 5% of children with primary enuresis and in only 1% of children with primary nocturnal enuresis. The reason for almost all primary enuresis is a delay in the maturation of urethral sphincter control. This immaturity may be prolonged by a psychologic overlay related to concerns about the problem on the part of parents and the child. Secondary enuresis usually is due to a psychologically stressful event or condition but also is more likely than primary enuresis to have an organic cause. A urinary tract infection is the most common organic etiology. Uncommon causes include chemical distal urethritis (e.g., from bubble bath), congenital anomalies (e.g., spina bifida), severe lower urinary tract obstruction (e.g., from posterior urethral valves, urethral cyst, or urethral duplication), ectopic ureter, diabetes mellitus or insipidus, and pelvic masses (e.g., presacral teratoma, fecal impaction, hydrocolpos).

In addition to incontinence, other related *clinical manifestations* of organic causes include dysuria, frequency, hematuria, straining on urination, dribbling, small-caliber stream, stress incontinence (with coughing, lifting, or running), gait disturbance, poor bowel control, and continuous dampness. A careful history and physical examination can rule out unusual causes. Urinalysis and a urine culture should be performed at the initial visit.

Treatment is usually not recommended before age 6 yr because spontaneous cure rates are high. Even after age 6 yr, the spontaneous cure rate for primary enuresis is 15%/yr; for secondary enuresis without an organic cause, spontaneous cure rates are also high.

Three commonly used treatments are counseling (Table 1–12), enuresis alarms, and imipramine. Enuresis alarms are the most effective treatment currently available. Cure rates are about 70%, with relapse rates of 10–15% in 5–15 yr olds. Complete success often takes several months. Imipramine has a high rapid initial response rate within the first week, but the relapse rate after discontinuation of the drug is so high that the long-term cure rate when the patient is taken off the drug is barely above the spontaneous cure rate. The dose of imipramine is 50 mg before bedtime for 8–12 yr olds and 75 mg for children over age 12 yr. After 1 mo without enuresis, the drug should be tapered over 2–4 wk. Untoward effects include anticholinergic

Table 1–12. Enuresis Counseling

Child assumes active, responsible role
  Keeps calendar of wet and dry nights
  Talks to physician
  Urinates just before bedtime
  Changes wet clothes and bedding

Fluids not given after dinner

Punishments and angry parental responses avoided

Positive reinforcement given for each dry night (star chart or other reward, depending on age)

Reassurance given about etiology and prognosis (aim is to remove blame and guilt)

symptoms, bone marrow suppression, and life-threatening accidental ingestions. Blood counts should be taken every 2–4 wk while the patient is on therapy.

References

Behrman RE (ed): Nelson Textbook of Pediatrics. 14th ed. Philadelphia, WB Saunders, 1992, Sec. 3.28.

Encopresis

Encopresis is incontinence of fecal material at any age when fecal continence is considered normal. In the United States, bowel control is usually achieved between 2 and 3 yr of age, and encopresis usually refers to regular fecal incontinence after age 4 yr. It involves a continuum from mild fecal soiling of underwear to the passage of larger amounts of fecal material. Encopresis has a prevalence of about 1% in 1st and 2nd graders; about 80% of those with encopresis are boys.

The *pathogenesis* of encopresis is based on retention of stool. The retention may be intermittent or partial, with the child having regular but incomplete defecation. With increasing retention, sensory feedback from the bowel is reduced, the rectal wall is stretched and loses contractile strength, and water absorption from fecal material increases, resulting in larger and harder feces. The result is a vicious circle in which the child has less control of his or her bowel movements.

Etiologic factors that contribute to the development of encopresis include constitutional predisposition for inefficient intestinal motility, overly aggressive and prolonged medical management (laxatives, enemas, and suppositories), dietary manipulation for perceived constipation, anal fissures and rashes that cause pain on defecation, and surgical procedures for imperforate anus and other anorectal conditions. Parental overreaction to irregular frequency or form of bowel movements may result in inappropriate use of medications or diet changes and/or counterproductive demands on the child. Not only may demands be impossible for the child to meet (i.e., he or she may not yet be ready for toilet training), but parental coercion may stimulate the negativism and resistance that characterize the toddler's budding autonomy. Toileting may be perceived as a negative experience by the child, who may withhold stool out of a need to exercise control or out of fear for the consequences of soiling. The resulting increased retention exacerbates the problem. During the preschool years, irrational fears of the toilet also often result in withholding. During the school years, rigid or hurried schedules or reluctance to use the school bathroom may cause alterations in bowel habits. At any age, psychosocial stresses or illness may cause a regression in toilet training or a change in bowel habits that may potentiate encopresis.

Although encopresis may be more prevalent in children with autism and other severe behavioral disorders, it usually occurs in children and families without significant psychopathology. However, encopresis may result in ridicule and shame for the child and family and carries a significant risk of secondary isolation, depression, and low self-esteem. Because parents and children may not spontaneously mention this problem during the interview, it should be specifically inquired about.

Diagnosis is based on a comprehensive assessment, with particular emphasis on a description of bowel patterns since birth, the age of onset of bowel-related symptoms, the effects of attempts to manage the symptoms, associations of the onset or exacerbations of symptoms with psychosocial stresses in the family, and the effects of the problem on the child and other family members. The child should be talked to directly about his or her perception of the problem and feelings about management plans. Hirschsprung disease is frequently considered in the differential diagnosis of encopresis (see Chapter 11).

A comprehensive approach to *treatment* is presented in Table 1–13. This approach involves reassurance about the commonness of the problem and an emphasis on the need for patience. Relapses are common, most often related to new or recurrent psychosocial stresses or illnesses. Refractory cases may involve complex underlying psychologic issues that warrant further investigation, organic disease that warrants re-evaluation, or inadequate evacuation of a chronic impaction.

Table 1–13. Management of Encopresis*

Treatment Phase	Treatment Program	Comments
Initial counseling	Education and "demystification" of the problem Removal of blame Establishment and explanation of treatment plan	Include diagram, review of colonic function, shared observation and x-ray views Emphasize need for intestinal "muscle building"

Initial catharsis
Inpatient
	High normal saline enemas (750 ml bid), 3–7 days
	Bisacodyl (Dulcolax) suppositories bid, 3–7 days
	Use of bathroom for 15 min after each meal
		Patient admitted when:
		    Retention is very severe
		    Home compliance likely to be poor
		    Parents prefer admission
		    Parental administration of enemas is inadvisable psychologically

At home	For moderate to severe retention, 3–4 cycles as follows:
	    Day 1: hypophosphate enemas (Fleet's Adult) twice
	    Day 2: bisacodyl (Dulcolax) suppositories twice
	    Day 3: bisacodyl (Dulcolax) tablet once
	For mild retention, senna or danthron, one tablet daily for one to two weeks
	Follow-up abdominal x-ray examination to confirm adequate catharsis
		Dosages or frequency may need alteration if child experiences excessive discomfort
		Admission should be considered if there is inadequate yield
		No lubricant during this phase

Maintenance regimen	Child sits on toilet twice a day at same times each day for 10 min each time Light mineral oil (at least 2 tablespoons) twice a day, usually for at least 4–6 mo Multiple vitamins, 2/day, between doses of mineral oil High-roughage diet: bran, cereal, vegetables, fruits Use of an oral laxative (senna or danthron) for 2–3 wk, then alternate days of mineral oil for 1 mo (given between doses); then laxative is discontinued; lubricant is continued	A kitchen timer can be helpful A chart with stars for sitting may be good for children less than 7 yr Bathroom reading encouraged Mineral oil can be put in juice, Coca Cola, or any other medium Vitamins to compensate for alleged problems with absorption secondary to mineral oil Diet should be applied but not to the point of coercion

Follow-up pattern	Visits every 4–10 wk, depending on severity, need for support, compliance, and associated symptoms
	Telephone availability to adjust doses when needed
	In case of relapse:
	    Check compliance
	    Use of oral laxative (e.g., Senokot) for 1–2 wk
	    Adjust dosage of mineral oil
	Counseling or referral for associated psychosocial and developmental issues
	Continuing use of demystification diagram to document progress
		Duration of treatment can be as long as 2–3 yr or as short as 6 mo
		Signs of relapse:
		    Excessive oil leaks
		    Large-caliber stools
		    Abdominal pain
		    Decreased frequency of defecation
		    Soiling
		Physician should spend time alone with child
		In patients who are slow to respond, physician should sustain optimism; persistence cures almost all cases (eventually)

* All dosages and frequencies are for an average-sized 7 yr old child. Appropriate adjustments should be made for smaller and larger patients.

(From Levine MD: Encopresis. *In* Levine MD, Carey WB, Crocker AC [eds]: Developmental-Behavioral Pediatrics. 2nd ed. Philadelphia, WB Saunders, 1992, p 394.)

References

Behrman RE (ed): Nelson Textbook of Pediatrics. 14th ed. Philadelphia, WB Saunders, 1992, Sec. 3.29, 13.13.

Toilet Training

Toilet training involves the mastery of bowel and urinary control while awake and asleep. The ages at which these tasks are mastered vary widely in different cultures, as well as within cultures (see the sections on Enuresis and Encopresis). The decision about when to start toilet training should be based on the following readiness signals: (1) dry periods lasting several hours; (2) interest in the potty chair; (3) desire to be changed when wet or dirty; and (4) ability to carry out a series of simple commands. Some general principles about approaching toilet training are as follows:

1. Anger or punishment for lack of performance on the potty chair or for accidents off the potty chair is usually counterproductive and inappropriate.
2. When the child resists sitting on the potty chair, allow her or him to get up and try again after a meal.
3. If resistance is persistent, postpone training for at least several weeks.
4. Power struggles should be avoided. The result may be stool retention, chronic constipation, encopresis, and/or strained parent–child relations. It is almost impossible to win a battle of wills with a toddler, and imposing the will of the adult may interfere with the child's developing autonomy and increase feelings of shame and doubt.
5. A key to successful toilet training is to approach it so that the child sees it as his or her own accomplishment.
6. The age at which daytime training is likely to be successful varies according to individual characteristics of the child: predictability of the child's elimination schedule; ability of the child to anticipate elimination and to understand the steps involved in toileting (getting to the bathroom on time, undressing, sitting on the potty chair, eliminating, wiping, flushing, and redressing); and motivation of the child to toilet train.

One of the many possible approaches to toilet training is the method presented in Table 1–14. This method works well for children with predictable elimination schedules. Children with irregular elimination schedules may have to be able to anticipate the need to go themselves before they can be trained. Complete daytime toilet training should be expected to take a long time. Success is sporadic initially, and occasional accidents are common long after toilet training is accomplished.

Table 1–14. Timing Method for Toilet Training

After demonstrating readiness signals, child introduced to potty chair.

Child initially sits on potty chair briefly, fully clothed.

Child then sits on potty chair with pants down for gradually increasing lengths of time (1 min, up to a maximum of 10 min).

Simple explanations of toileting procedure given repeatedly and emphasized by placing wet or soiled diapers in the potty.

Parent attempts to anticipate child's need to go (hence "timing method"), puts child on potty chair, and provides positive reinforcement for successful elimination on potty chair (praise, hug, star chart, stickers, or some other sufficiently motivating reward that can be given repeatedly).

References

Behrman RE (ed): Nelson Textbook of Pediatrics. 14th ed. Philadelphia, WB Saunders, 1992, Sec. 3.6, 3.15.
Brazelton TB: A child-oriented approach to toilet training. Pediatrics 29:121, 1962.

Recurrent Pain Disorders

Chronic, recurrent pain syndromes in childhood most commonly involve abdominal pain, headache, limb pain, or chest pain. It is unusual for children to present with more than one such pain syndrome at the same time, although they often may have had chronic, recurrent pain in a different location of the body in the past. An organic etiology is found in only about 10% of children. The diagnosis of psychogenic pain, however, should be based not only on the absence of adequate physical findings to explain the pain but also on evidence specific for the etiologic role of psychologic factors. The term "dysfunctional pain" is often used when no specific organic pathology or psychologic etiology is found. Most chronic recurrent pain syndromes fall into this latter category.

Diagnosis is based on a careful physical examination and history, including a comprehensive psychosocial assessment. In addition to the location, quality, and chronology of the pain, attention must be focused on the circumstances in which the pain is experienced. Signs and symptoms that increase the likelihood of an organic etiology include constant pain, pain awakening the child from sleep, well-localized pain, and physical findings like fever; weight loss; jaundice; changes in the color, consistency, or frequency of stools; and urinary tract symptoms.

It is important to distinguish between psychologic conditions that preceded and those that followed the onset of the recurrent pain syndrome, because evidence of psychologic stress usually is found by the time the child presents with a chronic problem. The nurturing responses of the family may provide secondary gain that prolongs the pain complaints. Alternatively, frustration with failure to find a specific cause may result in accusations of malingering and increased stress on the child that may create additional reasons for chronic pain. Diagnostic studies should be undertaken in response to specific findings that suggest an organic etiology.

Counseling is the primary treatment for the nonorganic diagnosis. Symptom diaries (including the events that immediately precede and follow the pain episode) are very helpful in the ongoing management of the problem as well as in the initial assessment. It is important to minimize secondary psychologic consequences of recurrent pain syndromes.

References

Behrman RE (ed): Nelson Textbook of Pediatrics. 14th ed. Philadelphia, WB Saunders, 1992, Sec. 6.53–6.54.

Levine MD, Rappaport LA: Recurrent abdominal pain in school children: The loneliness of the long-distance physician. Pediatric Clin North Am 31:969–991, 1984.

Failure to Thrive

Failure to thrive (FTT) is a term used to describe young children with inadequate weight gain, usually weight below the 3rd percentile on a standard growth chart. Because many of the children below the 3rd percentile are normal and some above it may have fallen from a much higher percentile and are failing to thrive, it is generally more meaningful to focus on percentile changes demonstrated over time. However, such changes can be misleading in the first year or two, when wide fluctuations in percentile position are not uncommon in normal children. For example, it is quite common for a child who is above the 75th percentile in weight in the first 6–9 mo to fall to the 50th percentile or lower from 9 to 18 mo and then to maintain that percentile position. When the percentile drop is great, it is helpful to compare the child's weight percentile to height and head circumference percentiles. It is not a concern when the weight falls from a disproportionately high percentile position

to a position consistent with height and head circumference. A fall to a disproportionately low weight is a cause for concern.

In the short term, a child who is failing to thrive will drop in weight percentile before dropping in height and head circumference. With chronic FTT, the height percentile also will fall but the head circumference is usually spared, unless the FTT is severe. FTT also may be defined as weight less than 80% of the median weight for height. Weight-by-height charts (see Figs. 1–7 and 1–13) are particularly helpful when adequate serial measurements are unavailable.

An etiologic approach to the *differential diagnosis* of FTT is presented in Table 1–15 along with some of the common causes. Almost every chronic and/or serious condition in childhood may cause FTT. It is the admitting diagnosis for 3–5% of children admitted to teaching hospitals. Berwick reported the following frequencies for FTT with uncertain etiology on admission: 44% environmental causes (psychosocial); 37% organic causes; and 19% no cause (or constitutional). The organic causes varied widely, with the most common being gastrointestinal, including cystic fibrosis, and neurologic.

In early infancy, feeding difficulties are the predominant cause of FTT, including lactation failure, inadequate feeding frequency or volume, and formula-mixing errors. A calorically inadequate diet at any age may be due to ignorance or neglect by the caregivers. It also may result from irregular caregiving arrangements that involve many caregivers, sometimes themselves children. Diet histories often do not coincide with actual diets, particularly when there are multiple caregivers. Even a competent mother simply may not know the actual intake of the child unless a detailed diary is kept by all caregivers.

Among children with FTT who are not hospitalized, the ratio of environmental to organic causes shifts further toward environmental causes. The diagnosis of an environmental cause should be based on observations of caregiver–child interactions, as well as on historic data from all important adults and from the child, if possible. Patterns frequently associated with nonorganic FTT include postpartum depression; maternal depression related to a significant loss (spouse or parent); a social environment characterized by many stresses and few social supports; and caregiver–child interactional patterns that are hostile, rejecting, or aloof.

History and observation are the most important aspects of the *diagnostic evaluation* of FTT. If possible, the attitudes and interactions of important caregivers with each other as well as with the child

Table 1–15. Etiology of Failure to Thrive (FTT)

Mechanism	Disorders
Nonorganic	
Psychosocial	Poor maternal–child interaction, poor feeding technique, psychologically disturbed mother, unusual maternal nutritional beliefs, errors in formula preparation, emotional deprivation, dwarfism, child neglect
Organic	
Inability to suck, swallow, or masticate	CNS pathology (psychomotor retardation), neuromuscular disease (Werdnig-Hoffmann, myotonia congenita)
Maldigestion, malabsorption	Cystic fibrosis, celiac disease, Schwachman-Diamond syndrome, chronic diarrhea
Poor nutrient utilization	Renal failure, renal tubular acidosis, inborn errors of metabolism
Vomiting	CNS abnormality (tumor, infection, increased pressure), metabolic toxin (inborn errors of amino or organic acid metabolism), intestinal obstruction (pyloric stenosis, malrotation), renal tubular disease
Regurgitation	Gastroesophageal reflux, hiatal hernia, rumination syndrome
Elevated metabolic rate	Thyrotoxicosis, chronic disease (bronchopulmonary dysplasia, heart failure), cancer, inflammatory lesions (SLE, inflammatory bowel disease, chronic infection), immunodeficiency diseases, burns
Reduced growth potential	Chromosomal disorders, primordial dwarfism, skeletal dysplasia, specific syndromes (fetal alcohol)

CNS = central nervous system; SLE = systemic lupus erythematosus.

should be observed or obtained by history. The presence of behavioral problems of the child or siblings (e.g., excessive crying, discipline problems, sleep disturbances, and feeding problems) often is associated with family dysfunction. *Clinical manifestations* in children with FTT caused by environmental deprivation include "frozen watchfulness," minimal smiling, decreased vocalization, resistance to being held, and self-stimulating rhythmic behaviors.

If a careful history and physical examination fail to identify a cause or clue that suggests specific diagnostic procedures, it is very unlikely that any tests will reveal a cause. In one study of children admitted to a teaching hospital with FTT of unknown etiology, less than 2% of tests performed during the hospitalization contributed to a diagnosis, and all of the positive tests were associated with a positive finding in the initial history and physical examination. Still, it is standard procedure to obtain a few screening tests: a complete blood count, urinalysis, serum electrolytes, and perhaps an erythrocyte sedimentation rate, calcium, thyroxine, and thyroid-stimulating hormone. If even mild gastrointestinal symptoms are present, then a stool culture, pH, reducing substances test, and guaiac test are indicated.

One common approach to FTT of unknown etiology, after outpatient attempts to manage the problem have failed, is to admit the child to the hospital and to observe him or her for weight gain after demonstrating adequate caloric intake. If the child gains weight, nonorganic FTT is assumed and steps are taken to monitor and support the environment as well as the child's nutrition after discharge. If the child fails to gain, an organic cause is more aggressively sought. However, environmental and organic factors can occur together. The increased environmental stresses faced by families of children with a chronic illness may adversely affect the adequacy of nutritional and psychologic nurturance of the child. Furthermore, children with nonorganic FTT may fail to gain weight in the hospital owing to adverse psychologic reactions to the strange and threatening environment and separation from even an inadequate parent. Table 1–16 presents data from one study demonstrating the time required in the hospital before catch-up weight gain was observed in children with caloric-deprivation FTT. Finally, children with nonorganic FTT may present with physical signs and symptoms due to nutritional deficiency, unusual diets, and perhaps neuroendocrine responses to stress (e.g., diarrhea, vomiting, depressed growth hormone levels, delayed bone age, iron deficiency, elevated serum transaminase levels, and glucose tolerance abnormalities).

Treatment of FTT by hospitalization of the child may be particularly stressful when the par-

Table 1–16. Time Required in Hospital for Accelerated Weight Gain in Children with Caloric-Deprivation FTT

Age less than 6 mo
  most gaining by 2–3 days
  all gaining by 9 days

Age 6–24 mo
  gaining by 2–17 days
  2 of 25 required more than 2 wk

Age 2 yr or more
  all gaining in 2–7 days

(Adapted from Ellerstein NS, Ostrov BE: Growth patterns in children hospitalized because of caloric-deprivation failure to thrive. Am J Dis Child 139:164–166, 1985.)

ent–child attachment is insecure. If the cause appears to be inadequate caloric intake, a reasonable initial ambulatory plan may be to provide dietary advice and have caregivers keep a detailed diary of feedings and the frequency, volume, and consistency of stools and vomitus. If the picture remains unclear and the child fails to exhibit catch-up growth within several weeks, hospitalization is necessary because adequate nutrition is crucial for brain development during the first 2 yr of life.

Table 1–17 presents a protocol for hospital management. Deferring investigations decreases the stress of the hospitalization, which may shorten the time required to achieve adequate caloric intake and thereby to test the hypothesis that the FTT is due to inadequate caloric intake. Because catch-up

Table 1–17. Hospital Protocol for FTT of Unknown Etiology

Defer all investigations for at least 1 wk (assuming no clues for organic etiology on comprehensive history and physical examination).

Aim to provide over 100% of the normal caloric requirements for the child's *ideal weight* (median weight for height).

Record the following data daily:
  Weight before breakfast (unclothed)
  Total calories consumed in the previous 24 hr
  Calories/kg of *ideal weight* in the previous 24 hr
  Output (stool, urine, vomitus)

Record observations of the child's behavior and interactions of the child with the parents and the staff.

Provide an organized program of stimulation, including regular affectionate interaction with adults.

Involve the parents from the start in the feeding and stimulation interventions.

Begin interdisciplinary evaluations on admission (e.g., social worker, nurse, nutritional support team or dietitian, behavioral/developmental specialist).

growth must be demonstrated, more calories should be provided than the normal requirements for the child's current depressed weight. A positive change in the mood of a child usually is followed by accelerated weight gain in 1–2 days. The parents should be involved in the development and implementation of the management plan.

The *prognosis* for children hospitalized for nonorganic FTT in the first 2 yr of life shows a high percentage of retardation (15–67%), school learning problems (37–67%), and behavioral disturbances (28–48%) at 3–11 yr of age. Continued FTT is a much less frequent problem.

References

Behrman RE (ed): Nelson Textbook of Pediatrics. 14th ed. Philadelphia, WB Saunders, 1992, Sec. 6.30.
Berwick DM: Nonorganic failure-to-thrive. Pediatr Rev 1: 265, 1980.

Child Abuse and Neglect

Child abuse is a frequent, serious problem that every state and the federal government have addressed by laws. The Child Abuse Prevention and Treatment Act (Public Law 93–247) defines child abuse and neglect as "the physical or mental injury, sexual abuse, negligent treatment, or maltreatment of a child under the age of eighteen by a person who is responsible for the child's welfare under circumstances which indicate that the child's health and welfare is harmed or threatened thereby." In most cases child abuse needs to be understood as a symptom of family dysfunction. Only by understanding the factors that contribute to its occurrence can a logical management plan be developed (Fig. 1–19).

Estimates of the *incidence* of child abuse and neglect vary widely, depending on the definition and the source. Approximately 1% of children are reported to be abused or neglected each year. Approximately two thirds of cases involved physical abuse, one fourth sexual abuse, 5% FTT due to underfeeding, and smaller percentages for other causes, including medical neglect, grossly inadequate supervision, intentional drugging or poisoning, and severe emotional abuse. Estimates of the incidence of child abuse based on household surveys range from 1 to 4 million cases/yr. Abuse is less likely to be reported if it involves children from white, nonpoor families; if the mother is alleged to be responsible for the abuse; and if the abuse is emotional rather than physical.

Physicians may be reluctant to report cases be-

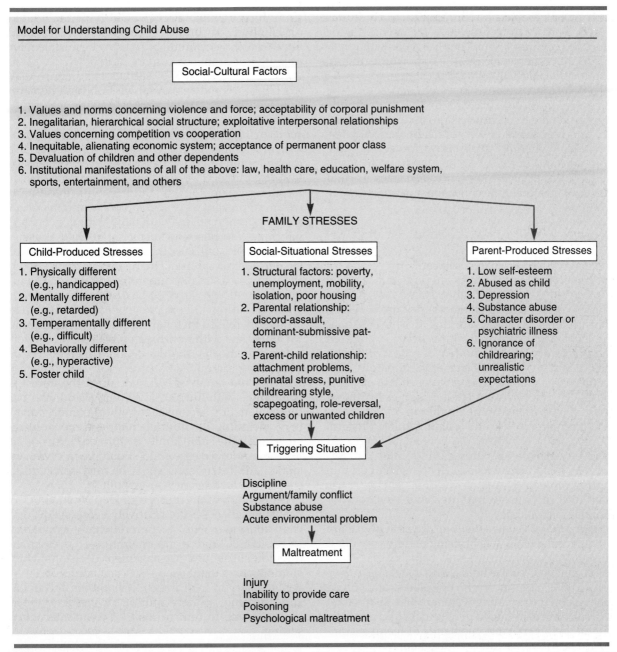

Model for Understanding Child Abuse

Social-Cultural Factors

1. Values and norms concerning violence and force; acceptability of corporal punishment
2. Inegalitarian, hierarchical social structure; exploitative interpersonal relationships
3. Values concerning competition vs cooperation
4. Inequitable, alienating economic system; acceptance of permanent poor class
5. Devaluation of children and other dependents
6. Institutional manifestations of all of the above: law, health care, education, welfare system, sports, entertainment, and others

FAMILY STRESSES

Child-Produced Stresses

1. Physically different (e.g., handicapped)
2. Mentally different (e.g., retarded)
3. Temperamentally different (e.g., difficult)
4. Behaviorally different (e.g., hyperactive)
5. Foster child

Social-Situational Stresses

1. Structural factors: poverty, unemployment, mobility, isolation, poor housing
2. Parental relationship: discord-assault, dominant-submissive patterns
3. Parent-child relationship: attachment problems, perinatal stress, punitive childrearing style, scapegoating, role-reversal, excess or unwanted children

Parent-Produced Stresses

1. Low self-esteem
2. Abused as child
3. Depression
4. Substance abuse
5. Character disorder or psychiatric illness
6. Ignorance of childrearing; unrealistic expectations

Triggering Situation

Discipline
Argument/family conflict
Substance abuse
Acute environmental problem

Maltreatment

Injury
Inability to provide care
Poisoning
Psychological maltreatment

Figure 1–19. Model for understanding child abuse. (From Bittner S, Newberger EH: Pediatric understanding of child abuse and neglect. Pediatr Rev 2:198, 1981. Copyright American Academy of Pediatrics, 1981.)

cause they are uncomfortable in the role of accuser, the antithesis of their usual role of compassionate helper, or because of time constraints, concern over possible court appearances, and lack of knowledge about the problem or how to proceed once child abuse is suspected. Laws that govern reporting attempt to overcome this reluctance by mandating the report of "suspected" abuse, by making physicians immune from suits related to a report made in good faith, and by making it the responsibility of protection agencies (not physicians) to determine whether abuse has actually occurred. Physicians thus can attempt to maintain a helping relationship with the family by telling them that they are obligated by law to make a report but that their aim is to help find ways to prevent a recurrence of the injury or condition. Some families react with anger or hurt, but others welcome the opportunity to find help for their difficult situation.

To detect less obvious cases of child abuse, the physician must be sensitive to the more subtle signs, and take the time to obtain an expanded history and behavioral observations. Because a determination of whether a report is warranted may take more time and/or expertise than the physician has, the use of a social worker who specializes in child abuse, or preferably a child abuse team, may be invaluable.

PHYSICAL ABUSE

Conservative estimates indicate that 1–2% of children in the United States are physically abused at some time during childhood and that 10% of injuries seen in a hospital emergency room in children under 5 yr of age are due to abuse. About one third of physical abuse cases occur in children under 1 yr of age and another one third between ages 1 and 6 yr. There are approximately 2000 deaths per year in the United States due to physical abuse. The abuser is a related caregiver in 90% of cases, a male friend of the mother in 5%, an unrelated babysitter in 4%, and a sibling in 1%. Physical abuse usually occurs in the context of increased social–environmental stresses and often is triggered by child behaviors such as persistent crying, wetting or soiling, spilling, or disobedience. Less than 10% of abusive parents have psychotic or criminal personalities.

Some *clinical manifestations* of physical abuse are unequivocal. Distinctive bruising patterns are often caused by blunt instruments, belts, cords, hand slaps, pinches, choke holds, and bites. Burn patterns from cigarettes, irons, hot plates, and forced submersion into scalding water are also distinctive. A circular burn limited to the buttocks and genitalia with no involvement of the hands or feet is incompatible with falling into or mistakenly entering a tub of hot water.

Usually, however, the presentation of child abuse is not so clear. Bruises, burns, and fractures may be accidental and often are dismissed as such without adequate consideration of other causes. Accidental bruises are most common over the forehead, anterior tibia, and bony prominences; bruises confined to the buttocks or lower back are most commonly caused by abuse. Anaphylactoid (Henoch-Schönlein) purpura may present with ecchymoses over the buttocks, but usually purpura

from organic etiologies does not have the limited distribution of bruising characteristic of child abuse. Healing cigarette burns may be mistaken for impetigo or atopic or contact dermatitis.

Some presentations of serious child abuse may not suggest the diagnosis at all. Subdural hematomas may be caused by violent shaking leading to the tearing of bridging cerebral vessels, in the absence of injury to the skull or scalp. Serious abdominal injuries may be caused by striking or squeezing the abdomen (e.g., rupture of the liver, spleen, intestines, or blood vessels; traumatic pancreatitis; or intramural hematomas); children with these injuries may present with signs and symptoms of an acute abdomen but may not have evidence of external trauma to raise the suspicion of child abuse.

Table 1–18 outlines the *diagnostic evaluation* for suspected child abuse. The history is crucial when the injury is not pathognomonic for abuse. The interviewer should strive to be a supportive listener while avoiding judgmental statements that may arouse increased defensiveness. After beginning the interview with nonthreatening general conversation, the focus should be on concrete details about how the injury occurred. Key questions are whether the family's explanation for the injury is compatible with the physical findings and whether the explanation is consistent among family members, including the injured child, and repeat interviews with the same family member. If old enough to be interviewed, the child should be interviewed alone. The interviewer must be very sensitive to the child's feelings of fear or guilt.

Description of the injury and identification of the probable cause are the relatively easy aspects of a child abuse work-up. A comprehensive evaluation of the family and social environment is essential to guide subsequent management decisions when child abuse is diagnosed. Hospital admission may be necessary to treat the child's injuries and to ensure the child's safety until it can be determined that it is safe to return home or to an alternative setting.

SEXUAL ABUSE

This injury involves engaging a child in sexual activities that the child often does not understand, to which the child cannot give informed consent, or that violate the sexual social taboos. This definition includes a broad range of sexual activities (e.g., exhibitionism, fondling, child pornography, and oral, anal, and genital contact), both inside and outside the family. Some reserve the term "sexual abuse" to refer to forced sexual contact between a

Table 1–18. Initial Diagnostic Evaluation for Suspected Child Abuse

History
Obtain separate histories from parents, other adults, and child (if possible)

Record history precisely
Record direct quotations
Clarify ambiguous statements
Use qualifiers like "the mother alleges that . . ." rather than "the child was . . ."

Record the following:
Date and time of evaluation
Date, time, and place of alleged abuse
Informant
How alleged abuse occurred and who allegedly caused it
History of past abuse

Physical Examination
Perform careful, complete examination

List bruises by site, size, shape, and color

Check the retina, eardrums, oral cavity, and genitalia for signs of occult trauma

Check bones and joints for tenderness and range of motion

Record height and weight percentiles

Obtain color photographs of injuries (include paper with patient's name, date, and time in the photograph)

Laboratory Test
Radiologic bone survey (skull, thorax, spine, long bones) for children under age 5 yr who are suspected victims of child abuse

Bleeding studies when bruising present (platelet count, bleeding time, prothrombin time [PT], and partial thromboplastin time [PTT])

Disposition
Consult immediately with social worker or child abuse team to arrange comprehensive multidisciplinary evaluation

Report to mandated agency if indicated

Inform parents of need to report and desire to be helpful

Hospitalize the child if further investigation necessary to determine safety of home and/or to treat injuries

Establish multidisciplinary follow-up plan (health and social services)

---

victim and perpetrator, while using the term "sexual misuse" for when a child is exposed to sexual stimulation inappropriate for the child's role in the family. **Incest** is sexual abuse by a close relative that involves intercourse. **Molestation** is sexual abuse by a stranger, with or without penetration. **Rape** involves forced genital contact. **Sexual assault** involves violent or nonviolent manual, oral, or genital contact with genitalia of the victim or the perpetrator. Activities that are considered to be normal sexual exploratory behavior among children of similar age may be considered sexual abuse or misuse if the ages are discrepant. There are at least 250,000 cases of sexual abuse per year in the United States, with the more serious and/or chronic forms affecting 1–3% of children. The majority of recognized sexual offenders are male, of whom about 20% are adolescents.

The *clinical manifestations* of sexual abuse may be more difficult to recognize than those of physical abuse. Early warnings may include simulation of sexual acts with dolls, inclusion of genitalia in drawings, precocious flirtation, and verbalization of concern about sexual molestation in general. Direct statements from children about abusive behavior should be taken seriously. Most sexually abused children are very reluctant to break the secrecy of the abuse because of fear and guilt; many who do make a statement recant it later. Many nonspecific behavioral problems may be associated with sexual abuse, including sleeping and eating disorders, school dysfunction, phobias, depression, acting out behaviors, conversion reactions, and suicide.

The presence in prepubertal children of genital and anal trauma or diseases that are usually sexually transmitted (e.g., gonorrhea, syphilis, lymphogranuloma venereum, trichomoniasis, genital herpes, and chlamydial infections) should raise a strong suspicion of sexual abuse. Recurrent urinary tract infections, recurrent nonspecific vaginitis, genital warts, or early pregnancy may also be the result of sexual abuse.

The diagnostic evaluation in Table 1–18 may need to be modified for sexual abuse. If it is clear that others also will need to interview the child (e.g., social worker, child protective worker, or police), it may be best to arrange a single, joint interview to obtain the initial detailed history because multiple histories are often traumatic for the child. Questions should be open ended and as nonjudgmental as possible. Dolls with body parts often involved in sexual abuse, drawings of a person or the family, and toys may help in the interview. Clarification of terminology frequently is necessary to be certain that the interviewer understands what the child means, and vice versa. If a girl is pubertal, a menstrual history should be obtained.

The physical examination often is easier for the child and the physician after a sensitive, supportive interview. If it must occur before the detailed history is obtained, the physician will need to obtain at least a brief history to guide the examination.

Particularly important points include the type and time of the alleged abusive act and subsequent events that may alter the presence of evidence (e.g., bathing, urinating, defecation, brushing teeth, or changing clothes). It is best to obtain this information from someone other than the child if there is not sufficient time to approach the sensitive questions gradually. The examination should proceed like a normal general one, with special attention to any evidence of physical abuse, trauma, or the presence of blood or semen on body parts or clothing. The knee–chest position may provide better visualization of the vagina and anus in prepubertal girls, although the lithotomy position is usually better as girls approach puberty. Wood lamp inspection of the body and clothing is indicated to look for the fluorescence of sperm. Laboratory evaluation for suspected sexual abuse is outlined in Table 1–19.

Treatment of venereal infections is discussed in Chapter 7. Pregnancy can be prevented within 72 hr of intercourse by giving two norgestrel and ethinyl estradiol (Ovral) tablets at the time of examination and two more 12 hr later. The physician will need the help of social workers and perhaps mental health professionals to immediately assess child and family functioning, the family's social environment, and their needs for services. A child victim will need extensive counseling. Hospital admission may be warranted for treatment of injuries, for mental health evaluation, for treatment, or to ensure safety. Subsequently, the effectiveness of health and social services to which the child and family have been referred should be monitored and close communication maintained among the professionals involved in the evaluation and continuing care of the family. Medical follow-up must ensure adequate treatment of injuries and infections; serology for syphilis should be rechecked in 6 wk.

References

Behrman RE (ed): Nelson Textbook of Pediatrics. 14th ed. Philadelphia, WB Saunders, 1992, Sec. 3.51–3.54, 10.17.
Emans SJ, Goldstein DP: The gynecologic examination of the prepubertal child with vulvovaginitis: Use of knee-chest position. Pediatrics 65:758–760, 1980.
Emans SJ: Pelvic examination of the adolescent patient. Pediatr Rev 4:307–312, 1983.
Kempe CH, Helfer RE (eds): The Battered Child. 3rd ed. Chicago, University of Chicago Press, 1980.
Krugman RD: Recognition of sexual abuse in children. Pediatr Rev 8:25–30, 1986.

Separation from One or Both Parents

HOSPITALIZATION

About 30% of children are hospitalized at least once during childhood, and about 5% have multiple hospital admissions. Along with separation from parents, hospitalization stresses include the illness itself (with discomfort, pain, fear, uncertainty, parental anxiety), separation from almost everything that is familiar (siblings, home, friends, school, customary routines), and exposure to many strange and threatening experiences (painful and uncomfortable procedures, many new people, sick or disabled people experiencing pain and emotional upset).

Hospitalization of a child can result in (1) distress during the hospitalization, (2) disturbance on return home, and (3) long-term sequelae. Distress during hospitalization is most marked between 6 mo and 4 yr of age. It is related to the degree of separation from all people to whom the child is attached, lack of opportunity to form new attachments (large numbers of frequently changing caregivers), and the strangeness of the environment. On returning home, many children exhibit regressive, withdrawn, ambivalent, or labile behavior.

Table 1–19. Laboratory Evaluation of Sexually Abused Child

Motile sperm
  Wet mount of vaginal specimen (mouth, rectum, if indicated)
  Cervical mucus aspirate

Infection
  Gonococcal cultures (vagina, cervix, rectum, throat)
  Gram stain of vaginal specimen for bacteria (e.g., gonococcus, *Gardnerella vaginalis*)
  KOH preparation of vaginal specimen for *Candida*
  Wet preparation of vaginal specimen for *Trichomonas*
  Other cultures of vagina or cervix (e.g., for *Chlamydia*, *Candida*, herpes)
  Syphilis serology (initially and 6 wk later)
  HIV tests

Serum or urine pregnancy test (if child is pubertal)

Specimens for police report (if indicated)
  Air-dried slide specimens from the vagina, cervix, rectum, and mouth (can be tested for sperm antibodies, blood, acid phosphatase)
  Fingernail scrapings for blood or fabric particles if a struggle took place
  Collection of loose hairs or threads of fabric from body and clothing

These difficult behaviors can be a source of great frustration and anguish for parents who are eager to comfort their sick child, but who are also stressed and fatigued. Parents should be warned to expect these behaviors, helped to understand their child's insecurity and fear of further separation from the parent, and counseled to provide increased nurturing. Multiple or prolonged hospitalizations carry an increased risk for long-term behavioral disturbance, especially among children from disadvantaged families.

Prolonged and serious illnesses in children place great stress on the parents (marital relationships, parenting of siblings, and work performance) and siblings, who are often neglected to some degree while the parents are consumed by the care of and anxiety over the sick child. Even with conditions that are judged as relatively mild by health care providers, the behavior of the parents toward the sick child may be altered for a long time after the illness resolves. Common problems include difficulties with separations, infantilization, preoccupation with bodily functions, and decreased school achievement.

DIVORCE

The problems associated with divorce are usually chronic and often devastating for both the children and the parents. Divorce is usually not a single event but a sequence of difficult changes and adjustments that span years. For years prior to divorce, children may be exposed to family turmoil that may include violent arguments and physical violence, including that between their parents, other family members, and perhaps themselves. Alternatively, some children, particularly young ones, may be completely unaware that a problem exists until one of the parents leaves. For the parents, the period between the separation and the formal divorce can be particularly acrimonious, making it very difficult for them to help the children cope with their losses, fears, and disruptions in the usual pattern of family life.

Complicating the family's emotional adjustment to the divorce are the untoward economic effects experienced by many of these families. Often ex-husbands fail to provide child support payments. Women, who are usually the custodial parents, may lack the education, job skills, or experience to get adequately compensated and secure jobs. When a mother who has remained in the home to care for a preschool child must start work, that child suffers a second loss. The custodial parent also must assume household responsibilities that

previously were shared. In addition, relocation to cheaper housing often is necessary, frequently involving a loss of friends and familiar school and neighborhood. Worsening parent–child relations often result from these additional stresses. It is usually not until after the first year of divorce that reduced tension and an increased sense of well-being begin to emerge in the children of divorce. Because the majority of divorced women and men remarry, there will be further periods of new adjustments as step-parents and often step-children join the family.

The most important determinant of initial responses of children to divorce is the age of the child (Table 1–20). In the long term, over one third of children are psychologically troubled and distressed 5 yr after the divorce. The most frequent clinical finding is depression. Poor psychologic adjustment in children is more likely when parental fighting continues and when they remain in the custody of a lonely, depressed, or emotionally disturbed mother.

Children who are told about the divorce before the actual separation, and who are reassured that

Table 1–20. Assistance Related to the Age of the Child

Age	Common Reactions of Child	Role of Physician
2–5 years	Regression, irritability, sleep disturbance	Encourage restabilization of household and bedtime routines Reassure child Urge restoration of contact with departed parent
6–8 years	Open grieving, feelings of rejection	Support maintenace of child's relationship to both parents; reassure child
9–12 years	Fear, anger at one or both parents	Express interest and availability to child
Adolescence	Worried about own future, depressed and/or acting-out behavior	Offer opportunity for private discussion

(From Wallerstein JS: Separation, divorce, and remarriage. *In* Levine MD, Carey WB, Crocker AC [eds]: Developmental-Behavioral Pediatrics. 2nd ed. Philadelphia, WB Saunders, 1992, p 140.)

they will continue to see both parents, are calmer at the time of separation. Children should be told the details about what their living arrangements and daily routines will be after the separation. They also need to be told repeatedly that they did not cause the divorce and that their efforts cannot mend it. Young children may be told that the divorce is necessary to bring an end to fighting or unhappiness between the parents. Older children may have more specific questions that should be answered simply without going beyond a concrete, superficial response unless questioned further. Children need to be assured that neither parent expects them to take sides, and they need to be allowed to love both parents. They also need to be allowed to express and vent feelings of anger, sadness, and disappointment. There is a continuing need for reassurances after the separation. Children who receive additional attention from grandparents, family, and friends do better than those who do not.

References

Behrman RE (ed): Nelson Textbook of Pediatrics. 14th ed. Philadelphia, WB Saunders, 1992, Sec. 3.16–3.19.

Green M, Solnit AJ: Reactions to the threatened loss of a child: A vulnerable child syndrome. Pediatrics 34: 58–66, 1964.

Hetherington EM: Divorce: A child's perspective. Am Psychol 34:851–858, 1979.

Rutter M: Separation experiences: A new look at an old topic. Pediatrics 95:147–154, 1979.

Sleep Disorders

Sleep patterns in children follow a typical developmental sequence, with the gradual increase of deep sleep and the development of regular sleep cycles. Sleep stages are defined by electroencephalographic (EEG), electromyographic, and electrooculographic characteristics, such as waking, rapid eye movement (REM), and non-REM sleep. Most infants (up to 70%) will sleep through the night (at least 5 hr at a stretch) by 3 mo post-term, at which time they have assumed schedules of about four sleep periods within 24 hr. Premature infants take longer to assume the patterns typical of full-term infants. Most children experience a point later in the first year of life, often associated with an intercurrent illness, when they begin to wake at night again, sometimes falling into patterns of night waking that persist for years and that require behavioral interventions for correction.

Common sleep disruption disorders may be or-

ganic in nature or related to environmental factors that usually are easily remedied once their features are recognized. Table 1–21 lists several common sleep disruption patterns and their treatments. When schedules need to be regularized, imposing a routine bedtime and naptime for the child, along with a usual presleep routine, and firmly but supportively maintaining it despite protests can be very successful. When parental work and life-styles result in children being awakened early and going to bed late, the schedule must be arranged so that the child gets enough sleep. In children with delayed sleep phase onset, the circadian clock is probably set so that the child is not ready for sleep at the prescribed bedtime; treatment involves either gradually moving the bedtime backward 15–30 min/day or forward by 2–3 hr/night over a week.

Obstructive sleep apnea occurs in children as well as in adults and frequently is associated with a predisposing physical condition such as tonsillar hypertrophy. It is characterized by snoring, may be associated with enuresis and/or obesity, and also may be associated with hyperactivity and school dysfunction in some children. Weight reduction and otolaryngologic surgery may be indicated.

Night terrors (pavor nocturnus), bedwetting (enuresis), and sleepwalking are common deep sleep phenomena that are developmentally normal and usually do not represent pathologic processes. Similarly, head rolling, head banging, and rocking are seen in many normal children between 9 mo and 3 yr of age and usually are benign, self-limited phenomena. If they persist or are associated with other developmental lags, they should be further evaluated.

References

Behrman RE (ed): Nelson Textbook of Pediatrics. 14th ed. Philadelphia, WB Saunders, 1992, Sec. 3.30.

Ferber R: Sleep disorders. In Levine MD, Casey WD, Crocker AC (eds): Developmental-Behavioral Pediatrics. 2nd ed. Philadelphia, WB Saunders, 1992, pp 398–406.

Mendelson WB, Gillin JC, Wyatt RJ: Human Sleep and Its Disorders. New York, Plenum Press, 1977.

Mental Retardation

Mental retardation (MR) is significantly subaverage general intellectual functioning for a child's developmental stage, existing concurrently with deficits in adaptive behavior. MR is defined statistically as tested cognitive performance that is 2 standard deviations below the mean (roughly below the 3rd

Table 1–21. Childhood Sleep Disruption Disorders

Type	Cause	Symptoms	Treatment
Organic			
Colic	Unknown	Crying, irritability	Rocking, pacifier, nursing Support until resolution
Medications	Stimulants Bronchodilators Anticonvulsants	Failure to fall asleep; restless sleep	Adjust dosage/timing; change medication
Illness	Any chronically irritating disorder (e.g., otitis, dermatitis, asthma, esophageal reflux)	Painful crying out	Treat disease symptomatically
CNS disorders	Variable; rule out seizures	Decreased sleep	Evaluate environment Sedatives as last resort
Parasomnias			
Sleepwalking, sleep terrors	Stage IV (deep) sleep instability	Awakening 1–3 hr after falling asleep	Reassurance; protective environment
Confusional arousals		Intense crying, walking, disorientation, talking	
Enuresis	? Stage IV instability Metabolic disease (e.g., diabetes) Urinary tract infection Urinary anatomic anomaly	Bedwetting	Rule out medical conditions Fluid limitation Prebed voiding Behavioral approaches (bell and pad) Emotional support Medication (e.g., imipramine) Reassurance
Sleep–Wake Schedule Disorders			
Irregular sleep–wake pattern	No defined schedule	Variable waking and sleeping	Regularize schedule
Regular but inappropriate sleep–wake schedule	Napping at wrong times Prematurely eliminated nap	Morning sleepiness Night wakenings	Rework schedule
Delayed sleep phase	Late sleep onset with resetting of circadian rhythm	Late sleep onset Morning sleepiness Not sleepy at bedtime	Enforce wake-up time Gradually move bedtime earlier or keep awake overnight to create drowsy state
Environmental and Psychosocial Factors			
Inappropriate sleep-onset associations	No defined bedtime routine Child falls asleep in conditions different from those of the rest of the night	Night wakings requiring intervention	Regularize routine Minimize nocturnal parental response
Excessive nocturnal fluid	Child gets food/drink with each awakening	Night waking wet or wanting drink	Gradually decrease nocturnal fluid
Inconsistent limit setting	Parental anxiety	Delayed bedtime Excessive expression of "needs" by child	Modify parental behavior to improve limit setting Gradually increase limits
Anxieties; fears	Separation anxieties	Night waking Refusal to sleep	Reassurance when appropriate Counseling in severe cases
Social disruptions	Family stressors	Night waking Refusal to sleep	Family counseling Regularize routines

Table 1–22. Levels of Mental Retardation

Level of Retardation	Stanford-Binet IQ Score	WISC-III IQ Score	Educational Label
Mild	67–52	70–55	"Educable (EMR)"
Moderate	51–36	54–40	"Trainable (TMR)"
Severe	35–20	39–25	} "Untrainable"*
Profound	Below 20	Below 24	

* No one is considered untrainable today.
WISC-III = Wechsler Intelligence Scale for Children–3rd ed.

percentile) of the general population. This implies that as many as 7.5 million persons in the United States can be characterized as retarded; clinical estimates range from 2.2 to 10 million (the higher number includes persons with so-called borderline intelligence and poor social adaptation). About 60,000 retarded individuals live in public residential facilities.

Levels of MR from IQ scores derived from two typical tests are shown in Table 1–22. These categories do not necessarily reflect the actual functional level of the tested individual. In school, a child with mild MR may, because of poor social (adaptive) abilities, be better served in a class for children defined as "trainable," whereas another child who tests in the moderate range of retarda-

Table 1–23. Mechanisms of Developmental Disabilities*

Disorder	Total Mentally Retarded Group (%)
Hereditary disorders: preconceptual origin, variable expression, multiple somatic effects, frequently a progressive course Inborn errors of metabolism (e.g., Tay-Sachs disease, Hurler disease, phenylketonuria) Other single gene abnormalities (e.g., muscular dystrophy, neurofibromatosis, tuberous sclerosis) Chromosomal aberrations, including translocation, fragile X syndrome Polygenic familial syndromes	5
Early alterations of embryonic development: sporadic events affecting embryogenesis, phenotypic changes, usually a stable developmental handicap Chromosomal changes, including trisomy (e.g., Down syndrome) Prenatal influence syndromes (e.g., intrauterine infections, drugs, alcohol, unknown forces)	32
Other pregnancy problems and perinatal morbidity: impingement on progress of fetus during last two trimesters or on newborn, neurologic abnormalities frequent, handicap stable or occasionally worsening Fetal malnutrition and placental insufficiency Perinatal difficulties (e.g., prematurity, hypoxia, trauma)	11
Acquired childhood diseases: acute modification of developmental status, variable potential for functional recovery Infection (e.g., encephalitis, meningitis) Cranial trauma Other (e.g., cardiac arrest, intoxications)	4
Environmental and social problems: dynamic influences, operational throughout development, commonly combined with other handicaps Deprivation Parental neurosis, psychosis Childhood neurosis Childhood psychosis	18
Unknown causes: no definite hereditary, gestational, perinatal, acquired, or environmental issues or else multiple elements present	

* Mental retardation, cerebral palsy, seizure disorders, and sensory handicaps.
(Adapted from Crocker AC, Nelson RP: Mental retardation. *In* Levine MD, Carey WB, Crocker AC [eds]: Developmental-Behavioral Pediatrics. 2nd ed. Philadelphia, WB Saunders, 1992, p 502.)

tion but who has especially good language abilities may be more stimulated in a class for children defined as "educable." Current practice supports the position that persons who perform in the severe or profound ranges of MR are capable of responding to some educational interventions as well.

The etiology of the central nervous system (CNS) insult resulting in MR may relate to genetic disorders, teratogenic influences, perinatal insults, acquired childhood disease, and environmental/social factors (Table 1–23). Although a single organic cause may be found, each individual's performance should be considered a function of the interaction of environmental influences on the person's organic substrate. Thus, it is common for a retarded child to have behavioral difficulties resulting from both the retarding condition itself and the family's reaction to the child and his or her condition. In general, more severe forms of retardation can be traced to biologic factors, and the earlier the retardation is recognized the more severe the deviation from normal is likely to be. The pattern of an individual's development can aid in making a diagnosis, but at any given point in time it may be very difficult to predict future performance accurately.

In approaching the diagnosis of MR, the first step is to provide interdisciplinary evaluations to identify functional strengths and weaknesses. Expertise from several disciplines is needed to characterize the child functionally for purposes of medical and habilitative therapies (see the sections on assessment and intervention). Once the developmental lags have been identified, the history and physical examination may suggest the point in development at which a CNS insult may have taken place and minimize the need for laboratory tests. Almost one third of mentally retarded individuals do not have readily identifiable reasons for their disabilities. However, in many cases, enough factors can be ruled out to allay the guilt and anxiety of families as to their responsibility in causing the defect.

References

Behrman RE (ed): Nelson Textbook of Pediatrics. 14th ed. Philadelphia, WB Saunders, 1992, Sec. 3.58.

Crocker AC, Nelson RP: Mental retardation. In Levine MD, Carey WB, Crocker AC (eds): Developmental-Behavioral Pediatrics. 2nd ed. Philadelphia, WB Saunders, 1992, pp 500–509.

Vision Impairment

Significant visual impairment is a problem in many children. Partial vision (defined as visual acuity between 20/70 and 20/200) occurs in 1 in 500 schoolchildren in the United States, with about 35,000 children having visual acuity between 20/200 and total blindness. "Legal blindness" is defined as distant visual acuity of 20/200 in the better eye or a visual field that subtends an angle not greater than 20 degrees. Although this definition allows for considerable residual vision, such impairment can be a major barrier to optimal educational development.

The most common *etiology* of severe visual impairment in children is retinopathy of premature infants (see Chapter 6). Congenital cataracts due to a variety of causes occur in 1:250 newborn infants and can result in significant amblyopia; they are also associated with other ocular abnormalities and developmental disabilities. Optic atrophy, retinal degeneration (Leber congenital amaurosis and retinitis pigmentosa), retinoblastoma, and congenital glaucoma are other common causes of significant visual impairment in childhood.

Diagnosis commonly is made between 4 and 8 mo of life based on parental suspicions aroused by unusual behavior, such as lack of smiling in response to appropriate stimuli or motor delays when reaching for an object. Fixation and visual tracking behavior can be seen in most children by 6 wk post-term and by many infants at birth. This behavior can be assessed by moving a brightly colored object or the examiner's face across the visual field of a quiet but alert infant at a distance of 1 ft. The eyes should be examined for red reflexes and pupillary reactions to light, although optical alignment should not be expected until the child is beyond the newborn period. Persistent nystagmus is abnormal at any age. If abnormalities are seen, referral to an ophthalmologist should be made.

The developmental implications of visual impairment are many. Perceptual development is abnormal in terms of body image, and imitative behavior such as smiling is delayed. Delays in mobility may occur in children who are visually impaired from birth, although their postural milestones usually are achieved appropriately. Social bonding with the parents also is limited. Stereotypic behaviors ("blindisms") occur in these children and may at times be self-injurious, requiring intensive behavioral interventions to reduce trauma to eyes, periorbital structures, or other body parts.

Treatment for children with vision impairments is aimed at maximizing available visual skills and developing compensatory methods for individualized education. Classroom settings may be augmented with resource room assistance to present material in a nonvisual format; some schools utilize consultations with an experienced teacher of the blind. Segregated programs sometimes are necessary in training for mobility and for multiply handicapped individuals. Fine motor activity development, listening skills, and Braille reading and writing are intrinsic to successful educational intervention with the child with severe visual impairment.

References

Behrman RE (ed): Nelson Textbook of Pediatrics. 14th ed. Philadelphia, WB Saunders, 1992, Sec. 22.1–22.4.

Davidson PW: Vision impairment. In Levine MD, Carey WB, Crocker AC (eds): Developmental-Behavioral Pediatrics. 2nd ed. Philadelphia, WB Saunders, 1992, pp 519–526.

Nelson LB: The visually handicapped child. Pediatr Rev 6: 173–182, 1984.

Hearing Impairment

The clinical significance of hearing loss varies with its type (conductive vs. sensorineural), its frequency distribution, and its severity as measured in number of decibels (Table 1–24). The most common *cause* of mild to moderate hearing loss in children is a conduction abnormality due to middle ear disease. This abnormality may have significant impact on the development of speech and other aspects of language, particularly if there is chronic fluctuating middle ear fluid. Sensorineural hearing loss is more common as an etiologic factor as hearing loss becomes more severe. The age of onset of the hearing loss may suggest the etiology as well. Other causes of deafness are congenital infection with rubella or cytomegalovirus, meningitis, birth asphyxia, perinatal complications such as kernicterus, ototoxic drugs such as aminoglycoside anti-

Table 1–24. Neurodevelopmental-Behavioral Complications of Hearing Loss

Severity of Hearing Loss	Possible Etiologic Origins	Complications			Types of Therapy
		Speech–Language	*Educational*	*Behavioral*	
Slight 15–25 dB (ASA)	Serous otitis media Perforation of tympanic membrane Sensorineural loss Tympanosclerosis	Difficulty with distant or faint speech	Possible auditory learning dysfunction May reveal a slight verbal deficit	Usually none	May require favorable class setting, speech therapy, auditory training Possible value in hearing aid
Mild 25–40 dB (ASA)	Serous otitis media Perforation of tympanic membrane Sensorineural loss Tympanosclerosis	Difficulty with conversational speech over 3–5 ft May have limited vocabulary and speech disorders	May miss 50% of class discussions Auditory learning dysfunction	Psychologic problems May act inappropriately if directions are not heard well Acting-out behavior Poor self-concept	Special education resource help Hearing aid Favorable class setting Lip reading instruction Speech therapy
Moderate 40–65 dB (ASA)	Chronic otitis media Middle ear anomaly Sensorineural loss	Conversation must be loud to be understood Defective speech Deficient language use and comprehension	Learning disability Difficulty with group learning or discussion Auditory processing dysfunction Limited vocabulary	Emotional and social problems Behavioral reactions of childhood Acting out Poor self-concept	Special education resource or special class Special help in speech–language development Hearing aid and lip reading Speech therapy
Severe 65–95 dB (ASA)	Sensorineural loss Middle ear disease	Loud voices may be heard 2 ft from ear. Identification of environmental sounds Defective speech and language No spontaneous speech development if loss present before 1 yr	Marked educational retardation Marked learning disability Limited vocabulary	Emotional and social problems that are associated with handicap Poor self-concept	Full-time special education for deaf children Hearing aid, lip reading, speech therapy Auditory training Counseling
Profound 95 dB or more (ASA)	Sensorineural or mixed loss	Relies on vision rather than hearing Defective speech and language Speech and language will not develop spontaneously if loss present before 1 yr	Marked learning disability owing to lack of understanding of speech	Congenital and prelingually deaf may show severe emotional underdevelopment	As above Oral and manual communication Counseling

(From Gottlieb MI: Otitis media. In Levine MD, Carey WB, Crocker AC, Gross RT [eds]: Developmental-Behavioral Pediatrics. Philadelphia, WB Saunders, 1983, p 469.)

biotics, and tumors and their treatments. Genetic deafness may be either dominant or recessive in inheritance pattern; this is the main cause of hearing impairment in schools for the deaf. In Down syndrome, there is a predisposition to both conductive loss due to middle ear infection and sensorineural loss due to cochlear disease.

Screening of children who are at risk may allow for early appropriate intervention. Hearing can be screened by means of an office audiogram, but other techniques are needed (e.g., auditory evoked brain stem potential) for the young, neurologically immature or impaired, behaviorally difficult, or severely cognitively impaired child. The typical audiologic *assessment* will include pure tone audiometry over a variety of sound frequencies (pitches), especially over the range of frequencies in which most

speech takes place. The response to actual speech at various volumes (decibel levels) is also tested. **Tympanometry** is used in the assessment of middle ear function and the evaluation of tympanic membrane compliance for pathology in the middle ear, such as fluid, ossicular dysfunction, and eustachian tube dysfunction. For the young infant or less cooperative child who nevertheless can consistently turn his or her eyes to sound stimuli, pure tone and speech audiometry can be done in a sound field, with and without masking of one ear at a time. A list of indications for referral is shown in Table 1–8.

Treatment of hearing impairment may be medical or surgical. The audiologist may believe that amplification is indicated, in which case hearing aids can be tuned to preferentially amplify the fre-

Table 1–25. Language Disorders, Evaluative Techniques, and Interventions

Disorder	Etiology	Evaluative	Treatment
Disorders of Resonance			
Hypernasality	Increased air through nose due to incompetent velopharyngeal seal	Examine for clefts (open or submucous)	ENT, dental evaluation Functional therapy
Hyponasality	Decreased air through nose due to mucosal or lymphoid obstruction of nasal passage	Look in nose for edema Look for tonsillar or adenoidal hypertrophy	ENT evaluation Speech therapy not indicated
Disorders of Voice			
Abnormality of voice quality, pitch, or loudness	Vocal nodules Voice misuse Prolonged endotracheal intubation Neuropathy Nonmalignant tumors Laryngeal trauma Anxiety	History and physical Listen to and describe voice quality Laryngoscopy, direct and indirect	Voice therapy Surgical intervention, when needed Antihistaminic medications for allergy
Disorders of Fluency			
Stuttering	Normal development Response to anxiety Neurogenic (aphasic disorders)	History from family Speech observation Speech pathology evaluation in presence of severe stutter, attempts to hide behavior, avoidance of speaking, muscle tension	Observation in mild cases Speech therapy referral in moderate–severe cases Psychologic evaluation if emotional stressors present Decrease stress of speaking, slow pace of conversation
Disorders of Receptive/Expressive Language			
Auditory attention Auditory discrimination Narrative organization Syntax abnormalities Vocabulary problems Word-finding problems	Hearing loss Neurogenic causes Unknown (functional problem in isolation) Social/cultural factors	General: History and physical Oral examination Speech pathology evaluation	Speech therapy

ENT = ear, nose, and throat.

quency ranges in which the patient has decreased acuity. Educational intervention typically includes speech–language therapy and manual communication. For some children with significant language impairments, manual communication may be used as an adjunct to aid in language concept formation (Total Communication), even in the absence of severe hearing impairment. Even with amplification, many hearing-impaired children demonstrate deficits in processing information presented through the auditory pathway, requiring special educational services to aid in reading and other academic skills. Cochlear implants may be of benefit to some children.

Speech and Language Impairment

Among the most common and difficult developmental problems is the child with speech delay. The most common causes are MR, hearing impairment, social deprivation, and oral–motor abnormalities. If a problem is suspected based on screening, such as the Denver Developmental Screening Test (DENVER II) or the Early Language Milestone Scale, a referral to a specialized hearing and speech center should be arranged.

Language development may be characterized by progress in both receptive and expressive areas of auditory and visual functioning. Simply assessing speech quality, although important, does not suffice for identification of significant language impairments. A child with severe motor impairments may, for example, have speech delays but have normal auditory reception and understanding, whereas a deaf child may lack the capability of speech and be unresponsive to auditory stimuli but have excellent communication abilities via the visual pathway (Table 1–25).

References

Behrman RE (ed): Nelson Textbook of Pediatrics. 14th ed. Philadelphia, WB Saunders, 1992, Sec. 22.19.
Bashir AS, Stark RE, Graham JM: Communicative disorders. In: Levine MD, Carey WB, Crocker AC (eds): Developmental-Behavioral Pediatrics. 2nd ed. Philadelphia, WB Saunders, 1992, pp 557–568.
Resnick TJ, Allen DA, Rapin I: Disorders of language development: Diagnosis and intervention. Pediatr Rev 6: 85–92, 1984.

Cerebral Palsy

The term "cerebral palsy" (CP) includes a variety of nondegenerating neurologic disabilities caused

Table 1–26. Etiologic Classification of Cerebral Palsy

Developmental anomalies
  Disorders of neuronal migration (polymicrogyria)
    Spastic diplegia

  Schizencephalies (double porencephalies)
    Double or bilateral hemiplegia

Congenital infection (TORCH)

Perinatal trauma
  Intracerebral hemorrhage, cerebral infarction, or both
    Spastic states

Metabolic disorders in perinatal period
  Hypoxia-ischemia
    Premature infant
      Spastic diplegia
    Full-term infant
      Spastic states
      Choreoathetosis
      Ataxia

  Hypoglycemia
    Spastic states

  Hyperbilirubinemia
    Choreoathetosis

TORCH = toxoplasmosis, other (syphilis, hepatitis, zoster), rubella, cytomegalovirus, and herpes simplex.
(Adapted from Eiben RM, Crocker AC: Cerebral palsy within the spectrum of developmental disabilities. In Thompson GH, Rubin IL, Bilenker RM [eds]: Comprehensive Management of Cerebral Palsy. New York, Grune & Stratton, 1983, p 20).

by abnormal CNS development and/or injuries in the prenatal and perinatal period that result in abnormalities of motor function. The incidence is about 7:1000 live births and the prevalence is about 500 cases/100,000 population. Significant cognitive handicap is also present in 30–70% of children with CP.

The *causes* of CP are presented in Table 1–26.

The *clinical manifestations* are varied but several distinct patterns can be identified.

Spastic diplegia (10–33%) typically occurs in low-birth-weight infants; it is related to cerebral asphyxia, with or without intraventricular hemorrhage from the immature germinal matrix. The lower extremities are more involved than the upper, with increased muscle tone (spasticity), increased deep tendon reflexes, and a Babinski reflex. Seizures may be present along with other impairments such as learning disabilities and language problems. Severe mental retardation is less common than in other forms of CP. Hip, knee, and ankle contractures can interfere with subsequent ambulation.

Spastic quadriplegia (9–43%) involves all four

extremities. It is associated with low birth weight and severe asphyxial insults, MR, seizures, and feeding difficulties. Scoliosis and other orthopedic problems are much more common in this type of CP.

Spastic hemiplegia (25–40%) is associated with the situations just described but also may be due to cerebrovascular insults such as embolic phenomena or vascular malformations. Seizures are common, but cognitive function may be spared because only one side of the brain is involved. Motor impairments and language processing difficulties can be significant.

Extrapyramidal CP (9–22%) is characterized by hypotonia, choreoathetosis, and dystonic movements occurring later in life. It has been closely associated with the development of kernicterus and has become less common with aggressive management of neonatal hyperbilirubinemia (see Chapter 6). There are fewer seizures and more normal cognitive function than in other forms of CP, although hearing impairment is more common and motor speech disorders may mimic retardation.

Atonic CP is associated with marked hypotonia, brisk reflexes, and severe cognitive delays. It easily can be confused with other spastic forms of CP that also may include hypotonia early in their course. The presence of brisk reflexes helps differentiate atonic CP from hypotonic disorders not originating in the CNS, such as muscular dystrophy or Werdnig-Hoffmann disease.

Mixed forms (9–22%) of CP are due to combinations of insults to multiple cerebral areas, and typically are associated with more complications, including sensory deficits, seizures, and cognitive/perceptual impairments.

Prognosis in CP depends on the individual's spectrum of disability and on the type and intensity of habilitative intervention.

Treatment depends on the pattern of dysfunction that is present. Physical and occupational therapies can facilitate optimal positioning and movement patterns, increasing function of the affected parts. Management of seizures, orthopedic impairments, and sensory impairments will aid in providing optimal educational stimulation. Family support is essential to allow for emotional growth.

References

Behrman RE (ed): Nelson Textbook of Pediatrics. 14th ed. Philadelphia, WB Saunders, 1992, Sec. 20.49.

Taft LT, Matthews WS: Cerebral palsy. *In* Levine MD, Carey WB, Crocker AC (eds): Developmental-Behavioral Pediatrics. 2nd ed. Philadelphia, WB Saunders, 1992, pp 527–533.

School Dysfunction

The inability to function normally in school may be caused by a variety of problems (Table 1–27). This dysfunction may itself result in somatic complaints such as headache, abdominal pains, sleep disorders, and other problems. Learning disabilities and the attention deficit disorders are particularly important causes of school dysfunction that are discussed here.

LEARNING DISABILITIES

Learning disabilities occur in 5–15% of school-age children. Parents may become aware of behavioral difficulties that may interfere with learning in the preschool years when a child demonstrates hyperactivity and inattention, but usually learning disabilities do not become evident until the child enters the primary grades. Teachers then may identify weaknesses in specific areas of school performance or behavior that interfere with learning. The physician may be asked to evaluate the child for evidence of neurologic impairment or other medical illness.

Clinical manifestations usually are not identified by vision and hearing screening. In an extended neurologic examination, markers of neurologic immaturity ("soft signs") and gross and fine motor incoordination may be observed. These findings are physical concomitants that suggest that many learning disabilities are neurologically based at some level; the findings should be used only in conjunction with other tests to describe the child's strengths and weaknesses. They are not predictive

Table 1–27. Causes of School Dysfunction

Systemic medical illness

Learning disability

Medication effects (e.g., chronic administration of bronchodilators, anticonvulsants, decongestants)

Anxiety due to social and emotional factors (e.g., child abuse/neglect, sexual abuse, parental divorce)

Sensory impairments

Classroom–student mismatch (e.g., language barriers, classwork too simple, classwork too hard)

Attention deficit disorder

Occult seizure activity

Environmental toxins (e.g., lead poisoning)

of learning disorders, because they may occur in the absence of educational disability. An expanded neurodevelopmental examination can better describe skills, whereas specialized psychoeducational testing must be done to characterize particular learning disabilities.

ATTENTION DEFICIT DISORDER

The diagnosis of attention deficit disorder (ADD) is based on the presence of a complex of behaviors that characterize the child as inattentive, easily distracted, overactive, and impulsive to such an extent that his or her behavior interferes with the ability to function socially and academically. Restlessness and fidgetiness (hyperactivity) are common but not essential concomitants of this syndrome. Specific learning disabilities also are commonly associated, and some children may display aggressive or oppositional behavior.

The *clinical manifestations* of ADD usually are obvious to teachers. Inattentiveness is demonstrated by failure to complete tasks once begun, failure to grasp directions, and making errors through inattention rather than lack of understanding of the material presented. "Impulsivity" refers to the child's difficulty in controlling reactions and responses when he or she faces uncertainty or the need to attend carefully. Impulsive children commonly act without thinking, shifting quickly from one activity to another, and often exhibit the right behavior at the wrong time, such as calling out in class with an inappropriate answer. They often get into trouble with their peers because they seem "socially inept." Distractibility presents as a reaction to environmental noises or visual stimuli that others can ignore. Distractible children also may be distracted by their own bodies, clothing, or other objects (e.g., touching clothes or hair or running their hands over furniture or walls).

Overactivity, although the most noticeable feature of ADD, is not uniformly present. Children with ADD and ADD with hyperactivity (ADHD) commonly can be observed swinging their legs, rocking their bodies, tapping fingers, or making odd noises. In more obvious cases, they may be in near-constant motion, darting around the room, often ignoring their own or others' safety. ADD has a male-to-female ratio of 4:1. Girls more typically present with inattention but without hyperactivity.

The physical examination typically is normal, although there may be a suggestion of neurologic immaturity. Cranial imaging and EEG are not of benefit in diagnosing or treating ADD or other forms of school dysfunction. They should be performed only when seizures or focal neurologic findings are suggested by history and physical examination.

Some infants and preschool children who are later characterized as having ADD are colicky, irritable, and occasionally more active than their peers, spending a shorter time than normal playing with a given toy and requiring more supervision than other children.

As the child with ADD ages, neurologic maturation may result in symptomatic improvement. However, adolescents who had ADD in their early school years often continue to demonstrate school dysfunction, as well as low self-esteem and social inappropriateness.

Primary *treatment* of the child with ADD combines pharmacologic and environmental interventions. However, such management often is complicated by the presence of associated learning disabilities that require specific educational interventions. Moreover, many such children have developed emotional reactions to what may be years of social inappropriateness and school dysfunction, and both family behavior patterns and the child's psychologic reactions must be assessed to avoid continuation of undesirable stereotyping. The beneficial effects of medication are decreased significantly in the presence of unaddressed emotional or educational needs.

Table 1–28. Stimulant Medications Used for Treatment of Attention Deficits

Generic Name	Brand Name	Preparations	Range of Daily Dose (Average)	Onset of Action	Duration of Action	Comments
Methylphenidate	Ritalin	Tablets: 5, 10, 20 mg; 20-mg sustained release	5–60 mg (10–30) (0.3–1.0 mg/kg)	30 min	3–5 hr 4–8 hr	Not recommended below 6 yr
Dextroamphetamine	Dexedrine	Tablets: 5 mg; sustained-release capsules: 5, 10, 15 mg	5–40 mg (5–20)	30 min	3–5 hr	Not recommended below 3 yr
Pemoline	Cylert	Tablets: 18.75, 37.5, 75 mg	18.75–112.5 mg (56.25–75)	2–4 hr (may not see clinical results until 3–4 wk of therapy)	"Long-acting"	Not recommended below 6 yr

The drugs most commonly used in treating ADD are presented in Table 1–28. They are presumed to have their neuropharmacologic effects on dopaminergic neurons in the brain stem reticular activating system. Such psychostimulants are most effective when used in conjunction with behavior modification techniques. Major side effects of these drugs are sleep and appetite impairment, elevation of pulse rate and blood pressure, rebound overactivity, irritability on withdrawal of the medication, and attentional overfocusing. Motor tics may be exacerbated by these drugs. The child should play an active role in decisions about medications in terms of administration and monitoring the effect of the drug, both to give the child a measure of control in managing his or her problem and to avoid noncompliance.

There are no significant beneficial effects of specific dietary interventions in children with ADD or other forms of school dysfunction.

References

Behrman RE (ed): Nelson Textbook of Pediatrics. 14th ed. Philadelphia, WB Saunders, 1992, Sec. 3.39, 3.55.

Klein RG: Prognosis of attention deficit disorder and its management in adolescence. Pediatr Rev 8:216–222, 1987.

Levine MD: Attentional variation and dysfunction. In Levine MD, Carey WB, Crocker AC (eds): Developmental-Behavioral Pediatrics. 2nd ed. Philadelphia, WB Saunders, 1992, pp 468–474.

Levine MD: Maladaptation to school. In Levine MD, Carey WB, Crocker AC (eds): Developmental-Behavioral Pediatrics. 2nd ed. Philadelphia, WB Saunders, 1992, pp 495–499.

Chronic Disease

Chronic diseases may be characterized by long-term disability, a variable relapsing course, or a gradual declining course. Some examples of such disorders include arthritis, asthma, autism, traumatic brain injury, cerebral palsy, chronic renal failure, congenital heart disease, cystic fibrosis, diabetes mellitus, mental retardation, visual impairments, seizure disorders, sickle cell disease, leukemia, acquired immunodeficiency syndrome, hearing impairment, neural tube defects, cleft palate/lip, hemophilia, and phenylketonuria. The goal in managing such patients is to maximize their potential for productive adult functioning and for a high quality of life by treating the primary disease and aiding the patient and family to deal with the stresses incurred because of the disease. The factors that influence responses to chronic diseases include disease-related factors (such as pain, treatment, and visibility of condition), age of onset, age and developmental level of the child, and family attitudes and stress.

Whenever a chronic disease is diagnosed, family members typically go through grieving processes similar to those seen at the time of death, including anger, denial, negotiation in an attempt to forestall the inevitable, and depression. However, because the child with the chronic disease is a constant reminder of the object of this grief, it may take family members a long time to accept the condition. Understanding and support on the part of the physician can facilitate this process by sharing both the known and the unknown and by allaying guilty feelings and fear. In order to minimize denial, it is helpful to confirm the family's observations about the child. Once the diagnosis has been presented, the family may not be able to absorb any further information, so written material and the option for further discussion at a later date should be offered.

When children with chronic diseases are acutely ill, treatment becomes a common goal for all concerned. However, as stabilization takes place and the child is not "cured," it is important that the family not feel abandoned by staff who are involved in the case. There are predictable times in the course of a chronic illness when stress is greatest (Table 1–29).

A major goal of care for the family of the child with a chronic disease is that the family and child feel in control of the situation. Although in the acute health care setting the locus of control is with the medical management team, as the child moves into a more routine home-based life the control should shift to the family and the child. Treatment plans should be organized to allow for the greatest degree of normalization of the child's life.

Among chronic diseases, the most difficult with which to deal are those with major multiple system involvement, such as spina bifida, severe cerebral palsy, cystic fibrosis, sickle cell disease, inborn

Table 1–29. Predictable Crises and Stress in the Medical Course of Chronic Disease

Onset and diagnosis
Disease-specific, emotionally distressing medical symptoms
Hospitalization(s)
Response to appearance of initial major complication
Confrontation with significant therapeutic choices
Failure(s) of an expected therapeutic response
Threat of imminent death

(From Hamburg BA: Chronic illness. In Levine MD, Carey WB, Crocker AC, Gross RT [eds]: Developmental-Behavioral Pediatrics. Philadelphia, WB Saunders, 1983, p 456.)

metabolic errors, and a variety of congenital anomaly syndromes. The combination of sensory, motor, and cognitive handicap and emotional/behavioral abnormality is a particularly difficult problem, requiring multiple medical and habilitative specialists. The primary physician may assume the role of coordinator of care.

References

Behrman RE (ed): Nelson Textbook of Pediatrics. 14th ed. Philadelphia, WB Saunders, 1992, Sec. 3.57.

Gortmaker SL, Sappenfield W: Chronic childhood disorders: Prevalence and impact. Pediatr Clin North Am 31: 3–18, 1984.

Perrin JM: Chronic illness. In Levine MD, Carey WB, Crocker AC (eds): Developmental-Behavioral Pediatrics. 2nd ed. Philadelphia, WB Saunders, 1992, pp 304–308.

Swartz DR: Dealing with chronic illness in childhood. Pediatr Rev 6:67–73, 1984.

Autism and Psychoses in Childhood

These rare disorders may have a distinctive early onset in infancy and preschool years or an adultlike presentation in older children.

Early **infantile autism** is a disorder of unknown cause and poor prognosis that usually is characterized by significant impairment of the child's ability to relate to people, including parents. It affects 0.7–4.5:10,000 children. *Clinical manifestations* typically indicate that, as an infant, the autistic child was noticeably "uncuddly," with delayed or absent smiling. Later the young child may spend hours in solitary play and be withdrawn in the presence of other children or adults and indifferent to attempts to communicate. Ritualistic behavior and compulsive routines are characteristic, and the interruption of this behavior may invoke tantrum or rage reactions. Eye contact is minimal or absent. Head banging, teeth grinding, rocking, diminished responsiveness to pain and external stimuli, and even self-mutilation may be noted. Speech often is delayed and, when present, frequently is dominated by echolalia, pronoun reversal, nonsense rhyming, and other unusual language forms. The child's IQ is difficult to evaluate because of language and socialization deficits and often falls in the functional retarded range by conventional testing. Suspicion of this diagnosis requires referral to a specialist for further evaluation and treatment. A relationship between autism and schizophrenia has been suspected, but these children rarely go on to develop classic schizophrenic symptoms.

The onset of affective psychosis and schizophrenia in older children resembles that in adults. The same diagnostic criteria are applied but must be interpreted in terms of the developmental stage of the child. Long-term psychiatric care often is required for these chronic disorders.

References

Behrman RE (ed): Nelson Textbook of Pediatrics. 14th ed. Philadelphia, WB Saunders, 1992, Sec. 3.43–3.46.

Brent DA, Puig-Antich J, Rabinovitch H: Major psychiatric disorders in childhood and adolescence. In Levine MD, Carey WB, Crocker AC (eds): Developmental-Behavioral Pediatrics. 2nd ed. Philadelphia, WB Saunders, 1992, pp 569–588.

Larsson EV, Luce SC, Anderson SR, et al: Autism. In Levine MD, Carey WB, Crocker AC (eds): Developmental-Behavioral Pediatrics. 2nd ed. Philadelphia, WB Saunders, 1992, pp 534–542.

Pediatric Nutrition and Nutritional Disorders

Andrew M. Tershakovec
Virginia A. Stallings

2

Proper nutrition is central in promoting the normal growth and development of children. Rapidly growing infants, children, and maturing adolescents have specific but not necessarily fixed requirements for macronutrients (protein, fat, carbohydrates, fluids) and micronutrients (vitamins, trace elements, minerals). Pathophysiologic mechanisms present during various disease states may adversely affect nutritional status, thus retarding growth and development even in the presence of normal recommended intakes of both macro- and micronutrients. Diseases associated with inflammation (infectious diseases, systemic lupus erythematosus, inflammatory bowel disease), trauma (fractures, burns), malignancy, malabsorption (cystic fibrosis, celiac disease, sprue), inborn errors of metabolism (galactosemia, maple syrup urine disease), and chronic cardiopulmonary insufficiency (heart failure, bronchopulmonary dysplasia) place additional stress on nutritional balance, may alter energy and nutrient needs, and thus may require nutrient supplementation or special diets. These disease processes may limit the genetic potential and may even modify the eventual expression of growth.

Nutritional disorders are not confined to children living in areas of famine and starvation. Deficiencies and excesses of nutrient intake are common problems among infants and children in the United States, as evidenced by the continued existence of iron-deficiency anemia and the increasing rate of childhood obesity, respectively. Furthermore, specific nutritional deficiency syndromes are relatively common among low-birth-weight infants, children with malabsorption (cystic fibrosis, short bowel syndrome, cholestatic jaundice), breast-fed infants of strict vegetarian parents, and acutely or chronically ill hospitalized children with multiorgan system dysfunction requiring intensive care (Fig. 2–1).

BODY COMPOSITION AND GROWTH

Nutrition plays a central role in growth and the changing body composition. Growth and maturation begin at the moment of conception and cease with the end of puberty. Prenatal growth is part of a continuous developmental and genetic process modified by maternal variables; during postnatal growth this process is more dependent on family, socioeconomic, and environmental factors. The normal growth patterns after birth are shown in Figures 1–2 through 1–14. The velocity (rate of change) of body mass and length accretion is greater at 32 wk gestation (15 kg/yr and 65 cm/yr, respectively) than in any subsequent period, including puberty. Growth in length reflects the differential growth of the head, trunk, and long bones of the legs (see Fig. 1–15). Head size increases most rapidly after 28 wk of gestation and ceases before 2 yr of age. The trunk increases during the same period but continues to lengthen at a slower rate from 2 yr through puberty. The legs grow fastest during the period covering the last 14 wk of a gestation through the first 6 mo of life (18 cm/yr). This rate exceeds that of leg growth in male puberty (4 cm/yr). Linear growth and mass growth are differentially reduced by malnutrition but synchronously increased by obesity. (See Chapters 1 and 17 for measurement of growth.)

Height and weight measurements provide only a crude estimation of body composition. Organ weights increase with maturation; some organs assume a smaller proportion of body mass (brain), while the percentage of body mass that is composed of muscle and adipose tissue increases (Fig. 2–2). Little adipose tissue is deposited during early fetal development, but a rapid deposition occurs during the last 3 mo of gestation. The term infant's

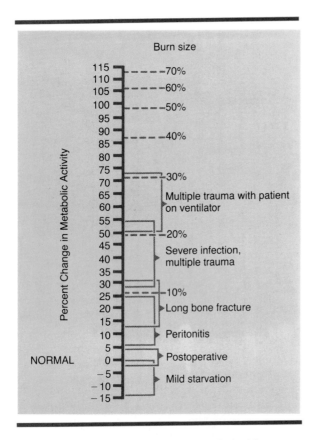

Figure 2–1. Increased energy needs with stress. (Adapted from Witmore D: The Metabolic Management of the Critically Ill. New York, Plenum, 1977; *In* Walker W, Watkins J [eds]: Nutrition in Pediatrics: Basic Science and Clinical Application. Boston, Little, Brown & Co Inc, 1985, p 873.)

body contains approximately 20–25% adipose tissue, 80% of which is subcutaneous and 20% visceral. After early infancy, the percentage of fat decreases to 15% until the acceleration during pubertal growth. During puberty the proportion of fat increases to 20–30% in the average girl. The largest tissue of the body is skeletal muscle, which makes up 25% of body mass during fetal life and increases to 45% in the adult. The rate of increase is greatest between birth and 5 yr, with an additional small increase in boys at puberty.

Different organ systems develop at different times and different rates. Seventy-five percent of brain growth is completed by 3 yr of age and 90% by 7 yr; the reproductive system grows little until puberty. The effect of malnutrition on development depends on the stage of development. Because the brain develops early, it is relatively protected from malnutrition in later childhood;

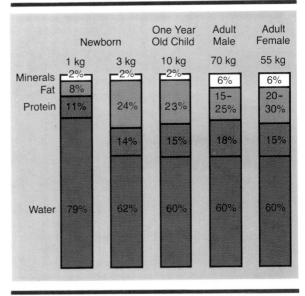

Figure 2–2. The changes in the proportions of body composition with growth. (Adapted from Pencharz P: Body composition and growth. *In* Walker W, Watkins J [eds]: Nutrition in Pediatrics: Basic Science and Clinical Application. Boston, Little, Brown & Co Inc, 1985, p 81.)

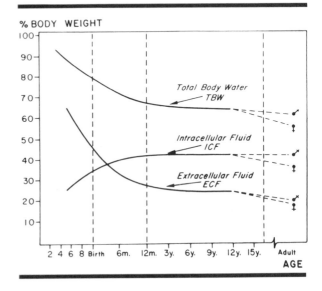

Figure 2–3. Change with age in total body water and its major subdivisions. (Data from Friis-Hansen. Body water compartments in children: Changes during growth and related changes in body composition. Pediatrics 28:169, 1961. *In* Winters RW [ed]: The Body Fluids in Pediatrics. Boston, Little, Brown & Co Inc, 1973, p 100.)

delayed puberty is seen in malnourished adolescents.

The embryo contains 95% water, which decreases to 80% at 28 wk gestation. During the 3rd trimester, as significant fat (which is anhydrous) is deposited, the proportion of body water decreases further to 72%. By 8 yr of age, it has reached the adult proportion of 60%. The extracellular fluid compartment is substantially greater than the intracellular fluid compartment during fetal life. Before 6 mo of age, intracellular fluid increases and extracellular fluid decreases so the components become equal. This trend continues so that, by adulthood, the intracellular fluid compartment has twice the volume of the extracellular compartment (Fig. 2–3). The relatively high extracellular fluid volume in the young infant results in a vulnerability to abnormal fluid losses during illness.

DIET OF THE NORMAL INFANT

In the first 4–6 mos of life, human milk or, more often, various infant formulas can provide complete nutrition to the growing infant. However, breast milk is the recommended source of nutrition for almost all children. Nonetheless, very few infants are exclusively breast fed beyond 2–3 mos of age. Every effort should be made to encourage and promote breast feeding.

Although infant formulas simulate the composition of human milk, human milk has several subtle nutritional and nonnutritional advantages over infant formula. From a practical point of view, breast milk does not need to be warmed, is ready to serve, does not need a clean water supply, is generally free of micro-organisms, and does not need a clean serving container. These issues are significant concerns in less developed areas of the world. Breast feeding also encourages maternal–infant bonding. Human milk reduces the incidence of cow's milk protein allergy, eczema, and various infections and contains protective bacterial and viral antibodies (immunoglobulin A) and macrophages. Although the iron content of human milk is relatively low, the iron is more biologically available than that in cow's milk. Human milk also contains lactoferrin, an iron-binding whey protein that inhibits the growth of *Escherichia coli*. In addition, there are other nutrients contained in breast milk that are not present in most formulas (e.g., cholesterol, taurine, nucleotides), whose function or importance is not well understood. Breast feeding is recommended for 6–12 mo.

The alternative to human milk is iron-fortified

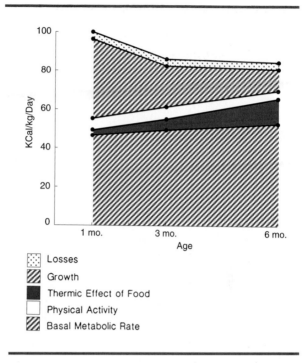

Figure 2–4. Energy requirements of infants. (From Waterlow JC. Basic concepts in the determination of nutritional requirements of normal infants. *In* Tsang RC, Nichols BL [eds]: Nutrition during infancy. Philadelphia, Hanley and Belfus, Inc, 1988, p 6.)

formula, which permits adequate growth of most infants. No supplements are needed with such formulas. Cow's milk should not be introduced until after the 1st year of life.

After 4–6 mo, solid foods (beikost) and juices are introduced (using these nutrient sources initiates *weaning*), progressively replacing some of the calories and nutrients provided by human milk or formula. Although the growth rate of the child is decreasing, energy needs for greater activity increase (Fig. 2–4). A relatively high-fat and calorically dense diet (milk) still is needed to deliver adequate calories. Nutritional supplements become an important source of some nutrients (iron) in the second 6 mo of life.

The chemical composition of lean body mass (LBM) changes with growth. The concentrations of nitrogen and potassium increase and the concentration of chloride decreases as the relationship between extracellular and intracellular water compartments changes. After the 7th mo of gestation, the fall in total extracellular sodium is counterbalanced by an increase in total sodium in bone. Calcium is confined primarily to bone, but phosphorus

Table 2–1. Food and Nutrition Board, National Academy of Sciences–National Research Council Recommended Dietary Allowances, RDA (Revised 1989)*

Category	Age (yr) or Condition	Weight† kg	Weight† lb	Height† cm	Height† in	Protein (g)	Fat-Soluble Vitamins Vitamin A (μg RE)‡	Vitamin D (μg)§	Vitamin E (mg α-TE)‖	Vitamin K (μg)
Infants	0.0–0.5	6	13	60	24	13	375	7.5	3	5
	0.5–1.0	9	20	71	28	14	375	10	4	10
Children	1–3	13	29	90	35	16	400	10	6	15
	4–6	20	44	112	44	24	500	10	7	20
	7–10	28	62	132	52	28	700	10	7	30
Males	11–14	45	99	157	62	45	1000	10	10	45
	15–18	66	145	176	69	59	1000	10	10	65
	19–24	72	160	177	70	58	1000	10	10	70
	25–50	79	174	176	70	63	1000	5	10	80
	51+	77	170	173	68	63	1000	5	10	80
Females	11–14	46	101	157	62	46	800	10	8	45
	15–18	55	120	163	64	44	800	10	8	55
	19–24	58	128	164	65	46	800	10	8	60
	25–50	63	138	163	64	50	800	5	8	65
	51+	65	143	160	63	50	800	5	8	65
Pregnant						60	800	10	10	65
Lactating	1st 6 mo					65	1300	10	12	65
	2nd 6 mo					62	1200	10	11	65

* The allowances, expressed as average daily intakes over time, are intended to provide for individual variations among most normal persons as they live in the United States under usual environmental stresses. Diets should be based on a variety of common foods in order to provide other nutrients for which human requirements have been less well defined.

† Weights and heights of Reference Adults are actual medians for the U.S. population of the designated age, as reported by NHANES II. The median weights and heights of those under 19 years of age were taken from Hamill et al. (1979). The use of these figures does not imply that the height-to-weight ratios are ideal.

‡ Retinol equivalents. 1 retinol equivalent = 1 μg retinol or 6 μg β-carotene.

§ As cholecalciferol. 10 μg cholecalciferol = 400 IU of vitamin D.

‖ α-Tocopherol equivalents. 1 mg d-α-tocopherol = 1 α-TE.

¶ 1 NE (niacin equivalent) is equal to 1 mg of niacin or 60 mg of dietary tryptophan.

(From Recommended Dietary Allowances. 10th ed., National Academy Press, 1989, pp 15–17.)

is an equally important constituent of soft tissues. During the first 2 mo of gestation, the phosphorus concentration is greater than that of calcium. Skeletal calcification begins thereafter, and body calcium concentration increases more rapidly than that of phosphorus. At term, 98% of body calcium concentration, 80% of phosphorus, and 60% of magnesium are in bones. During the adolescent growth period, a male accumulates 12 kg of protein, 1.2 kg of calcium, 0.7 kg of phosphorus, 26 g of magnesium, 4 g of iron, and 1.5 g of zinc. These nutrients are accumulated in specific tissues, which cease to grow when they reach a size proportional to the total body length and mass. The genetic coordination of tissue accretion is remarkable, but various dietary deficiencies may become rate limiting for any of these growth processes.

Energy and nutrient requirements generally are proportional to LBM; these requirements increase as children grow and attain more LBM. Because women have proportionally more fat mass and less LBM, their requirements usually are less than those of men. For some nutrients, women have equal (vitamin C) or greater (iron) needs than men. To meet the recommended dietary allowance (RDA), a woman needs to ingest a more nutrient-dense diet than a man. Thus women are at risk for deficiencies of some of those specific nutrients.

References

Behrman RE (ed): Nelson Textbook of Pediatrics. 14th ed. Philadelphia, WB Saunders, 1992, Sec. 3.1–3.10.

Widowson EM: Growth and body composition in childhood. In Brunser O, Carrazza FR, Gracey M, et al (eds): Clinical Nutrition of the Young Child. New York, Raven Press, 1984, pp 1–14.

Nutrient Needs (Tables 2–1 and 2–2)

The *minimum daily requirement* (MDR) of a nutrient is set at a level of consumption below which

Water-Soluble Vitamins							Minerals						
Vitamin C (mg)	Thiamin (mg)	Ribo-flavin (mg)	Niacin (mg NE)¶	Vitamin B_6 (mg)	Folate (µg)	Vitamin B_{12} (µg)	Calcium (mg)	Phos-phorus (mg)	Mag-nesium (mg)	Iron (mg)	Zinc (mg)	Iodine (µg)	Selenium (µg)
30	0.3	0.4	5	0.3	25	0.3	400	300	40	6	5	40	10
35	0.4	0.5	6	0.6	35	0.5	600	500	60	10	5	50	15
40	0.7	0.8	9	1.0	50	0.7	800	800	80	10	10	70	20
45	0.9	1.1	12	1.1	75	1.0	800	800	120	10	10	90	20
45	1.0	1.2	13	1.4	100	1.4	800	800	170	10	10	120	30
50	1.3	1.5	17	1.7	150	2.0	1200	1200	270	12	15	150	40
60	1.5	1.8	20	2.0	200	2.0	1200	1200	400	12	15	150	50
60	1.5	1.7	19	2.0	200	2.0	1200	1200	350	10	15	150	70
60	1.5	1.7	19	2.0	200	2.0	800	800	350	10	15	150	70
60	1.2	1.4	15	2.0	200	2.0	800	800	350	10	15	150	70
50	1.1	1.3	15	1.4	150	2.0	1200	1200	280	15	12	150	45
60	1.1	1.3	15	1.5	180	2.0	1200	1200	300	15	12	150	50
60	1.1	1.3	15	1.6	180	2.0	1200	1200	280	15	12	150	55
60	1.1	1.3	15	1.6	180	2.0	800	800	280	15	12	150	55
60	1.0	1.2	13	1.6	180	2.0	800	800	280	10	12	150	55
70	1.5	1.6	17	2.2	400	2.2	1200	1200	320	30	15	175	65
95	1.6	1.8	20	2.1	280	2.6	1200	1200	355	15	19	200	75
90	1.6	1.7	20	2.1	260	2.6	1200	1200	340	15	16	200	75

signs of deficiency develop. The *RDA* is set at 2–6 times the MDR and takes into consideration modifications needed for weight, sex, age, pregnancy, and lactation. The RDA for nutrients usually is greater than 2 standard deviations above the mean requirement for each food group, while it is at the mean for energy requirements. Some nutrients have no RDA and thus recommendations are based on quantities known to be safe within a given adequate range (Table 2–2). Caloric needs may be determined by resting energy expenditure plus energy needed for exercise, both of which are determined by oxygen consumption. More often caloric needs are estimated by the following rule of thumb: 100 kcal/kg for the first 10 kg, 50 kcal/kg for the next 10–20 kg, and 20 kcal/kg for weight above 20 kg (see Chapter 6).

Breast Feeding

Mothers should decide before delivery whether to breast feed or bottle feed their infants. When breast feeding is chosen, they should be assisted to develop appropriate feeding skills and practices. The ultimate goal is to produce sufficient milk to breast feed an infant for 6–12 mo (see Table 6–23 for composition of human milk).

BEGINNING BREAST FEEDING

The mother should be comfortable and the infant positioned so that nothing interferes with mouth-to-breast contact. The breast from which the infant nurses should be supported with the opposite hand, with the thumb and index fingers above the nipple to allow the infant easy access to the nipple. The *rooting reflex* should be explained to the parents to make initiation of breast feeding easier. The nipple should be stroked against the infant's cheek nearest the nipple. The infant will turn toward the nipple (rooting reflex) and open the mouth, allowing the introduction of the nipple and areola. The entire nipple and most of the areola should be placed in the infant's mouth. The infant "latches on" by compressing the lips. The mechanics of normal suckling include: (1) suction of 4–6 cm of the areola, (2) compression of the nipple against the palate, (3) stimulation of milk ejection by initial rapid non-nutritive sucking, and (4) extraction of milk from the lactiferous sinuses by a slower suck–swallow rhythm of approximately 1/sec. The infant is removed from the breast by placing a clean finger between the baby's gums and the areola to release suction. The mean feeding frequency is 8–12 times/day during the first 2 wk.

EXCLUSIVE BREAST FEEDING

Breast feeding is the recommended method for feeding normal infants during the first 6 mo of life. By making the mother aware of possible nursing problems that may arise shortly after hospital dis-

Table 2–2. Estimated Safe and Adequate Daily Dietary Intakes of Selected Vitamins and Minerals*

| Category | Age (years) | Vitamins | | Trace Elements† | | | | |
		Biotin (μg)	Pantothenic Acid (mg)	Copper (mg)	Manganese (mg)	Fluoride (mg)	Chromium (μg)	Molybdenum (μg)
Infants	0–0.5	10	2	0.4–0.6	0.3–0.6	0.1–0.5	10–40	15–30
	0.5–1.0	15	3	0.6–0.7	0.6–1.0	0.2–1.0	20–60	20–40
Children and adolescents	1–3	20	3	0.7–1.0	1.0–1.5	0.5–1.5	20–80	25–50
	4–6	25	3–4	1.0–1.5	1.5–2.0	1.0–2.5	30–120	30–75
	7–10	30	4–5	1.0–2.0	2.0–3.0	1.5–2.5	50–200	50–150
	11+	30–100	4–7	1.5–2.5	2.0–5.0	1.5–2.5	50–200	75–250
Adults		30–100	4–7	1.5–3.0	2.0–5.0	1.5–4.0	50–200	75–250

* Because there is less information on which to base allowances, these figures are not given in the main table of RDA and are provided here in the form of ranges of recommended intakes.

† Because the toxic levels for many trace elements may be only several times usual intakes, the upper levels for the trace elements given in this table should not be habitually exceeded.

(From Recommended Dietary Allowances. 10th ed, National Academy Press, 1989, p 284.)

charge, many cases of lactation failure may be averted. *Colostrum*, a high protein and low fat and lactose product, is produced in small amounts during the first few postpartum days. It seems to have some nutritional value but primarily has important immunologic and maturational properties. Primiparous women usually experience breast engorgement on the 3rd postpartum day; the breasts become hard and are painful, the nipples become nonprotractile, and the mother's temperature may increase slightly. Enhancement of milk flow is the best management. If severe engorgement occurs, areolar rigidity may prevent the infant from grasping the nipple and areola. Attention to proper "latch on" and hand expression of milk assist drainage. The first appetite spurt of the infant is noted at 8–10 days of life by an increase in the demand for nursing, which serves to stimulate the production of a greater volume of milk. Hydration status is an index of the adequacy of intake. A well-hydrated infant voids 6–8 times/day. Each voiding should soak, not merely moisten, a diaper. Parents should be advised to contact the pediatrician if the infant voids less than 6 times/day. Telephone follow-up is valuable during the interim between discharge and the first pediatric visit in order to monitor the progress of lactation. Initial weight loss in the neonatal period is greater in the breast-fed than in the bottle-fed infant, but birth weight generally is regained by 2 wk of age.

The duration of nursing ranges from 4–20 min per breast. Longer nursing may be an adaptation to inadequate milk production or ineffective "latch on." Eighty percent of milk is consumed in the first 4 min of nursing at each breast. Milk volume increases rapidly during the first 2 wk after parturition. Women who breast feed their infants exclusively produce approximately 750 mL/day. This level of production is maintained for at least 4–6 mo, but milk volume declines in response to decreased nursing after solid foods have been added to the infant's diet.

The characteristics of the stools of breast-fed infants often alarm mothers. Stool frequencies of normal breast-fed infants range from one at each nursing to one per week. Stools are unformed, yellow, brown, or green, and seedy in appearance.

In the newborn period, elevated concentrations of bilirubin occur more often in breast-fed infants than in formula-fed infants. Feeding frequency during the first 3 days of life of breast-fed infants is related inversely to the serum level of bilirubin; frequent feedings stimulate meconium passage and excretion of bilirubin. The use of water supplements in breast-fed infants has no effect on serum bilirubin levels. If the concentration of serum bilirubin rises sufficiently to be of clinical concern, formula feedings should be substituted, which may prevent an increase in bilirubin levels. A temporary discontinuation of breast feeding for 24–72 hours is of diagnostic value in identifying *breast milk jaundice* (Chapter 6). Slight elevations in serum bilirubin commonly are observed when breast feeding is resumed, and a less severe level of jaundice may persist for several weeks. No detrimental effects of breast milk jaundice have been reported. If temporary formula feeding is introduced, the mother's milk production can be maintained by manual milk expression.

SUPPLEMENTATION

Breast-fed term infants require supplementation with vitamin K (intramuscular ×1) at birth; thereafter they require vitamin D and fluoride. Iron or iron-fortified formula should be added at 4–6 mo of life. Vitamin B_{12} should be included if the mother is a strict vegan. Formula and/or water supplements in addition to breast milk are not necessary for term breast-fed infants. Supplementary formula feedings in this period usually are needed for feeding difficulties and/or lactation failure. When nursing from an artificial nipple, the infant positions the tongue differently than when breast feeding. If the infant has difficulty breast feeding after nursing from a bottle, the mother should make certain that the infant's mouth is positioned well over the areola.

Iron-fortified infant formula should be used as supplementary feedings, if such feedings are given to the infant under 12 mo of age. Alternatively, the working mother may express her milk and store it frozen for use by other caregivers.

After 4–6 mo of age, solid foods may be added to the diet. After 6 mo of age, the nutrients often found somewhat lacking in the diet of the exclusively breast-fed infant are likely to be protein, iron, and zinc; total calories may be lacking as well. Thus, the most appropriate first food to add to the diet of exclusively breast-fed infants may be iron-fortified (rice) cereals.

COMMON BREAST-FEEDING PROBLEMS

If a lactating woman reports fever, chills, and malaise, mastitis should be considered. Treatment includes frequent and complete emptying of the breast. Breast feeding should not be stopped because the mother's mastitis has no adverse effects on the breast-fed infant. Antibiotic therapy is indicated. Untreated mastitis may progress to a breast abscess. If an abscess is diagnosed, breast feeding should be discontinued from the affected breast until the condition is successfully treated. Milk expression from the affected breast should continue, but the milk should be discarded.

Maternal infections of active tuberculosis, syphilis, human immunodeficiency virus, typhoid, rubella, mumps, cytomegalovirus, or herpes are contraindications to breast feeding. When the mother has active tuberculosis or syphilis, breast feeding may be continued after initiating therapy.

The mother should be advised against the use of unprescribed drugs, including alcohol, nicotine, caffeine, or "street drugs." No medications (including over-the-counter drugs) should be taken without consulting a physician. Table 2–3 shows effects of selected maternal drugs on the breast-fed infant.

Table 2–3. Effect of Maternal Drugs on the Breast-Fed Infant

Drug	Effect	Comment
Amoxicillin	None	Safe
Antimetabolites	Carcinogenic	Contraindicated
Aspirin	Rare complication of bleeding	Usually safe
Atenolol	None	Probably safe
Bromocriptine	Suppresses lactation	Avoid
Carbamazepine	Unknown	Probably safe
Cascara	Colic, diarrhea	Avoid
Chloramphenicol	Gray baby syndrome	Contraindicated
Codeine	Lethargy	Usually safe
Diazepam	Lethargy, apnea	High doses contraindicated
Digoxin	None	Safe
Ergot	Gangrene, vasospasm	Contraindicated
Furosemide	None	Safe
Gold salts	Hepatonephrotoxicity	Contraindicated
Meperidine	Lethargy	Avoid
Methimazole	Hypothyroidism	Contraindicated
Metoprolol	None	Probably safe
Metronidazole	Carcinogenic?	Contraindicated
Phenindione	Hemorrhage	Contraindicated
Phenobarbital	Lethargy	Usually safe
Phenytoin	None	Safe
Prednisone	None	Probably safe
Propoxyphene	Lethargy	Usually safe
Propranolol	None	Probably safe
Propylthiouracil	Usually none; rare goiter	Probably safe
Radioactive material	Carcinogenic	Discontinue breast feeding 1–2 wk
Tetracycline	Discolored teeth	Contraindicated

References

Behrman RE (ed): Nelson Textbook of Pediatrics. 14th ed. Philadelphia, WB Saunders, 1992, Sec. 4.10.
Freed G: Breast-feeding. JAMA 269:243, 1993.
Lawrence R: Breastfeeding. 2nd ed. St. Louis, CV Mosby, 1985.

Weaning Foods

Substitutes for and supplements to human milk are regarded as weaning foods in this section.

COW'S MILK–BASED FORMULAS

Such formulas (see Table 6–23) are composed of reconstituted, skimmed cow's milk or a mixture of skimmed cow's milk and electrolyte-depleted cow's milk whey or casein proteins. The fat used in infant formulas is a mixture of soy, palm, coconut, corn, oleo, or safflower oils; all contain lactose. Modern cow's milk–based formulas are equivalent to human milk in that they promote growth during the first 6 mo of life. Complete cow's milk–based infant formulas are used as *substitutes* for breast milk for infants whose mothers choose not to or cannot breast feed, as *supplements* for breast-fed infants whose mothers choose to omit occasional feedings, or as *complementary* feedings if breast feeding alone does not result in normal growth or other signs of malnutrition are present. Breast milk fortifiers (whey–casein protein, corn syrup–lactose, butterfat, minerals) also are available for use in special situations (premature infants when breast milk is inadequate for growth).

SOY FORMULA

Soy protein–based formulas are used if cow's milk–based formula intolerance occurs either from protein hypersensitivity or from lactose intolerance. These formulas are nutritionally sound and safe alternatives to cow's milk–based formulas (see Table 6–23). The soy protein is supplemented with l-methionine to improve its nutritional qualities. The carbohydrate in soy formulas is sucrose, glucose oligomers (smaller molecular weight corn starches), or a mixture of the two. The fat mixture is similar to that used in cow's milk formulas.

Soy protein formulas do not prevent the development of allergic disorders in later life, and clinical intolerances to soy milk proteins or cow's milk occur with equal frequency (see Chapter 11). Soy protein formulas can be recommended for use in vegetarian families choosing not to serve animal protein formulas and in the management of galactosemia and primary and secondary lactose intolerance. Although safe for the normal child, soy-based formula has been associated with protein-losing enteropathy in patients with cystic fibrosis and with neonatal rickets in premature infants. Too often soy and other "special" formulas are used indiscriminately to "treat" poorly evaluated patients with colic, formula intolerance, or more serious diseases.

PREMATURE INFANT FORMULAS (See Chapter 6)

THERAPEUTIC FORMULAS

The composition of infant formulas has been further modified to meet specific therapeutic requirements (Table 6–23). Therapeutic formulas designed to avoid digestive insufficiency or protein hypersensitivity contain hydrolyzed casein, whole casein, or soy protein as a source of amino acids. These formulas are also lactose free; some contain glucose oligomers and soluble starches, and some contain medium-chain triglycerides. Modular formulas allow stepwise introduction of specific carbohydrates and fats into the diet in a logical sequence for the purpose of therapeutic feeding trials. Modular formulas are nutritionally incomplete, are often hyperosmolar, and should be used only under close professional supervision.

WHOLE COW'S MILK

Whole cow's milk should not be introduced into the diet before the age of 1 yr. The high solute load of cow's milk, its low iron content, and the potential to create cow's milk protein intolerance if ingested before 12 mo make it inappropriate to use earlier. Cow's milk protein intolerance may cause gross or microscopic intestinal bleeding leading to iron deficiency.

BABY FOODS

Commercially prepared or homemade foods fulfill the nutritional needs of the infant. Such foods are introduced at 4–6 mo. Because infant foods are calorically less dense than milk, they do not "fatten up" an infant. Furthermore, oropharyngeal coordination is immature before 3 mo. Vitamin- and mineral-enriched dry cereals are used as a source of calories (~375 calories/100 g), vitamins, and minerals (particularly iron) to supplement the diet of infants whose needs for these nutrients are not met by human milk, formula, or other milks. The manufacture of infant dry cereals involves the enzymatic hydrolysis of cereal flour and heat to precook and gelatinize the starches. Cereals are mixed with milk, water, or juice and later with fruits. To help identify possible allergies or food intolerances that may arise from adding new foods to the diet, single-grain cereals (rice, oatmeal, and barley) are recommended as starting cereals. Mixed cereal (oat, corn, wheat, soy) provides greater variety to older infants. High-protein cereal (soy, oat, wheat) offers the advantages of low cost and high protein in addition to variety.

Puréed fruits, vegetables, and meats are available in containers that provide an appropriate serving size. The caloric ranges are 40–80 calories/container for vegetables and 90–100 calories/container for fruit. Fruit and vegetable juices provide a maximum of only 4% of the total caloric intake of infants. The juices are strained, homogenized, and supplemented with vitamin C to achieve a uniform nutrient level that is equivalent to that of fresh orange juice. Excessive milk (>24 oz/day) or juice intake should be avoided in infants over 1 yr of age, because they may reduce the intake of nutritionally important solid foods. Foods with high allergic potential that should be avoided during early infancy include fish, peanuts, egg whites, and various food additives.

References

Behrman RE (ed): Nelson Textbook of Pediatrics. 14th ed. Philadelphia, WB Saunders, 1992, Sec. 4.11–4.12.

Nichols BL: Infant feeding practices. *In* Tsang RC, Nichols BL (eds): Nutrition during Infancy. Philadelphia, Hanley and Belfus, Inc, 1988, pp 367–377.

Nichols BL, Nichols VN: Nutrition during early development. *In* Linder MC (ed): Nutritional Biochemistry and Metabolism. New York, Elsevier Scientific Publishing Co, 1985, pp 255–283.

DIET OF THE NORMAL CHILD AND ADOLESCENT

Nutrient needs for children and adolescents are shown in Table 2–2.

OBESITY

Pathology. In infants and children of normal weight, increases in adipocyte size account for most of the increase in adipose mass during the first year of life. The total adipocyte number increases slowly between 6 mo and 2 yr of age and remains stable until 8–10 yr, when an increase in size and number occurs in association with puberty. Obese children have larger fat cells than normal-weight controls and have increased numbers of adipocytes.

Epidemiology. Although there are familial tendencies toward leanness or obesity, the critical issue is the extent to which such trends are due to similar genetic or environmental influences. When comparing adopted twin pairs, up to 80% of the variance in weight for height or skinfold thickness may be explicable on the basis of genotype. A strong relationship exists between the body mass index of adoptees and their biologic parents; a poor relationship exists between adoptees and their adoptive parents.

Maternal obesity has been associated with increased adipose tissue in the newborn. Children from families in which either one or both parents are obese are susceptible to adult obesity (approximately 40% risk if one parent is obese; 80% if both are obese). There is a modest correlation between excessive weight gain or weight-gain velocity during the 1st yr of life and later obesity. However, overweight infants usually do not become obese children. Most obese infants and children do not become obese adults. The risk of obesity persisting to adulthood increases with a more advanced age of onset (adolescence vs. infancy) and severity of obesity (100% adult obesity if the child weighs greater than 180% of his or her ideal body weight).

Clinical Manifestations. Complications of obesity often are noted during the preadolescent and teenage years (Table 2–4). During these periods children develop increasing awareness of body types and generate negative stereotypic characteristics toward obesity. Medical complications usually are related directly to the degree of obesity and resolve with weight reduction.

The *diagnosis* of obesity is made by determining the percent deviation from the ideal body weight for height after adjusting for age. An actual weight greater than 120% of the ideal weight is considered obese. However, weight-for-height deviations may result in a muscular person incorrectly being identified as obese. Therefore, caliper measurement of triceps skinfold thickness is a more accurate, readily available method for assessing adiposity; a measurement greater than the 85th percentile is considered obese. In addition to obtaining anthropometric data, the history and physical examination should be directed toward identifying the many potential complications noted among obese

Table 2–4. Complications of Obesity

Complication	Effects
Psychosocial	Peer discrimination, teasing, reduced college acceptance, isolation, reduced job promotion*
Growth	Advanced bone age, increased height, early menarche
Central nervous system	Pseudotumor cerebri
Respiratory	Sleep apnea, pickwickian syndrome, infection
Cardiovascular	Hypertension, cardiac hypertrophy, ischemic heart disease,* sudden death*
Orthopedic	Slipped capital femoral epiphysis, Blount disease
Metabolic	Insulin resistance, type II diabetes mellitus, hypertriglyceridemia, hyperchloesterolemia, gout,* hepatic steatosis,* polycystic ovary disease, pancreatitis
Malignancy	Endometrial,* breast,* prostate,* colon*

* Complications unusual until adulthood.

patients (Table 2–4) in addition to specific diseases associated with obesity (Table 2–5).

Treatment   Obesity is difficult to treat, and management often includes a combination of education, behavior modification, exercise, and diet. A balanced diet consisting of an approximately 30% decrease in the previous caloric intake (total calories 1000–1500) is an appropriate starting point for most obese patients. Dietary fat and thus calories are reduced; portion size and meal patterns also are modified. More severe dietary restriction, such as the very-low-calorie diet or "protein modified fast," may be needed when life-threatening complications such as alveolar hypoventilation, sleep apnea, or significant hypertension are present. Such restrictive diets require close supervision; supplementation with potassium, magnesium, calcium, and multiple vitamins; and the use of high-quality protein sources. Surgical therapy for morbid obesity includes gastric stapling or ileal bypass, but is rarely indicated in children or adolescents.

Prevention.   There is no recognized method of prevention, although increasing exercise and decreasing fat intake possibly are helpful. Despite constant energy intake/unit weight, there are large differences among normal children for rate of fat accumulation. Thus, an "appropriate" level of calories for a given child may be difficult to specify. Dietary recommendations, therefore, should be based on an acceptable rate of growth, rather than on a fixed number of calories per kilogram of body weight.

References

Behrman RE (ed): Nelson Textbook of Pediatrics. 14th ed. Philadelphia, WB Saunders, 1992, Sec. 4.20.

Danforth E, Sims EAH: Obesity and efforts to loss weight. N Engl J Med 327:1947, 1992.

Table 2–5. Diseases Associated with Childhood Obesity*

Syndrome	Manifestations
Alstrom syndrome	Hypogonadism, retinal degeneration, deafness, diabetes mellitus
Carpenter syndrome	Polydactyly, syndactyly, cranial synostosis, mental retardation
Cushing syndrome	Adrenal hyperplasia or pituitary tumor
Frohlich syndrome	Hypothalamic tumor
Hyperinsulinism	Nesidioblastosis, pancreatic adenoma, hypoglycemia, Mauriac syndrome (poor diabetic control)
Laurence-Moon-Bardet-Biedl syndrome	Retinal degeneration, syndactyly, polydactyly, hypogonadism, mental retardation; autosomal recessive
Muscular dystrophy	Late onset of obesity
Myelodysplasia	Spina bifida
Prader-Willi syndrome	Neonatal hypotonia, normal growth immediately after birth, small hands and feet, mental retardation, hypogonadism; some have partial deletion of chromosome 15
Pseudohypoparathyroidism	Variable hypocalcemia, cutaneous calcifications
Turner syndrome	Ovarian dysgenesis, lymphedema, web neck; XO chromosome

* These diseases represent less than 5% of cases of childhood obesity.

Garrow JS: Treating obesity: The first law of thermodynamics still holds. BMJ 302:803, 1991.

Must A, Jacques PF, Dallal GE, et al: Long-term morbidity and mortality of overweight adolescents: A follow up of the Harvard Growth Study of 1922 to 1935. N Engl J Med 327:1350, 1992.

EATING DISORDERS

Anorexia Nervosa

The prevalence of anorexia nervosa has been estimated to be 1–5% in teenage girls. The female-to-male ratio is approximately 20:1 and shows a familial pattern. The cause of anorexia nervosa is unknown.

The *clinical manifestations* of weight loss usually begin with moderate efforts to lose weight, which accelerate into a fear of obesity and a preoccupation with becoming thin (Tables 2–6 and 2–7). Predisposing factors include perfectionist behavior, low self-esteem, and, in 40% of cases, a history of being mildly overweight. An almost invariable feature of anorexia nervosa is the patient's pleasure in the achievement of low weight for personal and emotional reasons. Any weight gain generates severe anxiety; weight loss reduces this anxiety. Vitamin and nutrient deficiency disorders are infrequently observed. Nonetheless, scalp hair loss is common; fine lanugo-like hair grows on the face and the trunk. The skin becomes rough, scaly, and petechial. Two types of dieting prevail: the fasting, abstaining, or restricting type, and the so-called bulimic type. In the bulimic type of dieting, binge eating initially occurs in spurts but gradually becomes a habit. Binge eating ends with self-induced vomiting, either alone or in combination with laxative and/or diuretic abuse as a means to get rid of excess weight. Intense compulsive exercise is another weight-control method.

Table 2–6. Diagnostic Criteria for Anorexia Nervosa

Refusal to maintain minimal normal body weight for age and height

Weight loss leading to body weight 15% below expected or failure to have expected weight gain during growth leading to weight 15% below expected

Disturbance of body image: feels fat despite emaciation

Intense fear of becoming obese, even with progressive weight loss

Absence of at least three consecutive menstrual cycles when expected to occur

No known physical illness to account for weight loss

Additional features include bradycardia, osteopenia, delayed gastric emptying, lymphopenia, low voltage on electrocardiogram, decreased 1-sec forced expiratory volume (FEV_1), hypothermia, myopathy, neuropathy, and, if severe, organic brain syndrome.

Endocrine changes are starvation induced (Table 2–7; see also Table 2–11). For most patients, amenorrhea, which occurs when body weight drops below the normal range, is due to low plasma luteinizing hormone levels, which result in reduced ovarian stimulation, low estradiol levels, and nonmeasurable progesterone levels. The hypothalamic–pituitary–thyroid axis changes are identical to those in marasmic patients. The cortisol production rate is elevated. When dexamethasone is administered, plasma cortisol levels are not suppressed. Weight gain to the normal premorbid level reverses all the endocrine changes in patients with anorexia nervosa. The *differential diagnosis* includes Addison disease, hyperthyroidism, diabetes mellitus, malignancy (including brain tumors), drug abuse, primary depression, schizophrenia, and obsessive–compulsive disorders.

Treatment requires a multidisciplinary approach consisting of a feeding program and individual and family therapy. Therapy is difficult because the patients and families involved often deny the severity of the illness and may conceal symptoms. Goals of therapy are to restore normal function and body weight and to re-establish normal eating patterns. Adequate nutrition is of lifesaving importance in the acutely ill, severely underweight patient, but weight restoration and refeeding require the patient's cooperation if this therapy is to succeed. Discussion and negotiation of a detailed treatment contract with the patient and the parents is essential before treatment begins. The first step is to restore body weight; the patient's weight should be increased to more than 80% of normal levels for height and age. This is accomplished by voluntary intake of regular foods or of a nutritional formula ingested orally or by nasogastric tube. Occasionally parenteral nutrition is indicated to improve the nutritional status to a safe level. During the second step, the patient is given freedom to gain weight at a personal pace. Hospitalization is indicated when weight loss exceeds 25% of ideal body weight; personal/family dynamics place the patient at excessive risk for suicide or abuse; metabolic disturbances (dehydration, hypokalemia, severe dysrhythmias, severe recurrent induced vomiting or laxative abuse) are noted; or outpatient therapy fails.

Antidepressant drug therapy (desipramine, flu-

Table 2–7. Comparative Characteristics of Anorexia Nervosa and Bulimia Nervosa

Characteristics	Anorexia Nervosa	Bulimia Nervosa
Intense preoccupation with food	Yes	Yes
Weight loss	Severe	Fluctuates
Female	90–95%	90–95%
Family history	+ for anorexia nervosa	+ for depression
Methods of weight control	Severe food restrictions, emesis, exercise	Restriction and binges with self-induced vomiting and diuretic and/or laxative purging
Guilt/shame	None	Yes
Denial	Yes	None
Personality	Withdrawn/asexual	Outgoing/heterosexual
Onset (age)	Bimodal (13–14 yr and 17–18 yr)	17–25 yr
Endocrinopathy/metabolism	Amenorrhea, increased growth hormone, osteoporosis, hypercarotenemia, hypothermia	Menstrual irregularities, hypokalemia
Cardiovascular complications	Bradycardia, hypotension, arrhythmias	Ipecac toxicity
Gastrointestinal	Constipation, elevated hepatic enzymes	Gastric dilation and rupture, Mallory-Weiss syndrome, esophagitis, parotid enlargement, dental enamel erosion
Psychiatric	Depression, suicide, obsessional fears	Impulsive behaviors, alcohol–drug addictions, depression, suicide

oxitine, clomipramine) may be indicated for depressed patients; the latter two drugs may improve obsessive–compulsive traits. An appetite stimulant, such as cyproheptadine, also may be helpful. The *prognosis* includes a 3–5% mortality (suicide, malnutrition) rate, the development of bulemic symptoms (30%), and persistent problems (20%).

Bulimia Nervosa

The diagnostic indicators in the behavior of a patient with bulimia nervosa are binge-eating episodes and the loss of control during overeating (Table 2–8). Although often considered a symptom of anorexia nervosa, the term "bulimia" also is applied to a distinct eating disorder. Previous dieting is usually a precondition for the development of bulimia. It occurs in young women of normal weight or in slightly overweight women. The prevalence may be as high as 5% of female college students; the female-to-male ratio is 10:1. In the fully developed syndrome, binge eating is precipitated by a variety of conditions. During these episodes patients tend to consume large volumes of "forbidden" foods that are high in carbohydrate and fat

Table 2–8. Diagnostic Criteria for Bulimia Nervosa

Recurrent episodes of binge eating (rapid consumption of large food quantities in short time periods); at least two episodes a week for 3 mo

Overconcern with body shape and weight

Three of the following:
  Consumption of high-caloric, easily ingested food during a binge
  Inconspicuous eating during a binge
  Termination of binge by abdominal pain, self-induced vomiting, sleep, or social interruption
  Repeated attempts to lose weight by restrictive diets, cathartics, diuretics, or self-induced vomiting
  Frequent weight fluctuations of more than 4.5 kg due to binges and fasts

Awareness of abnormal eating patterns and fear of being unable to stop eating voluntarily; lack of control during binges

Depression and self-deprecating thoughts after binge

Exclusion of anorexia nervosa or known physical causes of bulimic episodes

content; others may eat leftovers of unpalatable foods. The food is consumed rapidly and secretly without dwelling on the taste. Vomiting eventually becomes coupled to binge eating. Most patients overeat with the forethought of vomiting afterward. Most metabolic abnormalities are the result of excessive vomiting (see Table 2–7). The excessive use of laxatives or diuretics also increases the risks of metabolic disturbance, such as hypokalemia.

Compared to patients with anorexia nervosa, patients with bulimia are more likely to present with personality disturbances, impulse control difficulties (stealing, drug abuse, sexual promiscuity), personal and family history of affective disorders, and a positive response to antidepressant therapy. These patients often feel embarrassed, guilty, and ashamed of their secret addiction. Repetitive binge eating and vomiting can result in salivary gland enlargement, esophagitis, fluid and electrolyte imbalance, callus formation on knuckles due to abrasion from teeth while vomiting was induced, and erosion of dental enamel. Ipecac abuse (to induce emesis) may cause cardiomyopathy.

A combination of nutritional, educational, and self-monitoring techniques is employed to increase awareness of the maladaptive behavior, after which efforts are made to change the eating behavior. Antidepressants have a place in the treatment of bulimia. Suicide occurs in up to 5% of patients, with many more patients attempting suicide.

References

Behrman RE (ed): Nelson Textbook of Pediatrics. 14th ed. Philadelphia, WB Saunders, 1992, Sec. 10.14.

Fairburn CG: Bulimia nervosa. BMJ 300:485, 1990.

Patton G: The course of anorexia nervosa. BMJ 299:139, 1989.

ARTERIOSCLEROSIS (SEE CHAPTER 5 FOR FAMILIAL HYPERLIPOPROTEINEMIA)

Evidence suggests the utility of adult cardiovascular disease prevention beginning in children. Elevated low-density lipoprotein (LDL) cholesterol levels are associated with heart disease in adults; dietary modification reduces LDL cholesterol levels in adults and children. The childhood origin of atherosclerosis is suggested by finding vascular atherosclerotic lesions in young soldiers killed in the Korean and Viet Nam wars and in autopsies of younger children. Childhood cholesterol levels are associated with subsequent cholesterol levels and heart disease in adulthood. Given the known influences (diet, exercise, smoking) on LDL cholesterol and the development of heart disease and the resistance of many adults to behavioral intervention, children should be encouraged to adopt healthier life-styles to reduce the risk of atherosclerotic heart disease. The prudent or Step-One diet (Table 2–9) is proposed for all children over 2 yr of age, and especially those with elevated cholesterol levels, whereas the Step-Two diet is reserved for those with more significant elevations in LDL cholesterol that have not responded to the original dietary intervention. Drug therapy is reserved for older children (generally over 10 yr) with very severe elevations in LDL cholesterol after failing 6–12 mo of dietary management. Drug therapy in children should be considered only after consultation with a pediatric lipid specialist.

Several questions have been raised about the safety and efficacy of dietary interventions in children. Some children fail to thrive when put on very-low-fat, low-calorie diets by well-meaning but misguided parents. Dietary intervention should be

Table 2–9. Characteristics of Step-One and Step-Two Diets for Lowering Blood Cholesterol

Nutrient	Recommended Intake	
	Step-One Diet	*Step-Two Diet*
Total fat	Average of no more than 30% of total calories	Same
Saturated fatty acids	Less than 10% of total calories	Less than 7% of total calories
Polyunsaturated fatty acids	Up to 10% of total calories	Same
Monounsaturated fatty acids	Remaining total fat calories	Same
Cholesterol	Less than 300 mg/day	Less than 200 mg/day
Carbohydrates	About 55% of total calories	Same
Protein	About 15–20% of total calories	Same
Calories	To promote normal growth and development and to reach or maintain desirable body weight	Same

(From National Cholesterol Education Program. Report of the Expert Panel on Blood Cholesterol Levels in Childhood and Adolescents. Pediatrics 89(suppl):556, 1992.)

Table 2–10. Cutpoints of Total and Low-Density Lipoprotein (LDL) Cholesterol for Dietary Intervention in Children and Adolescents with a Family History of Hypercholesterolemia or Premature Cardiovascular Disease

Category	Total Cholesterol (mg/dL)	LDL Cholesterol (mg/dL)	Dietary Intervention
Acceptable	<170	<110	Recommended population eating pattern
Borderline	170–199	110–129	Step-One Diet prescribed, other risk factor intervention
High	≥200	≥130	Step-One Diet prescribed, then Step-Two Diet if necessary

(From National Cholesterol Education Program. Report of the Expert Panel on Blood Cholesterol Levels in Childhood and Adolescents. Pediatrics 89(suppl):556, 1992.)

undertaken with appropriate guidance (a registered dietitian with pediatric experience) to ensure that the diet has sufficient calories and nutrients for growth while fulfilling the guidelines of the prudent diet.

There is concern about the psychosocial consequences of labeling children as hypercholesterolemic (i.e., the development of the "sick child" role). To avoid this, intervention programs should focus on the positive changes the child and family can make to help limit their risk. Another concern is the mislabeling of children based on a single or inaccurate screening test as a result of inherent biologic and laboratory variability in cholesterol testing. Any measure of cholesterol should be completed with adequate quality assurance; repeated measurements help define a child's lipid status (Table 2–10).

The current National Cholesterol Education Program guidelines recommend screening children with a positive family history of early (before 55 yr of age) cardiovascular disease or hypercholesterolemia (>240 mg/dL). Those children with unknown histories or other cardiovascular risk factors may be screened at the physician's discretion. To prevent heart disease, it is also important to focus on lifestyle interventions to minimize other risk factor—smoking, hypertenion, obesity, diabetes mellitus, and physical inactivity.

References

Behrman RE (ed): Nelson Textbook of Pediatrics. 14th ed. Philadelphia, WB Saunders, 1992, Sec. 8.20–8.35.

Committee on Nutrition: Statement on cholesterol. Pediatrics 90:469, 1992.

National Cholesterol Education Program: Report of the expert panel on blood cholesterol levels in children and adolescents. Pediatrics 89:525, 1992.

Polonsky SM, Bellet PS, Sprecher DL: Primary hyperlipidemia in a pediatric population: Classification and effect of dietary treatment. Pediatrics 91:92, 1993.

PITFALLS IN CHILD AND ADOLESCENT NUTRITION

When dietary intakes are compared with recommendations (see Tables 2–1 and 2–2), the intake of preschool children in the United States is deficient in zinc. The deficiency is profound in the diets of children living in families of low socioeconomic status (70% in 1–3 yr olds and 79% in 4–5 yr olds). Calcium intake is inadequate (82%) in these children unless the families participate in federal food stamp programs. Iron intake tends to be inadequate (65%) in children between 1 and 3 yr of age in the United States. The incidence of iron-deficiency anemia is decreasing in the United States in part as a result of participation in the Women, Infants and Children (WIC) program, but is still significant. Dietary iron deficiency is the major nutritional risk for the 1–2 yr age group. Latent calcium and zinc deficiencies are likely to be buffered by adaptive mechanisms; however, the presence of illness may precipitate clinical signs and symptoms of deficiency.

In the United States 20% of all children and 50% of all black and Hispanic children live in families of low socioeconomic status. Among those families who participate in federal assistance programs, 2–3 times the expected number of children have weight-for-height measurements below the 5th percentile. This problem is evident in infants from 3 mo through the 2nd yr of life. Surveillance of growth velocity is essential in this population, and evidence for macro- and micronutrient deficiencies should be sought in all children placed below the 5th percentile of weight-for-height measurements.

References

Fisher KD, Bennett RB (eds): A Report of the Scientific Community's Views on Progress in Attaining the Public Health Service National Nutrition Goals for 1990. Bethesda, MD, Federation of American Societies for Experimental Biology, 1986, pp 27–38.

Nationwide Food Consumption Survey: Continuing Survey of Food Intakes by Individuals. Women 19–50 Years and Their Children 1–5 Years, 1 Day. Washington, DC, US Department of Agriculture, 1985, pp 40–41, 66–77.

MACRONUTRIENT DEFICIENCIES

Worldwide, protein–energy malnutrition (PEM) is a leading cause of death among children under 5 yr of age. PEM is a spectrum of conditions due to varying proportions of protein and calorie deficiencies. Primary PEM is due to social or economic factors that result in lack of food. Secondary PEM occurs in children with various diseases associated with increased caloric requirements (infection, cancer), increased caloric loss (malabsorption, cystic fibrosis), reduced calorie intake (anorexia, cancer, oral intake restriction, social factors), or a combination of these three variables.

Marasmus

Marasmus is the most common form of primary PEM and is due to severe caloric depletion. Many secondary forms of marasmic PEM are associated with diseases such as cystic fibrosis, tuberculosis, cancer, acquired immunodeficiency syndrome, or celiac disease.

The principal *clinical manifestation* in a child with severe malnutrition is emaciation with a body weight below 60% of that expected for age or below 70% of the ideal weight for height. Although growth stunting may be observed with longer term malnutrition, the ratio of observed to expected weight to height reveals a reduction in body mass exceeding that of any coexisting growth stunting. Visible loss of muscle mass and subcutaneous tissue is confirmed by inspection or palpation and quantified by anthropometric measurements. The head appears large but generally is proportional to the body length. Edema usually is absent. The skin is dry and thin, and the hair is thin and sparse and easily pulled out. Marasmic children are apathetic and weak. Bradycardia and hypothermia signify severe and life-threatening malnutrition. Atrophy of the filiform papillae of the tongue is common, and monilial stomatitis is frequent. Recent weaning of the child or inappropriate weaning practices and chronic diarrhea are common findings in developing countries.

Role of Chronic Diarrhea

Malnutrition often is associated with chronic diarrhea, as a result of the effects of malnutrition on the gastrointestinal tract (mucosal atrophy, secondary malabsorption) and the increased susceptibility to viral, bacterial, protozoal, and parasitic infections related to a secondary T and B cell immunodeficiency state. Recurrent episodes of diarrhea treated with prolonged periods of fasting or oral electrolyte solutions reduce caloric intake and contribute to malnutrition. Diarrhea may worsen during rehabilitation (in 10–20% of children) as a result of excessive refeeding or formula intolerance (transient lactose or monosaccharide malabsorption or milk protein intolerance). Nonetheless, cow's milk formulas are used routinely to rehabilitate malnourished children with good results. In very severe cases of diarrhea, malabsorption, and malnutrition, intravenous refeeding may be necessary.

Kwashiorkor

Kwashiorkor, presenting with pitting edema that starts in the lower extremities and ascends with increasing severity, is due to inadequate protein intake in the face of fair to good caloric intake. It is common in developing countries if children are weaned to low-protein foods, but also may be a complication of critical illness (burns, cancer, acute and chronic infections, multiorgan system failure, inflammatory bowel disease, anorexia nervosa, and postoperative surgery) when inadequate amounts of protein are provided for a prolonged time.

The major *clinical manifestation* of kwashiorkor is that the body weight of the child ranges from 60–80% of the expected weight for age; weight may not represent the nutritional status because of the presence of edema. Physical examination reveals a relative maintenance of subcutaneous adipose tissue and a marked atrophy of muscle mass. Edema varies from a minor pitting of the dorsum of the foot to generalized edema accompanied by involvement of the eyelids and scrotum. The hair is sparse, easily pluckable, and appears dull brown, red, or yellow–white. Adequate protein intake restores hair color (flag sign). Skin changes are common and range from hyperpigmented hyperkeratosis to an erythematous macular rash on the trunk and extremities. In its most severe form, a superficial desquamation occurs over pressure surfaces. Angular cheilosis and the atrophy of the filiform papillae of the tongue are common. Monilial stomatitis is frequent. Examination of the abdomen reveals a large, soft liver with an indefinite edge. Lymphatic tissue is atrophic. Chest examination reveals basilar rales. The abdomen is distended and the bowel sounds are hypoactive.

Treatment of Malnutrition

The basal metabolic rate and immediate nutrient needs during malnutrition are decreased. When nutrients are provided, the metabolic rate increases, stimulating anabolism and thus increasing nutrient requirements. The malnourished child may have compensated for vitamin and mineral deficiencies with lower metabolic and growth rates; refeeding may unmask these deficiencies. Furthermore, the gastrointestinal tract may not tolerate a rapid increase in intake. Nutritional rehabilitation, therefore, should be initiated and advanced slowly to minimize these complications. Fluid and solute load must be monitored to avoid stressing the compromised myocardial function. The caloric intake should be kept stable until the edema begins to resolve.

Calories can be safely initiated at 20% above the child's recent intake. If no estimate of the caloric intake is available, 50–75% of the normal energy requirement is safe. Caloric intake can be increased 10–20%/day, with monitoring for electrolyte imbalances, poor cardiac function, edema, or feeding intolerance. If these occur, further caloric increases are not made until the status stabilizes. Caloric intake is increased until appropriate regrowth is initiated. This may require 150% or more of the recommended calories for an age-matched well-nourished child. Protein needs also are increased as anabolism begins and are provided in proportion (10–20%) to the caloric intake.

In most cases, cow's milk–based formulas are tolerated and provide an appropriate mix of nutrients. Other easily digested foods, appropriate for the age, also may be introduced slowly. If feeding intolerance occurs, lactose-free or, rarely, other regimens (parenteral nutrition) may be considered (see Marasmus). During 2–3 wk of dietary rehabilitation and rapid growth, a hypermetabolic "nutritional recovery syndrome" may develop that is characterized by postprandial diaphoresis, hepatic glycogenesis, and eosinophilia.

Vitamin and mineral intake in excess of the RDA is provided to account for the increased requirements. Potassium, phosphorus, calcium, and magnesium status is carefully monitored. Potassium, as a major component of lean body tissue, is needed during growth and healing; serum levels may decrease dangerously in response to a glucose load, with subsequent insulin-induced transcellular shift of potassium. Phosphorus is needed for phosphorylated intermediates because it becomes "trapped" intracellularly by such phosphorylation in response to a glucose load, increased anabolism, and increased metabolic rate. Magnesium, a cofactor for adenosine triphosphatase, is needed when the metabolic and anabolic rates increase. Hypomagnesemia blunts the parathyroid response to hypocalcemia, which may be due to the vitamin D and calcium deficiencies associated with malnutrition (see Chapter 17). Electrolyte imbalances can further alter cardiac function, exacerbating heart failure. Overzealous refeeding has been documented to cause life-threatening abnormalities of these and other nutrients.

Complications of Malnutrition

Malnourished children are more susceptible to infection, especially sepsis, pneumonia, and gastroenteritis. Hypoglycemia is common after periods of severe fasting but also may be a sign of sepsis. Apnea may be associated with hypoglycemia. Hypothermia may signify infection or, with bradycardia, may signify a decreased metabolic rate to conserve energy. Bradycardia and poor cardiac output predispose the malnourished child to heart failure, which is exacerbated by acute fluid or solute loads. Vitamin deficiencies also can complicate malnutrition. Vitamin A deficiency is common in the developing world and is an important cause of altered immune response and increased morbidity (infections, blindness) and mortality (especially measles). Depending on the age of onset and the duration of the malnutrition, such children may suffer permanent growth stunting (malnutrition in utero, infancy, adolescence) and delayed development (malnutrition in infancy). Environmental (social) deprivation may interact with the effects of the malnutrition to further impair development and cognitive function.

References

Behrman RE (ed): Nelson Textbook of Pediatrics. 14th ed. Philadelphia, WB Saunders, 1992, Sec. 4.15–4.18.

Torún B, Viteri F: Protein-energy malnutrition. In Shils ME, VR Young (eds): Modern Nutrition in Health and Disease. 7th ed. Philadelphia, Lea & Febiger, 1988, pp 746–773.

PATHOPHYSIOLOGY OF MACRONUTRIENT DEFICIENCIES

PEM represents a complex interrelationship among reduced protein and calorie intake, inciting events such as weaning or gastrointestinal infection, and the complications associated with PEM and infection. The child's adaptation to reduced

Table 2–11. Summary of Selected Hormonal Changes and Their Main Metabolic Effects Usually Seen in Severe PEM

Hormone	Influenced in PEM by	Hormonal Activity in		Metabolic Effects of Changes in PEM
		Energy Deficit	*Protein Deficit*	
Insulin	Low food intake (↓ glucose) (↓ amino acids)	Decreased	Decreased	↓ muscle protein synthesis ↓ lipogenesis ↓ growth
Growth hormone	Low protein intake (↓ amino acids) Reduced somatomedin synthesis	Normal or moderately increased	Increased	↑ visceral synthesis ↓ urea synthesis ↑ lipolysis
Somatomedins	Low protein intake?	Variable	Decreased	↓ muscle and cartilage protein synthesis ↓ collagen synthesis ↓ lipolysis ↓ growth ↑ production of growth hormone
Epinephrine	Stress of food deficiency, infections (↓ glucose)	Normal but can increase	Normal but can increase	↑ lipolysis ↑ glycogenolysis inhibits insulin secretion
Glucocorticoids	Stress of hunger Fever (↓ glucose)	Increased	Normal or moderately increased	↑ muscle protein catabolism ↑ visceral protein turnover ↑ lipolysis ↑ gluconeogenesis
Aldosterone	↓ blood volume ↑ extracellular K? ↓ serum Na?	Normal	Increased	↑ sodium retention and ↑ water retention contribute to appearance of edema
Thyroid hormones	?	T_4 normal or decreased; T_3 decreased	T_4 usually decreased; T_3 decreased	↓ glucose oxidation ↓ basal energy expenditure ↑ reverse T_3
Gonadotropins	Low protein intake? Low energy intake?	Decreased	Decreased	Delayed menarche

↓ = low or reduced; ↑ = high or increased.
(From Shils M, Young V: Modern Nutrition in Health and Disease. 7th ed. Philadelphia, Lea & Febiger, 1988.)

protein and calorie intake is typical for that of starvation, and secondary immune dysfunction and continued exposure to infectious diseases increase the morbidity and mortality of PEM.

ENDOCRINE ADAPTATION

The hormonal responses to malnutrition are noted in Table 2–11. The net effects of nutrient deficiency and these hormonal events are to reduce (spare) tissue glucose utilization and to increase alternate fuel mobilization and use (proteolysis, lipolysis, ketogenesis). Initially, free fatty acids and ketones may spare proteolysis, but with profound deficiencies muscle breakdown continues and net protein synthesis is reduced.

METABOLIC SUBSTRATES

There are several stages of metabolic adaptation in PEM. The first is a reduction in voluntary energy expenditure, the second is a reduction in the gain of body mass and length, and the last is a reduction in resting energy expenditure. The marasmic form

of malnutrition results in a more striking reduction in resting energy expenditure than the reduction produced by kwashiorkor.

Inadequate macronutrient intake, especially when amplified by concurrent infection, results in growth arrest. Normal nitrogen balance may be sustained if protein intake has not been exceeded by excessive nitrogen losses; in both healthy children and those with PEM, the efficiency of nitrogen balance is greater than 95%. Protein turnover is a measure of total endogenous protein synthesis and degradation. In normal adults, the rate of turnover is influenced only modestly by starvation, but in children with kwashiorkor the rate of turnover is strikingly reduced. In contrast, turnover rates in normal children are increased in response to the stress of an infection.

The turnover of individual proteins is reduced under modest dietary restrictions. In both well-nourished and malnourished children, a reduced protein intake results in a few days in reduced rates of albumin synthesis and, later, if the reduction continues, in decreased concentrations of serum transferrin, retinol-binding protein, and prealbumin. The synthesis of hepatic acute-phase proteins, such as C-reactive protein, nonetheless is preserved under these conditions. In addition to the hepatic synthetic adaptations, there is increased degradation of muscle proteins. In the marasmic child, these mechanisms maintain the plasma levels of free amino acids and hepatic secretory proteins. In the child with kwashiorkor, the adaptation fails to maintain serum amino acids and hepatic protein synthesis, and the plasma levels of branched-chain amino acids decrease. In marasmus, the urea synthesis and concentration are normal, but in kwashiorkor, urea levels are below 7 mg/dL, reflecting a reduced amino acid pool. Hepatic steatosis occurs in patients with kwashiorkor owing to a failure to synthesize and secrete hepatic triglyceride-transporting proteins.

Macronutrient deficiency and specific infections (e.g., measles and rotavirus) also decrease the rate of synthesis of pancreatic enzymes and intestinal mucosa brush-border hydrolases, which can retard later dietary rehabilitation.

Body water content is increased in kwashiorkor owing to reduced adipose tissue mass and fluid retention. Blood osmolality and serum sodium concentrations may be low, and serum concentrations of potassium and magnesium may be reduced. Total body magnesium and potassium are reduced in all malnourished children owing to loss of muscle mass. In kwashiorkor, there also are defects in the maintenance of the normal sodium–potassium membrane gradients in soft tissues. Calcium and phosphorus are uniformly low, but tetany is rare. Concentrations of serum zinc and copper are strikingly reduced in kwashiorkor but are normal in marasmus. If adequate micronutrient dietary supplements are not provided, serum zinc and copper concentrations fall rapidly during nutritional rehabilitation.

References

Frenk S: Metabolic adaptation in protein-energy malnutrition. J Am Coll Nutr 5:371–381, 1986.
Waterlow JC: Metabolic adaptation to low intakes of energy and protein. Annu Rev Nutr 6:495–526, 1986.

IMMUNE FUNCTION

Cell-mediated immunity is depressed in PEM. Severely malnourished children fail to respond to tuberculin or *Candida albicans* skin tests, which reveals an inability of their system to demonstrate prior sensitization. They also do not react to dinitrofluorobenzene sensitization, indicating that noncommitted lymphocytes are unresponsive.

Thymic, lymph node, tonsil, and splenic tissues are atrophic in malnourished children. Total circulating lymphocytes are reduced, indicating a reduction of the thymus-derived cells, or T lymphocytes; the T lymphocytes present have a poor response to in vitro mitogenic stimulation. Vitamin A deficiency produces a reduced CD4/CD8 ratio and total CD4 naive T cells. This immunocompromised status improves with dietary rehabilitation; functional recovery occurs within 2 wk and the total lymphocyte count recovers within 4 wk.

The concentration of bursa-derived cells, or B lymphocytes, in lymphoid tissues and in peripheral blood is normal. Immunoglobulin (Ig) synthesis is increased, as reflected in elevated total circulating IgA, IgM, IgG, IgD, and IgE levels. The concentrations are greater in children with kwashiorkor than in those with marasmus. The quantitative antibody response to vaccines for yellow fever, influenza, and typhoid is reduced, although the response to cholera vaccine is not. The recovery of antigenic response is dependent on adequate protein intake. Malnourished children have reduced secretory IgA (sIgA) levels in nasal washings, duodenal fluids, and tears despite the elevated serum IgA. The reduction is reflected by the diminished response of sIgA to measles and polio vaccines. The loss of secretory immunity may contribute to an increase in respiratory and intestinal infections.

The response of polymorphonuclear (PMN) leukocytes to chemotactic stimulation is normal, but that of the macrophages is reduced in PEM. The PMN leukocytes are able to phagocytize bacteria but have reduced ability to kill *Staphylococcus aureus, E. coli,* and *C. albicans.*

Patients with kwashiorkor have reduced hemolytic complement (CH50) titers because of the presence of anticomplementary serum factors. Titers return to normal after a week of dietary rehabilitation. All PEM subjects have depressed concentrations of specific complement factors (C1q, C1s, C3, C5, C6, C8, C9, and C3PA). The levels of C1q, C6, and C8 are more profoundly depressed in kwashiorkor but respond to dietary therapy within 4 wk. Levels of C9 may remain low for several months. Recovery of complement levels occurs more quickly in children who receive diets with adequate protein.

INFECTION

A triangle of interactions exists among host defenses, infection, and macronutrient malnutrition. PEM may be initiated by primary dietary deficiencies or by illnesses that induce a secondary dietary deficiency. Infections induce anorexia and increase caloric requirements owing to hypermetabolism during the febrile response. Contributing infections may be bacterial (*E. coli* enteritis, pneumococcal pneumonia), viral (rotavirus, measles), protozoal (malaria, giardia), or due to intestinal helminths (roundworms, flukes, tapeworms). The result is catabolism and a loss of body nutrient stores, leading to clinical malnutrition. The impaired host defenses associated with PEM are important factors in determining the frequency and severity of infection. Gastrointestinal infections also exacerbate intestinal malabsorption, mucosal atrophy, and micronutrient losses.

References

Keusch GT, Farthing MJG: Nutrition and infection. Annu Rev Nutr 6:131–154, 1986.
Suskind RM: Malnutrition and the immune response. *In* Suskind RM (ed): Textbook of Pediatric Nutrition. New York, Raven Press, 1981, pp 241–254.

MICRONUTRIENT DEFICIENCIES

The etiologies of micronutrient deficiencies are diverse and relate to unusual diets; various malabsorption or maldigestion syndromes; drugs that alter nutrient absorption, metabolism, and excretion or that compete with vitamin action; and various genetic disorders associated with specific nutrient metabolic defects (Tables 2–12 and 2–13).

Water-Soluble Vitamins

ASCORBIC ACID

The first recognized micronutrient deficiency disease was that of ascorbic acid (vitamin C). The principal forms of vitamin C are L-ascorbic acid and the oxidized form dehydroascorbic acid. Ascorbic acid accelerates hydroxylation reactions in many biosynthetic reactions. The needs of full-term infants for ascorbic acid are calculated by estimating the availability of this vitamin in human milk. Commercially available cow's milk–based formulas are fortified to a comparable level of 5.5 mg/dL (8 mg/100 kcal). Formulas adapted for preterm infants contain ascorbic acid concentrations of from 7 to 30 mg/dL.

A deficiency of ascorbic acid results in the clinical manifestations of **scurvy**. Infantile scurvy presents with irritability, bone tenderness with swelling, and pseudoparalysis of the legs; it may be seen if

Table 2–12. Etiology of Vitamin and Nutrient Deficiency States

Etiology	Deficiency
Diet	
Vegans (strict)	Protein, vitamins B_{12}, D, riboflavin
Breast-fed infant	Vitamins K, D
Cow's milk–fed infant	Iron
Bulimia, anorexia nervosa	Electrolytes, other deficiencies
Parenteral alimentation	Essential fatty acid, trace elements
Alcoholism	Calories, vitamin B_1, B_6, folate
Medical Problems	
Malabsorption syndromes	Vitamins A, D, E, K, zinc, essential fatty acids
Cholestasis	Vitamins E, D, K, A, zinc, essential fatty acids
Medications	
Sulfonamides	Folate
Phenytoin, phenobarbital	Vitamins D, K, folate
Mineral oil	Vitamins A, D, E, K
Antibiotics	Vitamin K
Isoniazid	Vitamin B_6
Antacids	Iron, phosphate, calcium
Digitalis	Magnesium, calcium
Penicillamine	Vitamin B_6
Specific Mechanisms	
Transcobalamine II or intrinsic-factor deficiency	Vitamin B_{12}
Other digestive enzyme deficiencies	Carbohydrate, fat, protein
Menke kinky hair syndrome	Copper
Acrodermatitis enteropathica	Zinc
Reduced direct sunlight	Vitamin D

infants are fed unsupplemented cow's milk in the 1st yr of life. Subperiosteal hemorrhage, hyperkeratosis of hair follicles, and a succession of mental changes characterize the progression of the illness. Anemia, secondary to decreased iron absorption or to abnormal folate metabolism, also is seen in chronic scurvy. *Treatment* is recorded in Table 2–14.

THIAMINE

Vitamin B_1 functions as a coenzyme in biochemical reactions related to carbohydrate metabolism, to decarboxylation of alpha-keto acids and pyruvate, and to transketolase reactions of the pentose pathway. Thiamine also is involved in the decarboxyl-

Table 2–13. Characteristics of Vitamin Deficiencies

Vitamin	Purpose	Deficiency	Comments	Source
Water soluble				
Thiamine (B$_1$)	Coenzyme in ketoacid decarboxylation (e.g., pyruvate → acetyl-CoA transketolase reaction)	*Beri-beri:* polyneuropathy, calf tenderness, heart failure, edema, ophthalmoplegia	Inborn errors of lactate metabolism; boiling milk destroys B$_1$	Liver, meat, milk, cereals, nuts, legumes
Riboflavin (B$_2$)	FAD coenzyme in oxidation–reduction reactions	Anorexia, mucositis, anemia, cheilosis, nasolabial seborrhea	Photosensitizer	Milk, cheese, liver, meat, eggs, whole grains, green leafy vegetables
Niacin (B$_3$)	NAD coenzyme in oxidation–reduction reactions	*Pellagra:* photosensitivity, dermatitis, dementia, diarrhea, death	Tryptophan is a precursor	Meat, fish, liver, whole grains, green leafy vegetables
Pyridoxine (B$_6$)	Cofactor in amino acid metabolism	Seizures, hyperacusis, microcytic anemia, nasolabial seborrhea, neuropathy	Dependency state; deficiency secondary to drugs	Meat, liver, whole grains, peanuts, soybeans, meat
Pantothenic acid	Coenzyme A in Krebs cycle	None reported	—	Meat, vegetables
Biotin	Cofactor in carboxylase reactions of amino acids	Alopecia, dermatitis, hypotonia, death	Bowel resection, inborn errors of metabolism and ingestion of raw eggs	Yeast, meats; made by intestinal flora
B$_{12}$	Coenzyme for 5-methyl-tetrahydrofolate formation; DNA synthesis	Megaloblastic anemia, peripheral neuropathy, posterior lateral column disease, vitiligo	Vegans; fish tapeworm; transcobalamine or intrinsic factor deficiencies	Meat, fish, cheese, eggs
Folate	DNA synthesis	Megaloblastic anemia	Goat milk deficient; drug antagonists; heat inactivates	Liver, greens, vegetables, cereals, cheese
Ascorbic acid (C)	Reducing agent; collagen metabolism	*Scurvy:* irritability, purpura, bleeding gums, periosteal hemorrhage, aching bones	May improve tyrosine metabolism in preterm infants	Citrus fruits, green vegetables; cooking destroys it
Fat soluble				
A	Epithelial cell integrity; vision	Night blindness, xerophthalmia, Bitot spots, follicular hyperkeratosis	Common with protein–calorie malnutrition; malabsorption	Liver, milk, eggs, green and yellow vegetables, fruits
D	Maintain serum calcium, phosphorus levels	*Rickets:* reduced bone mineralization	Prohormone of 25- and 1,25-vitamin D	Fortified milk, cheese, liver
E	Antioxidant	Hemolysis in preterm infants; areflexia, ataxia, ophthalmoplegia	May benefit patients with G6PD deficiency	Seeds, vegetables, germ oils, green leafy vegetables
K	Post-translation carboxylation of clotting factors II, VII, IX, X and proteins C, S	Prolonged prothrombin time; hemorrhage; elevated PIVKA (protein induced in vitamin K absence)	Malabsorption; breast-fed infants	Liver, green vegetables; made by intestinal flora

FAD = flavin adenine dinucleotide; G6PD = glucose-6-phosphate dehydrogenase; NAD = nicotinamide adenine dinucleotide.

ation of branched-chain amino acids. Loss of the vitamin occurs during milk pasteurization and sterilization. The thiamine content of commercial formulas for full-term and preterm infants is 59–156 μg/100 kcal and 100–250 μg/100 kcal, respectively.

Infantile beriberi occurs between 1 and 4 mo of life in breast-fed infants whose mothers have a thiamine deficiency, in infants with protein–calorie malnutrition, in infants receiving unsupplemented hyperalimentation fluid, or in infants receiving boiled milk. Acute cardiac symptoms and signs predominate. Anorexia, apathy, vomiting, restlessness, and pallor progress to dyspnea, cyanosis, and death from congestive heart failure. Infants with beriberi have a characteristic aphonic cry; they appear to be crying but no sound is uttered. *Treatment* is noted in Table 2–14.

RIBOFLAVIN

Vitamin B$_2$ is a constituent of two coenzymes, riboflavin-5′-phosphate and flavin-adenine dinucleotide, which are essential components of glutathione reductase and xanthine oxidase and which are involved in electron transport. A deficiency of riboflavin affects glucose, fatty acid, and amino acid metabolism. Riboflavin and its phosphate are decomposed by exposure to light and by strong alkaline solutions. The intake of riboflavin from standard infant formulations, which contain

Table 2–14. Recommended Daily Dose Ranges for Treatment of Vitamin-Related Diseases

Vitamin	Treatment of Vitamin Deficiency	Treatment of Deficiency in Patients with Malabsorption	Treatment of Dependency Syndrome
A (IU)	5000–10,000	10,000–25,000	—
D (IU)	400–5000	4000–20,000	50,000–200,000
Calcifediol (μg)	—	20–100	50–100
Calcitriol (1,25-$(OH)_2$-D) (μg)	—	1–3	1–3
E (IU)	—	100–1000	—
K (mg)	1*	5–10*	—
Ascorbic acid (C)(mg)	250–500	500	—
Thiamine (mg)	5–25	5–25	25–500
Riboflavin (mg)	5–25	5–25	—
Niacin (mg)	25–50	25–50	50–250
B_6 (mg)	5–25	2–25	10–250
Biotin (mg)	0.15–0.3	0.3–1.0	10
Folic acid (mg)	1.0	1.0	—†
B_{12} (μg)	—*	—*	1–40

* To be used parenterally as needed.
† To be used only in conjunction with multivitamin mixtures.
(From AMA Council on Scientific Affairs: Vitamin preparations as dietary supplements and as therapeutic agents. JAMA 257: 1929–1936, 1987. Copyright 1987, American Medical Association.)

147–156 μg/100 kcal, is significantly greater than from human milk (uniform throughout lactation and averaging 49 μg/100 kcal). The processes of pasteurization, evaporation, and condensation of milk do not destroy riboflavin.

Ariboflavinosis is characterized by angular stomatitis, glossitis, cheilosis, seborrheic dermatitis around the nose and mouth, and eye changes that include reduced tearing, photophobia, corneal vascularization, and formation of cataracts. Subclinical riboflavin deficiencies have been found in diabetic subjects, children from low socioeconomic families, children with chronic cardiac disease, and infants undergoing prolonged phototherapy for hyperbilirubinemia. *Treatment* is noted in Table 2–14.

NIACIN

Niacin consists of the compounds nicotinic acid and nicotinamide (niacinamide). Nicotinamide, the predominant form of the vitamin, functions as a component of the coenzymes nicotinamide adenine dinucleotide (NAD) and nicotinamide adenine dinucleotide phosphate (NADP). Niacin is involved in multiple metabolic processes, including fat synthesis, intracellular respiratory metabolism, and glycolysis. When determining the needs for niacin, the content of tryptophan in the diet must be considered because it is converted to niacin. Niacin is stable in foods and can withstand heating and prolonged storage. The concentration of niacin in human milk remains stable throughout lactation and averages 0.29 mg/100 kcal. Approximately 70%

of the total niacin equivalents in human milk are derived from tryptophan. Infants fed commercial formula receive 0.8–1.2 mg of preformed niacin/ 100 kcal. The deficiency disease **(pellagra)** is characterized by weakness, lassitude, dermatitis, inflammation of mucous membranes, diarrhea, vomiting, dysphagia, and, in severe cases, dementia. *Treatment* is noted in Table 2–14.

VITAMIN B_6

Vitamin B_6 refers to three naturally occurring pyridines: pyridoxine (pyridoxol), pyridoxal, and pyridoxamine; the phosphates of the latter two pyridines are metabolically and functionally interrelated and are converted in the liver to the coenzyme form, pyridoxal-5-phosphate. The metabolic functions of vitamin B_6 include interconversion reactions of amino acids, conversion of tryptophan to niacin and serotonin, metabolic reactions in the brain, carbohydrate metabolism, immune development, and the biosynthesis of heme and prostaglandins. The pyridoxal and pyridoxamine forms of the vitamin are destroyed by heat; heat treatment has been responsible for vitamin B_6 deficiency and seizures in infants fed improperly processed formulas. For this reason, heat-stable pyridoxine is presently used for the fortification of milk. The vitamin B_6 content in human milk reflects the mother's nutritional status. The concentration of B_6 in milk obtained from mothers whose intake exceeds the RDA is 18 μg/100 kcal. The range of vitamin B_6 concentrations in cow's milk–based formulas routinely used for full-term infants (59–62 µg/ 100 kcal) satisfies the recommended allowances. Goat's milk is deficient in vitamin B$_6$. Full-term infants become B$_6$ deficient when fed human milk containing 9–12 µg/100 kcal.

Dietary deprivation or malabsorption of vitamin B$_6$ in children results in hypochromic microcytic anemia, vomiting, diarrhea, failure to thrive, listlessness, hyperirritability, and seizures. Children receiving isoniazid may require additional B$_6$ because the drug binds to the vitamin. *Treatment* is noted in Table 2–14.

BIOTIN

Biotin has coenzyme functions in the metabolism of fat and carbohydrate (e.g., it is a component of several carboxylase enzymes). Biotin is synthesized by intestinal bacteria, and thus a deficiency state is uncommon. The average biotin concentration in mature human milk is 0.9 µg/100 kcal. Biotin deficiencies have been reported when it was omitted from parenteral alimentation solutions. Deficiency of *biotinidase*, the enzyme needed for conservation of metabolically active biotin, produces biotin deficiency. *Clinical manifestations* of biotin deficiency include anorexia, nausea, glossitis, pallor, mental changes, alopecia, and a fine maculosquamous dermatitis, which becomes exfoliative. Antibiotics may increase biotin requirements by decreasing enteric synthesis of the vitamin, and the protein avidin, in raw eggs, binds biotin. *Treatment* is noted in Table 2–14.

References

Behrman RE (ed): Nelson Textbook of Pediatrics. 14th ed. Philadelphia, WB Saunders, 1992, Sec. 4.22–4.28.
Guthrie HA: Water-soluble vitamins. *In* Introductory Nutrition. St. Louis, Times Mirror/Mosby College Publishing, 1989, pp 381–448.

Fat-Soluble Vitamins

VITAMIN A

The basic constituent of the vitamin A group is retinol. Ingested plant carotene or animal-tissue retinol esters release retinol after hydrolysis by pancreatic and intestinal enzymes. Chylomicron-transported retinol esters are stored in the liver as retinol palmitate. Retinol is transported from the liver to target tissues by retinol-binding protein (RBP). After delivering free retinol to the target tis-

sues, the RBP is excreted by the kidney. Diseases of the kidney diminish excretion of RBP, whereas liver parenchymal disease or malnutrition lowers the synthesis of RBP. The uptake of retinol by target tissues is facilitated by specific cellular binding proteins. In the eye, retinol is metabolized to form rhodopsin; the action of light on rhodopsin is the first step of the visual process. Retinol also influences the growth and differentiation of epithelia and serves as a cofactor in glycoprotein synthesis. Retinoic acid can substitute for retinol in all functions except those for maintaining tissue growth and vision. The retinol content of human milk averages 50 µg/dL; that of formulas averages 100–200 µg/dL.

Vitamin A deficiency in humans appears in a group of ocular signs termed **xerophthalmia.** The earliest symptom is night blindness, which is followed by xerosis of the conjunctiva and cornea. Untreated, xerophthalmia can result in ulceration, necrosis, keratomalacia, and a permanent corneal scar. Clinical and subclinical vitamin A deficiencies are associated with immunodeficiency, increased risks of infection, especially measles, and increased risk of mortality, especially in developing nations. *Treatment* is noted in Table 2–14. Hypervitaminosis A also has serious sequelae, including dry skin, alopecia, headaches, and hepatotoxicity. Death may occur (Table 2–15).

VITAMIN E

There are eight naturally occurring compounds with vitamin E activity. The most active of these, α-tocopherol, accounts for 90% of the vitamin E present in human tissues and is commercially available as an acetate or succinate. The other compounds of importance are β- and γ-tocopherol, which possess 33% and 10%, respectively, of the activity of α-tocopherol.

In humans, vitamin E acts as a biologic antioxidant by inhibiting the peroxidation of polyunsaturated fatty acids (PUFA) present in cell membranes. It scavenges free radicals generated by the reduction of molecular oxygen and by the action of oxidative enzymes. In the process, the α-tocopherol is oxidized to a quinone, which is excreted in the urine.

Human milk has a lower content of α-tocopherol and a lower ratio of vitamin E to PUFA than do currently utilized formulas. Nevertheless, term and preterm infants have higher serum α-tocopherol levels when fed human milk. The vitamin E requirement is increased in diets having high concentrations of PUFA or iron, both of which facilitate

Table 2–15. Toxic Effects of Vitamins

Vitamin	Effects	Comments
Fat Soluble		Toxicity noted at lower multiples of RDA than water-soluble vitamins
A		
Acute	Lethargy, headache, papilledema, bulging fontanel	Megadoses used to prevent cancer,* treat acne
Chronic	Scaly dry skin, alopecia, sore tongue, hyperostoses, anorexia, increased intracranial pressure (pseudotumor cerebri); teratogenic	Consumption of polar bear liver; toxicity with chronic 20,000–50,000 IU/24 hr
D		
Acute	Hypercalcemia, muscle weakness, anorexia, emesis, headache, polyuria	Hypercalcemia produces arrhythmias, hypertension, renal water wasting
Chronic	Nephrocalcinosis, bone pain, vascular calcification, renal insufficiency; idiopathic infantile hypercalcemia	Toxicity with chronic 3000–4000 IU/24 hr
E	Muscle weakness, diarrhea, antagonism of vitamin K, enhanced anticoagulant drug action	Megadoses used to improve libido*; toxicity with 300–800 IU/24 hr
K	Water-soluble analogues produce neonatal jaundice	Menadione induces neonatal hemolysis
Water Soluble		
C	Uricosuria, oxalate stones, G6PD-deficient hemolysis, rebound scurvy in infants; false-positive test for glycosuria; false-negative test for hematochezia	Prevention of upper respiratory tract infections*
Niacin	Histamine release, ulcers, asthma, flushing, pruritus, gout, hepatotoxic	Orthomolecular treatment of schizophrenia*; toxicity with 200–1000 mg/24 hr
Pyridoxine (B$_6$)	Peripheral sensory neuropathy; fetal–neonatal dependency and seizures	Treat depression* and premenstrual syndrome*; toxicity with 2–6 g/24 hr
Tryptophan	Eosinophilia, myositis, fasciitis, scleroderma	Treat depression* and premenstrual syndrome*; possible toxic metabolite; toxicity with 0.5–4.0 g/24 hr

* No established benefit.
G6PD = glucose-6-phosphate dehydrogenase.

membrane peroxidation and generation of free radicals.

Because colostrum contains high concentrations of vitamin E, the blood tocopherol of breast-fed term infants increases within a few days after birth and remains in the normal adult range of 1.46 ± 0.63 mg/dL until weaning. Term infants who are fed formulas low in vitamin E have low blood levels of α-tocopherol (<0.8 mg/dL) for many months. Complete formulas are fortified to contain a minimum of 0.3 IU of vitamin E/100 kcal and 0.7 IU of vitamin E/g of linoleic acid.

Tocopherol deficiency occurs in children with prolonged and profound fat malabsorption secondary to biliary atresia, cystic fibrosis, and abetalipoproteinemia; these children may develop a syndrome of progressive sensory and motor neuropathy late in the 1st decade of life. Deficient preterm infants at 1–2 mo of age develop hemolytic anemia characterized by an elevated reticulocyte count, an increased sensitivity of the erythrocytes to hemolysis in hydrogen peroxide, peripheral edema, and thrombocytosis. All the abnormalities are corrected after oral vitamin E therapy (Table 2–14). Toxicity due to excess vitamin E is noted in Table 2–15.

VITAMIN D

Cholecalciferol (D$_3$) is the mammalian form of vitamin D and is produced by ultraviolet irradiation of inactive precursors in the skin. Ergocalciferol (D$_2$) is derived from plants. Both require further metabolism to become active and are of equivalent potency. Clothing, lack of sunlight exposure, and skin pigmentation decrease the generation of vitamin D in the epidermis and dermis. Vitamin D (D$_2$

and D$_3$) is metabolized in the liver to calcidiol, or 25-(OH)-D; this metabolite, which has little intrinsic activity, is transported by a plasma-binding globulin to the kidney, where it is converted to the most active metabolite calcitriol, or 1,25-(OH)$_2$-D. The molecular action of 1,25-(OH)$_2$-D results in a decrease in the mRNA for collagen in bone and an increase of the concentration of messenger RNA for vitamin D–dependent calcium-binding protein in the intestine (directly mediating increased intestinal calcium transport). Calcium transport is mediated by the specific local synthesis of the intestinal vitamin D–dependent calcium-binding protein. The antirachitic action of vitamin D probably is mediated by provision of appropriate concentrations of calcium and phosphate in the extracellular space of bone and by enhanced intestinal absorption of these minerals. The direct effect of vitamin D on bone is probably similar to that of parathyroid hormone and results in bone resorption. Vitamin D also may have a direct anabolic effect on bone. 1,25-(OH)$_2$-D also has direct feedback to the parathyroid gland and inhibits secretion of parathyroid hormone.

The most prevalent form of vitamin D measured in plasma, 25-(OH)-D, ranges from 10 to 60 ng/mL. The values vary with dietary intake, sunlight (ultraviolet light) exposure, and body stores. The serum concentration of 1,25-(OH)$_2$-D ranges from 18 to 60 ng/mL.

Vitamin D deficiency appears as **rickets** in children and as osteomalacia in postpubertal adolescents. Inadequate direct sun exposure and vitamin D intake are sufficient causes, but other factors (e.g., high cereal intake, a vegetarian diet, or various drugs [phenobarbital, phenytoin]) also may produce rickets.

The *pathophysiology* of rickets results from defective bone growth, especially marked at the epiphyseal cartilage matrix, which fails to mineralize. The uncalcified osteoid results in a wide, irregular zone of poorly supported tissue, the rachitic metaphysis. This soft, rather than hardened, zone produces many of the skeletal deformities through compression and lateral bulging or flaring of the ends of bones.

The *clinical manifestations* of rickets are most common during the first 2 yr of life and require several months of a vitamin D–deficient diet to become evident. Craniotabes is due to thinning of the outer table of the skull, which feels to the touch like a Ping-Pong ball when compressed. Enlargement of the costochondral junction (rachitic rosary) and thickening of the wrists and ankles may be palpated. The anterior fontanel is enlarged, and its closure may be delayed. In advanced rickets, there may be scoliosis and exaggerated lordosis. Bowlegs or knock knees may be evident in older infants, and greenstick fractures may be observed in long bones.

The *diagnosis* of rickets is based on a dietary history of poor vitamin D intake and little exposure to direct ultraviolet sunlight. The serum calcium usually is normal but may be low, the serum phosphorus level always is reduced, and the serum alkaline phosphatase activity is elevated. When serum calcium levels decline below 7.5 mg/dL, tetany may occur. 24,25-(OH)$_2$-D levels are undetectable and serum 1,25-(OH)$_2$-D levels are below 7 ng/mL. Characteristic roentgenologic changes of the distal ulna and radius include widening, concave cupping, and frayed, poorly demarcated ends. The increased space between the distal ends of the radius and ulna and the metacarpal bones is the enlarged, nonossified metaphysis.

The *treatment* of vitamin D–deficiency rickets and osteomalacia is indicated in Table 2–14. Breast-fed infants born of mothers with adequate vitamin D stores usually maintain adequate serum 1,25-(OH)$_2$-D levels for the first 6 mo, but they may subsequently develop rickets if they are not exposed to the sun or do not receive supplementary vitamin D. Toxic effects of vitamin D are noted in Table 2–15.

VITAMIN K

The plant form of vitamin K is phylloquinone or vitamin K$_1$. Another form, menaquinone or vitamin K$_2$, is one of a series of compounds with unsaturated side chains synthesized by the intestinal bacteria. Plasma factors II (prothrombin), VII, IX, and X in the cascade of blood coagulation factors depend on vitamin K for synthesis and for post-translational conversion of precursor proteins of these plasma factors. The post-translational conversion of glutamyl residues to γ-carboxyglutamic acid residues of a prothrombin molecule creates effective calcium-binding sites, making the protein active.

Other vitamin K–dependent proteins include proteins C, S, and Z in plasma and γ-carboxyglutamic acid (gla)–containing proteins in kidney, spleen, lung, uterus, placenta, pancreas, thyroid, thymus, testes, and bone. Bone contains a major vitamin K–dependent protein, osteocalcin, as well as lesser amounts of other glutamic acid–containing proteins.

Phylloquinone is absorbed from the intestine and transported by chylomicrons. The rarity of dietary vitamin K deficiency in humans with normal intestinal function suggests that the absorption of menaquinones is possible. Vitamin K deficiency has been observed in subjects with impaired fat absorption caused by obstructive jaundice, pancreatic insufficiency, and celiac disease; often these problems are combined with the use of antibiotics that change intestinal flora. Absorption of vitamin K also may be inhibited by mineral oil and high dietary intakes of vitamins A and E. The phylloquinone content of mature human milk averages 2.1 ng/mL, not different from that of colostrum samples. Average concentrations of phylloquinones are 11.5 ng/mL in supplemental soy-based formulas and 55–58 ng/mL in cow's milk formulas.

Hemorrhagic disease of the newborn, a disease primarily of breast-fed infants, occurs at 2–10 days of life in those who do not receive prophylactic vitamin K on the first day of life. The recommended preventive dose is 0.5–1.0 mg. Hemorrhagic disease of the newborn usually is marked by generalized ecchymoses, gastrointestinal hemorrhage, or bleeding from a circumcision or umbilical stump; intracranial hemorrhage is uncommon (see Chapter 6).

References

Behrman RE (ed): Nelson Textbook of Pediatrics. 14th ed. Philadelphia, WB Saunders, 1992, Sec. 4.21–4.33.
Guthrie HA: Fat-soluble vitamins. *In* Introductory Nutrition. St. Louis, Times Mirror/Mosby College Publishing, 1989, pp 339–378.

MINERALS

Calcium

Ninety-nine percent of calcium is in the skeleton; the remaining 1% is in extracellular fluids, intracellular compartments, and cell membranes. The 1% nonskeletal calcium serves a role in nerve conduction, muscle contraction, blood clotting, and membrane permeability. There are two distinct bone calcium phosphate pools, a large crystalline form and a smaller amorphous phase. Bone calcium constantly turns over, with concurrent bone resorption and formation. Bone mass peaks in the late 2nd to 3rd decade and is influenced by prior and concurrent dietary calcium intake, exercise, and hormone status (testosterone, estrogen).

Dietary calcium intake depends on the consumption of dairy products. The calcium equivalent of 1 cup of milk is 3/4 cup plain yogurt, 1½ oz cheddar cheese, 2 cups ice cream, 4/5 cup almonds, and 2½

oz sardines. Other sources of calcium include some leafy green vegetables (broccoli, kale, collards), lime-processed tortillas, and calcium-precipitated tofu.

There is no classical calcium deficiency syndrome, because blood and cell levels are closely regulated. The body can mobilize skeletal calcium and increase the absorptive efficiency of dietary calcium. *Osteoporosis* is characterized by diminished quantity of bone that is histologically normal. Osteoporosis is rare in childhood and related to protein–calorie malnutrition, vitamin C deficiency, steroid therapy, immobilization and disuse, osteogenesis imperfecta, or severe calcium deficiency (premature infants; see Chapter 6). The cause of osteoporosis in postmenopausal women is multifactorial. The primary method of prevention is to ensure maximum peak bone mass by providing optimal calcium intake during childhood and adolescence. Bone mineral status can be monitored by single- and dual-energy photon densitometry and dual-energy x-ray absorptiometry.

No adverse effects are observed in adults on dietary calcium intakes of up to 2.5 g/day. Nonetheless, there is concern that high intakes may increase the risk for urinary stone formation, constipation, and decreased renal function and inhibit intestinal absorption of other minerals (iron, zinc).

References

Behrman RE (ed): Nelson Textbook of Pediatrics. 14th ed. Philadelphia, WB Saunders, 1992, Sec. 6.6.
Guthrie HA: Macronutrient elements. *In* Introductory Nutrition. St. Louis, Times Mirror/Mosby College Publishing, 1989, pp 261–277.

Nutritional Anemia (also see Chapter 14)

The recognition of anemia in infancy requires knowledge of normal age- and birth weight–related changes in hemoglobin concentration. Reference values are given in Table 14–2.

IRON-DEFICIENCY ANEMIA

In infancy, the major causes of iron-deficiency anemia are a dilution of body iron by rapid growth and an iron-poor diet. Blood loss results in more severe iron-deficiency anemia than is seen with the other two causes. Blood loss may be caused by conditions such as fetal–maternal transfusion, placenta previa, rupture of umbilical vessels, and twin–twin transfusion. Intestinal bleeding may be due to the ingestion of fresh cow's milk in early infancy or, rarely, pulmonary hemosiderosis, a bleeding Meckel diverticulum, esophagitis, or peptic ulcer. The removal of blood for laboratory studies in infants requiring intensive care also may result in iron-deficiency anemia.

Iron is used in the synthesis of hemoglobin, myoglobin, and enzyme iron. Iron-deficiency anemia occurs when a lack of iron is sufficient to restrict the production of hemoglobin and its concentration falls below the normal range. Body iron content is regulated primarily through modulation of iron absorption, which depends on the state of body iron stores, the form and amount of iron in foods, and the mixture of foods in the diet. Iron excretion occurs through the feces.

There are two categories of iron in food. The first is *heme iron*, present in hemoglobin and myoglobin; it is supplied by meat and rarely accounts for more than a quarter of the iron ingested by infants. The absorption of heme iron is relatively efficient and is not influenced by other constituents of the diet. The second category is *nonheme iron*, which represents the preponderance of iron intake and exists in the form of salts. The absorption of nonheme iron is determined by the composition of consumed foods. The fractional intestinal absorption of the small amount of iron in human milk is 50%, in contrast to 10% of iron absorbed from unfortified cow's milk formula and 4% absorbed from iron-fortified cow's milk formula. About 4% of the iron from iron-fortified infant dry cereals is absorbed. Enhancers of nonheme iron absorption are ascorbic acid, meat, fish, and poultry. Inhibitors are bran, polyphenols (including the tannates in tea), and phosphate. During pregnancy, iron is efficiently transported from the maternal circulation to the fetus, and transport is not impaired by maternal iron-deficiency anemia. In the *term infant,* there is little change in total body iron and little need for exogenous iron before 4 mo of age. Iron deficiency is rare among term infants during the first 4 mo, unless there has been substantial blood loss.

After 4 mo of age, iron reserves become marginal for the remainder of infancy. From 4 to 12 mo, an average of 0.9 mg of iron/24 hr must be absorbed from the diet to provide 0.7 mg/24 hr for growth and 0.2 mg/24 hr to balance normal fecal losses. In term infants who receive unfortified cow's milk formula, depletion of storage iron occurs as early as 4 mo of age, as indicated by low serum ferritin concentrations (10 µg/liter). Breast-fed infants rarely deplete their iron stores until after 6 mo of age. In the absence of iron fortification or supplementation, iron stores eventually become inadequate in breast-fed infants at the age when solid foods are added to the diet. *Premature infants* have a lower amount of stored iron since significant amounts of iron are transferred from the mother in the third trimester. In addition, their postnatal iron needs are greater because of rapid rates of growth.

Term breast-fed infants need an alternative source of iron after 4–6 mo of age. Some recommend ferrous sulfate supplementation, while others introduce iron containing solid foods. Iron fortified formula is the only alternative for breast milk in the under 1 yr old child.

Premature infants fed human milk may develop iron-deficiency anemia unless they receive iron supplements of 2 mg of iron/kg/24 hr. Formula-fed preterm infants should receive iron-fortified formula by approximately 1 or 2 mo of age. Evidence of vitamin E deficiency may occur among low-birth-weight infants fed iron-fortified formula prior to 1–2 mo of age.

The *diagnosis* of iron-deficiency anemia is established by the presence of a microcytic hypochromic anemia, low serum ferritin, low serum iron, reduced transferrin saturation, normal to elevated red cell width distribution (RDW), and enhanced iron-binding capacity. The mean corpuscular volume (MCV) and red cell indices are reduced, and the reticulocyte count is between 0 and 1%. Iron deficiency may be present without anemia (see Chapter 14). Clinical manifestations are noted in Table 2–16.

Treatment of iron-deficiency anemia requires changes in the diet to provide adequate iron as well as the administration of 2–6 mg iron/kg/24hr (as ferrous sulfate). Reticulocytosis is noted within 3–7 days of starting treatment, and the hemoglobin may rise as rapidly as 0.25–0.40 g/dL/24 hr; usually half-correction is achieved after 2 wk and two thirds correction after 4 wk. Oral treatment should be continued for 5 mo. Rarely, intramuscular or intravenous iron therapy is needed if oral iron cannot be given or compliance is poor. Such parenteral therapy has the risk of anaphylaxis.

MEGALOBLASTIC ANEMIA

In infancy, these rare anemias are caused by folate deficiency, vitamin B_{12} deficiency, and inborn errors of metabolism. *Folate deficiency,* which may result from a low dietary intake, malabsorption, or vitamin–drug interactions, can develop within a few weeks of birth because infants require 10 times as much folate as adults per kilogram of body weight but have scant stores of folate in the newborn period. The recommended intake varies be-

Table 2–16. Characteristics of Mineral Deficiencies

Mineral	Function	Manifestations of Deficiency	Comments	Sources
Iron	Heme-containing macromolecules (e.g., hemoglobin, cytochrome, myoglobin)	Anemia, spoon nails, reduced muscle and mental performance	History of pica, cow's milk, gastrointestinal bleeding	Liver, eggs, grains
Copper	Redox reactions (e.g., cytochrome oxidase)	Hypochromic anemia, neutropenia, osteoporosis, hypotonia, hypoproteinemia	Inborn error, Menke kinky hair syndrome	Liver, oysters, meat, nuts, grains, legumes, chocolate
Zinc	Metalloenzymes (e.g., alkaline phosphatase, carbonic anhydrase, DNA polymerase; wound healing	*Acrodermatitis enteropathica;* poor growth, acro-orificial rash, alopecia, delayed sexual development, hypogeusia, infection	Protein–calorie malnutrition; weaning; malabsorption syndromes	Meat, grains, cheese, nuts
Selenium	Antioxidant Glutathione peroxidase	Keshan cardiomyopathy in China	Endemic areas; long-term TPN	Meat, vegetables
Chromium	Insulin cofactor	Poor weight gain, glucose intolerance, neuropathy	Protein–calorie malnutrition, long-term TPN	Yeast, breads
Fluoride	Strengthen dental enamel	Caries	Supplementation during tooth growth, narrow therapeutic range, fluorosis may cause staining of the teeth	Seafood, water
Iodine	Thyroxine, tri-iodothyronine production	Simple endemic goiter *Myxedematous cretinism:* congenital hypothyroidism *Neurologic cretinism:* mental retardation, deafness, spasticity, normal T_4 level at birth	Endemic in New Guinea, the Congo; endemic in Great Lakes area prior to iodized salt	Seafood, iodized salt, most food in nonendemic areas

TPN = total parenteral nutrition.

tween 30 and 65 μg/day. **Heat-sterilizing** home-prepared formula can decrease the folate content by half. **Evaporated milk** has less than 20 μg of folate per reconstituted liter. **Goat's milk** has less than 6 μg/L. Folate deficiency has been reported in healthy low-birth-weight infants fed formulas based on heated or boiled evaporated or pasteurized milk. In proprietary infant formulas, the presence of ascorbic acid decreases the loss of folic acid. Infants fed human milk or proprietary cow's milk formulas are not at risk of nutritional folate deficiency.

Very-low-birth-weight infants should be given supplemental folate to support their rapid growth, especially until their milk or formula volume intake provides adequate folate. Folate deficiency due to malabsorption may occur with chronic diarrhea. The conjugated polyglutamate forms of folate in the diet may not be digested to the monoglutamate form that can be absorbed. Diarrhea also interferes with the normal enterohepatic circulation of folate. Patients with chronic hemolysis (sickle cell anemia, thalassemia) require extra folate to avoid deficiency caused by increased red blood cell production.

Folate deficiency should be suspected when hypersegmented neutrophils and/or elevation of the MCV to about 100 fL is noted. The diagnosis is confirmed by the determination of both serum and red cell folate and serum vitamin B_{12}. A therapeutic dose of folate (0.5–1.0 mg of pteroylglutamic acid/24 hr, 10 or more times the daily allowance) is given when the diagnosis of folate deficiency is established (Table 2–14). Treatment is monitored by the reticulocyte response and by the rise in hemoglobin and hematocrit, responses similar to those noted during the iron treatment of iron-deficiency anemia. Folate therapy may mask the hematologic manifestations of vitamin B_{12} deficiency.

VITAMIN B_{12} DEFICIENCY

Early diagnosis and treatment of this rare disorder in childhood are important because of the danger of irreversible neurologic damage. Most cases in childhood result from a specific defect in absorption (see Tables 2–12 and 2–13). Such defects include congenital pernicious anemia (absent intrinsic factor), juvenile pernicious anemia (autoimmune), and deficiency of transcobalamin II transport. Intestinal resection, small bowel bacterial overgrowth, or the fish tapeworm *Diphyllobothrium latum* also causes vitamin B_{12} deficiency. An exclusively breast-fed infant ingests approximately 0.3 μg of vitamin B_{12}/24 hr, unless the mother is a strict vegetarian. The absorption of vitamin B_{12} depends on the formation of a complex between the vitamin and a mucoprotein, intrinsic factor. The complex is absorbed in the distal ileum. In the plasma, vitamin B_{12} is bound to a specific serum transport protein, transcobalamin II. The vitamin is stored in the liver. These stores are large in the newborn and are rarely depleted before 1 yr of age.

Depression of serum vitamin B_{12} below 100 pg/mL and the appearance of hypersegmented neutrophils are the earliest *clinical manifestations* of deficiency. Late findings of vitamin B_{12} deficiency are similar to the findings of folate deficiency and include megaloblastic anemia, leukopenia, and thrombocytopenia. Neurologic manifestations include peripheral neuropathy, posterior column signs, dementia, and eventual coma; these signs do not occur in folate deficiency, but administration of folate in excess of 0.1 mg/24 hr to vitamin B_{12}–deficient individuals aggravates the neurologic manifestations.

Diagnosis is made by history and the presence of a macrocytosis accompanied by a megaloblastic bone marrow. Serum folate is normal, but red cell folate may be reduced with vitamin B_{12} deficiency. Serum vitamin B_{12} is reduced. Patients with vitamin B_{12} deficiency also have increased urine levels of methylmalonic acid.

In nondietary deficiencies, a Schilling test must be performed to identify those patients with pernicious anemia and bacterial overgrowth. Vitamin B_{12} (radiolabeled) is ingested, and 2 hr later a flushing intravenous dose of 1 mg of vitamin B_{12} is given. If less than 7% of radiolabeled vitamin B_{12} is excreted in urine, the test is repeated with the addition of oral intrinsic factor. Normal excretion following intrinsic factor confirms the diagnosis of pernicious anemia (absent endogenous intrinsic factor). If urinary excretion of labeled vitamin B_{12} remains below 7% in 24 hr, an intestinal lesion such as bacterial overgrowth may be present; pretreatment with antibiotics and repetition of the test with subsequent normal results confirms the diagnosis.

Most cases of vitamin B_{12} deficiency in infants and children are not of dietary origin and require *treatment* throughout life. An intramuscular dose of 50–100 µg is used to initiate therapy. Maintenance therapy consists of repeated monthly intramuscular injections.

References

Behrman RE (ed): Nelson Textbook of Pediatrics. 14th ed. Philadelphia, WB Saunders, 1992, Sec. 16.9–16.11.
Dallmann PR: Nutritional anemia of infancy: Iron, folic acid and vitamin B_{12}. *In* Tsang RC, Nichols BL (eds): Nutrition During Infancy. Philadelphia, Hanley and Belfus, Inc, 1988, pp 216–235.

Trace Elements

Trace element deficiencies are important clinical syndromes in persons with malabsorption and/or on parenteral nutrition. Many of these elements have a narrow therapeutic range and may cause toxicity.

COPPER

Copper, as a constituent of many enzymes, is involved in energy production via oxidative phosphorylation, in the protection of cell membranes against oxidative damage, in the oxidation of iron released from storage, in erythropoietin synthesis, and in cerebral protein and myelin deposition. Some of the better known cuproenzymes are cytochrome oxidase, superoxide dismutase, ceruloplasmin, ferroxidase II, lysyl oxidase, tyrosinase, and dopamine β-hydroxylase.

Because copper is present in most foods (Table 2–16), adequate intake levels are easily achieved. Large amounts of copper are deposited in the fetal liver during the 3rd trimester and gradually are depleted when ceruloplasmin synthesis and secretion begin. Transcuprein is the predominant vehicle of copper transport to the liver in the portal circulation. The liver of term infants contains a copper concentration 10–20 fold greater than that in the liver of adults. After its uptake from the portal circulation, copper is bound to hepatic metallothionein, from which it is released for enzyme synthesis in mitochondria and cytosol, transferred to the nuclei, and then incorporated into ceruloplasmin, which is released into the plasma compartment. Copper in plasma is found in four fractions: transcuprein and albumin, each 15%; ceruloplasmin, 60%; and various low-molecular-weight components, 10%. Synthesis and secretion in the liver occur with ceruloplasmin-bound copper, the preferred transport form to other tissues (e.g., brain, muscle, and bones). Copper breakdown products normally are sequestered in lysosomes and excreted in bile; copper overload may occur in patients with cholestasis. Urinary excretion of copper normally is minimal.

Serum levels of copper and ceruloplasmin are low at birth and remain low for several weeks in preterm infants. Levels rise, however, as ceruloplasmin synthesis begins between the 6th and 12th postnatal weeks, varying with the gestational age of the infant. Concentrations are not affected by the levels of oral copper intake.

Copper deficiency first was reported in infants recuperating from PEM whose diet was based on cow's milk. It also has been noted in infants and patients receiving total parenteral nutrition containing inadequate amounts of copper, with chronic antacid use, and after ingesting large amounts of zinc. The clinical manifestations of copper deficiency may be traced to the specific cuproenzyme affected—depigmentation (hair, skin) and tyrosinase; hypothermia, hypotonia, and cytochrome C; altered elastin and collagen and lysyl oxidase deficiency; central nervous system degeneration (hypotonia, psychomotor retardation) and dopamine-β-hydroxylase. Other signs include apnea, scurvy-like hemorrhage, blood vessel rupture, failure to thrive, flaring of anterior ribs, fractures, osteoporosis, periosteal reaction, metaphyseal spurs, hypercholesterolemia, edema, diarrhea, altered glucose tolerance, anemia, and neutropenia.

Wilson disease is an autosomal-recessive disease (1:200,000 births) of unknown etiology characterized by increased copper deposition in brain, liver, kidney, and cornea and low serum copper and ceruloplasmin levels. Hepatic failure with cirrhosis, hepatitis, Fanconi renal syndrome, hemolytic anemia, Kayser-Fleischer corneal pigmented rings, and neurologic signs such as behavioral problems, tremor, spasticity, and poor fine motor control are noted after the age of 5 yr. Treatment is a low-copper diet and lifelong chelation therapy with D-penicillamine.

Menke kinky hair syndrome, a lethal X-linked condition of unknown etiology, is characterized by decreased intestinal copper transport, low serum copper and ceruloplasmin levels, and increased copper in fibroblasts and urine. Manifestations include hypotonia, myoclonic seizures, spasticity, failure to thrive, steely depigmented hair, osteoporosis, and arterial tortuosity. There is no specific therapy.

Excessive copper intake is associated with **Indian childhood cirrhosis.** Copper *toxicity* may produce nausea, hemolysis, and hepatic necrosis.

ZINC

Zinc is important in protein metabolism and synthesis, in nucleic acid metabolism, and in the stabilization of cell membranes. Zinc metalloenzymes include erythrocyte carbonic anhydrase, alcohol dehydrogenase, carboxypeptidases A and B, alkaline phosphatase, DNA and RNA polymerase, various dehydrogenases, and retinene reductase (Table 2–16); many other enzymes use zinc as a cofactor.

Dietary zinc is absorbed (20–80%) in the duodenum and proximal small intestine. In zinc sufficiency, an increasing zinc pool triggers synthesis of intestinal mucosal metallothionein, which binds intracellular zinc. Protein-bound zinc and human milk zinc are the most readily absorbed forms of the mineral. Histidine and cysteine facilitate absorption, whereas phytase and fiber inhibit it. Excess dietary copper, iron, or cadmium decreases zinc absorption by competing for cellular uptake and metallothionein binding. After cellular uptake, the metal is secreted into the portal circulation, where it binds primarily to albumin. Zinc transported from the intestine is taken up rapidly by the liver, pancreas, kidneys, and spleen. Excretion occurs through fecal losses. Dietary requirements vary from 1.0 to 3.1 mg of zinc/day for 2 mo old infants. Zinc requirements for term infants receiving parenteral nutrition have been estimated at 100 μg/kg/day. In the presence of ongoing losses, such as chronic diarrhea, requirements can drastically increase.

The original account of *zinc deficiency dwarfism* syndrome was described in a group of children with low levels of zinc in their hair, poor appetite, diminished taste acuity, hypogonadism, and short stature.

Acute acquired zinc deficiency may occur in patients receiving parenteral alimentation without zinc supplementation and in premature infants fed human milk. Transient zinc deficiency rarely has been reported in full-term, breast-fed infants. Mild clinical manifestations of zinc deficiency in infants include failure to thrive, and in children and adolescents include decreased growth velocity, anorexia, and hypogeusia. Moderately severe manifestations include delayed sexual maturation, rough skin, pica, and hepatosplenomegaly, and the severe signs include acral and periorificial skin lesions, failure to thrive, diarrhea, mood changes, alopecia, night blindness, and photophobia.

Acrodermatitis enteropathica is an autosomal recessive disorder that begins within 2–4 wk of weaning infants from breast milk. It is characterized by an acute perioral and perianal dermatitis, alopecia, and failure to thrive. The disease is due to severe zinc deficiency from an undefined but specific defect of intestinal zinc absorption. Plasma zinc levels are reduced, and serum alkaline phosphatase activity is low. Treatment is with oral zinc supplementation (1 mg/kg/24 hr).

Zinc *excess* produces nausea, emesis, abdominal pain, headache, vertigo, and seizures.

SELENIUM

The only well-defined function of selenium is as part of the enzyme glutathione peroxidase (GSHPx), one of the enzyme systems that, with catalase, superoxide dismutase, and vitamin E, protects cells from oxidative damage by destroying cytosolic hydrogen peroxide (Table 2–16). Selenium is well absorbed. The primary route of excretion is in the urine. An intake greater than 1.5 µg/kg/24 hr prevents a fall in blood selenium levels in young infants. Concentrations in human milk reflect selenium levels in the mother. The intake of selenium by exclusively breast-fed infants is approximately 10 µg/24 hr, compared with 7 µg/24 hr by formula-fed infants. Infants and children who receive total parental nutrition may have a rapid drop of blood selenium levels unless adequate amounts are provided in the solution (approximately 1 µg/kg of body weight).

A *selenium deficiency syndrome* (Keshan disease) has been reported in rural China and is characterized by necrosis and fibrosis of the myocardium, which results in potentially fatal acute or chronic heart failure. Those most at risk include infants, young children, and women of child-bearing age. Supplementation with 1 mg of selenium daily has been effective in preventing new cases. Fatal cardiomyopathy has been reported in adults on long-term total parenteral nutrition and in a 2 yr old child whose diet was very low in both selenium and animal protein. Blood selenium levels below 40 ng/mL in orally fed preterm infants also are associated with increased erythrocyte fragility. Muscle pain, myopathy, and nail bed changes may occur.

IODINE

Iodine is an integral part of the thyroid hormones (Table 2–16). Circulating iodine is taken up avidly by the thyroid gland, where it is bound to thyroglobulin, an iodinated glycoprotein, from which the hormones thyroxine (T_4) and tri-iodothyronine (T_3) are formed. In iodine deficiency, the synthesis and release of thyroid hormones are decreased, low blood levels of T_4 and T_3 result, and the feedback mechanism involving the thyroid–hypothalamus–pituitary axis is stimulated. This sequence of events produces an increased output of thyroid-stimulating hormone (TSH) by the pituitary, which ultimately results in enlargement of the thyroid gland, or **goiter**.

Ingested iodine is readily absorbed; the main route of excretion is in the urine. Fifty percent of an adequate iodine intake is retained by healthy infants. A daily dietary intake of 40 µg for infants from birth to 6 mo, increased to 50 µg for infants from 6 to 12 mo, is recommended. The minimum intake by an exclusively breast-fed infant is 22 µg/24 hr, but this is well above the minimum estimated requirement of 1 µg/kg/24 hr. Infant formulas contain at least 5 µg of iodine/100 kcal, and most formulas for both full- and preterm infants supply 2–3 times this amount. For infants of iodine-sufficient mothers, additional iodine is not necessary during short-term intravenous feeding. Because of its potential for toxicity, all sources of iodine to the infant should be considered before supplementation is initiated.

Moderate *iodine deficiency* may produce a euthyroid state accompanied by hyperplasia and hypertrophy of the thyroid gland or goiter. Severe dietary iodine deficiency results in hypothyroidism. **Endemic cretinism** is seen in the same geographic areas as endemic goiter and may be characterized by ataxia, spasticity, deaf–mutism, and mental retardation with or without short stature, and little or no impairment of thyroid function. This variant affecting the nervous system is probably due to early fetal iodine deficiency. The **myxedematous type** of cretinism is characterized by retarded growth, delayed mental and sexual function, and the presence of myxedema in the absence of abnormal neurologic signs. This variant may be due to late fetal and postnatal iodine deficiency, which results in low thyroid hormone levels, elevated TSH concentration, and markedly delayed bone age. Both syndromes are prevented by iodine supplementation. *Excessive* iodine treatment may produce thyrotoxicosis or goiter.

FLUORIDE

Dental enamel is strengthened when fluoride is substituted for hydroxyl ions in the hydroxyapatite crystalline mineral matrix of the enamel. The resulting fluorapatite is more resistant to both chemical and physical damage. Fluoride is incorporated into the enamel during the mineralization stages of tooth formation and also by surface interaction after the tooth has erupted. Fluoride is similarly incorporated into bone mineral and may protect against osteoporosis later in life. Approximately 80% of fluoride in foods and fluids is absorbed; as much as 97% is absorbed from soluble supplements such as sodium fluoride. Fluoride is excreted mainly in the urine, with less than 10% of the intake appearing in the feces.

In the formula-fed infant, the need for supplementation depends on the type of formula used.

Commercial formulas now are made with defluorinated water and contain low amounts of fluoride. An infant who receives only ready-to-feed formula should be given supplemental fluoride. The fluoride content of human milk is low, 5–15 ng/mL, and intakes by exclusively breast-fed infants are about 4–15 μg/day in optimally fluoridated areas. Breast-fed infants should receive fluoride supplements, especially if breast fed longer than 6 mo. Fluoride levels of the water supply to which the child is exposed should be determined before prescribing fluoride supplements. Fluorosis commonly stains the teeth. Fluoride supplementation is unlikely to provide additional protection for the preterm infant and may cause toxicity.

References

Behrman RE (ed): Nelson Textbook of Pediatrics. 14th ed. Philadelphia, WB Saunders, 1992, Sec. 4.6, 19.14.

Casey CE, Walravens PA: Trace elements. *In* Tsang RC, Nichols BL (eds): Nutrition during Infancy. Philadelphia, Hanley and Belfus, Inc, 1988, pp 190–215.

DIETARY MANAGEMENT DURING ILLNESS

Nutritional Assessment

Pediatric nutritional assessment includes consideration of medical and nutrition history, dietary intake, factors that alter nutrient utilization and absorption, physical examination (including growth patterns and current anthropometry), and laboratory assessment. The assessment is used to define nutritional status (Fig. 2–5) and nutrient needs in children. Macronutrient depletion can be assessed by comparing height, weight, and head circumference measurements of the patient with normal standards. Recent weight loss or failure of normal growth is an important consideration. A low percentage of expected weight for height suggests recent macronutrient deficiency (usually calories), whereas low height for age suggests chronic deficiency. Loss of body fat is measured by determining triceps skinfold thicknesses, and loss of muscle mass is reflected in reduced arm circumference measurements corrected for skinfold thicknesses. Measurements of the triceps skinfold and the circumference of the upper arm are made midpoint in the distance between the palpated head of the humerus and the bony prominence of the elbow on the extensor (dorsal) surface when the elbow is flexed 90 degrees. Additional physical signs are noted in Table 2–17. Useful laboratory tests include

DATE:______ DIAGNOSIS:______
PT. AGE:______ PT. SEX:______ DIET ORDER:______
ALLERGIES:______ RDA FOR AGE: CALORIES______ PROTEIN______
______ DIETITIAN:______

ANTHROPOMETRIC DATA
HEIGHT (cm):______ WEIGHT (kg):______ HEAD CIRCUMFERENCE (cm):______
TRICEPS SKINFOLD (mm):______ ARM CIRCUMFERENCE (cm):______
ARM MUSCLE AREA (mm²):______
CLINICAL DATA
HEMOGLOBIN (g/dl):______ BUN (mg/dl):______ ALBUMIN (g/dl):______
LEUKOCYTE COUNT/mm³:______ DIFFERENTIAL: LYMPHOCYTES (%):______
TOTAL LYMPHOCYTES/mm³:______
URINARY CREATININE (mg/24 hr)______

BODY SIZE	HEAD CIRCUMFERENCE (mm)	5	10	50	90	95	PERCENTILE
BODY SIZE	HEIGHT (cm)/AGE	5	10	50	90	95	PERCENTILE
BODY SIZE	WEIGHT (kg)/HEIGHT	5	10	50	90	95	PERCENTILE
FAT	TRICEPS SKINFOLD (mm)	5	15	50	85	95	PERCENTILE
MUSCLE PROTEIN	ARM MUSCLE AREA (cm³)	5	15	50	85	95	PERCENTILE
MUSCLE PROTEIN	CREATININE HEIGHT INDEX (24-hr creatinine excretion / standard for height)	60%	80%	85%	90%	95%	
VISCERAL PROTEIN	ALBUMIN (g/dl)	2.8	3.5	4.0	4.5	5.0	
VISCERAL PROTEIN	TOTAL LYMPHOCYTES (mm³)	1000	1500	2000	2500	3000	
VISCERAL PROTEIN	SKIN TEST (mm) □SK/SD□DT□CANDIDA □OTHER:______	2	5	10	15	20	
		Depleted	LOW	NORMAL			

Figure 2–5. Nutritional assessment form. Nutritional data for the patient are recorded and graphed on this form. Values falling in the area labeled "Depleted" are considered abnormal and those in the adjacent column borderline. (From Merritt RJ, Sinatra FR, Smith GA: Nutritional support of the hospitalized child. Adv Nutr Res Vol 5: 77–103, 1983.

measurement of hepatic secretory proteins in serum (Table 2–18). Albumin, retinol-binding protein, prealbumin, and transferrin are depleted during inadequate protein or calorie intake. Albumin is affected by non-nutritional influences; these other proteins have a shorter half-life and reflect recent macronutrient intake (days to weeks). Reduced total lymphocyte count and a failure of T-cell function are reflected in anergy in skin tests.

The nutritional management of the ill patient is accomplished by enteral or parenteral feeding. Priority should be given to oral feedings, followed by intragastric, duodenal, or jejunal tube delivery, peripheral intravenous infusions, and finally central intravenous infusions. The complexity and expense of nursing and dietary care increase exponentially with the progression through this management sequence. The immunologic and metabolic effects of malnutrition make the delayed in-

Table 2–17. Physical Signs of Nutritional Deficiency Disorders

System	Sign	Deficiency
General appearance	Reduced weight for height	Calories
Skin/hair	Pallor	Anemias (iron, B_{12}, vitamin E, folate, and copper)
	Edema	Protein, thiamine
	Nasolabial seborrhea	Calories, protein, vitamin B_6
	Dermatitis	Riboflavin, essential fatty acids, biotin
	Photosensitivity dermatitis	Niacin
	Acrodermatitis	Zinc
	Follicular hyperkeratosis (sandpaper-like)	Vitamin A
	Depigmented skin	Calories, protein
	Purpura	Vitamins C, K
	Scrotal, vulval dermatitis	Riboflavin
	Alopecia	Zinc, biotin, protein
	Depigmented, dull hair	Protein, calories, copper
Subcutaneous tissue	Decreased	Calories
Eye (vision)	Adaptation to dark	Vitamins A, E, zinc
	Color discimination	Vitamin A
	Bitot spots, xerophthalmia, keratomalacia	Vitamin A
	Conjunctival pallor	Nutritional anemias
	Fundal capillary microaneurysms	Vitamin C
Face, mouth, neck	Angular stomatitis	Riboflavin, iron
	Cheilosis	Vitamins B_6, niacin, riboflavin
	Bleeding gums	Vitamins C, K
	Atrophic papillae	Riboflavin, iron, niacin
	Smooth tongue	Iron
	Red tongue (glossitis)	Vitamins B_6, B_{12}, niacin, riboflavin, folate
	Parotid swelling	Protein
	Caries	Fluoride
	Anosmia	Vitamins A, B_{12}, zinc
	Hypogeusia	Vitamin A, zinc
	Goiter	Iodine
Cardiovascular	Heart failure	Thiamine, selenium, nutritional anemias
Genital	Hypogonadism	Zinc
Skeletal	Costochondral beading	Vitamins D, C
	Subperiosteal hemorrhage	Vitamin C, copper
	Cranial bossing	Vitamin D
	Wide fontanel	Vitamin D
	Epiphyseal enlargement	Vitamin D
	Craniotabes	Vitamin D, calcium
	Tender bones	Vitamin C
	Tender calves	Thiamine, selenium
	Spoon-shaped nails (koilonychia)	Iron
	Transverse nail lines	Protein
Neurologic	Sensory, motor neuropathy	Thiamine, vitamins E, B_6, B_{12}
	Ataxia, areflexia	Vitamin E
	Ophthalmoplegia	Vitamin E, thiamine
	Tetany	Vitamin D, Ca^{2+}, Mg^{2+}
	Retardation	Iodine, niacin
	Dementia, delirium	Vitamin E, niacin, thiamine

Table 2–18. Screening Tests for Nutritional Deficiency Disorders*

Test	Deficiency
Hemoglobin + RBC indices	Iron, folate, vitamins B_{12}, B_6, copper
Lymphocyte count	Protein, calories
Delayed hypersensitivity skin tests	Protein, calories
Retinol-binding protein prealbumin, transferrin	Protein, calories
Albumin	Protein; affected by fluids, renal and hepatic dysfunction
Calcium, phosphate	Vitamin D
Prothrombin time	Vitamin K
Thyroxine	Iodine
Bone radiographs	Iodine, vitamins D and C copper
Alkaline phosphate	Zinc
Ceruloplasmin	Copper

* Specific assays are available for most vitamins. Macronutrients and trace elements are determined when indicated by the history and physical examination and screening tests.

RBC = red blood cell count.

troduction of adequate feeding a clinical risk that must be aggressively addressed.

Reference

Gibson RS: Principles of Nutritional Assessment. New York, Oxford University Press, 1990.

Grand RJ, Sutphen JL, Dietz WH (eds): Pediatric Nutrition. Boston, Butterworth, 1987, pp 395–420.

Enteral Nutrition

Contraindications to oral feeding are an obstructive ileus, gastric retention, intestinal perforation, anatomic obstruction, severe acute gastrointestinal hemorrhage, and severe diet-induced diarrhea. In all other conditions, feeding should begin with a diet appropriate for age given first in diluted form or in a limited amount. When tolerance is established, there should be as rapid a progression as reasonable toward full concentration and nutritional adequacy. The rate of this progression is governed by gastrointestinal tolerance as determined by emesis, abdominal distention, and diarrhea.

When intestinal digestion is abnormal or when protein hypersensitivity is suspected, an *oligomeric* or elemental enteral product can be utilized. In older children this commonly is administered by a continuous intragastric drip because of the objectionable taste. Some of these products have an in-creased osmolarity and may produce intestinal luminal water sequestration if delivered into the jejunum at rates adequate to meet nutrient requirements. The level of tolerance for oligomeric diets varies with each patient and the etiology of the gastrointestinal disease. Glucose polymers, medium-chain and long-chain triglycerides, and oligopeptides are available when needed for specific patients. Care must be taken to ensure the overall quality of the therapeutic diet. In moderately to severely affected patients, enteral feeding should be supplemented with peripheral intravenous nutrition until acceptable nutrient absorption and weight gain are established.

A number of complications can occur as a consequence of enteral feeding. Enteral catheter complications include erosion of the nasal septum, displacement of the catheter tip into the esophagus, lung, or duodenum, and perforation of the gastric wall. Silastic catheters reduce irritation and the likelihood of perforation. A percutaneously placed gastrostomy feeding tube should be considered for long-term enteral feeding.

Parenteral Nutrition

Total parenteral nutrition (TPN) is indicated when enteral nutrients cannot meet the nutritional needs for normal growth. Enteral nutrition is preferred, because it is more physiologic, less expensive, and associated with fewer complications. Often, the parenteral nutrition supplements the enteral intake until the latter route provides sufficient nutrients for growth. Indications for TPN include congenital gastrointestinal anomalies, severe necrotizing enterocolitis, short bowel syndrome, and intractable diarrhea unresponsive to enteral alimentation. TPN also is useful in patients with trauma, burns, malignant disease, multiple organ system failure, and severe inflammatory bowel disease. Generally, TPN by peripheral venous access is instituted first, with central access established when peripheral access becomes unavailable. In patients who need long-term TPN, a central venous line will be placed early in the course of care. With few exceptions (e.g., marked fluid limitations), adequate nutritional support can be provided by either central or peripheral line TPN. Intravenous nutrient solutions provide all of the protein, calorie, electrolyte, vitamin, mineral (except iron), trace element, and essential fatty acid requirements. The nonprotein calories are provided by both carbohydrates (dextrose) and a 20% lipid emulsion.

PERIPHERAL INTRAVENOUS (IV) NUTRITION

Peripheral TPN is based on a 10–12% dextrose solution with 2–3% amino acids solution to provide about 0.8–2.0 g protein/kg/24 hr for older children, 1.5–3.0 g/kg/24 hr for full-term and older infants, and 2.5–3.5 g/kg/24 hr for preterm infants. The caloric density of glucose and amino acid–based solutions is limited by the solution's osmolality (10% glucose = 550 mOsm). Solutions with greater than 600 mOsm/L cause phlebitis of peripheral veins. The high caloric density but low osmolar lipid emulsion usually provides additional calories in excess of the 3–5% of total calories needed to prevent essential fatty acid deficiency. The rate of lipid infusion is initiated at 0.5–1.0 g/kg/24 hr but is advanced to 2–4 g/kg/24 hr. Intravenous caloric requirement is approximately 10% less than the enteral requirement because of the omission of the caloric expenditure for the thermic effect of feeding (see Chapter 6).

CENTRAL VENOUS NUTRITION

Central TPN primarily differs from peripheral TPN in the dextrose concentration; usually 20% vs. 10% with peripheral TPN. In situations with severe fluid limitations and/or lipid intolerance, up to 25–30% dextrose may be used centrally. The silicon-rubber cuffed catheter is surgically placed in a branch of the subclavian or jugular vein, tunnelled subcutaneously to an exit site on the anterior chest wall, and threaded to the superior vena cava into the right atrium. The high blood flow in central veins reduces the risks of the hyperosmolar solutions. The lipid infusion ranges from the minimal 3–5% of calories to 2–4 g/kg/24 hr, as needed to meet the caloric requirements. The protein (amino acid), vitamin, and trace mineral intakes are individualized for the patient.

Careful monitoring of the venous line site and placement, fluid and electrolyte balance, growth, and metabolic response are essential to the safety and efficacy of TPN. *Laboratory evaluation* includes measurement of blood glucose, urea nitrogen, creatinine, calcium, phosphorus, magnesium, bilirubin, albumin, liver enzymes, and triglyceride. These are obtained prior to initiation of TPN and weekly during infusion. Serum triglycerides are monitored as the amount of lipids infused is increased from 2 g/kg/24 hr to the level required for caloric needs (3–4 g/kg/24 hr).

Table 2–19. Potential Complications of Total Parenteral Alimentation

Catheter-Related	Metabolic
Superior vena cava syndrome (thrombosis)	Hypoglycemia (infusion stopped)
Pulmonary thromboembolism	Hyperglycemia (hyperosmolar state)
Pulmonary hypertension	Hyperaminoacidemia (↑ protein intake)
Pneumothorax	Hyperammonemia (↑ protein intake)
Pleural effusions (extravasated solution)	Azotemia (↑ protein intake)
Cardiac arrhythmias	Hypoalbuminemia (↓ protein intake)
Pericardial effusion	Essential fatty acid deficiency
Mural thrombosis (cardiac)	Hypertriglyceridemia
Intramyocardial infusion	Carnitine deficiency
Tricuspid valve injury	Vitamin deficiencies (biotin)
Hemorrhage	Acanthocytosis (lipids)
Flocculation precipitation of nutrients	
	Systemic
Infections	Cholestasis (hepatic dysfunction)
Staphylococcal *(S. aureus, S. epidermidis)* sepsis	Fatty infiltration (liver, monocytes, lung; intralipid)
Candida sepsis	Altered myocardial function (phosphate, calcium depletion)
Malasseziza furfur (intralipid)	Intestinal mucosal atrophy
Aspergillosis sepsis	Platelet dysfunction (intralipid)
Entry, exit site, tract infections	?Hemolysis (intralipid)
Contaminated solutions (rare organisms)	Osmotic diuresis (glucose)
	Metabolic bone disease (osteopenia)
Electrolyte (minerals)	Isosmolar coma (protein, glucose)
Hyponatremia	Increased deposition of body fat
Hypernatremia	Increased extracellular fluid space
Hypokalemia	White blood cell dysfunction (phosphate depletion, lipids)
Hypophosphatemia	Poor sucking, swallowing (NPO)
Hypomagnesemia	
Metabolic acidosis	
Trace mineral deficiency (Zn, Cu)	
Aluminum toxicity	

Complications of TPN are categorized as metabolic, technical (catheter related), or infectious (Table 2–19). *Hepatobiliary dysfunction* is seen in some patients who require long-term (>2 wk) TPN. Cholestasis is associated with conjugated hyperbilirubinemia, modest elevation in the hepatocellular enzymes, and, rarely, irreversible hepatic failure. Although several factors (fasting, toxic amino acids) have been implicated in the pathogeneses of hepatobiliary dysfunction, no single causal factor has been identified. The diagnosis of TPN-induced cholestasis is one of exclusion; other causes of hyperbilirubinemia must be considered, such as sepsis, structural abnormalities, α_1-antitrypsin deficiency, cystic fibrosis, viral hepatitis, and inborn errors of metabolism (galactosemia, tyrosinemia). The development of cholestasis increases the urgency to establish enteral support and discontinue TPN as soon as enteral intake is adequate. To avoid infection, the catheter site is cleaned with aseptic solutions by trained personnel; entry into the system is avoided and if necessary is performed with sterile technique.

Delays in behavioral development may result from the long-term administration of enteral nasogastric or parenteral feedings to young infants, in part because the development of oral feeding patterns is bypassed. The opportunity for non-nutritive sucking (i.e., the provision of a pacifier) may prevent this complication. When the infant has not learned to suck or swallow, a team approach is required to teach the infant these functions.

References

Behrman RE (ed): Nelson Textbook of Pediatrics. 14th ed. Philadelphia, WB Saunders, 1992, Sec. 4.9–4.14, 6.14.

Warner BW: Parenteral nutrition in the pediatric patient. *In* Fisher JE (ed): Total Parenteral Nutrition. Boston, Little Brown, 1991, pp 299–322.

Wilson SE: Pediatric enteral feedings. *In* Grand RJ, Sutphen JL, Dietz WH (eds): Pediatric Nutrition. Boston, Butterworths, 1987, pp 771–788.

Zlotkin SH, Stallings VA, Pencharz PB: Total parenteral nutrition in children. Pediatr Clin North Am 32:2, 1985.

The Acutely Ill Child

Bradley P. Fuhrman

3

Much of pediatric practice is dedicated to helping the child make the transition from the intrauterine environment through infancy, childhood, and adolescence to adulthood. When a patient has a serious illness that interrupts this progression, the responsible practitioner tries first to localize the disease to a particular organ system, then make a diagnosis, and finally provide subsequent treatment. The practice of medicine, as it applies to the acutely ill child, has evolved from a diagnosis-driven system to one recognizing key physiologic derangements in organ systems. This activity may require aggressive supportive care, with or without providing specific therapy based on a diagnosis.

The initial approach to the acutely ill child is basically a problem of triage. Decisions must be made about hospitalization and the need for intensive care. In nonacute situations, the physician takes a detailed history, does a complete physical examination, gathers laboratory studies, and arrives at a diagnosis, which ultimately leads to a treatment plan. However, when confronted with an immediate, life-threatening illness, the physician must make decisions regarding therapeutic intervention expeditiously, based on very limited information.

Common causes of death among children over 1 mo of age include sudden infant death syndrome, serious trauma (motor vehicle accidents, child abuse, violence), burns, toxic ingestions, severe infections (meningitis), metabolic disorders (diabetic ketoacidosis), and the consequences of the treatment of congenital anomalies (congenital heart disease) or malignancy (immunosuppression, bone marrow transplantation). The initial focus in treating these acutely ill children is to correct their abnormal physiology, and then to try to make a specific diagnostic evaluation. For example, the child with hypotension, tachycardia, and poor perfusion, by definition, has poor cardiac output. The physician intervenes immediately to improve circulation, thereby restoring oxygen delivery to tissues. In initially trying to stabilize the patient, it is more

important to recognize the pathophysiology than it is to determine whether the poor cardiac output is due to infection, trauma, congenital anomaly, metabolic derangements, or respiratory illness. *Basic supportive cardiopulmonary care is initiated prior to making a definitive diagnosis.* Therapy is directed at the physiologic manifestations of the illness, which means implementing an approach similar to that required for establishing priorities during cardiopulmonary resuscitation: sequentially stabilizing *A*irway, *B*reathing, and *C*irculation, and then providing *D*rugs or targeted pharmacologic intervention.

Objective data are used both to assess the response to stabilization procedures and to make the ultimate diagnosis. Such data require ongoing *monitoring of vital organ functions*, including brain, heart, kidney, bone marrow, lung, and liver. By using a combination of monitoring and therapeutic interventions, the physician is able to anticipate the further progression of the illness and can manage ongoing physiologic derangements (Table 3–1).

DRUG THERAPY IN THE ACUTELY ILL CHILD

The goal of pharmacotherapy for the critically ill child is to achieve a specific effect. The physician needs to appreciate that such goals are limited to the augmentation, ablation, or modulation of normal physiologic processes, because drugs cannot create physiologic responses that are not intrinsic to the patient.

Two important groups of factors determine the efficacy of drug therapy (Table 3–2): *pharmacokinetic* determinants relate to the absorption, distribution, metabolism, and excretion of the drug, and *pharmacodynamic* determinants reflect the drug's mechanism of action and their safety profiles. Effective therapy will be achieved if the selected drug has

Table 3–1. Elements of Acute Care

Examine

Initial assessment followed by complete and systematic evaluation

Focus examination on areas of chief complaints

Synthesize findings to plan further evaluation

Monitor

Vital signs

Physiologic parameters required to:
  1) make diagnosis, and/or
  2) ascertain response to therapy or progression of disease

Prospectively determine allowable limits for changes in monitored parameters; generate and record objective data to guide therapy

Intervene

Prior to initiating therapy, determine therapeutic goals and endpoints

Initiate therapy based on recognized pathophysiologic derangements

Adjust therapeutic strategies to individual patient needs

Use objective data to guide alterations in therapy

Anticipate

Requires understanding of the underlying pathophysiology

Always plan for the "worst-case" scenario

Use data obtained through examination and monitoring to update prognostic impressions continually

---

favorable pharmacokinetic and pharmacodynamic properties.

In treating infants and children, drug selection and action are confounded by normal growth and development. Various developmental changes affect each phase of pharmacokinetics, as well as drug–receptor interactions and drug safety profiles. Changes in gastric acidity and gastrointestinal motility affect the rate and extent of oral drug *absorption*. Once absorbed, the *distribution* of drug into tissues is influenced by several factors. In the newborn period, it is influenced by the presence of fetal albumin, which has binding characteristics that differ from those of adult albumin. Also in neonates, endogenous substances such as bilirubin and elevated free fatty acids may displace drugs from their albumin-binding sites. Finally, drug distribution in neonates is affected profoundly by the changes in extracellular fluid volume that occur during normal maturation. At birth, water may account for up to 80% of the infant's total body weight, whereas in adults the extracellular fluid volume comprises only 60% of the total body weight. This may account, in part, for the higher dosages that infants and young children require for effects to be obtained, compared with doses required by adults, when assessed on a milligram-per-kilogram basis.

Drug *metabolism* accounts for the major differences in interindividual responses to drugs. In addition, marked changes in the drug-metabolizing enzymes in the liver occur during early infancy and then again at the time of adolescence, when sex differences in drug metabolism may be due to changes in steroid hormone levels. These changes in drug metabolism coincide with the changes in drug *excretion* by the kidney, which relate to the maturation of both glomerular filtration and tubular secretion (see Chapter 16).

Changes in the pharmacodynamics of drugs may result from developmental changes in receptor number and affinity or in receptor–effector coupling, so that a certain dosage producing particular therapeutic as well as adverse effects will change

Table 3–2. Pharmacokinetic Considerations in Critically Ill Children

Absorption Phase

Altered gastric emptying

Decreased gastrointestinal blood flow, ileus

Altered gastric pH; exogenous buffers—antacids, H_2-receptor antagonists, maturity

Time delay

Altered biliary function

Distribution Phase

Hemodynamic instability

Inflammation

Decreased protein synthesis/increased protein loss

Synthesis of acute-phase reactants

Extravascular fluid collections—ascites, pleural effusions

Drug interactions

Maturational changes of extracellular fluid space (see Chapter 2)

Metabolism Phase

Hemodynamic instability

Hypoxemia

Substrate deficiencies

Polypharmacy—drug interactions

Use of hormones and autacoids as pharmacologic rather than physiologic agents

Enzyme maturational changes in biotransformation

Excretion Phase

Altered vascular volume

Altered renal blood flow (illness, maturation)

Hypoxemia

Nephrotoxic agents

Altered hepatic function (illness, maturation)

as the newborn progresses from infancy through childhood to adolescence and adulthood. This continuum of changing pharmacokinetics and pharmacodynamics related to growth and development is complicated further by the impact of the various physiologic derangements during an acute illness (Table 3–2).

Pharmacodynamic alterations in critically ill children may result from vascular volume and electrolyte derangements and from the effects of acute alterations in acid–base status. Moreover, acutely ill patients generate endogenous substances that alter drug responsiveness, and the long-term use of certain hormones and autacoids may result in the down-regulation of their various receptors. Finally, patients who already are seriously ill are less likely to tolerate the potential side effects of various drugs, so that the safety profile of the drugs employed in a critical care setting may be altered drastically.

The superposition of acute illness on a developmental program controlling drug biodisposition and response presents a challenge to the development of effective therapeutic strategies. One strategy, the *target-concentration strategy*, consists of an attempt to achieve specific plasma levels of a drug. Therapeutic principles include an awareness of drug pharmacokinetics and active metabolites, having predetermined expectations of the manifestations of drug efficacy and toxicity, awareness of appropriate sampling times for drug levels, treating the patient and *not* the drug level, and, if inconsistencies develop, re-evaluating and re-examining the patient. This strategy often is applied to drugs used chronically to treat illnesses having intermittent clinical manifestations. Examples of such problems include reversible reactive airway disease, seizure disorders, and cardiac arrhythmias. Implementing this strategy requires effective use of the drug analysis laboratory (Table 3–3). The tar-

Table 3–3. Prerequisites for Therapeutic Drug Monitoring

The analytic method must be specific, sensitive, accurate, and available in an appropriate time frame

The active drug and important metabolites are measured

Development of tolerance at receptor sites does not occur

Concentration of drug in serum is proportional to the concentration of drug at receptor sites

There must be reasonably good correlation between concentration and therapeutic effects

The therapeutic range must be well defined

Proper care is taken in interpretation of values

Table 3–4. Drugs Amenable to Therapeutic Monitoring for Drug Toxicity

Antibiotics
Aminoglycosides—gentamicin, tobramycin, amikacin
Chloramphenicol
Vancomycin

Immunosuppression
Methotrexate
Cyclosporine

Antipyretics
Acetaminophen
Salicylate

Other
Digoxin
Lithium
Theophylline

geted concentrations may relate either to drug efficacy or to toxicity and generally are based on data obtained from large populations rather than from individual patients.

The types of drugs that lend themselves to the target-concentration strategy are those manifesting a wide interindividual variation in drug absorption, distribution, or elimination (Table 3–4). Therapeutic monitoring for drug efficacy is possible for theophylline, anticonvulsants (phenytoin, phenobarbital, valproate, carbamazepine ethosuximide), and antiarrhythmic agents (procainamide and its metabolite NAPA, quinidine, lidocaine, amiodarone). This strategy also is useful for administering drugs having a narrow therapeutic index and for those designed to attain relatively sustained and constant effects over a long period of time. Such a strategy can be considered only when the concentrations of drug in the plasma relate directly to clinical effects of the drug that can be monitored. Knowing the therapeutic range and toxic level for each drug and the average values for absorption, distribution, and elimination of the drug permits intelligent use of serum drug levels. The pathophysiologic conditions that alter these parameters and the extent of this alteration also must be appreciated.

The *target-effect strategy* is the second approach to the drug treatment of acutely ill children. Two principles are essential to its application: the first is the dose–response relationship (i.e., the concept that most drugs show increasing clinical or adverse effects with increasing doses); the second is that, prior to the initiation of therapy, there must be a well-defined clinical endpoint (e.g., the physician prescribing the drug must have a reasonable understanding of the drug's pharmacodynamic ac-

Table 3–5. Drugs for Employing a Target-Effect Strategy in Critically Ill Children

Catecholamines—dopamine, dobutamine, epinephrine, isoproterenol, norepinephrine, terbutaline

Vasodilators—nitroglycerine, nitroprusside, hydralazine, angiotensin-converting enzyme inhibitors

Anticoagulants—heparin, warfarin

Beta-lactam antibiotics—penicillins, cephalosporins, carbapenems, monobactams

Anxiolytics, sedatives—diazepam, lorazepam, midazolam, morphine, fentanyl, chloral hydrate, secobarbital

Oxygen

Diuretics—furosemide, bumetanide, chlorothiazide, metolazone

tion, including its side effects). There must also be a reasonable understanding of the impact of both ontogeny and disease on these pharmacodynamic actions. Finally, before therapy begins, a system must be set in place to monitor both the efficacy and toxicity of the drug.

The target-effect strategy is particularly appropriate to the intensive care setting (Table 3–5). For example, if oxygen is being used as a drug to attempt to increase a patient's oxygen saturation in the presence of respiratory failure, the approach is to choose a clinically acceptable oxygen saturation level (e.g., >90%) and to increase the inspired oxygen concentration serially until the patient is receiving the desired oxygen saturation or until the patient is inspiring 100% oxygen. The essence of drug dosing using the target-effect strategy is to increase the dosage until the desired therapeutic effect is achieved, but if sequential increases produce no increased effect and the therapeutic effect has not been achieved or if drug toxicity supervenes, changing the drug rather than adding different drugs to the regimen is the appropriate response.

References

Behrman RE (ed): Nelson Textbook of Pediatrics. 14th ed. Philadelphia, WB Saunders Co., 1992, Sec. 6.55.
Blumer J: Principles of drug disposition in the critically ill child. *In* Fuhrman B, Zimmerman J (eds): Pediatric Critical Care. St Louis, CV Mosby, 1992, pp 1055–1072.
Reynolds DJM, Aronson JK: Making the most of plasma drug concentration measurements. BMJ 306:48, 1993.
Snodgrass WR: Selected aspects of pediatric intensive care unit clinical pharmacology. Curr Opin Pediatr 3:314, 1991.

PAIN MANAGEMENT

The critically ill neonatal, child, or adolescent patient may experience pain, discomfort, and anxiety resulting from injury, surgery, and invasive procedures (intubation, bone marrow aspiration, central venous line placement) or during life-sustaining mechanical ventilation. Pain may be manifested as verbal or visible discomfort, crying, agitation, tachycardia, hypertension, and tachypnea. The physician has a commitment to relieve discomfort and treat pain. Common pharmacologic agents employed to manage acute and chronic pain are noted in Table 3–6.

References

Behrman RE (ed): Nelson Textbook of Pediatrics. 14th ed. Philadelphia, WB Saunders, 1992, Sec. 6.54.
Brill JE: Control of pain. Crit Care Clin 8:203, 1992.
Lebovitz DJ, Blumer JL: Sedation and analgesic therapy for critically ill children. Curr Opin Pediatr 4:305, 1992.

MAJOR TRAUMA

Epidemiology

Accidents account for almost 50% of the deaths in children 1–14 yr of age. Almost 50% of these are due to motor vehicle accidents. A majority of the rest are due to falls (25–30%) and burns (10–15%). Gunshot wounds, assaults, and ingestions account for 5–10% of pediatric trauma. More than one half of trauma fatalities occur at the scene of the accident rather than at secondary sites to which the victim may be transported, such as hospitals or the home. Children with blunt and penetrating thoracoabdominal injuries account for 82% of the deaths; many of these children are in critical condition on arrival at the hospital.

Education for Preventing Accidental Trauma

The recognition that much of the morbidity and mortality are determined at the scene of the accident has stimulated the development of prevention measures throughout the country, including decreasing the speed limit to 55 mph, imposing more stringent automobile safety standards, mandating the use of child automobile restraining devices, promoting cardiopulmonary resuscitation (CPR) training, and the more frequent use of the Heimlich maneuver for the choking victim. The number of Regional Poison Control Centers also has grown

Table 3–6. Pharmacologic Management of Pain

Agent	Comments
Nonopioid Analgesia	

Nonsteroidal anti-inflammatory drugs (NSAIDs)
  Ibuprofen
  Naprosyn
  Tolectin
  Ketorolac (only IV preparation)
	Greater efficacy than acetaminophen, equal to or greater than oral opioids. Opioid and NSAID combination reduces opioid tolerance and enhances analgesia. *Chronic complications:* decreased glomerular filtration rate; fluid retention, gastrointestinal ulceration; bleeding; perforation. No abuse potential but has ceiling effect.

Acetaminophen	Potency equivalent to aspirin; less than NSAIDs. *Acute ingestion:* hepatic toxicity.
Opioid Analgesia	

Pure agonists
  Morphine
  Codeine
  Fentanyl, alfentanil, sufentanil
	Have no ceiling effect (e.g., higher dose, greater analgesia) and greater *side effects* (respiratory depression, sedation, miosis, nausea, histamine release–pruritis, decreased gut motility, constipation, increased sphincter of Oddi tone, urinary retention, biliary spasm). Opioid abstinence syndrome if withdrawn quickly. High abuse potential.

Partial agonists/agonist–antagonists
  Pentazocine
  Nalbuphine
  Butorphanol
  Buprenorphine
  Propoxyphene
  Methadone
	May produce dysphoria, acute withdrawal symptoms if given with pure agonist opioids. Possible reduced biliary spasm.

Meperidine	No histamine release, possibly decreased biliary spasm. Toxic, active metabolite—normeperidine—produces seizures.
Sedative–Hypnotics	

Benzodiazepines
  Diazepam
  Midazolam (short-acting)
  Lorazepam (long-acting)
	Produce anxiolysis, sedation, muscle relaxation, amnesia; useful in combination with opioids for painful procedures or postoperative pain. Tolerance possible. *Acute complications:* apnea, decreased blood pressure, decreased myocardial function.

Other agents Ketamine	Produces dissociative anesthesia, analgesia, amnesia, increased heart rate, increased blood pressure, increased bronchial secretions (decreased with atropine), bronchodilation and emergent delirium, hallucinations, vivid dreams (reduced with benzodiazepines). Contraindicated with increased intracranial pressure.
Propofol	Rapid onset, lipophilic. May decrease cardiovascular function.
Chloral hydrate	Predominantly sedative, weak analgesia. *Toxicity* includes emesis, gastrointestinal bleeding, esophageal stricture, hepatic dysfunction, arrhythmias, decreased blood pressure, and possible carcinogenesis.
Tricyclic antidepressants	Useful as adjuvant analgesia for chronic pain (e.g., cancer pain).
Carbamazepine	Useful as adjuvant for various chronic neuralgias.

(Data from Med Lett 35:1, 1993; Committee on Drugs AAP, Guidelines for monitoring and management of pediatric patients during and after sedation for diagnostic and therapeutic procedures. Pediatrics 89:1110, 1992; Brill JE: Control of pain. Crit Care Clin 8:203, 1992; Zetter LK, Anderson CT, Schechter NL: Pediatric pain: Current status and new directions. Curr Prob Pediatr 20: 411, 1990.)

throughout the country, providing the lay public and medical professionals with information regarding toxic ingestions and exposures. Other primary prevention efforts have included fire safety programs, water safety and swimming programs, and legislative efforts to require the reporting of suspected child abuse and to control the temperature of hot water in order to prevent children from being scalded.

Providing Prehospital Care

The care of trauma patients may be divided into three phases. The first and most important is the

Table 3–7. Children Requiring Pediatric Trauma Center Care

Patients with serious injury to more than one system

Patients with one system injury who require intensive care unit

Patients with signs of shock who require more than one transfusion

Patients with fracture complicated by suspected neurovascular compartment injury

Patients with fracture of axial skeleton

Patients with two or more long bone fractures

Patients with potential replantation of an extremity

Patients with suspected or actual spinal cord or column injuries

Patients with head injury with any one of the following:
  Orbital or facial bone fracture
  Cerebrospinal fluid leaks
  Altered state of consciousness
  Changing neural signs
  Open head injuries
  Depressed skull fracture
  Requiring intracranial pressure monitoring

Patients suspected of requiring ventilator support

prehospital phase, which may take place at the scene of the trauma or en route to the hospital and which consists of two types of activities. The first is taking a *primary survey* of injuries and initiating basic life support measures (see ABCDEs below). The first priority in responding to a trauma victim includes resuscitating from cardiopulmonary arrest, controlling hemorrhage, treating shock, and providing direct attention to major thoracic, abdominal, and head injuries. The specific elements of this treatment overlap with the treatment the patient receives on arrival at the hospital's receiving facility and will be discussed subsequently. The *secondary survey* involves a more detailed assessment for specific injuries (maxillofacial, chest, ab-

domen, extremity, cranial). The second priority involves treating burns and skeletal injuries, and the third priority focuses on treating minor injuries.

The second activity in the prehospital phase involves the appropriate triage of the trauma victim to the emergency room, the intensive care unit, or directly to the operating room (Table 3–7).

Evaluating and Managing the Trauma Patient in the Emergency Department

On the patient's arrival at the emergency room, an organized and synchronized response must be initiated by the responding team, based on the priorities and directives of the pediatric general surgeon. The most appropriate objective scoring system for evaluating the degree of trauma and prognosis in children is the Pediatric Trauma Score (Table 3–8).

The initial approach to patients in the Emergency Department focuses on the *ABCDEs of emergency care* as modified for trauma from the ABCs of cardiopulmonary resuscitation: "A" stands for *airway*, accompanied by *cervical spine control*. Effective care of the traumatized child should ensure immobilization. If there is a question regarding cervical spine stability, orotracheal intubation should be performed with the neck immobilized in the neutral position. Nasotracheal intubation may be contraindicated in facial trauma or basilar skull fracture, because the tube may enter the cranial vault. Cricothyrotomy also may be employed in instances of facial trauma or cervical spine fracture.

"B" stands for assessment of *breathing*, which is critical in the traumatized patient, even if an artificial airway is already in place. Ventilation can be assessed by observation, palpation, and auscultation, as a component of the primary survey. Major thoracic injuries (Table 3–9) must be assessed and treated immediately to ensure a successful resuscitation.

Table 3–8. Pediatric Trauma Score*

Category Component	+2	+1	−1
Size	>20 kg	10–20 kg	<10 kg
Airway	Normal	Maintainable	Unmaintainable
Systolic BP†	>90 mm Hg	50–90 mm Hg	<50 mm Hg
CNS	Awake	Obtunded/LOC	Coma/Decerebrate
Skeletal	None	Closed Fracture	Open/Multiple Fractures
Cutaneous/Wounds	None	Minor	Major/Penetrating

* If score <8, refer to Pediatric Trauma Center.
† If proper size BP cuff is not available: +2 = palpable pulse at wrist; +1 = palpable pulse at groin; −1 = no palpable pulse.
BP = blood pressure; CNS = central nervous system; LOC = loss of consciousness.
(Modified from Tepas J, Mollitt D, Talbert J, et al: The pediatric trauma score as a predictor of injury severity in the injured child. J Pediatr Surg 22:14, 1987.)

Table 3–9. Life-Threatening Chest Injuries

Tension Pneumothorax

One-way valve leak from lung parenchyma

Complete collapse with mediastinal and tracheal shift to side opposite the leak

Compromises venous return and decreases ventilation of other lung

Clinically, becomes manifest by respiratory distress, unilateral absent breath sounds, tracheal deviation, distended neck veins, tympany to percussion of involved side, cyanosis

Relieve first with needle aspiration, then chest tube drainage

Open Pneumothorax (sucking chest wound)

Effect on ventilation depends on size

Major Flail Chest

Usually due to blunt injury resulting in multiple rib fractures

Loss of bone stability of thoracic cage

Major disruption of synchronous chest wall motion

Mechanical ventilation and positive end-expiratory pressure required

Massive Hemothorax

Must be drained with large-bore tube

Initiate drainage only with vascular volume replacement

Cardiac Tamponade

Beck triad
  1) Decreased or muffled heart sounds
  2) Distended neck veins from increased venous pressure
  3) Hypotension with pulsus paradoxus (decreased pulse pressure during inspiration)

Must be drained

"C" stands for *circulation and hemorrhage control.* Control of bleeding is one of the primary responsibilities in the acute care of the traumatized child. Hemorrhage must be identified, then stopped, by using direct pressure, extremity tourniquets, or military antishock trousers (MAST) devices.

In trauma care, "D" stands for *disability,* which serves as a reminder to assess continually neurologic status, a condition that may be changing constantly. These changes may provide important diagnostic and therapeutic direction, as well as therapeutic direction. Head injury is present in 80% of all multiple trauma patients, and in 60% of pediatric cases the head is the most severely affected part of the body. The mortality in multiple trauma accompanied by head injury is 16%, compared with only 6% in the absence of significant head injury.

"E", for *exposure,* has been added to the mnemonic as a reminder that, in order to fully assess the patient, the child must be completely disrobed so that the entire body can be examined in detail.

The majority of deaths from trauma occur at the scene of the accident. These deaths occur to patients who receive injuries to the brain stem, head, aorta, heart, and high cervical spine. The next substantial group of deaths occurs within several hours of arrival in the emergency room; survival depends on the severity of shock at the time of presentation and the length of time the shock state was present. If the patient is taken to a center where definitive care can be provided and is stabilized within an hour of the time of the injury, the outcome is likely to be optimal. A final peak in mortality occurs days to weeks after the initial injury and results from severe, life-threatening complications because the injuries have not responded to medical and surgical management.

Specific Organ Injuries

The initial physical examination in the emergency department, which is augmented by screening laboratory data (Table 3–10), should provide

Table 3–10. Initial Laboratory Evaluation of the Major Trauma Patient

Hematology

Complete blood count
Platelet count
Prothrombin time
Activated partial thromboplastin time
Fibrinogen
Type and cross match

Urinalysis

Gross
Microscopic

Clinical Chemistry

Na, K, Cl, BUN, CO_2, glucose, calcium
Creatinine
Amylase
SGOT/SGPT

Radiology

Cervical spine films
AP chest roentgenogram
Roentgenograms of all apparent fractures
CT scans where indicated for head, chest, and abdominal trauma
IVP if urinalysis positive for blood

AP = anteroposterior; BUN = blood urea nitrogen; CT = computerized tomography; IVP = intravenous pyelogram; SGOT/SGPT = serum glutamic oxaloacetic transaminase/serum glutamic pyruvic transaminase.

information and direction for further diagnostic evaluation. When subsequently focusing on various organ systems, evaluating and treating severe *head injury* is given a high priority. Major trauma to the *chest and mediastinal structures* usually requires immediate surgical intervention; except for pulmonary contusion, these injuries have a significant mortality. The *musculoskeletal* also may require immediate attention. Fractures contribute most to the long-term morbidity associated with multiple trauma, and, if inappropriately assessed, may lead to loss of limb or life. There is approximately a 12% failure rate in the diagnosis of significant fractures in and around the time of injury. Most fractures may be managed by closed techniques.

HEAD TRAUMA (see Chapter 18)

ABDOMINAL TRAUMA

Perhaps no area of trauma management has undergone more rigorous changes in the past decade than the management of abdominal trauma. *Sharp penetrating trauma* must be distinguished from blunt trauma. The former accounts for less than 10% of pediatric abdominal trauma but more than 50% of adult abdominal trauma. Pediatric patients experiencing sharp penetrating trauma may be asymptomatic or in hypovolemic shock. Performing serial physical examinations is the primary method for obtaining information on which to base decisions regarding operative intervention. Abdominal computerized tomography (CT) scanning is invaluable in assessing intra-abdominal trauma. Gunshot wounds to the abdomen, an important category of abdominal trauma, involve multiple organs in 80% of cases and have a mortality rate of over 12%; operative exploration may be indicated when peritoneal irritation, hypovolemia, free air on plain film, or positive results of paracentesis (Table 3–11) are present.

Blunt abdominal trauma occurs far more often in children than does penetrating abdominal trauma. The most frequently injured organs, in descending order, are the colon, spleen, genitourinary tract,

Table 3–11. Criteria for a Positive Paracentesis

Free aspiration ≥10 mL gross blood
Turbid or bloody fluid that prevents reading newsprint
Free egress through indwelling urinary catheter or chest tube
Presence of >500 WBC/mL or >100,000 RBC/mL
Amylase >175 U/mL
Presence of gross stool or food debris

RBC = red blood cells; WBC = white blood cells.

intestine, liver, pancreas, pelvis, and major vessels. Optimal management of these injuries requires serial physical examinations. Operative intervention may be required in a patient whose vital signs are persistently unstable, even when there is no extravascular volume loss or no enlarging abdomen. The presence of peritoneal irritation or abdominal wall discoloration, together with signs of intravascular volume loss, indicates the need for laparotomy. Abdominal CT scan is an especially important adjunct in the patient who is unconscious as a result of a head injury. Using high-fluid volumes to resuscitate this type of patient may exacerbate brain swelling; therefore, CT scan or, if it is unavailable, paracentesis and early surgery may be the judicious approach in some children.

INJURY TO THE SPLEEN

Splenic injuries often are signaled by pain at the tip of the shoulder or in the left chest, accompanied by respiratory distress, nausea, and vomiting. A positive Kehr sign (pressure on the left upper quadrant eliciting left shoulder pain) also is strongly suggestive of this diagnosis. No other consistent clinical or laboratory findings suggest a splenic injury.

Nonoperative management of serious splenic injuries is the treatment of choice. This treatment includes intensive care and serial observation by CT, radionuclide scan, or follow-up ultrasound. Surgery is indicated for patients having an estimated blood loss greater than 40 mL/kg of transfused blood in 24–36 hr. The operative approach is often to repair the lesion rather than to remove the spleen, but splenectomy is required if the organ is totally separated from its blood supply; if a severe head injury exists for which rapid, high-volume circulatory support might be hazardous; or if an increase in blood loss of unknown cause has occurred in the presence of fecal contamination of the peritoneal contents. If a splenectomy is performed, patients should remain on penicillin prophylaxis for life and receive pneumococcal and *Haemophilus influenzae* vaccines because there is an increased morbidity and mortality owing to overwhelming sepsis in asplenic patients.

RENAL INJURY

The kidney commonly is injured by blunt abdominal trauma, and more than 40% of children with injured kidneys have other internal injuries. A young child's kidney is more vulnerable to trauma than an adult's because it is positioned more anteriorly in the peritoneal cavity, because the child's rib cage is more compliant, and because the child's abdominal muscle development is immature. In the child in whom minor trauma has led to major renal injury, congenital renal anomalies also should be suspected. The diagnosis of renal injury is based on history and physical examination, coupled with a urinalysis showing blood and increased protein levels. An intravenous pyelogram (IVP) may be diagnostic; however, CT scans also are useful. In more than 80% of the children with positive IVPs, simple monitoring is all that is required; in the remaining patients, surgery usually is indicated for falling hemoglobin, refractory shock, or bladder distention caused by clots.

LIVER TRAUMA

Major trauma to the liver is a serious cause of morbidity and accounts for 40% of all deaths associated with blunt abdominal trauma in children. Almost 90% of these injuries involve the right lobe of the liver, and they usually are diagnosed by the presence of pain in the right shoulder and right upper quadrant. Patients may have hypotension secondary to blood loss, but hematobilia is rare. The site of the traumatic lesion may determine its severity. Subcapsular hematomas are less serious than capsular tears, which, in turn, are less serious than minor or deep lacerations. Burst injuries, with or without major vascular injury, are the most severe of all traumatic injuries to the liver and almost invariably are fatal.

For most children experiencing liver trauma, conservative management is recommended. This management involves admission to an intensive care unit and monitoring by CT scan and follow-up ultrasounds. Operative management should be reserved for life-threatening situations.

INJURIES OF THE PANCREAS AND BILIARY TREE

Injuries of the pancreas and biliary tree are less common in children than in adults. Pancreatic injuries almost always are present in association with injury to overlying structures, including the stomach, duodenum, extrahepatic biliary tree, and spleen. Pancreatic injury generally is identified by diffuse abdominal tenderness, pain, and vomiting. A midepigastric mass also is variably present. Hemodynamic instability, secondary to retroperitoneal hemorrhage, may be the presenting sign. Hyperamylasemia may not occur until 3–5 days after the injury. In managing these patients, naso-gastric suction and parenteral nutrition are indicated. Surgical removal of part or all of the pancreas may be required in one third of the patients who develop a pseudocyst or a persistent fistula. CT scan or ultrasound detects pancreatic injury, abscess formation, or pseudocyst.

Injury to the biliary tree is evident in children through the appearance of hematobilia after right upper quadrant trauma. The diagnosis usually is confirmed by the presence of bile in the peritoneal cavity or retroperitoneal space. When these children do not present with an acute injury, their chronic course is characterized by anorexia, weight loss, the development of bilious ascites, jaundice, and acholic stools. Biliary tree injury generally requires prompt surgical repair once it is identified.

INTESTINAL INJURY

In children, injury to the intestine usually is associated with other injuries requiring surgical treatment. The risk of intestinal injury varies with the amount of intestinal contents. A full bowel is likely to shear more easily than an empty bowel, and the shearing occurs at points of fixation (i.e., the ligament of Treitz, the ileocecal valve, and the ascending and descending peritoneal reflections). Perforation is more common in the jejunum and ileum than in the colon or stomach. Pneumoperitoneum that exists in association with intestinal perforation occurs in only 20% of patients. Diagnosis often is established by paracentesis that is positive for bowel contents. Prompt surgical intervention is required.

References

Behrman RE (ed): Nelson Textbook of Pediatrics. 14th ed. Philadelphia, WB Saunders, 1992, Sec. 6.31–6.35.

Galat JA, Grisoni ER, Gauderer MWL: Pediatric blunt liver injury: Establishment of criteria for appropriate management. J Pediatr Surg 25:1162, 1990.

Ghajar J, Hariri RJ: Management of pediatric head injury. Pediatr Clin North Am 39:1093, 1992.

Kissoon N: Triage and transport of the critically ill child. Crit Care Clin 8:37, 1992.

Peclet MH, Newman KD, Eichelberger MR, et al: Thoracic trauma in children: An indicator of increased mortality. J Pediatr Surg 25:961, 1990.

Yurt RW: Triage, initial assessment, and early treatment of the pediatric trauma patient. Pediatr Clin North Am 39:1083, 1992.

BURNS

A significant proportion of children who have traumatic injuries are burned. Almost 1% of the population are burned or scalded each year; half of these patients require a temporary restriction of activity and one fourth are confined to bed during convalescence. Approximately 2.3:100,000 in the population die from burns annually.

Severe burns in children require admission to an experienced burn center to ensure that their unique needs are met. For example, it is important for their development that these children avoid social isolation as much as possible, and parents should be involved as far as feasible in both the acute and ongoing rehabilitative care.

Shock is common in children if the burn exceeds 12% of the total body surface area. For the same area of involvement, the physiologic sequelae in younger patients are much more severe than in older patients. Because the mortality rate from burns is significantly greater in children than in adults, the initial assessment of a child with a serious burn requires an early decision regarding resuscitation status.

The upper extremities are the areas most frequently involved in burns (71%), followed by the head and neck (52%). Scalding injuries (75%) are most common and inhalation injuries are least common in pediatric patients.

Classification

Burns usually are classified on the basis of four criteria: the depth of injury, the percent of body surface area involved, the location of the burn, and association with other injuries. Most burn surgeons recommend that the depth of injury be assessed solely on clinical criteria of appearance. *First degree burns* are superficial (epidermal damage), painful, and dry. They heal in 3–6 days. *Second-degree* or partial-thickness burns may be superficial (red, mottled, blistered, healing in 10–21 days) or deep dermal (pale, painful, yellow), resulting from immersion (21–28 days to heal) or flames (≥3 wk to heal and potentially scarring). The severest burns, *third-degree burns,* are full thickness and require grafts (if >1 cm in diameter). They are avascular and are characterized by coagulation necrosis.

A *severe burn* is one that covers greater than 15% of the body surface area or involves the face or perineum. Second- and third-degree burns of the

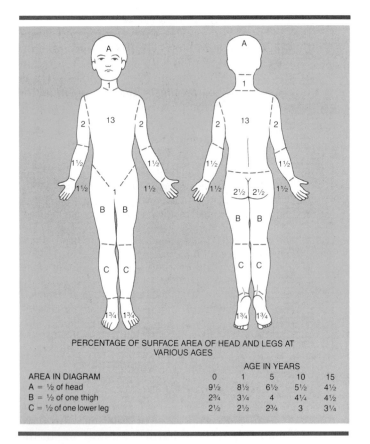

PERCENTAGE OF SURFACE AREA OF HEAD AND LEGS AT
VARIOUS AGES

AREA IN DIAGRAM	AGE IN YEARS				
	0	1	5	10	15
A = ½ of head	9½	8½	6½	5½	4½
B = ½ of one thigh	2¾	3¼	4	4¼	4½
C = ½ of one lower leg	2½	2½	2¾	3	3¼

Figure 3–1. This chart of body areas, together with the table showing the percentage of surface area of head and legs at various ages, can be used to estimate the surface area burned in a child. (From Solomon JR: Pediatric burns. Crit Care Clin 1:159–174, 1985.)

hands or feet, as well as circumferential burns of the extremities, also are classified as severe. Inhalation injuries resulting in bronchospasm and impaired pulmonary function also must be considered severe burns. A method for estimating the percentage of skin surface area involved in children of various ages is presented in Figure 3–1. The extent of skin involvement of older adolescent and adult patients is estimated as follows: each upper extremity, 9%; each lower extremity, 18%; anterior trunk, 18%; posterior trunk, 18%; the head, 9%; and the perineum, 1%.

The location of the burn is important in assessing the risk for disability. The risk is greatest when the face, eyes, ears, feet, perineum, or hands are involved. With partial-thickness burns, no disability generally results; however, full-thickness burns almost always result in permanent impairment. Inhalational injuries not only cause respiratory compromise but may result in difficulty in eating and drinking. Inhalational injuries also may be associated with burns of the face and neck.

Initial Evaluation

The triage decision for the physician caring for a burn patient is based on the extent of the burn, the body surface area involved, the type of burn, associated injuries, any complicating medical or social problems, and the availability of ambulatory management (Figure 3–2). The initial treatment requires removing the patient from the site of injury, cleansing away any chemical or injurious contactants, and removing the clothing. The next priority is airway management; the upper airway is susceptible to burn injury, whereas the subglottic space appears protected. Few signs of injury may be present initially, although facial burns, singed

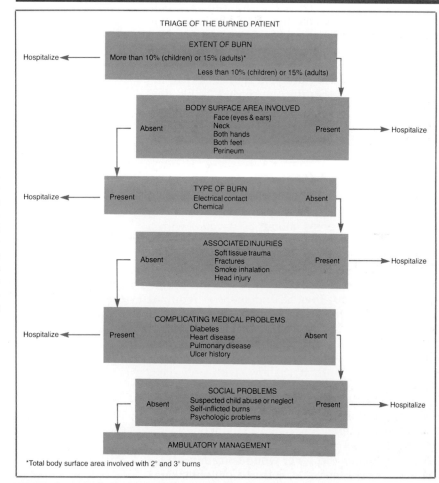

Figure 3–2. Triage of the burned patient. Additional considerations for hospitalization include involvement of major joints, third-degree burns of >5%, and poor guardianship at home regarding wound care. (From Wachtel TL: Epidemiology, classification, initial care and administrative considerations for critically burned patients. Crit Care Clin 1:3–26, 1985.)

nasal hairs or eyebrows, and acute inflammation of the oropharynx should suggest inhalation injury. Smoke inhalation may be associated with carbon monoxide toxicity; 100% oxygen should be given if hypoxia or inhalation is suspected. Hoarseness on vocalization also is consistent with a supraglottic injury. Some children with inhalation burns require endoscopy, an artificial airway, and mechanical ventilation.

Fluid and Electrolyte Management

The initial fluid and electrolyte support of the burned child is critical. The first priority is to support the circulating blood volume, which requires the administration of intravenous fluids to provide both maintenance fluid and electrolyte requirements and to replace ongoing burn losses. The amount of fluid required for resucitation and ongoing losses is considered to be 4 mL/kg/% body surface area involved. This fluid is designed to cover "third space" losses associated with capillary leaking. Lactated Ringer solution should be infused on day 1; urine output should be ≥1 mL/kg/hr. Half the estimated burn requirement is administered during the first 8 hr after admission, and the remaining burn fluid requirement is divided over the subsequent 16 hr. During the second 24 hr, dextrose water in 0.25 normal saline and 5% albumin (0.5 mL/kg/% burn over 6–8 hr) are substituted for this regimen.

Initial Wound Care

Wound care requires careful surgical management. The treatment is simple and noninvasive, and the involved areas should be covered with a sterile sheet. Wrapping with plastic, particularly for circumferential burns, may increase the child's comfort. Initial surgical attempts focus on relieving any pressure on the peripheral circulation by the developing eschar; then débridement is required for reclassifying the injury, a procedure that must occur prior to administering any topical therapy. Following débridement, burns are generally covered with silver sulfadiazine applied to fine-mesh gauze or, if the burn is shallow, with polymicin B–bacitracin–neomycin (Neosporin) ointment. Silver nitrate and mafenide acetate (painful, produces metabolic acidosis, penetrates eschar) are alternate antimicrobial agents. Such agents inhibit but do not prevent bacterial growth. Various grafts also have been used initially to cover wounds (cadaver allografts, porcine xenografts, cultured patient's keratinocytes). Full-thickness burns require skin auto-

Table 3–12. Complications of Burns

Problem	Treatment
Sepsis (*Staphylococcus aureus, Pseudomonas aeruginosa*)	Monitor for infection, avoid prophylactic antibiotics
Hypovolemia	Fluid replacement
Hypothermia	Adjust ambient temperature: dry blankets in field
Laryngeal edema	Endotracheal intubation, tracheostomy
Carbon monoxide poisoning	100% O_2
Cardiac dysfunction	Inotropic agents, diuretics
Curling gastric ulcers	H_2-receptor antagonist, antacids
Compartment syndrome	Escharotomy incision
Contractures	Physical therapy
Hypermetabolic state	Enteral and parenteral nutritional support
Renal failure	Supportive care, dialysis
Transient antidiuresis	Expectant management
Anemia	Transfusions as indicated
Psychologic trauma	Psychologic rehabilitation
Pulmonary infiltrates	
Burn injury	PEEP, ventilation, O_2
Pulmonary edema	Avoid overhydration, give diuretics
Pneumonia	Antibiotics
Bronchospasm	Beta agonist aerosols

PEEP = positive end-expiratory pressure.

grafting and artificial skin substitutes to eventually close. Burn management and rehabilitation are highly specialized and include recognizing many complications of burns (Table 3–12) and evaluating the wound and its cause for suspected child abuse or neglect.

Prevention

Over 600,000 children suffer burns each year; 94% occur in the home. Prevention is possible by using smoke and fire alarms, having identifiable escape routes and a fire extinguisher, and reducing hot water temperature to 120° F. Emersion full-thickness burns develop after 1 sec at 158° F, 5 sec at 140° F, 30 sec at 130° F, 60 sec at 127° F, 5 min at 122° F, and 10 min at 120° F.

References

Behrman RE (ed): Nelson Textbook of Pediatrics. 14th ed. Philadelphia, WB Saunders Co., 1992, Sec. 6.37.

Corvajal HF, Griffith JA: Burn and inhalation injuries. *In* Fuhrman BP, Zimmerman JJ (eds): Pediatric Critical Care. St. Louis, Mosby-Year Book, 1992, pp 1209–1220.

Finklestein JL, Schwartz SB, Madden MR, et al: Pediatric burns: An overview. Pediatr Clin North Am 39:1145, 1992.

Wachtel TL: Epidemiology, classification, initial care and administrative consideration for critically burned patients. Crit Care Clin 1:3–26, 1985.

POISONING

Ingestions

Accidental ingestions are most common in the 1–5 yr old age group, an incidence that reveals the young child's inquisitiveness and the adult's carelessness in leaving drugs and household chemicals within reach. In older children, drug overdoses (poisonings) most often are associated with suicide attempts. Most ingestions (88%) are accidental, occur in the home (92%), and produce no (82%) or minor (17%) toxicity; 0.01% are fatal. Common agents in young children include their family members' medication, cleaning or polishing solutions, plants, and cosmetics. Fatal childhood poisonings are due to carbon monoxide, medications, hydrocarbons, and pesticides. The fatal medication poisonings are from salicylates, tricyclic antidepressants, cardiovascular drugs, drugs of abuse, and pills containing iron.

CLINICAL ASSESSMENT

Poisoning usually is a diagnosis of exclusion, but the history and physical examination often provide sufficient clues to distinguish between toxic ingestion and organic disease (Table 3–13). The comatose child should be considered to have ingested a poison until proved otherwise. Because the comatose patient's history as well as physical examination may be unrevealing, using the toxicology laboratory to obtain information sometimes is helpful. Nonetheless, no toxicology screen can substitute for careful physical examination by someone who understands the signs and symptoms of various ingestions.

The diagnosis for a number of agents can be established based on evaluating the level of consciousness, determining the pupillary size, and validating the presence of muscle fasciculations, cardiac arrhythmias, seizures, or hypothermia. Certain complexes of symptoms and signs are relatively specific to a given class of drugs (Table 3–14). Even in the absence of an obvious toxidrome, a careful and thorough examination is helpful in suggesting a diagnosis of poisoning. It also is important to determine whether the patient's vital signs are unstable, which warrants immediate supportive cardiopulmonary care.

The recognition of additional clinical manifestations is helpful in determining poisoning involving a particular agent (Table 3–14). For example, an elevated body temperature may be related to sepsis or meningitis but also is typical of salicylate and anticholinergic overdose. The patient with an acute onset of jaundice or hepatic coma is not likely to have had a recent ingestion, but perhaps may be manifesting a delayed toxic presentation resulting from previous ingestion of a substance such as acetaminophen.

The patient's breath odors also may provide valuable clues to potential ingestions (see Table 3–13). A fruity smell may signify diabetic ketoacidosis, a silver polish smell is typical of cyanide, and a cleaning fluid–type odor is consistent with carbon tetrachloride ingestion. An evaluation of the lungs may reveal pulmonary edema, which can be due to tricyclic antidepressants, organophosphates, or methaqualone.

MAJOR PATTERNS OF PRESENTATION

The poisoned child can present with any one of six basic clinical patterns. *Coma* is perhaps the most striking but leads to the greatest confusion because the comatose child is unarousable and unresponsive. Coma may be due to trauma, a cerebrovascular accident, a global asphyxial event, meningitis, or poisoning; a careful history and clinical examination are required to distinguish among these alternatives. The rapid loss of brain stem function usually suggests a supratentorial lesion, whereas the persistence of the pupillary light reflex in the presence of diminished respiratory effort and diminished level of consciousness often indicates a metabolic insult to the brain. The level of consciousness in the latter condition often is depressed out of proportion to other neurologic signs. Decorticate posturing strongly suggests structural or metabolic disorders rather than toxic ingestions. Pinpoint pupils suggest either a pontine lesion or the toxic ingestion of opiates, organophosphates, phenothiazines, or chloral hydrate. Dilated pupils often are associated with tricyclic antidepressant overdoses (see Table 3–13). Structural lesions often may be

Table 3–13. Historic and Physical Findings in Poisoning

Odor

Bitter almonds	Cyanide
Acetone	Isopropyl alcohol, methanol, salicylate
Alcohol	Ethanol
Wintergreen	Methyl salicylate
Garlic	Arsenic, thallium, organophosphates
Violets	Turpentine

Ocular Signs

Miosis	Narcotics (except meperidine), organophosphates, muscarinic mushrooms, clonidine, phenothiazines, chloral hydrate, barbiturates (late), PCP
Mydriasis	Atropine, alcohol, cocaine, amphetamines, antihistamines, tricyclic antidepressants, cyanide, carbon monoxide
Nystagmus	Phenytoin, barbiturates, ethanol, carbon monoxide
Lacrimation	Organophosphates, irritant gas or vapors
Retinal hyperemia	Methanol
Poor vision	Methanol, botulism, carbon monoxide

Cutaneous Signs

Needle tracks	Heroin, PCP, amphetamine
Bullae	Carbon monoxide, barbiturates
Dry, hot skin	Anticholinergic agents, botulism
Diaphoresis	Organophosphates, nitrates, muscarinic mushrooms, aspirin, cocaine
Alopecia	Thallium, arsenic, lead, mercury
Erythema	Boric acid, mercury, cyanide, anticholinergics

Oral Signs

Salivation	Organophosphates, salicylate, corrosives, strychnine
Dry mouth	Amphetamine, anticholinergics, antihistamine
Burns	Corrosives, oxalate-containing plants
Gum lines	Lead, mercury, arsenic
Dysphagia	Corrosives, botulism

Intestinal Signs

Cramps	Arsenic, lead, thallium, organophosphates
Diarrhea	Arsenic, iron, boric acid
Constipation	Lead, narcotics, botulism
Hematemesis	Aminophylline, corrosives, iron, salicylates

Cardiac Signs

Tachycardia	Atropine, aspirin, amphetamine, cocaine, tricyclic antidepressants, theophylline
Bradycardia	Digitalis, narcotics, mushrooms, clonidine, organophosphates, beta-blockers, calcium channel blockers
Hypertension	Amphetamine, LSD, cocaine, PCP
Hypotension	Phenothiazines, barbiturates, tricyclic antidepressants, iron, beta-blockers, calcium channel blockers

Respiratory Signs

Depressed respiration	Alcohol, narcotics, barbiturates
Increased respiration	Amphetamines, aspirin, ethylene glycol, carbon monoxide, cyanide
Pulmonary edema	Hydrocarbons, heroin, organophosphates, aspirin

CNS Signs

Ataxia	Alcohol, antidepressants, barbiturates, anticholinergics, phenytoin, narcotics
Coma	Sedatives, narcotics, barbiturates, PCP, organophosphates, salicylate, cyanide, carbon monoxide, tricyclic antidepressants, lead
Hyperpyrexia	Anticholinergics, quinine, salicylates, LSD, phenothiazines, amphetamine, cocaine
Muscle fasciculation	Organophosphates, theophylline
Muscle rigidity	Tricyclic antidepressants, PCP, phenothiazines, haloperidol
Paresthesia	Cocaine, camphor, PCP, MSG
Peripheral neuropathy	Lead, arsenic, mercury, organophosphates
Altered behavior	LSD, PCP, amphetamines, cocaine, alcohol, anticholinergics, camphor

CNS = central nervous system; LSD = lysergic acid diethylamide; MSG = monosodium glutamate; PCP = phencyclidine.

Table 3–14. Toxic Syndromes

Agent	Manifestations
Acetaminophen	Nausea, vomiting, pallor, delayed jaundice–hepatic failure (72–96 hr)
Amphetamine, cocaine and sympathomimetics	Tachycardia, hypertension, hyperthermia, psychosis/paranoia, seizures, mydriasis, diaphoresis, piloerection, aggressive behavior
Anticholinergics	Mania, delirium, fever, red dry skin, dry mouth, tachycardia, mydriasis, urinary retention
Carbon monoxide	Headache, dizziness, coma, skin bullae, other systems affected
Cyanide	Coma, convulsions, hyperpnea, bitter almond odor
Ethylene glycol (antifreeze)	Metabolic acidosis, hyperosmolarity, hypocalcemia, oxalate crystalluria
Iron	Vomiting (bloody), diarrhea, hypotension, hepatic failure, leukocytosis, hyperglycemia, radiopaque pills on KUB, late intestinal stricture, *Yersinia* sepsis
Narcotics	Coma, respiratory depression, hypotension, pinpoint pupils, hyporeflexia
Cholinergics (organophosphates, nicotine)	Miosis, salivation, urination, diaphoresis, lacrimation, bronchospasm (bronchorrhea), muscle weakness and fasciculations, emesis, defecation, coma, confusion, pulmonary edema, bradycardia, reduced erythrocyte and serum cholinesterase, late peripheral neuropathy
Phenothiazines	Tachycardia, hypotension, muscle rigidity, coma, ataxia, oculogyric crisis, miosis, radiopaque pills on KUB
Salicylates	Tachypnea, fever, lethargy, coma, vomiting, diaphoresis, alkalosis (early), acidosis (late)
Tricyclic antidepressants	Coma, convulsions, mydriasis, hyperreflexia, arrhythmia (prolonged QT interval), cardiac arrest, shock

KUB = kidney–ureter–bladder roentgenogram.

accompanied by midpoint-fixed pupils or unilaterally dilated pupils and disturbances of ocular movement.

Hydrocarbon ingestion may result in *systemic and pulmonary* (locally by aspiration) *toxicity* (Table 3–15). Halogenated hydrocarbons or those with toxic additives have the greatest systemic toxicities and should be removed by lavage. Hydrocarbons with low viscosity, low surface tension, and high volatility pose the greatest risk for producing aspiration pneumonia, but, once swallowed, they pose no risk unless emesis is induced. Emesis or lavage should *not* be initiated in the child who has ingested volatile hydrocarbons.

Caustic ingestions may cause dysphagia, epigastric pain, oral mucosal burns, and low-grade fever. Patients with esophageal lesions may have no oral burns or may have significant signs and symptoms. Treatment depends on the agent ingested and the presence or absence of esophageal injury. **Alkali agents** may be solid, granular, or liquid (Liquid Drain-O, 9.5% NaOH; Liquid Plumber, 8% KOH). Both of the latter agents are tasteless and will produce full-thickness liquefaction necrosis of the esophagus or oropharynx. When the esophageal lesions heal, strictures form. There also is a long-term risk of esophageal carcinoma. Initial therapy includes diluting the agent with water and milk, but no attempt should be made to induce emesis or neutralize the alkali. Subsequent treatment includes antibiotics if there are signs of infection and dilation of late-forming (2–3 wk) strictures.

Ingested button batteries also may produce a

Table 3–15. Acute Hydrocarbon Risk Assessments

Systemic Toxicity Common*
Trichloroethane (spot remover), trichlorethylene, carbon tetrachloride, methylene chloride, benzene, hydrocarbon additives (camphor, heavy metals, insecticides, aniline), toluene

Local Toxicity by Aspiration Common,† Systemic Toxicity Uncommon
Mineral seal oil, signal oil, furniture polish, turpentine, gasoline, kerosene, charcoal lighter fluid, toluene

Nontoxic in 95% of Cases
Asphalt, tar, motor oil, mineral or liquid petroleum, lubricants, baby oil

* Chronic abuse of volatile hydrocarbons (e.g., sniffing) may cause ataxia, tremor, seizures, coma, myopathy, peripheral neuropathy, and renal tubular defects. Lead poisoning also is noted with abuse of lead-containing gasoline.
† Hydrocarbons of low viscosity (30–60 SSU), low surface tension, and high volatility have the greatest risk for inducing aspiration pneumonia.

caustic mucosal injury from NaOH, KOH, or mercuric oxide. If they pass to the stomach, no further therapy is needed because they are likely to be passed in the stool within a week. Those that do not pass through the esophagus may cause esophageal burns and erosion and should be removed with the endoscope.

Acid agents such as Lysol Toilet Bowl Cleaner (8.5% HCl) or Vanish Toilet Bowl Cleaner (65% sodium acid sulfate) injures the lungs (HCl fumes), oral mucosa, esophagus, and stomach. Because acids taste sour, children will immediately stop drinking the solution, thus limiting the injury. Acids produce a coagulation necrosis, which also limits the chemical from penetrating into deeper layers of the mucosa and, therefore, damages tissue less severely than alkali. The signs and symptoms and initial therapeutic measures (dilution, no emesis or neutralization) are similar to those for alkali ingestion.

The poisoned child also may present with *metabolic acidosis* (Table 3–16), which is assessed easily by measuring arterial blood gases, serum electrolytes, and urine pH. Determining serum sodium, potassium, chloride, glucose, urea nitrogen, and CO_2 levels permits the calculation of the serum anion gap (Chapter 16) and osmolality ($OSM = 2 \times Na + [glucose/18] + [BUN/2.8]$), which may be compared with measured osmolality. A difference of more than 10 between the measured and calculated osmolality, an **osmolal gap**, strongly suggests the presence of an unmeasured component, such as methanol or ethylene glycol. Because these ingestions require thorough assessment and prompt intervention, this approach allows a tentative diagnosis to be made pending access to the toxicology laboratory.

Rhythm abnormalities may be prominent signs of a variety of toxic ingestions, although ventricular arrhythmias are rare. Prolonged Q-T intervals may suggest phenothiazine or antihistamine ingestion, and widened QRS complexes are seen with tricyclic antidepressants and quinidine. Because many drug and chemical overdoses may lead to sinus tachycardia, it is not a useful or discriminating sign; sinus bradycardia, however, should suggest digoxin, cyanide, or beta-blocker ingestion. A full 12-lead electrocardiogram should be part of the initial evaluation in all patients suspected of suffering from ingestions (Table 3–17).

Gastrointestinal symptoms of poisoning include emesis, nausea, abdominal cramps, and diarrhea. These may be due to direct toxic effects on the intestinal mucosa or to systemic toxicity following absorption.

Table 3–16. Screening Laboratory Clues in Toxicologic Diagnosis

Metabolic Acidosis (Mnemonic = MUDPIES)

Methanol,* carbon monoxide	Isoniazid, iron
Uremia*	Ethanol,* ethylene glycol*
Diabetes mellitus*	Salicylates, starvation, seizures
Paraldehyde,* phenformin	

Hypoglycemia
Ethanol
Isoniazid
Insulin
Propranolol

Hyperglycemia
Salicylates
Isoniazid
Iron
Phenothiazine
Sympathomimetics

Hypocalcemia
Oxalate
Ethylene glycol
Fluoride

Radiopaque Substance on KUB (Mnemonic = CHIPPED)
Chloral hydrate, calcium carbonate
Heavy metals (lead, zinc, barium, arsenic, lithium, bismuth as in Pepto-Bismol)
Iron
Phenothiazines
Play-Doh, potassium chloride
Enteric-coated pills
Dental amalgam

* Indicates hyperosmolar condition.
KUB = kidney–ureter–bladder roentgenogram.

Seizures are the sixth major mode of presentation for children with toxic ingestions, but poisoning is an uncommon cause of afebrile seizures. When seizures do occur with intoxication, they may be life threatening and require aggressive therapeutic intervention (see Table 3–17).

INITIAL THERAPY

Supportive Care

Prompt attention must be given to protecting and clearing the airway, establishing effective breathing, and supporting the circulation (asystole, bradycardia, hypotension). This management sequence takes precedence over other diagnostic or therapeutic procedures. If there is a depressed level of consciousness and a toxic substance is suspected, glucose (1 g/kg IV), 100% oxygen, and nal-

Table 3–17. Drugs Associated with Major Modes of Presentation

Common Toxic Causes of Cardiac Arrhythmia	Causes of Coma	Common Agents Causing Seizures (Mnemonic = CAPS)
Amphetamine	Alcohol	Camphor
Antiarrhythmics	Anticholinergics	Carbon monoxide
Anticholinergics	Antihistamines	Cocaine
Antihistamines	Barbiturates	Cyanide
Arsenic	Carbon monoxide	
Carbon monoxide	Clonidine	Aminophylline
Chloral hydrate	Cyanide	Amphetamine
Cocaine	Hypoglycemic agents	Anticholinergics
Cyanide	Lead	Antidepressants (tricyclic)
Digitalis	Lithium	
Freon	Methemoglobinemia*	Pb (lead) (also lithium)
Phenothiazines	Methyldopa	Pesticide (organophosphate)
Physostigmine	Narcotics	Phencyclidine
Propranolol	Phencyclidine	Phenol
Quinine, quinidine	Phenothiazines	Phenothiazines
Theophylline	Salicylates	Proproxyphene
Tricyclic antidepressants	Tricyclic antidepressants	
		Salicylates
		Strychnine

* Causes of methemoglobinemia: amyl nitrite, aniline dyes, benzocaine, bismuth subnitrate, dapsone, primaquine, quinones, spinach, sulfonamides.

oxone should be administered. Laboratory studies helpful in the initial management include specific toxin–drugs assays, arterial blood gases, electrolytes, blood glucose, electrocardiogram, and the calculation of the anion or osmolar gap.

Gastric Decontamination

There is controversy about the most effective and safe means for gastric emptying and prevention of absorption of a toxic substance.

Syrup of ipecac has been suggested as the drug of choice for ensuring rapid gastric emptying in patients of all ages with an acute ingestion. Ipecac works best if given immediately ofter the ingestion (e.g., at home), removes more gastric contents than lavage, and is more effective for substances (pills) too large to be removed by lavage and those toxins not absorbed by activated charcoal. The delayed and prolonged emesis, especially if administered in the emergency room, may increase the risk of aspiration pneumonia and reduce the ability to administer the more effective activated charcoal. Doses of 15 mL (1 tablespoon) in children over the age of 1 yr and 30 mL (2 tablespoons) in adolescent and adult patients are effective in inducing emesis within 30 min of administration in 85–95% of patients. The response rate is improved to almost 100% if a second dose is given to those who failed to respond to the first dose. In children under 1 yr of age, self-administered toxic ingestions are rare,

but 1 mL/kg doses of syrup of ipecac have proved safe and effective.

It is recommended that syrup of ipecac be in the home of every family with children under the age of 12 yr, but it should be used only at the direction of a physician or the local poison control center. Syrup of ipecac is *contraindicated* in the comatose child, the child who has ingested a caustic agent, and the child less than 6 mo of age, and in the presence of a foreign body, absent bowel sounds (ileus), shock, increased intracranial pressure, hypertension, pregnancy, drugs with rapid onset of central nervous system depression, and certain volatile petroleum distillates.

Adverse reactions to syrup of ipecac are rare when it is used as directed and include mild diarrhea, lethargy, irritability, and fever. Syrup of ipecac has been abused by young adolescent patients with anorexia nervosa and bulimia. This type of chronic overdose has been associated with cardiomyopathy and death.

Gastric lavage is an alternative to syrup of ipecac for patients who go to the hospital. Lavage does not interfere with activated charcoal and should be used in potentially lethal ingestions or with toxins not absorbed by activated charcoal. The procedure involves placing a large-diameter tube into the stomach by either the nasal or oral route. Normal saline is recommended for lavage to prevent or minimize any electrolyte disturbances; cycles of 15 mL/kg are recommended, but large total volumes

(5–20 L) are required for effectively removing toxins.

In children presenting in coma, gastric lavage should be undertaken only following intubation with a cuffed endotracheal tube. No intubation is required for children who are awake. In the responsive but obtunded child, endotracheal intubation may be necessary prior to gastric intubation, and this decision will require clinical judgment. Lavage is *contraindicated* in children who ingest caustic materials or hydrocarbons and in the presence of neurologic symptoms (coma, seizures) likely to impair normal mechanisms that are protective of the airway.

Complications of gastric lavage include aspiration pneumonia, which appears secondary to vomiting during the lavage procedure, and laryngospasm with cyanosis, related to kinking of the lavage tube in the esophagus. Esophageal perforation also has been reported.

Activated charcoal, a binder, may be used as a primary gastric decontaminant with or without gastric emptying. Activated charcoal is prepared by pyrolyzing organic materials, such as wood pulp, and then activating them by exposing them to an oxidizing gas flow at a high temperature, which produces a fine network of pores.

Activated charcoal adsorbs a wide variety of organic materials from the gastrointestinal tract in a process that occurs within the first few minutes following administration. Because the surface area contained in the charcoal is large and because activated charcoal exhibits a relative affinity for certain compounds, it may prevent absorption of the toxin from the intestine. The charcoal also may serve as a reservoir for drugs removed from the blood that perfuses the intestine. Multiple doses of charcoal may enhance the elimination of numerous drugs that undergo enterohepatic recirculation, secretion across the gastric membranes into the bowel lumen, or continued prolonged absorption. Administering charcoal in divided doses over 72 hr is very effective in reducing the plasma half-life of phenobarbital, theophylline, digoxin, and methotrexate. An alternative to this intermittent dosing is administering the charcoal by continuous nasogastric infusion. Activated charcoal is ineffective against caustic or corrosive agents, hydrocarbons, alcohols, heavy metals (arsenic, lead, mercury, iron, lithium), glycols, and water-insoluble compounds. Charcoal interferes with *N*-acetylcysteine (NAC) therapy of acetaminophen ingestion; the therapy should be separated by 2 hr or twice the NAC given with the charcoal.

A dose of 15–30 g should be used for small chil-dren and a dose of 50–100 g for children over 12 yr of age; alternatively, 1–2 g/kg can be given safely and effectively. The acceptance of oral charcoal as a slurry in water is variable, but its poor palatability may cause problems, and thus a variety of maneuvers have been attempted to increase its acceptance, including flavoring, cocoa powders, sweeteners, thickeners, and presentation in soft drink cans. If these fail, the charcoal may be given by nasogastric intubation.

One of the difficulties encountered with using multiple doses of charcoal relates to the effects when it is combined with cathartic agents, such as sorbitol. Several charcoal preparations are prepackaged in a slurry with 70% sorbitol. The sorbitol may result in significant diarrhea and fluid and electrolyte loss. In contrast, using activated charcoal alone in children may cause constipation. When using multiple or continuous infusions of charcoal, the dose of sorbitol must be adjusted so that the amount being given is sufficient to prevent constipation, but not so much as to cause significant diarrhea. Hydration status must be rigorously monitored in these children. *Contraindications* include caustic or corrosive agents, an ileus, and poor control of the airway.

Catharsis alone (sorbitol, magnesium citrate) is an ineffective decontamination method. Whole-bowel irrigation is a new method to remove coalesced pills (iron igestion) and employs polyethylene glycol (Golytely) as a nonabsorbable cathartic.

ADDITIONAL THERAPY

After the initial resuscitation and gastric decontamination have been achieved, it is often difficult to determine whether or not further therapy is needed. There are basically three choices in the subsequent care of the child with a significant ingestion: (1) providing continued supportive care, (2) using specific antidotes where available, and (3) actively removing the toxin from the bloodstream. In order to make a rational decision regarding these options, a judgment should be made as to whether or not a drug causes tissue damage (methyl alcohol, aspirin, acetaminophen, theophylline, iron, ethylene glycol). Tissue damage is defined as an irreversible or slowly reversible structural or functional change in an organ system as a direct result of ingestion of a poison; this definition precludes indirect effects such as respiratory depression or hypotension. The decision should take into consideration the amount taken; the diagnostic assessment, including the condition of the patient at the time of presentation; and the natural history of the sus-

Table 3–18. Emergency Antidotes*

Poison	Antidote	Dosage	Comments
Acetaminophen	N-Acetylcysteine	140 mg/kg PO initial dose, then 70 mg/kg PO q4h × 17 doses	Most effective within 16 hr
Atropine	Physostigmine	Initial dose 0.01–0.1 mg/kg IV	Can produce convulsions, bradycardia
Benzodiazepine	Flumazenil	0.1–0.3 mg IV adult dose	Possible seizures, arrhythmias
Beta-blocking agents	Atropine Isoproterenol Glucagon	0.01–0.10 mg/kg IV 0.05–5 µg/kg/min IV infusion 1 mg IV	
Carbon monoxide	Oxygen	100%; hyperbaric O_2	Half-life of carboxyhemoglobin is 5 hr in room air but 1.5 hr in 100% O_2
Coumarin	Vitamin K	2.5–10 mg IV/IM	Monitor PT; FFP or plasma for acute bleeding; repeated vitamin K for super-warfarin
Cyanide	Amyl nitrite then sodium nitrite	1–2 pearls every 2 min Initially 0.33 mL (10 mg 3% sol)/kg IV	Methemoglobin–cyanide complex Causes hypotension; dosage assumes normal hemoglobin
	Sodium thiosulfate	25% solution; 1.65 mg/kg IV over 10 min	Forms harmless sodium thiocyanate
Digoxin, digitoxin	Digoxin-specific Fab antibody fragments	Dose based on serum digoxin concentration and body weight; 1 vial (40 mg) neutralizes 0.6 mg digoxin	With acute life-threatening ingestion, dose and serum concentration are unknown; give contents of 20 vials
Iron	Deferoxamine	Initial dose 15 mg/kg/hr IV	Deferoxamine mesylate—forms excretable ferrioxamine complex; hypotension
Isoniazid	Pyridoxime	1 mg/mg isoniazid	—
Lead	Edetate calcium (calcium disodium versenate [EDTA])	1500 mg/m^2/day × 5 days; divided q6h or by continuous infusion	May lower to 1000 mg/m^2/day if given with BAL; nephrotoxic
	BAL (British Anti-Lewisite [dimercaprol])	500 mg/m^2/day IM divided q4h × 3 days	May cause hypertension and sterile abscesses
	Penicillamine	20 mg/kg/day PO divided q8h	Requires weekly monitoring for hepatic and bone marrow toxicity; should not be used in the presence of ongoing ingestion
	2,3-dimercaptosuccinic acid (DMSA)	30 mg/kg/day PO tid × 5 days then 20 mg/kg/day PO bid × 14 days	Few toxic effects
Mercury, arsenic, gold	BAL (British Anti-Lewisite)	5 mg/kg IM as soon as possible	Each mL BAL in oil has dimercaprol, 100 mg in 210 mL (21%) benzyl benzoate, and 680 mL peanut oil—forms stable nontoxic excretable cyclic compound
Methyl alcohol (ethylene glycol)	Ethyl alcohol in conjunction with dialysis	1 mL/kg of 100% ethanol initially in glucose solution; maintain blood level of 100 mg/dL	Competes for alcohol dehydrogenase; prevents formation of formic acid and oxalates
Nitrites/ Methemoglobinemia†	Methylene blue	1–2 mg/kg IV, repeat in 1–4 hr if needed; treat for levels >30%	Exchange transfusion may be needed for severe methemoglobinemia; methylene blue overdose also causes methemoglobinemia
Opiates, Darvon, Lomotil	Naloxone	0.10 mg/kg IV, ET, SC, IM for children, up to 2 mg	Naloxone causes no respiratory depression (0.4 mg/ 1 mL ampule)
Organophosphates	Atropine	Initial dose 0.05–1.0 mg/kg IV	Physiologic: blocks acetylcholine; up to 5 mg IV every 15 min may be necessary in the critically ill adult patient
	Pralidoxime (2 PAM-chloride) (Protopam)	Initial dose 25–50 mg/kg IV	Specific: disrupts phosphate–cholinesterase bond; up to 500 mg/hr may be necessary in the critically ill adult patient
Tricyclic antidepressants	Sodium bicarbonate	To produce pH 7.5–7.55	—
Sympathomimetic agents	Blocking agents: phentolamine; beta-blocking agents; other antihypertensives		Must be used in a setting in which vital signs can be monitored effectively

* (Data from Haddad LM, Winchester JF (eds): Clinical Management of Poisoning and Drug Overdose. Philadelphia, WB Saunders, 1983; Kulig K: Initial management of ingestions of toxic substances. N Engl J Med 326:1677, 1992; Barkin R: Toxicologic emergencies. Pediatr Ann 19:629, 1990.)
† See Table 3–17 for causes of methemoglobinemia.

pected type of ingestion. All of these variables may be influenced by the child's prior clinical status or underlying medical problems. For example, in a patient with underlying severe hepatic or renal impairment, a more aggressive approach involving active removal might be selected, even though the ingestion ordinarily would require only the use of simple supportive care. It also should be kept in mind that, in the face of a chronic ingestion, an

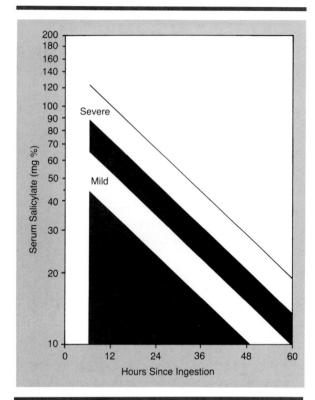

Figure 3–4. Nomogram relating serum salicylate concentration and expected severity of intoxication at various intervals following the ingestion of a single dose of salicylate. (From Done AK: Salicylate intoxication: Significance of measurements of salicylate in blood in cases of acute ingestion. Pediatrics 26:800, 1960.)

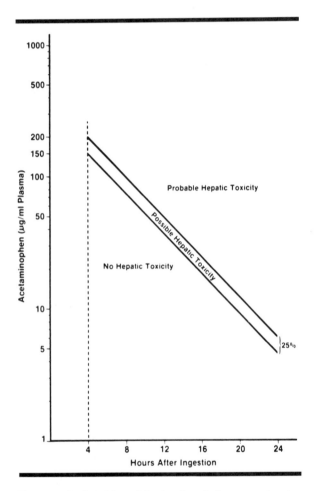

Figure 3–3. Semi-logarithmic plot of plasma acetaminophen levels versus time. Rumack-Matthew nomogram for acetaminophen poisoning. Cautions for use of this chart: (1) the time coordinates refer to time of ingestion; (2) serum levels drawn before 4 hr may not represent peak levels; (3) the graph should be used only in relation to a single, acute ingestion; and (4) the lower solid line, 25% below the standard nomogram, is included to allow for possible errors in acetaminophen plasma assays and estimated time from ingestion of an overdose. (Adapted from Rumack BH, Matthew H: Acetaminophen poisoning and toxicity. Pediatrics 55:871, 1975, with permission from the authors and the publisher.)

acute overdose may require a lower dosage of the drug to cause significant clinical toxicity.

For most common ingestions, continued supportive care and treatment directed toward specific complications are appropriate for otherwise healthy individuals. Specific antidotes should be used according to prescribed guidelines (Table 3–18). Active removal (hemoperfusion, dialysis) should be undertaken only for those toxins that may cause tissue damage, those that have been ingested by a patient already exhibiting confounding medical problems, or to avoid very prolonged supportive care.

Toxicology assays are important for some agents, not only for identifying the specific drug but also for providing guidance for therapy and help in anticipating complications and estimating the prognosis. Serum iron levels below 300 μg/dL usually are safe following iron ingestion, but levels of free iron above 600 μg/dL usually are associated

Table 3–19. Bites, Stings, and Envenomations

Species	Characteristics	Agents or Venoms	Treatment
Snakes			
Pit vipers: rattlesnake, copperhead, cotton mouth; triangular head, elliptical pupils, heat-sensing pits	Strike on provocation; site: hand, leg, foot; only 75% of bites have venom release; pain, swelling, ecchymosis ± coagulopathy, rhabdomyolysis, shock, weakness, hemolysis; bites of head and neck are most severe	Phospholipases, proteases, hyaluronidase, thrombin, Mojave (paralytic) toxin	Keep extremity dependent, immobilized; avoid ice, aspirin; mechanically extract venom; gentle tourniquet; treat shock; antivenom (polyvalent) if severe*; tetanus check†; antibiotics‡
Coral snake (cobra, mamba family)	Local pain and edema, hypesthesia, paresthesia, fasciculations, weakness, bulbar palsy, descending paralysis, respiratory paralysis	Paralytic toxin	Antivenom if severe*
Sea snake	Pinprick lesion, paralysis, myoglobinuria	Neurotoxin, phospholipase	Antivenom, antibiotics‡
Scorpions	Usually benign; local pain, tingling, hypesthesia; paralysis, agitation, seizures rare; tachycardia, hypertension	Sympathetic and parasympathetic nervous system toxin	No treatment unless severe, then antitoxin; propranolol for tachyarrhythmia
Hymenoptera			
See Chapter 8 for allergy and anaphylaxis			
Ticks	Paralysis (spring, summer); tick located in scalp, groin	Paralytic toxin in saliva	Remove tick with forceps or gauze by constant, gentle, upward motion; prevention: DEET, permethrins
Spiders			
Black widow	Punctate lesions, local erythema, and immediate pain, muscle rigidity, spasms, abdominal pain, periorbital edema, hypertension, diaphoresis; spider has red hourglass marking on abdomen; lives in moist dark outdoor sites	Polypeptides producing spontaneous motor neuron depolarization	Analgesics, diazepam, intravenous calcium; antivenom if severe*
Brown recluse	Fiddle shape over cephalothorax; lives in dark, indoor dry areas; necrotic painful, pruritic skin lesion; vesiculation, hemorrhage, and eschar formation; hemolysis, DIC, headache, seizures	Sphingomyelinase, protease, esterase, hyaluronidase, hemolysin	Wound débridement; ice; Dapsone; steroids(?)
Tarantula	Local pain, swelling, urticaria from hairs; usually benign	Polyamines, hyaluronidase	Analgesics, ice; remove hair with tape
Marine Envenomation			
Stingray	Defensive attack; laceration, puncture plus venom; pain, edema, bleeding, limb paralysis	Serotonin, phosphodiesterase	Antivenom, hot water immersion, surgical wound exploration
Jellyfish, Portuguese man-of-war	Burning, painful urticaria, pain, lymphadenopathy, anaphylaxis, fever, chills, muscle spasm, paralysis, hypotension	Bradykinin, histamine, hyaluronidase, phosphodiesterase	Remove tentacles, avoid fresh water; topical vinegar, corticosteroids, papain, isopropyl alcohol; calcium IV
Reptiles			
Gila monster	Local pain, edema, cyanosis, hypotension; animal jaws may clamp around the wound	Serotonin, phospholipase, protease, hyaluronidase	Analgesics, ice, immobilization; remove reptile
Toads	Salivation, cyanosis; seizures from placing toads in mouth	Bufotoxin	Supportive care
Mammals			
Humans	Directly from a bite or indirectly from a fist fight; laceration, swelling, erythema, cellulitis	*Eikenella corrodens, Streptococcus aureus,* streptococcal species	Débridement; tetanus check†; augmentin, nafcillin
Dogs	Swelling, erythema, cellulitis, lymphangitis; laceration, crush injury, tenosynovitis	*S. aureus,* streptococci; rabies	Débridement; tetanus check†; antibiotics per culture; rabies check
Cats	Laceration, swelling, cellulitis, osteomyelitis, tenosynovitis	*Pasteurella multocida, S. aureus,* streptococci; rabies	As for dogs; penicillin/ampicillin for *P. multocida*
Rats	Local pain, inflammation (common); rat bite fever (rare) with chills, fever, leukocytosis, rash, arthritis, abscesses, endocarditis, may relapse *(Streptobacillus moniliformis); Spirillum minus* produces suppurative bite lesion	Skin, mouth flora; no rabies; *Streptobacillus moniliformis; Spirillum minus;* plague, leptospirosis	Penicillin for rat bite fever
Raccoons, skunks, foxes	Laceration, pain, swelling	Rabies, plus mouth and skin flora	Rabies vaccine and rabies immunoglobulin; tetanus check†

* Types of antivenom that are prepared in animals (horse, goat) as hyperimmune serum and as foreign proteins may cause anaphylaxis.
† Tetanus check for all animal bites includes evaluation for need of tetanus immune globulin and booster vaccine.
‡ Antibiotics to treat human cutaneous and animal mouth flora.
DEET = diethyltoluamide; DIC = disseminated intravascular coagulation; ? = Effect unproved.
(Data from Banner W: Bites and stings in the pediatric patient. Curr Probl Pediatr 28:1, 1988; Auerbach PS: Marine environments. N Engl J Med 325:486, 1991; Gentile DA, Kennedy BC: Wilderness medicine for children. Pediatrics 88:967, 1991.)

with significant toxicity. Plasma levels of tricyclic antidepressants greater than 1000 ng/mL usually indicate a serious ingestion. The timing of the physician's testing of the plasma level relative to the time of the patient's ingesting the drug also is useful in predicting the severity of illness for acetaminophen (Fig. 3–3) and salicylate (Fig. 3–4). Patients with drug levels (related to the time after ingestion) in the serious zone warrant immediate treatment.

PREVENTING INGESTIONS

Most ingestions occur in the home, and the toxins involved are common household medications, household cleaning and work solutions, or vitamins. Accidental poisonings are more frequent in children under 5 yr of age, in boys, in families of low socioeconomic status, and during times of family disorganization; they occur most frequently in the kitchen, bathroom, or garage. Properly educating parents to use childproof medication containers, to store toxic substances in locked cabinets, and to label toxic chemicals properly is necessary for preventing ingestions. Kerosene and other toxic liquids should not be stored in soda pop bottles, and children should not come in contact with clothing exposed to pesticides. Old or unused medications should be discarded, and currently used medications should not be left on tabletops or in the mother's purse. If a child has ingested poison, the Poison Control Center should be called. All households should have 30 mL of syrup of ipecac available and ready to administer as directed by the Poison Center personnel or the physician.

Bites, Stings, and Envenomations

Toxic reactions to saliva or venom of living creatures or injuries caused by them are common and depend on exposure, provocation, and the species of specific indigenous insects or animals, or those encountered during travel. Most reactions produce local inflammation, with little progression or systemic manifestations. Some reactions may represent allergic responses to insect antigens (papular urticaria), whereas others may result in tissue necrosis, infection, paralysis, and death (Table 3–19).

References

Behrman RE (ed): Nelson Textbook of Pediatrics. 14th ed. Philadelphia, WB Saunders, 1992, Sec. 26.2–26.19.
Fine JS, Goldfrank LR: Update in medical toxicology. Pediatr Clin North Am 39:1031, 1992.

Kulig K: Initial management of ingestions of toxic substances. N Engl J Med 326:1677, 1992.
Litovitz T, Manoguerra A: Comparison of pediatric poisoning hazards: An analysis of 3.8 million exposure incidents. Pediatrics 89:999, 1992.
Vale JA, Proudfoot AT: How useful is activated charcoal? BMJ 306:78, 1993.

SHOCK

Shock may result from a number of relatively common childhood disorders, including gastroenteritis, diabetes, mellitus, trauma, infection, and accidental drug ingestion. The best opportunity to improve the clinical outcome of shock depends on early recognition and prompt, appropriate treatment.

Oxygen delivery is directly related to the arterial oxygen content (oxygen saturation, hemoglobin concentration) and cardiac output (Fig. 3–5). Changes in metabolic needs are met primarily by adjustments in cardiac output, which are determined by the amount of blood ejected from the left ventricle (stroke volume) and by the heart rate. Stroke volume is related to myocardial end-diastolic fiber length (preload), myocardial contractility (inotropy), and resistance of blood ejection from the ventricle (afterload) (see Chapter 13). In the young infant whose myocardium possesses relatively less contractile tissue, increased demand for cardiac output is met primarily by a neurally mediated increase in heart rate. In the older child and adult, cardiac output is most efficiently augmented by increasing stroke volume through neurohumorally mediated changes in vascular tone, resulting in increased venous return to the heart (increased preload), decreased arterial resistance (decreased afterload), and increased myocardial contractility.

Shock Syndromes (Table 3–20, Fig. 3–6)

HYPOVOLEMIC SHOCK

Acute hypovolemia is the most common cause of shock in pediatric patients and results from blood loss, from fluid and electrolyte depletion secondary to vomiting and diarrhea, from third space fluid losses due to capillary leak syndromes, and from pathologic renal fluid losses (Table 3–20). Hypovolemic shock is distinguished from other causes of shock by the presence of hypotension and tachycardia without signs of heart failure (such as hepatomegaly, rales, edema, jugular venous distention, or a gallop) or of sepsis (fever, leukocytosis, or focal

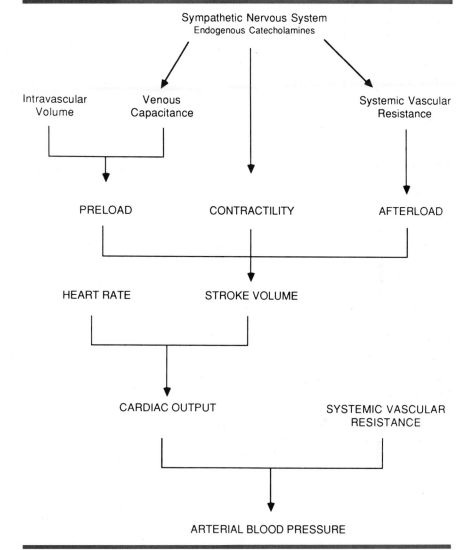

Figure 3–5. Determinants of cardiac output and arterial blood pressure. (From Witte MK, Hill JH, Blumer JL: Shock in the pediatric patient. Adv Pediatr 34:139–174, 1987. Reproduced with permission.)

infection). Reduced blood volume produces a decreased preload, stroke volume, and cardiac output. Recovery depends on the degree of hypovolemia and on the patient's pre-existing status; the prognosis is good, with a low mortality (<10%) in uncomplicated cases.

Compensatory mechanisms include increased sympathoadrenal activity, which produces increased heart rate and myocardial contractility. Neurohumorally mediated constriction of the arterioles and capacitance vessels also maintains blood pressure, augments venous return to the heart to improve preload, and redistributes blood flow from nonvital to vital organs. Increased heart rate may impair coronary blood flow and ventricular filling; elevated systemic vascular resistance increases myocardial oxygen consumption, resulting in poorer myocardial function. Intense systemic vasoconstriction and hypovolemia produce tissue ischemia, which impairs cell metabolism and releases potent vasoactive mediators from injured cells. The latter include arachidonic acid metabolites and vasoactive peptides, which change myocardial contractility, vascular tone, and membrane permeability.

DISTRIBUTIVE SHOCK

Abnormalities in the distribution of blood flow may result in profound inadequacies in tissue perfusion, even in the presence of a normal or high cardiac output. These maldistributions of flow usu-

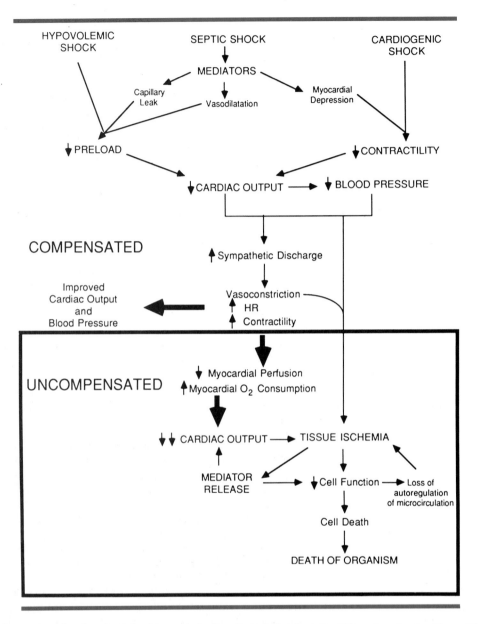

Figure 3–6. Sequence of pathophysiologic events in the clinical shock state. HR = heart rate. (From Witte MK, Hill JH, Blumer JL: Shock in the pediatric patient. Adv Pediatr 34:139–174, 1987. Reproduced with permission.)

ally result from abnormalities in vascular tone. *Septic shock* is the most common type of distributive shock in children, and it is commonly a complication of sepsis caused by gram-positive and gram-negative bacteria, as well as infection due to rickettsiae and viruses (Table 3–21, Fig. 3–7). Patients usually have fever, lethargy, petechiae or purpura, and an identified infectious focus. They often have tachycardia and poor peripheral perfusion, with cool, mottled extremities and poor capillary refill time. Hypotension, intense vasoconstriction, and a decreased cardiac index are present. Widespread cellular dysfunction, resulting from inadequate tissue perfusion in the early phases of shock, subsequently leads to diminishing organ function. In the early stages of shock, patients may be febrile and tachycardiac, with warm, flushed skin and poor urine output ("warm shock"). Systemic arterial blood pressure is normal, and cardiac output is normal or increased. The diagnosis of warm shock re-

Table 3–20. Classification of Shock and Common Underlying Causes

Type	Primary Circulatory Derangement	Common Causes
Hypovolemic	Decreased circulating blood volume	Hemorrhage Diarrhea Diabetes insipidus Diabetes mellitus Burns Adrenogenital syndrome Capillary leak syndrome
Distributive	Vasodilation → venous pooling → decreased preload Maldistribution of regional blood flow	Sepsis Anaphylaxis CNS/spinal injury Drug intoxication
Cardiogenic	Decreased myocardial contractility	Congenital heart disease Severe heart failure Arrhythmia Hypoxic/ischemic injuries Cardiomyopathy Metabolic derangements Myocarditis Drug intoxication Kawasaki disease
Obstructive	Mechanical obstruction to ventricular outflow	Cardiac tamponade Massive pulmonary embolus Tension pneumothorax Cardiac tumor
Dissociative	Oxygen not released from hemoglobin	Carbon monoxide poisoning Methemoglobinemia

CNS = central nervous system.

quires a high index of suspicion on the part of the physician and usually is made in the setting of an obvious predisposing condition, such as a known infection or immunosuppression (see Chapter 10).

In the systemic inflammatory response syndrome (Table 3–21, Fig. 3–7), bacterial products stimulate the elaboration of a wide variety of mediators. Endotoxins are bacterial cell wall lipopoly-

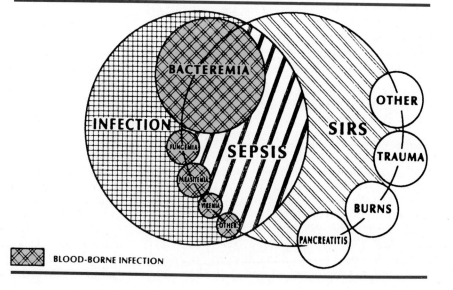

Figure 3–7. Interrelationship between various host responses to infections and other potential inflammatory injuries (burns, trauma). The systemic inflammatory response syndrome (SIRS) may be initiated by multiple inciting events; the inflammatory mediators released by these events initiate and perpetuate the SIRS. (American College of Chest Physicians/Society of Critical Care Medicine Consensus conference: Definitions for sepsis and organ failure and guidelines for the use of innovative therapies in sepsis. Crit Care Med 20:864, 1992.)

Table 3–21. Definitions of Related Infectious and Shock States

Infection: Microbial phenomenon characterized by an inflammatory response to the presence of microorganisms or the invasion of normally sterile host tissue by those organisms

Bacteremia: The presence of viable bacteria in the blood

Systemic Inflammatory Response Syndrome: The systemic inflammatory response to a variety of severe clinical insults. The response is manifested by two or more of the following conditions:
    Temperature >38°C or <36°C
    Heart rate >90 beats/min
    Respiratory rate >20 breaths/min or $Paco_2$ <32 torr (<4.3 kPa)
    WBC >12,000 cells/mm³, <4000 cells/mm³, or >10% immature (band) forms

Sepsis: The systemic response to infection. This systemic response is manifested by two or more of the following conditions as a result of infection:
    Temperature >38°C or <36°C
    Heart rate >90 beats/min
    Respiratory rate >20 breaths/min or $Paco_2$ <32 torr (<4.3 kPa)
    WBC >12,000 cells/mm³, <4000 cells/mm³, or >10% immature (band) forms

Severe Sepsis: Sepsis associated with organ dysfunction, hypoperfusion, or hypotension. Hypoperfusion and perfusion abnormalities may include, but are not limited to, lactic acidosis, oliguria, or an acute alteration in mental status

Septic Shock: Sepsis with hypotension, despite adequate fluid resuscitation, along with the presence of perfusion abnormalities that may include, but are not limited to, lactic acidosis, oliguria, or an acute alteration in mental status. Patients who are on inotropic or vasopressor agents may not be hypotensive at the time that perfusion abnormalities are measured

Hypotension: A systolic BP of <90 mm Hg* or a reduction of >40 mm Hg from baseline in the absence of other causes for hypotension

Multiple Organ Dysfunction Syndrome: Presence of altered organ function in an acutely ill patient such that homeostasis cannot be maintained without intervention

  * Adults.
  BP = blood pressure.
  (American College of Chest Physicians/Society of Critical Care Medicine Consensus conference: Definitions for sepsis and organ failure and guidelines for the use of innovative therapies in sepsis. Crit Care Med 20:864, 1992.)

saccharides that activate macrophage production of tumor necrosis factor (TNF) and interleukin-1 in addition to the complement, kinin, fibrinolytic, and coagulation pathways and result in the release of cellular histamine and prostaglandins. Additional inflammatory mediators include cytokines (interleukin-6), bioactive lipids (platelet-activating factor, leukotrienes), interferons, and the products of primary and secondary leukocyte granules. Direct injection of TNF produces cardiovascular, inflammatory, metabolic, hematologic, pulmonary, and renal abnormalities identical to those that occur in septic shock. The effect of TNF is blocked by neutralizing antibodies to TNF and only partially blocked by inhibition of prostaglandin synthesis. Most second mediators decrease vascular tone and increase vascular permeability, resulting in the maldistribution of blood flow. Arteriolar vasodilation (vasculopathy) results in reduced systemic vascular resistance, which serves to lower tissue perfusion pressure and impair coronary blood flow. The increased venous capacitance produced by venodilation results in venous stasis and decreased venous return to the heart. Mediator-induced changes in vascular permeability cause capillary leaks and loss of intravascular volume, which impair ventricular filling and thus cardiac output. Activated complement components and arachidonic acid metabolites promote leukocyte and platelet aggregation in capillary beds, producing obstruction to flow in the microcirculation. Vasculotoxins also directly depress cardiac output by decreasing intrinsic cardiac contractility or by inducing coronary vasospasm.

CARDIOGENIC SHOCK

This type of shock is due to an abnormality in myocardial function and is expressed as depressed myocardial contractility and cardiac output and poor tissue perfusion. Primary cardiogenic shock occurs in children having congenital heart disease. For example, infants who have shock due to ductal-dependent congenital heart disease are seen in the 1st mo of life after the ductus arteriosus closes. Heart failure precedes cardiogenic shock in most patients who have congenital heart disease (except hypoplastic left heart syndrome) and in those who have circulatory obstruction (e.g., coarctation of the aorta, critical pulmonary stenosis; see Chapter 13).

In cardiogenic shock, compensatory mechanisms may contribute to the progression of shock by further depressing cardiac function. Neurohumoral vasoconstrictor responses increase afterload and add to the work of the failing ventricle. Tachycardia impairs coronary blood flow and decreases myocardial oxygen delivery. Increased central blood volume caused by sodium and water retention and by incomplete emptying of the ventricles during systole results in elevated left ventricular volume and pressure, which impair subendocardial blood flow. Because of this self-perpetuating cycle, congestive heart failure progressing to death may be rapid. As compensatory mechanisms are overcome, the failing left ventricle produces increased ventricular end-diastolic volume and pressure, which leads to increased left atrial pressure, resulting in pulmonary edema. This sequence also contributes to right ventricular failure because of increased pulmonary artery pressure and increased right ventricular afterload. The liver usually enlarges, a gallop is present, and jugular venous distention may be noted. The spleen also may be enlarged. Because renal blood flow is poor, sodium and water are retained, contributing to the formation of peripheral edema. Generally, *treatment* of this kind of shock requires cardiotonic supportive drugs and diuretics to control the pulmonary edema. In cardiogenic shock that develops in infants and children with underlying cardiovascular disease, the *prognosis* is poor.

Cardiogenic shock also may occur in previously healthy children following a hypoxic–ischemic injury. In this circumstance, shock may be reversed by administering cardiotonic drugs.

OBSTRUCTIVE SHOCK

Obstructive shock results from the patient's inability to produce adequate cardiac output, despite normal intravascular volume and normal myocardial contractility, because the ventricular outflow is mechanically obstructed; the major cause of the obstruction is pericardial tamponade. Clinically, tamponade should be suspected in the setting of trauma or previous heart surgery whenever a patient has a narrow pulse pressure, a muffled heart tone, an enlarged heart as determined by percussion or roentgenogram, or electromechanical dissociation. Echocardiography may be diagnostic, but attempts at needle aspiration should not be delayed. The *treatment* is to clear the obstruction by performing emergency needle aspiration of the pericardial space.

DISSOCIATIVE SHOCK

This term describes conditions in which tissue perfusion is normal but oxygen cannot be utilized by the cells because the hemoglobin has an abnormal affinity for oxygen, preventing its release to the tissues (see Table 3–20).

Therapy for Shock

GENERAL PRINCIPLES

The key to therapy is the *recognition of shock* in its early state, when many of the hemodynamic and metabolic alterations may be reversible. Therapy for shock is directed largely at treating the signs and symptoms as they appear, rather than directly addressing the primary cause or mechanisms involved.

Therapy should minimize cardiopulmonary work while ensuring cardiac output, blood pressure, and gas exchange. Intubation plus mechanical ventilation improves oxygenation and decreases or eliminates work of breathing but may impede venous return if distending airway pressures (positive end-expiratory pressure, peak inspiratory pressure; see Chapter 6) are excessive. Blood pressure support is critical because the vasodilation in sepsis may reduce perfusion despite supranormal cardiac output.

Monitoring a child in shock or in impending shock requires maintaining access to the central venous circulation to record pressure measurements, to perform blood sampling, and to measure systemic blood pressure continuously through an indwelling arterial catheter. These measurements facilitate the estimation of preload and afterload. When it is critical to know the patient's left atrial pressure, it can be measured through a left atrial catheter connected to a pressure monitor or estimated by measuring pulmonary capillary wedge pressure by using a flow-directed balloon tip catheter. Directly measuring the cardiac index by thermodilution, injection of indocyanine green, or a Fick procedure also may be helpful. In addition, the management of shock requires monitoring arterial blood gases for oxygenation, ventilation (CO_2), and acidosis and frequently assessing sodium, potassium, calcium, magnesium, phosphorus, and blood urea nitrogen.

ORGAN-DIRECTED THERAPEUTICS

Cardiovascular Support

In general, shock states are characterized by some form of primary or secondary impairment of myocardial function. Therefore, efforts to improve cardiac output are a basic component of shock therapy. Cardiovascular therapy should be targeted at fluid resuscitation and improvement of myocardial output, heart rate and rhythm, preload, afterload, and contractility.

Fluid Resuscitation

Alterations in preload dramatically affect cardiac output. In hypovolemic and distributive shock, decreased preload significantly impairs cardiac output. However, in cardiogenic shock, an elevated preload contributes to pulmonary edema. Table 3–22 lists fluids available for volume resuscitation. Plasma volume may be restored successfully by using crystalloid solutions, provided that sufficient volumes are employed, but edema fluid may accumulate (as a result of capillary leakage) if excessive amounts are infused. This accumulation may be unavoidable but nonetheless may be associated with a good outcome. Colloids contain larger molecules that theoretically may stay in the intravascular space longer than crystalloid solutions, and thus colloids exert oncotic pressure and draw fluid out of the tissues into the vascular compartment.

Selecting fluids for resuscitation and for ongoing use is dictated by the clinical circumstances. Crystalloid volume expanders may be recommended as initial choices because they are effective and inexpensive. However, care must be exercised in treating cardiogenic shock with volume expansion, because the ventricular filling pressures may rise without improvement of the cardiac performance. Carefully monitoring cardiac output or central venous pressure helps guide safe volume replacement. In patients with significant cerebral edema, the need to improve cardiac output by fluid replacement should be balanced by the requirement to reduce intracranial pressure with the need to maintain an acceptable cerebral perfusion pressure

Table 3–22. Intravenous Fluids Available for Pediatric Volume Resuscitation

Crystalloids	Colloids
0.9% sodium chloride	5% human serum albumin in 0.9% sodium chloride
Ringer lactate	
Hypertonic saline (3%)	25% human serum albumin in 0.9% sodium chloride
	6% hydroxyethyl starch in 0.9% sodium chloride
	10% dextran 40 in 5% dextrose in water
	Fresh frozen plasma
	Whole blood

(mean blood pressure − intracranial pressure); intensive fluid resuscitation may increase intracranial pressure, exacerbating cerebral edema. Restoration of blood pressure and cardiac output have the highest priority in this situation.

Cardiotonic and Vasodilator Therapy

In an effort to improve cardiac output after volume resuscitation or when further volume replacement may be dangerous, a variety of cardiotonic and vasodilator drugs may be useful. Therapy is directed toward increasing myocardial contractility and decreasing left ventricular afterload, respectively. Currently, five sympathomimetic agents are available (Table 3–23), but the hemodynamic status of the patient dictates the choice of the agent.

Therapy usually is initiated with dopamine or dobutamine. Combinations of these agents are highly effective. In children who fail to respond to several increases in either the dopamine or dobutamine infusion rate, a more potent cardiotonic agent, such as epinephrine or norepinephrine, may be indicated.

In addition to the catecholamines, which may directly act on the heart to improve contractility, a group of vasodilator drugs is available that may improve cardiac performance by decreasing the resistance against which the heart must pump (i.e., they may decrease afterload). The greatest clinical experience has been with nitroprusside and nitroglycerine. Afterload reduction also occurs with dobutamine, isoproterenol, amrinone, and angiotensin-converting enzyme inhibitors. The use of these drugs may be particularly important in late shock, when vasoconstriction is prominent.

RESPIRATORY SUPPORT

The lung is a target organ for inflammatory mediators in shock and the systemic inflammatory response syndrome. Respiratory failure may develop rapidly and become progressive. Intervention requires endotracheal intubation and mechanical ventilation accompanied by the use of supplemental oxygen and positive end-expiratory pressure (PEEP). The *adult respiratory distress syndrome* may occur in children who are in shock (see Chapter 12). The mechanism underlying this syndrome is increased vascular permeability (noncardiogenic pulmonary edema) from the release of mediators. Vascular permeability, which results from direct damage to the alveolar–capillary endothelium, with leakage of proteaceous fluid into the interstitium and alveoli, may interfere with surfactant ac-

Table 3–23. Catecholamines Used for Cardiopulmonary Resuscitation

	Positive Inotrope	Positive Chronotrope	Direct Pressor	Indirect Pressor	Vasodilator
Dopamine	+ +	+	+/−	+ +	+ +*
Dobutamine	+ +	+/−	−	−	+
Epinephrine	+ + +	+ + +	+ + +	−	−
Isoproterenol	+ + +	+ + +	−	−	+ + +
Norepinephrine	+ + +	+ + +	+ + +	−	−

* Primarily splanchnic and renal in low doses (3–5 µg/kg/min).

tion and is treated with diuretics, cardiotonics, combinations of a diuretic and a colloid, and PEEP to prevent atelectasis and pulmonary edema. Severe cardiopulmonary failure may be managed with extracorporeal membrane oxygenation (ECMO; see Chapter 6).

RENAL SALVAGE

Poor urine output during shock may be due to acute tubular necrosis or to prerenal factors. Hypotension associated with shock may lead to acute renal failure. Prerenal azotemia may be due to poor cardiac output accompanied by decreased renal blood flow; however, severe hypotension may produce acute tubular necrosis (ATN). The former is corrected when blood volume deficits are replaced or myocardial contractility is improved, but ATN does not improve immediately once shock is corrected. Prerenal azotemia is associated with a serum blood urea nitrogen–creatinine ratio of greater than 10:1 and a urine sodium level below 20 mEq/L; ATN has a ratio of 10:1 and a urine sodium level of between 40 and 60 mEq/L (see Chapter 16). Aggressive fluid replacement often is necessary to improve oliguria associated with prerenal azotemia. Because the management of shock requires administering large volumes of fluid (often >50 mL/kg during resuscitation), maintaining urine output greatly facilitates patient management. Preventing ATN and the subsequent complications associated with acute renal failure (e.g., hyperkalemia, acidosis, hypocalcemia, edema) or treating electrolyte imbalances or ATN with continuous arteriovenous hemofiltration or conventional peritoneal and hemodialysis are of paramount importance. Thus, using pharmacologic agents to augment urine output is indicated once the intravascular volume has been replaced. The use of loop diuretics, such as furosemide and bumetanide, mannitol, or combinations of a loop diuretic and a thiazide may enhance urine output. Infusing doses of dopamine, which produce renal artery vasodila-

tion, also may improve urine output. Nevertheless, should hyperkalemia, refractory acidosis, hypervolemia, or the altered mental status associated with uremia occur, dialysis should be initiated. ATN is a self-limited condition that requires good supportive care to avoid potential complications until renal function improves, usually 3–7 days after the renal tubular injury.

References

Behrman RE (ed): Nelson Textbook of Pediatrics. 14th ed. Philadelphia, WB Saunders, 1992, Sec. 633–6.34, 12.14, 15.74.

Bone R: Toward an epidemiology and natural history of SIRS (systemic inflammatory response syndrome). JAMA 268:3452, 1992.

Carcillo J, Davis A, Zaritsky A: Role of early fluid resuscitation in pediatric shock. JAMA 266:1242, 1991.

Huskisson L: Intravenous volume replacement: Which and why? Arch Dis Child 67:649, 1992.

Ognibene F, Cunnion R: Mechanisms of myocardial depression in sepsis. Crit Care Med 21:6, 1993.

Witte MK, Hill JH, Blumer JL: Shock in the pediatric patient. Adv Pediatr 34:139–174, 1987.

Ziegler E: Tumor necrosis factor in humans. N Engl J Med 318:1533–1535, 1988.

CARDIOPULMONARY RESUSCITATION

Cardiopulmonary resuscitation rarely is needed in pediatric practice, and most infants and children who do need CPR have had an isolated respiratory arrest. Nevertheless, the ability to anticipate the need and thus recognize the child at risk for cardiopulmonary arrest and to initiate prompt and appropriate therapy for both cardiac and pulmonary complications may not only save the child's life but also preserve the quality of that sustained life.

Hypoxia plays a central role in most of the potential events leading to cardiopulmonary arrest in children. Furthermore, the presence of hypoxia leads to subsequent organ dysfunction or to ischemic damage, no matter what underlying illness affects the child. Hypoxia may be acute or chronic and may result from either an acquired or a congenital illness. In some children, abnormal pulmonary vasculature or congenital heart disease, leading to right-to-left shunting, contributes to tenuous oxygenation. Physicians should be acutely aware of the potential damage that hypoxia and the resulting ischemia may produce in susceptible organs (Table 3–24) so that their approach to an infant or a child experiencing cardiopulmonary arrest extends beyond CPR to include efforts to preserve vital organ function.

The goal in resuscitating the pediatric patient who has sustained a cardiopulmonary arrest should be to optimize cardiac output and tissue oxygen delivery, which may be accomplished by using artificial ventilation and chest compression, and the judicious administration of pharmacologic agents.

Pediatric and adult cardiopulmonary arrests are different in one important aspect: adult arrests tend to be sudden in onset, and asystole usually precedes respiratory arrest, whereas the child may go through a series of physiologic changes prior to the onset of asystole, and most often respiration ceases before or concurrently with the cardiopulmonary arrest. Therefore, a child who is at risk may be identified prior to the occurrence of cardiopulmonary arrest (Table 3–25); respiratory arrest may be anticipated and interventions started before asystole occurs.

Table 3–24. Target Organs for Hypoxic–Ischemic Damage

Organ	Effect
Brain	Seizures, cerebral edema, infarction, anoxic damage, SIADH, diabetes insipidus
Heart	Heart failure, myocardial infarct, tricuspid insufficiency
Lung and pulmonary vasculature	Adult respiratory distress syndrome
Liver	Infarction, necrosis, cholestasis
Kidney	Acute tubular necrosis, acute cortical necrosis
GI tract	Gastric ulceration, mucosal damage
Hematologic	Disseminated intravascular coagulation, symmetric, peripheral gangrene

GI = gastrointestinal; SIADH = syndrome of inappropriate secretion of antidiuretic hormone.

Table 3–25. Warning Signs and Symptoms Suggesting the Potential Need for Resuscitative Intervention*

CNS	Lethargy, irritability, obtundation, confusion
Respiratory	Apnea, grunting, nasal flaring, retracting, tachypnea, poor air movement
Cardiovascular	Arrhythmia, bradycardia, tachycardia, weak pulses, poor capillary refill, hypotension
Skin and mucous membranes	Mottling, pallor, cyanosis, diaphoresis, poor membrane turgor, dry mucous membranes

* One would seldom act if only one or two of these signs and symptoms were present, but the occurrence of several in concert foreshadows grave consequences. Intervention should be directed at the primary disorder.
CNS = central nervous system.

Airway

On recognizing that a clinical situation requiring resuscitation exists, the physician should first make sure that there is a patent airway, then should initiate means to *examine, monitor, intervene,* and *anticipate* in response to the situation. In children, airway patency often is compromised by a loss of muscle tone, allowing the mandibular block of tissue, including the tongue, the bony mandible, and the soft surrounding tissues, to rest against the posterior pharyngeal wall. In adult patients, such problems can be corrected by using manual head tilt maneuvers, but in infants and young children, this correction may result in the excessive overextension of the neck and further narrowing of the tracheal airway.

Pediatric patients requiring resuscitation should be endotracheally intubated. Once the endotracheal tube is in place, the child must be assessed again for breathing, which requires not only assessing respiratory movements but also performing auscultations of the trachea and chest to detect bilateral and symmetric breath sounds. If air exchange is not heard or cyanosis continues, then the position of the tube must be re-evaluated.

Breathing

The major role of endotracheal intubation is to ensure the delivery of adequate oxygen to the patient. Because hypoxemia is the final common pathway in pediatric arrests, providing oxygen is more important than correcting the respiratory acidosis that also develops. Thus, 100% oxygen, at a rate of 20 breaths/min, should be delivered through the tube using a tidal volume necessary to produce adequate chest rise and relieve cyanosis; this is usually equal to 10–15 mL/kg of body weight.

Once a patent airway is established and oxygenation and ventilation are maintained, many children will re-establish cardiac output. Thus, carefully reassessing the patient before proceeding with other mechanical and pharmacologic maneuvers is essential. This evaluation should include observing the color of the skin and mucous membranes and palpating both central and peripheral pulses. If cyanosis persists or the brachial or femoral pulses remain weak or absent, adequate circulation has not been re-established.

Circulation

A cardiac compression/respiratory ventilation ratio of 5:1 is optimal. Compressions usually are given between ventilations (e.g., at end expiration). The compression rate is 100/min.

Drugs (Table 3–26)

When mechanical means fail to re-establish adequate circulation, pharmacologic intervention is essential. Drug therapy during CPR is directed toward improving cardiac output and the delivery of oxygen to tissues. The special requirements of drugs used during CPR limit the number of potential routes for their administration. Administration through a central venous line is preferred. The effectiveness of peripheral intravenous administration is limited by poor circulation. Alternative routes for administration of some drugs are through the endotracheal tube or by intramedullary (bone marrow) infusion.

Table 3–26. Drug Doses for Cardiopulmonary Resuscitation

Drug	Indication	Dose
Adenosine	Supraventricular tachycardia	0.1–0.2 mg/kg; maximum 12 mg
Atropine	Supraventricular or junctional bradycardia Asystole?	0.02 mg/kg/dose (minimum dose 0.1 mg); up to 0.5 mg (child), 1.0 mg (adolescent); higher doses needed in anticholinesterase poisoning
Bicarbonate	Metabolic acidosis? Hyperkalemia	0.5–1 mEq/kg bolus, if metabolic acidosis present; ensure adequate ventilation
Bretylium	Ventricular tachycardia	5 mg/kg IV bolus; may repeat; may cause hypotension
Calcium	Hypocalcemia Hyperkalemia Wide QRS pattern?	25 mg/kg calcium chloride; stop if bradycardia occurs
Dobutamine	Inotropy	2–30 μg/kg/min
Dopamine	Inotropy Renal preservation	0.5–2 μg/kg/min splanchnic, renal dilation; 2–7 μg/kg/min inotrope; 7–20 μg/kg/min inotrope + pressor
Epinephrine	Chronotropy Inotropy Hypotension	0.01 mg/kg bolus; 0.05–2 μg/kg/min drip, inotrope + pressor; 0.1 mg/kg as subsequent doses if 0.01 mg/kg is ineffective; may cause subendocardial ischemia and arrhythmias
Fluid	Hypovolemia Sepsis	Use colloid or crystalloid tailored to patient's physiologic needs
Glucose	Hypoglycemia	2 mL/kg 10% dextrose; follow Dextrostix
Isoproterenol	Chronotropy Inotropy	0.05–1 μg/kg/min inotrope + vasodilator effects; chronotropic response may limit dose; may cause subendocardial ischemia and arrhythmias
Lidocaine	Ventricular tachycardia	1 mg/kg/bolus followed by 20–50 μg/kg/min continuous infusion; monitor serum concentration and widening of QRS for toxicity
Nitroprusside	Reduce systemic vascular resistance Hypertensive crisis	0.05–10.0 μg/kg/min by continuous infusion
Oxygen	Hypoxia	100%, humidified
Phenytoin	Ventricular tachycardia, digitalis-induced arrhythmias	15–20 mg/kg slow loading dose; titrate maintenance therapy to serum concentrations of 15–30 μg/mL

? = Controversial, uncertain, or unproven efficacy.

(Data from Committee on Drugs, AAP: Emergency drug doses for infants and children. Pediatrics 81:462, 1988; Anonymous: Pediatric advanced life support. JAMA 268:2262, 1992.)

Perhaps the most important agent employed during CPR in children is *oxygen*. Whenever possible, 100% oxygen should be administered through an endotracheal tube. Short exposures to high oxygen tensions cause little pulmonary toxicity, and high oxygen tensions may be required to reverse some of the reactive pulmonary vascular responses to poor cardiac output.

The use of buffers is the subject of considerable controversy. *Sodium bicarbonate* is the most commonly used buffer, but its risk may outweigh its potential benefits. One of the hallmarks of poor cardiac output is acidemia. In pediatric patients, however, this acidemia is primarily respiratory rather than metabolic. Judicious use of sodium bicarbonate to correct the metabolic component of the acidosis may be beneficial. However, the use of sodium bicarbonate in an attempt to correct what is primarily a respiratory problem can exacerbate respiratory acidosis by inducing the production of more CO_2. Sodium bicarbonate may produce hypernatremia, hyperosmolality, hypokalemia, metabolic alkalosis (shifting the oxyhemoglobin curve to the left and impairing tissue oxygen delivery), reduced ionized calcium level, and impaired cardiac function.

Catecholamines constitute the mainstay of therapy for CPR. They are administered both as boluses during the acute phases of resuscitation and by continuous infusions during the maintenance therapy involved in postresuscitative stabilization. Epinephrine is the primary agent employed. It is a catecholamine with mixed alpha- and beta-agonist properties. The alpha-adrenergic effects are most important during the acute phases, because of the alpha-induced increase in systemic vascular resistance that results in a greater pressure gradient across the coronary bed and an improved coronary blood flow.

When asystole is converted to ventricular fibrillation by catecholamine treatment, *electrical defibrillation* is indicated (Table 3–27). Bolus administration of lidocaine is recommended prior to defibrillation. Defibrillation should be distinguished from *cardioversion* of supraventricular tachycardias which also may compromise cardiac output. Cardioversion requires a lower starting dose and a synchronization of the discharge to the electrocardiogram to avoid discharging during a susceptible period, which may convert supraventricular tachycardia to ventricular tachycardia or fibrillation.

Table 3–27. Recommendations for Defibrillation and Cardioversion in Children

Defibrillation

Pretreat with 0.01 mg/kg epinephrine (1:10,000) IV

Place saline gauge or conduction jellied pad at apex and upper right sternal border

Use 4.5-cm diameter paddles for infants and 8–10-cm diameter paddles for children

Notify all participating personnel before discharging paddles so that no one is in contact with patient or bed

Begin with 2 W/sec/kg (2 J/kg)

If unsuccessful, double current (4 J/kg) and repeat rapidly ×3

Cardioversion

Determine mechanism of the predominant rhythm

Consider pretreatment with lidocaine, 1 mg/kg IV, for risk of inducing ventricular tachycardia and valium for sedation

For symptomatic supraventricular tachycardia, synchronize signal with electrocardiogram*

Choose paddles, position pads, and notify personnel as above

Begin with 0.5–1 W/sec/kg (J/kg)

If unsuccessful, double the current

* Consider adenosine first (see Table 3–26).

Pediatric CPR requires a careful integration of mechanical skills and pharmacotherapy (see Table 3–26). Intervention should commence in an anticipatory fashion, and the drug doses provided should serve as a guide rather than a limit to therapy. Resuscitative efforts should be directed toward preserving vital organ function and reversing ongoing tissue damage rather than simply starting the heart. This clinical strategy should continue into the postresuscitative period.

References

Anonymous: Neonatal resuscitation. JAMA 268:2276, 1992.

Anonymous: Pediatric advanced life support. JAMA 268:2262, 1992.

Anonymous: Pediatric basic life support. JAMA 268:2251, 1992.

Anonymous: Special resuscitation situations. JAMA 268:2242, 1992.

Behrman RE (ed): Nelson Textbook of Pediatrics. 14th ed. Philadelphia, WB Saunders, 1992, Sec. 6.33, 15.62–15.65.

Committee on Drugs, AAP: Emergency drug doses for infants and children. Pediatrics 81:462, 1988.

Genetic Disorders

4

R. Stephen S. Amato

Thousands of known inherited genetic conditions are found in humans. Genetic conditions are common causes of acute and chronic diseases that occur during fetal life, immediately at birth, or sometime during childhood. Genetic abnormalities may produce congenital malformations (e.g., trisomy 13 and 18), metabolic disturbances (e.g., phenylketonuria, galactosemia), specific organ dysfunction (e.g., mental retardation, congenital heart disease), or abnormalities of sexual differentiation (e.g., Turner syndrome). Approximately 1% of newborn infants will manifest monogenic diseases (e.g., cystic fibrosis, sickle cell anemia), and 0.5% will have chromosomal disorders (e.g., Down syndrome); 1–3% of children have diseases that are multifactorial in pathogenesis (e.g., congenital heart disease, spina bifida). Approximately 40% of childhood deaths are due to genetic disorders and birth defects.

GENE STRUCTURE AND FUNCTION

The human genome consists of approximately 100,000 genes. Each gene is a unique sequence of a deoxyribonucleic acid (DNA) macromolecule, which is arranged as a double-stranded chain of deoxyribose residues linked by complementary base pairs. The purine bases adenine and guanine are paired with hydrogen bonds to the pyrimidine bases thymine and cytosine, respectively. There are about 3 billion of these base pairs in the haploid human genome contained in the 23 chromosomes.

Double-stranded DNA must *replicate* to produce new copies of genetic material for daughter cells. *Transcription* is the process of initiating protein synthesis by reading the DNA and copying the future amino acid sequence encoded in the DNA onto a single strand of messenger ribonucleic acid (mRNA). Mature mRNA from the nucleus then affixes to cytoplasmic ribosomes, where the genetic message is *translated* into a polypeptide chain as amino acids are carried to the ribosome-mRNA

complex by transfer RNAs (tRNA), small RNA molecules that are specific for each amino acid.

Genes or fragments of DNA from specific genes can be cloned in the laboratory. Specific DNA probes can be labeled to identify the gene's DNA. Specific probes or characteristic *restriction fragment length polymorphisms* can be used to identify mutant or absent genes from patients with genetic disorders. A probe is a radioactively labeled single-stranded DNA fragment that selectively binds or hybridizes to complementary DNA of a specific gene, to part of the DNA sequence of a gene, or to parts of the DNA flanking the gene. The patient's DNA fragments are separated by gel electrophoresis. A single-stranded ^{32}P-labeled DNA probe then is hybridized to the patient's DNA. An x-ray plate then is exposed to the gel, which produces an autoradiograph, demonstrating the sites of ^{32}P-DNA binding.

Because each human chromosome has hundreds of thousands of base pairs, smaller workable units must be produced to identify genes. *Restriction endonucleases* are enzymes that recognize specific 4–8 base pair sequences and cleave DNA into smaller fragments at these specific sites. Each of the over 150 endonucleases will produce a reproducible and characteristic fragment pattern, which can be separated by size on an agarose gel. Mutations at the site of cleavage will change the fragmentation pattern, thus producing a restriction fragment length polymorphism. DNA from the agarose gel can be transferred to cellulose nitrate, where single-stranded DNA fragments can hybridize with probe DNA to identify the fragment containing the complementary DNA (cDNA). Hybridization of single-stranded DNA to DNA is called Southern blotting; hybridization of RNA to DNA is Northern blotting. The demonstration of antibody to protein bands is called Western blotting.

The combination of cDNA probes, restriction fragment length polymorphism, and Southern blotting has made it possible to diagnose genetic diseases, to clone genes, to add to our basic understanding of genetic diseases, to offer prenatal diagnoses, and, in the future, to treat certain genetic disorders by replacing the missing normal gene. Small quantities of genomic DNA can be amplified with the *polymerase chain reaction* (PCR). The PCR is a powerful tool for making many copies of a DNA or RNA segment, which simplifies subsequent analysis.

INHERITED CONDITIONS

Three basic mechanisms of inheritance exist for single-gene conditions. The three methods of human inheritance are dominant, recessive, and sex- or X-linked. Except for genes on the X and Y chromosomes in males, all genes are duplicated in a normal diploid individual. If a single copy of the gene (a single allele) has a detectable effect when present, the condition is said to be *dominant*. If the effect of the allele is inapparent when only one allele is present and is expressed if two identical alleles are present, the condition is described as *recessive*. If an individual has two identical alleles, the person is said to be homozygous for the gene. If an individual has two different alleles, the person is heterozygous for the gene in question. The effects of recessive conditions are observed only in homozygous persons, whereas the effects of dominant conditions are observed in the heterozygous individual. A person who is heterozygous for a hidden recessive allele is described as a *carrier*.

X-linked inheritance is a variation of dominant and recessive inheritance modified by the fact that males have only one X chromosome. Normal XY males will express any genes present on their X chromosome; they are *hemizygous* for genes on the X chromosome. Males also possess a Y chromosome that is passed from father to son (holandric distribution). The Y chromosome is important in determining maleness but appears to do little else.

MENDELIAN INHERITANCE AND CYTOGENETICS

Autosomal Dominant Inheritance

The ability to explain gene inheritance during genetic counseling requires an understanding of how a pattern of inheritance occurs. In autosomal dominant conditions (Table 4–1), if one parent displays a dominant condition and is heterozygous for the gene, each child has a 50% chance of receiving the gene's single allele and also of manifesting the condition. The *major histocompatibility complex* (MHC)

genes illustrate another important type of autosomal dominant inheritance (Fig. 4–1). These genes determine cell surface antigens (proteins) and are located in a cluster close to the middle of the short (p) arm of the number 6 chromosome. Three human leukocyte antigen (HLA) genes in the MHC are designated HLA-A, HLA-B, and HLA-C and code for class MHC proteins located on all nucleated cells and platelets. Each HLA gene has a large number of possible alleles; the alleles are designated by number. An unusual feature of the HLA system is that most of the individual alleles have an effect that can be detected on the leukocyte surface. When the effects of each different allele can be detected, the alleles are called "codominants." In this special case, the appearance of the condition produced by the genes (phenotype) corresponds to the allelic composition (genotype). HLA alleles (haplotypes) of gene A are A1, A2, A3, and so forth, continuing past A32; alleles of gene C are C1 to C8; and alleles of gene B are B1 to B49. The HLA genes A, B, and C are all codominant, so that an individual will have two alleles for each HLA gene site (A,C,B) and, thus, six detectable HLA alleles. (The actual sequence of the genes is A, C, B rather than in alphabetical order.)

Myotonic dystrophy, an autosomal dominant disorder, is unusual because a severe congenital form occurs by transmission from the mother and not the father. In addition, the disease demonstrates *anticipation*, the severity of the disease increases with each subsequent generation. Mutable expansion of a GCT triplet repeat in a 3′ untranslated region of the myotonic protein kinase gene develops with each meiosis (especially maternal), thus explaining the genetic anticipation or increasing severity in the next generation.

Autosomal Recessive Inheritance

In these conditions, the phenotype is expressed when identical alleles are present. For example, located on the distal segment of the q (long) arm of chromosome 12 is a gene for the enzyme phenylalanine hydroxylase. If an individual is homozygous for a gene that codes for an abnormal enzyme (or for a nonfunctional gene product) in this location, that person is not able to convert the essential amino acid phenylalanine to tyrosine. Under these circumstances, excess phenylalanine cannot be metabolized and will accumulate along with phenylalanine metabolic by-products to produce phenylketonuria (PKU). Elevated levels of phenylalanine can be neurotoxic and can lead to mental retardation (see Chapter 5). The risk of two carriers having

Table 4–1. Autosomal Dominant Diseases

	Frequency	Comments
Peutz-Jeghers disease		Mucocutaneous pigment, GI hamartoma
Huntington disease	1:2500	Chromosome 4 (short arm)
Adult polycystic kidney disease	1:1200	Chromosome 16 (short arm)
Neurofibromatosis	1:3000	Chromosome 17, 50% new mutations
Bilateral acoustic neuroma (neurofibromatosis II)	$1:1 \times 10^6$	Chromosome 22 (long arm)
Protein C deficiency	1:15,000	Gene cloned; chromosome 2 (short arm) spontaneous thrombosis
Hereditary angioedema (HANE) Type I (decreased protein) Type II (dysfunctional protein)	1:10,000	Deficiency of C1 esterase inhibitor, chromosome 11, idiomorphic variants
Hereditary hemorrhagic telangiectasia (Osler-Weber-Rendu disease)	1–2:100,000	Angiodysplasia
Myotonic dystrophy	1:25,000	Chromosome 19 (long arm)
Familial retinoblastoma	1:20,000	Multifocal tumor, chromosome 13, gene cloned
von Willebrand disease	1:100	Chromosome 12, male = female incidence
Tuberous sclerosis	1:29,900	Chromosome 19; adenoma sebaceum, seizures, retardation
Gilbert disease		Indirect hyperbilirubinemia
Hereditary spherocytosis	1:5000	Spectrin deficiency, some variants autosomal recessive
Marfan syndrome	1:20,000	Variable penetrance
Achondroplasia	0.5–1.5:10,000	90% new mutations
Alpha-1-antitrypsin deficiency	1:3000	Gene cloned: chromosome 14 cirrhosis, emphysema
Hyperlipidemia	1:500	Possible prevention of heart disease

GI = gastrointestinal.

a child with PKU is 1:4 (25%). Other autosomal recessive conditions are shown in Table 4–2.

Sex-Linked Inheritance

A sex-linked condition occurs when the gene locus appears on the X chromosome. There are many more sex-linked recessive conditions than sex-linked dominant conditions, and for this reason males are subject to a much larger number of inherited disorders than are females (Table 4–3). Hemophilia A, a sex-linked recessive condition, exemplifies this mode of inheritance. The gene for clotting factor VIII is located on the distal q arm of the X chromosome. An absence of normal factor VIII leads to "classic" hemophilia. When the maternal parent is a carrier for hemophilia (factor VIII deficiency), 50% of the male offspring will have hemophilia, and 50% of the female offspring will be carriers like their mothers.

An inspection of the segregation of the sex chromosomes also leads to other important conclusions. The daughters of a man with a sex-linked recessive condition such as hemophilia will all be "obligate carriers" for the condition. A male cannot pass a sex-linked condition to his sons, and, therefore, male-to-male transmission establishes an autosomal pattern of inheritance.

Males with hemophilia can be detected relatively easily, but it is difficult to identify carrier daughters of hemophilia, even using closely linked DNA polymorphisms or gene probes. One reason for the difficulty in detection relates to the very large size of the hemophilia gene; it includes 25 intervening sequences (introns) and 27,000 bases that code for the mRNA. Thus, there is the potential for a great number of deletions and mutations in many areas of the single gene, all leading to the same disease and making it difficult to interpret the results of gene probe tests. A second reason for difficulty in

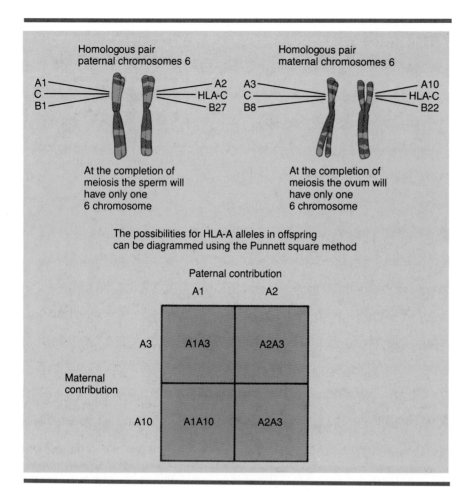

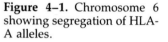

Figure 4–1. Chromosome 6 showing segregation of HLA-A alleles.

Table 4–2. Autosomal Recessive Diseases

	Frequency	Comments
Congenital adrenal hyperplasia (21-hydroxylase)	1:5000–15,000; 1:700 in Yupik Eskimo	Chromosome 6, linked to HLA groups
Phenylketonuria	1:14,000	Gene cloned; chromosome 12
Sickle cell anemia	1:625 in African Americans	Gene cloned; chromosome 11
Cystic fibrosis	1:2000 in whites	Gene cloned; chromosome 7
Gaucher disease	1:2500 in Ashkenazi Jews	Gene cloned; chromosome 1 (long arm)
Tay-Sachs disease	1:3000 in Ashkenazi Jews	Gene cloned; chromosome 15 (long arm)
Galactosemia	1:60,000	Gene cloned; chromosome 9 (short arm)
Infantile polycystic renal failure	1–2:14,000	Renal and hepatic cysts
Wilson disease	1:200,000	Gene cloned; chromosome 13 (long arm)
Fanconi anemia	?	Absent thumb, chromosomal breaks

HLA = human leukocyte antigen.

Table 4–3. X-Linked Recessive Disease

	Frequency	Comments
Lesch-Nyhan syndrome	1:100,000	Hypoxanthine-phosphoribosyl transferase
Ornithine transcarbamoylase deficiency	?	Gene cloned—milder disease in females
Duchenne muscular dystrophy	1:5000	Gene cloned—high spontaneous mutation rate
Hemophilia A + B	1:10,000	Gene cloned; factor replacement needed
Fragile X syndrome	1:2000	25% of mentally retarded males—macrocephaly, macro-orchidism, demonstrates anticipation
Bruton agammaglobulinemia	$1:1 \times 10^5$	Recurrent infections
Chronic granulomatous disease	$1:1 \times 10^6$	Recurrent infections, some variants autosomal recessive
Glucose-6-phosphate dehydrogenase deficiency	10% of American blacks	Oxidant-induced hemolysis
Color blindness	$1:1 \times 10^5$	

establishing the carrier state for sex-linked conditions in females stems from the natural inactivation of one X chromosome in females, a phenomenon called the **Lyon rule** (or Lyon hypothesis).

According to the Lyon rule, early in embryogenesis, one of the two X chromosomes in each cell of a female embryo is randomly inactivated, leaving just one in the active state. All of the subsequent cells developing from this active ancestor have the same active X chromosome. For most of the genes on the X chromosome, females display a phenomenon called *mosaicism*, in which some cells have one X active and other cells have the alternative X active. Therefore, unless there is a test for the presence of the gene itself, tests for sex-linked gene products are very difficult to interpret. In many cells, the inactive X chromosome often can be seen as the Barr body (a clump of heterochromatin) adjacent to the nuclear membrane. There is ordinarily one Barr body for every X chromosome exceeding the active X (normal females who are 46,XX have one Barr body; a female who is 47,XXX would have two Barr bodies).

A SEX-LINKED CONDITION WITH A CYTOGENETIC MARKER

A number of sex-linked conditions lead to mental retardation, and for many years it had been observed that there were many more males with mental retardation than comparably handicapped females. A chromosome marker called the **"fragile X,"** so named for a gap that can be induced on the distal q arm of the X chromosome, is present in many of these males. The condition is characterized by the fragile X marker (enhanced by special treatment of the cells in tissue culture); macro-orchidism in the postpubertal male; disproportionately severe delays in expressive language development; mild to moderate mental retardation; and, in general, a normal appearance, except occasionally for some superficial findings such as prominent ears.

Fragile X is another example of *anticipation*, with mutatable expansion of a CGG triplet repeat. This amplification occurs only during maternal meiosis, thus explaining transmission through carrier mothers and not through an unaffected "carrier" father. Amplification of CGG triplet repeats creates the heritable unstable element of the X chromosome.

Genes and Linkage

Adjacent genes on the same chromosome are likely to be inherited together unless another genetic event separates the genes from each other. In *recombination*, a genetic event that takes place in meiosis, segments of DNA are exchanged (crossing over) in a reciprocal fashion between homologous chromosomes. The chance of this happening generally is proportional to the distance between the loci. The unit that is used to describe the distance between loci is the "centimorgan." A centimorgan does not represent a specific physical distance; rather, it is a number that reflects the chance that recombination will occur between two linked genes. If two loci are separated by 10 centimorgans, recombination between the loci will occur about 10% of the time.

It is possible in a clinical situation to use the concept of linkage to determine genetic composition in a particular individual. If two genes are known to be linked in a given family and one of the genes is linked in a given family and one of the genes is detectable by its normal effect but the other, mutated gene is undetectable, the individual demonstrating that he or she has the linked normal gene might be assumed to have the deleterious one also. The degree of certainty of this assumption depends on the chance that recombination has not occurred between the gene loci.

By employing appropriate methodology using restrictive endonucleases to digest DNA, a mutated gene can be presumed to exist based on identification of the presence of a known closely linked DNA restrictive fragment polymorphism. The degree of certainty still is based on the chance for recombination occurring between the polymorphism and the mutated gene. The use of several closely linked polymorphic DNA fragments, especially those that flank the gene in question, can increase the certainty that recombination has not occurred and that the mutated gene is present. When the actual abnormal DNA sequence responsible for the mutated allele is known (through a probe) and can be tested for directly, there is no uncertainty.

Pedigree Analysis

Constructing a family pedigree is a quick way of surveying family history; the pedigree also helps to analyze the family visually for a specific pattern of inheritance. The conventional symbols used in pedigree construction are shown in Figure 4–2. *Autosomal dominant conditions* should occur in each generation and should not be passed on by individuals who do not manifest the condition (see Table 4–1). (An obvious exception would be an individual in whom there is no detectable expression of the gene, even though the gene is present.) Affected males should approximately equal affected females. An example is a pedigree of three generations affected with neurofibromatosis. Each child has a 50% chance (1:2 will be affected) of receiving the gene, and male-to-male transmission is present, excluding a sex-linked condition.

If a child is affected with a condition that is known to follow a dominant mode of inheritance but no family history can be constructed, several possibilities must be considered: (1) the child represents a new mutation; (2) a parent is affected but the expression cannot be detected; (3) the condition is genetically heterogeneic and in this family it follows another pattern of inheritance, such as an autosomal recessive pattern; (4) this condition is a *phenocopy* with another cause entirely; or (5) an identified parent is not the biologic parent.

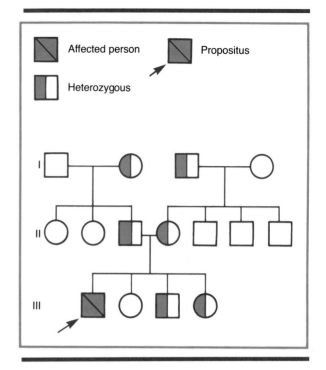

Figure 4–2. A pedigree showing an autosomal recessive pattern of inheritance.

Autosomal recessive conditions typically appear without an antecedent family history. Occasionally, the parents will be consanguineous (parents who have relatively close ancestors in common). Related persons have a greater chance of sharing the same hidden recessive genes than do unrelated persons. If a child is found to have a known autosomal recessive condition, the parents are carriers and the risk of recurrence for each subsequent child is 25%. Figure 4–2 shows a pedigree for autosomal recessive conditions (see Table 4–2).

An exception to the biparental carrier state in instances of autosomal recessive conditions has been discovered. This exception, called "uniparental disomy," must be considered as an occasional mechanism for explaining the occurrence of recessive conditions. In uniparental disomy, two chromosomes of a pair are derived from one parent. The pair of chromosomes are not just homologues but replicates of each other. This virtually ensures that all genes on the chromosomes will be homozygous. If a deleterious gene is present, a recessive condition will occur. (See *Chromosomal Imprinting*)

Sex-linked recessive conditions (Table 4–3) are far more common than sex-linked dominant conditions. Only boys are affected, and transmission is

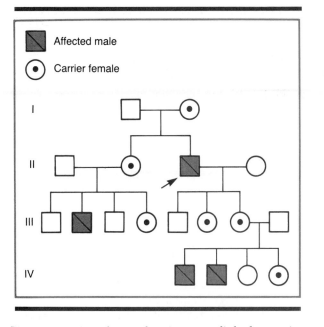

Figure 4–3. A pedigree showing a sex-linked recessive condition.

through the mother, who often has affected male relatives (brothers or maternal uncles). Figure 4–3 shows a typical pedigree.

Multifactorial Inheritance: Conditions with an Empiric Recurrence Risk

For genetic disease inherited by autosomal recessive and by dominant or sex-linkage patterns, the recurrence or inheritance risks are based on classic mendelian genetic laws. There is, however, no definitive genetic explanation for the inheritance of multifactorial genetic conditions. A large number of conditions occurring in children or adults seem to confer an increased risk of also occurring in parents, close relatives, and subsequent generations in the family. In this type of genetic disorder, it is postulated that a spectrum of genes confers a vulnerability for the condition in the individual and that some precipitating environmental factors interact to bring the condition about. By evaluating the reproductive outcomes of many families with similar conditions, a pooled empiric recurrence risk can be calculated. Most multifactorial disorders have a recurrence rate of 4–10%. Some have a sex predilection (e.g., pyloric stenosis in males and congenital dislocated hips in females), whereas others have a racial predilection (e.g., neural tube defects in whites or facial clefts in Orientals).

The *inheritance of birth defects* often is multifacto-

rial. It is likely that the causation of complex birth defects is heterogeneous and the defect may represent a final common pathway with many different causes. Congenital heart anomalies, neural tube defects, and cleft lip and cleft palate have empiric recurrence risks that exceed the general population risk, but the empiric recurrence risk is never as high as the recurrence risk for a classic specific gene disorder. Congenital heart anomalies affect about 5–10 infants per 1000 live births; the empiric recurrence is probably 5–10%. Neural tube defects such as anencephaly and meningomyelocele may affect as few as 1 infant per 1000 live births. There are significant differences in the prevalence of neural tube defects from area to area in the United States and from country to country; the incidence is higher in the United Kingdom and the Republic of Ireland than in the United States. The recurrence risk is 1–5%; however, recurrence risk can be lowered by preconception and early gestation maternal folic acid supplementation.

In evaluating multifactorial genetic conditions, studies of twins may differentiate genetic from environmental factors. If twins have a disorder in common, they are said to be in *concordance* for their disorder; if they differ, they are described as *discordant* for the finding. With multifactorial genetic disorders there is never 100% concordance, even in monozygotic twins (twins resulting from cleavage of a single egg). For example, concordance for all types of facial clefts is only about 33% in monozygotic twins and about 7% in dizygotic twins. Thus, other factors contribute to producing facial clefts.

Some multifactorial genetic diseases are associated with HLA types. Diabetes mellitus is associated with histocompatibility markers DR3 and DR4, whereas ankylosing spondylitis and postvenereal or enteric spondyloarthropathy are associated with HLA B27. Enteric spondyloarthropathy illustrates an interaction of environmental variables with a genetic predisposition to produce specific diseases.

Mitochondrial inheritance is another exception to Mendelian or nuclear inheritance. Many mitochondrial proteins and enzymes are determined by nuclear genes, but some (cytochrome system) are dependent on the mitochondrial chromosome. Mitochondria are derived from the maternal parent exclusively, and mutations in the mitochondrial chromosome can be expected to follow a maternal pattern of inheritance. Therefore, both sexes are equally likely to inherit a mitochondrial mutation; expression may vary depending on environmental and genetic factors. Leber optic neuropathy (sudden adult onset blindness; mtDNA mutation of electron transport); myoclonic epilepsy and ragged red fiber–MERRF (myoclonus, seizures, optic atrophy; mtDNA mutation of transfer RNA genes); mitochondrial myopathy, encephalopathy, lactic acidosis; stroke-like episodes–MELAS (emesis, hemiplegia, cortical blindness; mtDNA mutation of transfer RNA gene); and Kearns-Sayre syndrome (ophthalmoplegia, retinal degeneration, ataxia; mtDNA deletion) are examples of maternal inheritance because of a mitochondrial chromosome mutation.

Cytogenetics

Cytogenetics, the study of chromosome number and morphology, is an important part of the study of human inheritance.

It is possible to analyze the chromosomes of any cell capable of division. In a clinical setting, most cytogenetic analyses are performed using a mitotic-stimulating agent to cause division of peripheral blood lymphocytes placed in a tissue culture medium. Fibroblasts, bone marrow cells, and chorionic villi also can be used. Mitotic cells undergoing division are arrested in metaphase and ruptured, and the chromosomes spread out. Each pair of chromosomes has its own pattern of substructure that is expressed as a sequence of light and dark bands when the chromosomes are stained appropriately. The banding relates to the distribution of repetitive spacer DNA and nonrepetitive genomic DNA. These methods permit the identification of each pair of chromosomes and allow the chromosomes to be studied in detail; over 1000 bands can be detected for the diagnosis of deletions and duplications of parts of chromosomes. Banding techniques vary: Q banding is detected with quinacrine, G banding with Giemsa, and C banding when the centromere region is stained.

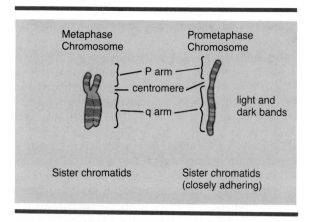

Figure 4–4. Chromosome morphology.

An understanding of cytogenetics and chromosomal abnormalities requires a special vocabulary and technology (Fig. 4–4).

CHROMOSOMAL ABNORMALITIES

Chromosomal abnormalities may arise de novo during gametogenesis, so that an individual can be conceived with a chromosomal abnormality without any prior family history. Chromosomal abnormalities and chromosomal rearrangements also can be present in a parent and passed to an offspring. Sometimes this is associated with a family history of multiple spontaneous abortions or a higher-than-chance frequency of giving birth to children with chromosomal abnormalities. Chromosomal abnormalities or rearrangements also can occur in somatic cells at any time. If they arise early in embryogenesis, they can give rise to a clone that may have adverse consequences for the mosaic individual. Chromosomal alterations that occur later in life also may have adverse consequences on health; a high percentage of malignant neoplasms are associated with chromosomal abnormalities when the constitutional karyotype of the individual is not normal.

Chromosomal abnormalities present at conception often lead to spontaneous abortion; about 50% of first trimester spontaneous abortions are chromosomally abnormal. Even the chromosomal abnormalities that are observed at term, such as trisomy 21 and Turner syndrome (45,X), represent only a fraction of the individuals conceived with these chromosomal problems. In general, abnormalities involving somatic chromosomes have a greater negative impact on the individual than do abnormalities of sex chromosomes.

Indications for obtaining chromosome studies include confirmation of a suspected chromosomal syndrome, multiple organ system malformations, significant developmental delays or mental retardation not otherwise explained, short stature or very delayed menarche in girls, infertility or a history of several spontaneous abortions, ambiguous genitalia, and advanced maternal age (the fetus should be tested). The only way to establish that an individual has a normal karyotype is to perform a chromosome analysis. Higher resolution banding studies have revealed subtle chromosomal alterations in a number of conditions.

Trisomy 21 (Down Syndrome)

Trisomy 21 is the most common autosomal chromosomal abnormality in humans. A detailed review of this condition serves as a helpful model for understanding other chromosomal abnormalities.

Trisomy 21 occurs in all areas of the world and among all racial groups. The prevalence is 1:800 live births. The incidence of this and other chromosomal aneuploidy increases in frequency with increasing maternal age; the incidence is 1:2000 at 20 yr and 2–5% above 40 yr. Many trisomy 21 conceptuses result in spontaneous abortion. At 20 wk of gestation, a fetus with trisomy 21 has few phenotypic findings to suggest the diagnosis; however, at term, most infants have clinical manifestations suggesting the diagnosis.

CYTOGENETICS

About 92% of children with Down syndrome have trisomy with an extra 21 chromosome present in all body cells, for a total chromosome count of 47. Chromosomal nondisjunction during *maternal meiosis* is responsible for 80–90% of cases of trisomy 21. About 5% of children have a translocation involving the 21 chromosome; the extra chromosome is attached to another chromosome, most often another acrocentric chromosome (chromosome numbers 13, 14, 15, 21, or 22), and the total chromosome count is 46. The majority of cases of trisomy due to translocation represent a new event. However, when a child is found to have trisomy owing to a translocation, parental karyotype analysis should be undertaken; it reveals a parent with a balanced translocation 20–40% of the time. If a parent has a balanced translocation, the other immediate family members should be studied to determine who may be at risk for having affected children. About 3% of the time mosaicism occurs; some cells display trisomy 21, but others have a normal karyotype.

CLINICAL MANIFESTATIONS

Infants born with trisomy 21 are the survivors of abnormal embryogenesis and fetal development. There is no clinical difference between children with translocation trisomy and those with simple trisomy. In children with mosaicism, the clinical consequences of trisomy depend on the location and percent of chromosomally normal cells. In many instances of mosaicism, the normal cells represent a minor clone that does not significantly alter the clinical manifestations. Cytogenetic analysis cannot predict the extent of organ malformation. Children with trisomy 21 have almost a 40% chance of congenital heart disease. Virtually all children with Down syndrome are smaller than their siblings and smaller than peer-age children. The intel-

Table 4–4. Clinical Findings That May Be Present with Trisomy 21*

Stature smaller than peer age group

Developmental delays

Congenital heart disease

Structural abnormalities of the bowel (tracheoesophageal atresia, duodenal atresia, annular pancreas, duodenal web, Hirschsprung disease)

Central hypotonia

Brachycephaly

Delayed closure of fontanels

Small midface, small (short) ears

Lax joints, including laxity of the atlantoaxial articulation (the latter predisposing the patient to C1–C2 dislocation)

Short, broad hands, feet, and digits; single palmar crease, clinodactyly

Exaggerated space between 1st and 2nd toe

Velvety, loosely adhering mottled skin in infancy; coarse skin in adolescence

Statistically increased risk for leukemia

Statistically increased risk for Alzheimer disease

* An individual may show any combination of these findings. There is no correlation between the number of physical findings and eventual level of mental performance. The increased risk for leukemia is significant but probably no greater than 1.0% for any individual. Alzheimer disease is relatively common in persons with trisomy 21 who die in middle adult life, but the frequency in all adults with Down syndrome is not known.

ligence is retarded, but the range of abilities is wide and approximates a bell-shaped curve shifted below the normal mean. Craniofacial manifestations include a small midface with upturned nose, epicanthal folds, brachycephaly, flat occiput, speckled iris (Brushfield spots), and palpebral fissures that slant down to the midline. The Oriental appearance of these infants led to the term "mongolism." Because of the small mandible and maxillae, the tongue may be prominent and the palate high and narrow. Eighty percent of infants with trisomy 21 are hypotonic at birth, but this feature often disappears with time. Table 4–4 lists some of the clinical findings that may be present in trisomy 21.

Other Autosomal Trisomies

Down syndrome accounts for the majority of chromosomal aneuploidy at birth. Trisomy 13 (1: 10,000) and trisomy 18 (1:8000) are other trisomies that can be differentiated by their spectra of clinical findings (Table 4–5). These trisomies have a higher

Table 4–5. Findings That May Be Present in Trisomy 13 and Trisomy 18

	Trisomy 13	Trisomy 18
Head and face	Scalp defects (cutis aplasia) Micro-ophthalmia, corneal abnormalities Cleft lip and palate (60–80%) Microcephaly Sloping forehead Holoprosencephaly (arhinencephaly) Capillary hemangiomas	Small and premature appearance Tight palpebral fissures Narrow nose and hypoplastic nasal alae Narrow bifrontal diameter Prominent occiput Micrognathia Cleft lip and/or palate
Chest	Congenital heart disease (VSD, PDA, ASD) 80%	Congenital heart disease (VSD, PDA, ASD) Short sternum
Extremities	Overlapping of fingers and toes (clinodactyly) Polydactyly Hypoplastic nails	Limited hip abduction Clinodactyly and overlapping of fingers: index over 3rd, 5th over 4th Rocker-bottom feet Hypoplastic nails
General	Developmental delays and pre- and postnatal growth retardation Renal abnormalities Nuclear projections in neutrophils	Developmental delays and pre- and postnatal growth retardation

ASD = atrial septal defect; PDA = patent ductus arteriosus; VSD = ventricular septal defect.

risk of spontaneous death in utero than does Down syndrome. Most children with these trisomies die in infancy; very few survive more than 1 yr. Definitive diagnosis is through chromosome analysis.

Recurrence Risk for Autosomal Chromosomal Abnormalities

If a mother is less than 35 yr of age, the recurrence risk for de novo chromosome abnormalities is about 1%. For couples in which the mother is over 35 yr, recurrence risk seems to approximate the empiric age risk.

Chromosomal Imprinting

The sex of the parent contributing a specific chromosome may affect the expression of some of the genes on the chromosome. *Imprinting* is a strong parental (chromosomal) influence on the expression of a particular gene. A small deletion of the q arm adjacent to the centromere of a number 15 chromosome appears to give rise to Prader-Willi syndrome (PWS), if the deletion is in the paternal 15 chromosome. An entirely different syndrome, Angelman syndrome, seems to result if the deletion is in the maternal 15 chromosome. Maternal chromosome 15 uniparental disomy also seems to result in PWS. It seems that a paternal 15 chromosomal area is necessary to prevent PWS.

SEX CHROMOSOME ABNORMALITIES

The clinical consequences of sex chromosome abnormalities in term infants are much less severe than those associated with autosomal chromosomal abnormalities. However, Turner syndrome has a dramatic association with fetal death. Its frequency is about 1 affected individual per 10,000 female live term births, but the condition may be present in almost 1% of female fetuses.

Turner Syndrome

This syndrome is associated with functional monosomy of the p arm of the X chromosome. The most common karyotype in Turner syndrome is 45,X with the second sex chromosome missing, but many affected females are mosaics. 45,X/46,XX is the most common mosaic, but 45,X/47,XXX and 45,X/46,XY also have been observed. Some females with Turner syndrome do have two X chromosomes, but in these instances one X has a missing p arm. The risk of Turner syndrome does not increase with advancing maternal age. These findings suggest an abnormality of embryonic cell division rather than fertilization by an abnormal gamete as the cause of Turner syndrome.

In utero mortality in Turner syndrome often is associated with severe and generalized edema and a cystic hygroma. If swallowing is obstructed, polyhydramnios results. In many instances of severe fetal edema, pulmonary effusions impair lung development. However, live-born infants have an excellent prognosis. The gonads are present at birth and appropriately infantile; during childhood they often regress and may be absent at puberty.

The main *clinical manifestations* of Turner syndrome are short stature (adult height less than 150 cm in the untreated woman), sexual infantilism, and the consequences of congenital anomalies. Females with Turner syndrome have an increased incidence of bicuspid aortic valve and coarctation of the aorta. Furthermore even in the absence of coarctation there is a higher frequency of hypertension later in life. In neonates there also may be carpal and/or pedal edema; this spontaneously resolves but may recur in adolescence when estrogen treatment is initiated. Additional features include a low hairline, webbed neck, widely spaced hypoplastic nipples, horseshoe kidney, and cubitus valgus of the elbow. Some children have problems with spatial relationships and geometric visual problem solving. As a consequence of having only one functional X chromosome, females with Turner syndrome display the same frequency of sex-linked conditions as do males with such conditions as hemophilia A or B.

Treatment of short stature has been successful using parenteral human growth hormone and oral anabolic steroids. Secondary sexual characteristics can be developed with estrogen or a combination of estrogen and progesterone (or their synthetic substitutes). A few girls will produce estrogen on their own, but most do not and have elevated gonadotropins. Girls who are mosaic for cells containing a Y chromosome should have their gonads removed in adolescence to eliminate the risk for later gonadal neoplasm. A few women have become pregnant and have carried to term (presumably each had functioning ovaries). Several women with Turner syndrome have had in vitro fertilization and have carried to term.

Klinefelter Syndrome

This syndrome occurs at a frequency of about 1:1000 live male infants, and the frequency at birth appears to increase with advancing maternal age. The typical karyotype is 47,XXY, but Klinefelter syndrome has occurred with multiple X chromosomes and one (or two) Y chromosomes. Infants and prepubertal boys are not identified owing to absence of recognizable clinical features. In the postpubertal male there is infertility resulting from hypogonadism, with hypospermia or aspermia. Gonadotropin levels usually are elevated unless

normal levels of testosterone are produced. Additional clinical manifestations may include mild mental retardation, long limbs, small penis, small and soft testes, and gynecomastia. Testosterone treatment may be indicated at adolescence.

Other Sex Chromosomal Abnormalities

Nature is extremely tolerant of variation in the sex chromosome composition. At least one normal X chromosome is essential for viability, but monosomy of the X chromosome, as in Turner syndrome, is compatible with normal but infertile life. Klinefelter syndrome and all its cytogenetic variants (47,XXY, 48,XXXY, 49,XXXXY, 48,XXYY, and others) are compatible with life, are not associated with elevated fetal loss, and also are associated with sterility. Klinefelter syndrome has been associated with personality disorders. Two other relatively frequent sex chromosomal abnormalities occur in humans—the karyotype 47,XXX (triple-X female) and the karyotype 47,XYY (the double-Y male). Each abnormality occurs with a frequency of about 0.1% and does not lead to sterility or to unique phenotypes. Because these karyotypes increase in frequency with maternal age, they are apt to be detected during prenatal diagnosis. The XYY male occasionally has been associated with antisocial behavior.

GENETIC COUNSELING

For the family, inherited conditions and chromosomal abnormalities can create long-term and expensive health problems (mental retardation, major correctable or noncorrectable congenital anomalies, and multispecialized comprehensive care hospitalization). The success in the prevention of environmentally caused illness, especially infectious diseases, has led to an increased focus on genetic diseases and birth defects as causes of infant mortality and childhood morbidity. Only some birth defects are inherited, but the scope of clinical genetics includes all conditions with a familial recurrence risk that is higher than normal. Genetic evaluation should be followed by genetic counseling to estimate the recurrence risk for the family and relatives. Often, treatment for a genetic condition can be started before a definitive diagnosis is made, but appropriate genetic counseling requires a correct diagnosis.

Genetic counseling is a process of family education about inherited conditions or conditions that may affect future children. It is initiated as soon as a person begins to be evaluated and continues for as long as the physician is in contact with the family. This responsibility to communicate also may extend into the indefinite future if a new treatment is found or if new methods for screening or for prenatal diagnosis become available. Birth defects, whether genetic or not, and genetic conditions have the potential for significant emotional impact on the family, often because of the potential for parental feelings of guilt. Because these disorders frequently occur without prior history, the family may not understand the nature of the condition and may develop maladaptive coping mechanisms, which will adversely affect the long-term outcome for the child. Genetic counseling can help the family understand the condition, cope with hidden fears and superstitions, and proceed with the process of dealing constructively with the problem. Genetic counseling should include a discussion in understandable terms of the nature of the condition and the mode of inheritance; if the condition is not inherited, this should be explicitly stated. The estimated recurrence risk, the possibilities for prenatal diagnosis, the prognosis, and the treatment alternatives also should be included in the counseling.

Recurrence Risk

Conditions inherited in mendelian fashion have a very precise recurrence risk that can be described and explained. An empiric risk for recurrence, if present, also should be explained to families. If there is no elevated recurrence risk, this should be explicitly stated. Couples should understand that no elevated recurrence risk is not the same as no risk.

Prenatal Diagnosis

The possibility for prenatal diagnosis should be discussed, even if it is not currently possible in a given case. A significant number of inherited disorders and virtually all chromosomal abnormalities can be diagnosed prenatally. With the use of fetal ultrasonography, many conditions with an empiric recurrence risk also can be diagnosed before birth.

Prognosis

Predictions for the outcome of a disease or the long-term development of a child are approximations at best. Specific predictions often are inappropriate, but the range and variation of a disease or condition can be described.

Treatment Alternatives

Inherent in the discussion of treatments is the necessity to review the risks and benefits of each alternative. Some treatments, of course, are dramatic and potentially lifesaving, such as the surgical correction of duodenal atresia. However, other less dramatic treatments include the recommendation for the avoidance of cigarette smoking in an individual with alpha-1-antitrypsin deficiency, or the dietary and medical management of a person with elevated cholesterol and an abnormal pattern of triglycerides and lipoproteins.

EVALUATION OF THE PATIENT: PROBLEMS OF HUMAN SIMILARITIES AND VARIATIONS

Evaluating an individual whose condition potentially is genetic is a challenging diagnostic problem. The pediatrician needs to consider a number of questions, such as: Is this a "known" inherited condition? Is it a chromosomal disorder? Is it a "known" syndrome (a combination of nonrandom findings that seem to be associated in affected individuals)? Is the condition due to a disruption of normal development? Is the condition one that can arise because of exposure to an environmental agent (viral, bacterial, chemical, physical)? Finally, is it a condition that may be inherited or that has an elevated recurrence risk, or is it one that is known to occur as a random event without elevated recurrence risk?

If there is a positive family history for the condition, the evaluation may be easier than if there is no history; however, many genetic conditions arise without a prior family history. Recessive conditions typically occur in a family without a prior history because most carriers are unaware of their status. New mutation dominant conditions also arise de novo, and even sex-linked conditions can occur as new mutations. In addition, minimal expressivity or nonpenetrance in other family members can result in a genetic condition without an apparent antecedent history. Genetic conditions or chromosomal disorders occur regardless of the general health of the mother or father.

In evaluating an individual child, several general points about heredity should be kept in mind. Children resemble their parents and other family members, although each individual will have a unique personal appearance. It is therefore a good idea to observe the appearance of parents and siblings.

There are also *group or racial similarities among individuals* that may need to be taken into account.

Similarity of appearance in population groups may be explained at least partially in the following manner. If we consider that each person has two parents, four grandparents, eight great-grandparents, and so on, the number of ancestors for a given generation can be calculated by raising 2 to the power represented by the number of generations the individual is removed from the ancestor. For example, if a person is separated from an ancestor in the 15th century by 20 generations, then one person would have to have 2^{20} ancestors if none of the 15th century ancestors were to be related to each other (2^{20} = 1,048,576 people). It is obvious that the population of the world in the 15th century was not large enough to provide each person presently living with an unduplicated set of ancestors. Groups originating from limited geographic areas must have had many ancestors in common. It is not surprising, therefore, that inbreeding and limited gene mixing are common among physically, socially, or religiously isolated populations (e.g., Amish, Ashkenazi Jews, and others).

There often is appreciable *variability among families with the same genetic disease*. The early discovery that sickle cell hemoglobin resulted from a point mutation leading to a single amino acid substitution in the beta chain of hemoglobin in every case of sickle cell disease encouraged geneticists to attribute specific gene disorders to identical changes in a single gene. Now we know that human genes are quite complex and that changes in different parts of the same gene can result in significant variation in the expression of the disease. It is probable that individuals homozygous for a recessive gene condition probably are actually heterozygous for specific alleles, but that both alleles are abnormal. Data extracted from studies of families with hemophilia A (factor VIII deficiency) indicate that most families have gene alterations specific only to that family. It is probable that inherited conditions will display many kinds of gene changes. Some changes will be quite specific and common to many families (as with the sickle cell point mutation), but differences in disease expression may depend on the modulating effects from other components of the genome. Other gene changes may be variable because the gene is affected in different ways by a plethora of mutational mechanisms, duplications, deletions, and frame shifts. Mechanisms relating to expressivity always can be expected to operate to alter the clinical condition.

Heterogeneity refers to the fact that a condition may have separate causes. The condition, disease, or phenotype may represent the final common pathway in an abnormal process. For example, if a patient is found to have a hemolytic anemia, there are numerous causes, some acquired and some inherited. Even if we limit the cause of the hemolytic anemia to an inherited hemoglobinopathy, there still are numerous abnormalities of hemoglobin synthesis to consider. These include thalassemia, hemoglobin SS, hemoglobin SC, and others. The concept of heterogeneity must be kept in mind in the practice of medicine as well as in the practice of genetics. In genetic heterogeneity, separate genetic mechanisms may produce the same phenotype.

Another important concept is *expressivity*, which refers to the extent to which an individual is phenotypically affected by a gene or genes. For example, some patients with sickle cell anemia have a mild clinical course due in part to persistent production of fetal hemoglobin. *Penetrance* refers to the difference between the persons with a gene composition who show the effects of the gene and those with the same gene composition who do not show the effects. If a gene has a penetrance of 80%, 8:10 persons with the gene can be expected to show some effects of the gene. It does not mean that a person with the gene will be 80% affected; a gene is either penetrant or not penetrant in an individual.

Pleiotropism means that one gene or pair of genes can have many effects on the individual. When the mechanism of action of the gene or genes is not known, it may be difficult to explain why a single gene pair can have so many different effects on the person. For example, without knowing the molecular and cellular pathology of sickle cell disease, the separate clinical manifestations of the condition would be difficult to explain on the basis of one homozygous gene pair because the effects seem so diverse. Persons with sickle cell disease would be described as having anemia, susceptibility to bacterial infections, renal disease, musculoskeletal pain, hand and foot swelling, and a predisposition to cerebral vascular accidents. When the molecular basis of the condition is understood, the multiple effects of the gene(s) make more sense.

EVALUATING AN INFANT WITH UNUSUAL PHYSICAL FINDINGS AND CLINICAL MALFORMATIONS

The challenge in physical diagnosis of an infant or child with unusual findings is describing as clearly as possible, in nonjudgmental terms, what is observed in the patient. Human variation is extensive but occurs on a continuum, with significant overlaps between what we call normal and what we term abnormal. The subset of genetics that deals with the study of structural defects that alter appearance is called *dysmorphology.*

During the evaluation of an infant with unusual physical findings, a careful history is important even if it proves to be negative. Measurements of height, weight, and head circumference are essential, as are careful observations, documented in detail, for syndrome identification. Judicious laboratory tests can identify metabolic acidosis quickly, and chromosome analysis may be helpful. Sonography and computerized tomography can identify internal abnormalities.

A variety of specific terms are used to describe discrete features or structures. Word descriptions also can serve; for example, one can say that the eyebrows meet in the midline or alternatively that *synophrys* is present. Table 4–6 lists a glossary of some additional terms used in clinical morphology. Syndromes are identified from the detailed description of unusual findings (Table 4–7). If an infant does not fit any specific condition, the child can be observed over time for growth, development, and physical changes that eventually may define the condition. In uncertain diagnostic situations, photographs can be helpful for discussion of the child with colleagues.

Throughout the physical examination, the taking of a family history, and each step of the evaluation, the physician should be compassionate, truthful, and respectful of patient, parents, and principles of the medical profession. Particularly, the physician should appreciate that diagnostic labels may produce untoward as well as beneficial effects on the family and, later, on the patient.

PRENATAL DIAGNOSIS AND GENETICS

Prenatal diagnosis is a process for evaluating the health status of a fetus as early in gestation as possible. It includes analysis of cells from the developing chorion frondosum sampled at the 8th embryonic wk (chorionic villus sampling, [CVS]), maternal serum analysis for alpha-fetoprotein (MSAFP) or other substances of fetal origin after the 16th men-

Table 4–6. A Glossary of Selected Terms Used in Dysmorphology

Terms Pertaining to the Face and Head

Brachycephaly	A head shape that is shortened from front to back along the sagittal plane; the skull is rounder than normal	Scaphocephaly	A head elongated from front to back in the sagittal plane; most normal skulls are scaphocephalic
Canthus	The lateral or medial angle of the eye formed by the junction of the upper and lower lids	Synophrys	Eyebrows that meet in the midline
		Telecanthus	A wide space between the medial canthi
Columella	The fleshy tissue of the nose that separates the nostrils	**Terms Pertaining to the Extremities**	
Glabella	Bony midline prominence of the brows	Brachydactyly	Short digits
Nasal alae	The lateral flaring of the nostrils	Camptodactyly	A digit that is bent or fixed in the direction of flexion (a "trigger finger"–type appearance)
Nasolabial fold	Groove that extends from the margin of the nasal alae to the lateral aspects of the lips	Clinodactyly	A crooked digit that curves toward or away from adjacent digits
Ocular hypertelorism	Increased distance between the pupils of the two eyes	Hypoplastic nail	The nail of a digit is unusually small
Palpebral fissure	The shape of the eyes based on the outline of the eyelids	Melia	A suffix meaning limb (e.g., amelia—missing limb; brachymelia—short limb)
Philtrum	The vertical groove in the midline of the face between the nose and the upper lip	Polydactyly	Six or more digits on an extremity
Plagiocephaly	A head shape that is asymmetric in the sagittal or coronal planes; this can result from asymmetry in suture closure or from asymmetry of brain growth	Syndactyly	Two or more digits are at least partially fused (can involve any degree of fusion, from webbing of skin to full bony fusion of adjacent digits)

Table 4–7. Causes of Congenital Malformations

Monogenic	(7.5% of serious anomalies) X-linked hydrocephalus Achondroplasia Ectodermal dysplasia Apert disease Treacher Collins syndrome (6% of serious anomalies)	Environmental agents	(% unknown) Polychlorinated biphenyls Herbicides Mercury Alcohol

Chromosomal	Trisomies 21, 18, 13
	XO, XXY
	Deletions 4p−, 5p−, 13q−,
	   18p−, 18q−
	Prader-Willi syndrome (50% have
	   deletion of chromosome 15)
		Medications	(% unknown)
			Thalidomide
			Diethylstilbestrol
			Phenytoin
			Warfarin
			Cytotoxic drugs
			Isotretinoin (vitamin A)
			D-Penicillamine
			Valproic acid

Maternal infection	(2% of serious anomalies)
	Intrauterine infections, (herpes
	   simplex, varicella-zoster, rubella,
	   toxoplasmosis)
		Unknown
		etiologies
			(60% of serious anomalies)

Maternal illness	(3.5% of serious anomalies) Diabetes mellitus Phenylketonuria Hyperthermia	Polygenetic	Anencephaly/spina bifida Cleft lip/palate Pyloric stenosis Congenital heart disease Hirschsprung disease
Uterine environment	(% unknown)	Sporadic syndrome complexes (anomalads)	CHARGE syndrome VATER syndrome DiGeorge syndrome Pierre Robin syndrome Williams syndrome Prune-belly syndrome

Deformation	Uterine pressure,
	   oligohydramnios: clubfoot,
	   torticollis, congenital hip
	   dislocation, pulmonary
	   hypoplasia, 7th nerve palsy		

Disruption	Amniotic bands, congenital
	   amputations, gastroschisis,
	   porencephaly, intestinal atresia		

Twinning	Conjoined twins, intestinal atresia, porencephaly		

CMV = cytomegalovirus; HIV = human immunodeficiency virus.

strual wk, ultrasound examination of the embryo/fetus during gestation, and analysis of amniotic fluid and/or amniotic cells removed by amniocentesis during the middle trimester of gestation (Table 4–8). During the 3rd trimester, assessments of amniotic fluid for lecithin/sphingomyelin ratio to determine fetal lung maturity, and the analysis of amniotic fluid for bilirubin to evaluate fetal hemolysis, also are part of prenatal diagnosis. (See Chapter 6.)

Genetic indications for prenatal diagnosis include parental age and the risk of a detectable genetic condition based on the history or a known carrier state (X-linked or autosomal recessive). MSAFP testing is indicated for every pregnant woman. Chromosome analysis of amniotic fluid is virtually 100% accurate in detecting chromosomal abnormalities (Table 4–8). The combination of ultrasound, amniotic fluid AFP analysis, and amniotic fluid acetylcholinesterase measurement is capable of detecting 95–98% of all neural tube defects. Hemoglobinopathies and a number of other gene disorders can be detected by DNA analysis or gene product (hemoglobin electrophoresis) assay (Table 4–8). Many birth defects occur without a prior history in couples not at identifiable risk; therefore, it is unlikely that all major congenital malformations will be identified unless all pregnant women receive antenatal ultrasonography.

Table 4–8. Prenatal Diagnosis

DNA analysis	Alpha-1-anitrypsin deficiency, thalassemia, sickle cell anemia, muscular dystrophy, hemophilia A, congenital adrenal hyperplasia, phenylketonuria
Enzyme assay	Tay-Sachs disease, galactosemia, Hunter syndrome, maple syrup urine disease, Wolman syndrome, Lesch-Nyhan syndrome, Gaucher disease, I-cell disease, Menkes disease
Chromosome disorders	Trisomy 13, 18, 21; chromosome deletions; Turner syndrome; Klinefelter syndrome; fragile X
Alpha-fetoprotein	
Elevated	Twins, neural tube defects, intestinal obstruction, congenital hepatitis, congenital nephrosis, impending fetal demise, omphalocele
Decreased	Trisomy 21, and possibly other chromosomal disorders
Ultrasonography	Hydrops fetalis, hydronephrosis, neural tube defects, intestinal obstruction, congenital heart disease, diaphragmatic hernia, gastroschisis, omphalocele, limb reduction anomalies, assessment of growth
Cordocentesis	Fetal anemia, fetal acid–base and oxygenation disorders, fetal hypoalbuminemia, thrombocytopenia, thalassemia, cells for DNA
Fetal skin biopsy	Albinism, epidermolysis bullosa, xeroderma pigmentosum

ENVIRONMENTAL AGENTS CAPABLE OF PRODUCING BIRTH DEFECTS

Many environmental agents have been alleged to produce birth defects, and it is best to consult the current literature and regional "hot lines" that are available for evaluating potential agents of embryo and fetal injury. If a structure has formed before the exposure, the agent cannot affect its formation. It is rare for an environmental agent to affect every exposed fetus, so most risks will be estimates of probable effects. Table 4–7 includes a list of some known environmental agents that present a risk to the developing fetus.

References

Behrman RE (ed): Nelson Textbook of Pediatrics. 14th ed. Philadelphia, WB Saunders, 1992, Sec. 7.1–7.36.

Caskey T: Disease diagnosis by recombinant DNA methods. Science 236:1223, 1987.

Hall J: Genomic imprinting and its clinical implications. N Engl J Med 326:827, 1992.

Jones K: Smith's Recognizable Patterns of Human Malformation. 4th ed. Philadelphia, WB Saunders, 1988.

Leppig KA, Werler MM, Cann CI, et al: Predictive value of minor anomalies. I. Association with major malformations. J Pediatr 110:531–536, 1987.

McKusick VA: Mendelian Inheritance in Man. 10th ed. Baltimore, Johns Hopkins, 1992.

Tarleton J, Saul R: Molecular genetic advances in fragile X syndrome. J Pediatr 122:169, 1993.

Wallace D: Mitochondrial genetics: A paradigm for aging and degenerative diseases? Science 256:628, 1992.

Williamson RA, Weiner CP, Patil S, et al: Abnormal pregnancy sonogram: Selective indication for fetal karyotype. Obstet Gynecol 69:15, 1987.

Inborn Errors of Metabolism

5

John F. Nicholson

The term "inborn errors of metabolism" was introduced by Garrod in 1908 to indicate recognizable abnormalities in human chemistry and postulated that all intrinsic and developmental abnormalities in humans were due to genetic abnormalities in chemical reactions. We now recognize a great number of such abnormalities, many of which are best considered in the context of specific organ systems (e.g., sickle cell disease and congenital adrenal hyperplasia). Garrod's term now usually is applied to intermediary metabolism, loosely defined as the chemistry of dietary organic compounds and of the fuels derived from them, to which are added multisystem genetic diseases of biochemical origin.

Each of these diseases is caused by a deficiency of enzymatic catalysis or of an enzyme that facilitates the transport of biologic substances. In general, failure of enzymatic function leads to the accumulation of a reactant, which may or may not have toxic effects (Table 5–1). The product of the blocked reaction, if not available otherwise, becomes deficient. Defects in transport can impair intestinal absorption of dietary constituents, renal tubular reabsorption of filtered compounds, and the disposition of compounds within the body and even within the cell (Table 5–2).

The molecular nature of the many defects that have been described is diverse. In some instances, therapeutic strategies can be developed to deal with specific defects. For some disorders, the chemical problem can be defined as failure of interaction between an enzyme and a cofactor, usually a vitamin, in which case provision of a large excess of the vitamin can lead to chemical and clinical correction of the defect (e.g., cobalamin-responsive methylmalonic acidemia). Other therapeutic strategies deal with basic pathogenetic mechanisms—reducing the toxic reactant and providing the deficient product. In galactosemia, dietary elimination of galactose can be helpful. This can be done safely because galactose residues necessary for the formation of glycoproteins, polysaccharides, and complex lipids can be synthesized readily by humans.

In contrast, treatment of phenylketonuria (PKU) requires reduction but not elimination of dietary phenylalanine, because phenylalanine cannot be synthesized by humans. In biotinidase deficiency, which impairs the recycling of biotin, supplementation of the diet with biotin is curative.

The following discussion concentrates on the diseases that are of general concern in the practice of pediatrics: diseases for which screening tests are performed in the neonatal period; those that enter into the differential diagnosis of hyperammonemia, hypoglycemia, and metabolic acidosis; disorders of lipoprotein metabolism that produce clinical disease in childhood; and metabolic diseases associated with dysmorphic syndromes.

GENERAL CONSIDERATIONS

Family History

Inherited metabolic disease frequently is discovered when the second child develops a particular clinical disorder. Consanguinity is common in the family history of such patients. When parents are closely related (e.g., first cousins), the possibility of two rare inherited disorders in a single child becomes significant. For this reason, correlation of clinical findings with a single genetic defect is suspect when the correlation is based solely on the product of a consanguineous union.

Failure to Thrive

Infants with inborn errors of metabolism frequently exhibit failure to thrive. Chemical clues to metabolic disease include hyperammonemia, hypoglycemia, acidosis, ketonuria, abnormalities in hepatic transaminases, and hyperbilirubinemia. Generally, metabolic defects severe enough to cause failure to thrive also produce readily recognizable chemical abnormalities.

Laboratory Tests

Plasma glucose, as measured by the usual laboratory methods, averages 80 mg/dL in the fasting

139

Table 5–1. Pathogenesis of Enzymatic Disorders

| Enzymatic Disorder | Reactant | | Product | | Clinical Disease |
	Accumulated	Toxic?	Not Made	Deficient?	
Galactosemia	Galactose-1-phosphate	Yes	UDP–galactose	No	Yes
Biotinidase deficiency	Lysyl biotin	No	Biotin	Yes	Yes
Essential fructosuria	Fructose	No	Fructose-1-phosphate	No	No

state, with a range of 60–100 mg/dL. During acute illness with temporary starvation, the blood glucose may fall to levels below 60 mg/dL in individuals who have no primary metabolic disorder. Therefore, it always is necessary to judge whether a given low value for blood glucose represents an appropriate physiologic adaptation or a true disorder. Autonomic manifestations (pallor, sweating, tremor, diplopia), seizures, and coma are clear manifestations of hypoglycemia as a disorder, whereas irritability and lethargy are defined as hypoglycemic in origin only when they respond dramatically to the administration of glucose. Hypoglycemia is an integral part of a number of metabolic diseases. (See Chapter 17). In some of these diseases, acidosis and/or hyperammonemia may so dominate the clinical picture that the serious effects on glucose homeostasis are neglected.

Plasma ammonia is present in very small concentrations (10–50 μmol/L) in normal fasting individuals. Blood samples should be collected on ice and analyzed within ½ hr because ammonia rises rapidly in such samples. In general, elevations of less than twice the upper limit of normal in acutely ill patients do not indicate a significant disorder of nitrogen elimination.

In older infants and children, *ketonuria* is a normal response to starvation but not to a normal overnight fast. In the neonate, ketonuria always is indicative of metabolic disease.

Urine screening tests for metabolic disease include the ferric chloride test (PKU, tyrosinosis, and others), the dinitrophenylhydrazine test (PKU, maple syrup urine disease), and the cyanide–nitroprusside test (homocystinuria, cystinuria). When the clinical manifestations suggest the diagnosis, these tests can be used as a basis for initiating therapy, but they should never be considered definitive. Abnormalities in the concentrations of metabolites in body fluids and urine can provide diagnoses that are sufficient for long-term management and genetic counseling, but definitive diagnosis is made only by demonstration of a specific enzymatic or transport deficiency.

DISORDERS OF METABOLISM FOR WHICH NEONATAL SCREENING IS PERFORMED

The purpose of neonatal screening is the detection and treatment of disorders during their preclinical phases. For PKU and homocystinuria, this strategy can be effectively carried out. Galactosemia and maple syrup urine disease (MSUD) usually do not remain subclinical for the time necessary to perform and report the tests.

Phenylketonuria

Phenylketonuria is an autosomal recessive disease that affects primarily the brain. It occurs in 1:10,000 persons. Classic PKU is the result of a defect in the hydroxylation of phenylalanine to form tyrosine (Fig. 5–1); the activity of phenylalanine hydroxylase in the liver is absent or greatly reduced.

Table 5–2. Pathogenesis of Disorders of Transport

Disease	Transport System	Organs or Organelles Affected	Pathogenesis
Cystinuria	Cystine/arginine Lysine/ornithine	Kidney/intestine	Cystine stone formation
Hartnup disease	Monocarboxylic monoamino acids	Kidney/intestine	Tryptophan malabsorption
Glycogen storage disease Ib	Glucose-6-phosphate	Microsome	Hypoglycemia Excess glucose-6-phosphate

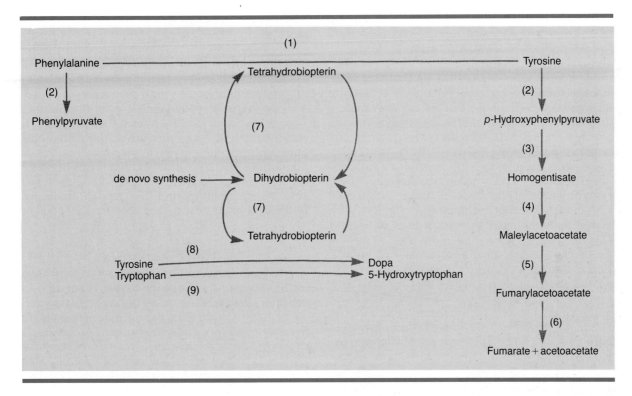

Figure 5–1. Metabolism of aromatic amino acids: (1) phenylalanine hydroxylase, (2) tyrosine transaminase, (3) *p*-hydroxyphenylpyruvate oxidase, (4) homogentisate oxidase, (5) maleylacetoacetate isomerase, (6) fumarylacetoacetate hydrolase, (7) dihydrobiopterin reductase, (8) tyrosine hydroxylase, (9) tryptophan hydroxylase.

A small percentage of phenylketonuric infants have a variant disorder, **malignant** PKU, that results from a defect in the synthesis or metabolism of tetrahydrobiopterin, the cofactor for phenylalanine hydroxylase and for other enzymes involved in the intermediary metabolism of aromatic amino acids.

Affected infants are normal at birth, and the only constant *clinical manifestation* of PKU is the evolution of severe mental retardation (IQ <30). In addition, children may have blond hair, blue eyes, eczema, and mousy odor of the urine. Infants whose disease is caused by an error in the synthesis or metabolism of tetrahydrobiopterin (2% of PKU) develop a progressive, lethal central nervous system disease, reflecting abnormalities in other neural enzymatic reactions for which tetrahydrobiopterin is necessary.

In classic PKU, the *diagnosis* is made by demonstrating:

1. Hyperphenylalaninemia—1.2 mM (20 mg/dL) or higher (normal approximately 0.06 mM, or 1 mg/dL) *and*
2. Normal or reduced plasma tyrosine (normal approximately 0.06 mM, or 1 mg/dL).

The screening test for PKU measures whole blood phenylalanine; elevations should be confirmed by column chromatography of plasma amino acids. It is necessary to demonstrate normal (or lower) levels of tyrosine in blood because the pathway for phenylalanine metabolism develops late in gestation, with the result that a significant percentage of premature infants and a few full-term infants have transient elevations in both phenylalanine and tyrosine during the neonatal period. This condition, **transient tyrosinemia**, carries much less risk of permanent sequelae than classic PKU.

Phenylpyruvic acid is present in the urine of phenylketonuric infants after the neonatal period and can be detected by adding a few drops of 10% ferric chloride to freshly voided urine. In the presence of phenylpyruvic acid, a deep green color develops immediately.

Malignant PKU is diagnosed by measuring dihydrobiopterin reductase in erythrocytes and analyzing biopterin metabolites in urine. Screening for malignant PKU is carried out in all hyperphenylalaninemic infants because there is no other way to differentiate the hyperphenylalaninemia due to deficiency of phenylalanine hydroxylase from that due to deficiency of tetrahydrobiopterin.

Achievement of normal intelligence is possible in most infants with classic PKU by *treatment* with a diet specifically restricted in phenylalanine begun within the first 3 wk of life. For infants with malignant PKU, restriction of dietary phenylalanine reduces plasma phenylalanine but does not ameliorate the clinical disease, which must be treated by replacement of the cofactor if biopterin synthesis is impaired and by neuropharmacologic agents if tetrahydrobiopterin reductase is deficient. Success in the management of malignant PKU is less predictable than that in the management of classic PKU.

In practice, a significant percentage of infants who are shown to be hyperphenylalaninemic by neonatal screening do not satisfy the chemical criteria for the diagnosis of classic PKU and do not satisfy the clinical criteria for malignant PKU. These infants are defined as having **hyperphenylalaninemia**. In some, plasma phenylalanine remains less than 0.6 mM (10 mg/dL) without therapeutic intervention, and in others, plasma phenylalanine can be maintained at that level by reducing dietary protein to 2 g/kg/day. A few require specific restriction of dietary phenylalanine to achieve "safe" (i.e., 0.4–0.6 mM or 7–10 mg/dL) levels in plasma.

The age, if any, at which the phenylalanine-restricted diet should be discontinued has not been determined. Recent studies indicate that continuance of the diet into late childhood is beneficial but also that different dietary strategies designed to ameliorate the maldistribution of amino acids in the brain are possible for treatment of the older child and adolescent. **Maternal hyperphenylalaninemia** constitutes a major problem requiring rigorous management prior to conception and throughout pregnancy to avoid fetal brain damage and microcephaly.

RELATED DISORDERS

Abnormalities in the catabolism of tyrosine can produce positive tests for phenylketones in the urine but not elevations in blood phenylalanine. Although **tyrosinemia** can occur as a nonspecific consequence of severe liver disease, it is the most striking finding in fumarylacetoacetate hydrolase deficiency (Fig. 5–1), a rare disease in which metabolites that accumulate as a result of the impaired reaction produce severe liver disease (bleeding disorders, hypoglycemia, hypoalbuminemia, elevated transaminases, cirrhosis) and defects in renal tubular function. There are two clinical forms of the disease, acute highly lethal liver disease in the first months of life, and chronic liver disease, frequently associated with rickets, that manifests itself later in infancy or childhood. A high proportion of patients develop hepatic malignancies in later childhood. *Treatment* includes a low-phenylalanine, low-tyrosine diet, NTBC (an inhibitor of the oxidation of para-hydroxyphenylpyruvic acid), and liver transplantation. There are more benign forms of hereditary tyrosinemia in which enzymes catalyzing tyrosine transamination and the oxidation of *para*-hydroxyphenylpyruvate are specifically deficient.

Homocystinuria

This autosomal recessive disease (1:200,000 live births) involving connective tissue, brain, and the vascular system is caused by deficiency of cystathionine beta-synthase. In the normal metabolism of the sulfur amino acids, methionine gives rise to cystine; homocysteine is a pivotal intermediate (Fig. 5–2). When cystathionine beta-synthase is deficient, homocysteine accumulates in the blood and appears in the urine. There also is enhanced reconversion of homocysteine to methionine, resulting

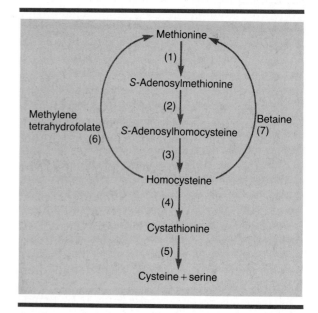

Figure 5–2. Metabolism of methionine and homocysteine: (1) methionine adenosyltransferase, (2) *S*-methyltransferase, (3) *S*-adenosylhomocysteine hydrolase, (4) cystathionine beta-synthase, (5) cystathionase, (6) homocysteine methyltransferase, (7) betaine-homocysteine methyltransferase.

in an increase in the level of methionine in the blood. The neonatal screening test most commonly used measures methionine in whole blood.

Through mechanisms not clearly understood, an excess of homocysteine produces a slowly evolving *clinical syndrome* that includes in its fully developed form dislocated lenses, the habitus of Marfan syndrome, malar flushing, and livedo reticularis. Arachnodactyly, scoliosis, pectus excavatum or carinatum, and genu valgum are features of the skeletal disorder. Mental retardation and/or psychiatric illness may be present. Major arterial or venous thromboses are a constant threat.

There are no neonatal manifestations of homocystinuria. Confirmation of the *diagnosis* requires demonstration of homocystine in blood and urine.

Treatment of homocysteinuria sometimes can be accomplished by giving, together with supplemental folate, large doses of pyridoxine (100–1000 mg/day) to provide a great excess of the cofactor for cystathionine beta-synthase. If pyridoxine therapy fails, the accumulation of homocysteine can be controlled by a diet restricted in methionine and supplemented with cystine and folate. The use of supplemental betaine, to stimulate the alternative pathway for resynthesis of methionine from homocysteine, also appears to have a role in the management of pyridoxine-unresponsive patients. The prognosis is good for infants whose plasma homocystine is controlled.

Galactosemia

This autosomal recessive disease (1:60,000 births) is caused by an extreme deficiency of the enzyme galactose-1-phosphate uridyltransferase (Fig. 5–3). *Clinical manifestations* are most striking in the neonate, who, when fed milk, generally exhibits evidence of liver failure (bilirubinemia, disorders of coagulation, hypoglycemia) and disordered renal tubular function (acidosis, glycosuria, aminoaciduria) and frequently develops cataracts. The neonatal screening test has limited usefulness for severely affected infants, because they may die before the test result is available. When neonatal manifestations are mild or nonexistent, failure to thrive may evolve. Major acute effects on liver and kidney function and the development of cataracts are limited to the first few years of life, but older children tend to have learning disorders, whether or not they were treated in infancy. Ovarian failure is a late sequela.

Laboratory manifestations depend to a large extent on dietary galactose. When galactose is ingested (generally as lactose), plasma galactose and erythrocyte galactose-1-phosphate are elevated. Hepatocellular enzymes (alanine aminotransferase and aspartate aminotransferase) rapidly increase in plasma. Elevations of plasma conjugated and unconjugated bilirubin follow quickly, as do reductions in coagulation factors synthesized by the liver. Hypoglycemia is frequent, and albuminuria always is present in infants with clinical disease. Galactose frequently is present in the urine and can be detected by a positive reaction for reducing substances (Clinitest tablets) but no reaction with glucose oxidase on urine strip tests. Absence of urinary reducing substance cannot be relied on to exclude the diagnosis. Renal tubular dysfunction may be evidenced by hyperchloremic metabolic acidosis. The *diagnosis* is made by demonstrating extreme reduction in erythrocyte galactose-1-phosphate uridylyltransferase.

Treatment by the elimination of dietary galactose results in rapid correction of abnormalities, but infants who are extremely ill prior to treatment may die before therapy is effective. In addition, galactosemic infants are at increased risk for severe neonatal *E. coli* infections.

Generally, it is possible to relax the dietary galactose restriction in later childhood. Congenital cataracts and mild brain damage have occurred even when galactosemic infants are treated from birth. For this reason dietary galactose is eliminated during pregnancy in mothers who have delivered galactosemic infants. Because the galactosemic fetus can synthesize galactose-1-phosphate, this therapeutic approach may have limited value.

RELATED DISORDERS

Galactokinase deficiency, an autosomal recessive disorder (1:250,000), also leads to the accumu-

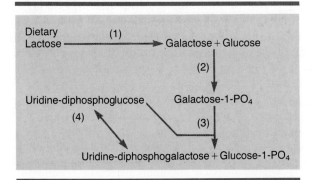

Figure 5–3. Pathway of galactose metabolism: (1) lactase (intestinal), (2) galactokinase, (3) galactose-1-phosphate uridylyltransferase, (4) uridine diphosphoglucose 4-epimerase.

lation of galactose in body fluids (Fig. 5–3), which results in the formation of galactitol (dulcitol) through the action of aldose reductase. Galactitol, acting as an osmotic agent, can be responsible for cataract formation and, rarely, for increased intracranial pressure. These are the only clinical manifestations. Persons homozygous for galactokinase deficiency develop cataracts in the neonatal period, whereas heterozygous individuals are at risk for cataracts as adults. *Treatment* is lifelong elimination of galactose from the diet.

Hereditary fructose intolerance in many ways is analogous to galactosemia. When fructose is ingested, deficiency of fructose-1-phosphate aldolase leads to the intracellular accumulation of fructose-1-phosphate with resultant emesis, hypoglycemia, and severe liver and kidney disease. Elimination of fructose and sucrose from the diet cures the clinical disease.

Fructosuria is analogous to galactokinase deficiency in that it is caused by fructokinase deficiency, but the defect in fructosuria is entirely harmless.

Maple Syrup Urine Disease

This autosomal recessive disease, more properly named branched-chain ketoaciduria, is caused by deficiency of the decarboxylase that initiates the degradation of the ketoacid analogues of the three branched-chain amino acids—leucine, isoleucine, and valine (Fig. 5–4).

Although intermittent and late-onset forms of the disease occur, clinical manifestations of the classic form typically begin within 1–4 wk of birth. Poor feeding, vomiting, and tachypnea commonly are noted, but the hallmark of the disease is profound depression of the central nervous system associated with alternating hypotonia and hypertonia (extensor spasms), opisthotonus, and seizures. The urine has the odor of maple syrup in most cases.

Laboratory manifestations include hypoglycemia and metabolic acidosis with elevation of the undetermined anions; the latter is due in part to plasma branched-chain organic acids and in part to the usual "ketone bodies," beta-hydroxybutyrate and acetoacetate. The branched-chain ketoacids, but neither the beta-hydroxybutyrate nor the acetoacetate, react immediately with 2,4-dinitrophenylhydrazine to form a copious white precipitate. This reaction is the basis for a urine screening test. Definitive *diagnosis* generally is made by demonstrating large increases in plasma leucine, isoleucine, and valine; diagnosis by analysis of organic acids also is possible.

If untreated, the disease is rapidly fatal. MSUD is *treated* by restricting the intake of branched-chain amino acids (all three are essential amino acids) to the amounts required for growth. In severely affected infants, peritoneal dialysis for removal of the branched-chain ketoacids can be life-saving. Treatment with special diets must be continued for life, and ordinary catabolic stresses, such as moderate infections, can precipitate clinical crises.

Biotinidase deficiency (see below) also is included in some programs for neonatal screening.

INBORN ERRORS CAUSING CLINICAL DISEASE IN THE NEONATE

Virtually all of the diseases that cause metabolic acidosis, hyperammonemia, or hypoglycemia can produce clinical manifestations in the neonate. Because the fetus can be considered to undergo perpetual dialysis against an optimized nutrient solution, the infant with an inborn error of metabolism typically seems normal at birth. As the infant adapts to extrauterine life and the oral intake of nutrients, chemical abnormalities appear and symptoms follow at an interval that reflects both the type and the severity of the inborn error. Clini-

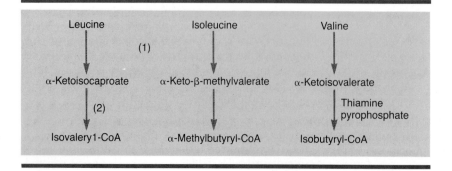

Figure 5–4. Metabolism of the branched-chain amino acids: (1) aminotransferases, (2) alpha-ketoacid dehydrogenase complex.

cal recognition can occur as early as the 3rd day of life and generally is possible within the 1st wk. Poor feeding, vomiting, tachypnea, and seizures are manifestations common to neonates with inborn errors of metabolism, but these also are manifestations of a variety of other diseases, including neonatal septicemia. The most characteristic manifestation of metabolic disease is depression of the central nervous system exhibited by inattention to feedings, lethargy, and hypotonia, occurring in the absence of signs of disease of a specific organ or of neonatal septicemia. Laboratory evaluation of arterial blood gases, liver function, plasma glucose and ammonia, and routine urinalysis, including a test for reducing substance, usually will provide clues that lead to a diagnosis.

Nonketotic Hyperglycinemia

This autosomal recessive disease is caused by a defect in the glycine cleavage system whereby glycine and serine are metabolically interconverted. As evidence that the fetus is affected by this disorder, malformations of the brain, most notably agenesis of the corpus callosum, are common.

Clinically the disease produces profound deterioration in central nervous system function early in the neonatal period: alternating hypertonia and hypotonia, seizures, respiratory depression, inattentiveness, coma, and death within the first weeks of life. The P_{CO_2} may be increased as a result of respiratory depression and hyperglycinemia may be present, but the *diagnosis* rests on the demonstration of greatly increased glycine in cerebrospinal fluid and of an abnormal ratio of glycine in cerebrospinal fluid to glycine in plasma.

No effective *treatment* has been developed, but seizures may be ameliorated by sodium benzoate, which lowers plasma glycine, and by diazepam, which competes with glycine for receptors in the central nervous system. Although the genetic disease has a uniformly poor *prognosis*, there is a self-limited form of neonatal nonketotic hyperglycinemia that can mimic the genetic disease clinically and chemically but resolves spontaneously with no apparent residual effects.

Hyperammonemia

Hyperammonemia can be considered to result from a failure of the liver to clear plasma ammonia. This failure can be caused mechanically by portal venous obstruction or chemically when an adequately perfused liver malfunctions, as occurs in hepatitis with cellular necrosis, in Reye syndrome with generalized hepatocellular dysfunction, and in a number of inborn errors of metabolism involving the synthesis of urea.

CLINICAL MANIFESTATIONS

Symptoms and signs depend on the underlying cause of the hyperammonemia, the age at which it develops, and its degree. Common constellations of findings in children are described in the following sections.

Severe Neonatal Hyperammonemia

Infants with complete genetic defects in urea synthesis, infants with *transient neonatal hyperammonemia* (see below), and, uncommonly, infants with defects in urea synthesis secondary to genetic disorders of organic acid metabolism can develop levels of blood ammonia 100 times normal (>1000 μmol/L) in the first days of life. Poor feeding, hypotonia, apnea, hypothermia, and vomiting rapidly give way to coma and intractable seizures. Death occurs within days if the condition is untreated.

Moderate Neonatal Hyperammonemia

Moderate neonatal hyperammonemia, in the range of 200–400 μmol/L, is associated with depression of the central nervous system, poor feeding, and vomiting, but seizures are not characteristic. This type of hyperammonemia may be caused by incomplete defects in urea synthesis and commonly is caused by disorders of organic acid metabolism that secondarily interfere with the elimination of nitrogen.

Clinical Hyperammonemia in Later Infancy and Childhood

Infants affected by defects in the urea cycle but who are not ill in the neonatal period may do well while receiving the low-protein intake of breast milk, but may later develop clinical hyperammonemia when dietary protein is increased or when catabolic stress occurs after the first few months of life. The clinical presentation is dominated by vomiting and lethargy, frequently progressing to coma. As protein intake is restricted by anorexia and vomiting, the sensorium clears and the infant recovers, only to develop symptoms again when the stimulus to hyperammonemia returns. Seizures are not typical of the disorder. During a crisis, plasma ammonia is usually 200–500 μmol/L, but when protein is restricted it becomes much lower and may even become normal. If the manifestations are not striking (i.e., there is no coma), the condition may go unrecognized for years. When a crisis occurs during an epidemic of influenza, the child mistakenly may be thought to have Reye syndrome.

Subclinical Hyperammonemia

Infants and children with chronic elevations of plasma ammonia at the level of 100–200 μmol/L often do not have symptoms or signs of the derangement.

Transient Neonatal Hyperammonemia

Affected infants do not have a genetic disease but develop striking hyperammonemia shortly after birth. Clinical manifestations may be extreme and include respiratory distress, apnea, and hypotonia. Exchange transfusion, hemofiltration, hemodialysis, or peritoneal dialysis may result in survival without neurologic sequelae. The etiology of this self-limited condition is unknown.

DEFECTS IN THE UREA CYCLE

Inherited enzymatic deficiencies have been described for each of the steps of urea synthesis (Fig. 5–5). The following discussion considers, as examples, only two of these, ornithine carbamoyltransferase (OCT) deficiency and argininosuccinic aciduria (argininosuccinic acid lyase deficiency).

Ornithine Carbamoyltransferase Deficiency

This disease is unique among the defects in the urea cycle in that it is sex linked. Although the defective enzyme may have low-level activity, it generally is nonfunctional, resulting in absent OCT activity in the affected male, who will die in the neonatal period if untreated. Affected females are heterozygous, with one affected cell line and one unaffected cell line; the relative preponderance of each line is randomly determined according to the Lyon hypothesis (see Chapter 4). Because the liver is a mosaic of affected and unaffected nests of cells, it is not possible to define by needle biopsy the degree of enzymatic deficiency in clinically affected females, but it seems likely that overall activity of OCT must be reduced to roughly 20% of normal or lower in order to produce clinical disease. Thus, *clinical manifestations* range from lethal disease in the male to clinical normalcy in a high percentage of females. Manifestations in clinically affected fe-

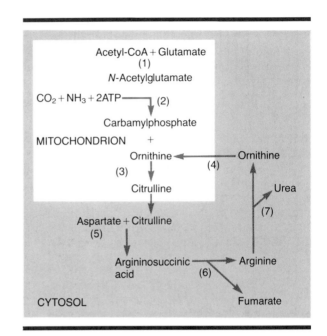

Figure 5–5. The urea cycle: (1) *N*-acetylglutamate synthetase, (2) carbamoylphosphate synthetase, (3) ornithine carbamoyltransferase (OCT), (4) ornithine translocator, (5) argininosuccinic acid synthetase, (6) argininosuccinic acid lyase, (7) arginase.

males include recurrent emesis, lethargy, mental retardation, and psychiatric problems. *Diagnosis* utilizes the fact that orotic acid, produced as a byproduct of carbamoyl phosphate, is excreted in greatly increased quantities in the urine (Fig. 5–5). The oroticaciduria, while much increased above normal, is not quantitatively significant for nitrogen excretion. Although some females heterozygous for the genetic defect excrete normal quantities of orotic acid, the majority of affected females excrete excess orotic acid when given allopurinol.

Argininosuccinic Aciduria

Argininosuccinic acid lyase deficiency results in accumulation of argininosuccinic acid in tissues and blood; however, because the acid is cleared readily by the kidney, it is best identified in the urine, where it is found in gram quantities. Because the synthesis of argininosuccinic acid serves to fix ammonia nitrogen, hyperammonemia is not present at all times in all patients. However, the defect disrupts the urea cycle, and depletion of ornithine can lead to severe hyperammonemia. Death in the neonatal period has been reported, as has symptomatic hyperammonemia in later infancy and childhood. Failure to thrive, hepatomegaly, friable hair (trichorrhexis nodosa), slow motor and mental development, and seizures are characteristic features of the disease, whether or not there is clinical hyperammonemia. Argininosuccinicaciduria is an autosomal recessive disease.

TREATMENT OF HYPERAMMONEMIA

Reduction of dietary protein is the most important treatment for hyperammonemia. During episodes of extreme hyperammonemia, protein intake is eliminated and intravenous glucose is given in sufficient quantity to suppress catabolism of endogenous protein. Because 20% of total urea production is accounted for by detoxification of ammonia generated by bacterial urease in the intestine, sterilization of the intestine can provide brief benefit during acute episodes of hyperammonemia. Long-term benefit is possible with lactulose, a disaccharide not digestible by humans, which is fermented to lactic acid by intestinal bacteria. The resultant reduction in pH inhibits the transluminal absorption of ammonia. Other treatment modalities include sodium benzoate and phenylacetic acid (or its precursor, phenylbutyric acid), which are excreted in the urine as conjugates of glycine and glutamine, respectively. It must be noted as well that arginine is an essential amino acid when arginine synthesis via the urea cycle is grossly impaired. When hyperammonemia is extreme, direct removal of ammonia usually is carried out. For this purpose, hemodialysis or hemofiltration is more effective than exchange transfusion or peritoneal dialysis.

Organic Acidoses

Metabolic acidosis is a state in which acidification of urine is inadequate to maintain normal acid–base balance. Renal tubular acidosis frequently occurs in inborn errors of metabolism and is the result of disordered acidification of urine. Intermediary metabolic acidosis is the result of an overload of metabolic acids to be excreted. The latter condition, acid overload, is characterized by acidosis, acid urine, normal renal function, and an increase in circulating acids manifested by an abnormally large anion gap. In normal plasma, the **anion gap** as calculated by the formula $[Na - (Cl + HCO_3)]$ is 10–15 mEq/L. Intermediary metabolic acidosis results in values that are frequently 30 mEq/L or more as a result of the accumulation of organic acids. Both renal failure as a primary disorder and renal hypoperfusion associated with dehydration may increase the anion gap. Anion gaps exceeding 25 mEq/L usually do not occur in simple dehydration. However, for a given child, it may be necessary to defer evaluation of the anion gap until rehydration has been accomplished.

STARVATION KETOSIS AND KETOTIC HYPOGLYCEMIA

The most common circumstance in which acidosis is found in children is starvation associated with vomiting in the course of a viral illness. The clinical manifestations are those of the causative illness (see Chapters 2 and 11); the acidosis is mild, is associated with ketonuria, and promptly responds to the administration of carbohydrate. In this normal response to starvation, the blood glucose is relatively low (generally 50–70 mg/dL, but occasionally lower), and no symptoms referable to hypoglycemia appear (see Chapter 17).

In contrast, ketotic hypoglycemia is a common but abnormal condition in which tolerance for fasting is impaired to the extent that symptomatic hypoglycemia with seizures and/or coma occurs when the child encounters a ketotic stress. The stress may be significant (e.g., a viral infection with vomiting) or minor (e.g., a prolongation by several hours of the normal overnight fast). Ketotic hypoglycemia generally first appears in the 2nd yr of life. It occurs in otherwise healthy children and usually is treated by frequent snacks and the provision of glucose during periods of stress. Manifestations typically are limited to the first 5–6 yr of life. Carbohydrate tolerance, gluconeogenesis, and hormone responses characteristically are normal.

LACTIC ACIDOSIS

In most tissues, glucose is oxidized to CO_2 and H_2O, with pyruvate as an intermediate (Fig. 5–6). Interference with mitochondrial oxidative processes results in an accumulation of pyruvate. Because lactate dehydrogenase is ubiquitous and because the equilibrium catalyzed by this enzyme greatly favors lactate over pyruvate, accumulation of pyruvate results in lactic acidosis. The most common interference with mitochondrial oxidation is oxygen deficiency owing to anoxia and/or poor perfusion. Hence, one expects lactic acidosis in the event of cardiac arrest, shock, severe cyanosis, and profound congestive heart failure. Poisons such as cyanide, sulfide, and CO, which, like anoxia, block the terminal reaction of the mitochondrial respiratory chain, also produce lactic acidosis (see also Chapter 16).

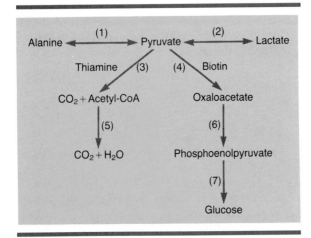

Figure 5–6. Metabolism of pyruvate and lactate: (1) alanine aminotransferase, (2) lactate dehydrogenase, (3) pyruvate dehydrogenase, (4) pyruvate carboxylase, (5) Krebs cycle, (6) phosphoenolpyruvate carboxykinase, (7) reverse glycolysis.

Defects of the respiratory chain also can produce lactic acidosis. Given the complexity of the respiratory chain, it is not surprising that the defects described are varied in type and cause, some showing autosomal recessive inheritance, some showing mitochondrial (maternal) inheritance, and some showing no apparent inheritance pattern. Myopathy is very frequent, often showing ragged red fibers on muscle biopsy. Three striking entities are Kearns-Sayre syndrome (ophthalmoplegia, retinal degeneration, and ragged red fibers), MERRF (myoclonic epilepsy with ragged red fibers), and MELAS (myopathy, encephalopathy, lactic acidosis, strokes). Alpers syndrome (degenerative disease of gray matter with seizures) and Leigh disease (subacute necrotizing encephalomyelopathy) are similar in molecular pathogenesis but clinically manifest primarily in the central nervous system.

Lactic acidosis also can occur when specific reactions of pyruvate are impaired. For practical purposes pyruvate has three fates:

1. Transamination with glutamate to form alanine for protein synthesis; the reaction is catalyzed by alanine aminotransferase.
2. Dehydrogenation and decarboxylation to form acetyl-coenzyme A (CoA); the reaction is catalyzed by the pyruvate dehydrogenase complex (PDH).
3. Carboxylation to form oxaloacetate; the reaction is catalyzed by pyruvate carboxylase (PC).

Formation of alanine is the least important, quantitatively speaking. The PDH reaction is the first step

in pyruvate oxidation, and the PC reaction initiates gluconeogenesis. Inborn defects in both PDH and PC have been described. For *PDH deficiency* the spectrum of reported clinical disease ranges from intractable, lethal acidosis in the first months of life to episodes of ataxia that improve with substitution of fat for carbohydrate in the diet. PDH deficiency also has been noted in some cases of Leigh disease. *PC deficiency* can produce a rapidly lethal neonatal disease that has as one of its elements hyperammonemia secondary to deficiency of aspartate, the product of transamination of oxaloacetate. Other infants with milder deficiencies show metabolic acidosis and mental retardation. In practice, the initial clinical manifestations associated with lactic acidosis due to inborn errors of metabolism frequently are nonspecific. The evaluation of the patient therefore must encompass a broad spectrum of both primary and secondary possibilities.

Treatment is limited for most mitochondrial defects, although disorders of gluconeogenesis may be treated with frequent carbohydrate feeding. Acidosis should be corrected (Chapter 16).

DISORDERS OF THE PROPIONATE PATHWAY

Propionyl-CoA, a major catabolic metabolite of amino acids and lipids, is converted to succinyl-CoA in a series of reactions called the propionate pathway (Fig. 5–7). A key step in the sequence is the formation of succinyl-CoA from methylmalonyl-CoA, the cofactor for which is 5'-deoxyadenosyl cobalamin; this cofactor is the product of a series of reactions involving cobalamin (vitamin B_{12}). Defects in most steps of this pathway have been described, and all produce the **ketotic hyperglycinemia syndrome**. The specific entities are named for specific defects (e.g., propionic acidemia, methylmalonic acidemia, beta-ketothiolase deficiency).

The *clinical manifestations* of ketotic hyperglycinemia, which can begin in the neonatal period, consist of intermittent (1) ketoacidosis, (2) hyperglycinemia, (3) neutropenia, (4) thrombocytopenia, (5) hyperammonemia, and (6) hypoglycemia. After the first months of life, there is generally mild to moderate metabolic acidosis owing to the accumulation of the acid whose metabolism is impaired. Crises involving the intermittent elements of the syndrome occur during periods of catabolic stress but also may occur without an apparent precipitating event. During periods of neutropenia, the risk of serious bacterial infection is increased. Failure to thrive and impaired development are very com-

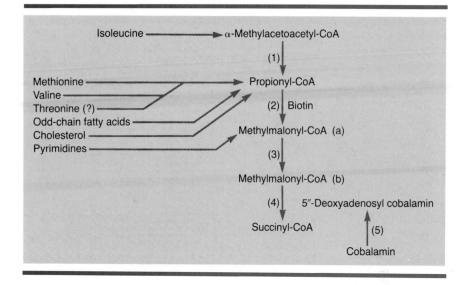

Figure 5–7. The propionate pathway: (1) ketothiolase, (2) propionyl-CoA carboxylase, (3) methylmalonyl-CoA isomerase, (4) methylmalonyl-CoA mutase, (5) cobalamin metabolic pathway.

mon. The syndrome, caused by any of the reported defects, is inherited as an autosomal recessive.

Treatment with massive doses of vitamin B_{12} is helpful in some cases of methylmalonic acidemia. For the remainder, management includes the restriction of dietary protein or of the specific amino acid precursors of propionyl-CoA (isoleucine, valine, methionine, threonine). Carnitine supplementation is indicated. Because intestinal bacteria produce a significant quantity of propionate, antibacterial treatment to reduce the population of bacteria in the gut has some beneficial effect in propionic acidemia and B_{12}-unresponsive methylmalonic acidemia.

ISOVALERICACIDEMIA

This acidemia is similar in its clinical manifestations to those associated with defects in the propionate pathway. Two significant differences are that infants with isovalericacidemia have a "sweaty feet" odor and that glycine therapy is beneficial through enhancement of the formation of isovalerylglycine, a relatively harmless conjugate of isovaleric acid (Fig. 5–8).

Recurrent Reye Syndrome

Recurrent episodes of encephalopathy with evidence of liver dysfunction can occur in a number of metabolic diseases, notably those affecting the urea cycle and disorders of fatty acid metabolism. The normal response to deprivation of food is mobilization and utilization of stored fats. Oxidation

of fatty acids released from adipose tissues is catalyzed by several acyl-CoA dehydrogenases whose activities vary with the chain lengths of the fatty acids (Fig. 5–9). Inherited defects in each of these dehydrogenases have been reported, the best characterized being medium-chain acyl-CoA dehydrogenase. The clinical disease in this deficiency is the result of failure to oxidize fatty acids completely. The following are chemical consequences:

1. Fatty acids not oxidized are excreted in the urine, in part as carnitine esters, producing carnitine depletion.
2. Because beta-oxidation of fatty acids is blocked prior to acetoacetyl-CoA, production of ketone bodies is severely impaired.
3. In the event of food deprivation, glucose cannot be

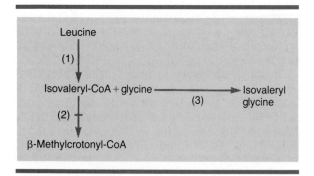

Figure 5–8. Metabolism in isovalericacidemia: (1) leucine catabolic pathway (transamination and decarboxylation), (2) isovaleryl-CoA dehydrogenase, (3) glycine acyltransferase.

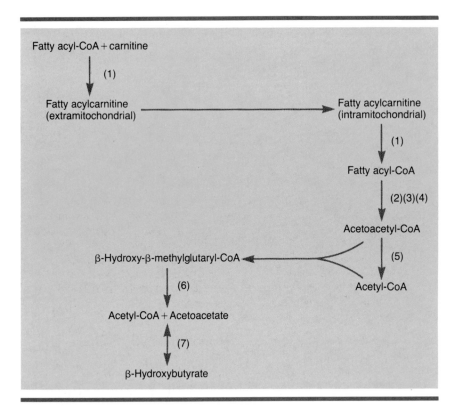

Figure 5–9. Scheme of fatty acid catabolism and ketone body formation: (1) carnitine acyl-CoA dehydrogenases, (2) long-chain fatty acyl-CoA dehydrogenase, (3) medium-chain fatty acyl-CoA dehydrogenase, (4) short-chain fatty acyl-CoA dehydrogenase, (5) ketothiolase, (6) hydroxymethylglutaryl-CoA lyase, (7) hydroxybutyrate dehydrogenase.

spared by fatty acid and ketone body oxidation in a normal manner and hypoglycemia develops rapidly. Encephalopathy results at least in part from hypoglycemia and hypoketonemia. Toxic effects of the unmetabolized medium-chain fatty acids also may contribute to the clinical manifestations.

Hydroxymethylglutaryl-CoA lyase deficiency produces similar clinical manifestations because the blocked reaction is necessary for ketone body production and because carnitine depletion can occur through the excretion of carnitine esters of the organic acids that accumulate as a result of the defect (Fig. 5–9).

Clinical manifestations include episodic periods of emesis, lethargy, coma, and hypoglycemia. Manifestations of secondary systemic carnitine deficiency also may be noted. Sudden infant death and Reye syndrome occurring in young infants in the same family also should suggest these metabolic disorders.

Diagnosis is suspected by the clinical picture and by nonketotic hypoglycemia. It is confirmed by analysis of urinary fatty acids and enzyme assay.

Treatment of these conditions is not very satisfactory, but a high-carbohydrate diet, frequent feed-ings, and carnitine supplementation generally are employed.

Carnitine Deficiency

Carnitine is a critically important cofactor in the transport of fatty acids across the mitochondrial inner membrane (Fig. 5–9). It is synthesized from lysine by humans and also is present in dietary red meat and dairy products. *Carnitine deficiency* was first described in 1973 and has come to be thought of as either primary (i.e., due to failure of normal synthesis or normal transport of carnitine) or secondary (i.e., due to the excretion of excessive amounts of carnityl esters of organic acids whose catabolism is genetically impaired). Primary carnitine deficiency has not been defined clearly, but there are numerous examples of secondary carnitine deficiency among the organic acidurias, most prominently in disorders of the propionate pathway and in disorders of the beta-oxidation of long- and medium-chain fatty acids. Manifestations of carnitine deficiency include failure to produce acetoacetic and beta-hydroxybutyric acids, hypoglycemia, lethargy, lassitude, muscle weakness, and cardiomyopathy. Treatment with carnitine has been dramatically effective in some cases and, in general, has facilitated the excretion of uncatabolizable organic acids.

Biotinidase Deficiency, Beta-Methylcrotonylglycinuria, and Holocarboxylase Deficiency

Biotin is a ubiquitous vitamin that is covalently linked to a number of carboxylases by holocarboxylase synthetase in a variety of tissues. Normal turnover of the carboxylases is accompanied by freeing of biotin for reutilization through the action of biotinidase. Inherited biotinidase deficiency greatly increases the dietary requirement for biotin, with the result that affected individuals can become biotin deficient while consuming normal diets. Clinical disease can appear in the neonatal period or be delayed until later infancy.

The *clinical manifestations* vary greatly—seizures, hypotonia, alopecia, skin rash, metabolic acidosis, and immune deficits—and undoubtedly are dependent on which enzyme(s) in which tissues bear the brunt of the biotin depletion. Because carboxylation is a critical reaction in the metabolism of or-

ganic acids, most patients with biotinidase deficiency excrete abnormal amounts of several organic acids, prominent among which is beta-methylcrotonylglycine. In addition to biotinidase deficiency, there also is an inherited deficiency of holocarboxylase synthetase, which gives rise to severe disease and to similar patterns of organic aciduria. Both conditions respond well to *treatment* with large (10–40 mg/day) doses of supplemental biotin.

Glycogen Storage Diseases

This group of disorders enters into the differential diagnoses of hypoglycemia and of hepatomegaly (Table 5–3). Glycogen is the storage form of glucose and is found most abundantly in the liver, where it serves to modulate blood glucose, and in muscles, where it facilitates anaerobic work.

Glycogen is synthesized from uridine–diphosphoglucose through the concerted action of glycogen synthetase and brancher enzyme (Fig. 5–10). Accumulation of glycogen is stimulated by insulin. Glycogenolysis occurs through a cascade phenomenon, initiated by epinephrine and/or glucagon and culminating in rapid phosphorolysis of glycogen to yield glucose-1-phosphate, accompanied by

Table 5–3. Glycogen Storage Diseases*

Disease	Affected Enzyme	Organs Affected	Clinical Syndrome	Neonatal Manifestations	Prognosis
Type 1 von Gierke	Glucose-6-phosphatase	Liver, kidney, GI tract, platelets	Hypolgycemia, lactic acidosis, hepatomegaly, hypotonia, slow growth, diarrhea, bleeding disorder, gout, hypertriglyceridemia, xanthomas	Hypoglycemia, lactic acidemia, liver may not be enlarged	Early death from hypoglycemia, lactic acidosis; may do well with supportive management; hepatomas occur in late childhood
Type II Pompe	Lysosomal α-glucosidase	All, notably striated muscle, nerve cells	Symmetric profound muscle weakness, cardiomegaly, heart failure, shortened PR interval	May have muscle weakness and/or cardiomegaly	Very poor; death in the 1st yr of life is usual; variants exist
Type III Forbes	Debranching enzyme	Liver, muscles	Early in course hypoglycemia, ketonuria, hepatomegaly that resolves with age; may show muscle fatigue	Usually none	Very good for hepatic disorder; if myopathy present, it tends to be like that of type V
Type IV Andersen	Branching enzyme	Liver, ? nerves	Hepatic cirrhosis beginning at several months of age; early liver failure	None	Very poor; death from hepatic failure before age 4 yr
Type V McArdle	Muscle phosphorylase	Muscle	Muscle fatigue beginning in adolescence	None	Good, with sedentary life-style
Type VI Hers	Liver phosphorylase	Liver	Mild hypoglycemia with hepatomegaly, ketonuria	Usually none	Probably good
Type VII Tarui	Muscle phosphofructokinase	Muscle	Clinical findings similar to type V	None	Similar to that of type V
Type VIII	Phosphorylase kinase	Liver	Clinical findings similar to type III, without myopathy	None	Good

* Except for hepatic phosphorylase kinase and muscle phosphoglycerate kinase, which are X linked, the remaining disorders are autosomal recessive.
GI = gastrointestinal.

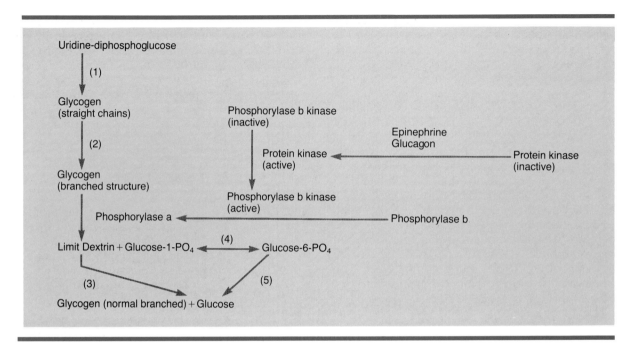

Figure 5–10. Glycogen synthesis and degradation: (1) glycogen synthetase, (2) brancher enzyme, (3) debrancher enzyme, (4) phosphoglucomutase, (5) glucose-6-phosphatase.

a lesser degree of hydrolysis of glucose residues from the branch points in glycogen molecules (Fig. 5–10). In the liver and kidneys, glucose-1-phosphate can give rise to free glucose through the actions of phosphoglucomutase and glucose-6-phosphatase. The latter enzyme is not present in muscles.

Glycogen storage diseases fall into four categories:

1. Those that predominantly affect the liver and have direct influence on blood glucose (types I, VI, and VIII).
2. Those that predominantly involve muscles and affect the ability to do anaerobic work (types V and VII).
3. Those that can affect both the liver and muscles and directly influence both blood glucose and muscle metabolism (type III).
4. Those that affect various tissues but have no direct effect on blood glucose or on the ability to do anaerobic work (types II and IV).

In general, the *diagnosis* of hepatic glycogen storage disease can be made noninvasively by testing the response of blood glucose and lactate to glucagon (type I shows no rise in glucose, but a striking increase in lactate), by assaying enzymes (debrancher, brancher, phosphorylase, phosphorylase kinase) in white blood cells, and by analyzing the structure of glycogen in erythrocytes. Type IV

is best diagnosed by liver biopsy. Glycogen storage disease involving muscles can be assessed by electromyography (pathognomonic changes in type II), by measurement of the response of blood lactate to ischemic exercise (little change in type V as opposed to the normal brisk rise), and by muscle biopsy.

Treatment of hepatic glycogen storage is aimed at maintaining satisfactory blood glucose levels. This usually is not difficult, except in glucose-6-phosphatase deficiency (type I), the treatment for which requires nocturnal intragastric feedings of glucose during the 1st yr or two of life. Thereafter, snacks of uncooked cornstarch may be satisfactory. No specific treatment exists for the diseases of muscle that impair ischemic exercise. For both of the lethal glycogenoses (types II and IV), enzyme replacement has been attempted without success. Liver transplantation has been carried out successfully for severe hepatic glycogen storage disease.

Familial Hyperlipoproteinemia

In *type I hyperlipoproteinemia* (familial hypertriglyceridemia), autosomal recessive deficiency of lipoprotein lipase leads to the accumulation of chylomicrons in serum. Serum cholesterol may exceed 1000 mg/dL, but low-density lipoprotein (LDL) cholesterol is normal or low; serum is grossly milky, with an easily visible layer of chylomicrons. This condition is rarer than type II disease. *Clinical manifestations* of type I disease include eruptive xanthomata and periodic episodes of severe abdominal pain (pancreatitis), which may begin in infancy as colic. A diet very low in fat resolves the xanthomatosis and reduces the risk of the painful crises, which are sometimes fatal. Atherosclerotic disease does not occur.

In *type II hyperlipoproteinemia* (familial hypercholesterolemia) hepatic clearance of LDL cholesterol is impaired because of genetic defects related to the LDL receptor. This results in large elevations in serum cholesterol (>500 mg/dL) in homozygous individuals and lesser elevations in heterozygotes. The *clinical manifestations* of the disease include tendinous xanthomata and early atherosclerotic cardiovascular disease; angina pectoris and myocardial infarction may occur during late childhood and adolescence in homozygous individuals. The serum of affected subjects is clear.

Metabolic Diseases Associated with Dysmorphic Syndrome

Most children who have inborn errors of metabolism are not dysmorphic, and conversely, most dysmorphic children do not have currently recognized inborn errors of metabolism. Exceptions include homocystinuria, which can produce Marfan syndrome (see above), the glutaricacidurias, Zellweger syndrome, and the lysosomal storage diseases.

TYPE I GLUTARICACIDURIA

This is produced by deficiency of glutaryl-CoA dehydrogenase activity (Fig. 5–11). *Clinical manifes-*

tations include macrocephaly, which may be present at birth; dystonia, which characteristically develops after 6 mo of age; and recurrent acute episodes of hepatic dysfunction, acidosis, hypoglycemia, and hyperammonemia (i.e., recurrent Reye syndrome). Intelligence is much less affected than motor function. There is no satisfactory treatment for this condition, which shows autosomal recessive inheritance.

TYPE II GLUTARICACIDURIA

This clinical disease is produced by a defect in the transfer of electrons from flavine adenine nucleotides to the electron transport chain, caused by a deficiency of either electron transport flavoprotein or electron transfer flavoprotein–ubiquinone oxidoreductase (Fig. 5–11). When the enzyme essentially is nonfunctional, congenital anomalies are common—renal cysts, facial abnormalities, rocker-bottom feet, and hypospadias. Severely affected infants develop hypoglycemia without ketosis, metabolic acidosis, and the odor of sweaty feet soon after birth, and may die within the neonatal period. Less severely affected infants may develop a more episodic recurrent Reye-like illness. Skeletal and cardiac myopathy can be prominent in this complex, pansystemic disease, the manifestations of which may be delayed in some cases to adult life. *Treatment* generally has not been effective in infants, but riboflavin in large doses (100–300 mg/day) has benefited some patients with late-onset disease. Because of the biochemical complexity of glutaricaciduria type II, the inheritance of the disease cannot be stated with certainty, but the evidence available favors autosomal recessive inheritance for all reported cases.

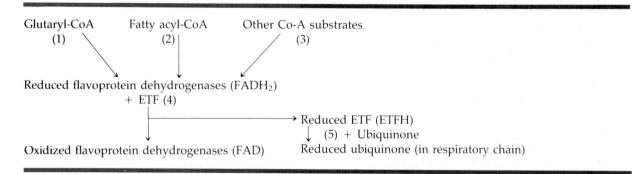

Figure 5–11. Scheme of flavoprotein metabolism with reference to glutaricaciduria types I and II: (1) glutaryl-CoA dehydrogenase (deficient in glutaricaciduria type I), (2) fatty acyl-CoA dehydrogenases, (3) other flavoprotein dehydrogenases, (4) electron transfer flavoprotein (ETF) (deficiency results in glutaricaciduria type II), (5) ETF–ubiquinone oxidoreductase (deficiency results in glutaricaciduria type II).

Table 5–4. Lysosomal Storage Diseases

Disease (Eponym)	Enzyme(s) Deficient	Clinical Onset	Dysostosis Multiplex	Cornea	Retina
Mucopolysaccharidoses (MPS)					
MPS I (Hurler)	α-L-Iduronidase	~1 yr	Yes	Cloudy	—
MPS II (Hunter)	Iduronate-2-sulfatase	1–2 yr	Yes	Clear	Retinitis, papilledema
MPS (Sanfilippo)	One of several degrading heparan SO₄s	2–6 yr	Mild	Clear	—
MPS IV (Morquio)	Galactose-6-sulfatase or β-galactosidase	2 yr	No, dwarfism deformities	Faint clouding	—
MPS VI (Maroteaux-Lamy)	N-Acetylgalactosamine-4-sulfatase	2 yr	Yes	Cloudy	—
MPS VII (Sly)	β-Glucuronidase	Variable neonatal	Yes	± Cloudy	—
Lipidoses					
Glucosylceramide lipidosis 1 (Gaucher 1)	Glucocerebrosidase	Any age	No	Clear	Normal
Glucosylceramide lipidosis 2 (Gaucher 2)	Glucocerebrosidase	Neonatal to 2nd yr	No	Clear	Normal
Sphingomyelin lipidosis A (Niemann-Pick A)	Sphingomyelinase	1st mo	No	Clear	Cherry-red spots (50%)
Sphingomyelin lipidosis B (Niemann-Pick B)	Sphingomyelinase	1st mo or later	No	Clear	Normal
GM₂ gangliosidosis (Tay-Sachs)	Hexosaminidase A	3–6 mo	No	Clear	Cherry-red spots
Generalized gangliosidosis (Infantile GM₁)	β-Galactosidase	Neonatal	Yes	Clear	Cherry-red spots (50%)
Metachromatic leukodystrophy	Arylsulfatase A	1–2 yr	No	Clear	Normal
Fabry disease	α-Galactosidase (cerebrosidase)	Childhood, adolescence	No	Cloudy by slit lamp	—
Galactosyl ceramide lipidosis (Krabbe)	Galactocerebroside β-galactosidase	Early months	No	Clear	Optic atrophy
Wolman disease	Acid lipase	Neonatal	No	Clear	Normal
Farber lipogranulomatosis	Acid ceramidase	1st 4 mo	No	Usually clear	Cherry-red spots (12%)
Mucolipidoses (ML) and clinically related diseases					
ML I (Sialidosis II)	Neuraminidase	Neonatal	Yes	Cloudy	Cherry-red spots
ML I (Sialidosis I)	Neuraminidase	8 yr and older	No	Clear	Cherry-red spots
ML II (I-cell disease)	Mannosyl phosphotransferase	Neonatal	Yes	Late clouding	—
ML III (Pseudo-Hurler polydystrophy)	Mannosyl phosphotransferase	4 yr	Yes	Late clouding	Normal
Multiple sulfatase deficiency	Many sulfatases	1–2 yr	Yes	Usually clear	Usually normal
Aspartylglycosaminuria	Aspartylglucosaminidase	6 mo	Yes	Clear	Normal
Mannosidosis	α-Mannosidase	Neonatal	Yes	Cloudy	—
Fucosidosis	α-L-Fucosidase	Neonatal	Yes	Clear	May be pigmented

CNS = central nervous system; WBC = white blood cell.

Liver, Spleen	CNS Findings	Stored Material in Urine	WBC/Bone Marrow Findings	Comment	Multiple Forms
Both enlarged	Profound loss of function	Acid mucopolysaccharide	Alder-Reilly bodies (WBC)	Kyphosis	Yes—Schei and compounds
Both enlarged	Slow loss of function	Acid mucopolysaccharide	Alder-Reilly bodies (WBC)	X linked	Yes
Liver ± enlarged	Rapid loss of function	Acid mucopolysaccharide	Alder-Reilly bodies (WBC)	—	Several types biochemically
—	Normal	Acid mucopolysaccharide	Alder-Reilly bodies (WBC)	—	Yes
Normal in size	Normal	Acid mucopolysaccharide	Alder-Reilly bodies (WBC)	—	Yes
Both enlarged	± Affected	Acid mucopolysaccharide	Alder-Reilly bodies (WBC)	Nonimmune hydrops	Yes
Both enlarged	Normal	No	Gaucher cells in marrow	Bone pain fractures	Variability is the rule
Both enlarged	Profound loss of function	No	Gaucher cells in marrow	—	Yes
Both enlarged	Profound loss of function	No	Foam cells in marrow	—	Yes
Both enlarged	Normal	No	Foam cells in marrow	—	Yes
Normal	Profound loss of function	No	Normal	—	Yes
Both enlarged	Profound loss of function	No	Inclusions in WBC	—	Yes
Normal	Profound loss of function	No	Normal	—	Yes
Liver may be large	Normal	No	Normal	X linked	No
Normal	Profound loss of function	No	Normal	Storage not lysosomal	Yes
Liver enlarged	Profound loss of function	No	Inclusions in WBC	—	Yes
May be enlarged	Normal or impaired	Usually not	—	Arthritis, nodules, hoarseness	Yes
Both enlarged	Profound affectation	Oligosaccharide	Yes	—	Yes
Normal in size	Seizures	Oligosaccharide	Sometimes	—	Probably
Both often enlarged	Profound loss of function	Oligosaccharide	No	—	No
Normal in size?	Modest loss of function	Oligosaccharide	No	—	No
Both enlarged	Profound loss of function	Acid musopoly-saccharide	Alder-Reilly bodies (WBC)	—	No
Early, not late	Profound loss of function	Aspartylglucosamine	Inclusions	Develop cataracts	No
Liver enlarged	Profound loss of function	Generally no	Inclusions	Cataracts	Yes
Both enlarged	Profound loss of function	No	Inclusions	—	Yes

ZELLWEGER SYNDROME

This autosomal recessive disease (1:100,000 births) is also known as cerebrohepatorenal syndrome. In Zellweger syndrome, peroxisomes are absent, as are normal peroxisomal functions, which include the oxidation of very-long-chain fatty acids. Affected infants have high foreheads, flat orbital ridges, widely open fontanels, hepatomegaly, and hypotonia. Other anomalies are common. Failure to thrive, seizures, and nystagmus develop early, and death occurs within the 1st yr. The disease is not treatable, and its pathogenesis is unclear. *Neonatal adrenoleukodystrophy* and *infantile Refsum syndrome* are related peroxisomal disorders.

LYSOSOMAL STORAGE DISEASES

There are at least a hundred diseases now characterized as disorders of lysosomal function. Most of these diseases are associated with at least some degree of dysmorphism.

Lysosomes are ubiquitous cellular organelles that degrade various cellular constituents by hydrolysis, thus allowing the components of these cellular constituents to be (re)utilized. Absence of one or more hydrolytic activities leads to accumulation of nondegraded cellular material within the lysosome. Because tissues vary greatly in the rate of synthesis and degradation of specific constituents, the absence of a specific hydrolase affects one tissue more than another. If the stored material turns over (i.e., is degraded) rapidly under normal circumstances, the disease is likely to become manifest earlier than if the stored material turns over very slowly under normal circumstances.

Given the permutations of lysosomal hydrolases, cellular constituents, and tissues, it is not surprising that the known disease entities are large in number and increasing rapidly. Clinically, all of them are progressive, although some only slowly so. Defects of bones and joints with evolution of gargoylism or dysmorphic dwarfism (skeletal dysplasia), increasing hepatosplenomegaly, gingival hyperplasia, degenerative disease of the central nervous system, clouding of the corneae, and changes in retinal pigmentation are common manifestations in the group as a whole.

Some "rules of thumb" can help in the approach to a specific patient:

1. *Dysostosis multiplex* (gargoylism) is pathognomonic of mucopolysaccharide storage.
2. Macular cherry-red spots, seen on funduscopic examination, are pathognomonic of storage disease affecting the brain and specifically indicate lipid storage.
3. Rapid development of clinical manifestations over the first months of life often implies deficiency of more than one hydrolytic activity and frequently is associated with storage of both mucopolysaccharide and lipid.

Table 5–4 presents information regarding some of the known storage diseases, the more prominent of which are noted by boldface type. Unless otherwise indicated, the disorder is an autosomal recessive trait.

References

Azeu CG, et al: Intellectual development in 12-year-old children treated for phenylketonuria. Am J Dis Child 145:35, 1991.

Behrman RE (ed): Nelson Textbook of Pediatrics. 14th ed. Philadelphia, WB Saunders, 1992, Sec. 8.1–8.48.

Berry GT, Yudkoff M, Segal S: Isovaleric acidemia: Medical and neurodevelopmental effects of long-term therapy. J Pediatr 113:58, 1988.

Hudak ML, Jones MD Jr, Brusilow SW: Differentiation of transient hyperammonemia of the newborn and urea cycle enzyme defects by clinical presentation. J Pediatr 107:712, 1985.

Lindstedt S, Holme E, Lock EB, et al: Treatment of hereditary tyrosinaemia type 1 by inhibition of 4-hydroxyphenylpyruvate dioxygenase. Lancet 340:813, 1992.

Scriver CR, Beaudet AL, Valle D (eds): The Metabolic Basis of Inherited Disease. 6th ed. New York, McGraw-Hill Book Co, 1989.

Wagoner DD, Buist NR, Donnell GN: Long-term prognosis in galactosemia: Results of a survey of 350 cases. J Inherit Metab Dis 13:802, 1990.

Fetal and Neonatal Medicine

6

Robert M. Kliegman

The optimal care of both low- and high-risk newborn infants depends on knowledge of the family history, the history of prior and current pregnancies, and the events of labor and delivery. Thus, neonatal medicine, although focused on the care of the infant after birth, requires a continuum of understanding of the physiology of normal pregnancy; placental and fetal growth, function, and maturity; and any extrauterine or intrauterine pathologic events that affect the mother, placenta, or fetus. These latter adverse effects, which may result in an untoward neonatal outcome, often are interrelated and include such significant influences as poor maternal nutrition, poverty, physical or psychologic stresses, extremes of maternal age (<16 yr, >35 yr), black race, medical illness present prior to pregnancy, obstetric complications during the antepartum and intrapartum periods, and the inherent genetic predisposition of the fetus.

The late fetal and early neonatal period is the time of life exhibiting the highest mortality rate of any age interval. *Perinatal mortality* refers to fetal deaths occurring from the 20th wk of gestation until the 7th (or 28th) day after birth and is expressed as number of deaths per 1000 live births. Intrauterine fetal death represents 40–50% of the perinatal mortality rate. Such infants, defined as stillborn, are born without a heart rate and are apneic, limp, pale, and cyanotic. Many have evidence of maceration, pale peeling skin, corneal opacification, and very soft cranial contents. The *neonatal mortality rate* includes all infants dying during the period beginning after birth and continuing up to the first 28 days of life, and also is expressed as number of deaths per 1000 live births. Modern neonatal intensive care has delayed the mortality of many newborn infants who have life-threatening diseases, so that they survive the neonatal period only to die of their original diseases or of complications of therapy sometime after the 28th day of life. This delayed mortality occurs during the *postneonatal period*, which begins after 28 days of life and extends to the end of the 1st yr of life. The *infant*

mortality rate encompasses both the neonatal and the postneonatal periods and also is expressed as number of deaths per 1000 live births. The infant mortality rate in the United States declined in 1990 to 9.1:1000; the rate for black infants was 18.6:1000.

The most common causes of perinatal and neonatal death are recorded in Table 6–1. Overall, congenital anomalies and diseases of the premature infant are the most significant etiologies of neonatal mortality.

Low-birth-weight (LBW) infants, defined as those having birth weights of less than 2500 g, represent a disproportionately large component of the neonatal and infant mortality rates. Although these infants comprise only about 7% of all births, they account for two thirds of all neonatal deaths. *Very-low-birth-weight* (VLBW) infants, weighing less than 1500 g at birth, represent only about 1% of all births but account for 50% of neonatal deaths. In comparison with infants weighing 2500 g or more, LBW infants are 40 times more likely to die in the neonatal period, and VLBW infants have a 200-fold higher risk of neonatal death. In contrast to improvements in the infant mortality rate, there has been no recent improvement in the LBW rate. The LBW rate is one of the major reasons why the infant mortality of the United States is high compared with that of other large, modern, industrialized countries. If one calculates birth weight–specific mortality rates, the United States has one of the highest survival rates, but, because of the large number of LBW infants, the total infant mortality remains high.

Maternal factors associated with a LBW infant caused by premature birth or intrauterine growth retardation include a previous LBW birth, low socioeconomic status, low level of educational achievement, no antenatal care, maternal age less than 16 yr or greater than 35 yr, short time interval between pregnancies, cigarette smoking, alcohol and illicit drug abuse, physical or psychologic stresses, unmarried status, low prepregnancy

Table 6–1. Major Causes of Perinatal and Neonatal Mortality

Fetus	Preterm Infant	Full-term Infant
Placental insufficiency	Respiratory distress syndrome/	Congenital anomalies
Intrauterine infection	bronchopulmonary dysplasia	Birth asphyxia
Severe congenital malformations	Severe immaturity	Infection
Umbilical cord accident	Intraventricular hemorrhage	Meconium aspiration pneumonia
Abruptio placentae	Congenital anomalies	Persistent fetal circulation
Hydrops fetalis	Infection	
	Necrotizing enterocolitis	

weight (<45 kg or 100 lb) and poor weight gain during pregnancy (<10 lb), and black race. Race is especially significant because LBW and VLBW rates for black women are twice those for white women. In addition, the neonatal and infant mortality rates are also 2-fold higher among black infants. These racial differences are explained only in part by poverty.

In addition to the sociodemographic variables associated with LBW, there are specific identifiable medical causes of preterm birth (Table 6–2). Many of these factors interrelate with poverty and thus may be a final common pathway by which a disadvantaged extrauterine environment becomes expressed as preterm labor. Nevertheless, factors such as uterine anomalies, hydrops fetalis, and most medical illnesses are not seen more frequently

in blacks or in patients of lower socioeconomic status.

A comprehensive and multidisciplinary approach is required to identify and care for the high-risk pregnancy and to achieve the optimal neonatal outcome. Appropriate communication between the perinatal obstetrician and the pediatrician is essential. Additionally, the pediatrician must have a detailed up-to-date understanding of relevant perinatal obstetrics.

References

Behrman RE (ed): Nelson Textbook of Pediatrics. 14th ed. Philadelphia, WB Saunders, 1992, Sec. 5.3, 9.15–9.17.

Collins J: Disparate black and white neonatal mortality rates among infants of normal birth weight in Chicago: A population study. J Pediatr 120:954, 1992.

Kliegman R, Rottman C, Behrman R: Strategies for the prevention of low birth weight. Am J Obstet Gynecol 162:1073, 1990.

Wegman M: Annual summary of vital statistics—1990. Pediatrics 88:1081, 1991.

PERINATAL OBSTETRICS

Risk Assessment

Pregnancies associated with perinatal morbidity or mortality are considered high risk, and their identification is an essential component of obstetric care. These high-risk pregnancies may result in intrauterine fetal death, intrauterine growth retardation, congenital anomalies, excessive fetal growth, birth asphyxia and trauma, prematurity (birth before 38 wk) or postmaturity (birth of 42 wk or more), neonatal disease, or the long-term risks of cerebral palsy, mental retardation, and chronic sequelae of neonatal intensive care. Between 10% and 20% of women can be considered high risk at some time during their pregnancy. Although some obstetric complications are first seen during labor and delivery and cannot be predicted prior to parturition, many of these high-risk problems are present prior to labor and delivery. Overall, 50%

Table 6–2. Identifiable Causes of Preterm Birth

Fetal
Fetal distress
Multiple gestation
Erythroblastosis
Nonimmune hydrops fetalis
Congenital anomalies

Placental
Placenta previa
Abruptio placentae

Uterine
Bicornuate uterus
Incompetent cervix (premature dilation)

Maternal
Pre-eclampsia
Chronic medical illness (e.g., cyanotic heart disease)
Infection (e.g., group B streptococcus, herpes simplex, syphilis, chorioamnionitis)
Drug abuse (e.g., cocaine)

Other
Premature rupture of membranes
Hydramnios
Iatrogenic (e.g., cesarean section)
Trauma/surgery
Diethylstilbestrol exposure during mother's gestation

of perinatal mortality and morbidity results from pregnancies identified as high risk prior to delivery. Following identification, measures can be instituted to prevent complications, to provide intensive fetal surveillance, and to initiate appropriate treatments of the mother and fetus.

Maternal factors associated with high-risk status include the previously mentioned factors associated with LBW births. Additional maternal factors may be identified from past pregnancies. A history of premature birth, intrauterine fetal death, multiple gestation, intrauterine growth retardation, congenital malformation, explained or unexplained neonatal death, birth trauma, pre-eclampsia, gestational diabetes, grand multipara status (5 or more pregnancies), or cesarean section is associated with additional risk for the subsequent pregnancy.

Pregnancy complications during the current gestation that increase risk include placenta previa, abruptio placentae, pre-eclampsia, diabetes, oligo- or polyhydramnios, multiple gestation, blood group sensitization, abnormal level of alpha-fetoprotein, hydrops fetalis, trauma or surgery, abnormal fetal presentation (breech), exposure to prescribed or illicit drugs, prolonged labor, cephalopelvic disproportion, prolapsed cord, fetal distress, prolonged or premature rupture of membranes, and exposure to rubella, cytomegalovirus, herpes simplex, human immunodeficiency virus, toxoplasmosis, syphilis, and gonorrhea.

Medical complications associated with increased risk for maternal and fetal morbidity and mortality include maternal diabetes, chronic hypertension, congenital heart disease (especially with right-to-left shunting, Eisenmenger complex), glomerulonephritis, collagen vascular disease (especially systemic lupus erythematosus with or without antiphospholipid antibodies), lung disease such as cystic fibrosis, severe anemia such as sickle cell anemia, hyperthyroidism, myasthenia gravis, idiopathic thrombocytopenic purpura, inborn errors of metabolism such as maternal phenylketonuria, and malignancy. Furthermore, inheritance of maternal autosomal recessive genes such as those for cystic fibrosis, galactosemia, and sickle cell anemia place the newborn infant at increased risk for complications of these diseases that may become manifest in utero, in the newborn, or in the older infant.

OBSTETRIC COMPLICATIONS ASSOCIATED WITH FETAL OR NEONATAL RISK

Vaginal bleeding in the 1st or early 2nd trimester may be due to a threatened or actual spontaneous abortion. If pregnancy continues, the fetus may be at increased risk for congenital malformations or chromosomal disorders. Vaginal bleeding that is painless, is not associated with labor, and occurs in the late 2nd or, more likely, the 3rd trimester often is due to placenta previa. Bleeding develops as the placental mass overlies the internal cervical os, which may produce maternal hemorrhagic shock, necessitating transfusions, and premature delivery. Painful vaginal bleeding is often the result of retroplacental hemorrhage and separation of an abruptio placentae. Associated findings may be hydramnios, twin gestation, and pre-eclampsia. Fetal asphyxia will ensue as the retroplacental hematoma causes placental separation that interferes with fetal oxygenation. Both types of bleeding are associated with fetal blood loss. However, neonatal anemia may be more common with placenta previa.

Abnormalities of the volume of amniotic fluid, resulting in oligohydramnios or polyhydramnios, are associated with increased fetal and neonatal risk. **Oligohydramnios** is associated with intrauterine growth retardation and with major congenital anomalies, particularly of the fetal kidneys. Bilateral renal agenesis results in a specific deformation syndrome (*Potter syndrome*) that is indicated by clubfeet, characteristic compressed facies, low-set ears, scaphoid abdomen, and diminished chest wall size that is accompanied by pulmonary hypoplasia and, often, pneumothorax. Uterine compression in the absence of amniotic fluid retards lung growth, and patients with this condition die of respiratory failure rather than of renal insufficiency. Twin–twin transfusion syndrome (donor) and complications from amniotic fluid leakage also are associated with oligohydramnios. Oligohydramnios (amniotic ultrasound fluid index ≤ 5 cm) increases the risk of fetal distress during labor (meconium-stained fluid, variable decelerations); the risk may be reduced by saline amnioinfusion during labor.

Polyhydramnios may be acute and may be associated with premature labor, maternal discomfort, and respiratory compromise. More often, polyhydramnios is chronic and is associated with diabetes, immune or nonimmune hydrops fetalis, multiple gestation, trisomy 18 or 21, and major congenital anomalies. Anencephaly, hydrocephaly, and meningomyelocele are neurologic problems associated with reduced fetal swallowing, whereas esophageal and duodenal atresia and cleft palate interfere with swallowing and gastrointestinal fluid dynamics. **Hydrops fetalis** may be due to Rh or other blood group incompatibilities with intrauterine hemolysis of fetal erythrocytes by maternal immunoglobulin IgG sensitized antibodies crossing the placenta. Hydrops is characterized by fetal edema, ascites, hypoalbuminemia, and congestive heart failure. Causes of **nonimmune hydrops** include fetal supraventricular tachycardia, fetal anemia (resulting from bone marrow suppression), nonimmune hemolysis, twin–twin transfusion, severe congenital malformation, intrauterine infections, congenital neuroblastoma, inborn errors of metabolism (storage diseases), fetal hepatitis, nephrotic syndrome, and pulmonary lymphangiectasia. Twin–twin transfusion syndrome (recipient) also may be associated with polyhydramnios. Polyhydramnios in many other patients is due to unknown causes. If severe, polyhydramnios may be managed with bed rest, indomethacin, or amniocentesis.

Premature rupture of the membranes, which occurs in the absence of labor, and *prolonged rupture of the membranes* for greater than 24 hr are both associated with an increased risk of maternal or fetal infection (chorioamnionitis) and preterm birth. Typically, group B streptococcus, *Escherichia coli*, and *Listeria monocytogenes* are associated with fetal infection, although *Mycoplasma hominis*, *Ureaplasma urealyticum*, *Chlamydia trachomatis*, and anaerobic bacteria of the vaginal flora also have been implicated in infection of the amniotic fluid. The risk of serious fetal infection increases as the length of the time between rupture and labor (latent period) increases, especially if the period is greater than 24 hr.

Multiple gestation is associated with increased risk resulting from polyhydramnios, premature birth, intrauterine growth retardation, abnormal presentation (breech), congenital anomalies (such as intestinal atresia, porencephaly, and single umbilical artery), intrauterine fetal demise, birth asphyxia, and the **twin–twin transfusion syndrome.** The latter syndrome is seen only in monozygotic twins who share a common placenta and who demonstrate an arteriovenous connection between their circulations. The fetus on the arterial side of this shunt serves as the blood donor, which results in its fetal anemia, growth retardation, and oligohydramnios. The recipient, or venous-side twin, is larger or discordant in size, is plethoric and polycythemic, and may demonstrate polyhydramnios. Weight differences of 20% and hemoglobin differences of 5 g/dL confirm the diagnosis. In addition to the twin–twin transfusion syndrome, the birth order of twins affects morbidity by increasing the risk of the second-born twin for breech position, birth asphyxia, birth trauma, and respiratory distress syndrome.

Overall, twinning is observed in 1:80 pregnancies, and 80% of all twin gestations are dizygotic twins. The diagnosis of the type of twins can be determined by placentation, sex, fetal membrane structure, and, if necessary, tissue typing.

Toxemia of pregnancy, or pre-eclampsia–eclampsia, is a disorder of unknown but probably vascular etiology that may result in maternal hypertension, uteroplacental insufficiency, intrauterine growth retardation, intrauterine asphyxia, maternal seizures, and possible maternal death. Toxemia is more common in primiparous women and in women with twin gestation, chronic hypertension, or diabetes mellitus.

MEDICAL PROBLEMS DURING PREGNANCY ASSOCIATED WITH FETAL OR NEONATAL RISK

Medical diseases presenting during pregnancy can affect the fetus directly or indirectly (Table 6–3). Various immunologically mediated diseases affecting maternal tissues are due to autoantibodies; such antibodies also may cross the placenta. Because IgG immunoglobulins are transported actively across the placenta during the last half of the 3rd trimester, all IgG class antibodies will be present in the fetus. Pathologic antibodies can affect the same tissue in the fetus as in the mother. Other maternal illnesses, such as severe pulmonary disease (cystic fibrosis), cyanotic heart disease, and sickle cell anemia, may reduce oxygen availability to the fetus, whereas severe hypertensive or diabetic vasculopathy can result in uteroplacental insufficiency.

Diabetes mellitus that develops during pregnancy (gestational diabetes), or diabetes that is present before pregnancy, adversely influences fetal and neonatal well-being. The effect on the fetus depends in part on the severity of the diabetic state in terms of age of onset of diabetes, duration of treatment with insulin, and the presence of arterial disease. Poorly controlled maternal diabetes results in maternal hyperglycemia, which in turn, because glucose levels in the fetus are slightly lower than but directly proportional to maternal glucose values, produces fetal hyperglycemia that stimulates the fetal pancreas, resulting in hyperplasia of the islets of Langerhans. Fetal hyperinsulinemia, which acts as a fetal growth hormone in the last trimester, results in increased fat and protein synthesis and fetal macrosomia, producing a fetus that is large for gestational age. After birth, hyperinsulinemia persists, resulting in fasting neonatal hypoglycemia. Strictly controlling maternal diabetes during pregnancy and avoiding hyperglycemia

Table 6–3. Maternal Diseases Affecting the Fetus or Neonate

Disorder	Effects	Mechanism
Cyanotic heart disease	Intrauterine growth retardation	Low fetal oxygen delivery
Diabetes mellitus		
Mild	Large for gestational age, hypoglycemia	Fetal hyperglycemia—produces hyperinsulinemia; insulin promotes growth
Severe	Growth retardation	Vascular disease, placental insufficiency
Drug addiction	Intrauterine growth retardation, neonatal withdrawal	Direct drug effect, plus poor diet
Endemic goiter	Hypothyroidism	Iodine deficiency
Graves disease	Transient thyrotoxicosis	Placental immunoglobulin passage of thyrotropin receptor antibody
Hyperparathyroidism	Hypocalcemia	Maternal calcium crosses to fetus and suppresses fetal parathyroid gland
Hypertension	Intrauterine growth retardation, intrauterine fetal demise	Placental insufficiency, fetal hypoxia
Idiopathic thrombocytopenia	Thrombocytopenia	Nonspecific platelet antibodies cross placenta
Isoimmune neutropenia or thrombocytopenia	Neutropenia or thrombocytopenia	Specific antifetal neutrophil or platelet antibody crosses placenta following sensitization of mother
Malignant melanoma	Placental or fetal tumor	Metastasis
Myasthenia gravis	Transient neonatal myasthenia	Immunoglobulin to acetylcholine receptor crosses the placenta
Myotonic dystrophy	Neonatal myotonic dystrophy	Autosomal dominant with genetic anticipation
Obesity	Macrosomia, hypoglycemia	Unknown
Phenylketonuria	Microcephaly, retardation	Elevated fetal phenylalanine levels
Renal transplant	Intrauterine growth retardation	Uteroplacental insufficiency
Rh or other blood group sensitization	Fetal anemia, hypoalbuminemia, hydrops, neonatal jaundice	Antibody crosses placenta directed at fetal cells with antigen
Systemic lupus erythematosus	Congenital heart block, rash, anemia, thrombocytopenia, neutropenia, stillbirth	Antibody directed at fetal heart, red and white blood cells, and platelets; lupus anticoagulant

during labor and delivery prevent macrosomic fetal growth and neonatal hypoglycemia, respectively. Additional problems of the diabetic mother and her fetus and newborn are noted in Table 6–4.

In addition to the fetus' being directly affected by maternal illnesses, both the fetus and the newborn may be adversely affected by the medications used to treat those maternal illnesses. These effects may appear as teratogenesis (Table 6–5) or as an adverse metabolic, neurologic, or cardiopulmonary adaptation to extrauterine life (Table 6–6).

Acquired infectious diseases of the mother also may affect the fetus or newborn adversely. Chronic carriage of hepatitis B virus results in neonatal transmission that, in turn, results in chronic or acute neonatal infection. Syphilis, rubella, and toxoplasmosis have been associated with fetal or neonatal infection resulting in serious sequelae, along with *Listeria*, herpes simplex virus type II, cytomegalovirus, parvovirus, human immunodeficiency virus, varicella-zoster virus, and other viral, bacterial, or protozoan agents.

Table 6–4. Problems of the Diabetic Pregnancy

Maternal
Ketoacidosis
Hypoglycemia
Pre-eclampsia
Polyhydramnios
Retinopathy

Neonatal
Prematurity
Macrosomia and birth trauma
Birth asphyxia
Respiratory distress syndrome
Transient tachypnea of newborn
Hypoglycemia
Hypocalcemia
Polycythemia
Unconjugated hyperbilirubinemia
Congenital malformations
Cardiac septal hypertrophy
Small left colon syndrome
Renal vein thrombosis
Intrauterine fetal death

Table 6–5. Common Teratogenic Drugs

Drug	Results
Alcohol	Fetal alcohol syndrome, microcephaly, congenital heart disease
Aminopterin	Mesomelia, cranial dysplasia
Coumarin	Hypoplastic nasal bridge, chondrodysplasia punctata
Isotretinoin (Accutane)	Facial and ear anomalies, congenital heart disease
Lithium	Ebstein anomaly
Methyl mercury	Microcephaly, blindness, deafness, retardation
Penicillamine	Cutis laxa syndrome
Phenytoin (Dilantin)	Hypoplastic nails, intrauterine growth retardation, typical facies
Radioactive iodine	Fetal hypothyroidism
Stilbestrol (DES)	Vaginal adenocarcinoma during adolescence
Streptomycin	Deafness
Testosterone-like drugs	Virilization of female
Tetracycline	Enamel hypoplasia
Thalidomide	Phocomelia
Trimethadione	Congenital anomalies, typical facies
Valproate	Spina bifida

Table 6–6. Maternal Drugs Affecting Neonatal Status

Drug	Effects
Anesthetics	Central nervous system depression
Angiotensin-converting enzyme inhibitors	Oligohydramnios, renal failure
Barbiturates	Central nervous system depression
Bromides	Rash
Cocaine	Preterm birth, growth retardation, learning disabilities
Coumarin derivatives	Bleeding
Indomethacin	PFC?, bleeding
Intravenous fluids Salt free	Hyponatremia
High glucose loads	Hypoglycemia
Iodides	Goiter
Local anesthetic: "caines"	Bradycardia, neonatal seizures
Magnesium sulfate	Respiratory depression, meconium plug
Morphine (Demerol)	Central nervous system depression, apnea, hypotonia
Naphthalene and nitrofurantoin	Hemolytic anemia in glucose-6-phosphate dehydrogenase deficiency
Oxytocin	Hyponatremia, hyperbilirubinemia
Phenobarbital	Vitamin K deficiency
Phenytoin (Dilantin)	Bleeding, vitamin K deficiency
Propranolol	Hypoglycemia?, apnea?
Reserpine	Nasal stuffiness, drowsiness, poor temperature control
Sulfonamides	Bilirubin displaced from albumin binding, kernicterus
Tolbutamide	Hypoglycemia
Thiazides	Thrombocytopenia?
Vitamin K analogues (excessive amounts)	Jaundice

PFC = persistent fetal circulation.

Assessment of Fetal Well-being and Maturity

FETAL GROWTH

Fetal growth can be assessed clinically by determining the fundal height of the uterus through bimanual examination of the gravid abdomen. In addition, ultrasonographic measurement of the fetal biparietal diameter, femur length, and abdominal circumference all have been employed to estimate fetal growth. A combination of these measurements will predict fetal weight accurately. Deviations from the normal fetal growth curve are associated with high-risk conditions.

Intrauterine growth retardation is present when fetal growth stops and, with time, falls below the 5th percentile of growth for gestational age or when growth proceeds slowly but the absolute size remains less than the 5th percentile (Fig. 6–1). Growth retardation may result from fetal causes producing reduced innate growth potential, such as fetal rubella infection, primordial dwarfing syndromes, chromosomal abnormalities, and congenital malformation syndromes. Placental causes include villitis, placental tumors, chronic abruptio placentae, twin–twin transfusions, and placental insufficiency. Maternal causes of intrauterine growth retardation include severe peripheral vascular diseases that reduce uterine blood flow, such as chronic hypertension, diabetic vasculopathy, and pre-eclampsia–eclampsia. Additional maternal causes include reduced nutritional intake, alcohol or drug abuse, cigarette smoking, and uterine con-

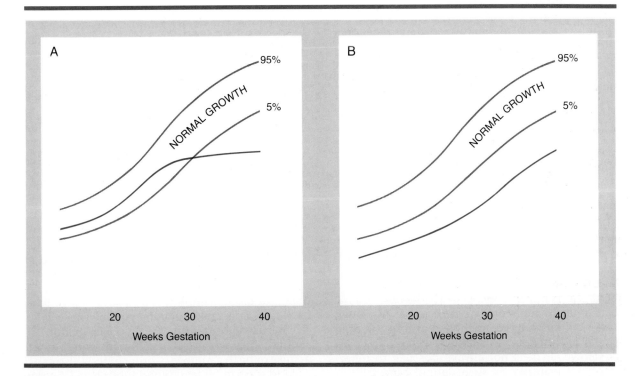

Figure 6–1. Hypothetical fetal growth curves depicting two patterns of intrauterine growth retardation. *A*, In this pattern, there is normal fetal growth during the 20th to 30th week of gestation. Thereafter, fetal growth stops and the fetal growth parameter (biparietal diameter, abdominal circumference, femur length) falls below 5%. This "late flattening" pattern is noted in the donor twin involved in a twin–twin transfusion syndrome, in a fetus supplied by poor maternal nutrition, and in those growing within an environment of maternal pre-eclampsia. Catch-up growth is common after delivery from the adverse in utero environment. *B*, Fetal growth parameters are persistently below 5%. These fetuses demonstrate continued growth, albeit at a reduced rate. Fetuses with this "low-profile" pattern may have reduced growth potential, as noted in those with intrauterine viral infections, chromosome disorders, or malformation syndromes. Fetuses born to mothers who themselves were small for gestational age and who demonstrate reduced prepregnancy weight often have this characteristic growth profile. Some of these fetuses are normal in all other parameters except that they exhibit reduced intrauterine growth.

Table 6–7. Problems of the Intrauterine Growth-Retarded Infant

Intrauterine fetal death
Perinatal asphyxia
Meconium aspiration pneumonia
Cold stress
Hypoglycemia
Polycythemia–hyperviscosity

straint noted predominantly in mothers of small stature with a low prepregnancy weight and reduced weight gain during pregnancy. The outcome of intrauterine growth retardation of the fetus or newborn depends on the cause of the reduced fetal growth and the associated complications after birth (Table 6–7). Fetuses subjected to chronic intrauterine hypoxia as a result of uteroplacental insufficiency are at an increased risk for birth asphyxia, polycythemia, and hypoglycemia. Fetuses with reduced tissue mass resulting from chromosomal or multiple congenital anomaly syndromes have poor outcomes based on the prognosis for the particular syndrome. Fetuses born to small mothers or fetuses with poor nutritional intake usually do well and may demonstrate catch-up growth after birth.

FETAL MATURITY

Fetal size can be determined accurately by using ultrasonographic techniques. Unfortunately, fetal size does not always correlate with functional or structural maturity. The need to determine maturity is critical when a decision has been made to deliver a fetus because of fetal distress or severe maternal pre-eclampsia. Fetal gestational age may be determined accurately based on a correct estimate of the last menstrual period. Furthermore, clinically relevant landmark dates can be used to determine gestational age, because the first audible heart tones by fetoscope are detected at 18–20 wk (12–14 wk by Doppler methods), and quickening of fetal movements is usually perceived at 18–20 wk. However, it is not always possible to determine fetal maturity by such dating, especially in high-risk situations such as preterm labor or in the case of diabetic pregnancy.

Fetal pulmonary maturity may be determined through examination of the phospholipid profile present in the amniotic fluid. Surfactant, a combination of surface active phospholipids and proteins, is produced by the maturing fetal lung and eventually is secreted into the amniotic fluid. The amount of surfactant in amniotic fluid is a direct reflection of surface active material in the fetal lung and can be used to predict the presence or absence of pulmonary maturity. Because dipalmityl phosphatidylcholine, or lecithin, is a principal component of surfactant, the determination of lecithin in amniotic fluid is used to predict a mature fetus. Lecithin concentration increases with increasing gestational age, commencing at 32–34 wk (see Respiratory Distress Syndrome: Lung Development).

ASSESSMENT OF FETAL WELL-BEING

Methods employed to assess fetal well-being prior to the onset of labor attempt to identify the fetus at risk for asphyxia or the fetus currently experiencing hypoxia who is already compromised by uteroplacental insufficiency. The *oxytocin challenge test* simulates uterine contractions by an infusion of oxytocin sufficient to produce three contractions in a 10-min period. The development of periodic fetal bradycardia out of phase with uterine contractions (late deceleration) is a positive test and predicts the fetus at risk. The *nonstress test* examines the heart rate response to fetal body movements: heart rate increments of greater than 15 beats/min, lasting 15 sec, are reassuring. If two such episodes occur in 20 min, the test is considered reactive (vs. nonreactive) and the fetus is not at risk. Additional signs of fetal well-being include fetal breathing movements, gross body movements, fetal tone, and the presence of amniotic fluid pockets of greater than 1 cm as noted by ultrasound. The **biophysical profile** combines the nonstress test with these four parameters and offers the most accurate fetal assessment.

Doppler examination of the fetal aorta can permit identification of decreased or reversed diastolic blood flow, which is associated with increased peripheral vascular resistance, fetal hypoxia, and placental insufficiency. *Cordocentesis* (percutaneous umbilical blood sampling) can provide fetal blood for PO_2, pH, lactate, and hemoglobin. These values can be used to identify the hypoxic, acidotic, or anemic fetus who is at risk for intrauterine fetal demise or birth asphyxia. Cordocentesis also can be used to determine fetal blood type, platelet count, microbial culture, antibody titer, and rapid karyotype.

In the high-risk pregnancy the fetal heart rate should be monitored continuously along with uterine contractions during labor. Fetal heart rate abnormalities include baseline tachycardia (greater than 160 beats/min as a result of anemia, beta-sympathomimetic drugs, maternal fever, hyperthyroidism, arrhythmia, or fetal distress); baseline bradycardia (less than 120 beats/min as a result of fetal distress, complete heart block, or local anesthetics); or reduced beat-to-beat variability (flattened tracing resulting from fetal sleep, tachycardia, atropine, sedatives, prematurity, or fetal distress). In addition, periodic changes of the heart rate relative to the tracing of uterine pressure will help determine the presence of hypoxia and acidosis caused by uteroplacental insufficiency or maternal hypotension (late or type II decelerations) or by umbilical cord compression (variable decelerations). In the presence of severe decelerations (any late or repeated prolonged variable), a fetal scalp blood gas level should be obtained to assess fetal acidosis. A scalp pH of less than 7.20 is serious and indicates fetal hypoxic compromise. A pH between 7.20 and 7.25 is in a borderline zone and warrants repeating the test.

Delivery Room Care: Resuscitation

The approach to the birth of an infant, just like the approach to any other medical situation, requires a detailed history (Table 6–8). Knowing the mother's risk factors (e.g., demographic risks and past and present medical illnesses, including a drug history, the prior pregnancy, and the problems of the current pregnancy) enables the delivery room team to anticipate problems that may occur after birth. Furthermore, the history of a woman's labor and delivery can reveal events that could lead to complications adversely affecting either the mother or neonate, even when the pregnancy was previously considered low risk. Anticipating the need to resuscitate a newborn because of its fetal distress increases the likelihood of resuscitating that infant successfully.

Table 6–8. Components of the Perinatal History

Demographic Social Information	**Present Pregnancy**
Age	Current gestational age
Race	Method of assessing gestational age
Sexually transmitted diseases, hepatitis, AIDS	Fetal surveillance (OCT, NST, biophysical profile)
Illicit drugs, cigarettes, ethanol abuse	Ultrasonography (anomalies, hydrops)
Immune status (syphilis, rubella, blood group)	Amniotic fluid analysis (L/S ratio)
Occupational exposure	Oligohydramnios–polyhydramnios
	Vaginal bleeding
Past Medical Diseases	Preterm labor
Chronic hypertension	Premature (prolonged) rupture of membranes (duration)
Heart disease	Pre-eclampsia
Diabetes mellitus	Urinary tract infection
Thyroid disorders	Colonization status (herpes simplex, group B streptococcus)
Hematologic/malignancy	
Collagen vascular disease (SLE)	Medications–drugs
Genetic history—inborn errors of metabolism, bleeding, jaundice	Acute medical illness/exposure to infectious agents
Drug therapy	Fetal therapy
Prior Pregnancy	**Labor and Delivery**
Abortion	Duration of labor
Intrauterine fetal demise	Presentation—vertex, breech
Congenital malformation	Vaginal versus cesarean section
Incompetent cervix	Spontaneous labor versus augmented or induced with oxytocin (Pitocin)
Birth weight	Forceps delivery
Prematurity	Presence of meconium-stained fluid
Twins	Maternal fever/amnionitis
Blood group sensitization/neonatal jaundice	Fetal heart rate patterns (distress)
Hydrops	Scalp pH
Infertility	Maternal analgesia, anesthesia
	Nuchal cord
	Apgar score/methods of resuscitation
	Gestational age assessment
	Growth status (AGA, LGA, SGA)

AGA = average for gestational age; AIDS = acquired immunodeficiency syndrome; LGA = large for gestational age; L/S = lecithin/sphingomyelin ratio; NST = nonstress test; OCT = oxytocin challenge test; SGA = small for gestational age; SLE = systemic lupus erythematosus.

TRANSITION FROM FETAL TO NEONATAL PHYSIOLOGY

Oxygen transport across the human placenta results in a gradient between the maternal and the fetal PaO$_2$. Although fetal oxygenated blood has a low PaO$_2$ compared with that of adults and infants, the fetus is not anaerobic. Fetal oxygen uptake and oxygen consumption are similar to neonatal rates of oxygen utilization, even though the thermal environments and activity levels of fetuses and neonates differ significantly. Furthermore, the oxygen content of fetal blood is almost equal to that of older infants and children, because fetal blood has a much higher concentration of hemoglobin.

Fetal hemoglobin (two alpha and two gamma chains) has a higher affinity for oxygen than adult hemoglobin does, thus facilitating oxygen transfer across the placenta. The fetal hemoglobin–oxygen dissociation curve thus is shifted to the left of the adult curve (Fig. 6–2); at the same PaO$_2$, fetal hemoglobin will be more saturated than adult hemoglobin. However, because fetal hemoglobin functions on the steep, lower end of the oxygen saturation curve (PaO$_2$ 20–30 mm Hg), oxygen unloading to the tissue is not deficient. In contrast, at the higher oxygen concentrations present in the placenta, oxygen loading is enhanced. In the last trimester, fetal

hemoglobin production begins to decrease and adult hemoglobin production begins to increase, becoming the only hemoglobin available to the newborn by 3–6 mo of life. At this time, the fetal hemoglobin dissociation curve has shifted to the adult position (Fig. 6–2).

A portion of the well-oxygenated umbilical venous blood returning to the heart from the placenta perfuses the liver; the remainder bypasses the liver through a shunt, the ductus venosus, and enters the interior vena cava. This oxygenated blood in the vena cava constitutes 65–70% of venous return to the right atrium. The crista dividens in the right atrium directs one third of this vena caval blood across the patent foramen ovale to the left atrium, where it is subsequently pumped to the coronary, cerebral, and upper extremity circulations by the left ventricle. Venous return from the upper body combines with the remaining two thirds of the vena caval blood in the right atrium and then is directed to the right ventricle. This mixture of venous low-oxygenated blood from the upper and lower body enters the pulmonary artery, from which only 8–10% of it is pumped to the pulmonary circuit. The remaining 80–92% of the right ventricular output bypasses the lungs through a patent ductus arteriosus and enters the descending aorta. The amount of blood (8–10%) flowing to the pulmonary system is low because vasoconstriction produced by medial muscle hypertrophy of the small-sized pulmonary arterioles and fluid in the fetal lung increase vascular resistance to blood flow. Pulmonary artery tone also responds to hypoxia, hypercapnia, and acidosis by vasoconstriction, a response that may further increase pulmonary vascular resistance.

The ductus arteriosus remains patent in the fetus owing to low PaO$_2$ levels and dilating prostaglandins (i.e., PGE$_2$). Cardiac circulation in utero is similar to two pumps connected and operating in parallel arrangement, but after birth the ventricular arrangement resembles a "series" connection. In utero, the right ventricle is the dominant ventricle, pumping 65% of the combined ventricular output, which is a very high volume (450 mL/kg/min) compared with that pumped by the older infant's right ventricle (200 mL/kg/min).

The transition of the circulation occurring between the fetal and neonatal periods involves the phasing out of the low-resistance circulation of the placenta, the onset of air respiration and reduction of the pulmonary arterial resistance, and the closure of shunts that were used in utero. When the umbilical cord is clamped, the low-pressure system of the placenta is eliminated, increasing systemic

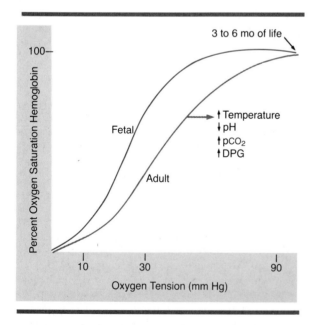

Figure 6–2. Hemoglobin–oxygen dissociation curves. The position of the adult curve depends on the binding of adult hemoglobin to 2,3-diphosphoglycerate (DPG), temperature, carbon dioxide tension (pCO$_2$), and hydrogen ion concentration (pH).

blood pressure. Venous return from the placenta is reduced, thus also decreasing right atrial pressure. When the breathing process begins, air replaces lung fluid, maintaining the functional residual capacity. Fluid leaves the lung, in part, through the trachea and is either swallowed or squeezed out during vaginal delivery. The pulmonary lymphatic and venous systems reabsorb the remaining fluid.

Most normal infants require very little pressure to "open" the lungs after birth (5–10 cm H_2O); a few infants require greater opening pressures (20–30 cm H_2O). With the onset of breathing, pulmonary vascular resistance falls, due in part to the mechanics of breathing and in part to the elevated arterial oxygen tensions. The increased blood flow to the lungs results in a greater quantity of pulmonary venous blood returning to the left atrium; left atrial pressure now exceeds right atrial pressure, and the foramen ovale closes. As the flow through the pulmonary circulation increases and the arterial oxygen tensions become elevated, the ductus arteriosus begins to constrict. In the term infant, this constriction functionally closes the ductus arteriosus within 1 day after birth. A permanent closure requires thrombosis and fibrosis, which may take several weeks. In the premature infant, the ductus arteriosus is less sensitive to the effects of oxygen, and, if circulating levels of vasodilating prostaglandins are elevated, the ductus arteriosus may remain patent. This patency is a common problem in the premature infant exhibiting the respiratory distress syndrome.

Ventilation, oxygenation, and normal pH and Pco_2 levels immediately reduce pulmonary artery vasoconstriction by causing smooth muscle relaxation. Remodeling of the medial muscle hypertrophy will begin at birth and continue for the next 3 mo, resulting in a further reduction of pulmonary vascular resistance and a further increase of pulmonary blood flow. Infants with a ventricular septal defect (VSD) usually do not develop a significant left-to-right shunt and congestive heart failure until pulmonary vascular resistance declines. Thus, term infants with a VSD become ill between 2 and 3 mo of age. Premature infants have not developed a full complement of pulmonary arteriole medial muscle and thus have a more rapid decline of the pulmonary vascular resistance. Because of a more rapid decline of pulmonary artery pressure, the preterm infant with a VSD develops left-to-right shunting and symptoms sooner than does the term infant, often prior to discharge from the nursery. Persistence or aggravation of pulmonary vasoconstriction caused by acidosis, hypoxia, hypercapnia, hypothermia, polycythemia, asphyxia, shunting of

blood from the lungs, or pulmonary parenchymal hypoplasia results in persistent pulmonary hypertension or a persistent fetal circulation (see Persistent Fetal Circulation). Failure to replace pulmonary alveolar fluid completely with air can result in respiratory distress (see Transient Tachypnea of the Newborn).

ASPHYXIA: RESUSCITATION (see also Hypoxic–Ischemic Encephalopathy)

Fetal or neonatal hypoxia, hypercapnia, poor cardiac output, and a metabolic acidosis can result from one or a number of many conditions affecting the fetus, the placenta, or the mother. Whether in utero or after birth, asphyxia-caused hypoxic–ischemic brain injury results from reduced gaseous exchange through the placenta or through the lungs, respectively. Asphyxia associated with severe bradycardia or cardiac insufficiency will reduce or eliminate tissue blood flow, resulting in ischemia. The fetal and neonatal circulatory systems respond to reduced oxygen availability by shunting the blood preferentially to the brain, heart, and adrenal glands and away from the intestine, kidney, lung, and skin. When severe hypoxia and hypercapnia occur in utero, placental blood flow also is reduced. The response to asphyxia also is characterized by (1) release of catecholamines (predominantly norepinephrine) from the adrenal glands; (2) transient hypertension and tachycardia followed by bradycardia and shock, which are both mediated in part from the chemoreceptors and baroreceptors; (3) production of a mixture of respiratory and metabolic acidosis; and (4) hypoxemia. The metabolic acidosis is due to the combined effects of poor cardiac output secondary to hypoxic depression of myocardial function, systemic hypoxia, and tissue anaerobic metabolism. With severe or prolonged intrauterine or neonatal asphyxia, multiple vital organs will be affected (Table 6–9).

Many conditions that contribute to fetal or neonatal asphyxia are the same medical or obstetric problems associated with the high-risk pregnancy (Table 6–10). Maternal diseases that interfere with uteroplacental perfusion, such as chronic hypertension, pre-eclampsia, or diabetes mellitus, place the fetus at risk for intrauterine asphyxia. Both maternal epidural anesthesia and the development of the vena caval compression syndrome may produce maternal hypotension, which decreases uterine perfusion. Maternal medications given to relieve pain during labor may cross the placenta and

Table 6–9. Effects of Asphyxia

System	Effect
Central nervous system	Hypoxic–ischemic encephalopathy, IVH, cerebral edema, seizures, hypotonia, hypertonia
Cardiovascular	Myocardial ischemia, poor contractility, tricuspid insufficiency, hypotension
Pulmonary	Persistent fetal circulation, respiratory distress syndrome
Renal	Acute tubular or cortical necrosis
Adrenal	Adrenal hemorrhage
Gastrointestinal	Perforation, ulceration, necrosis
Metabolic	Inappropriate ADH, hyponatremia, hypoglycemia, hypocalcemia, myoglobinuria
Integument	Subcutaneous fat necrosis
Hematology	Disseminated intravascular coagulation

ADH = antidiuretic hormone; IVH = intraventricular hemorrhage.

depress the infant's respiratory center, resulting in apnea at the time of birth.

Fetal conditions associated with asphyxia usually do not become manifest until delivery, when the infant must initiate and sustain ventilation, which requires an intact respiratory drive from the centers for respiration in the medulla. In addition, the upper and lower airways must be patent and unobstructed. The alveolus must be free from foreign material such as meconium, amniotic fluid debris, and infectious exudate, which increase airway resistance, reduce lung compliance, and result in respiratory distress and hypoxia (Table 6–10). Some very immature infants weighing less than 1000 g at birth may be unable to expand their lungs, even in the absence of pneumonia or other obvious signs of central nervous system dysfunction. Their compliant chest wall and surfactant deficiency may result in poor air exchange at birth, retractions, hypoxia, and apnea. Usually, more mature newborn infants do not manifest apnea in the delivery room as a sign of the respiratory distress syndrome.

Any condition resulting in hypoxia in the delivery room may cause apnea, because the newborn infant, particularly the preterm infant, responds paradoxically to hypoxia by developing apnea rather than by developing tachypnea, as occurs among adults. Episodes of intrauterine asphyxia also may depress the neonatal central nervous system. If recovery of the fetal heart rate occurs as a result of improved uteroplacental perfusion, fetal hypoxia and acidosis may resolve. Nonetheless, if the effect on the respiratory center is more severe, the newborn infant may not initiate an adequate ventilatory response at birth and thus will undergo another episode of asphyxia.

The *Apgar examination*, a rapid scoring system based on physiologic responses to the birth process, is a very good method for assessing the need to resuscitate a newborn infant (Table 6–11). At intervals of 1 min and 5 min after birth, each of the five physiologic parameters is observed or elicited by a qualified examiner. Full-term infants with a normal cardiopulmonary adaptation should score 8–9 at 1 and 5 min. Apgar scores of 4–7 require close attention to determine whether the infant's status will improve and to ascertain whether any pathologic condition resulting from labor or deliv-

Table 6–10. Etiology of Birth Asphyxia

Type	Example
Intrauterine	
Hypoxia–ischemia	Uteroplacental insufficiency, abruptio placentae, prolapsed cord, maternal hypotension, unknown
Anemia–shock	Vasa previa, placenta previa, fetomaternal hemorrhage, erythroblastosis
Intrapartum	
Birth trauma	Cephalopelvic disproportion, shoulder dystocia, breech presentation, spinal cord transection
Hypoxia–ischemia	Umbilical cord compression
Postpartum	
Central nervous system depression	Maternal medication, trauma, previous episodes of fetal hypoxia–acidosis
Congenital neuromuscular disease	Congenital myasthenia gravis, myopathy
Infection	Consolidated pneumonia, shock
Airway disorder	Choanal atresia, severe obstructing goiter, laryngeal webs
Pulmonary disorder	Severe immaturity, pneumothorax, pleural effusion, diaphragmatic hernia, pulmonary hypoplasia
Renal disorder	Pulmonary hypoplasia/pneumothorax

Table 6–11. Apgar Score

Signs	Points		
	0	1	2
Heart rate	0	<100/min	>100/min
Respiration	None	Weak cry	Vigorous cry
Muscle tone	None	Some extremity flexion	Arms, legs well flexed
Reflex irritability	None	Some motion	Cry, withdrawal
Color of body	Blue	Pink body, blue extremities	Pink all over

ery or residing within the newborn is contributing to the low Apgar score. By definition, an Apgar of 0–3 is either a cardiopulmonary arrest or a condition due to severe bradycardia, hypoventilation, and/or central nervous system depression. Most low Apgar scores are due to difficulty in establishing adequate ventilation and not to primary cardiac pathology. Infants with the most severe types of complex congenital heart disease (such as lethal hypoplastic left heart syndrome) do not have low Apgar scores because of their cardiac lesion. Low Apgar scores may be due to fetal hypoxia or to other factors listed in Table 6–10. Most infants with low Apgar scores respond to assisted ventilation by face mask or by endotracheal intubation and usually do not need emergency medication.

Resuscitation of the newborn infant having a low Apgar score follows the same systematic sequence (see Cardiopulmonary Resuscitation in Chapter 3) as that for resuscitation of older patients, but in the newborn period this simplified ABC approach requires some qualification. Although "A" stands for securing a patent airway by clearing amniotic fluid or meconium by suctioning, "A" should also remind us about "anticipation" and the need for knowing the events of pregnancy, labor, and delivery. This history also should include knowledge of fetal distress, fetal heart rate and acid–base status, abnormal position, vaginal bleeding, blood group sensitization, and ultrasonographic evidence of hydrops or congenital malformations, because such knowledge may modify the approach to the airway. For example, evidence of a diaphragmatic hernia and a low Apgar score indicate that immediate endotracheal intubation is required. If a mask and bag are used, gas will enter both the lung and the stomach, and the latter may act as an expanding mass in the chest that compromises respiration. Knowing the blood group sensitization and that

fetal hydrops has occurred with pleural effusions may indicate the need for bilateral thoracentesis to evacuate the pleural effusions, so that adequate ventilation can be established.

"B" represents breathing. If the patient is apneic or hypoventilates and remains cyanotic, artificial ventilation should be initiated. It should be performed with a well-fitted mask that is attached to an anesthesia bag and a manometer to prevent very high pressures from being given to the newborn infant. One hundred percent oxygen should be given through the mask. If the infant does not revive, an endotracheal tube should be placed through the vocal cords and then attached to the anesthesia bag and manometer and 100% oxygen administered. The pressure generated should begin at 20–25 cm H_2O, with a rate of 60 breaths/min. An adequate response to ventilation is indicated by good chest rise, return of breath sounds, well-oxygenated color, heart rate returning to the normal range (120–160 beats/min), and, later, by increased muscle activity and wakefulness. The usual recovery after a cardiac arrest is, first, a return to a normal heart rate. After that, cyanosis disappears and the infant will appear well perfused. An infant may remain limp and be apneic for a prolonged time after return of cardiac output and correction of acidosis.

For the asphyxiated newborn infant, breathing should initially be briefly delayed if there is meconium-stained amniotic fluid. If the meconium is not cleared from the oropharyngeal and tracheal airways, it may be disseminated into the lungs, producing a severe **aspiration pneumonia.** If meconium is noted in the amniotic fluid, the oropharynx should be suctioned by the birth attendant once the head is delivered. After the birth of the infant, the oral cavity should be suctioned again; the vocal cords then should be visualized with a laryngoscope and the infant intubated with suction applied while the tube is below the vocal cords. If meconium is noted below the cords, intubation should be repeated quickly to clear the remaining meconium. During this time, the infant should not be stimulated to breathe nor should positive-pressure ventilation be applied.

"C" represents circulation and external cardiac massage. If artificial ventilation does not improve the bradycardia, if asystole is present, or if peripheral pulses cannot be palpated, external cardiac massage should be performed at a rate of 100–120 beats per minute. External cardiac massage usually is not needed, because most infants in the delivery room respond to ventilation.

"D" represents the administration of drugs. If

bradycardia that is unresponsive to ventilation persists or if asystole is present, drugs should be added to the process of resuscitation. Intravenous epinephrine (1:10,000, 0.1–0.3 mL/kg) should be given through an umbilical venous line, or epinephrine may be injected into the endotracheal tube. Intracardiac injection of epinephrine is not necessary. Additional medications for resuscitation may include 1–2 mEq/kg of sodium bicarbonate (0.5 mEq/mL) if acidosis is prolonged; calcium gluconate (2–4 mL/kg of 10% solution) if there is evidence of hypocalcemia; or a rapid infusion of fluids if poor perfusion suggests hypovolemia. Before administering medications in the presence of electrical–mechanical dissociation, it is important to determine whether there is a pneumothorax, because this is a very common cause of electrical cardiac activity unaccompanied by palpable pulses or blood pressure. Transillumination of the thorax, using a bright light through each of the two sides of the thorax and over the sternum, may suggest pneumothorax if one side transmits more light than the other. There also are decreased breath sounds over a pneumothorax and a shift of the heart tones away from the side of a tension pneumothorax.

If central nervous system depression in the infant is thought to be due to analgesic medications, such as meperidine, that were given to the mother, naloxone (Narcan) can be given to the infant as a specific antidote. Prior to administering this drug, however, the ABCs should be followed carefully, and naloxone should be given only after full resuscitation has been completed.

Other Neonatal Emergencies in the Delivery Room

CYANOSIS

Acrocyanosis (blue color of the hands and feet with pink color of the rest of the body) is common in the delivery room and not of clinical concern. *Central cyanosis* of the trunk, mucosal membranes, and tongue can occur in the delivery room or at any time after birth and is always a manifestation of a serious underlying condition. Central cyanosis can be due to problems in many different organ systems, although cardiopulmonary diseases are the most common (Table 6–12). Respiratory distress syndrome, sepsis, and cyanotic heart disease are the three most common causes of cyanosis among infants admitted to a neonatal intensive care unit. A systematic evaluation for these and other causes of cyanosis is required for every cya-

notic infant after prompt administration of oxygen, with or without assisted ventilation as indicated.

LIFE-THREATENING CONGENITAL MALFORMATIONS (Table 6–13)

Various congenital anomalies can interfere with vital organ function after birth. Some malformations, such as choanal atresia or other lesions obstructing the airway, may prevent ventilation. Intrathoracic lesions such as cysts or bowel that has herniated into the chest also interfere with respiration. Other malformations that obstruct the gastrointestinal system at the level of the esophagus, duodenum, ileum, or colon may result in aspiration pneumonia, intestinal perforation, or gangrene. Gastroschisis and omphalocele both are associated with intestinal necrosis and exposed bowel on the abdominal wall. Omphalocele also is associated with other malformations.

Many congenital malformations are obvious in the delivery room. By using fetal ultrasonography, the obstetrician is able to detect many serious congenital anomalies in utero. Immediate palliative medical or surgical treatment or corrective surgery must be planned for most infants with major congenital malformations. Prompt stabilization, as noted for the asphyxiated infant, is essential. In addition, specific attention must be given to the particular problems associated with the malformation.

SHOCK

Shock in the delivery room is manifested by cyanosis, pallor, poor capillary refilling time, unpalpable pulses, hypotonia, and, eventually, cardiopulmonary arrest. Cyanosis in the presence of pallor, with or without purpuric ecchymosis, is very suggestive of shock. Blood loss prior to or during labor and delivery is a common cause of shock in the delivery room. Blood loss may be due to a fetal–maternal hemorrhage, placenta previa, vasa previa, a twin–twin transfusion, or displacement of blood from the fetus to the placenta as during asphyxia, hence the term *asphyxia pallida*. Hemorrhage into a viscus such as the liver or spleen may be noted in macrosomic infants, and hemorrhage into the cerebral ventricles may produce shock and apnea in preterm infants. Finally, anemia, hypoalbuminemia, hypovolemia, and shock at birth are common manifestations of Rh immune hydrops. Diseases causing nonimmune hydrops also can result in fetal anemia and hypovolemia.

Severe intrauterine bacterial sepsis may present

Table 6–12. Differential Diagnosis of Neonatal Cyanosis

System/Disease	Mechanism
Pulmonary	
Respiratory distress syndrome	Surfactant deficiency
Sepsis, pneumonia	Inflammation, pulmonary hypertension ARDS
Meconium aspiration pneumonia	Mechanical obstruction, inflammation, pulmonary hypertension
Persistent fetal circulation	Pulmonary hypertension
Diaphragmatic hernia	Pulmonary hypoplasia, pulmonary hypertension
Transient tachypnea	Retained lung fluid
Cardiovascular	
Cyanotic heart disease with decreased pulmonary blood flow	Right-to-left shunt as in pulmonary atresia, tetralogy of Fallot
Cyanotic heart disease with increased pulmonary blood flow	Right-to-left shunt as in D-transposition, truncus arteriosus
Cyanotic heart disease with congestive heart failure	Right-to-left shunt with pulmonary edema and poor cardiac output as in hypoplastic left heart and coarctation of aorta
Heart failure alone	Pulmonary edema and poor cardiac contractility as in sepsis, myocarditis, supraventricular tachycardia, or complete heart block; high-output failure as in PDA or vein of Galen or other arteriovenous malformation
Central Nervous System	
Maternal sedative drugs	Hypoventilation
Asphyxia	CNS depression
Intracranial hemorrhage	CNS depression, seizure
Neuromuscular disease	Phrenic nerve palsy; hypotonia, hypoventilation, pulmonary hypoplasia
Hematologic	
Acute blood loss	Shock
Chronic blood loss	Congestive heart failure
Polycythemia	Pulmonary hypertension
Methemoglobinemia	Low-affinity hemoglobin or red blood cell enzyme defect
Metabolic	
Hypoglycemia	CNS depression, congestive heart failure
Adrenogenital syndrome	Shock (salt-losing)

CNS = central nervous system; PDA = patent ductus arteriosus; ARDS = adult respiratory distress syndrome.

with septicemic shock in the delivery room or immediately after transfer to the nursery. Typically, these infants are mottled, hypotonic, and cyanotic and have diminished peripheral pulses. They have a normal hemoglobin concentration and usually manifest neutropenia, thrombocytopenia, and disseminated intravascular coagulation. Peripheral symmetric gangrene (purpuric rash) often is a sign of hypotensive shock among infants with severe congenital bacterial infections.

Treatment of newborn infants with shock should include the management approaches used for the sick infant, which are discussed in the section on asphyxia and resuscitation. Problems may be anticipated through knowledge of the infant's immune status, evidence of hydrops, or suspicion of intrauterine infection. Stabilization of the airway, institution of respiratory support, and external cardiac massage are essential. Hypovolemic shock should be managed with repeated boluses of 10–15 mL/kg of either normal saline or albumin. If severe immune hemolysis is predicted, blood typed against the mother's blood should be available in the delivery room and should be given to the newborn infant if signs of anemia and shock are present. Thereafter, all blood should be cross-matched with both the infant's and the mother's blood prior to transfusion. Vasoactive drugs, such as dopamine, dobutamine, and epinephrine may improve cardiac output and tissue perfusion.

Table 6–13. Common Congenital Anomalies

Name	Manifestations
Choanal atresia	Respiratory distress in delivery room, apnea, unable to pass nasogastric tube through nares
Diaphragmatic hernia	Scaphoid abdomen, bowel sounds present in chest, respiratory distress
Tracheoesophageal fistula	Polyhydramnios, aspiration pneumonia, excessive salivation, unable to place nasogastric tube in stomach
Intestinal obstruction: volvulus, duodenal atresia, ileal atresia	Polyhydramnios, bile-stained emesis, abdominal distention
Gastroschisis/omphalocele	Polyhydramnios; intestinal obstruction
Renal agenesis/Potter syndrome	Oligohydramnios, anuria, pulmonary hypoplasia, pneumothorax
Hydronephrosis	Abdominal masses
Neural tube defects: anencephalus, meningomyelocele	Polyhydramnios, elevated alpha-fetoprotein; decreased fetal activity
Down syndrome (trisomy 21)	Hypotonia, congenital heart disease, duodenal atresia
Ductal-dependent congenital heart disease	Cyanosis, murmur

BIRTH INJURY

Birth injury refers to both avoidable and unavoidable injury to the fetus during the birth process. Birth asphyxia has been discussed in a previous section. Other traumatic injuries due to mechanical forces applied to the infant during parturition are discussed here.

Caput succedaneum is a diffuse, edematous, often dark swelling of the soft tissue of the scalp that extends across the midline and suture lines. In infants delivered from a face presentation, soft tissue edema of the eyelids and face is an equivalent phenomenon. Caput succedaneum may be seen after prolonged labor in both full-term and premature infants. Molding of the head often is associated with caput succedaneum and is the result of pressure induced from overriding the parietal and frontal bones against their respective sutures.

A *cephalhematoma* is a subperiosteal hemorrhage that does not cross the suture lines surrounding the respective bones. A linear skull fracture rarely may be seen underlying a cephalhematoma. With time, the cephalhematoma may organize, calcify, and form a central depression.

Infants with cephalhematoma and caput succedaneum require no specific treatment. Occasionally, a premature infant may develop a massive scalp hemorrhage. This *subgaleal bleeding* and the bleeding noted from a cephalhematoma may cause indirect hyperbilirubinemia that requires treatment with phototherapy.

Retinal and *subconjunctival hemorrhages* are common but usually are small and insignificant, requiring no treatment.

Spinal cord or spine injuries may occur in the fetus, from the hyperextended "star gazing" posture, and in infants following excessive rotational (at C3-4) or longitudinal (at C7-T1) force transmitted to the neck during vertex or breech delivery. Fractures of vertebrae are rarer and may cause direct damage to the spinal cord that results in transection and permanent sequelae or hemorrhage, edema, and neurologic signs. Occasionally, a snapping sound indicative of cord transection rather than vertebral displacement is heard at the time of delivery. Neurologic dysfunction usually includes complete flaccid paralysis, absent deep tendon reflexes, and absence of responses to painful stimuli below the lesion. Painful stimuli may elicit reflex flexion of the legs. Infants with spinal cord injury often are flaccid, apneic, and asphyxiated, all of which may mask the underlying spinal cord transection. With time, these infants will develop bowel and bladder problems, spasticity, and hyperreflexia.

Injury to the nerves of the *brachial plexus* may result from excessive traction on the neck, producing paresis or complete paralysis, depending on the nerve roots involved. **Erb-Duchenne paralysis** involves the 5th and 6th cervical nerves. The infant cannot abduct the arm at the shoulder, externally rotate the arm, or supinate the forearm. The usual picture is one of painless adduction, internal rotation of the arm, and pronation of the forearm. There is an absent Moro reflex on the involved side; the hand grasp is intact. A **phrenic nerve palsy** (C3, 4, and 5) may result in diaphragmatic paralysis and respiratory distress. An elevated diaphragm caused by nerve injury must be differentiated from elevation resulting from eventration caused by congenital weakness or absence of diaphragm muscle. **Klumpke paralysis** is due to injury to the 7th and 8th cervical nerves and the 1st thoracic nerve, resulting in a paralyzed hand and, if the sympathetic nerves are injured, ipsilateral Horner syndrome (ptosis, miosis). Complete arm and hand paralysis is noted with damage to C5, 6, 7, and 8 and T1. Treatment of brachial plexus injury is supportive and includes positioning to avoid contractures. Active and passive range-of-motion exercises also may be of benefit. If the deficit persists, nerve grafting may be beneficial.

Facial nerve injury may be due to compression of the 7th nerve between the facial bone and the mother's pelvic bones or the physician's forceps. This peripheral nerve injury is characterized by an asymmetric crying face whose normal side, including the forehead, moves in a regular manner. The affected side is flaccid, the eye will not close, the nasolabial fold is absent, and the side of the mouth droops at rest. When there is a central injury to the facial nerve, only the lower two thirds of the face is involved (not the forehead). Complete agenesis of the facial nucleus results in a central facial paralysis; when this is bilateral, as in **Möbius syndrome**, the face appears expressionless. There is no treatment for these injuries, but there often is some spontaneous recovery.

Fractures of the cranium are rare, are usually linear, and require no treatment other than observation for very rare delayed (1-3 mo) complications (e.g., leptomeningeal cyst). Depressed **skull** fractures are unusual but may be seen with complicated forceps delivery. Fractures of the **clavicle** usually are unilateral and are noted in macrosomic infants following shoulder dystocia. Often a snap is heard following a difficult delivery, and the infant presents with an asymmetric Moro response and decreased movement of the affected side. The prognosis is excellent; many infants require no treatment or a simple figure-of-8 bandage to immobilize the bone. **Extremity** fractures are less common than those of the clavicle and involve the humerus more often than the femur. Treatment requires immobilization and a triangular splint bandage for the humerus and traction suspension of the legs for femoral fractures. The prognosis is excellent. Fractures of the **facial bones** are rare, but dislocation of the cartilaginous part of the nasal septum out of the vomeral groove and columella is common. Manifestations include feeding difficulty, respiratory distress, asymmetric nares, and a flattened, laterally displaced nose. Treatment reduces the dislocation by elevating the cartilage back into the vomeral groove.

Visceral trauma to the liver, spleen, or adrenal gland is noted in macrosomic infants and in very premature infants, with or without breech or vaginal delivery. Rupture of the liver with subcapsular hematoma formation may result in anemia, hypovolemia, shock, hemoperitoneum, and disseminated intravascular coagulation. Infants with anemia and shock who are suspected of having an intraventricular hemorrhage but who have a normal head ultrasound examination should be evaluated for hepatic or splenic rupture. Adrenal hemorrhage may be asymptomatic, as noted by a high incidence of normal infants with calcified adrenal glands. Nonetheless, if severe, infants with adrenal hemorrhage may present with a flank mass, jaundice, and hematuria, with or without shock.

TEMPERATURE REGULATION

In utero thermoregulation of the fetus is performed by the placenta, which acts as an efficient heat exchanger. Fetal temperature is, nonetheless, higher than the mother's temperature. If maternal temperature becomes elevated during a febrile illness or on exposure to environmental heat, fetal temperature will increase further. Thus, the immediate temperature at birth of an infant born to a febrile mother with chorioamnionitis will be elevated regardless of the presence of infection in the infant, unless the infant has cooled in the delivery room.

After birth, the newborn infant begins life covered by amniotic fluid and situated in a cold environment (20–25° C). An infant's skin temperature may fall 0.3° C/min, and the core temperature may decline 0.1° C/min in the delivery room. In the absence of an external heat source, the infant will have to increase metabolism substantially to maintain body temperature.

Heat loss occurs by four basic mechanisms. In the cold delivery room, the wet infant loses heat predominantly by evaporation (cutaneous and respiratory loss when wet or in low humidity), radiation (loss to nearby cold solid surfaces), and convection (loss to air current). Once the infant is dry, radiation, convection, and conduction (loss to object in direct contact with infant) are important causes of heat loss. After birth, all high-risk infants should be dried immediately to eliminate evaporative heat losses (Table 6–14). Furthermore, a radiant or convective heat source should be provided for these high-risk infants. Normal term infants should be dried and wrapped in a blanket.

The ideal environmental temperature is the *neutral thermal environment*, the ambient temperature resulting in the lowest rate of heat produced by the infant while maintaining normal body temperature. The neutral thermal environmental temperature decreases with increasing gestational age and

Table 6–14. General Management Strategies for Sick Newborns

Procedure	Rationale
Warmth in a neutral thermal environment	Avoids cold stress, minimizes oxygen consumption
Humidification	Reduces insensible water losses
Intravenous fluids and glucose	Maintains fluid balance, avoids dehydration, hyperbilirubinemia, prevents prerenal azotemia, prevents hypoglycemia, provides supplemental calories to support oxygen consumption
Oxygen	Treats hypoxia, supports oxygen consumption, prevents cell injury and death
Monitor blood gases	Avoids hyperoxic retinal injury and hypoxic brain injury, guides treatment with mechanical ventilation

increasing postnatal age. Ambient temperatures below the neutral thermal environment first result in increasing rates of oxygen consumption for heat production, which is designed to maintain normal body temperature. If the ambient temperature falls further or if oxygen consumption cannot increase sufficiently (as a result of hypoxia, hypoglycemia, or drugs), the core body temperature falls.

Heat production by the newborn infant is created predominantly by *nonshivering thermogenesis* from chemical reactions of adenosine triphosphate (ATP) hydrolysis in specialized areas of tissue containing brown adipose tissue. Brown fat is highly vascular, contains many mitochondria per cell, and is situated around large blood vessels, resulting in rapid heat transfer to the circulation. The vessels of the neck, thorax, and interscapular region are common locations of brown fat. These tissues also are innervated by the sympathetic nervous system, which serves as a primary stimulus for heat production by brown adipose cells. Shivering does not occur in newborn infants.

Severe *cold injury* in the infant will be manifested by acidosis, hypoxia, hypoglycemia, apnea, bradycardia, pulmonary hemorrhage and a pink skin color. The latter is due not to adequate oxygenation but rather to trapping of oxygenated hemoglobin in the cutaneous capillaries. Many of these infants appear dead, but most will respond to treatment and recover. Milder degrees of cold injury in the delivery room may contribute to metabolic acidosis and hypoxia after birth. Conversely, hypoxia will delay heat generation in cold-stressed infants. Treatment of severe hypothermia should include resuscitation and rapid warming of both core (lung, stomach) and external surfaces. Fluid resuscitation also is needed to treat the hypovolemia seen in many of these infants. Reduced core temperature (32–35° C) in the immediate newborn period often requires only external warming with a radiant warmer or incubator, or both.

Exposure to ambient temperatures above the neutral thermal environment results in *heat stress* and an elevated core temperature. Sweating is uncommon in newborn infants and may be noted only on the forehead. Excessive environmental temperatures may result in heat stroke or in the hemorrhagic shock encephalopathy syndrome.

Routine Delivery Room Care

Once the cardiopulmonary transition from fetal to newborn life has successfully occurred and no acute life-threatening conditions exist, routine delivery room or postpartum room care should be provided. Silver nitrate (1%) instilled into both eyes (without being washed out) is an indicated effective therapy for the prevention of neonatal gonococcal ophthalmia, which can result in severe panophthalmitis and subsequent blindness. Silver nitrate may produce a chemical conjunctivitis with a mucopurulent discharge and is not effective against *Chlamydia trachomatis*. Therefore, many hospitals use erythromycin drops to prevent neonatal gonococcal and chlamydial eye disease.

Bacterial colonization of the newborn may begin in utero when the fetal membranes have been ruptured prior to or during labor. Most infants become colonized after birth and acquire the bacteria present in the mother's genitourinary system, such as staphylococcus, *E. coli*, and clostridial species. Colonization is common at the umbilicus, skin, nasopharynx, and intestine. Antiseptic skin and/or cord care is routine in most nurseries to prevent spread of pathologic bacteria from baby to baby and to prevent disease in the individual baby. Staphylococcal bullous impetigo, omphalitis, diarrhea, and systemic disease may result from colonization with virulent *Staphylococcus aureus*. For term infants, washing of the skin with 3% hexachlorophene may avoid serious staphylococcal disease; preterm infants may absorb hexachlorophene and develop neurotoxicity. Triple dye may be applied to the umbilical cord to effectively reduce its colonization with gram-positive bacteria.

Vitamin K prophylaxis should be given to all infants to prevent hemorrhagic disease of the newborn.

References

Behrman RE (ed): Nelson Textbook of Pediatrics. 14th ed. Philadelphia, WB Saunders, 1992, Sec. 9.1–9.29.

Blickstein I: The twin–twin transfusion syndrome. Obstet Gynecol 76:714, 1990.

Gibbs RS, Romero R, Hillier SL, et al: A review of premature birth and subclinical infection. Am J Obstet Gynecol 166:1515, 1992.

Hickok DE, Mills M, Western Collaborative Perinatal Group: Percutaneous umbilical blood sampling: Results from a multicenter collaborative registry. Am J Obstet Gynecol 166:1614, 1992.

James DK, Parker MJ, Smoleniec JS: Comprehensive fetal assessment with three ultrasonographic characteristics. Am J Obstet Gynecol 166:1486, 1992.

Luck CA: Value of routine ultrasound scanning at 19 weeks: A four year study of 8849 deliveries. BMJ 304:1474, 1992.

Marlow N: Do we need an Apgar score? Arch Dis Child 67:765, 1992.

Out JH, Bruinse HW, Christiaens CGML, et al: A prospective, controlled multicenter study on the obstetric risks of pregnant women with antiphospholipid antibodies. Am J Obstet Gynecol 167:26, 1992.

Smedler A-C, Faxelius G, Bremme K, et al: Psychological development in children born with very low birth weight after severe intrauterine growth retardation: A 10-year follow-up study. Acta Paediatr 81:197, 1992.

Strong TH Jr, Getzler G, Sarno AP, et al: Prophylactic intrapartum amnioinfusion: A randomized clinical trial. Am J Obstet Gynecol 162:1370, 1990.

PHYSICAL EXAMINATION AND GESTATIONAL AGE ASSESSMENT

The first physical examination of the newborn infant serves many important purposes. It may be a general physical examination of a well baby or an examination to determine the cause of various manifestations of neonatal diseases. Because the transition from fetal to neonatal life requires significant cardiopulmonary adjustments, problems in this transition may be detectable immediately in the delivery room or during the 1st day of life. Effects of the labor and delivery resulting from asphyxia, drugs, or birth trauma also may become evident by physical examination. Furthermore, the first newborn examination is an important way to detect congenital malformations or deformations (see Table 6–13). Congenital malformations are due to many different causes—for example, to chromosomal trisomies, teratogens, or recognizable syndromes without identifiable causes. Significant congenital malformations may be present in as many as 1–3% of all births. Congenital deformations are due to compression of fetal parts by the uterus, usually in the absence of amniotic fluid. Thus, some cases of clubfoot are due to compression of the fetal foot by the uterine wall (see Chapter 19).

The *general appearance* of the infant should be evaluated first. Signs such as cyanosis, nasal flaring, intercostal retractions, and grunting suggest pulmonary disease. Meconium staining of the umbilical cord, nails, and skin suggests fetal distress and the possibility of aspiration pneumonia (see below). The level of spontaneous activity, passive muscle tone, quality of the cry, and apnea are useful screening signs to evaluate the state of the nervous system initially.

The examination should then proceed with an assessment of *vital signs*, particularly heart rate (the normal rate is 120–160 beats/min), respiratory rate (the normal rate is 30–60 breaths/min), temperature (usually done initially per rectum and later as an axillary measurement), and blood pressure (often reserved for sick infants). In addition, length, weight, and head circumference should be measured and plotted on growth curves to determine whether growth is normal, accelerated, or retarded for the specific gestational age.

Gestational age is determined by assessing various physical signs (Fig. 6–3) and neurologic characteristics (Fig. 6–4) that vary according to fetal age and maturity. Physical criteria that mature with advancing fetal age include increasing firmness of the pinna of the ear, increasing size of the breast tissue, decreasing lanugo hair over the back, and decreasing opacity of the skin. Neurologic criteria that mature with gestational age include increasing flexion of the legs, hips, and arms; increasing tone of the flexor muscles of the neck; and decreasing laxity of the joints. These signs are determined during the 1st day of life and are assigned scores. The cumulative score is correlated with a gestational age, which is usually accurate to within 2 wk (Fig. 6–5).

Gestational age assessment permits the detection of abnormal fetal growth patterns, thus aiding in predicting the neonatal complications of largeness or smallness for gestational age. Infants born at a weight greater than the 90th percentile for their age are considered **large for gestational age** (LGA). Risks associated with being LGA include all the

EXTERNAL SIGN	SCORE				
	0	1	2	3	4
Edema	Obvious edema of hands and feet; pitting over tibia	No obvious edema of hands and feet; pitting over tibia	No edema		
Skin texture	Very thin, gelatinous	Thin and smooth	Smooth; medium thickness; rash or superficial peeling	Slight thickening; superficial cracking and peeling, especially on hands and feet	Thick and parchmentlike; superficial or deep cracking
Skin color (infant not crying)	Dark red	Uniformly pink	Pale pink; variable over body	Pale; only pink over ears, lips, palms, or soles	
Skin opacity (trunk)	Numerous veins and venules clearly seen, especially over abdomen	Veins and tributaries seen	A few large vessels clearly seen over abdomen	A few large vessels seen indistinctly over abdomen	No blood vessels seen
Lanugo (over back)	No lanugo	Abundant, long and thick over whole back	Hair thinning, especially over lower back	Small amount of lanugo and bald areas	At least half of back devoid of lanugo
Plantar creases	No skin creases	Faint red marks over anterior half of sole	Definite red marks over more than anterior half; indentations over less than anterior third	Indentations over more than anterior third	Definite deep indentations over more than anterior third
Nipple formation	Nipple barely visible; no areola	Nipple well defined, areola smooth and flat; diameter <0.75 cm	Areola stippled, edge not raised; diameter <0.75 cm	Areola stippled, edge raised, diameter >0.75 cm	
Breast size	No breast tissue palpable	Breast tissue on one or both sides <0.5 cm diameter	Breast tissue both sides; one or both 0.5 to 1.0 cm	Breast tissue both sides; one or both >1 cm	
Ear form	Pinna flat and shapeless, little or no incurving of edge	Incurving of part of edge of pinna	Partial incurving whole of upper pinna	Well-defined incurving whole of upper pinna	
Ear firmness	Pinna soft, easily folded, no recoil	Pinna soft, easily folded, slow recoil	Cartilage to edge of pinna, but soft in places, ready recoil	Pinna firm, cartilage to edge; instant recoil	
Genitalia Male	Neither testis in scrotum	At least one testis high in scrotum	At least one testis down in scrotum		
Female (with hips half abducted)	Labia majora widely separated; labia minora protruding	Labia majora almost cover labia minora	Labia majora completely cover labia minora		

Figure 6–3. Physical criteria to estimate gestational age. (From Dubowitz L, Dubowitz V: Gestational Age of the Newborn. Reading, MA, Addison-Wesley, 1977.)

risks of the infant of a diabetic mother (see Table 6–4) and risks associated with postmaturity. Infants born at a weight less than the 10th percentile for their age (some growth curves use less than two standard deviations or the 5th percentile) are **small for gestational age** (SGA) and have intrauterine growth retardation. Problems associated with the SGA infant include congenital malformations in addition to those problems listed in Table 6–7.

The *skin* should be evaluated for pallor, plethora, jaundice, cyanosis, meconium staining, petechiae, ecchymoses, congenital nevi, and neonatal rashes. Vasomotor instability with cutis marmorata, telangiectasia, phlebectasia (intermittent mottling with venous prominence), and acrocyanosis (feet and hands) is normal in the premature infant. Acrocyanosis also may be noted in the healthy term infant in the first days after birth. The **harlequin color change** is a striking transient but normal sign of vasomotor instability and divides the body from head to pubis through the midline into equal halves of pink and pale color. The skin is covered with fine immature **lanugo hair**, which disappears by term gestation. **Hair tufts** over the lumbosacral spine suggest a spinal cord defect. **Vernix caseosa**, a soft, white, creamy layer covering the skin in preterm infants, disappears by term. Post-term infants often have peeling, parchment-like skin. **Mongolian spots** are transient dark blue– to black-pigmented macules seen over the lower back and buttock in 90% of black, Indian, and oriental infants. **Nevus simplex**, or pink macular hemangiomas, are common, usually transient, and noted on the back of the neck, eyelids, and forehead. **Nevus flammeus**, or the **port-wine stain**, commonly is seen on the face and should cause the examiner to consider the Sturge-Weber syndrome (trigeminal angiomatosis, convulsions, and ipsilateral intracranial

NEURO-LOGIC SIGN	SCORE					
	0	1	2	3	4	5
POSTURE						
SQUARE WINDOW	90°	60°	45°	30°	0°	
ANKLE DORSI-FLEXION	90°	75°	45°	20°	0°	
ARM RECOIL	180°	90-180°	<90°			
LEG RECOIL	180°	90-180°	<90°			
POPLIT-EAL ANGLE	180°	160°	130°	110°	90°	<90°
HEEL TO EAR						
SCARF SIGN						
HEAD LAG						
VENTRAL SUSPEN-SION						

Figure 6–4. Neurologic criteria to estimate gestational age to be used with physical findings. (From Dubowitz L, Dubowitz V: Gestational Age of the Newborn. Reading, MA, Addison-Wesley, 1977.)

"tram-line" calcifications). **Capillary hemangiomas** are raised red lesions, whereas **cavernous hemangiomas** are deeper, blue-colored masses. Both increase in size after birth, only to resolve when the infant is 1–4 yr of age. When enlarged, these hemangiomas may produce high-output heart failure or platelet trapping and hemorrhage. **Erythema toxicum** is an erythematous, papular–vesicular rash common to neonates that develops after birth and has eosinophils in the vesicular fluid. **Pustular melanosis**, more common in black

infants, may be seen at birth and consists of a small, dry vesicle on a pigmented brown macular base. Both erythema toxicum and pustular melanosis are benign lesions but may mimic more serious conditions such as the vesicular rash of disseminated herpes simplex or the bullous eruption of *Staphylococcus aureus* impetigo. Tzanck smear, Gram stain, Wright stain, direct fluorescent antibody stain, and appropriate cultures may be needed to distinguish these rashes. Other common characteristic rashes include **milia**, yellow-white epidermal cysts of the pilosebaceous follicles that are noted on the nose, and **miliaria** (prickly heat), which is caused by obstructed sweat glands. **Edema** may be present in preterm infants but should also suggest hydrops fetalis, sepsis, or lymphatic disorders.

The *skull* may be elongated and molded after a prolonged labor, but this resolves 2–3 days after

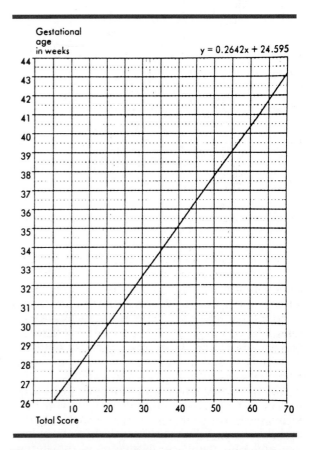

Figure 6–5. Score graph to determine gestational age. After adding the score from the physical criteria to that from the neurologic examination, the total score correlates with gestational age within ± 2 wk. (From Dubowitz L, Dubowitz V: Gestational Age of the Newborn. Reading, MA, Addison-Wesley, 1977.)

birth. The sutures should be palpated to determine the width and the presence of premature fusion, or **cranial synostosis**. The anterior and posterior fontanel should be soft and nonbulging, with the anterior larger than the posterior. A **large fontanel** is associated with hydrocephalus, hypothyroidism, rickets, and other disorders. Soft areas away from the fontanel are **craniotabes**; these lesions have a Ping-Pong ball–like feeling and may be due to in utero compression. The skull should be examined carefully for signs of trauma or lacerations from internal fetal electrode sites or fetal scalp pH sampling; abscess formation may develop in these areas. (See Birth Injury for discussion of **caput succedaneum** and **subgaleal hemorrhage**.)

The *face* should be inspected for dysmorphic features such as epicanthal folds, hypertelorism, preauricular tags or sinuses, low-set ears, long philtrum, and cleft lip or palate. Facial asymmetry may be due to 7th nerve palsy, and head tilt due to torticollis. The *eyes* should open spontaneously, especially in an upright position. Coloboma, megalocornea, and microphthalmia should suggest other malformations or intrauterine infections. A cornea greater than 1 cm in diameter also may be seen in congenital glaucoma, uveal tract dysgenesis, and storage diseases. Conjunctival and retinal hemorrhages are common and usually of no significance. The pupillary response to light is present at 28 wk of gestation, and the **red reflex** of the retina is demonstrated easily. A white reflex, or **leukocoria**, is abnormal and may be due to cataracts, ocular tumor, severe chorioretinitis, persistent hyperplastic primary vitreous, or retinopathy of prematurity.

The *mouth* should be inspected for the presence of natal teeth, clefts of the soft and hard palate and uvula, and micrognathia. White, shiny multiple transient epidermal inclusion cysts (Epstein pearls) on the hard palate are normal. Hard marble-sized masses in the buccal mucosa are usually transient idiopathic fat necrosis. The *tympanic membranes* are dull, gray, opaque, and immobile. These findings may persist for 1–4 wk and should not be confused with otitis media.

The *neck* appears short and symmetric. Abnormalities include midline clefts or masses due to thyroglossal duct cysts or to goiter and lateral neck masses (or sinuses), which are, in turn, due to branchial clefts. Other masses include cystic hygromas and hemangiomas. Shortening of the sternocleidomastoid muscle with a fibrous "tumor" over the muscle produces head tilt and asymmetric facies (**neonatal torticollis**). The Arnold-Chiari malformation and cervical spine lesions also produce torticollis. Edema and webbing of the neck should

suggest Turner syndrome. Both clavicles should be palpated for fractures.

Examination of the *chest* includes inspection of the chest wall to identify asymmetry resulting from absence of the pectoralis muscle and inspection of the breast tissue to determine gestational age and to detect a breast abscess. Both males and females may have breast engorgement and produce milk; milk expression should not be attempted. **Supernumerary nipples** may be bilateral and occasionally are associated with renal anomalies.

Examination of the *lungs* includes observations of the rate, depth, and nature of intercostal or sternal retractions. Breath sounds should be equal on both sides of the chest, and rales should not be heard after the first 1–2 hr of life. Diminished or absent breath sounds on one side should suggest **pneumothorax**, collapsed lung, pleural effusion, or diaphragmatic hernia. Shift of the cardiac impulse away from a tension pneumothorax and diaphragmatic hernia and toward the collapsed lung is a helpful physical finding to differentiate these disorders. **Subcutaneous emphysema** of the neck or chest also suggests a pneumothorax, whereas bowel sounds auscultated in the chest in the presence of a scaphoid abdomen suggest a diaphragmatic hernia.

The position of the *heart* in infants is more midline than in older children. The first heart sound is normal, whereas the second heart sound may not be split in the 1st day of life. Decreased splitting of the second heart sound is noted in persistent fetal circulation, transposition of the great vessels, and pulmonary atresia. **Heart murmurs** are common in the delivery room and during the 1st day of life. Most of these murmurs are transient and due to closure of the ductus arteriosus, peripheral pulmonary stenosis, or a small VSD. Pulses should be palpated in the upper and lower extremities, usually over the brachial and femoral arteries. Blood pressure in the upper and lower extremities should be measured in all patients with a murmur or heart failure. An upper-to-lower extremity gradient of more than 10–20 mm Hg suggests coarctation of the aorta.

In the *abdomen*, the liver may be palpable 2 cm below the right costal margin, whereas the spleen tip may be felt less frequently. A left-sided liver suggests situs inversus and the asplenia syndrome. Both kidneys should be palpable in the 1st day of life with gentle deep palpation. The first urination occurs during the 1st day of life in over 95% of normal term infants. **Abdominal masses** may represent hydronephrosis, dysplastic–multicystic kidney disease, ovarian cysts, intestinal duplication, neuroblastoma, or mesoblastic nephroma; masses should be evaluated immediately with ultrasound. Abdominal distention may be due to intestinal obstructions such as ileal atresia, meconium ileus, midgut volvulus, imperforate anus, or Hirschsprung disease. Meconium stool is passed normally within 48 hr of birth in 99% of term infants. The anus should be patent. An imperforate anus is not always visible; therefore, the first temperature should be taken carefully with a rectal thermometer. The abdominal wall musculature may be absent, as in prune-belly syndrome, or weak, resulting in diastasis recti. **Umbilical hernias** are common among black infants. The umbilical cord should be inspected to determine the presence of two arteries and one vein and the absence of a urachus or a herniation of abdominal contents, as occurs with an **omphalocele**. The latter is associated with extraintestinal problems such as genetic trisomies and hypoglycemia (Beckwith-Wiedemann syndrome). Bleeding from the cord should suggest a coagulation disorder, and a chronic discharge may be a granuloma of the umbilical stump or, less frequently, a draining omphalomesenteric cyst. Erythema around the umbilicus is **omphalitis** and may cause portal vein phlebitis and portal hypertension. The herniation of bowel through the abdominal wall 2–3 cm lateral to the umbilicus is a **gastroschisis**.

The appearance of the *genitalia* varies with gestational age. At term, the testes should be descended into a well-formed pigmented and rugated scrotum. The testes occasionally are in the inguinal canal; this is more common among preterm infants, as is **cryptorchidism**. Scrotal swelling may represent a transient hydrocele, in utero torsion of the testes, or, rarely, dissected meconium from meconium ileus and peritonitis. Hydroceles are clear and readily seen by transillumination, whereas testicular torsion in the newborn may present as a painless dark swelling. The urethral opening should be at the end of the penis. Epispadias or hypospadias alone should not raise concern about pseudohermaphroditism. However, if no testes are present in the scrotum and hypospadias is present, problems of sexual development should be suspected. Circumcision should be deferred with hypospadias, because the foreskin is needed for the repair. The prepuce is often too tight to retract in the neonatal period. The female genitalia normally may reveal a milky white or blood-streaked vaginal discharge as a result of maternal hormone withdrawal. Mucosal tags of the labia majora are common. Distention of an **imperforate hymen** may produce **hydrometrocolpos** and a lower midline abdominal mass as a result of an enlarged uterus. Clitoral enlargement with fusion of the labial–scrotal folds (labia majora) suggests adrenogenital syndrome or exposure to masculinizing maternal hormones.

Examination of the *extremities* should include assessment of length, symmetry, and presence of hemihypertrophy, atrophy, polydactyly, syndactyly, simian creases, absent fingers, overlapping fingers, rocker-bottom feet, clubfoot, congenital bands, and amputations.

The *spine* should be examined for evidence of a dermal sinus tract above the gluteal folds, congenital scoliosis (due to hemivertebra), and soft tissue masses such as a lipoma or meningomyelocele.

The *hips* should be examined for congenital dysplasia (dislocation). Gluteal fold asymmetry or leg length discrepancy is a suggestive sign of this condition, but the examiner should perform the **Barlow test** and the **Ortolani maneuver** to evaluate the stability of the hip joint. These tests determine whether the femoral head can be displaced from the acetabulum (Barlow test) and then replaced (Ortolani maneuver). The examiner's long finger is placed over the greater trochanter, and the thumb is placed medially just distal to the long finger. With the thighs held in midabduction, the femoral head is pulled out of the acetabulum by lateral pressure of the thumb and by rocking the knee medially. The reverse maneuver is performed by pressing the long finger on the greater trochanter and rocking the knee laterally. A "clunking" sensation is palpated when the femoral head leaves and returns to the acetabulum.

The *neurologic* examination should include assessment of active and passive tone, level of alertness, primary neonatal (primitive) reflexes, deep tendon reflexes, spontaneous motor activity, and cranial nerves (retinal examination, extraocular muscle movement, masseter power as in sucking, facial motility, hearing, and tongue function). Primary newborn reflexes include the **Moro reflex** (present at birth, gone between 3–6 mo), which is elicited by sudden slight dropping of the supported head from a slightly raised supine position. This slight drop should elicit opening of the hands and extension and abduction of the arms, followed by upper extremity flexion and a cry. The **palmar grasp** is present as early as 28 wk of age and gone by 4 mo of age. **Deep tendon reflexes** may be brisk in the normal newborn; 10–20 beats of ankle clonus are normal. The **Babinski sign** is extensor or upgoing. The sensory examination can be evaluated by withdrawal of an extremity, grimace, and cry in response to painful stimuli. The **rooting reflex**, or the turning of the head toward light tactile stimulation of the perioral area, is present as early as 32 wk of age.

References

Aladjem S, Vidyasagar D: Atlas of Perinatology. Philadelphia, WB Saunders, 1982.

Behrman RE (ed): Nelson Textbook of Pediatrics. 14th ed. Philadelphia, WB Saunders, 1992, Sec. 9.2–9.4, 9.17.

Illingworth R: The Normal Child. 10th ed. Edinburgh, Churchill Livingstone, 1991.

Leppig K, Werler M, Cann C, et al: Predictive value of minor anomalies. I. Association with major malformations. J Pediatr 110:530, 1987.

RESPIRATORY DISORDERS

Approach to the Patient

Respiratory distress that becomes manifest by tachypnea, intercostal retractions, reduced air exchange, cyanosis, grunting, and flaring of the ala nasi is a nonspecific response to serious illness. Not all of the disorders producing neonatal respiratory distress are primary diseases of the lungs. The differential diagnosis of respiratory distress includes pulmonary, cardiac, hematologic, infectious, anatomic, and metabolic disorders that may directly or indirectly involve the lungs (see Tables 6–12 and 6–15). Surfactant deficiency causes the *respiratory distress syndrome*, resulting in cyanosis and tachypnea; *infection* produces pneumonia demonstrated by interstitial or lobar infiltrates; *meconium aspiration* results in chemical pneumonitis with pulmonary hypertension; *hydrops fetalis* causes anemia and hypoalbuminemia with high-output heart failure and pulmonary edema; and congenital or acquired *pulmonary hypoplasia* causes pulmonary hypertension and pulmonary insufficiency. It also is useful to differentiate the common causes of respiratory distress according to gestational age (Table 6–15).

In addition to the specific therapy of the individual disorder, the supportive care and evaluation of the infant with respiratory distress can be applied universally to all the problems mentioned earlier (see Tables 6–14 and 6–16). Blood gas monitoring and interpretation are key components of general respiratory care. Treatment of hypoxemia requires knowledge of normal values. In term infants, the arterial PaO_2 is 55–60 mm Hg at 30 min of life, 75 mm Hg at 4 hr, and 90 mm Hg by 24 hr. Preterm infants have slightly lower values. $PaCO_2$ levels should be between 35 and 40 mm Hg, and the pH should be 7.35–7.40. It is imperative that arterial blood gas analysis be performed in all infants with significant respiratory distress, whether or not cyanosis is perceived. Cyanosis becomes evident when there are 5 g of unsaturated hemoglobin; thus anemia may interfere with the perception of cyanosis. Jaundice also may interfere with the appearance of cyanosis. Capillary blood gas determinations are useful in determining blood pH and PCO_2. Because of the nature of the heel-stick capillary blood gas technique, venous blood may mix with arterial blood, resulting in falsely low blood PaO_2 readings. Serial blood gases may be monitored by an indwelling arterial catheter placed through the umbilical artery to the aorta at the level of the T6-10 or the L4-5 vertebrae. This placement avoids catheter occlusion of the celiac (T12), superior mesenteric (T12-L1), renal (Ll-2), and inferior mesenteric arteries (L2-3). Another method for monitoring blood gases is to combine capillary blood gas techniques with noninvasive methods used to monitor oxygen (e.g., pulse oximetry or transcutaneous oxygen diffusion [$TcPO_2$]).

Metabolic acidosis, defined as a reduced pH (<7.25) and bicarbonate concentration (<18) accompanied by a normal or low PCO_2, may be due to hypoxia or to insufficient tissue perfusion; the origin of the disorder may be pulmonary, cardiac, infectious, renal, hematologic, nutritional, or iatro-

Table 6–15. Etiology of Respiratory Distress

Preterm Infant	Full-Term Infant	Preterm and Full-Term Infant
Respiratory distress syndrome	Meconium aspiration pneumonia	Bacterial sepsis
Erythroblastosis fetalis	Persistent fetal circulation	Transient tachypnea
Nonimmune hydrops	Polycythemia	Spontaneous pneumothorax
		Congenital anomalies (e.g., diphragmatic hernia)
		Congenital heart disease
		Pulmonary hypoplasia
		Viral infection (e.g., herpes simplex, CMV)
		Inborn metabolic errors

CMV = cytomegalovirus.

Table 6–16. Initial Laboratory Evaluation of Respiratory Distress

Test	Rationale
Chest roentgenogram	To determine reticular granular pattern of RDS; to determine presence of pneumothorax, cardiomegaly, life-threatening congenital anomalies
Arterial blood gas	To determine severity of respiratory compromise, hypoxemia, hypercapnia, and type of acidosis; the severity determines treatment strategy
Complete blood count	Hemoglobin/hematocrit to determine anemia and polycythemia; white blood cell count to determine neutropenia/sepsis; platelet count and smear to determine DIC
Buffy coat smear	For Gram stain of bacteria
Blood culture	To recover potential pathogen
Blood glucose	To determine presence of hypoglycemia, which may produce or occur simultaneously with respiratory distress; to determine stress hyperglycemia
Echocardiogram, electrocardiogram	In the presence of a murmur, cardiomegaly, refractory hypoxia; to determine structural heart disease or PFC

DIC = disseminated intravascular coagulation; PFC = persistent fetal circulation; RDS = respiratory distress syndrome.

genic. The initial approach to metabolic acidosis is to determine the cause and treat the pathophysiologic problem. This approach may include, as in the sequence of therapy for hypoxia, increasing the inspired oxygen concentration, applying continuous positive airway pressure nasally using oxygen as the gas, or initiating mechanical ventilation using positive end-expiratory pressure and oxygen. Hypotension produced by hypovolemia requires fluids and circulatory support. If metabolic acidosis persists despite specific therapy, sodium bicarbonate (1–2 mEq/kg/dose) may be given by slow intravenous infusion and repeated as needed.

Respiratory acidosis, defined as an elevated P_{CO_2} and reduced pH without a reduction in the bicarbonate concentration, may be due to pulmonary insufficiency or central hypoventilation. Most disorders producing respiratory distress can result in hypercapnia. Treatment requires assisted ventilation but *not* sodium bicarbonate. If central nervous system depression of respirations is due to placental passage of narcotic analgesics, assisted ventilation is instituted first, and then the central nervous system depression is reversed by naloxone.

Mixed metabolic/respiratory acidosis is common and requires combined therapy. Other acid–base disturbances such as metabolic alkalosis and respiratory alkalosis are uncommon in the neonatal period, unless caused by diuretics or by ventilator-induced hyperventilation, respectively.

Respiratory Distress Syndrome (Hyaline Membrane Disease)

LUNG DEVELOPMENT

An appreciation of lung development is basic to understanding the pathophysiology of respiratory distress syndrome (RDS). The lungs develop from an outpouching of the embryonic gut at 24 days of gestation. By 12 wk the trachea, bronchi, lobes, pulmonary artery, and pleura are present; at this time, there are no air spaces and the lung appears "glandular." The airways become cannulized, the terminal respiratory air spaces develop, and, by 26–28 wk of gestation, the alveoli appear and the capillary network has proliferated. The number of alveoli at birth continues to increase until early childhood, resulting in an 11-fold increase in the air–tissue interface. The lining of the alveolus consists of 90% type I cells and 10% type II cells. After 20 wk of gestation, the type II cells contain vacuolated, osmophilic, lamellar inclusion bodies, which are packages of surface-active material (Fig. 6–6). This lipoprotein *surfactant* is 90% lipid and is composed predominantly of saturated phosphatidylcholine (dipalmityl phosphatidylcholine, or lecithin) but also contains phosphatidylglycerol, other phospholipids, and neutral lipids. The surfactant proteins (SP), SP-A, SP-B, and SP-C, are packaged into the lamellar body and contribute to surface-active properties and recycling of surfactant. Surfactant prevents atelectasis by reducing surface tension at low lung volumes when it is concentrated at end-expiration as the alveolar radius decreases; surfactant contributes to lung recoil by increasing surface tension at larger lung volumes when it is diluted during inspiration as the alveolar radius increases. Without surfactant, surface tension forces are not reduced and atelectasis develops during end-expiration as the alveolus collapses.

The timing of surfactant (lecithin) production in quantities sufficient to prevent atelectasis depends

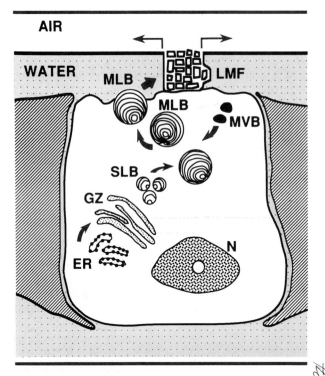

Figure 6–6. Proposed pathway of synthesis, transport, secretion, and reuptake of surfactant in the type II alveolar cell. Phospholipids are synthesized in the smooth endoplasmic reticulum (ER). The glucose/glycerol precursor may be derived from lung glycogen or circulating glucose. Phospholipids and surfactant proteins are packaged in the Golgi apparatus (GZ), emerge as small lamellar bodies (SLB), coalesce to mature lamellar bodies (MLB), migrate to the apical membrane, and are released by exocytosis into the liquid hypophase below the air–liquid interface. The tightly coiled lamellar body unravels to form the lattice (tubular) myelin figure (LMF), the immediate precursor to the phospholipid monolayer at the alveolar surface. Reuptake by endocytosis forms multivesicular bodies (MVB), which recycle surfactant. The enzymes, receptors, transporters, and surfactant proteins are controlled by regulatory processes at the transcriptional level in the nucleus (N). Corticosteroid and thyroid hormones are regulatory ligands that may accelerate surfactant synthesis. (From Hansen T, Corbet A: Lung Development and Function. *In* Taeusch HW, Ballard R, Avery ME [eds]: Diseases of the Newborn. 6th ed. Philadelphia, WB Saunders, 1991.)

on an increase in fetal cortisol levels that begins between 32 and 34 wk of gestation. Between 34 and 36 wk, sufficient surface-active material is produced by the type II cells in the lung, is secreted into the alveolar lumen, and is excreted into the amniotic fluid. Thus, the concentration of lecithin in amniotic fluid indicates fetal pulmonary matur-

ity. Because quantitation of lecithin is difficult to perform, the ratio of lecithin (which increases with maturity) to sphingomyelin (which remains constant during gestation) (L/S ratio) is determined. A ratio of 2:1 usually indicates pulmonary maturity. The presence of minor phospholipids such as phosphatidylglycerol also is indicative of fetal lung maturity and may be useful in situations in which the L/S ratio is borderline or possibly affected by maternal diabetes, which reduces lung maturity. Alternately, a "shake test" may be performed on the amniotic fluid to examine the stability of the bubbles maintained by surface-active material after shaking diluted amniotic fluid in a test tube.

CLINICAL MANIFESTATIONS OF RDS

Respiratory distress syndrome is due to a deficiency of pulmonary surfactant that results in atelectasis, a decreased functional residual capacity, arterial hypoxemia, and respiratory distress. In addition to the developmental deficiency, surfactant synthesis may be reduced as a result of hypovolemia, hypothermia, acidosis, and hypoxemia. These factors also produce pulmonary artery vasospasm, which may contribute to respiratory distress syndrome in larger premature infants who have developed sufficient pulmonary arteriole smooth muscle to produce vasoconstriction. Surfactant deficiency–induced atelectasis causes alveoli to be perfused but not ventilated, which results in a pulmonary shunt and hypoxemia. As atelectasis increases, the lungs become increasingly difficult to expand and lung compliance decreases. Because the chest wall of the premature infant is very compliant, the infant attempts to overcome decreased lung compliance with increasing inspiratory pressures, resulting in retractions of the chest wall. The sequence of decreased lung compliance and chest wall retractions results in poor air exchange, an increased physiologic dead space, alveolar hypoventilation, and hypercapnia. A vicious cycle of hypoxia, hypercapnia, and acidosis acts on type II cells to reduce surfactant synthesis and, in some infants, on the pulmonary arterioles to produce pulmonary hypertension.

Pathologic examination of the lung reveals atelectasis and acidophilic pink membranes (hyaline membranes) lining the air spaces. Hyaline membrane formation results from transudation of fluid through the capillary endothelium into the surfactant-deficient alveolus.

The infants at greatest risk for RDS are premature and have an immature L/S ratio. The incidence of RDS increases with decreasing gestational age.

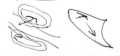

Table 6–17. Acute Deterioration in RDS

Pneumothorax
Extubation
Endotracheal tube in right main stem bronchus
Mucous plug in endotracheal tube
Pulmonary hemorrhage
Intraventricular hemorrhage
Pneumopericardium
Sepsis
Intra-abdominal hemorrhage (liver, spleen, adrenal)

Nonetheless, only 30–60% of infants between 28 and 32 wk of gestation develop RDS. Other risk factors include delivery of a previous preterm infant with RDS, an infant of a diabetic mother, hypothermia, asphyxia, male sex, Caucasian race, being a second twin, and delivery by cesarean section without labor.

Signs of RDS may develop immediately in the delivery room in very immature infants at 26–30 wk of gestation. However, some more mature infants (34 wk of gestation) may not show signs of RDS until 3–4 hr after birth. Manifestations of RDS include cyanosis, tachypnea, nasal flaring, intercostal and sternal retractions, and a whining, crying, moaning sound called grunting. The latter sign is due to partial closure of the glottis during expiration, resulting in higher end-expiratory airway pressures that may ameliorate atelectasis. Atelectasis is well documented by the chest radiograph, which demonstrates a ground-glass haze in the lung surrounding air-filled bronchi (the air bronchogram). Severe RDS may demonstrate an airless lung field or a "whiteout" on roentgenogram, even obliterating the distinction between the atelectatic lungs and the heart.

During the first 72 hr, infants with RDS have increasing distress and hypoxemia. Infants with severe RDS develop edema, apnea, and respiratory failure necessitating mechanical ventilation. Thereafter, uncomplicated cases demonstrate a spontaneous improvement that often is heralded by diuresis and a marked resolution of edema. Complications include those noted in Table 6–17 plus the development of a patent ductus arteriosus and bronchopulmonary dysplasia. The differential diagnosis of RDS includes diseases associated with cyanosis and respiratory distress (see Tables 6–12 and 6–15).

PREVENTION AND TREATMENT OF RDS

Essential preventive measures for RDS include avoiding premature birth from either elective cesar-

ean section or premature labor. In addition, prevention of cold stress, birth asphyxia, and hypovolemia reduces the risk of RDS and its severity. If premature delivery is unavoidable, the antenatal administration of corticosteroids to the mother (and thus to the fetus) may stimulate fetal lung production of surfactant, but this approach requires multiple doses for at least 48 hr, the most effective time for administration being between 28 and 32 wk of gestation.

After birth, RDS may be prevented or its severity reduced by the intratracheal administration of synthetic or natural surfactants to premature infants with immature amniotic L/S ratios. Synthetic (lecithin, tyloxapol, hexadecanol) or natural (lecithin-fortified extract of cow lungs) surfactant also can be administered repeatedly during the course of RDS in patients receiving endotracheal intubation, mechanical ventilation, and oxygen therapy. Additional management includes the general supportive and ventilation care discussed in Tables 6–14, 6–16, and 6–18.

The Pa_{O_2} should be maintained between 60 and 70 mm Hg and pH kept above 7.25–7.28. An increased concentration of warm and humidified inspired oxygen administered by an oxygen hood may be all that is needed for larger premature infants. If hypoxemia (Pa_{O_2} <50 mm Hg) is present and the needed inspired O_2 concentration is 70–100%, continuous positive airway pressure (nasal CPAP) should be added at a distending pressure of 8–10 cm H_2O. If respiratory failure ensues (P_{CO_2} >60 mm Hg, pH <7.20, and Pa_{O_2} <50 on 100% O_2), mechanical ventilation using a respirator is indicated. Conventional rate (25–60 breaths/min), high-frequency jet (150–600 breaths/min), and oscillator (900–3000 breaths/min) ventilators each have been successful in managing respiratory failure due to severe RDS. Suggested starting settings on a conventional ventilator include: fraction of inspired oxygen (FiO_2), 60–100%; peak inspiratory pressure (PIP), 20–25 cm H_2O; positive end-expiratory pressure (PEEP), +5 cm H_2O; and a rate of 20–40 breaths/min. The inspiratory-to-expiratory time (I:E) ratio is 1:1.2 to 1:2.0.

In response to persistent hypercapnia, alveolar ventilation (tidal volume minus dead space times rate) must be increased. This may be achieved by increasing the ventilator's rate or by increasing the tidal volume, which is the gradient between PIP and PEEP. In response to hypoxia, the inspired oxygen content may be increased. Alternately, the degree of oxygenation is dependent on the mean airway pressure (Paw). Paw is directly related to PIP, PEEP, flow, and I:E ratio. Increased Paw may

Table 6–18. Ventilator Management of RDS

Setting	Result	Rationale	Risks
↑ FiO$_2$	↑ Po$_2$	↑ Alveolar O$_2$	Oxygen toxicity
↑ PIP	↑ Po$_2$ ↓ Pco$_2$	↑ $\overline{\text{Paw}}$ ↑ Tidal volume	Pneumothorax, barotrauma, ↓ cardiac output?
↑ PEEP	↑ Po$_2$	↑ $\overline{\text{Paw}}$	↑ Pco$_2$ by ↓ tidal volume ↓ Cardiac output?
↑ Rate	↓ Pco$_2$	↑ Alveolar ventilation	↓ Expiratory time causes gas trapping
↑ I:E ratio	↑ Po$_2$	↑ $\overline{\text{Paw}}$	↓ Expiratory time causes gas trapping

FiO$_2$ = fraction of inspired oxygen; I:E = inspiratory to expiratory time ratio; $\overline{\text{Paw}}$ = mean airway pressure; PEEP = positive end-expiratory pressure; PIP = peak inspiratory pressure.

improve oxygenation by improving lung volume, thus enhancing ventilation–perfusion matching (Table 6–18).

Because of the difficulty in distinguishing sepsis and pneumonia from RDS, broad-spectrum parenteral antibiotics (ampicillin and gentamicin) are administered for 72 hr, pending the recovery of an organism from a previously obtained blood culture.

COMPLICATIONS OF RDS

Patent Ductus Arteriosus

The ductus arteriosus constricts after birth in normal term infants in response to an elevated Pao$_2$. The ductus arteriosus in the preterm infant is less responsive to vasoconstrictive stimuli, in part as a result of the persistent vasodilatory effect of prostaglandins (PGE$_2$); this decreased vasoconstriction response, combined with hypoxemia during RDS, may result in a persistently patent ductus arteriosus (PDA) that may create a shunt between the pulmonary and systemic circulations. During the acute phase of RDS, pulmonary arterial vasoconstriction and increased pressure are due to hypoxia, hypercapnia, and acidosis. Therefore, the pulmonary and systemic pressures may be equal, and flow through the ductus may be small or bidirectional. When RDS improves and pulmonary vascular resistance declines, flow through the ductus arteriosus increases in a left-to-right direction. Significant systemic-to-pulmonary shunting may result in heart failure and pulmonary edema. Excessive intravenous fluid administration may increase the incidence of a symptomatic PDA. The infant's respiratory status deteriorates owing to increased lung fluid, hypercapnia, and hypoxemia. In response to poor blood gases, the infant is subjected to higher inspired oxygen concentrations and higher peak inspiratory ventilator pressures, both of which damage the lung (see Bronchopulmonary Dysplasia).

Clinical manifestations of a PDA usually become apparent on the 3rd–5th day of life. Because the left-to-right shunt is to a low-pressure circulation from one of high pressure, the pulse pressure widens; a previously inactive precordium now demonstrates a very active precordial impulse, and the peripheral pulses become easily palpable and bounding. The murmur of a PDA may be continuous in systole and diastole, but usually only the systolic component is auscultated. Heart failure and pulmonary edema result in rales and hepatomegaly. A chest roentgenogram demonstrates cardiomegaly and pulmonary edema; a two-dimensional echocardiogram demonstrates patency, whereas Doppler studies demonstrate markedly increased left-to-right flow through the ductus.

Treatment of a PDA during RDS includes an initial period of fluid restriction and diuretic administration. If after 24–48 hr there is no improvement, indomethacin, a prostaglandin synthetase inhibitor, is administered (0.2 mg/kg) intravenously every 12 hr for three doses. Thereafter the drug is administered at 0.1–0.2 mg/kg every 24 hr for 5 days. This has been most successful in closing the PDA among premature infants in the first 2 wk of life, when prostaglandins may still be playing a significant role in maintaining ductal patency. Contraindications to using indomethacin include thrombocytopenia (<50,000), bleeding, serum creatinine measuring more than 1.8 mg/dL, and oliguria. Because 20–30% of infants do not respond initially to indomethacin and, of those who do, the PDA reopens in 10%, a repeated course of indomethacin or surgical ligation is required in a significant number of patients.

Pulmonary Air Leaks

High PIPs and PEEPs may cause overdistention of alveoli in localized areas of the lung. Rupture of the alveolar epithelial lining may produce **pulmo-**

nary interstitial emphysema (PIE) as gas dissects along the interstitial space and the peribronchial lymphatics. Extravasation of gas into the parenchyma reduces lung compliance and worsens respiratory failure. Gas dissection into the mediastinal space produces a **pneumomediastinum**, occasionally with gas dissecting into the subcutaneous tissues around the neck, causing **subcutaneous emphysema**. Alveolar rupture adjacent to the pleural space produces a **pneumothorax** (see Physical Examination and Gestational Age Assessment). If the gas is under tension, the pneumothorax shifts the mediastinum to the opposite side of the chest, producing hypotension, hypoxia, and hypercapnia. A pneumothorax may be *diagnosed* by unequal transillumination of the chest and may be confirmed by chest roentgenogram. *Treatment* of a symptomatic pneumothorax requires inserting a pleural chest tube connected to negative pressure or to an underwater drain. Prophylactic or therapeutic use of exogenous surfactant has reduced the incidence of pulmonary air leaks.

Pneumothorax also is observed following vigorous resuscitation, meconium aspiration pneumonia, pulmonary hypoplasia, and diaphragmatic hernia. Spontaneous pneumothorax may be seen in less than 1% of deliveries and may be associated with renal malformations.

Pneumopericardium is a severe life-threatening condition that may cause cardiac tamponade. Systemic gas embolism is another rare but lethal complication of mechanical ventilation.

Bronchopulmonary Dysplasia

Oxygen concentrations over 40% are toxic to the neonatal lung. Oxygen-mediated lung injury results from the generation of superoxides, H_2O_2, and oxygen-free radicals, which disrupt membrane lipids. Mechanical ventilation with high peak pressures produces barotrauma, compounding the damaging effects of high inspired oxygen levels. Most patients develop bronchopulmonary dysplasia (BPD) following ventilation for RDS that may have been complicated by PDA or PIE. Failure of RDS to improve after 2 wk and the need for mechanical ventilation and oxygen therapy at 1 mo of age are characteristic of patients with RDS who develop BPD. Infants weighing less than 1000 g who require mechanical ventilation for poor respiratory drive in the absence of RDS also may develop BPD.

The roentgenographic appearance of BPD may go through phases characterized initially by lung opacification and, subsequently, by development of cysts accompanied by areas of overdistention and atelectasis, giving the lung a sponge-like appearance. The histopathology of BPD reveals interstitial edema, atelectasis, mucosal metaplasia, interstitial fibrosis, necrotizing obliterative bronchiolitis, and overdistended alveoli.

The *clinical manifestations* of BPD are oxygen dependence, hypercapnia, compensatory metabolic alkalosis, pulmonary hypertension, and the development of right-sided heart failure. Increased airway resistance with reactive airway bronchoconstriction also is noted, and is treated with bronchodilating agents. Severe chest retractions produce very negative interstitial pressure that draws fluid into the interstitial space. These chest retractions, together with cor pulmonale, cause fluid retention necessitating fluid restriction and administration of diuretics.

Patients with BPD may require *treatment* with mechanical ventilation for many months. To reduce the risk of subglottic stenosis, a tracheotomy may be indicated. To reduce oxygen toxicity and barotrauma, ventilator settings are reduced to maintain blood gases with slightly lower Pa_{O_2} (50 mm Hg) and higher Pa_{CO_2} (50–75 mm Hg) than for infants during the acute phase of RDS. Dexamethasone therapy may reduce inflammation and enhance weaning of patients from mechanical ventilation.

Retinopathy of Prematurity (Retrolental Fibroplasia)

This disorder is caused by the acute and chronic effects of oxygen toxicity on the developing blood vessels of the premature infant's retina. The completely vascularized retina of the term infant is not susceptible to retinopathy of prematurity (ROP). ROP is a leading cause of blindness for VLBW infants (<1500 g). Excessive arterial oxygen tensions produce vasoconstriction of the immature retinal vasculature in the first stage of this disease, which is followed by vaso-obliteration if the duration and extent of hyperoxia are prolonged beyond the time when vasoconstriction is reversible. The subsequent proliferative stages are characterized by extraretinal fibrovascular proliferation, forming a ridge between the vascular and avascular portions of the retina, and by the development of neovascular tufts. In mild cases, vasoproliferation is noted at the periphery of the retina. Severe cases may have neovascularization involving the entire retina, retinal detachment resulting from traction on vessels as they leave the optic disk, fibrous proliferation behind the lens producing leukocoria, and synechiae displacing the lens forward and resulting in glaucoma. Both eyes usually are involved, but severity may be asymmetric.

The incidence of ROP may be reduced by careful monitoring of arterial blood gases in all patients receiving oxygen. Although there is no absolutely safe Pa_{O_2}, it is wise to keep the arterial O_2 between 50 and 70 torr in premature infants. Cryotherapy may be used for vitreous hemorrhage or for severe progressive vasoproliferation. Surgery is indicated for retinal detachment. Less severe stages of ROP resolve spontaneously without visual impairment in the majority of patients.

Transient Tachypnea of the Newborn

Transient tachypnea of the newborn (TTN) is a self-limited condition characterized by tachypnea, mild retractions, and occasional grunting, usually without signs of severe respiratory distress. Cyanosis, when present, usually requires no more than 30–40% O_2. TTN usually is noted in larger premature infants and in term infants born by cesarean section without prior labor. The infant of a diabetic mother or the infant with poor respiratory drive as a result of placental passage of analgesic drugs is also at risk. Chest roentgenograms show prominent central vascular markings, fluid in the lung fissures, overaeration, and, occasionally, a small pleural effusion. Air bronchograms and a reticulogranular pattern are not seen in TTN, and their presence would suggest another pulmonary process such as RDS or pneumonia. TTN may be due to retained lung fluid and/or slow resorption of lung fluid.

Meconium Aspiration Syndrome

Meconium-stained amniotic fluid is seen in 10–15% of predominantly term, growth-retarded, and post-term deliveries. Although passage of meconium into amniotic fluid is very common among infants born in the breech presentation, meconium-stained fluid should be considered a sign of fetal distress for infants born in all presentations. Fetal scalp pH should be determined and biophysical evaluation should be done to assess the well-being of the fetus. The presence of meconium in the amniotic fluid suggests in utero asphyxia, hypoxia, and acidosis.

An additional risk is aspiration of amniotic fluid contaminated with particulate meconium. Aspiration may occur in utero in a distressed, gasping fetus, but more often meconium is aspirated into the lung immediately after delivery. Over 50% of infants born with meconium-stained fluid have meconium in the trachea at the time of birth. Half of these infants will develop abnormal chest roentgenograms demonstrating a very high incidence of pneumonia and pneumothoraces.

Meconium aspiration pneumonia is characterized by tachypnea, hypoxia, hypercapnia, and small airway obstruction that results in a ball-valve effect, producing air trapping, overdistention, and extra-alveolar air leaks. Complete small airway obstruction produces atelectasis. Within 24–48 hr, a chemical pneumonia develops in addition to the mechanical effects of airway obstruction. The chest roentgenogram demonstrates patchy infiltrates, overdistention, flattening of the diaphragm, increased anteroposterior diameter, and a very high incidence of pneumomediastinum and pneumothoraces. Quite unexpectedly, many symptomatic infants with severe hypoxia demonstrate a completely normal-appearing chest film. The condition of these infants with severe pulmonary hypertension is very similar to that of infants with persistent fetal circulation (PFC). Comorbid diseases include those associated with in utero asphyxia that initiated the passage of meconium (see Table 6–9).

Treatment of meconium aspiration includes general supportive care and mechanical ventilation. Infants with a PFC-like presentation should be treated for PFC. If severe hypoxia does not subside with conventional or high-frequency ventilation, extracorporeal membrane oxygenation (ECMO) may be beneficial.

Prevention of meconium aspiration syndrome includes careful in utero monitoring to avoid asphyxia. When meconium-stained fluid is observed, the obstetrician should suction the oropharynx of the infant before delivering the rest of the infant's body. After birth the infant's oropharynx should be suctioned, the vocal cords visualized, and the area below the vocal cords suctioned to remove meconium from the trachea. This procedure could be repeated 2–3 times as long as meconium is present, prior to either stimulating the infant to breathe or initiating artificial ventilation (see Asphyxia: Resuscitation). Saline intrauterine amnioinfusion during labor may reduce the incidence of aspiration and pneumonia.

Persistent Fetal Circulation (Primary Pulmonary Hypertension)

This disorder is characterized by severe hypoxemia without evidence of parenchymal lung or structural heart disease that also may cause right-to-left shunting. PFC often is seen in term or post-term infants who are asphyxiated or who have had meconium-stained fluid. The chest roentgenogram usually demonstrates normal lung fields rather than the expected infiltrates and hyperinflation that may accompany massive meconium aspiration pneumonia. Additional problems that may result in PFC include congenital pneumonia, hyperviscosity–polycythemia, congenital diaphragmatic hernia, pulmonary hypoplasia, hypoglycemia, and hypothermia. Total anomalous venous return associated with obstruction of blood flow may produce a clinical picture that includes severe hypoxia and that is indistinguishable from PFC; chest roentgenogram, however, reveals severe pulmonary venous engorgement and a small heart; echocardiography or cardiac catheterization will confirm the diagnosis.

PFC is characterized by significant right-to-left shunting through a patent formen ovale, through a PDA and through intrapulmonary channels. The pulmonary vasculature often demonstrates hypertrophied arterial wall smooth muscle, suggesting that the process of or predisposition to PFC began in utero as a result of previous periods of fetal hypoxia. After birth, hypoxia, hypercapnia, and acidosis exacerbate pulmonary artery vasoconstriction, resulting in further hypoxia and acidosis. In addition to pulmonary hypertension, some infants with PFC develop extrapulmonary manifestations as a result of asphyxia (see Table 6–9). Myocardial injuries include heart failure, transient mitral insufficiency, and papillary muscle or myocardial infarction. Thrombocytopenia, right atrial thrombi, and pulmonary embolism also may be noted.

The *diagnosis* of PFC may be confirmed by echocardiogram, which demonstrates elevated pulmonary artery pressures and sites of right-to-left shunting. Echocardiography also is helpful to rule out structural congenital heart disease and transient myocardial dysfunction.

Treatment of PFC includes general supportive care in addition to correction of hypotension, anemia, and acidosis and the management of complications associated with asphyxia. If myocardial dysfunction is present, dopamine or dobutamine will be needed. The most important therapy for PFC is mechanical ventilation. Reversible mild pulmonary hypertension may respond to conventional ventilator settings (Table 6–18). However, patients with severe PFC do not always respond to conventional therapy and may require hyperventilation to reverse pulmonary vasoconstriction by reducing P_{CO_2} to 20 mm Hg and increasing pH to 7.5–7.6. Paralysis with pancuronium may be needed to assist such vigorous ventilation. Occa-

sionally, tolazoline (Priscoline, 1 mg/kg dose) is given in an attempt to chemically dilate the pulmonary artery, thereby improving oxygenation, but tolazoline is a nonselective alpha-adrenergic blocking agent that may decrease both pulmonary and systemic blood pressures, thus producing systemic hypotension. If mechanical ventilation and supportive care are unsuccessful in improving oxygenation, the patient may be a candidate for ECMO. Infants who require very high ventilator settings, marked by an alveolar-to-arterial oxygen gradient greater than 620 mm Hg, have a high mortality rate and may benefit from ECMO. Inhaled nitric oxide (NO) is a promising new therapy for PFC. NO is an endogenous endothelium derived vessel relaxing factor which may reduce pulmonary vasoconstriction.

Apnea

Apnea is defined as the cessation of pulmonary airflow for a specific time interval, usually longer than 10–20 sec. Bradycardia often accompanies prolonged apnea. *Central apnea* refers to a complete cessation of airflow and respiratory efforts with no chest wall movement; *obstructive apnea* exhibits no airflow but the chest wall movements continue. A combination of these two events, *mixed apnea*, is the most frequent type. It usually begins as a brief episode of obstruction followed by a central apnea.

A careful evaluation to determine the cause should be performed immediately in any infant with apnea (Table 6–19). The incidence of apnea increases as gestational age decreases. Idiopathic apnea, a disease of premature infants, appears in the absence of any other identifiable disease states during the 1st week of life and resolves by 36 wk of postconceptional age (gestational age at birth + postnatal age). The premature infant's process of regulating respiration is especially vulnerable to apnea. For example, preterm infants respond paradoxically to hypoxia by developing apnea rather than by increasing respirations, as mature infants do. Poor tone of the laryngeal muscles also may result in collapse of the upper airway, leading to obstruction. Isolated obstructive apnea, the least common type of apnea, also may occur as a result of flexion or extreme lateral positioning of the premature infant's head, obstructing the soft trachea.

Treatment of apnea of prematurity includes administration of oxygen to hypoxic infants, transfusion of anemic infants, and physical cutaneous stimulation for mild apnea. Persistent apnea with bradycardia can be treated with methylxanthines, caffeine, or theophylline. Theophylline decreases

Table 6–19. Potential Causes of Neonatal Apnea

CNS	IVH, drugs, seizures, hypoxic injury
Respiratory	Pneumonia, obstructive airway lesions, atelectasis, extreme prematurity (<1000 g), laryngeal reflex, phrenic nerve paralysis, severe RDS, pneumothorax
Infectious	Sepsis, necrotizing enterocolitis, meningitis (bacterial, fungal, viral)
Gastrointestinal	Oral feeding, bowel movement, gastroesophageal reflux, esophagitis, intestinal perforation
Metabolic	↓ Glucose, ↓ calcium, ↓ P_{O_2}, ↓↑ sodium, ↑ ammonia, ↑ organic acids, ↑ ambient temperature, hypothermia
Cardiovascular	Hypotension, hypertension, heart failure, anemia, hypovolemia, change in vagal tone
Idiopathic	Immaturity of respiratory center, sleep state, upper airway collapse

CNS = central nervous system; IVH = intraventricular hemorrhage.

the incidence of apnea by acting as a central nervous system stimulant. Loading doses of 5 mg/kg followed by 1–2 mg/kg every 8–12 hr are sufficient. Elimination of theophylline is prolonged in preterm infants, and serum levels should be carefully monitored and maintained between 5 and 10 μg/mL. In the newborn infant, theophylline also is converted to caffeine, thus increasing its efficacy. Nasal CPAP of 3–5 cm H_2O also is an effective method of treating obstructive or mixed apneas; it may work by splinting the upper airway.

Miscellaneous Respiratory Disorders

Pulmonary hypoplasia becomes manifest as severe respiratory distress in the delivery room that progresses rapidly to pulmonary insufficiency. The lungs, which are very small, develop pneumothoraces with normal resuscitative efforts. A small chest size roentgenographically, joint contractures, and early onset of pneumothoraces, often bilateral, are early clues to the diagnosis. Pulmonary hypertension results from the decreased lung mass and hypertrophy of pulmonary arteriole muscle.

Pulmonary hypoplasia may be due to asphyxiating thoracic dystrophies (a small, bony chest wall) or to decreased amniotic fluid volume that causes uterine compression of the developing chest wall, thus inhibiting lung growth. The latter failure of lung development may be associated with renal agenesis (Potter syndrome) or with a chronic leak of amniotic fluid from ruptured membranes. Isolated agenesis of one lung (usually the left lung) often is asymptomatic and familial. In contrast, serious pulmonary hypoplasia is noted in patients with a *diaphragmatic hernia*. Herniated bowel interferes with lung growth and also results in hypertrophy of the muscle layers of small pulmonary arteries, producing pulmonary hypertension. Pneumothoraces are common. Treatment of a diaphragmatic hernia requires surgical evacuation of the chest and repair of the diaphragmatic defect. Respiratory care is similar to that for patients with PFC.

Neuromuscular diseases that interfere with fetal breathing movements also may produce pulmonary hypoplasia (e.g., congenital anterior horn cell disease [Werdnig-Hoffmann syndrome]).

Another cause of bilateral pulmonary hypoplasia is *hydrops fetalis* (see Obstetrical Complications Associated with Fetal or Neonatal Risks). Hydrops from any cause is characterized by anasarca, ascites, and pleural and pericardial effusions. Bilateral pleural effusions act as space-occupying masses that interfere with lung growth, resulting in pulmonary hypoplasia.

References

Behrman RE (ed): Nelson Textbook of Pediatrics. 14th ed. Philadelphia, WB Saunders, 1992, Sec. 9.17–9.19, 9.30–9.40, 14.1–14.3, 14.76.

Carter JM, Gerstmann DR, Clark RH, et al: High-frequency oscillatory ventilation and extracorporeal membrane oxygenation for the treatment of acute neonatal respiratory failure. Pediatrics 85:159, 1990.

Gibson DL, Sheps SB, Uh SH, et al: Retinopathy of prematurity-induced blindness: Birth weight-specific survival and the new epidemic. Pediatrics 86:405, 1990.

Hammerman C, Aramburo MJ: Prolonged indomethacin therapy for the prevention of recurrences of patent ductus arteriosus. J Pediatr 117:771, 1990.

Jeffries IP: The problems of tiny infants. Int Pediatr 5:305, 1990.

Merritt TA: Factors to consider when selecting a surfactant. Neo Intens Care May/June:30, 1992.

Northway WH Jr: Bronchopulmonary dysplasia: Twenty-five years later. Pediatrics 89:969, 1992.

Robertson PA, Sniderman SH, Laros RK Jr, et al: Neonatal morbidity according to gestational age and birth weight from five tertiary care centers in the United States, 1983 through 1986. Am J Obstet Gynecol 166:1629, 1992.

Upton CJ, Milner AD, Stokes GM: Upper airway patency during apnoea of prematurity. Arch Dis Child 67:419, 1992.

Wiswell TE, Henley MA: Intratracheal suctioning, systemic infection and the meconium aspiration syndrome. Pediatrics 89:203, 1992.

HEMATOLOGIC DISORDERS

Anemia

Embryonic hematopoiesis begins by the 20th day of gestation and is evidenced as blood islands in the yolk sac. In mid-gestation, erythropoiesis occurs in the liver and spleen; the bone marrow becomes the predominant site in the last trimester. Hemoglobin concentration increases from 8–10 g/dL at 12 wk to 16.5–18.0 g/dL at 40 wk. Fetal red blood cell production is responsive to erythropoietin, and the concentration of this hormone is increased with fetal hypoxia and anemia. After birth, hemoglobin levels increase transiently at 6–12 hr and then decline to 11 g/dL at 3–6 mo. The prematurely born infant, who is less than 32 wk of gestational age, has lower hemoglobin concentration and a more rapid postnatal decline of hemoglobin level, which achieves a nadir 1–2 mo after birth. Fetal and neonatal red blood cells have a shorter half-life (70–90 days) and a higher mean corpuscular volume (110–120 fL) than adult cells. Infants demonstrate a reticulocytosis of between 5% and 12% during the first days of life. Hemoglobin and hematocrit levels are higher in neonatal capillary samples obtained by skin pricks than they are in central venous or arterial samples.

In the fetus, *hemoglobin synthesis* in the last two trimesters of pregnancy produces fetal hemoglobin F, composed of two alpha chains and two gamma chains. Immediately prior to term, the infant begins to synthesize beta-hemoglobin chains; thus the term infant should have some adult hemoglobin (two alpha chains and two beta chains). Fetal hemoglobin represents 60–90% of hemoglobin at birth, and the levels decline to adult levels of less than 5% by 4 mo of age.

The time of presentation of hemoglobinopathy depends on the timing of chain synthesis. Thus alpha-thalassemia caused by a 4-gene defect produces no alpha chains and presents as severe anemia and hydrops (Bart hemoglobin, composed of four gamma chains). Hemoglobin H is due to a thalassemia 3-gene defect resulting in four beta chains, and appears with hemolysis and anemia in the infant. In contrast, infants with beta chain abnormalities such as Cooley anemia (beta-thalassemia major) and sickle cell anemia do not manifest anemia in the neonatal period.

The *blood volume* of the term infant is approximately 85 mL/kg. The placenta and umbilical vessels contain approximately 20–30 mL/kg of additional blood that, if clamping or milking ("stripping") of the umbilical cord is delayed at birth, can transiently increase neonatal blood ume and hemoglobin levels for the first 3 days (life. Delayed clamping increases the risk for polycythemia, increased pulmonary vascular resistance, hypoxia, and jaundice but improves glomerular filtration. Early clamping may result in anemia, a cardiac murmur, poor peripheral perfusion but lower pulmonary vascular pressures, and less tachypnea. To avoid both situations, cord clamping should be performed at approximately 30 sec after birth. Hydrostatic pressure affects blood transfer between the placenta and the infant at birth, and an undesired fetal-to-placental transfusion will occur if the infant is situated above the level of the placenta.

The *physiologic anemia* noted at 3–6 mo of age in term infants and at 1–2 mo of age in preterm infants is associated with undetectable erythropoietin levels. Although hemoglobin levels decline during this period, an increase in tissue oxygen becomes available as a result of the production of hemoglobin A, which releases oxygen to the tissues (hemoglobin A becomes unsaturated) at a higher P_{O_2} than does hemoglobin F. (See the oxygen dissociation curve of hemoglobin A in Fig. 6–2 and also Transition from Fetal to Neonatal Physiology.)

Symptomatic anemia in the newborn period may be due to blood loss, decreased red cell production, or hemolysis (Table 6–20). Anemia from *blood loss* at birth is manifested by two patterns of presentation, depending on the rapidity of blood loss. Acute blood loss following fetomaternal hemorrhage, rupture of the umbilical cord, placenta previa, and internal hemorrhage is characterized by pallor, diminished peripheral pulses, and shock. There are no signs of extramedullary hematopoiesis and no hepatosplenomegaly. The hemoglobin content and serum iron levels initially are normal, but the hemoglobin levels decline during the subsequent 24 hr. Chronic blood loss due to chronic fetomaternal hemorrhage or a twin–twin transfusion presents with marked pallor, heart failure, hepatosplenomegaly with or without hydrops, a low hemoglobin level at birth, a hypochromic microcytic blood smear, and decreased serum iron stores. Fetomaternal bleeding occurs in over 50% of all pregnancies, with fetal blood losses ranging between 1 and 50 mL. The diagnosis of fetomaternal hemorrhage is confirmed by the acid elution test of Kleihaur and Betke; pink fetal red blood cells are observed and counted in the mother's peripheral blood smear because fetal hemoglobin is resistant to acid elution; adult hemoglobin is eluted, leaving discolored maternal cells.

Anemia due to decreased production of red blood cells appears at birth with pallor, a low reticu-

eonatal Medicine

Table 6–20. Etiology of Neonatal Anemia

lood Loss	Decreased Production	Hemolysis
ternal bleed	Perinatal–congenital infections	Rh
revia	Anemia of prematurity	ABO
placentae		Minor groups
...–twin transfusion		
Vasa previa	Parvovirus	RBC enzyme deficiency
Rupture of umbilical cord	Diamond-Blackfan syndrome	Hemoglobinopathy
Hepatic hematoma	Osteopetrosis	RBC membrane disorders
Splenic hematoma	Congenital leukemia	Disseminated intravascular coagulopathy
Nuchal cord	Congenital neuroblastoma	Maternal autoimmune disorder (SLE)
Retroperitoneal hemorrhage	Sideroblastic anemia	Perinatal–congenital infections
	Postintrauterine transfusions	

RBC = red blood cell; SLE = systemic lupus erythematosus.

locyte count, and absence of erythroid precursors in the bone marrow (Table 6–20). There may be associated physical anomalies (see Chapter 14).

Immunologically mediated *hemolysis* in utero may result in **erythroblastosis fetalis**, or the fetus may be spared and **hemolytic disease** may appear in the newborn infant. Hemolysis of fetal erythrocytes is due to blood group differences between the sensitized mother and fetus, resulting in the production of maternal IgG antibodies directed against an antigen on fetal cells. All mothers with type O blood have isohemagglutinins, which are IgM antibodies. Because IgM does not cross the placenta, there is no risk of hemolysis.

ABO blood group incompatibility with neonatal hemolysis develops only if the mother has IgG antibodies from a previous exposure to A or B antigens. These IgG antibodies cross the placenta by active transport and affect the fetus or newborn. Sensitization of the mother to fetal antigens may have occurred by previous transfusions or by conditions of pregnancy that result in transfer of fetal erythrocytes into the maternal circulation, such as 1st trimester abortion, an ectopic pregnancy, amniocentesis, or even a normal pregnancy. The risk of fetomaternal transfusion is increased by manual extraction of the placenta and by version (external or internal) procedures.

ABO incompatibility with sensitization usually does not cause fetal disease other than very mild anemia. However, it may produce **hemolytic disease of the newborn** that is manifested as significant anemia and hyperbilirubinemia (see below). Because many mothers who are blood group O have IgG antibodies to A and B prior to pregnancy, the firstborn infant of A or B blood type may be

affected. In contrast to Rh disease, ABO hemolytic disease does not become more severe with subsequent pregnancies. Hemolysis with ABO incompatibility is less severe than hemolysis in Rh-sensitized pregnancy because the anti-A or -B antibody may bind to nonerythrocytic cells that contain A or B antigen or because fetal erythrocytes have fewer A or B antigenic determinants than they have Rh sites. ABO incompatibility is the most common cause of isoimmune hemolysis of the newborn infant.

Erythroblastosis fetalis classically is due to Rh blood group incompatibility. Rh-negative women do not develop natural IgM antibodies, and most Rh-negative women have no anti-Rh antibodies at the time of their first pregnancy. The Rh antigen system consists of five antigens, C, D, E, c, and e; the d type is not antigenic. In 90% of Rh-sensitized cases, the D antigen of the fetus sensitizes the Rh-negative (d) mother, resulting in IgG antibody production during the first pregnancy. A Du antigen is another Rh antigen that on initial assessment tests as Rh negative. Du mothers are Rh positive and thus are not at risk for sensitization.

Because most mothers are not sensitized to Rh antigens at the start of pregnancy, Rh erythroblastosis fetalis is usually a disease of the second and subsequent pregnancies. The first affected pregnancy results in an antibody response in the mother detected during antenatal screening with the Coombs test and determined to be anti-D antibody. The first affected newborn may demonstrate no serious fetal disease and may manifest hemolytic disease of the newborn only by the development of anemia and hyperbilirubinemia (see below). Subsequent pregnancies result in an increasing severity of response by having an earlier onset of hemolysis in utero. Fetal anemia, heart failure, and hypoalbuminemia result in **fetal hydrops**, which is characterized by ascites, pleural and pericardial effusions, and anasarca. There is a high risk of fetal death.

The *management* of the pregnancy complicated by Rh sensitization depends on the severity of hemolysis, its effects on the fetus, and the maturity of the fetus at the time it becomes affected. The severity of the hemolysis can be assessed by the quantity of bilirubin transferred from the fetus to the amniotic fluid, quantified by spectrophotometric analysis of the optical density (at 450 nm) of amniotic fluid. Bilirubin levels in normal pregnancies are higher at earlier gestational ages and decrease as the fetus matures.

Three zones of optical densities with decreasing slopes toward term gestation have been developed to predict the severity of the illness. The high-optical-density zone 3 is associated with severe hemolysis; fetuses in the lower zones probably are not affected. If a fetus's optical density measurement for bilirubin falls into zone 3 and the fetus has pulmonary maturity as determined by the L/S ratio, it should be delivered and treated in the neonatal intensive care unit. If the lungs are immature and the fetus is between 22 and 33 wk of gestational age, an intrauterine transfusion with O negative blood, either into the peritoneal cavity or into the umbilical vein, is indicated and may have to be repeated until pulmonary maturity is reached or fetal distress is detected. Indications for fetal intravascular transfusion in sensitized fetuses between 22 and 32 wk of gestational age include a fetal hematocrit of less than 25%, hemoglobin of less than 8 g/dL, fetal hydrops, and fetal distress too early in gestation for delivery and successful management with neonatal intensive care. Intravascular intrauterine transfusion corrects fetal anemia, improves the outcome of severe hydrops, and reduces the need for postnatal exchange transfusion but is associated with neonatal anemia as a result of continued hemolysis plus suppressed erythropoiesis.

Prevention of sensitization of the mother carrying an Rh-positive fetus is possible by treating her during gestation (after 28 wk) and within 72 hr after birth with anti–Rh-positive immune globulin (RhoGAM). The dose of RhoGAM (300 μg) is based on the ability of this amount of anti–Rh-positive antibody to bind all the possible fetal Rh-positive erythrocytes entering the maternal circulation during the fetal-to-maternal transfusion at birth (~30 mL). RhoGAM may bind Rh-positive fetal erythrocytes or interfere with maternal anti–Rh-positive antibody production by another unknown mechanism.

RhoGAM is effective only in preventing sensitization to the D antigen. Other blood group antigens that can cause immune hydrops and erythroblastosis include Rh C, E, Kell, and Duffy.

Nonimmune causes of hemolysis in the newborn include *red cell enzyme deficiencies* of the Embden-Meyerhof pathway, such as pyruvate kinase or glucose-6-phosphate dehydrogenase deficiency. *Red cell membrane disorders* are another cause of nonimmune hemolysis. Hereditary spherocytosis is inherited as a severe autosomal recessive form or less severe autosomal dominant form and is due to a deficiency of the red blood cell membrane protein spectrin.

Hemoglobinopathies such as thalassemia are another cause of nonimmunologically mediated hemolysis (Table 6–20).

DIAGNOSIS AND MANAGEMENT OF NEONATAL ANEMIA

Hemolysis in utero due to any cause may produce a spectrum of clinical manifestations at birth. Severe hydrops with anasarca, heart failure, and pulmonary edema may prevent adequate ventilation at birth, resulting in asphyxia. Infants affected with hemolysis in utero have hepatosplenomegaly and pallor and become jaundiced within the first 24 hr after birth. Less severely affected infants manifest pallor and hepatosplenomegaly at birth and develop jaundice subsequently. Patients with ABO incompatibility often are asymptomatic and without physical signs at birth and develop mild anemia with jaundice during the first 24–72 hr of life.

Because hydrops, anemia, and jaundice are secondary to many diverse causes of hemolysis, *a laboratory evaluation is needed in all patients with hemolysis.* A complete blood count, blood smear, reticulocyte count, blood type, and direct Coombs test (to determine the presence of antibody-coated red blood cells) should be performed in the initial evaluation of all infants with hemolysis. Reduced hemoglobin levels, reticulocytosis, and a blood smear characterized by polychromasia and anisocytosis are expected with isoimmune hemolysis. Spherocytes are commonly observed with ABO incompatibility. The determination of the blood type and the Coombs test identify the responsible antigen and antibody in immunologically mediated hemolysis.

In the absence of a positive Coombs test and blood group differences between the mother and fetus, causes of nonimmune hemolysis must be considered. Red cell enzyme assays, hemoglobin electrophoresis, or red cell membrane tests (osmotic fragility; spectrin assay) should be performed. Internal hemorrhage also may be associated with anemia, reticulocytosis, and jaundice when the hemorrhage reabsorbs; ultrasonographic evaluation of the brain, liver, spleen, or adrenal gland may be indicated when nonimmune hemolysis is suspected. Shock is more typical in patients with internal hemorrhage, whereas heart failure may be seen with severe anemia from hemolytic diseases. Evaluation of a possible fetomaternal hemorrhage should include the Kleihaur-Betke test.

The *treatment of neonatal anemia* is transfusion of cross-matched red blood cells. If immune hemolysis is present, the cells to be transfused must be cross-matched against both maternal and neonatal plasma. Acute volume loss may necessitate resuscitation with nonblood products such as saline or albumin if blood is not available; packed red blood cells can be given subsequently. Ten to 15 mL/kg of packed red blood cells should be sufficient to correct anemia and any remaining blood volume deficit. Cytomegalovirus (CMV)-seronegative blood should be given to CMV-seronegative infants, and all blood products should be screened for human immunodeficiency virus, hepatitis B, and syphilis. Recombinant erythropoietin (supplemented with iron) may reduce the need for transfusions necessitated by anemia of prematurity.

Hyperbilirubinemia

Hemolytic disease of the newborn is a common cause of neonatal jaundice. Nonetheless, because of the immaturity of the pathways of bilirubin metabolism, many newborn infants without evidence of hemolysis become jaundiced.

Bilirubin is produced by the catabolism of hemoglobin in the reticuloendothelial system. The tetrapyrrol ring of heme is cleaved by heme oxygenase to form equivalent quantities of biliverdin and carbon monoxide. Because no other biologic source of carbon monoxide exists, the excretion of this gas is stoichiometrically identical to the production of bilirubin. Biliverdin is converted to bilirubin by biliverdin reductase. One gram of hemoglobin produces 35 mg of bilirubin. Sources of bilirubin other than circulating hemoglobin represent 20% of bilirubin production; these sources include inefficient (shunt) hemoglobin production and lysis of precursor cells in bone marrow. Compared with adults, newborn infants have a 2- to 3-fold greater rate of bilirubin production (6–10 mg/kg/24 hr vs. 3 mg/kg/24 hr). This is due, in part, to an increased red blood cell mass (higher hematocrit) and a short-ened erythrocyte half-life of 70–90 days, compared with the 120-day erythrocyte half-life in adults.

Bilirubin produced following hemoglobin catabolism is lipid soluble, is unconjugated, and reacts as an indirect reagent in the van den Bergh test. Indirect-reacting, unconjugated bilirubin is toxic to the central nervous system and is insoluble in water, thus limiting its excretion. Unconjugated bilirubin binds to albumin on specific bilirubin binding sites; 1 g of albumin binds 8.5 mg of bilirubin in the newborn. If the binding sites become saturated or if a competitive compound binds at the site, displacing bound bilirubin, free bilirubin will be available to enter the central nervous system. Organic acids such as free fatty acids and drugs such as sulfisoxazole can displace bilirubin from its binding site on albumin.

Bilirubin dissociates from albumin at the hepatocyte and becomes bound to a cytoplasmic liver protein "Y" (ligandin). Hepatic conjugation results in the production of bilirubin diglucuronide, which is water soluble and capable of biliary and renal excretion. The enzyme UDP–glucuronyl transferase is the rate-limiting step of bilirubin conjugation. The concentrations of ligandin and glucuronyl transferase are lower in the newborn infant, particularly in the premature infant, as compared with older children.

Conjugated bilirubin gives a direct reaction in the van den Bergh test. Most conjugated bilirubin is excreted through the bile into the small intestine and is eliminated in the stool. However, some bilirubin may undergo hydrolysis back to the unconjugated fraction by intestinal glucuronidase and then may be reabsorbed (enterohepatic recirculation). In addition, bacteria in the neonatal intestine do not convert bilirubin to urobilinogen or stercobilinogen, which is excreted in urine and stool and usually limits bilirubin reabsorption. Delayed passage of meconium, which contains bilirubin, also may contribute to the enterohepatic recirculation of bilirubin.

Bilirubin is produced in utero by the normal fetus and by the fetus affected by erythroblastosis fetalis. Indirect, unconjugated, lipid-soluble fetal bilirubin is transferred across the placenta and subsequently becomes conjugated by maternal hepatic enzymes. The placenta is impermeable to conjugated water-soluble bilirubin. Fetal bilirubin levels become only mildly elevated in the presence of severe hemolysis, but may increase when hemolysis produces fetal hepatic inspissated bile stasis and conjugated hyperbilirubinemia. Maternal indirect (but not direct) hyperbilirubinemia also may increase fetal bilirubin levels.

Table 6–21. Etiology of Unconjugated Hyperbilirubinemia

	Hemolysis Present	Hemolysis Absent
Common	*Blood group incompatibility:* ABO, Rh, Kell, Duffy *Infection*	Physiologic jaundice, breast milk jaundice, internal hemorrhage, polycythemia, infant of diabetic mother
Rare	*Red cell enzyme defects:* glucose-6-phosphate dehydrogenase, pyruvate kinase *Red cell membrane disorders:* spherocytosis, ovalocytosis *Hemoglobinopathy:* thalassemia	Deficiency of glucuronyl transferase enzyme (Crigler-Najjar syndrome), pyloric stenosis, hypothyroidism, immune thrombocytopenia, Gilbert disease

ETIOLOGY OF INDIRECT UNCONJUGATED HYPERBILIRUBINEMIA (Table 6–21)

Physiologic jaundice is a common cause of hyperbilirubinemia among newborn infants. It is a diagnosis of exclusion after careful evaluation has ruled out more serious causes of jaundice, such as hemolysis, infection, or metabolic diseases. Physiologic jaundice is due to many factors that are normal physiologic characteristics of the newborn infant: increased bilirubin production resulting from an increased red blood cell mass, shortened red blood cell half-life, and hepatic immaturity of ligandin and glucuronyl transferase. Physiologic jaundice may be exaggerated among Greek and Oriental infants.

The clinical pattern of physiologic jaundice in term infants includes a peak indirect-reacting bilirubin level of no more than 12 mg/dL on the 3rd day of life. In premature infants, the peak is higher (15 mg/dL) and occurs later (5th day).

The peak level of indirect bilirubin during physiologic jaundice may be higher in breast milk–fed infants that in non-breast milk–fed infants (15–17 mg/dL vs. 12 mg/dL). This may be due, in part, to the decreased fluid intake of the former. Jaundice is unphysiologic or pathologic if it is evident on the 1st day of life, if the bilirubin level increases more than 0.5 mg/dL/hr, if the peak bilirubin is greater than 13 mg/dL in term infants, if the direct bilirubin fraction is greater than 1.5 mg/dL, or if hepatosplenomegaly and anemia are present.

Crigler-Najjar syndrome is a serious permanent deficiency of glucuronyl transferase that results in severe indirect hyperbilirubinemia. The autosomal dominant variety responds to enzyme induction by phenobarbital, producing an increase in enzyme activity and a reduction of bilirubin levels. The autosomal recessive form does not respond to phenobarbital and manifests as persistent indirect hyperbilirubinemia, which often results in kernicterus (see below).

Breast milk feeding may be associated with unconjugated hyperbilirubinemia without evidence of hemolysis during the 1st to 2nd wk of life. Bilirubin levels rarely increase to above 20 mg/dL. Interruption of breast feeding for 1–2 days results in a rapid decline of bilirubin levels that do not increase significantly after breast feeding is resumed. Breast milk may contain an inhibitor of bilirubin conjugation or increase the enterohepatic recirculation of bilirubin because of breast milk glucuronidase.

Jaundice on the first day of life is always pathologic, requiring immediate attention to establish the cause. Early onset often is due to hemolysis, internal hemorrhage (cephalhematoma, hepatic or splenic hematoma), or infection (Table 6–21). Infection also is often associated with direct-reacting bilirubin (see below) resulting from perinatal congenital infections or to bacterial sepsis.

Physical evidence of jaundice is observable in infants when the bilirubin levels reach 5–10 mg/dL, versus only 2 mg/dL in adults. Once jaundice is observed, the laboratory evaluation for hyperbilirubinemia should include a total bilirubin measurement to determine the magnitude of hyperbilirubinemia. Bilirubin levels in excess of 5 mg/dL on the 1st day of life or in excess of 13 mg/dL thereafter in term infants should be evaluated further with indirect and direct bilirubin levels, blood typing, Coombs test, complete blood count, blood smear, and reticulocyte count. These tests should be done prior to the treatment of hyperbilirubinemia with phototherapy or exchange transfusion. In the absence of hemolysis or evidence for either the common or the rare causes of nonhemolytic indirect hyperbilirubinemia, the diagnosis is either physiologic or breast milk jaundice. Jaundice present after 2 wk of age is pathologic and suggests a direct reacting hyperbilirubinemia.

Direct-reacting hyperbilirubinemia should be evaluated according to the diagnostic categories noted in Table 6–22. Direct-reacting bilirubin (composed mostly of conjugated bilirubin) is not neurotoxic to the infant but signifies a serious underlying disor-

Table 6–22. Etiology of Conjugated Hyperbilirubinemia

Common
Hyperalimentation cholestasis
CMV infection
Other perinatal congenital infections (TORCH)
Inspissated bile from prolonged hemolysis
Neonatal hepatitis
Sepsis

Uncommon
Hepatic infarction
Inborn errors of metabolism (galactosemia, tyrosinosis)
Cystic fibrosis
Biliary atresia
Choledochal cyst
Alpha-1-antitrypsin deficiency
Hepatitis B
Alagille syndrome (arteriohepatic dysplasia)
Byler disease

CMV = cytomegalovirus; TORCH = toxoplasmosis, other, rubella, cytomegalovirus, herpes simplex.

der involving cholestasis or hepatocellular injury. The diagnostic evaluation of patients with direct-reacting hyperbilirubinemia includes liver enzyme determinations (serum glutamic oxaloacetic transaminase, alkaline phosphatase, serum glutamic pyruvic transaminase, gamma-glutamyltranspeptidase), bacterial and viral cultures, metabolic screening tests, hepatic ultrasonography, sweat chloride test, and, occasionally, liver biopsy. The treatment of disorders manifested by direct bilirubinemia is specific for those diseases that are noted in Table 6–22. They do not respond to phototherapy or exchange transfusion.

KERNICTERUS

Lipid-soluble, unconjugated, indirect bilirubin fraction is toxic to the developing central nervous system, especially when indirect bilirubin concentrations are high and exceed the binding capacity of albumin. Kernicterus results when indirect bilirubin is deposited in brain cells, disrupting neuronal metabolism and function, especially in the basal ganglia. Indirect bilirubin may cross the blood–brain barrier because of its lipid solubility; other theories propose that a disruption of the blood–brain barrier permits entry of a bilirubin-albumin or free bilirubin–fatty acid complex.

Kernicterus usually is noted at an excessively high bilirubin level for gestational age. Term infants usually do not develop kernicterus when their bilirubin levels are below 20 mg/dL. The incidence of kernicterus increases as serum bilirubin

levels increase above 20 mg/dL. Kernicterus may be noted at bilirubin levels below 20 mg/dL in the presence of sepsis, meningitis, hemolysis, asphyxia, hypoxia, hypothermia, hypoglycemia, bilirubin displacing drugs, and prematurity. Very immature infants weighing less than 1000 g have developed kernicterus when their bilirubin levels are less than 10 mg/dL.

The earliest *clinical manifestations* of kernicterus include lethargy, hypotonia, poor Moro response, and poor feeding. A high-pitched cry and emesis also may be present. Later signs include bulging fontanel, opisthotonic posturing, pulmonary hemorrhage, fever, hypertonicity, paralysis of upward gaze, and seizures. Infants with severe cases of kernicterus die in the neonatal period. Spasticity resolves in surviving infants, who may later manifest nerve deafness, choreoathetoid cerebral palsy, mental retardation, enamel dysplasia, and discoloration of teeth as permanent sequelae. Kernicterus may be prevented by avoiding excessively high indirect bilirubin levels and by avoiding conditions or drugs that may displace bilirubin from albumin. Very early signs of kernicterus occasionally may be reversed by immediately instituting an exchange transfusion (see below).

THERAPY OF INDIRECT HYPERBILIRUBINEMIA

Phototherapy is an effective and relatively safe method for reducing indirect bilirubin levels, particularly when initiated before serum bilirubin increases to levels associated with kernicterus. In term infants, phototherapy is begun when indirect bilirubin levels are between 15 and 18 mg/dL. Phototherapy is initiated in premature infants when bilirubin is at lower levels to avoid bilirubin reaching the high concentrations requiring exchange transfusion. Both blue lights and white lights are effective in reducing bilirubin levels.

Phototherapy acts by producing nontoxic photoisomers from the native bilirubin deposited in the skin. Unconjugated bilirubin (IX) is in the 4Z,15Z configuration (referring to the arrangement of atoms around the respective double bonds). Phototherapy causes a photochemical reaction producing the reversible, more water-soluble isomer 4Z,15E bilirubin IX. This configurational isomer is excreted readily in an unconjugated form in bile and is one of the mechanisms of the action of phototherapy. Another photochemical reaction results in the rapid production of lumirubin, a more water-soluble isomer than the aforementioned isomer, that does not spontaneously revert to unconjugated native bilirubin and also can be excreted in urine.

Complications of phototherapy include an increased insensible water loss, diarrhea, and dehydration. Additional problems include macular–papular red skin rash, lethargy, masking of cyanosis, nasal obstruction due to eye pads, and the potential for retinal damage. Skin bronzing may be noted in infants with direct-reacting hyperbilirubinemia. Infants with mild hemolytic disease of the newborn occasionally may be successfully managed with phototherapy for hyperbilirubinemia, but care must be taken to follow these infants for the late occurrence of anemia from continued hemolysis.

Exchange transfusion usually is reserved for infants with dangerously high indirect bilirubin levels who are at risk for kernicterus. As a rule of thumb, a level of 20 mg/dL indirect reacting bilirubin is the "exchange number" for infants weighing over 2000 g. Asymptomatic infants with physiologic or breast milk jaundice may not require exchange transfusion unless the indirect bilirubin level approaches 25 mg/dL. The exchangeable level of indirect bilirubin for other infants may be estimated by calculating 10% of the birth weight in grams; thus a 1500-g infant's level would be 15 mg/dL. Infants weighing less than 1000 g usually do not warrant an exchange transfusion until the bilirubin exceeds 10 mg/dL.

Small infusions of whole blood cross-matched with that of the mother and infant are alternated with a withdrawal of an equivalent quantity of the infant's blood, which is discarded. Depending on the size of the infant, aliquots of 5–20 mL per cycle are withdrawn and infused, with the total procedure lasting 45–90 min. The total amount of blood exchanged is equal to twice the infant's blood volume, calculated as: weight (kg) $\times$ 85 mL/kg $\times$ 2. This volume should remove 85% of the infant's red blood cells (the source of bilirubin), maternal antibodies, and exchangeable tissue indirect bilirubin. The exchange transfusion usually is performed through an umbilical venous catheter placed in the inferior vena cava or, if free flow is obtained, at the confluence of the umbilical vein and the portal system. Serum bilirubin levels immediately after the exchange transfusion decline to levels that are about one half those prior to the exchange; levels rebound 6–8 hr later as a result of continued hemolysis and redistribution of bilirubin from tissue stores. Complications of exchange transfusion include problems resulting from the blood (transfusion reaction, metabolic instability, infection), the catheter (vessel perforation, hemorrhage), or the procedure (hypotension, necrotizing enterocolitis). Unusual complications include thrombocytopenia and graft-versus-host disease. Continuation of phototherapy may alleviate the necessity for subsequent exchange transfusions.

Polycythemia (Hyperviscosity Syndrome)

Polycythemia is an excessively high hematocrit (65% or more), resulting in hyperviscosity that produces symptoms related to vascular stasis, hypoperfusion, and ischemia. As the hematocrit increases from 40 to 60%, there is a very small increase of the blood viscosity. Once the central hematocrit increases above 65%, the blood viscosity begins to increase markedly and symptoms may appear. Neonatal erythrocytes are less filterable or deformable than adult erythrocytes, a fact that further contributes to hyperviscosity. A central venous hematocrit of 65% or more is noted in 3–5% of infants. Infants at special risk for polycythemia are term and post-term SGA infants, infants of diabetic mothers, infants with delayed cord clamping, and those having neonatal hyperthyroidism, adrenogenital syndrome, trisomy 21, twin–twin transfusion syndrome (recipient), and Beckwith-Wiedemann syndrome. In some infants, polycythemia may reflect a compensation for prolonged periods of fetal hypoxia from placental insufficiency; these infants have increased erythropoietin levels at birth.

Polycythemic patients appear plethoric or ruddy and may develop acrocyanosis. Symptoms are due to the increased red cell mass and to vascular compromise. Thus seizures, lethargy, and irritability reflect abnormalities of microcirculation of the brain, whereas hyperbilirubinemia may be due to the poor hepatic circulation or to the increased amount of hemoglobin that is being broken down into bilirubin. Additional problems include respiratory distress and PFC resulting, in part, from elevated pulmonary vascular resistance. The chest roentgenogram often demonstrates cardiomegaly, increased vascular markings, pleural effusions, and interstitial edema. Other problems include necrotizing enterocolitis, hypoglycemia, thrombocytopenia, priapism, and feeding intolerance. Many of these complications also are related to the primary condition associated with polycythemia (e.g., SGA infants are at risk for hypoglycemia and PFC following periods of hypoxia in utero).

Long-term sequelae of neonatal polycythemia relate to neurodevelopmental abnormalities that may be prevented by treatment of symptomatic infants with partial exchange transfusion after birth. A partial exchange transfusion removes whole blood and replaces it with normal saline or albumin. The equation to calculate the volume exchanged is based on the central venous hematocrit (Hct), because peripheral hematocrits may be falsely elevated:

Volume to exchange (mL) =

$$\frac{\text{Blood volume (observed Hct} - \text{desired Hct)}}{\text{observed Hct}}$$

The desired hematocrit is 50% and the blood volume 85 mL/kg.

Coagulation Disorders

Disorders of coagulation are very common in the neonatal period. Hemorrhage during this time may be due to trauma, inherited permanent deficiency of coagulation factors, transient deficiencies of vitamin K–dependent factors, disorders of platelets, and disseminated intravascular coagulation (DIC) seen in sick newborn patients with shock or hypoxia. Thrombosis is also a potential problem in the newborn because of developmentally lower circulating levels of antithrombin III, protein C (a vitamin K–dependent protein that inhibits factors VIII and V), and the fibrinolytic system.

There is no placental passage of coagulation factors, and newborn infants have relatively low levels of the vitamin K–dependent factors II, VII, IX, and X. Contact factors XI and XII, prekallikrein, and kininogen also are lower in newborn infants than in adults. Fibrinogen (factor I), plasma levels of factors V, VIII, and XIII, and platelet count are within the adult normal range.

Because of the transient, relative deficiencies of the contact and the vitamin K–dependent factors, the *partial thromboplastin time* (PTT), which is dependent on factors XII, IX, VIII, X, V, II, and I, is prolonged in the newborn period. Preterm infants have the most marked prolongation of the PTT (50–80 sec) compared with term (35–50 sec) and older, more mature (25–35 sec) infants. The administration of heparin and the presence of DIC, hemophilia, and severe vitamin K deficiency prolong the PTT. The *prothrombin time* (PT), which is dependent on factors VII, X, V, II, and I, is a more sensitive test for vitamin K deficiency. The PT is only slightly prolonged in the term infant (13–20 sec) as compared with the preterm (13–21 sec) and the more mature patient (12–14 sec). Abnormal prolongations of the PT occur with vitamin K deficiency,

hepatic injury, and DIC. Levels of *fibrinogen* and *fibrin degradation products* are similar in infants and adults. The *bleeding time,* which reflects platelet function and number, is normal during the newborn period in the absence of maternal salicylate therapy.

Vitamin K is a necessary cofactor for the carboxylation of glutamate on precursor proteins, converting them into the more active coagulation factors II, VII, IX, and X; gamma-carboxyglutamic acid binds calcium, which is required for the immediate activation of factors during hemorrhage. There is no congenital deficiency of hepatic synthesis of these precursor proteins, but, in the absence of vitamin K, their conversion to the active factor is not possible. PIVKA (protein induced by vitamin K absence) levels increase in vitamin K deficiency and are helpful diagnostic markers; vitamin K administration rapidly corrects the coagulation defects, reducing PIVKA to undetectable levels.

Although most newborn infants are born with reduced levels of vitamin K–dependent factors, only a few develop hemorrhagic complications. Those infants at risk for **hemorrhagic disease of the newborn** have the most profound deficiency of vitamin K–dependent factors, and these factors decline further after birth. Because breast milk is a poor source of vitamin K, infants fed breast milk are also at increased risk for hemorrhage that usually occurs between the 3rd and 5th days of life. Bleeding usually ensues from the umbilical cord, circumcision site, intestines, scalp, mucosa, and skin, but internal hemorrhage places the infant at risk for fatal complications, such as intracranial bleeding.

Hemorrhage on the 1st day of life resulting from a deficiency of the vitamin K–dependent factors often is associated with administration to the mother of drugs that affect vitamin K metabolism in the infant. This early pattern of hemorrhage has been seen with maternal warfarin therapy and in infants of mothers receiving phenobarbital and phenytoin. Late bleeding also may occur, as late as 1–3 mo after birth, particularly among breast-fed infants. Vitamin K deficiency in the latter group should also raise suspicion about the possibility of vitamin K malabsorption resulting from cystic fibrosis or antibiotic suppression of the colonic bacteria that produce vitamin K.

Bleeding due to vitamin K deficiency may be *prevented* by administration of vitamin K to all infants at birth. Prior to routine administration of vitamin K, 1–2% of all newborn infants had developed hemorrhagic disease of the newborn. One intramuscular dose (1 mg) of vitamin K prevents vitamin K–deficiency bleeding. *Treatment* of bleeding resulting from vitamin K deficiency requires intravenous administration of 1 mg of vitamin K. If severe, life-threatening hemorrhage is present, fresh frozen plasma should also be given. Unusually high doses of vitamin K may be needed for hepatic disease and for maternal warfarin or anticonvulsant therapy.

CLINICAL MANIFESTATIONS AND DIFFERENTIAL DIAGNOSES OF BLEEDING

Bleeding disorders in the newborn may be associated with cutaneous bleeding such as cephalohematoma, subgaleal hemorrhage, ecchymosis, and petechiae. Facial petechiae are common in infants born by vertex presentation, with or without a nuchal cord, and usually are insignificant. Mucosal bleeding may appear as hematemesis, melena, or epistaxis. Internal hemorrhage results in organ-specific dysfunction such as seizures accompanied by intracranial hemorrhage. Bleeding from venipuncture or heel stick sites, circumcision sites, or the umbilical cord also is common.

The *differential diagnosis* depends, in part, on the clinical circumstances associated with the hemorrhage. In the sick newborn, the differential diagnosis should include DIC, hepatic failure, and thrombocytopenia. Thrombocytopenia may be secondary to consumption by trapping of platelets in a hemangioma (Kasabach-Merritt syndrome) or may be associated with perinatal, congenital, or bacterial infections, necrotizing enterocolitis (NEC), thrombotic endocarditis, persistent fetal circulation, organic acidemia, maternal pre-eclampsia, or asphyxia. Thrombocytopenia also may be due to peripheral washout of platelets following an exchange transfusion. Treatment of the sick infant with thrombocytopenia should be directed at the underlying disorder, supplemented by infusions of platelets and/or blood.

The etiologies of *DIC in the newborn infant* include hypoxia, hypotension, asphyxia, bacterial or viral sepsis, NEC, death of a twin while in utero, cavernous hemangioma, nonimmune hydrops, neonatal cold injury, neonatal neoplasm, and hepatic disease. The treatment of DIC should be focused primarily on the therapy of the initiating or underlying disorder. Supportive management of consumptive coagulopathy includes platelet transfusions and factor replacement with fresh frozen plasma. Heparin should be reserved for those infants with DIC who also demonstrate thrombosis.

Disorders of hemostasis in the well child are not associated with systemic disease in the newborn but reflect coagulation factor or platelet deficiency.

Hemophilia initially is associated with cutaneous or mucosal bleeding and no systemic illness. If bleeding continues, hypovolemic shock may develop. Bleeding into the brain, liver, or spleen may result in organ-specific signs and shock.

In the well child, *thrombocytopenia* may be part of a syndrome such as Fanconi anemia (hypoplasia, aplasia of thumb), the radial aplasia–thrombocytopenia (TAR) syndrome (thumbs present), or Wiskott-Aldrich syndrome. Various maternal drugs also may reduce the neonatal platelet count without producing other adverse effects. These drugs include sulfonamides, quinidine, quinine, and thiazide diuretics.

The most common causes of thrombocytopenia in the well newborn infant are transient isoimmune thrombocytopenia and transient neonatal thrombocytopenia in well infants born to mothers with idiopathic thrombocytopenic purpura (ITP). **Isoimmune thrombocytopenia** is due to antiplatelet antibodies produced by the PLA1-negative mother after her sensitization to specific paternal platelet antigen (PLA1 positive) expressed on the fetal platelet. This response to maternal-sensitized antibodies that produce isoimmune thrombocytopenia is analogous to the response that produces erythroblastosis fetalis. The maternal antiplatelet antibody does not produce maternal thrombocytopenia, but, after crossing the placenta, this IgG antibody binds to fetal platelets that are trapped by the reticuloendothelial tissue, resulting in thrombocytopenia. Infants with thrombocytopenia produced in this manner are at risk for developing petechiae, purpura, and intracranial hemorrhage after birth. Vaginal delivery may increase the risk for neonatal bleeding; thus cesarean section may be indicated. Specific treatment for severe thrombocytopenia ($<10,000$ platelets/mm^3) or significant bleeding is transfusion of maternal platelets. Because the antibody in isoimmune thrombocytopenia is directed against the fetal rather than the maternal platelet, plateletpheresis of the mother will yield sufficient platelets for carrying out a platelet transfusion to treat the affected infant. After one platelet transfusion, the infant's platelet count dramatically increases and usually remains in a safe range. Without treatment, thrombocytopenia resolves during the first month of life as the maternal antibody level declines. Treating the mother with intravenous immunoglobulin or the thrombocytopenic fetus with intravascular platelet transfusion (cordocentesis), is also effective.

Neonatal thrombocytopenia in infants born to women with ITP also is due to placental transfer of maternal IgG antibodies. In ITP, these autoantibodies are directed against all platelet antigens, and, therefore, both mother and newborn may have low platelet counts. The risks of hemorrhage in the infant born to the woman with ITP may be lessened by cesarean section and by treatment of the mother with corticosteroids. *Treatment* of the affected infant born to the woman with ITP may include prednisone and intravenous immunoglobulin. In an emergency, random donor platelets may produce a transient rise in the infant's platelet count. Thrombocytopenia will resolve spontaneously during the 1st month of life as maternal-derived antibody levels decline. Elevated levels of platelet-associated antibodies also have been noted in thrombocytopenic infants with sepsis and thrombocytopenia of unknown cause, who were born to mothers without demonstrable platelet antibodies.

The *laboratory evaluation of an infant* (well or sick) *with bleeding* must include a platelet count, blood smear, PTT, and PT. Isolated thrombocytopenia in a well infant should suggest immune thrombocytopenia. Laboratory evidence of DIC should include a markedly prolonged PTT and PT (minutes rather than seconds), thrombocytopenia, and a blood smear suggestive of a microangiopathic hemolytic anemia (burr or fragmented blood cells). Further evaluation will reveal very low levels of fibrinogen (below 100 mg/dL) and elevated levels of fibrin degradation products. Vitamin K deficiency will prolong the PT more than the PTT, whereas hemophilia resulting from factors VIII and IX deficiency will prolong only the PTT. Specific factor levels will confirm the diagnosis of hemophilia.

References

Andrew M, Castle V, Saigal S, et al: Clinical impact of neonatal thrombocytopenia. J Pediatr 110:457, 1987.

Behrman RE (ed): Nelson Textbook of Pediatrics. 14th ed. Philadelphia, WB Saunders, 1992, Sec. 9.44–9.49.

Carnielli V, Montini G, Da Riol R, et al: Effect of high doses of human recombinant erythropoietin on the need for blood transfusions in preterm infants. J Pediatr 121:98, 1992.

Ennever JF: Phototherapy in a new light. Pediatr Clin North Am 33:603, 1986.

Lynch L, Bussel JB, McFarland JG, et al: Antenatal treatment of alloimmune thrombocytopenia. Obstet Gynecol 80:67, 1992.

Swetnam SM, Yabek SM, Alverson DC: Hemodynamic consequences of neonatal polycythemia. J Pediatr 110:443, 1987.

van de Bor M, Ens-Dokkum M, Schreuder AM, et al: Hyperbilirubinemia in low birth weight infants and outcome at 5 years of age. Pediatrics 89:359, 1992.

von Kries R: Vitamin K prophylaxis—a useful public health measure? Pediatr Perinat Epidemiol 6:7, 1992.

Whittle MJ: Rhesus haemolytic disease. Arch Dis Child 67:65, 1992.

NUTRITION AND GASTROINTESTINAL DISORDERS

Nutrition and Feeding

All newborn infants require water and a source of calories during the 1st day of life. In healthy, full-term infants, breast milk and/or formula is given on the 1st day of life as the source of fluid and nutrients during enteric alimentation; sick and very premature infants usually are managed with intravenous alimentation. Enteric alimentation of sick infants often is delayed until after their acute illnesses have resolved because of the risk of abdominal distention or ileus, either of which may lead to regurgitation and subsequent aspiration pneumonia, and because of the risk of the development of necrotizing enterocolitis (NEC). Delay in the onset of intravenous and enteric alimentation may be associated with fluid and electrolyte abnormalities such as hypernatremia, azotemia, dehydration, oliguria, fever, hypoglycemia, and hyperbilirubinemia.

Full-term infants usually are provided with breast feeding or are fed formula by mouth during the first few hours after birth. Because premature infants before 32–34 wk of gestational age may not be able to coordinate the mechanisms for oral feeding, they usually are fed through a nasal or oral gastric tube. Such "gavage feedings" may be given continuously or intermittently by gravity drip every 1–3 hr. Subsequently, oral feedings are started when the infant can coordinate sucking, cheek and tongue movement, uvula closure of the nasopharynx, and epiglottal closure of the larynx; has acquired the esphageal motility to propel the milk feeding to the stomach; and has developed a gag reflex.

Problems of enteric alimentation are common in premature infants; these problems are due to immaturity of the gastrointestinal tract and to systemic disease states that alter gastrointestinal function. They include gastroesophageal reflux, gastric stasis and retention of formula, abdominal distention and ileus, failure to defecate, and a variety of abnormalities related to the composition of milk. Premature infants also may develop bradycardia during enteral feedings, in part because of a reduced arterial oxygen content and gastric distention. Reflux of gastric contents may cause laryngospasm or aspiration pneumonia; both are

Table 6–23. Composition of Breast Milk and Infant Formulas

	Breast Milk (per dL)	Standard Formula (per dL)	Premature Formula (per dL)	Soy Formula (per dL)	Nutramigen (per dL)	Pregestimil (per dL)
Calories (kcal)	67–72	67	67–81	67	67	67
Protein (g)	1.2	1.5	2.0–2.4	2.0	1.9	1.9
(% calories)	(6%)	(9%)	(12%)	(12%)	(11%)	(11%)
Whey/casein protein ratio	80/20	60/40, 18/82	60/40	Soy protein	Casein hydrolysate, amino acid premix	Casein hydrolysate plus L-cystine, L-tyrosine, L-tryptophan
Fat (g)	4.5	3.6	3.4–4.6	3.6	2.6	3.8
(% calories)	(56%)	(50%)	(45%)	(48%)	(35%)	(48%)
MCT* (%)	0	0	40–50%	0	0	20% Corn oil/60% MCT
Carbohydrate (g)	6.8	6.9–7.2	8.5–8.9	6.8	9.1	6.9
(% calories)	(38%)	(41%)	(42%)	(40%)	(54%)	(41%)
Source	Lactose	Lactose	Lactose/glucose polymers, corn syrup	Corn syrup, sucrose	Sucrose, tapioca starch	Corn syrup solids, corn starch, dextrose
Minerals (per L)						
Calcium (mg)	340	420–550	750–1440	700	635	640
Phosphorus (mg)	140	280–390	400–720	500	475	430
Sodium (mEq)	7.0	6.5–8.3	6.5–15	13	14	12
Vitamin D (IU)	Variable	400	510–1200	400	400	400
Osmolality (mOsm/L)	273	300	250–310	240–260	290	290
Renal solute load (mOsm/L)	75	100–126	122–150	126	175	125
Comments	Reference standard, deficient in vitamin K; may be deficient in Na⁺, Ca²⁺, protein, vitamin D for VLBW	Risk of milk protein intolerance, gastrointestinal bleeding, anemia, wheezing, eczema	Specifically fortified with additional protein, Ca²⁺, P, Na⁺, vitamin D, and MCT oil	Useful for lactose and milk protein intolerance; may develop soy protein intolerance; VLBW develop rickets	Useful for lactose and milk protein intolerance	Useful for malabsorption states, lactose and milk protein intolerance

Comments column chemical notations: Na$^+$, Ca^{2+}.

* MCT = medium chain triglycerides.

associated with hypoxia, apnea, and bradycardia. Excessively large volumes of formula fed rapidly over a short time have been associated with the development of NEC. Problems associated with feeding tubes include erosive esophagitis, bowel perforation, fat malabsorption, and abnormal bacterial colonization of the upper intestine. There also may be a temporary loss of the ability to feed directly by mouth, if gavage or intravenous feeding is of long duration.

The composition of commonly used formulas and the indications for the initiation of *special infant formulas* are presented in Table 6–23. Breast milk is often the standard milk fed to newborn infants and serves as a nutritional reference point for comparison with other infant formulas.

The caloric requirements of the newborn infant include energy for growth, for regulation of body temperature, and for maintenance (replacement and turnover) of body macromolecules (Table 6–24). When fed 100–120 kcal/kg/24 hr, the infant

should gain 10–30 g/24 hr. The energy required for tissue synthesis is a small proportion, and that required for storage as macromolecules is a large proportion, of the energy required for growth. Energy partitioning for synthesis and storage depends on the composition of the new tissue; fat synthesis requires more calories than protein synthesis. Net deposition of new tissue macromolecules (depositing 20–30% fat and 10–12% protein) requires 4–6

Table 6–24. Neonatal Caloric Requirements

Source	Kcal/Kg/24 Hr
Maintenance	50
Growth	25–35
Activity	0–15
Cold stress	0–10
Specific dynamic action (caloric cost of food)	10
Nutrient losses (stool)	10–20
Total	95–120

kcal/g tissue. Energy requirements may be spared for tissue synthesis if the infant is kept warm in a neutral thermal environment to avoid cold stress–induced energy utilization.

The *protein requirement* of the breast-fed, full-term infant may be as little as 1.5–2.0 g/kg/24 hr. Colostrum has a higher protein content than breast milk, which may contain as little as 0.9 g/dL. Standard formula for older premature infants and for full-term infants provides more protein than breast milk (see Table 6–23); growing infants consuming 150 mL/kg/24 hr will have a protein intake of 2.25 g/kg/24 hr. Preterm infants may have an increased requirement for protein to support growth but may develop an elevated blood urea nitrogen level, hyperaminoacidemia, hyperammonemia, and metabolic acidosis when fed casein-predominant (80%) formula or when fed greater than 4.5 g/kg/24 hr total proteins. The **late metabolic acidosis of prematurity** probably is due, in part, to increased endogenous acid production from casein-containing formula (high in sulfur and acidic amino acids). This disorder is characterized by metabolic acidosis and reduced weight gain in VLBW infants. Treatment includes substitution of a ''humanized'' whey-predominant formula and oral $NaHCO_3$.

All infants have an absolute requirement for the essential amino acids. Preterm infants also have an additional requirement for cystine and tyrosine because of immaturity of the enzymes required to convert cystathionine and phenylalanine to these amino acids. In addition, histidine and taurine also may be essential for the premature infant.

Fat absorption by the newborn infant may be reduced as a result of a small bile salt pool and a low pancreatic lipase activity. The latter may be compensated for by breast milk and lingual and gastric lipase activities. Reduced bile salt concentrations will be exacerbated by cholestatic jaundice. With the exception of human milk fat, animal fats are not well absorbed. Corn or soy oils are better tolerated, as are medium-chain triglycerides that do not require bile salts for absorption. Three to 5% of the total calories should be in the form of essential fatty acids. Provision of linolenic and linoleic acids (unsaturated fatty acids) will provide precursors for arachidonic acid and prostaglandin synthesis, thus avoiding **essential fatty acid deficiency**. The latter is characterized by growth failure, dermatitis, reduced pigmentation, and hypotonia. Excessive intake of polyunsaturated fatty acids may produce hemolysis by overcoming the antioxidant mechanisms of the erythrocyte. The provision of additional vitamin E may prevent this hemolysis.

Forty percent of milk calories are derived from *carbohydrates* (see Table 6–23). There is no absolute requirement for specific carbohydrates; however, both glucose and galactose can produce glycogen and prevent hypoglycemia. Lactose, a disaccharide of glucose and galactose, is the natural carbohydrate of human milk and of most formulas. Preterm infants have not developed normal full-term levels of the intestinal mucosal enzyme lactase, which is necessary to digest lactose. Malabsorption of lactose may result in watery, acidic stools from the production of organic acids by colonic bacteria. These organic acids may be absorbed and contribute to the development of late metabolic acidosis of prematurity. Newborn infants with gastrointestinal injury frequently develop lactose intolerance and require lactose-free formula. Because of the developmental immaturity of lactase activity, formulas for premature infants usually contain glucose polymers that will be digested by pancreatic amylase.

Vitamin deficiency is rare in the immediate newborn period. Breast-fed infants of strict vegan mothers may develop vitamin B_{12} deficiency, and infants fed goat's milk may become folate deficient. Vitamin D deficiency may be seen in infants of mothers with osteomalacia and in infants with cholestatic jaundice. Vitamin D deficiency also may be a contributing factor to osteopenia of prematurity (see below). Preterm infants may need more vitamin C to improve tyrosine metabolism. Vitamin E deficiency in the immediate newborn period may be due to an excess of oxidants such as iron and an abundance of oxidizable polyunsaturated fatty acids. Vitamin E deficiency of the premature infant may result in edema, anemia, reticulocytosis, and thrombocytosis. Vitamin K deficiency has been discussed under hemorrhagic disease of the newborn.

Trace element deficiency is unusual in formula-fed infants. It usually occurs during unsupplemented total parenteral alimentation. Copper deficiency was common before the addition of trace elements to intravenous alimentation solutions and manifests as anemia, neutropenia, and periosteal bone formation. Zinc deficiency may be noted during total intravenous alimentation or among breast-fed infants whose mothers have low zinc levels in their milk. These infants have alopecia, growth failure, and dermatitis around the anus and on the hands and feet. Iron deficiency rarely is manifested during the 1st mo of life. Prophylactic iron therapy should be started when preterm infants double their birth weight and in term infants after the 6th mo of life; therapy for both should be in the form of iron-fortified formula and cereal or ferrous sulfate solution.

Fluid Requirements

Fluid balance in the normal, growing infant is always positive because of the high water content present during cellular growth. Oral feedings, intravenous solutions, or a combination of the two is the usual source of fluid intake. Water from oxidation is an additional internal source of small quantities of water (10 mL/kg/24 hr). Fluid intake is required because of continuous insensible, urine, and stool water losses (Table 6–25). Excessive fluid intake may predispose the premature infant to a PDA, congestive heart failure, BPD, NEC, hyponatremia, and edema. Too little fluid intake will result in dehydration, azotemia, hyperbilirubinemia, and hypernatremia.

The correct amount of fluid intake depends on the size of the infant, the postnatal age, and coexistent diseases affecting fluid balance. On the 1st day of life, most infants should receive 60–80 mL/kg/24 hr of fluid. On subsequent days, this amount should be increased to 100–140 mL/kg/24 hr. Fluid intake greater than 150–160 mL/kg/24 hr has been associated with PDA, BPD, and NEC, and should be avoided unless there are excessive free water needs as a result of large insensible water losses. Hydration can be assessed by monitoring serum blood urea nitrogen (BUN), Na^+, urine output,

and urine specific gravity (see below). Rising serum Na^+, BUN, and urine specific gravity with weight loss suggest dehydration and a free water deficit.

Fluid balance in the newborn infant is tenuous because of very high rates of insensible water losses and immature renal function. Prior to 34 wk of gestation, the premature infant has a greatly reduced glomerular filtration rate (GFR). Although the GFR increases after 34 wk of age, the rate of filtration is still below adult values, even in full-term infants. Sodium reabsorption is reduced in the full-term infant and even more reduced in the preterm infant. Because of this, the fractional excretion of sodium is higher in the VLBW infant (up to 4%) than in the full-term infant or older child (less than 2.0%). Thus, although the required sodium intake in the term infant is 1–3 mEq/kg/24 hr, the VLBW infant may require 3–5 mEq/kg/24 hr to prevent sodium wasting and hyponatremia. The newborn infant also has a limited ability to excrete a diluted or a concentrated urine. Maximum urinary concentrating ability of the newborn is 600–700 mOsm/L compared with 1200–1400 mOsm/L in the adult. Urine osmolality should be maintained between 50 and 300 mOsm/L, which corresponds to a urine specific gravity of 1.003–1.012; overhydration is a risk when urine osmolality is below 20–30 mOsm/L. The immature kidney also is limited in its capacity to excrete excessive solute, which may result in diminished excretion of sodium and other components of the renal solute load (also known as ash components of formula). Additional signs of immaturity of renal function in the newborn include reduced $NaHCO_3$ reabsorption, diminished capacity to acidify the urine, and reduced excretion of drugs such as the aminoglycosides.

Table 6–25. Components of Fluid Losses

Source	Significance
Insensible water loss (IWL)	Varies with gestational and postnatal age; greatest in youngest, most immature 2–3 mL/kg/hr vs. term 0.5–0.8 mL/kg/hr; phototherapy, radiant warmer, low humidity increase IWL; ventilation, humidity, inner-plastic warmer shield decrease IWL
Urine output	Necessary to excrete obligate renal solute load; renal solute increases with fasting or a high-protein, high-electrolyte-containing formula; neonate has narrow range of urine concentration and diluting ability
Sweat	Uncommon in newborn; term infants sweat if overheated, with visible perspiration on forehead
Stool loss	Not a variable when on total parenteral alimentation; increased stool water loss with phototherapy and diarrhea

Parenteral Alimentation
See Chapter 2.

Gastrointestinal Diseases
OBSTRUCTION

See Chapter 11.

GASTROINTESTINAL HEMORRHAGE

See Chapter 11.

Gastrointestinal Perforation
Perforation of the small intestine associated with ileal atresia and cystic fibrosis results in sterile peri-

tonitis in utero (meconium peritonitis). After birth, bacterial colonization of the intestines results in a combined bacterial and chemical peritonitis following a postnatal perforation. Neonatal intestinal perforation may be traumatic (iatrogenic), idiopathic (stomach), drug induced (dexamethasone, indomethacin), or associated with gastrointestinal obstruction.

Necrotizing enterocolitis is the most common cause of intestinal perforation during the neonatal period, but not all cases of NEC result in perforation. Patients with NEC are usually premature infants who are receiving oral feedings and have recovered from previous diseases of prematurity. The onset of symptoms is usually in the 1st wk of life but may be delayed 1–2 mo after birth. The *clinical manifestations* of NEC include abdominal distention and tenderness, rectal bleeding, and a septic shock–like appearance. Abdominal roentgenograms reveal pneumatosis intestinalis and intrahepatic venous gas. Because epidemics of NEC are common and blood cultures are positive in 30% of patients, the *treatment* of NEC includes the initiation of broad-spectrum antibiotics as well as gastrointestinal decompression with a nasogastric tube and parenteral alimentation to put the bowel at rest. All newborn patients with evidence of intestinal perforation, such as pneumoperitoneum, require exploratory laparotomy.

References

Behrman RE (ed): Nelson Textbook of Pediatrics. 14th ed. Philadelphia, WB Saunders, 1992, Sec. 4.9–4.12, 6.11–6.26, 9.41–9.43, 13.28–13.33.

Cepero-Akselrad AE, Ramirez-Seijas F, Castaneda AM, et al: Acute renal failure in the newborn. Int Pediatr 5:328, 1990.

Costarino AT Jr, Gruskay JA, Corcoran L, et al: Sodium restriction versus daily maintenance replacement in very low birth weight premature neonates: A randomized, blind therapeutic trial. J Pediatr 120:99, 1992.

Hawdon JM, Platt MPW, Aynsley-Green A: Patterns of metabolic adaptation for preterm and term infants in the first neonatal week. Arch Dis Child 67:357, 1992.

Kliegman R: Models of the pathogenesis of necrotizing enterocolitis. J Pediatr 117:S2, 1990.

Kliegman R, Aucott S, Kosek M: Nutritional support of the neonate: Alternate fuels and routes of administration. *In* Cowett R (ed): *Principles of Perinatal-Neonatal Metabolism.* New York, Springer-Verlag, 1991.

METABOLIC DISORDERS

Hypoglycemia

Hypoglycemia is common during the neonatal period. Infants in many categories are at risk for

Table 6–26. Risk Factors for Neonatal Hypoglycemia

Factors	Mechanism
Common	
Prematurity	Limited glycogen stores
Infant of a diabetic mother	Hyperinsulinism
Intrauterine growth retardation	Limited glycogen stores, hyperinsulinism
Asphyxia–perinatal stress	Depleted glycogen stores
Hypothermia	Increased glucose utilization
Starvation	Depleted glycogen stores
Large for gestational age	Possible hyperinsulinism
Infant of obese mother	Possible hyperinsulinism
Maternal medications (tocolytics, propranolol, chlorpropamide, high-glucose infusion in labor)	Possible hyperinsulinism
Uncommon	
Erythroblastosis fetalis	Hyperinsulinism
Beckwith-Wiedemann syndrome	Hyperinsulinism
Islet cell adenoma	Hyperinsulinism
Nesidioblastosis	Hyperinsulinism
Familial hyperinsulinism	Hyperinsulinism
Polycythemia	Increased glucose utilization/decreased production
Sepsis	Increased glucose utilization
Inborn errors of metabolism	Decreased glycogenolysis, gluconeogenesis or utilization of alternate fuels
Growth hormone deficiency	Increased glucose utilization, decreased gluconeogenesis
Adrenal insufficiency	Decreased glucose production (gluconeogenesis)

neonatal hypoglycemia (Table 6–26). Serum glucose levels in healthy term infants are rarely less than 35 mg/dL between 1 and 3 hr of age, less than 40 mg/dL between 3 and 24 hr of age, and less than 45 mg/dL thereafter. Lower glucose levels among term or preterm infants suggest hypoglycemia. Alternately, symptoms compatible with hypoglycemia that respond to glucose infusions but with a higher glucose level are also considered to represent hypoglycemia.

Hypoglycemia in the **infant of a diabetic mother** is due to persistent hyperinsulinemia and a decreased ability to produce glucose (from glycogen) during neonatal fasting (see Medical Problems during Pregnancy Associated with Fetal or Neonatal Risk, and Table 6–4). Poorly controlled maternal diabetes produces maternal and, hence, fetal hyperglycemia, which stimulates the fetal beta cells of the pancreas to produce large quantities of insulin. After birth, hyperinsulinemia persists, suppressing fasting hepatic glucose production (from glycogenolysis). Hyperinsulinemia also suppresses lipolysis and reduces levels of free fatty acids. Oxidation of fatty acids is an important source of energy after birth, as noted by a decline of the respiratory quotient from 1 at birth to 0.8 at 2–3 hr after birth. If free fatty acid mobilization is reduced, there is less alternate fuel available for oxidation. In normal infants, free fatty acid metabolism spares glucose utilization and helps prevent hypoglycemia.

Infants with **intrauterine growth retardation** develop hypoglycemia as a result of reduced tissue stores of glycogen and fat. Thus glucose availability and fatty acid oxidation may be attenuated, resulting in a reduced total body energy production. The reduced level of oxygen consumption increases markedly with the provision of exogenous fuels during enteric feedings.

The *clinical manifestations* of neonatal hypoglycemia usually are noted on the 1st or 2nd day of life and vary from asymptomatic patients to those with central nervous system and cardiopulmonary disturbances. Hypotonia, lethargy, apathy, poor feeding, jitteriness, and seizures are common. Congestive heart failure, tachycardia, cyanosis, pallor, diaphoresis, apnea, and hypothermia are additional manifestations. Because many of these symptoms and signs are not specific for hypoglycemia, systemic (congenital heart disease, sepsis, intraventricular hemorrhage) or other metabolic (hypocalcemia, hypomagnesemia, narcotic withdrawal) disorders must be considered. Hypoglycemia also may be seen in association with other diseases such as complex cyanotic heart disease and asphyxia (see Chapter 17).

The occurrence of hypoglycemia can be anticipated and may be *prevented* by identification of a high-risk population (Table 6–26). Newborn infants who are at risk but who are asymptomatic and have no contraindications for oral feeding should be breast fed or given formula within the 1st few hours of birth. When early feedings are not possible because of concomitant cardiopulmonary disease, 10% glucose should be given intravenously. All asymptomatic newborn infants who are at risk should be monitored with serial capillary blood glucose levels during the first day of life; a low glucose value on the Chemstrip should be confirmed by serum glucose determination.

Treatment of hypoglycemia requires an initial intravenous bolus infusion of 200–400 mg/kg (2–4 mL/kg) of 10% glucose solution that rapidly raises blood glucose to the physiologic range; it should be followed immediately by a continuous infusion of 8 mg/kg/min of glucose. If hypoglycemia recurs, the bolus is repeated and the glucose infusion rate is incrementally increased to maintain physiologic glucose concentrations. The *prognosis* of symptomatic neonatal hypoglycemia with seizures is poor and is associated with abnormal neurointellectual development. The prognosis for other forms of hypoglycemia is better. Infants with nesidioblastosis often require surgical resection of the majority of the pancreas, if medical management with diazoxide or somatostatin fails.

Hypocalcemia

Hypocalcemia is common among sick and premature newborn infants. Most infants are born with calcium levels that are higher in cord blood than in maternal blood because of active placental transfer of calcium to the fetus. Fetal calcium accretion in the third trimester approaches 150 mg/kg/24 hr, and fetal bone mineral content doubles between 30 and 40 wk of gestation. All infants have a slight decline of serum calcium levels after birth that reach trough levels at 24–48 hr, the point at which hypocalcemia usually occurs. Total serum calcium levels of less than 7 mg/dL and ionized calcium levels of less than 3.0–3.5 mg/dL are considered hypocalcemic.

The *etiology* of hypocalcemia varies with the time of onset and the associated illnesses of the child. **Early neonatal hypocalcemia** occurs in the first 3 days of life and is often asymptomatic. Transient hypoparathyroidism and a reduced parathyroid response to the usual postnatal decline of serum calcium levels may be responsible for hypocalcemia among premature infants and infants of diabetic mothers. Congenital absence of the parathyroid gland and DiGeorge syndrome also have been associated with hypocalcemia. Hypomagnesemia (<1.5 mg/dL) may be seen simultaneously with hypocalcemia, especially in infants of diabetic mothers. Treatment with calcium alone will not relieve symptoms or increase serum calcium levels unless the hypomagnesemia also is treated. Sodium bicarbonate therapy, phosphate release from cell necrosis, transient hypoparathyroidism, and hypercalcitoninemia may be responsible for early neonatal hypocalcemia associated with asphyxia. Early-onset hypocalcemia associated with asphyxia often occurs with seizures as a result of the hypoxic–ischemic encephalopathy and/or hypocalcemia. **Late neonatal hypocalcemia**, or **neonatal tetany**, often is due to ingestion of high-phosphate–containing milk or the inability to excrete the usual phosphorus in commercial infant formula (see Table 6–23). Hyperphosphatemia (>8 mg/dL) usually occurs in infants with hypocalcemia after the 1st week of life. Vitamin D deficiency states and malabsorption also have been associated with late onset hypocalcemia.

The *clinical manifestations* of hypocalcemia and hypomagnesemia include apnea, muscle twitching, seizures, laryngospasm, **Chvostek sign** (facial muscle spasm when the side of the face over the 7th nerve is tapped), and **Trousseau sign** (carpopedal spasm induced by partial inflation of a blood pressure cuff). The latter two signs are rare in the immediate newborn period. On occasion, congestive heart failure has been associated with hypocalcemia.

Neonatal hypocalcemia may be *prevented* by administering intravenous or oral calcium supplementation at a rate of 25–75 mg/kg/24 hr. Early asymptomatic hypocalcemia of preterm infants and infants of diabetic mothers often resolves spontaneously. Symptomatic hypocalcemia should be treated with 2–4 mL/kg of 10% calcium gluconate given intravenously slowly over 10–15 min; a continuous infusion of 75 mg/kg/24 hr of elemental calcium then should be administered. If hypomagnesemia is associated with hypocalcemia, 50% magnesium sulfate, 0.1 mL/kg, should be given by intramuscular injection and repeated every 8–12 hr.

The *treatment* of late hypocalcemia includes immediate management as in early hypocalcemia plus the initiation of low-phosphate-containing formula feedings. Subcutaneous infiltration of intravenous calcium salts can cause tissue necrosis; oral supplements are hypertonic and may irritate the intestinal mucosa.

Osteopenia or Metabolic Bone Disease of Prematurity

The rate of fetal bone mineralization is not always maintained by the prematurely born infant fed breast milk or standard formula. Bone undermineralization or frank rickets may develop and result in pathologic fractures, altered growth, and respiratory insufficiency. Osteopenia predominantly is noted in infants weighing less than 1000 g and in infants with chronic diseases of prematurity such as BPD after the first 2–3 mo of life. Roentgenographic signs include bone demineralization and fractures. Serum alkaline phosphatase levels always are elevated, sometimes 2–3 times normal. The causes are not established but may include dietary deficiency of calcium and phosphate, vitamin D deficiency, copper deficiency, aluminum toxicity, diuretic-induced hypercalciuria, cholestatic jaundice–induced malabsorption of calcium, and altered metabolism of vitamin D. *Prevention* may be possible with a formula containing higher concentrations of calcium, phosphate, and vitamin D (see Table 6–23). *Treatment* consists of dietary supplementation with calcium, phosphate, and if indicated, vitamin D.

Neonatal Drug Addiction and Withdrawal

Infants may become passively and physiologically addicted to medications or to drugs of abuse (heroin, methadone, barbiturates, tranquilizers, and amphetamines) taken by the mother during pregnancy and, subsequently, have signs and symptoms of neonatal withdrawal. Many of these pregnancies are at high risk for other complications related to intravenous drug abuse, such as hepatitis, acquired immunodeficiency syndrome, and syphilis. In addition, the LBW rate and the long-term risk for the sudden infant death syndrome are higher in the infants of these high-risk women.

Neonatal withdrawal signs and symptoms usually begin at 1–5 days of life with maternal heroin abuse and at 1–4 wk with maternal methadone addiction. Manifestations of withdrawal include sneezing, yawning, ravenous appetite, emesis, diarrhea, fever, diaphoresis, tachypnea, high-pitched cry, tremors, jitteriness, poor sleep, poor feeding, and seizures. The illness tends to be more severe during methadone withdrawal. The initial management includes swaddling in blankets in a quiet, dark room. When hyperactivity is constant and irritability interferes with sleeping and feeding or when diarrhea or seizures are present, pharmacologic treatment is indicated. Seizures usually are treated with phenobarbital. The other symptoms may be managed with replacement doses of a narcotic (usually tincture of opium) to calm the infant; weaning from narcotics may be prolonged over 1–2 mo.

Cocaine abuse during pregnancy is associated

with preterm labor, abruptio placenta, neonatal irritability, intraventricular hemorrhage, and decreased attentiveness. Usually no treatment is needed.

References

Baker L, Thornton PS, Stanley CA: Management of hyperinsulinism in infants. J Pediatr 119:755, 1991.

Behrman RE (ed): Nelson Textbook of Pediatrics. 14th ed. Philadelphia, WB Saunders, 1992, Sec. 9.54–9.57, 8.59.

Burton BK: Inborn errors of metabolism: The critical diagnosis in early infancy. Pediatrics 79:359, 1987.

Kliegman R: Problems in metabolic adaptation: Glucose, calcium and magnesium. In Klaus M, Fanaroff A (eds): Care of the High Risk Neonate. 4th ed. Philadelphia, WB Saunders, 1993.

Koo WWK, Sherman R, Succop P, et al: Fractures and rickets in very low birth weight infants: Conservative management and outcome. J Pediatr Orthop 9:326, 1989.

Rivers RPA: Neonatal opiate withdrawal. Arch Dis Child 61:1236, 1986.

Singer L, Garber R, Kliegman R: Neurobehavioral sequelae of fetal cocaine exposure. J Pediatr 119:667, 1991.

NEONATAL INFECTIOUS DISEASE (see also Chapter 10 and Appendix)

Systemic and local infections (pneumonia, cutaneous, ocular, and meningeal infections) are common in the newborn period. Infection may be acquired in utero through the transplacental or transcervical routes and during and after birth. Ascending infection through the cervix, with or without rupture of the amniotic fluid membranes, may result in amnionitis, funisitis (infection of the umbilical cord), congenital pneumonia, and sepsis. The bacteria responsible for ascending infection of the fetus are common bacterial organisms of the maternal genitourinary tract such as group B streptococcus, *Escherichia coli*, and *Klebsiella*. Herpes simplex II also causes ascending infection that, at times, may be indistinguishable from bacterial sepsis. Syphilis and *Listeria monocytogenes* are acquired by transplacental infection.

Maternal humoral immunity may protect the fetus against some neonatal pathogens, such as group B streptococcus and herpes simplex type II. Nonetheless, various deficiencies of the neonatal antimicrobial defense mechanism probably are more important than maternal immune status as a contributing factor for neonatal infection, especially in the LBW infant. The incidence of sepsis is approximately 1:1500 in full-term infants and 1:250

in preterm infants. The 6-fold higher rate of sepsis among preterm infants compared with term infants relates both to the preterm infants' more immature immunologic system and to their prolonged period of hospitalization, which holds the added risk of nosocomially acquired infectious diseases.

Preterm infants prior to 32 wk of gestational age have not received the full complement of maternal antibodies (IgG), which cross the placenta by active transport predominantly in the latter half of the 3rd trimester. In addition, although LBW infants may generate IgM antibodies, their own IgG response to infection is reduced. These infants also have deficiencies of the alternate and, to a smaller degree, the classic complement activation pathways, which result in diminished complement-mediated opsonization. Newborn infants also demonstrate a deficit in phagocytic migration to the site of infection (e.g., to the lung) and in the bone marrow reserve pool of leukocytes. In addition, in the presence of suboptimal activation of complement, neonatal neutrophils ingest and kill bacteria less effectively than do adult neutrophils. Furthermore, neutrophils from sick infants seem to have an even greater deficit in bacterial killing capacity than do phagocytic cells from normal neonates.

Defense mechanisms against viral pathogens also may be deficient in the newborn infant. Neonatal antibody-dependent cell-mediated immunity by the natural killer lymphocytes is deficient in the absence of maternal antibodies and in the presence of reduced interferon production; reduced antibody levels occur in premature infants and in infants born during a primary viral infection of the mother, such as with herpes simplex II or cytomegalovirus. In addition, antibody-independent cytotoxicity also may be reduced in lymphocytes of newborn infants.

Neonatal Sepsis

Neonatal sepsis presents during three periods. **Early-onset sepsis** often begins in utero and usually is due to infection by the bacteria in the mother's genitourinary tract. These organisms include group B streptococcus, *E. coli, Klebsiella, Listeria monocytogenes*, and nontypable *H. influenzae*. Most infected infants are premature and show nonspecific cardiorespiratory signs such as grunting, tachypnea, and cyanosis at birth. Risk factors for early-onset sepsis include vaginal colonization with group B streptococcus, prolonged rupture of the membranes (>24 hr), amnionitis, maternal fever or leukocytosis, fetal tachycardia, and preterm birth. Black race and male sex are unexplained additional risk factors for neonatal sepsis.

Early-onset sepsis (birth to 8 days) is an overwhelming multiorgan system disease frequently manifested by respiratory failure, shock, meningitis (30%), DIC, acute tubular necrosis, and symmetric peripheral gangrene. Profound neutropenia, hypoxia, and hypotension may be refractory to treatment with broad-spectrum antibiotics, mechanical ventilation, and vasopressors such as dopamine and dobutamine. In the initial stages of early-onset septicemia in the preterm infant, it is often very difficult to differentiate sepsis from the respiratory distress syndrome. Because of this difficulty, most premature infants with respiratory distress syndrome receive-broad spectrum antibiotics.

Infants with early-onset sepsis should be *evaluated* by blood and cerebrospinal fluid (CSF) cultures; and by CSF Gram stain, cell count, protein, and glucose determinations. Buffy coat Gram stain or methylene blue stain also may help identify bacteria. Normal newborn infants generally have an elevated CSF protein content (100–150 mg/dL) and may have as many as 25 white blood cells (mean $9/mm^3$), which are 75% lymphocytes in the absence of infection. Some infants with neonatal meningitis caused by group B steptococcus do not have an elevated CSF leukocyte count but demonstrate micro-organisms on Gram stain of the spinal fluid. In addition to identification of the organism by culture, other methods to identify the pathogenic bacteria include the determination of bacterial antigen in samples of blood, urine, or spinal fluid by methods such as counterimmunoelectrophoresis or latex agglutination. Serial complete blood counts should be performed to identify neutropenia, an increased number of immature neutrophils (bands), and thrombocytopenia. C-reactive protein levels are often elevated in neonatal patients with bacterial sepsis.

A chest roentgenogram also should be obtained to determine the presence of pneumonia. Arterial blood gases should be monitored to detect hypoxemia and metabolic acidosis that may be due to hypoxia, shock, or both. Blood pressure, urine output, central venous pressure, and peripheral perfusion should be monitored to determine the need to treat septic shock with fluids and vasopressor agents.

A combination of ampicillin and gentamicin for 10–14 days is effective *treatment* against most organisms responsible for early-onset sepsis. If meningitis is present, the treatment is extended to 21 days, or 14 days after a negative CSF culture. Persistently positive spinal fluid culture is common with neonatal meningitis caused by gram-negative organisms, even with appropriate antibiotic treatment, and may be present for 2–3 days after antibiotic therapy. If gram-negative meningitis is present, some authorities continue to treat with an effective penicillin derivative plus an aminoglycoside, whereas others change to a 3rd-generation cephalosporin. Treatment with high-dose penicillin (250,000 U/kg/24 hr) is appropriate for group B streptococcus meningitis.

Late-onset sepsis (8–28 days) usually occurs in the healthy full-term infant who was discharged in good health from the normal newborn nursery. *Clinical manifestations* may include lethargy, poor feeding, hypotonia, apathy, seizures, bulging fontanel, fever, and direct-reacting hyperbilirubinemia. In addition to bacteremia, hematogenous seeding may result in focal infections such as meningitis (75%), osteomyelitis (group B streptococcus, *Staphylococcus aureus*), arthritis (gonococcus, *S. aureus*, *Candida albicans*, gram-negative bacteria), and urinary tract infection (gram-negative bacteria).

The *evaluation* of infants with late-onset sepsis is similar to that for those with early-onset sepsis, with special attention given to a careful physical examination of the bones (infants with osteomyelitis may present with pseudoparalysis) and to the laboratory examination and culture of urine obtained by sterile suprapubic aspiration or urethral catheterization. Late-onset sepsis may be due to the same pathogens as early-onset sepsis, but those infants presenting late in the neonatal period also may have infections caused by the pathogens usually found in older infants (*Haemophilus influenzae*, *Streptococcus pneumoniae*, *Neisseria meningitidis*).

Because of the increased rate of resistance of *H. influenzae* to ampicillin, some centers begin treatment with ampicillin and a 3rd generation cephalosporin when sepsis occurs in the last week of the 1st mo of life. The treatment for late-onset neonatal sepsis and meningitis is the same as that for early-onset sepsis (see above).

Nosocomially acquired sepsis (8 days to discharge) occurs predominantly among premature infants in the neonatal intensive care unit (NICU), and many of these infants have been colonized with the multidrug-resistant bacteria indigenous to the NICU. Frequent treatment with broad-spectrum antibiotics for sepsis and the presence of central venous indwelling catheters, endotracheal tubes, umbilical vessel catheters, and electronic monitoring devices increase the risk for such serious bacterial infection. Epidemics of bacterial or viral sepsis, bacterial or aseptic meningitis, staphylococcal bullous skin infections, cellulitis, pneumo-

Table 6–27. Perinatal Congenital Infections (TORCH)

Agent	Maternal Epidemiology	Neonatal Features
Toxoplasma gondii	Heterophil-negative mononucleosis Exposure to cats or raw meat or immunosuppression High-risk exposure at 10–24 weeks gestation	Hydrocephalus, abnormal spinal fluid, intracranial calcifications, chorioretinitis, jaundice, hepatosplenomegaly, fever Many infants asymptomatic at birth *Treatment:* pyrimethamine plus sulfadiazine

Rubella virus	Unimmunized seronegative mother; fever ± rash
	Detectable defects with infection:
	   by 8 wk, 85%
	   9–12 wk, 50%
	   13–20 wk, 16%
	Virus may be present in infant throat for 1 yr
	Prevention: vaccine
		Intrauterine growth retardation, microcephaly, microphthalmia, cataracts, glaucoma, "salt and pepper" chorioretinitis, hepatosplenomegaly, jaundice, PDA, deafness, blueberry muffin rash, anemia, thrombocytopenia, leukopenia, metaphyseal lucencies, B- and T-cell deficiency
		Infant may be asymptomatic at birth

Cytomegalovirus	Sexually transmitted disease: primary genital infection may be asymptomatic Heterophil-negative mononucleosis; infant may have viruria for 1–6 yr	Sepsis, intrauterine growth retardation, chorioretinitis, microcephaly, periventricular calcifications, blueberry muffin rash, anemia, thrombocytopenia, neutropenia, hepatosplenomegaly, jaundice, deafness, pneumonia Many asymptomatic at birth *Prevention:* CMV-negative blood products
Herpes simplex type II virus	Sexually transmitted disease (STD): primary genital infection may be asymptomatic; intrauterine infection rare, acquisition at time of birth more common	*Intrauterine infection:* chorioretinitis, skin lesions, microcephaly *Postnatal:* encephalitis, localized or disseminated disease, skin vesicles, keratoconjunctivitis *Treatment:* acyclovir
Varicella-zoster virus	Intrauterine infection with chickenpox during first trimester Infant develops severe neonatal varicella with maternal illness 5 days prior to or 2 days after delivery	Microphthalmia, cataracts, chorioretinitis, cutaneous and bony aplasia/hypoplasia/atrophy, cutaneous scars Zoster as in older child *Prevention of neonatal* condition with VZIG *Treatment of ill neonate:* acyclovir
Treponema pallidum syphilis	Sexually transmitted disease Maternal primary asymptomatic: painless "hidden" chancre Penicillin, not erythromycin, *prevents* fetal infection	Presentation *at birth* as nonimmune hydrops, prematurity, anemia, neutropenia, thrombocytopenia, pneumonia, hepatosplenomegaly *Late neonatal* as snuffles (rhinitis), rash, hepatosplenomegaly, condylomata lata, metaphysitis, cerebrospinal fluid pleocytosis, keratitis, periosteal new bone, lymphocytosis, hepatitis *Late onset*—teeth, eye, bone, skin, CNS, ear *Treatment:* penicillin
Parvovirus	Etiology of fifth disease; fever, rash, arthralgia in adults	Nonimmune hydrops, fetal anemia *Treatment:* in utero transfusion
Human immunodeficiency virus (HIV)	AIDS; most mothers are asymptomatic and HIV positive; high-risk history: prostitute, drug abuse, married to bisexual, or hemophiliac	AIDS symptoms develop between 3 and 6 mo of age in 25–40%; failure to thrive, recurrent infection, hepatosplenomegaly, neurologic abnormalities *Management:* Intravenous immunoglobulin, trimethoprim–sulfamethoxazole, AZT
Hepatitis B virus	Vertical transmission common; may result in cirrhosis, hepatocellular carcinoma	Acute neonatal hepatitis; many become asymptomatic carriers *Prevention:* HBIG, vaccine
Borrelia burgdorferi	Lyme disease, erythema chronicum migrans, meningitis, arthritis, carditis *Maternal treatment:* penicillin, ceftriaxone	Prematurity, rash, cortical blindness, fetal death?
Neisseria gonorrhoeae	STD, infant acquires at birth *Treatment:* cefotaxime, ceftriaxone	Gonococcal ophthalmia, sepsis, meningitis *Prevention:* silver nitrate, erythromycin eye drops *Treatment:* intravenous ceftriaxone
Chlamydia trachomatis	STD, infant acquires at birth *Treatment:* oral erythromycin	Conjunctivitis, pneumonia *Prevention:* erythromycin eye drops *Treatment:* oral erythromycin
Mycobacterium tuberculosis	Positive PPD skin test, recent converter, positive chest roentgenogram, positive family member *Treatment:* INH and rifampin ± ethambutol	Congenital rare septic pneumonia; acquired primary pulmonary TB; asymptomatic, follow PPD *Prevention:* INH, BCG, separation *Treatment:* INH, rifampin, pyrazinamide
Trypanosoma cruzi (Chagas disease)	Central South American native, immigrant, travel Chronic disease in mother	Failure to thrive, heart failure, achalasia *Treatment:* nifurtimox

AIDS = acquired immunodeficiency syndrome; AZT = azidothymidine; BCG = bacillus Calmette-Guerin; CNS = central nervous system; HBIG = hepatitis B immune globulin; INH = isoniazid; PPD = purified protein derivative; TB = tuberculosis; VZIG = varicella-zoster immune globulin.

nia (bacterial, adenovirus, respiratory syncytial virus), and diarrhea (staphylococcal, enteroviral, rotavirus, and enteropathogenic *E. coli* and associated NEC) are not uncommon in the NICU or even in the nursery for well babies.

The initial *clinical manifestations* of nosocomial infection in the premature infant may be subtle and include apnea and bradycardia, temperature instability, abdominal distention, and poor feeding as early signs. In the later stages, there may be shock, DIC, worsening respiratory status, and local reactions such as omphalitis, eye discharge, diarrhea, or bullous impetigo.

The *treatment* of nosocomially acquired sepsis depends on the indigenous microbiologic flora of the particular hospital and their antibiotic sensitivities. Because *S. aureus* (occasionally methicillin resistant), *Staphylococcus epidermidis* (usually methicillin-resistant) and gram-negative pathogens are common nosocomial bacterial agents in many nurseries, a combination of vancomycin or nafcillin with gentamicin is appropriate. The dose and interval for administering all aminoglycosides, such as gentamicin, vary with postnatal age and birth weight. In addition, treatment with aminoglycosides for more than 3 days is an absolute indication for monitoring serum peak and trough concentrations to optimize therapy and to avoid ototoxicity and nephrotoxicity. Persistent signs of infection despite antibacterial treatment should suggest candidal sepsis.

Perinatal Congenital (TORCH) Infections

The acronym "TORCH" represents a generic group of parasitic, bacterial, and viral pathogens that produce congenital or perinatally acquired infections. TORCH stands for *t*oxoplasmosis, *o*ther, *r*ubella, *c*ytomegalovirus (CMV), and *h*erpes simplex. The "other" is an increasing number of agents responsible for fetal infection, such as syphilis, varicella zoster, parvovirus, human immunodeficiency virus (HIV), hepatitis B virus, and *Borrelia burgdorferi.*

Many of the *clinical manifestations* of TORCH infections are similar and include intrauterine growth retardation, nonimmune hydrops, anemia, thrombocytopenia, jaundice, hepatosplenomegaly, chorioretinitis, and congenital malformations. Some of the unique manifestations and epidemiologic characteristics of these infections are noted in Table 6–27.

Evaluation of patients suspected of having TORCH infections should include attempts to iso-

late the organism by culture (rubella, CMV, herpes simplex II, gonorrhea, *Mycobacterium tuberculosis*); to identify the antigen of the pathogen (hepatitis B, *Chlamydia trachomatis*); and to identify specific fetal production of antibodies (IgM or increasing titer of IgG for *Toxoplasma*, syphilis, parvovirus, HIV, *Borrelia*).

Treatment is not always available, specific, or effective. Nonetheless, some encouraging results have been reported for preventing the disease and for specifically treating the infant once the correct diagnosis is made (Table 6–27).

References

Behrman RE (ed): Nelson Textbook of Pediatrics. 14th ed. Philadelphia, WB Saunders, 1992, Sec. 9.58–9.75.

Best J, Sutherland S: Diagnosis and prevention of congenital and perinatal infections: TORCH screening should be discouraged. BMJ 30:888, 1990.

Dorfman DH, Glaser JH: Congenital syphilis presenting in infants after the newborn period. N Engl J Med 323: 1299, 1990.

Gibbs RS, Hall RT, Yow MD, et al: Consensus: Perinatal prophylaxis for Group B streptococcal infection. Pediatr Infect Dis J 11:179, 1992.

Gladstone IM, Ehrenkranz RA, Edberg SC, et al: A ten-year review of neonatal sepsis and comparison with the previous fifty-year experience. Pediatr Infect Dis J 9:819, 1990.

Grose C, Itani O, Weiner CP: Prenatal diagnosis of fetal infection: Advances from amniocentesis to cordocentesis—congenital toxoplasmosis, rubella, cytomegalovirus, varicella virus, parvovirus and human immunodeficiency virus. Pediatr Infect Dis J 8:459, 1989.

Whitley R, Arvin A, Prober C, et al: A controlled trial comparing vidarabine with acyclovir in neonatal herpes simplex virus infection. N Engl J Med 324:444, 1992.

NEONATAL NEUROLOGY AND OUTCOME

The neonatal central nervous system is anatomically and functionally immature. Although division of cerebral cortical neuronal cells stops during the 2nd trimester of pregnancy, glial cell growth, dendritic arborization, myelination, and cerebellar neuronal cell number continue to increase beyond term gestation and into infancy. At birth, the human newborn spends more time asleep (predominantly rapid-eye-movement or active sleep) than in a wakeful state and is totally dependent on adults. Primitive reflexes, such as the Moro, grasp, stepping, rooting, sucking, and crossed extensor reflexes, are readily elicited and are normal for this age. In addition, the newborn infant has a wealth of cortical functions that are less easily demonstrated (e.g., the ability to extinguish repetitive or painful stimuli and to show visual preference for new or novel objects); the newborn also has the capacity for attentive eye fixation and differential responses to the mother's voice.

During the perinatal period, many pathophysiologic mechanisms can adversely and permanently affect the developing brain. These include prenatal events, such as hypoxia, ischemia, infections, malformations, maternal drugs, and coagulation disorders, and postnatal events, such as birth trauma, hypoxia–ischemia, inborn errors of metabolism, hypoglycemia, hypothyroidism, hyperthyroidism, polycythemia, hemorrhage, and meningitis.

Neonatal Seizures

Seizures during the neonatal period may be due to multiple causes with characteristic historic and clinical manifestations. Seizures due to *hypoxic–ischemic encephalopathy* (postasphyxial seizures), a common cause of seizures in the full-term infant, usually occur 12–24 hr after a history of birth asphyxia and often are refractory to conventional doses of anticonvulsant medications. Postasphyxial seizures also may be due to metabolic disorders associated with neonatal asphyxia, such as hypoglycemia and hypocalcemia. *Intraventricular hemorrhage* (IVH) is a common cause of seizures in premature infants and often occurs between 1 and 3 days of age. Seizures with IVH are associated with a bulging fontanel, hemorrhagic spinal fluid, anemia, lethargy, and coma. Seizures due to *hypoglycemia* often occur when blood glucose levels decline to the lowest postnatal value (e.g., 1–2 hr of age or after 24–48 hr of poor nutritional intake) (Table 6–26). Seizures due to *hypocalcemia* and *hypomagnesemia* develop among high risk infants and respond well to calcium and/or magnesium therapy.

Seizures noted in the delivery room often are due to direct *injection of local anesthetics* into the fetal scalp (associated with transient bradycardia and fixed dilated pupils), severe *anoxia*, or *congenital brain malformation*. Seizures after the first 5 days of life may be due to *infection* or *drug withdrawal*. Seizures associated with lethargy, acidosis, and a family history of infant deaths may be due to an *inborn error of metabolism*. An infant whose parent has a history of a neonatal seizure also is at risk for benign *familial seizures*. In an infant who appears well, a sudden onset of seizures on days 1–3 that are of short duration and that do not recur often is due to a *subarachnoid hemorrhage*. Focal seizures often are due to local cerebral infarction.

Seizures often may be difficult to differentiate from benign jitteriness or from tremulousness in infants of diabetic mothers, in infants with narcotic withdrawal syndrome, and in infants after an episode of asphyxia. In contrast to seizures, jitteriness and tremors are sensory dependent, elicited by stimuli, and interrupted by holding the extremity. Seizure activity becomes manifest by coarse, fast and slow clonic activity, whereas jitteriness is characterized by fine, very rapid movement. Seizures may be associated with abnormal eye movements such as tonic deviation to one side. The electroencephalogram (EEG) often will demonstrate seizure activity when the clinical diagnosis is uncertain. It is often difficult to identify seizures in the newborn period because the infant, especially the LBW infant, usually does not demonstrate the tonic–clonic major motor activity typical of the older child (Table 6–28). Subtle seizures are a very common manifestation among newborn infants. The subtle signs of seizure activity include apnea, eye deviation, tongue thrusting, eye blinking, and staring. Continuous bedside EEG monitoring can help identify subtle seizures.

The *diagnostic evaluation* of infants with seizures should include an immediate determination of capillary blood glucose levels with Chemstrip. In addition, determination of blood concentrations of sodium, calcium, glucose, and bilirubin should be obtained. When infection is suspected, appropriate cultures should be obtained. After the seizure has stopped, a careful examination should be done to identify signs of increased intracranial pressure, congenital malformations, and systemic illness. In the absence of signs of elevated intracranial pressure, a lumbar puncture should be performed. If the diagnosis is not apparent at this point, further evaluation should include computerized tomogra-

Table 6–28. Classification of Neonatal Seizures

Type	Manifestations
Subtle	Eye deviation, blinking, mouth movements, apnea, fluctuation of vital signs
Focal clonic	Localized jerking movement
Multifocal clonic	Multiple random clonic movements
Tonic	Extensor posturing with tonic eye deviation
Myoclonic	Synchronized single or multifocal rapid jerks Hypsarrhythmia on EEG possible
Tonic–clonic	Less common than in older children

phy or cerebral ultrasound and tests to determine the presence of an inborn error of metabolism. The latter determinations are especially important in infants with unexplained lethargy, coma, acidosis, ketonuria, or respiratory alkalosis.

The *treatment* of neonatal seizures may be specific, such as treatment of meningitis or the correction of hypoglycemia, hypocalcemia, hypomagnesemia, hyponatremia, and vitamin B_6 deficiency or dependency. In the absence of an identifiable cause, therapy should include an anticonvulsant agent such as 20–30 mg/kg of phenobarbital, 10–20 mg/kg of phenytoin (Dilantin), or 0.1–0.3 mg/kg of diazepam (Valium), followed by one of the two longer acting drugs. Treatment of status epilepticus requires repeated doses of phenobarbital and may also require a diazepam or paraldehyde drip titrated to clinical signs.

The long-term outcome for neonatal seizures usually is related to the underlying cause and to the primary pathology such as hypoxic–ischemic encephalopathy, meningitis, drug withdrawal, stroke, or hemorrhage.

Intracranial Hemorrhage

Intracranial hemorrhage may be confined to one anatomic area of the brain, such as the subdural, subarachnoid, periventricular, intraventricular, intraparenchymal, or cerebellar region. **Subdural hemorrhages** are seen in association with birth trauma, cephalopelvic disproportion, forceps delivery, LGA, infants and postnatal head trauma. The subdural hematoma does not always cause symptoms immediately after birth, but with time the red blood cells undergo hemolysis, and water is drawn into the hemorrhage because of the high oncotic pressure of protein, resulting in an expanding symptomatic lesion. Anemia, vomiting, seizures, and macrocephaly may occur in the 1–2 mo old infant with a subdural hematoma. Child abuse also should be suspected, and appropriate diagnostic evaluation undertaken to identify other possible signs of skeletal or soft tissue injury. Occasionally, a massive subdural hemorrhage in the neonatal period is due to rupture of the vein of Galen or to an inherited coagulation disorder such as hemophilia. These infants present with shock, seizures, and coma. The treatment of all subdural hematomas is surgical evacuation.

Subarachnoid hemorrhages may be spontaneous or associated with hypoxia and bleeding from a cerebral arteriovenous malformation. Seizures are a common presenting manifestation, and the prognosis depends on the underlying injury.

The treatment is directed at the seizure and the rare occurrence of posthemorrhagic hydrocephalus.

Periventricular hemorrhage and intraventricular hemorrhage are common among VLBW infants, and the risk decreases with increasing gestational age. Up to 50% of infants under 1500 g have evidence of intracranial bleeding. The *pathogenesis* for these hemorrhages is unknown (they usually are not due to coagulation disorders), but the initial site of bleeding may be the weak blood vessels in the periventricular germinal matrix. The vessels in this area have poor structural support and may rupture and hemorrhage because of passive changes in cerebral blood flow occurring with the variations of blood pressure that sick premature infants often exhibit (failure of autoregulation). In some sick infants, these blood pressure variations are the only identifiable etiologic factors. In others, the disorders that may cause the elevation or depression of blood pressure or that interfere with venous return from the head (venous stasis) increase the risk of IVH; these disorders include asphyxia, pneumothorax, mechanical ventilation, hypercapnia, hypoxemia, prolonged labor, breech delivery, PDA, heart failure, intravenous therapy with blood volume–expanding agents such as albumin, and therapy with hypertonic solutions such as sodium bicarbonate.

Most periventricular and intraventricular hemorrhages occur in the first 3 days of life. It is unusual for IVH to occur after the 5th day of life. The *clinical manifestations* include seizures, apnea, bradycardia, lethargy, coma, hypotension, metabolic acidosis, anemia not corrected by blood transfusion, bulging fontanel, and cutaneous mottling. Many infants with small hemorrhages (grade 1 or 2) are asymptomatic; those with larger hemorrhages (grade 4) often have a catastrophic event that rapidly progresses to shock and coma.

The *diagnosis* of IVH is confirmed and the severity graded by ultrasonographic examination through the anterior fontanel. Grade 1 IVH is confined to the germinal matrix; grade 2 is an extension of grade 1, with blood noted in the ventricle without ventricular enlargement; grade 3 is an extension of grade 2 with ventricular dilation; and grade 4 has blood in dilated ventricles and in the cerebral cortex, either contiguous with or distant from the ventricle. Grade 4 hemorrhage has a poor prognosis, as does the development of periventricular small echolucent cystic lesions, with or without porencephalic cysts and posthemorrhagic hydrocephalus. Periventricular cysts often are noted after the resolution of echodense areas in the periventricular white matter and may correspond to the development of periventricular leukomalacia that may be a precursor to cerebral palsy. Extensive intraparenchymal echodensities represent hemorrhagic necrosis, are associated with a high mortality rate, and have a very poor neurodevelopmental prognosis for survivors.

Treatment of the acute hemorrhage involves standard supportive care, including ventilation for apnea and blood transfusion for shock. Posthemorrhagic hydrocephalus may be managed with serial daily lumbar punctures, external ventriculostomy tube, or permanent ventricular–peritoneal shunt. The latter often is delayed as a result of the very high protein content of the hemorrhagic ventricular fluid.

Hypoxic–Ischemic Encephalopathy (see also Asphyxia: Resuscitation)

Conditions known to reduce uteroplacental blood flow or to interfere with spontaneous respiration result in perinatal hypoxia, in lactic acidosis, and, if severe enough to reduce cardiac output or to cause cardiac arrest, in ischemia. The combination of the reduced availability of oxygen for the brain that occurs from hypoxia and the diminished or absent blood flow to the brain that occurs from ischemia results in reduced glucose for metabolism and in an accumulation of lactate that produces local tissue acidosis. After reperfusion, hypoxic–ischemic injury also may be complicated by cell necrosis and vascular endothelial edema, reducing blood flow distal to the involved vessel. Typically, hypoxic–ischemic encephalopathy in the term infant is characterized by cerebral edema, cortical necrosis, and involvement of the basal ganglia, whereas in the preterm infant it is characterized by periventricular leukomalacia. Both lesions may result in cortical atrophy, mental retardation, and spastic quadriplegia or diplegia.

The *clinical manifestations* and characteristic course of hypoxic–ischemic encephalopathy vary according to the severity of the injury (Table 6–29). Infants with severe stage 3 hypoxic–ischemic encephalopathy are usually hypotonic, although occasionally they appear hypertonic and hyperalert at birth. As cerebral edema develops, brain functions become affected in a descending order; cortical depression produces coma, whereas brain stem depression results in apnea. As cerebral edema progresses, refractory seizures begin between 12 and 24 hr after birth. At this time, the infant has no signs of spontaneous respirations, is hypotonic, and has diminished or absent deep tendon reflexes.

Stage 3 survivors have a high incidence of seizures and serious neurodevelopmental handicaps. The outcome of severe asphyxia also depends on other organ system injury (see Table 6–9). Another indicator of poor prognosis is time of onset of spontaneous respiration as estimated by Apgar score. Infants with Apgar scores of 0–3 at 10 min have a 20% mortality and a 5% incidence of cerebral palsy; if the score remains this low by 20 min, the mortality increases to 60% and the incidence of cerebral palsy rises to 57%.

Neonatal Hypotonia

Decreased tone, floppiness, or hypotonia in the newborn infant may be transient and resolve without future problems or may be due to serious per-

Table 6–29. Hypoxic–Ischemic Encephalopathy in Term Infants

Signs	Stage 1	Stage 2	Stage 3
Level of consciousness	Hyperalert	Lethargic	Stuporous
Muscle tone	Normal	Hypotonic	Flaccid
Tendon reflexes/clonus	Hyperactive	Hyperactive	Absent
Moro reflex	Strong	Weak	Absent
Pupils	Mydriasis	Miosis	Unequal, poor light reflex
Seizures	None	Common	Decerebration
EEG	Normal	Low voltage changing to seizure activity	Burst suppression to isoelectric
Duration	<24 hr if progresses, otherwise may remain normal	24 hr to 14 days	Days to weeks

(Modified from Sarnat HB, Sarnat MS: Neonatal encephalopathy following fetal distress. A clinical and electroencephalographic study. Arch Neurol 33:696, 1976.)

manent disease originating in the central nervous system, spinal cord, anterior horn cell, neuromuscular junction, or muscle. Diseases of the *brain* producing hypotonia may be due to hypoxic–ischemic encephalopathy, IVH, meningitis, metabolic toxins (organic acids, ammonia), or centrally acting drugs. The infant does not appear alert and has a weak cry, seizures, normal deep tendon reflexes, and an abnormal EEG.

Spinal cord lesions often are due to trauma or malformation and present in an alert-looking child with a strong cry, decreased deep tendon reflexes, reduced spontaneous movement below the cord lesions, and a normal EEG. *Anterior horn cell disease,* such as Werdnig-Hoffmann disease, is indicated by an alert-appearing infant with hypotonia, tongue fasciculations, absent deep tendon reflexes, reduced muscle mass, and a neurogenic electromyogram (EMG) and muscle biopsy.

Neuromuscular junction disease, such as neonatal transient myasthenia gravis (in a child born to a woman with myasthenia gravis), is indicated by an alert infant with a weak cry, ophthalmoplegia, ptosis, normal deep tendon reflexes, an abnormal EMG, and a positive physostigmine test.

Muscle disease may have onset prior to or immediately after birth and may be due to congenital muscular dystrophy, congenital myotonia, glycogen storage disease, mitochondrial defects, congenital lactic acidosis, or other myopathies. The infant with muscle disease is alert and has a good cry but also displays decreased muscle mass, contractures, myopathic EMG, characteristic muscle biopsy, and elevated serum creatine phosphokinase (CPK), with or without diminished deep tendon reflexes.

Respiratory difficulty is present in many of these conditions; the infants have difficulty swallowing secretions, which they may aspirate, or they may develop respiratory failure as a result of weakness of the respiratory muscles. The evaluation of infants with hypotonia should include a family history of myasthenia gravis, myotonic dystrophy, muscular dystrophy, inheritable myopathies, and the existence of previous infants with metabolic diseases. Laboratory examinations depend on the history and physical examination and may include metabolic tests for organic acids and carnitine, muscle and head ultrasound, nerve conduction, EMG, serum CPK, physostigmine test, and muscle biopsy, with specific attention to electron microscopy. Chromosomal analysis also is helpful for diagnosing hypotonic infants with Prader-Willi syndrome, which has a deletion of the long arm of chromosome 15.

References

Bada HS, Korones SB, Perry EH, et al: Mean arterial blood pressure changes in premature infants and those at risk for intraventricular hemorrhage. J Pediatr 117:607, 1990.

Behrman RE (ed): Nelson Textbook of Pediatrics. 14th ed. Philadelphia, WB Saunders, 1992, Sec. 9.10, 9.13, 9.22–9.25, 9.28–9.29, 20.17–20.21.

Hakeem VF, Wallace SJ: EEG monitoring of therapy for neonatal seizures. Dev Med Child Neurol 32:858, 1990.

Sinha SK, D'Souza SW, Rivlin E, et al: Ischaemic brain lesions diagnosed at birth in preterm infants: Clinical events and developmental outcome. Arch Dis Child 65: 1017, 1990.

Ventriculomegaly Trial Group: Randomised trial of early tapping in neonatal posthaemorrhagic ventricular dilatation. Arch Dis Child 65:3, 1990.

Volpe JJ: Neurology of the Newborn. Philadelphia, WB Saunders, 1987.

OUTCOME AND FOLLOW-UP OF LBW OR PREMATURE INFANTS

Most LBW infants survive neonatal illnesses without long-term sequelae. Over 90% of infants weighing more than 1500 g survive, whereas as many as 40% of infants weighing as little as 750 g survive. Between 10% and 25% of survivors have mild developmental problems, and 5–10% have severe developmental problems; the smallest at birth are at greatest risk. Long-term sequelae include retinopathy of prematurity with blindness, hearing loss, hydrocephalus, microcephaly, mental retardation, cerebral palsy (spastic diplegia), chronic pulmonary insufficiency (BPD), short bowel syndrome (post-NEC), and growth failure.

Many infants demonstrate transient neonatal hypotonia, which resolves by 8 mo "corrected age" and is not associated with future problems. However, it is difficult to diagnose cerebral palsy before this age, and all hypotonic infants should be considered at high risk until proved otherwise. Additionally, many VLBW infants have learning disabilities that may result in poor school performance or school failure. Although IQ often relates to adverse events affecting the central nervous system during the neonatal period, the intelligence of premature infants also is influenced directly by poor maternal socioeconomic status.

Most infants with cerebral palsy are not preterm infants or term infants with birth asphyxia. Perinatal causes account for less than 10% of older infants who have severe mental retardation. Furthermore, although 10–25% of VLBW infants demonstrate some handicap, the vast majority of these infants are functional and able to attend regular schools.

References

Behrman RE (ed): Nelson Textbook of Pediatrics. 14th ed. Philadelphia, WB Saunders, 1992, Sec. 9.32, 20.49.

Low JA, Simpson LL, Ramsey DA: The clinical diagnosis of asphyxia responsible for brain damage in the human fetus. Am J Obstet Gynecol 167:11, 1992.

McCormick MC, Brooks-Gunn J, Workman-Daniels K, et al: The health and developmental status of very low-birth-weight children at school age. JAMA 267:2204, 1992.

Resnick MB, Roth J, Ariet M, et al: Educational outcome of neonatal intensive care graduates. Pediatrics 89:373, 1992.

Scottish Low Birthweight Study Group: The Scottish Low Birthweight Study: I. Survival, growth, neuromotor and sensory impairment. Arch Dis Child 67:675, 1992.

Scottish Low Birthweight Study Group: The Scottish Low Birthweight Study: II. Language attainment, cognitive status, and behavioural problems. Arch Dis Child 67a: 682, 1992.

Stanley JF, Watson L: Trends in perinatal mortality and cerebral palsy in Western Australia, 1967 to 1985. BMJ 304: 1658, 1992.

Adolescent Medicine

7

Richard E. Kreipe
Elizabeth R. McAnarney

ADOLESCENT GROWTH AND DEVELOPMENT

Adolescence refers to the passage from childhood to adulthood, whereas puberty refers to those biologic changes that lead to reproductive capacity. The events of puberty occur in a predictable sequence, but the timing of the initiation and the velocity of these changes are highly variable among individuals. The integration of pubertal changes into the adolescent's self-concept is crucial to normal adolescence.

Even "normal" conditions such as acne or dysmenorrhea deserve treatment because the adolescent may perceive them as serious problems. Providers of adolescent health care must be familiar with adolescent growth and development, the specific context in which these changes are occurring, and the manifestations of disease during adolescence.

Physical Growth and Development of Adolescents

FEMALES

Soon after adipose deposition and changes in the bony pelvis widen the contour of the hips, females experience budding of the breasts (thelarche) and the appearance of dark, straight pubic hair over the mons veneris (adrenarche) (Fig. 7–1). These latter two changes, occurring at about 11 yr of age (range 8–13 yr), mark the Tanner II stage of pubertal development. Breast development proceeds to the Tanner V (adult) stage over approximately the next 4 yr, but these changes can occur during a period as short as 18 mo or may take as long as 9 yr. The progression of the growth of pubic hair to the Tanner V (adult) stage takes about 2½ yr on average,

ranging from 1½ to 3½ yr. About 1 yr after the initiation of breast development, during the Tanner III stage, females experience a very rapid increase in their height (Fig. 7–2). The peak of this growth spurt should precede the onset of menstruation (menarche) in normal individuals. Thus, menarche is a relatively late pubertal event, usually occurring approximately 6 mo after the growth spurt, during or just prior to Tanner IV stage of breast development.

MALES

Boys also experience a regular sequence of physical changes during puberty but lack any milestone as obvious as breast development or menarche. Nocturnal emissions (wet dreams) can be considered the male counterpart of menstruation, first appearing during Tanner III stage, but they are not as regular as the menses. From 11 to 13 yr of age, the average boy is shorter than the average girl, so it is often erroneously assumed that boys begin puberty 2 yr later than girls. Boys begin puberty only about 6 mo later than girls. However, the growth spurt is a late event in the male pubertal sequence, in contrast to the relatively early female growth spurt (Fig. 7–3).

Testicular enlargement indicates a transition from Tanner I to Tanner II stage (Fig. 7–4). It begins at about 11½ yr of age (ranging from 9½ to 13½ yr), only a few months later than breast budding in females. Within a year of testicular enlargement, penile enlargement commences, marking the Tanner III stage. This is usually preceded by the appearance of pubic hair at the base of the penis, followed by growth of axillary hair. Completion of testicular growth can occur any time between 13½ and 17 yr of age. Penile lengthening and widening begin normally between 10½ and 14½ yr of age;

PUBERTAL DEVELOPMENT IN SIZE OF FEMALE BREASTS

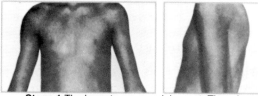

Stage 1 The breasts are preadolescent. There is elevation of the papilla only.

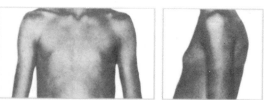

Stage 2 Breast bud stage. A small mound is formed by the elevation of the breast and papilla. The areolar diameter enlarges.

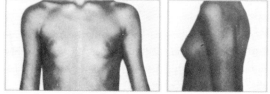

Stage 3 There is further enlargement of breast and areola with no separation of their contours.

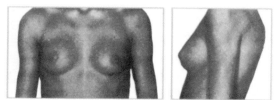

Stage 4 There is a projection of the areola and papilla to form a secondary mound above the level of the breast.

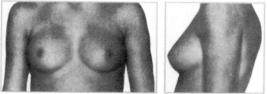
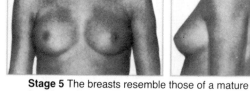

Stage 5 The breasts resemble those of a mature female as the areola has recessed to the general contour of the breast.

PUBERTAL DEVELOPMENT OF FEMALE PUBIC HAIR
Stage 1 There is no pubic hair.

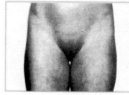
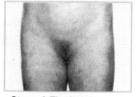
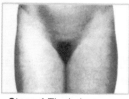
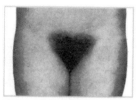

Stage 2 There is sparse growth of long, slightly pigmented, downy hair, straight or only slightly curled, primarily along the labia.

Stage 3 The hair is considerably darker, coarser, and more curled. The hair spreads sparsely over the junction of the pubes.

Stage 4 The hair, now adult in type, covers a smaller area than in the adult and does not extend onto the thighs.

Stage 5 The hair is adult in quantity and type, with extension onto the thighs.

Figure 7–1. Typical progression of female pubertal development. (Adapted from Tanner JM: Growth at Adolescence. 2nd ed. Oxford, Blackwell Scientific Publications, 1962. Reprinted with permission of Ross Laboratories, Columbus, OH 43216, from Assessment of Pubertal Development, © 1986 Ross Laboratories.)

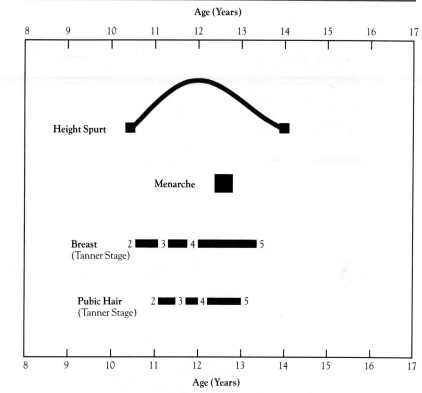

Figure 7–2. Sequence of pubertal events—average American female. (Adapted from Brookman RR, Rauh JL, Morrison JA, et al: The Princeton Maturation Study, 1976, unpublished data for adolescents in Cincinnati, Ohio. Reprinted with permission of Ross Laboratories, Columbus, OH 43216, from Assessment of Pubertal Development, © 1986 Ross Laboratories.)

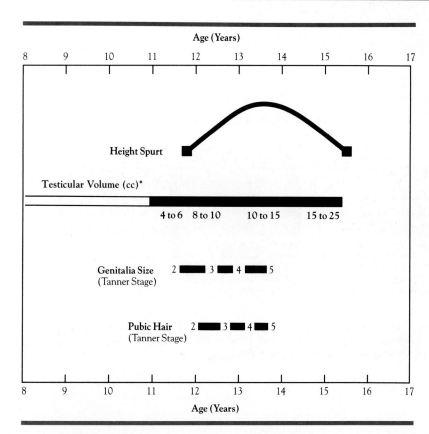

Figure 7–3. Sequence of pubertal events—average American male. *Testicular volume less than 4 cc using orchidometer (Prader Beads) represents prepubertal stage. (Adapted from Brookman RR, Rauh JL, Morrison JA, et al: The Princeton Maturation Study, 1976, unpublished data for adolescents in Cincinnati, Ohio. Reprinted with permission of Ross Laboratories, Columbus, OH 43216, from Assessment of Pubertal Development, © 1986 Ross Laboratories.)

PUBERTAL DEVELOPMENT IN SIZE OF MALE GENITALIA

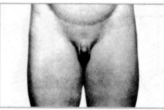

Stage 1 The penis, testes, and scrotum are of childhood size.

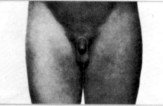

Stage 2 There is enlargement of the scrotum and testes, but the penis usually does not enlarge. The scrotal skin reddens.

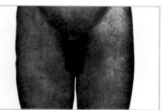

Stage 3 There is further growth of the testes and scotum and enlargement of the penis, mainly in length.

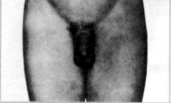

Stage 4 There is still further growth of the testes and scrotum and increased size of the penis, especially in breadth.

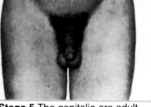

Stage 5 The genitalia are adult in size and shape.

PUBERTAL DEVELOPMENT OF MALE PUBIC HAIR
Stage 1 There is no pubic hair.

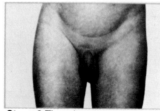

Stage 2 There is sparse growth of long, slightly pigmented, downy hair, straight or only slightly curled, primarily at the base of the penis.

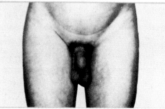

Stage 3 The hair is considerably darker, coarser, and more curled. The hair spreads sparsely over the junction of the pubes.

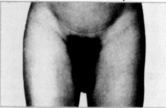

Stage 4 The hair, now adult in type, covers a smaller area than in the adult and does not extend onto the thighs.

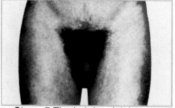

Stage 5 The hair is adult in quantity and type, with extension onto the thighs.

Figure 7–4. Typical progression of male pubertal development. (Adapted from Tanner JM: Growth at Adolescence. 2nd ed. Oxford, Blackwell Scientific Publications, 1962. Reprinted with permission of Ross Laboratories, Columbus, OH 43216, from Assessment of Pubertal Development, © 1986 Ross Laboratories.)

development of the penis reaches the Tanner V stage between 12½ and 16½ yr of age. The growth spurt, as previously noted, is a relatively late event in males but normally is initiated from 10½ to 16 yr of age and is completed by 13½–17½ yr of age, depending on the individual. Growth does continue at a slower pace for several years after the spurt.

REPRODUCTIVE ENDOCRINOLOGY

Puberty is initiated following the release from inhibition of the medial–basal hypothalamic neurons, which secrete gonadotropin-releasing hormone. A release of inhibition by negative feedback from gonadal steroids stimulates the pituitary. Gonadotropin-releasing hormone secretion results in the pulsatile release of luteinizing hormone (LH) and follicle-stimulating hormone (FSH) from the pituitary gland. This occurs initially during sleep and, later in puberty, throughout wakefulness. Pituitary secretion of gonadotropins initiates gonadal growth and maturation. Ovarian estradiol and testicular testosterone affect breast and penis growth,

respectively. Both hormones augment linear growth. Adrenarche (onset of pubic hair development) is mediated by adrenal androgens in females and testosterone in males.

PRECOCIOUS PUBERTY

See Chapter 17.

CHANGES ASSOCIATED WITH PHYSICAL MATURATION

The Tanner stage is a marker of biologic maturity that can be related to both specific laboratory value changes and certain conditions (Tables 7–1 and 7–2). For example, higher hematocrit values in adolescent males than in adolescent females are due to greater androgenic stimulation of the bone marrow, not to loss through menstruation. Alkaline phosphatase levels in both males and females increase during puberty because there is rapid bone turnover, especially during the growth spurt. Worsening of scoliosis is especially common in ad-

Table 7–1. Correlates of Female Pubertal Maturation

	Tanner Stage				
	1	2	3	4	5
Hematocrit (%)					
White *mean*	39.1	39.2	39.6	39.2	39.2
range	36.1–42.1	37.1–41.3	37.0–42.2	36.9–41.6	36.2–42.2
Black *mean*	37.3	38.9	39.0	38.4	38.7
range	34.6–39.9	35.7–42.1	35.2–42.6	34.9–42.8	35.9–41.5
Alkaline phosphatase (IU/L) (serum)					
White *mean*	70	89	76	33	38
range	51–90	49–134	36–108	16–60	23–76
Black *mean*	84	95	86	44	31
range	69–108	65–138	26–148	18–144	13–70
Short female with growth potential		+			
Short female with limited growth potential				+	+ +
Slipped capital femoral epiphysis		+	+ +		
Acute worsening of scoliosis		+	+ + +		
Osgood-Schlatter disease		+	+		
Oral contraceptive prescription				+	+ +
Diaphragm prescription					+
Acute worsening of straight back syndrome		+	+ +	+	
Acute vulgaris		+	+ +	+ +	
Physiologic leukorrhea			+		
Gonococcal vaginitis	+				
Gonococcal cervicitis		+	+	+	+
Regression of virginal breast hypertrophy					+
Timing of breast reduction or rhinoplasty					+

+ = possible; + + = more likely than +; + + + = most likely.
(Data from Copeland KC, Brookman RR, Rauh JL: Assessment of Pubertal Development. Columbus, Ross Laboratories, 1986; and Daniel WA: Growth at adolescence: Clinical correlates. Semin Adolesc Med 1:15–24, 1985.)

Table 7–2. Correlates of Male Pubertal Maturation

	Tanner Stage				
	1	*2*	*3*	*4*	*5*
Hematocrit (%)					
White *mean*	39.5	39.8	40.9	42.3	43.8
range	37.1–41.8	36.7–42.8	38.2–43.5	39.7–44.8	41.1–46.4
Black *mean*	37.7	38.4	39.7	41.1	42.7
range	35.2–40.2	36.0–40.9	37.3–42.0	38.3–43.8	39.6–45.9
Alkaline phosphatase (IU/L) (serum)					
White *mean*	72	77	101	75	58
range	54–110	42–106	53–141	41–158	21–120
Black *mean*	77	94	122	116	75
range	43–130	53–204	46–240	32–228	23–228
Short male with growth potential		+			
Short male with limited growth potential				+	+ +
Slipped capital femoral epiphysis		+	+ +		
Acute worsening of scoliosis		+	+ + +		
Osgood-Schlatter disease		+	+		
Acute worsening of straight back syndrome		+	+ +	+	
Gynecomastia		+	+ +		
Acne vulgaris		+	+ +	+ +	
Orchiopexy timing	+				
Timing of rhinoplasty					+

+ = possible; + + = more likely than +; + + + = most likely.
(Data from Copeland KC, Brookman RR, Rauh JL: Assessment of Pubertal Development. Columbus, Ross Laboratories, 1986; and Daniel WA: Growth at adolescence: Clinical correlates. Semin Adolesc Med 1:15–24, 1985.)

olescent females at the Tanner II and III stages, during the growth spurt.

PSYCHOLOGIC GROWTH AND DEVELOPMENT OF ADOLESCENTS (see Table 7–3)

See Chapter 1.

References

Behrman RE (ed): Nelson Textbook of Pediatrics. 14th ed. Philadelphia, WB Saunders, 1992, Sec. 3.9.
McAnarney ER, Kreipe RE, Orr DP, Comerci GD (ed): Textbook of Adolescent Medicine, Philadelphia, WB Saunders, 1992, Secs. 2 and 3.

ADOLESCENT HEALTH CARE

Overview

Adolescents present many challenges to health care providers because their physical symptoms often are related to psychosocial rather than biologic disorders. Nonetheless, adolescents frequently have chronic medical illnesses (Table 7–4), psychosocial problems, and unique causes of mortality specific for this age group (Table 7–5). Non-compliance with medical regimens is common. Limit-testing in the clinical setting and an adolescent's occasional insistence on confidentiality can threaten therapy. Adolescents and their families usually respond well to health care that is based on respect, with attention to the adolescent's individual developmental needs (see Table 7–3).

Adolescent health care ideally is provided in a setting where the self-conscious adolescent feels comfortable. Sufficient time and privacy should be allowed so that the adolescent and the clinician can discuss adequately sensitive topics such as physical growth and development, medical and psychologic concerns, substance use, sexuality, and personal goals.

THE INTERVIEW

The successful interview of an adolescent resembles a conversation between two persons with a great many interests in common. Developmental principles are applied so that the interview of early adolescents is directed toward specific questions that concrete-thinking adolescents understand. The interview of late adolescents is directed toward open-ended questions that conceptually competent and rationalizing late adolescents understand (see Table 7–3—Thinking).

Table 7–3. Developmental Characteristics Related to Adolescent Health Care Needs

Task	Characteristics	Health Care Needs
10–14 Year Olds		
Puberty	Wide variation in rapid physical changes; self-consciousness	Confidentiality; privacy
Independence	Ambivalence	Support for growing autonomy
Identity	Am I normal? peer group	Reassurance and positive attitude
Thinking	Concrete operational; egocentric; imaginary audience; focus on present	Emphasis on immediate consequences of actions
15–16 Year Olds		
Puberty	Females ahead of males; chronic illness may delay puberty	Emotional support for adolescents who vary from "normal"
Independence	Limit testing; noncompliance; "experimental" behaviors; dating	Consistency; limit-setting
Identity	Who am I?; introspection; global issues	Nonjudgmental acceptance; gentle reality testing
Thinking	Concrete → formal operational; personal fable; experiments with ideas	Problem solving; decision making; education
17–20 Year Olds		
Puberty	Adult appearance; slow change	Minimal needs except in chronic illness
Independence	Ambivalence about real independence, separation/individuation from family	Support
Identity	Who am I with respect to others, sexuality, education, job?	Encouragement of identity allowing maximal growth
Thinking	Formal operational; contemplation of future; introspection; commitments	Approach as adult, but recognize that adolescent still changing

CONFIDENTIALITY

There may be specific issues that adolescents prefer not to have discussed with their parents, but some issues cannot be kept confidential because of their serious adverse health consequences (e.g., suicidal ideation). Thus, it is important that clinicians caring for adolescents follow certain guidelines regarding confidentiality (Table 7–6) and discuss the issue of confidentiality at the onset.

Occasionally, an adolescent insists on absolute confidentiality. The clinician's decision whether or not to enter into this agreement depends on the reason for the request, the adolescent's developmental age, and whether this request is for one or multiple visits. Usually one can see an adolescent once for exploration of a problem, but it is important to make it clear from the outset, particularly for an early adolescent who lives at home, that there may be a need to involve the parents.

LEGAL ISSUES

Each adolescent health care provider should know the laws of the state and the policies of the institution(s) in which the physician practices. The law confers certain rights on adolescents, allowing them to receive health services without parental permission (Table 7–7).

CHAPERONS

It is often stated that a female chaperon should be present during the examination of a female by a male physician. In general, early adolescents may want a parent present, but middle adolescents and late adolescents usually prefer to be seen alone or with a chaperon of the same sex. A choice should be offered if one is available.

Well Adolescent Care

The guidelines of the American Academy of Pediatrics for health supervision should be followed (Table 7–8).

EARLY ADOLESCENCE (10–14 YR OLD)

New guidelines will be forthcoming in the near future from the federal government. Physical

Table 7–4. Prevalence of Common Chronic Illnesses of Children and Adolescents

Illness	Prevalence
Pulmonary	
Asthma	3–5%
Cystic fibrosis	1:2500 white, 1:17,000 black
Neuromuscular	
Cerebral palsy	2:1000
Mental retardation	3%
Seizure disorder	3:1000
Auditory–visual defects	10–30%
Traumatic paralysis	2:1000
Scoliosis	5% males, 10% females
Migraine	10%
Endocrine–Nutrition	
Diabetes mellitus	2:1000
Obesity	10%
Anorexia nervosa	0.5–1%
Bulimia	1% (young adolescence), 5–10% 19–20 yr
Dysmenorrhea	10%
Acne	80%

(Modified from Gortmaker S, Sappenfield W: Chronic childhood disorders; prevalence and impact. Pediatr Clin North Am 31:3, 1984.)

Table 7–5. Leading Causes of Death in Adolescents

Etiology	Comments
Accidents	Automobile, drug-related
Homicide	Drug-related, guns
Suicide	Males successful more often than females
Cancer	Leukemia, lymphoma, Hodgkin disease, bone, central nervous system

Table 7–6. Guidelines for Confidentiality in Adolescent Health Care

Based on principles of adolescent growth and development (see Table 7–3)

Assumes a developing ability of the adolescent to take responsibility for his or her own health care that will culminate in full adult responsibility

Reflects mutual respect and trust between adolescent and health care provider

Extends to both the adolescent and the adolescent's parents (i.e., parental communication also is privileged)

Should be relative, the scope determined by the individual situation

Should be discussed with patient and parent(s) at the outset of adolescent health care

Table 7–7. Legal Rights of Minors

Age of majority (≥ 18 yr of age in most states)

Exceptions in which health care services can be provided to a minor*:
  Emergency care (life-threatening condition, or condition in which a delay in treatment would significantly increase the likelihood of morbidity)

Diagnosis and treatment of sexuality-related health care

Diagnosis and treatment of drug-related health care

Emancipated minors (physically and financially independent of family; Armed Forces; married; childbirth)

Mature minors (able to comprehend the risks and benefits of evaluation and treatment)

All exceptions should be clearly documented in health record

* Determined by individual state laws.

changes and behavior related to the physical changes of puberty are the major characteristics of this substage. The history focuses on an overall appraisal of the early adolescent's physical and psychosocial health.

MIDDLE ADOLESCENCE (15–16 YR OLD)

Independence and a global sense of identity are the major characteristics of this substage. The history focuses on the middle adolescent's interactions with family, school, and peers. High-risk behaviors as a result of experimentation are common.

LATE ADOLESCENCE (17–20 YR OLD)

Individuality and planning for the future are the major characteristics of this substage. The content of the visit is similar to that of the visit with the middle adolescent, but greater emphasis is placed on the late adolescent's responsibility for his or her health. Transfer of health care to a physician who cares for adults and the details of that transfer are discussed during this visit.

Pelvic Examination

An unhurried approach that emphasizes patient comfort helps ensure a successful evaluation. Comfort is maximized by using a padded examination table with stirrups, by keeping the examination room and instruments warm, and by performing the examination soon after the adolescent is ready. Control is afforded by allowing her to choose a su-

Table 7–8. Guidelines for Adolescent Health Supervision Visits of the American Academy of Pediatrics

Early Adolescent (10–14 Yr Old)	Middle Adolescent (15–16 Yr Old)	Late Adolescent (17–20 Yr Old)
Interview with parent(s)		
General questions or concerns	General questions or concerns	Parents generally not interviewed unless specifically indicated
Family stresses and communication	Family stresses and communication	
Schoolwork and friends	Schoolwork and friends	
Mood and attitude	Dating, discipline, and privileges	
Interview with patient		
Health concerns	Health concerns	Health concerns
Eating habits	Eating habits	Eating habits
Sports, hobbies	Sports, hobbies	Sports, hobbies
Adjustment to junior high school	Adjustment to senior high school	Plans after graduation
Friends/dating	Friends/dating	Friends/dating
Home environment	Home environment	Home environment
Sexuality	Sexuality	Sexuality
Tobacco, drugs, alcohol	Tobacco, drugs, alcohol	Alcohol, drugs, tobacco
Feelings: worry, sadness, anger, anxiety	Feelings: worry, sadness, anger, anxiety	Feelings: worry, sadness, anger, anxiety
Chores in home	Work in/outside of home	Work outside of home
Physical examination (patient alone, chaperon may be indicated for younger patients requiring pelvic examination):		
Height/weight plotted on curve	Height/weight plotted on curve	Height/weight
Vision/hearing screening	Vision/hearing screening	Vision/hearing screening
Blood pressure	Blood pressure	Blood pressure
Tanner stage/external genital examination	Tanner stage/external genital examination	Tanner stage/external genital examination
Gynecomastia/breast asymmetry	Gynecomastia	Periodontal health
Scoliosis screen	Scoliosis screen	Skinfold thickness
Skinfold thickness, acne	Skinfold thickness, acne	Sports fitness screening
Self-examination of breast/testes, if mature	Self-examination of breast/testes	Self-examination of breast/testes
Sports fitness screening	Sports fitness screening	Pelvic examination
Pelvic examination if menstrual problem or sexually active	Pelvic examination if menstrual problem or sexually active	
Procedures		
Hematocrit (optional)	Hematocrit (optional)	Hematocrit (optional)
Tuberculin if indicated	Tuberculin if indicated	Tuberculin if indicated
Rubella titer if none previously	Rubella titer if none previously	Rubella titer if none previously
If sexually active, screen for gonorrhea and syphilis (STS/GC), Papanicolaou (PAP) smear	If sexually active, STS/GC screen, PAP smear	STS/GC screen and PAP smear in sexually active females
Human immunodeficiency virus (HIV) screening if at risk	HIV screening if at risk	Cholesterol/triglycerides in high-risk individuals
		HIV screening if at risk
Immunizations		
Check immunization status	Check immunization status	Check immunization status
Mumps, measles vaccine if none previously	Tetanus–diphtheria (Td) booster q 10 years	Td booster q 10 years
Rubella vaccine for nonimmune females if not pregnant	Mumps, measles vaccine if none previously	Mumps, measles vaccine if none previously
Hepatitis B vaccine, if not done previously	Rubella vaccine for nonimmune females if not pregnant	Rubella vaccine for nonimmune females if not pregnant
	Hepatitis B vaccine, if not done previously	Hepatitis B vaccine, if not done previously
Anticipatory guidance		
Health habits (smoking, diet, safety, substance use)	Health habits (smoking, diet, seat belt/helmet use, substance use, sexually transmitted disease/pregnancy prevention)	Health habits (diet, seat belt/helmet use, substance use, sexually transmitted disease/pregnancy prevention)
Social interaction	Social interaction	Social interaction
Academic activities	Academic activities	Plans for the future
Interaction with parents	Interaction with parents/adults	Independent adult life-style
Responsibility as a lifelong function	Responsibility as a lifelong function	Responsibility as a lifelong function

(Modified from American Academy of Pediatrics: Guidelines for Health Supervision II. Elk Grove Village, IL, American Academy of Pediatrics, 1988.)

pine or partially sitting position, by maintaining eye contact with the physician, by being told the importance of the examination, by being informed of all maneuvers before they are performed, by being informed of normal and abnormal findings, and by being encouraged to ask questions before, during, or after the examination.

Inspection of the genitalia includes evaluation of the pubic hair, labia majora and minora, clitoris, urethra, and hymenal ring. Bimanual palpation of the cervix, uterus, fallopian tubes, and ovaries should follow the speculum examination because the lubricant needed to assist insertion of the fingers interferes with samples obtained for microscopic and microbiologic evaluation. A Huffman or Pedersen speculum should be used with young virginal females; a nonvirginal introitus frequently will admit a small- to medium-sized adult speculum. The speculum should be warmed and lubricated with water and inserted gently. Visualization of the vaginal walls and cervical os will allow for the collection of appropriate specimens for Papanicolaou (PAP) smear, culture, Gram stain, and saline wet mount.

References

American Academy of Pediatrics: Guidelines for Health Supervision. II. Elk Grove Village, IL, American Academy of Pediatrics, 1988.

Behrman RE (ed): Nelson Textbook of Pediatrics. 14th ed. Philadelphia, WB Saunders, 1992. Sec. 10.22.

English A: Legal aspects of care. In McAnarney ER, Kreipe RE, Orr DP, Comerci GD (eds): Textbook of Adolescent Medicine. Philadelphia, WB Saunders, 1992, pp 164–171.

Kreipe RE, McAnarney ER: Psychosocial aspects of adolescent medicine. Semin Adolesc Med 1:33–45, 1985.

Hofmann AD: A rational policy toward consent and confidentiality in adolescent health care. J Adolesc Health Care 1:9–17, 1980.

NORMAL VARIANTS OF PUBERTY

Breast Asymmetry

In normal females, one breast may develop before or more rapidly than the other, usually resulting in slight asymmetry of size or Tanner stage. This can still be a source of concern for the early pubertal adolescent. The patient should be reassured that the asymmetry should become less noticeable as maturation progresses. The physical examination reveals no masses or discharge, although tenderness can occur in the breast-bud stage. A true breast mass is most commonly a be-

Table 7–9. Etiology of Breast Masses in Adolescents

Classic or juvenile fibroadenoma (70%)
Abscess
Fibrocystic breast disease
Fat necrosis
Lipoma
Intraductal papilloma
Cystosarcoma phylloides (low-grade malignancy)
Carcinoma (very rare)

nign fibroadenoma or cyst; cancer is exceedingly rare at this age (Table 7–9). Biopsy or surgery is contraindicated for asymmetry, but, together with cyst aspiration, either procedure is indicated for any true breast mass.

Physiologic Leukorrhea

During puberty, endogenous estrogen production stimulates glandular proliferation of the endometrium, often resulting in a vaginal discharge that usually occurs just prior to menarche, in Tanner stage III. The discharge usually is scant (although staining of the underwear is common), thin, mucoid, clear to milky, and neither pruritic nor foul smelling. Characteristics other than these require further evaluation. Physiologic leukorrhea is associated with a few white blood cells and microscopic evidence of the maturational effect of estrogen on the vaginal epithelium. Pathogens are not present in cultures. Physical examination reveals only the changes of midpuberty, without evidence of introital trauma or inflammation. Rubbing due to self-consciousness or masturbation may result in mild erythema, but abrasions or tears should raise concern about sexual abuse. Unless specifically indicated, pelvic examination generally is not necessary.

Irregular Menses

In the year following menarche, the menses often are irregular. Both the interval between periods and the duration of periods may vary as the hypothalamic–pituitary–ovarian system matures. On the average, it takes 18 mo to complete the first 12 menstrual periods. During most of that time, most females are infertile because of anovulation in more than half of the periods. Anovulatory periods often are irregular, with prolonged heavy bleeding but without midcycle or menstrual pain. However, some adolescents ovulate with their first cycle, as indicated by the fact that pregnancy can occur before menarche. The irregularity of early postmenarchal periods can be inconvenient, but treatment with birth control pills should be avoided. Reassurance, education about menstrual physiol-

Table 7–10. Etiology of Gynecomastia

Klinefelter syndrome
Testicular feminization
Hormone-secreting tumors
Hypohyperthyroidism
Cirrhosis
Drugs (amphetamines, cimetidine, digitalis, estrogens, opiates, ketoconazole, spironolactone, tricyclic antidepressants)
Familial gynecomastia

ogy, and awaiting more regular periods usually suffice.

Gynecomastia

Breast enlargement in the male is termed "gynecomastia." It is usually a benign, self-limited condition, noted in 50–60% of boys during early adolescence. Gynecomastia may be associated with Klinefelter or other syndromes and with certain medications (Table 7–10). Typical findings include

Table 7–11. Differential Diagnosis of Primary Amenorrhea

Etiology	History	Breast Development	Female Genitalia	Karyotype	FSH	Prolactin	Thyroid
Hypothalamic							
Physiologic delay	Positive family history of delayed puberty	Delayed	Normal	Normal (46, XX)	Low/normal	Normal	Normal
Nutritional	History of dietary restriction, severe systemic diseases, or malabsorption	Delayed	Normal	Normal	Low/normal	Normal	Normal
Gonadotropin-releasing hormone (GnRH) deficiency	Anosmia (Kallmann syndrome); acquired or congenital anatomic lesions	Delayed	Normal	Normal	Low/normal	Normal	Normal
Pituitary							
Hypopituitarism	Other signs and symptoms of hypopituitarism	Variable	Normal	Normal	Low	Normal	Low/normal
Gonadal							
Chromosomally incompetent ovarian failure	Wide range of phenotypic expression of Turner syndrome	Delayed	Normal	45, XO or mosaic	High	Normal	Normal
Chromosomally competent ovarian failure	May be congenital or acquired	Delayed	Small uterus	Normal	High	Normal	Normal
Uterine							
Congenital absence of uterus (Rokitansky syndrome)	May have associated renal anomalies	Normal	Absent uterus + varying degrees of vaginal dysgenesis	Normal	Normal	Normal	Normal
Vaginal							
Imperforate hymen	May have abdominal pain, pelvic, "mass"	Normal	Bulging hymen	Normal	Normal	Normal	Normal
Biosynthetic/Hormone Defects							
Hypothyroidism	May simulate pituitary tumor	Delayed	Normal	Normal	Low/normal	High	Low
Hyperprolactinemia	May not have galactorrhea	Normal	Normal	Normal	Low/normal	High	Normal
Hypercortisolism	Other signs and symptoms of Cushing syndrome	Normal	Normal	Normal	Low/normal	Normal	Normal
Androgen excess (polycystic ovarian disease)	Hirsutism, virilization	Minimal	Normal	Normal	LH high	Normal	Normal
Androgen resistance (testicular feminization)	Male pseudohermaphroditism	Normal	Absent uterus, shallow vagina, no pubic hair	46,XY	Low/normal	Normal	Normal

the appearance of a 1–3-cm, round, freely mobile, often tender, firm mass immediately beneath the areola during Tanner stage III. Large, hard or fixed enlargements and masses associated with any nipple discharge warrant further investigation. Reassurance that the condition is self-limited is usually the only treatment required. If the condition worsens and is associated with psychologic morbidity, pharmacologic treatment with bromocriptine may be used. Surgical treatment with reduction mammoplasty rarely is indicated.

Short Stature (Constitutionally Delayed Puberty)

See Chapter 17.

References

Beach RK: Breast disorders. In McAnarney ER, Kreipe RE, Orr DP, Comerci GD (eds): Textbook of Adolescent Medicine. Philadelphia, WB Saunders, 1992, pp 720–728.

Behrman RE (ed): Nelson Textbook of Pediatrics. 14th ed. Philadelphia, WB Saunders Co., 1992, Sec. 10.18–10.19.

Braunstein GD: Gynecomastia. N Engl J Med 328: 490–495, 1993.

Copeland KC: Variations in normal sexual development. Pediatr Rev 8:47–55, 1986.

PROBLEMS RELATED TO ADOLESCENT SEXUALITY

Menstrual Disorders

Lack of menstrual periods and irregularity of menstrual periods are among the most common complaints of early adolescents. As regular ovulatory cycles become established, painful menstruation becomes more frequent. Amenorrhea, dys-

Table 7–12. Differential Diagnosis of Secondary Amenorrhea

Etiology	History	Physical Examination	Galactorrhea
Hypothalamic			
Weight loss	Simple dieting; anorexia nervosa	Low weight, blood pressure, pulse, temperature	No
Weight gain	Overeating	Moderate to severe obesity	No
Exercise	Running >25 mi/wk, ballet	Physically healthy if weight normal	No
Stress	Family, school, peer problems	Normal	No
Chronic illness	Severe systemic illness	Signs of chronic illness	No
Idiopathic	Negative	Normal	No
Medication	Phenothiazines; oral contraceptive	No distinctive physical findings	Often
Pituitary			
Destructive lesions	Symptoms of hypopituitarism	Signs of pituitary failure or tumor	No
Gonadal			
Ovarian failure	Radiation, surgery	Signs of estrogen deficiency	No
Polycystic ovarian disease	May have oligomenorrhea	Obesity, hirsutism and virilization	No
Uterine			
Synechiae (Asherman syndrome)	Uterine curettage, endometritis	Normal	No
Hormonal/Metabolic			
Pregnancy	Highly variable, may deny sexual intercourse	Breast engorgement, weight gain	No
Hyperprolactinemia	Medications; may be negative	Usually normal physical examination	Often
Androgen excess	Concerns about virilization	Hirsutism, virilization	No
Hypothyroidism	Symptoms of ↓ thyroid	May be normal	Often
Hypercortisolism	Symptoms of ↑ cortisol	Signs of Cushing syndrome	Often

functional uterine bleeding, and dysmenorrhea constitute the most common menstrual disorders in adolescents.

AMENORRHEA

Primary amenorrhea refers to a lack of menstruation by age 16 yr in the presence of breast development or by age 14 yr in the absence of breast development (most females have menarche within 2 yr of breast development). *Secondary amenorrhea* refers to the cessation of previously regular menstruation for more than 3 consecutive months any time after menarche. Within the first year after menarche such irregularity of menses should be considered physiologic.

Amenorrhea may be due to functional or anatomic abnormalities of the hypothalamus, pituitary, ovary, or uterus, and may result in inadequate

hormonal stimulation of the endometrium, unresponsiveness of the endometrium to hormones, or obstruction to the flow of tissue and blood during endometrial shedding. The differential diagnosis of primary or secondary amenorrhea is broad (Tables 7–11 and 7–12). Physiologic immaturity, stress, exercise, and abnormal dietary patterns are usually the cause of amenorrhea. Secondary amenorrhea often is due to pregnancy.

The history and physical examination (Tables 7–13 and 7–14) provide the most valuable information and should guide the laboratory evaluation of any abnormality of vaginal bleeding, including amenorrhea. Thus, women with short stature and other stigmata of Turner syndrome should have chromosomal analysis, whereas those with signs of hypothyroidism, adrenogenital syndrome, or diabetes should be evaluated with specific tests for these diseases. If the patient with amenorrhea has

Pelvic Examination	Prolactin	Thyroid	Response to Progesterone Challenge	Gonadotropins
Normal	Normal	Normal	Bleeding	Low/normal
Normal	Normal	Normal	Bleeding	Low/normal
Normal	Normal	Normal	Bleeding	Low/normal
Normal	Normal	Normal	Bleeding	Low/normal
Normal	Normal	Normal	Bleeding	Low/normal
Normal	Normal	Normal	Bleeding	Low/normal
Normal	Normal/high	Normal	Bleeding	Low/normal
Normal	Normal/high	Normal/low	No Bleeding	Low
Normal	Normal	Normal	No bleeding	High FSH
Enlarged ovaries	Normal	Normal	Bleeding	High LH
Normal	Normal	Normal	No bleeding	Normal
Enlarged uterus; soft, cyanotic cervix	Normal	Normal	No bleeding	Low/normal
Normal	High	High	Bleeding	Low/normal
Clitoromegaly	Normal	Normal	Bleeding	Low/normal
Normal	Normal/high	Normal/high	Bleeding	Low/normal
Normal	Normal/high	Normal/high	Bleeding	Low/normal

Table 7–13. History and Review of Systems in Abnormal Vaginal Bleeding

History	
Bleeding	How long; how much (number of pads or tampons per day); color (bright red or brown): presence of clots or tissue; cramping; bleeding from other sites (nose, gingiva, after tooth extraction or surgery); relationship to intercourse?
Menstrual	Age of menarche; frequency, duration, amount; last menstrual period (dates of last 3 episodes of bleeding); dysmenorrhea, spotting, mid-cycle pain?
Sexual	Sexual activity; sexual abuse; masturbation with foreign objects; sexually transmitted diseases; pelvic surgery; previous pregnancies, abortions (spontaneous or terminated pregnancies), dyspareunia; sharp pain during intercourse?
Contraceptive use	What kind, how often, any used since last period; missed contraceptive pills?
Medications	All prescription or over-the-counter medications, drug abuse
Illnesses	Recent, chronic, bleeding disorders, cancers?
Family	Bleeding disorders, diethylstilbestrol (DES) exposure, thyroid disease?
Diet	Anorexia, bulimia, crash diets, diet medications?
Exercise	Amount, frequency, competition, kind?
Review of Systems	
General	Fatigue, weight loss, fever, chills, anorexia
Skin	Dry, ecchymosis, petechiae, acne
Hair	Dry, hair loss, brittle, hirsutism
Head/ENT	Visual changes, nosebleeds, gingival bleeding with flossing or brushing
Neck	Swelling or lumps, shoulder pain
Breasts	Soreness, enlargement, galactorrhea
Abdominal	Tenderness, swelling, waistband tight, pain
Genitourinary	Bleeding, dysuria, vaginal discharge, foreign body, trauma, abuse, hematuria, frequency, urgency
Gastrointestinal	Nausea, vomiting, diarrhea, rectal bleeding, mucus, cramps, tenesmus
CNS	Syncope or presyncope, headaches, fatigue
Endocrine	Weight change, nervousness, irritability, change in school performance, heat or cold intolerance

CNS = central nervous system; ENT = ear–nose–throat.
(From Anderson MM, Irwin CE, Snyder DL: Abnormal vaginal bleeding in adolescents. Pediatr Ann 15:697–707, 1986.)

normal secondary sex characteristics but no evidence of androgen excess (e.g., adrenogenital syndrome), pregnancy, or metabolic (e.g., thyroid disease) or uterine (imperforate hymen) pathology, the presence or absence of estrogen effect should be determined.

Superficial vaginal epithelial cells, representing greater than 10% of the cells on PAP smear obtained from the lateral vaginal wall, indicate the presence of estrogen, as does ferning of cervical mucus. Withdrawal bleeding 1–7 days after the injection of 100 mg of progesterone in oil or the administration of medroxyprogesterone, 10 mg PO bid × 5 days, indicates estrogen priming of the endometrium and an intact hypothalamic-pituitary-ovarian axis (positive progesterone challenge). Withdrawal bleeding is reassuring and indicates that regular menses will begin soon. Absence of estrogen effect requires further evaluation and determination of LH/FSH levels. In the absence of estrogen effects, low levels of LH/FSH indicate hypothalamic–pituitary pathology, such as a prolactin-secreting tumor. High gonadotropin levels indicate primary ovarian failure, such as in Turner syndrome (gonadal dysgenesis).

DYSFUNCTIONAL UTERINE BLEEDING

Normal periods are 28 ± 7 days apart, measured from the first day of one to the first day of the next period. Flow is usually not more than 6 days. Excessive flow may be quantified by the use of more than 6 pads or 10 tampons per day for more than 8 days; however, the frequency of pad change varies greatly among women. Excessive bleeding may cause iron-deficiency anemia and, rarely, hypovolemia.

Dysfunctional uterine bleeding, one of the few conditions in adolescent health care diagnosed by exclusion, is any abnormal pattern of endometrial shedding not caused by an underlying pathologic process (Table 7–15). Anovulation occurs in 75% of cases. Without production of progesterone by the corpus luteum, unopposed estrogen production can result in two abnormal patterns of bleeding: mild breakthrough bleeding due to insufficient es-

Table 7–14. Physical Examination in the Evaluation of Abnormal Vaginal Bleeding

General Physical Examination

Growth	Height, weight, obesity, overly thin
Vital signs	Heart rate and blood pressure changes with position, temperature
Skin	Ecchymosis, petechiae, pigmentation, pallor, sweating, capillary refill, striae, acne
Hair	Texture, amount, distribution, hirsutism, balding, low hair line
Eyes	Lid lag, proptosis, funduscopic examination (hemorrhages), visual fields
Nose/throat	Mucous membrane bleeding, petechiae, pallor
Neck	Enlarged thyroid, nodes, web neck
Breasts	Galactorrhea, Tanner stage
Cardiovascular	
Heart	Heart rate, murmurs
Pulses	Presence in extremities
Abdomen	Tenderness, masses, organomegaly, rebound
Rectal	Tone, blood, masses, fissures
Neurologic	Deep tendon reflexes, mental status, cranial nerves, visual fields
Nodes	Generalized lymphadenopathy

Pelvic Examination

External examination	Tanner stage; male vs. female hair pattern; clitoromegaly, discharge, condyloma, lacerations, erythema
Speculum examination	
Vagina	Erythema, punctate hemorrhages, discharge; rotate speculum to look for lacerations, masses, condyloma
Cervix	Color, discharge, punctate hemorrhages, tissue, erosion, friability, condyloma, polyps, abnormal shape
Bimanual examination	Palpate vaginal wall for masses or lacerations; cervical motion tenderness; softening of the cervix or uterocervical junction; adnexal tenderness or masses; size and shape of ovaries; uterine size, shape, and position; uterine tenderness
Laboratory evaluation	Cervical cultures for gonorrhea and *Chlamydia*, cervical smear for Gram stain, vaginal smears for potassium hydroxide (yeast, whiff test), saline (clue cells, *Trichomonas*), vaginal pH, cervical cytology (Papanicolaou [PAP] smear)

(From Anderson MM, Irwin CE, Snyder DL: Abnormal vaginal bleeding in adolescents. Pediatr Ann 15:697–707, 1986.)

trogen levels to support a proliferated endometrium, and heavy, prolonged, sometimes life-threatening menses resulting from lack of sufficient progesterone to stop menstrual flow by myometrial and vascular contractions. Once regular ovulatory cycles have continued for 1 yr, irregular bleeding usually indicates an organic abnormality.

Because dysfunctional uterine bleeding can be diagnosed only after excluding underlying pathology (Table 7–16), one must be cautious in evaluating and treating this condition. A thorough history and physical examination with pelvic examination should be combined with laboratory evaluation that minimally includes testing for pregnancy, gen-

Table 7–15. Definitions of Abnormal Patterns of Menstrual Flow

Pattern	Regularity of Cycles	Interval between Cycles	Flow Amount	Flow Duration	Flow Timing
Amenorrhea	—	—	Absent >3 months	—	—
Hypomenorrhea	Regular	28 ± 7 days	Decreased	Normal	Normal
Menorrhagia (hypermenorrhea)	Regular	28 ± 7 days	Increased	Normal	Normal
Metrorrhagia (spotting)	Irregular	Normal	Decreased	Decreased	Intermenstrual as well as menstrual
Menometrorrhagia	Irregular	Decreased	Increased	Increased	Variable
Oligomenorrhea	Regular	>35 days	Decreased	Decreased	Variable
Polymenorrhea	Regular	<21 days	Decreased	Decreased	Variable

Table 7–16. Differential Diagnosis of Abnormal Uterine Bleeding

Etiology	History	Pelvic Examination	Pregnancy Test	Coagulation Tests	Cervical Cultures
Complications of Pregnancy					
Threatened abortion	Abdominal cramps	Enlarged uterus	Positive	Normal	Negative
Ectopic pregnancy	Abdominal pain; syncope	Enlarged adnexa	Positive	Normal	Negative
Systemic Conditions					
Coagulation defects					
Secondary to liver disease	Chronic or severe acute liver disease	Normal	Negative	Abnormal	Negative
Secondary to blood dyscrasia	Leukemia	Normal	Negative	Thrombocytopenia	Negative
Primary coagulopathy	von Willebrand disease	Normal	Negative	Abnormal bleeding time	Negative
Hypothyroidism	Symptoms of ↓ thyroid; may be normal	Normal	Negative	Normal	Negative
Hyper- or hypocortisolism	Symptoms of ↑ or ↓ cortisol	Normal	Negative	Normal	Negative
Medications					
Birth control pills	Low-dose estrogen; noncompliance	Normal	Negative	Normal	Negative
Aspirin	Aspirin ingestion	Normal	Negative	Abnormal bleeding time	Negative
Pelvic Lesions					
Ovarian cyst	Abdominal pain	Tender, enlarged ovary	Negative	Normal	Negative
Endometriosis	Dysmenorrhea	Tender uterus	Negative	Normal	May be + for STD
Foreign body (IUD, retained tampon)	May have forgotton to remove tampon	Signs of foreign body	Negative	Abnormal if associated with toxic shock syndrome	May be + for *Staphylococcus aureus*
Cervicitis	Sexually transmitted disease (STD) contact	Severe inflammation	Negative	Normal	May be + for STD
Trauma	External genitalia may be normal	Signs of trauma	Negative	Normal	Negative
Diethylstilbesterol (DES) exposure	Maternal DES during pregnancy	Vaginal adenosis	Negative	Normal	Negative
Tumor	Often asymptomatic	Mass	Negative	Normal	Negative
Hypothalamic					
Anovulatory cycles	Symptoms related to anovulation	Normal	Negative	Normal	Negative
Stress	Family, school, peer problems; abnormal body image	Normal	Negative	Normal	Negative

ital infections, and thyroid and coagulation dysfunction and a complete blood count.

Approximately 20% of adolescent menorrhagia is caused by coagulation disorders, with an additional 10% related to other types of pathology. If underlying pathology is discovered, treatment should be directed at the primary disorder as well as at the secondary menstrual dysfunction. Unpredictable, heavy, and prolonged menses may seriously impair an adolescent's ability to attend school and function socially. Thus, the health care provider must attend to these equally important psychosocial dysfunctions and provide appropriate treatment.

Treatment of dysfunctional uterine bleeding is essential if there are heavy menstrual periods. The aim is to normalize the imbalance between estrogen and progesterone. Birth control pills (e.g., Lo-Ovral or Ortho-Novum) are effective and have a rapid onset. In rare patients with uncontrollable bleeding, uterine curettage may be indicated. In the presence of a bleeding disorder (e.g., von Willebrand disease), estrogen may raise the level of factor VIII. Treatment with iron is also important for women with continued excessive blood loss.

DYSMENORRHEA

Dysmenorrhea refers to cramping lower abdominal pains during the first 1–3 days of flow in a menstrual period. Painful uterine cramps are experienced by 65% of adolescent girls and are the leading cause of short-term school absenteeism among female students. Secondary dysmenorrhea is pain due to pelvic pathology (such as endometriosis, intrauterine device use, benign tumors, or anatomic abnormalities). Primary dysmenorrhea is more common and is not associated with a specific underlying structural problem. These two types of dysmenorrhea usually can be distinguished by history and physical examination (including pelvic examination) without the need for surgical or laboratory evaluation.

The treatment of secondary dysmenorrhea is directed at the underlying pathology. Endometriosis, which is becoming increasingly recognized as a common cause of secondary dysmenorrhea, requires treatment with birth control pills or danazol. Primary dysmenorrhea is associated with myome-trial contractions related to local prostaglandin activity in the early phases of shedding of the endometrium. Because prostaglandin production is related to progesterone produced by the corpus luteum after ovulation, painful menstruation is associated with ovulatory cycles. Effective medical therapy is directed primarily at inhibiting the synthesis or action of prostaglandins (Table 7–17). Hormonal regulation with oral contraceptive pills can be tried if these approaches are not beneficial. Failure to respond to these regimens increases the likelihood of unrecognized pelvic pathology.

References

Anderson MM, Irwin CE, Snyder DL: Abnormal vaginal bleeding in adolescents. Pediatr Ann 15:697–707, 1986.
Behrman RE (ed): Nelson Textbook of Pediatrics. 14th ed. Philadelphia, WB Saunders, 1992, Sec. 10.18.
Caufriez A: Menstrual disorders in adolescence: Pathophysiology and treatment. Hormone Res 36:156–159, 1991.
Emans SJH, Goldstein DP: Pediatrics and Adolescent Gynecology. 3rd ed. Boston: Little, Brown and Co, 1990.
Sanfilippo JS: Adolescent gynecologic practice. Pediatr Ann 15:499–541, 1986.

Pregnancy

Approximately 1 million American women less than 20 yr old become pregnant annually. In 1987, there were 472,623 births to women less than 20 yr of age, of which 64% were from nonmarital unions. Approximately 400,000 abortions are performed annually on American women less than 20 yr of age. Adolescent pregnancy is associated with premature birth, increased postneonatal mortality, child abuse, subsequent maternal unemployment,

Table 7–17. Treatment of Primary Dysmenorrhea

Severity	Characteristics	Treatment
Mild	Mild cramps Little interference with daily activities No systemic symptoms	Ibuprofen, 400 mg PO q.i.d. *OR* Naproxen sodium, 550 mg PO, then 275 mg q.i.d. treatment most effective if initiated at least 24 hr before menses begin Aspirin, 650 mg PO q.i.d.
Moderate	Moderate cramps Interference with daily activities No systemic symptoms	Treatment for mild dysmenorrhea, *AND* Cyclic combination oral contraceptive pills
Severe	Severe cramps Restriction of activities for several days each mo Systemic symptoms	Treatment for moderate dysmenorrhea *AND* Re-evaluation for organic pathology, such as benign tumors, endometriosis, or anatomic abnormalities

and poor maternal educational achievement. Most adolescents should not be considered high biologic risks, and in the presence of appropriate prenatal care, good nutrition, and social support and the absence of sexually transmitted diseases, the pregnant adolescent should have the same chance of delivering a healthy full-term infant as do adult women of similar sociodemographic background.

DIAGNOSIS

Adolescent pregnancy most commonly is associated with secondary amenorrhea. Loss of menstrual periods in the adolescent should be presumed to be due to pregnancy until proved otherwise, because adolescent pregnancy is prevalent and because, frequently, the pregnant adolescent delays seeking a diagnosis until several periods have been missed. However, serious consequences may result from a delayed diagnosis. Pregnant early adolescents often are seen with other symptoms, such as vomiting, vague pains, or deteriorating behavior. They may report normal periods. Pregnancy during early adolescence may result from rape or incest, and the patient may deny ever having had intercourse. Because of the varied presentations of adolescent pregnancy, a thorough menstrual history should be obtained in all menstruating females. Sensitive laboratory tests for the beta-subunit of the human placental chorionic gonadotropin allow for diagnosis approximately 7–10 days after conception.

DECISION ABOUT PREGNANCY

If pregnancy is confirmed, dating of the gestation should be done immediately. Most clinicians will not consider abortion after 20–24 wk of gestation. Pregnancy options include continuation of the pregnancy (the patient either keeps the infant or surrenders it for adoption) and termination of the pregnancy. During early adolescence, the clinician should urge the girl to involve the family in the decision, because the adolescent may not be mature enough to make the decision alone.

Continuation of the Pregnancy

Adolescents who desire to carry their pregnancies to term require early, consistent, and comprehensive prenatal care by professionals. Although less than 5% of adolescents who deliver put their babies up for adoption, this is an important option to discuss. Pregnancy is the most common cause of dropping out of school for females. Special attention should be given to keeping the adolescent in school, both during and after pregnancy.

Termination

If the pregnant adolescent chooses to terminate her pregnancy, she should be referred immediately to a setting in which abortion services are rendered. The choice of an abortion procedure depends on the gestational age of the fetus. The procedures include menstrual extraction, suction curettage, and intra-amniotic instillation of hypertonic saline or prostaglandin. In the future "chemical" termination with mifepristone (RU486) in combination with prostaglandin will be available in the United States as a safe and effective form of abortion. Psychosocial support should be available for adolescents who choose abortion.

PREVENTION

An estimated 70% of unmarried 19 yr old women and 80–90% of unmarried young men in the United States have had sexual intercourse. Sexual activity often is initiated without birth control. For those young people who initiate coitus, knowledge about and use of contraception is critical. Because unintended, unwanted pregnancy can be associated with significant psychosocial morbidity for the adolescent mother, the adolescent father, and the child, prevention should be a primary goal. Reliable methods include the following, which are summarized in Table 7–18.

Abstinence

This remains the most commonly used and ideal adolescent birth control method. It is free, 100% effective, and has no side effects. Unfortunately, it requires a degree of self-control, self-assuredness, and self-esteem not found in all adolescents. For those who choose to be sexually active, some form of birth control should be offered, because there is a 70% chance that a regularly sexually active adolescent will become pregnant within a year without birth control.

Birth Control Pills

Birth control pills have the lowest failure rate of any nonsurgical contraceptive method if taken regularly. The combined estrogen–progesterone pill prevents the LH surge, thus inhibiting ovulation. Contraindications are listed in Table 7–18. Following complete history and physical examination, in-

Table 7–18. Birth Control Methods for Adolescents

Method	Advantages	Product	Contraindications	Pregnancy Rate	Side Effects/Problems
Birth Control Pills (BCP)	Used properly, optimum protection ↓ Dysmenorrhea ↓ Risk of fibrocystic breast disease, cystic ovarian disease ↓ Risk of pelvic inflammatory disease ↓ Risk of ovarian, endometrial cancer	Combined BCPs: 30–35 μg of ethinyl estradiol or its equivalent (50 μg of mestranol) and a progestin Mini-pills: progestin only	*Absolute:* Pregnancy Active liver disease with abnormal liver function tests Thrombophlebitis/ thrombotic disease Undiagnosed uterine bleeding Breast, uterine cancer Congenital hyperlipidemia *Relative:* Hypertension Migraine headache Sickle cell disease Active gallbladder disease or mononucleosis	~1/100 women-years	*Common:* Noncompliance Nausea Weight gain Breast tenderness Fluid retention Break-through bleeding Postpill amenorrhea Acne No protection against AIDS *Uncommon, but serious and rare in adolescence:* Thromboembolic phenomena Cardiovascular sequelae (stroke, hypertension)
Homonal injections/implants					
Medroxyprogesterone (Depo-Provera)	Compliance Effective	150 mg IM q 3 months	Breast tumors?	~0.2–0.6/100 women/ year	Menstrual irregularity Amenorrhea IM injection
Levonorgestrel (Norplant)	Compliance Effective	Subcutaneous implants	Obesity	~0.4–0.6/100 women/ year	Menstrual irregularity Amenorrhea Minor surgery to place and to remove
Barrier Methods					
Condoms	Inexpensive, few side effects No prescription needed Male method Protection against sexually transmitted diseases (STDs), including AIDS (especially latex condoms)	Condom (used with vaginal foam or with spermicidal lubricant)	Inability of adolescent to plan ahead and use method effectively	~2–10/100 women-years	Interruption of coitus Proper use Motivation Allergy to rubber in condom Only water-based lubricants
Diaphragm	Safe and effective Cream, jelly available without prescription Protection against STDs Use only when needed	Arcing, coil, flat spring diaphragm fitted by health professional—used with contraceptive cream or jelly	Inability of adolescent to plan ahead and use method properly	~1.9–2.3/100 women-years	Preparation for coitus Proper use and motivation Toxic shock syndrome "Messiness" Recurrent cystitis
Intrauterine device (IUD)	Compliance not necessary Effective	Progesterone- or copper-impregnated device placed by physician in uterine cavity	Multiple sexual partners History of pelvic inflammatory disease or infection Uterine abnormalities Pregnancy	~2/100 women-years	*High incidence of:* Pelvic inflammatory disease among nulliparous women Ectopic pregnancies Extrusion Heavy bleeding

AIDS = acquired immunodeficiency syndrome.
(Data from Greydanus DE, McAnarney ER: Contraception in the adolescent: Current concepts for the pediatrician. Pediatrics 65:1–2, 1980; Med Lett 34:111, 1992; NEJM 328:1543, 1993; and Emans SJH, Goldstein DP, Pediatric and Adolescent Gynecology. 3rd ed. Boston, Little, Brown, & Co, 1990.)

cluding pelvic examination (assuming the adolescent female has regular menses and understands the risks and benefits of utilizing oral contraceptives), she can be started on birth control pills on the first Sunday after her next menstrual period. During the first month of taking birth control pills, an alternative method of birth control should be used. Pills containing 30–35 μg of ethinyl estradiol (or the equivalent) and a progestin in packs of 28 pills are prescribed first.

Common side effects include nausea, breast tenderness, fluid retention, and breakthrough bleeding (especially if pills are missed). Some adolescents discontinue using the pill because they attribute normal weight gain to the contraceptive. It is therefore best to avoid mentioning weight gain as a side effect. If bleeding occurs in the early part of the cycle, it may be necessary to prescribe pills with increased estrogenic activity. If breakthrough bleeding occurs late in the cycle, a pill with more progestational activity can be prescribed. Before any change in pills, however, one should ask "How often do you forget to take your pills?" If the adolescent has forgotten to take the pill for 1 day, two pills may be taken on the subsequent day. If 2 days were missed, two pills may be taken on the 2 subsequent days. If 3 or more days are missed, the adolescent should use another form of birth control for the rest of this cycle and the next cycle while resuming regular pill use.

Emergency postcoital contraception may be effective if given within 72 hr (2–3% failure rate). Treatment consists of 100 μg ethinyl estradiol and 1 mg norgestrel administered twice, 12 hr apart.

Condoms/Foam

When used with spermicidal foam in a conscientious manner, the effectiveness of the condom as a means of birth control can approach that of oral contraceptives. Advantages of this method include availability without a prescription and the prevention of sexually transmitted diseases, particularly human immunodeficiency virus (HIV) infections if latex condoms are used regularly.

Diaphragm

The diaphragm must be appropriately fitted to the individual adolescent female, and spermicidal jelly or cream must be used with each act of intercourse. There are few side effects from the diaphragm, but adequate use requires comfort with manipulating one's own genitalia. For the more mature older adolescent who has sex infrequently, it is often the best method.

Hormonal Injections/Implants

Intramuscular injection of 150 mg of medroxyprogesterone acetate (Depo-Provera) every 3 months is an effective form of birth control now approved for use in adolescents. Subdermal implantation of capsules containing levonorgestrel (Norplant, Capronor) provides effective contraception for adolescents for up to five years or until removed. These forms of pregnancy prevention offer the advantage of not requiring use at each sexual encounter, minimizing problems of non-

compliance. The main side effects are irregular menses, including amenorrhea (see Table 7-18).

Intrauterine Device

The intrauterine device (IUD) is a highly effective but less attractive means of birth control for adolescents because of an increased risk of pelvic inflammatory disease, ectopic pregnancy, and possibly infertility. Its use should be considered only in the older, parous adolescent with one sexual partner and no history of pelvic infection.

Coitus Interruptus

Withdrawal is a common method of adolescent birth control used by sexually active adolescents, but it is ineffective because sperm often are released into the vagina prior to ejaculation or because withdrawal of the penis occurs after ejaculation.

Rhythm Method (Periodic Coital Abstinence)

There are few data supporting the use of the rhythm method in adolescents. Their irregular menses and misunderstanding of the timing of ovulation may not allow optimal use.

References

Behrman RE (ed): Nelson Textbook of Pediatrics. 14th ed. Philadelphia, WB Saunders, 1992, Sec. 10.15–10.16.
Emans SJH, Goldstein DP: Pediatric and Adolescent Gynecology. 3rd ed. Boston, Little and Brown Co, 1990.
Greydanus DE: Contraception. In McAnarney ER, Kreipe RE, Orr DP, Comerci GD (eds): Textbook of Adolescent Medicine. Philadelphia, WB Saunders, 1992, pp 676–688.
Stevens-Simon C, McAnarney ER: Adolescent pregnancy. In McAnarney ER, Kreipe RE, Orr DP, Comerci GD (eds): Textbook of Adolescent Medicine. Philadelphia, WB Saunders, 1992, pp 689–695.

Sexually Transmitted Diseases

Adolescents have one of the highest rates of sexually transmitted diseases (STDs). Compared with adults, sexually active adolescents are less likely to use any contraceptive method, are more likely to come into contact with an infected sexual partner, are less likely to receive health care when they develop an STD, are more likely to believe that they cannot develop an STD, and are less compliant with treatment once an STD is discovered. In addition, there may be biologic factors that make adolescents more susceptible to certain STDs, such as *Chlamydia trachomatis*. STDs are associated with significant psychologic and biologic morbidity. Early diagnosis and treatment are important to prevent medical complications and infertility. Primary prevention of STDs should be a goal for all adolescent health care providers.

DIFFERENTIAL DIAGNOSIS

Numerous pathogens are capable of being transmitted venereally, often asymptomatically. How-ever, there are a limited number of clinical presentations of STD (Tables 7–19 through 7–22). Genital ulcers occur with both syphilis and herpes simplex type 2. Genital warts or pubic lice cause nonulcerative external genital lesions or symptoms that are usually quite distressing to the adolescent. Candidal genital infection usually is not sexually transmitted but can cause severe external genital inflammation. Vaginal discharge can be noted in infection with *Candida albicans*, *Trichomonas vaginalis*, and *Gardnerella vaginalis*. Urethritis in the male and cer-

Table 7–19. Features of Sexually Transmitted Diseases Characterized by Genital Ulcers in Adolescents

	Chancroid	Genital Herpes	Syphilis	Granuloma Inguinale (Donovanosis)
Agent	*Haemophilus ducreyi*	Herpes simplex virus (HSV) 1, 2	*Treponema pallidum*	*Calymmato-bacterium granulomatis*
Incubation (days)	3–10	4–14	10–90	8–80
Systemic Findings	None	Headache, fever, malaise, myalgia in ⅓ of cases	Fever, rash, malaise, anorexia, arthralgia, adenopathy	Local spread only
Inguinal Lymphadenopathy	Early , rapid, tender, and unilateral Suppuration likely	Early, bilateral, tender, no suppuration	Late, bilateral, nontender, no suppuration	Lymphatic obstruction Pseudoadenopathy
Primary Lesion	Papule to pustule	Vesicle	Papule	Papule
Ulcer Characteristics				
Number	<3	Multiple	1 or more	1 or more, may coalesce
Edges	Ragged, undermined	Reddened, ragged	Distinct	Rolled, distinct
Depth	Deep	Shallow	Shallow	Raised
Base	Necrotic	Red, smooth	Red, smooth	Beefy red, clean
Secretion	Pus, blood	Serous	Serous	None
Induration	None	None	Firm	Firm
Pain	Often	Usual	None	None
Diagnosis				
Serology	None	Complement fixation Ab rise only in 1° HSV	VDRL, ART, RPR, FTA-ABS	None
Isolation	Aspirate of node, swab of ulcer on selective medium	Viral culture + in 48 hrs	No in vitro test; rabbit inoculation	None
Microscopic	Gram-negative pleomorphic rods	PAP smear; Tzanck smear; direct FA	Darkfield examination	Staining of ulcer biopsy material for "Donovan" bodies
Treatment (Consider Treating Sexual Partners)	Aspirate fluctuant nodes Avoid incision and drainage Erythromycin 0.5 g PO q.i.d. ×10 days *OR* TMP/SMX, PO b.i.d. double-strength tab ×10 days *OR* Ceftriaxone, 250 mg IM ×1 dose	Acyclovir, 200 mg PO 5× day ×7–10 day Soaks to keep lesions clean and dry; no occlusive ointments Avoid contacting lesions: use handwashing, gloves, condoms	*Early:* Benzathine penicillin G, 2.4 million U, IM ×1 *OR* Tetracycline, 0.5 g PO q.i.d. ×15 days Repeat VDRL *Late:* (>1 yr duration) Benzathine penicillin G, 2.4 million U, IM q7d ×3 *OR* Tetracycline, 0.5 g PO q.i.d. ×30 days Avoid contact with lesions	Tetracycline, 0.5 g PO q.i.d. ×10 days

ART = automated reagin test; FA = fluorescent antibody; FTA-ABS = fluorescent treponemal antibody absorption; RPR = rapid plasma reagin; TMP/SMX = trimethoprim/sulfamethoxazole; VDRL = Venereal Disease Research Laboratory.

(Data from Abramowicz M [ed]: Drugs for sexually transmitted diseases. Med Lett 33:119, 1991; and 1989 STD treatment guidelines, Centers for Disease Control. MMWR 38(Suppl 8): S1–S43, 1989.)

Table 7–20. Features of Sexually Transmitted Diseases Characterized by Nonulcerative External Genital Symptoms in Adolescents

	Genital Warts	Vulvovaginal Candidiasis	Pediculosis Pubis (Crabs)
Agent	Human papillomavirus	*Candida albicans*	*Phthirus pubis*
Incubation (days)	30–90	Uncommon sexual transmission	5–10
Presenting complaints	Genital warts are seen or felt	Vulvar itching, discharge	Pubic itching, lice may be seen; sexual partner has "crabs"
Signs	Firm, gray to pink, single or multiple, fimbriated, painless excrescences on vulva, introitus, vagina, cervix, perineum, anus	Inflammatory of vulva, with thick, white, "cottage cheese" discharge, pH <5 Friable mucosa that easily bleeds	Eggs (nits) at base of pubic hairs, lice may be visible Excoriated, red skin, 2° infection
Clinical associations	Cervical neoplasia	Birth control pills, diabetes, antibiotics can lead to overgrowth	
Diagnosis	Clinical appearance; most infections asymptomatic	KOH: hyphae Gram stain: gram-positive hyphae Nickerson medium for culture	History and clinical appearance
Treatment (may need to treat sexual partner)	Cryotherapy with liquid nitrogen or cryoprobe Topital 10–25% podophyllin to external warts ONLY, washed off after 4 hr, repeated weekly; not used during pregnancy Electrodesiccation, or excision for internal, massive, or unresponsive warts Recombinant human interferon-alpha intralesion therapy	Miconazole or clotrimazole cream via applicator intravaginally, h.s. 3–7 days Lower dose estrogen BCPs, glucose control, d/c systemic antibiotics	1% permethrin creme rinse *OR* 1% gamma-benzene hexachloride shampoo *OR* Pyrethrin/piperonyl shampoo, or lotion May need to repeat

BCP = birth control pills; d/c = discontinue; 2° = secondary.
(Data from Abramowicz M [ed]: Drugs for sexually transmitted diseases. Med Lett 33:119, 1991; and 1989 STD treatment guidelines, Centers for Disease Control. MMWR 38(Suppl 8): S1–S43, 1989.)

vicitis or pelvic inflammatory disease in the female can result from infection with *Neisseria gonorrhoeae*, *C. trachomatis*, or both.

GONORRHEA

This is one of the most commonly reported STDs among adolescents; the most rapid rise in incidence is in the 15–19 yr old age group. The gram-negative diplococcus gains entry via the urethra, the periurethral Skene glands, the labial Bartholin glands, cervix, anus, pharynx, or conjunctiva. Purulent extension to the endometrium, fallopian tubes, and peritoneum is called **pelvic inflammatory disease** (PID), whereas perihepatitis with involvement of the liver capsule in females is termed the **Fitz-Hugh–Curtis syndrome**. In males, the prostate and epididymis also can be affected. Dissemination to the joints, skin, meninges, and endocardium can occur by the hematogenous route. Many patients may be asymptomatic or have only mild symptoms, such as vaginal or urethral discharge.

Several points are important to remember when determining the treatment for an individual patient infected with *N. gonorrhoeae* (Table 7–22). First, no form of penicillin is recommended for uncomplicated urethral, epididymal, endocervical, or rectal gonorrhea. Penicillin has been replaced by cefoxitin or ceftriaxone and doxycycline. Second, pharyngeal and rectal infection without other site involvement can be treated with ceftriaxone without the addition of doxycycline. Third, at least 30% of patients with gonococcal cervicitis, urethritis, proctitis, or epididymitis have a concomitant infection with *C. trachomatis*, which necessitates combined therapy for *C. trachomatis* in these syndromes (Table 7–22). Fourth, doxycycline, which is effective against both these agents, is teratogenic and should not be given to pregnant females but often can be replaced by erythromycin. Fifth, penicillinase-producing *N. gonorrhoeae* that also are resistant to doxycycline and erythromycin are being reported with increased frequency, necessitating alternative treatment. Sixth, the compliance with outpatient treatment for PID is so poor that many authorities recommend treating all adolescent patients as inpatients.

Chlamydia

This is becoming the most frequently diagnosed bacterial STD in adolescents (Tables 7–19 and 7–22). Chlamydia may be a more important pathogen than *N. gonorrhoeae*, accounting for most cases of nongonococcal mucopurulent cervicitis and urethritis; it has an equal if not a greater capability to result in severe sequelae, such as female infertility, PID, and **Reiter syndrome** (conjunctivitis, uveitis, urethritis, buccal ulceration, peripheral arthritis, sacroiliitis, keratoderma blennorrhagia, and HLA-B27). Serovar L1–3 produces lymphogranuloma venereum, whereas serovars B and D–K are associated with genital infections such as mucopurulent cervicitis, urethritis, proctitis, epididymitis, salpingitis, endometritis, and perihepatitis. These latter serovars also cause neonatal conjunctivitis and infantile pneumonia. Diagnosis by either culture, direct immunofluorescent antibody, or enzyme-linked immunoassay or radioimmunoassay is increasingly available. Treatment of milder infections can be done in an ambulatory setting. However, erythromycin frequently causes gastric upset, resulting in noncompliance, and doxycycline is teratogenic. A single oral dose of azithromycin (1g) is also effective therapy for uncomplicated chlamydial genital infections.

Table 7–21. Features of Syndromes with Vaginal Symptoms in Adolescents

	Physiologic Leukorrhea (Normal)	Trichomoniasis	Nonspecific Bacterial Vaginosis (*Gardnerella vaginalis*–associated Vaginitis)
Agent	Normal flora	*Trichomonas vaginalis*	*Gardnerella vaginalis* and anaerobes
Incubation (days)	—	3–28	Not sexually transmitted
Predominant Symptoms			
Itching	None	Mild to moderate	None to mild
Discharge	Minimal	Moderate to severe	Mild to moderate
Pain	None	Mild	Uncommon
Discharge			
Amount	Small	Profuse	Moderate
Color	Clear, milky	Yellow–green or gray	Gray
Consistency	Flocculent	Frothy	Homogeneous
Viscosity	Thin	Thin	Thin
Foul odor	None	None	Yes
Amine odor c̄/KOH	None	Possible	Characteristic fish odor
pH	<4.5	>5.0	>4.5
Vulvar			
Inflammation	None	Common	Uncommon
Vaginal			
Infammation	None	Usual	None to mild
Discharge	Nonadherent	Nonadherent	Adherent
Tenderness	None	Common	Minimal
Cervical	Normal	"Strawberry" hemorrhages	Normal
Bimanual Exam	Normal	Normal	Normal
Microscopic Findings			
Saline drop	Squamous and few white blood cells (WBCs)	Motile flagellates, slightly larger than WBCs, and WBCs	Squamous cells studded with bacteria ("clue cells") and WBCs
Potassium hydroxide	Negative	*Trichomonas* killed	Amine odor
Gram stain	Gram-positive and -negative rods and cocci	*Trichomonas* killed	Predominance of gram-negative rods
Culture	Mixed flora with *Lactobacillus* predominant	No standard culture for *Trichomonas*	Lactobacilli, *Gardnerella vaginalis*, anaerobes Gas chromatography for metabolic products
Treatment	Reassurance	Metronidazole, 2 g PO ×1, if not pregnant Avoid alcohol for 24 hr Treat sexual partner Clotrimazole, 100 mg intravaginal at night ×7 days if pregnant	Metronidazole, 500 mg PO b.i.d. ×7 days if not pregnant *OR* Clindamycin 300 mg PO b.i.d. ×7 days Treat sexual partner only if recurrent

(Data from Abramowicz M [ed]: Drugs for sexually transmitted diseases. Med Lett 33:119, 1991; and 1989 STD treatment guidelines, Centers for Disease Control. MMWR 38 (Suppl 8): S1–S43, 1989.)

Table 7–22. Features of Syndromes Characterized by Mucopurulent Cervicitis, Urethritis, or Pelvic Inflammatory Disease

	Gonorrhea	Chlamydia
Agent	*Neisseria gonorrhoeae*	*Chlamydia trachomatis*
Incubation (days)	3–14	5–12
Possible Presentations	The following possible presentations apply to both gonorrhea and chlamydiosis:	
	Female	*Male Partner*
	Asymptomatic	Asymptomatic
	Urethritis	Urethritis
	Skenitis/bartholinitis	Epididymo-orchitis
	Pelvic inflammatory disease	Proctitis
		Pharyngitis
	Anorectal/pharyngeal	
	Disseminated (arthritis, dermatitis, endocarditis, meningitis)	
Typical Findings in Mucopurulent Cervicitis or Urethritis	Cervical erythema, friability, ectopy, with thick, creamy discharge (penile discharge in males)	Cervical erythema, friability, ectopy, with thick, creamy discharge (penile discharge in males)
	Mucopus >10 polymorphonuclear cells (PMNs) per high power field (hpf)	Mucopus >10 PMNs/hpf
	Gram-negative intracellular diplococci	May coexist with gonorrhea
	Mild cervical tenderness	Mild cervical tenderness
Typical Findings in Pelvic Inflammatory Disease (PID)	Onset day 3–10 of menstrual period	
	Lower abdominal pain (95%)	
	Adnexal tenderness, mass (95%)	
	Pain on cervical motion (95%)	
	Fever (35%)	
	Mucopurulent cervical discharge (variable)	
	Menstrual irregularities (variable)	
	Nausea, vomiting (variable)	
	Weakness, syncope, dizziness (variable)	
	Perihepatitis (5%) (may be seen without PID)	
	Laparoscopy: Definitive diagnosis = salpingitis	
	Pelvic ultrasound: Thickened adnexal structures	
	↑ Sedimentation rate (65%)	
	↑ White blood count (45%)	
Important Differential Diagnoses in PID	Ectopic pregnancy	
	Ovarian cyst (torsion, rupture)	
	Septic abortion	
	Urinary tract infection	
	Appendicitis	
	Mesenteric adenitis	
	Inflammatory bowel disease	
Laboratory Studies	Gram stain in cervicitis: 60% sensitivity, 95% specificity; diagnostic in males	Tissue culture
	Culture-fastidious organism, selective medium	Antigen detection
	Gonozyme, antigen detection	1) Fluorescent antibody
	VDRL for syphilis	2) Enzyme-linked immunoassay
		3) DNA hybridization
Treatment Uncomplicated cervicitis, urethritis	Ceftriaxone, 250 mg IM ×1 or Cefixime, 400 mg PO	Doxycycline 0.1 g PO b.i.d. ×7 days
	PLUS	*OR*
	Doxycycline, 100 mg PO b.i.d. ×7 days	Tetracycline, 0.5 g PO q.i.d. ×7 days
	OR	*OR*
	Tetracycline, 0.5 g PO q.i.d. ×7 days	Erythromycin, 0.5 g PO q.i.d. ×7 days
		OR
		Azithromycin, 1.0 g PO ×1 dose
Pharyngitis/anal (men)	Ceftriaxone 250 mg IM ×1	

Continued

Table 7–22. *(Continued)*

	Gonorrhea	Chlamydia
PID		
Outpatient	Ceftriaxone 250 mg IM ×1 *OR* Cefoxitin 2 g IM ×1 with provenecid 1.0 g PO *PLUS* Doxycycline 0.1 g PO b.i.d. ×10–14 days or tetracycline 0.5 g PO q.i.d. Re-examination within 48 hr and at end of treatment	
Inpatient	Cefoxitin, 2 g IV q.i.d., + doxycycline, 100 mg IV b.i.d., for at least 4 days or until cultures dictate change *FOLLOWED BY* Doxycycline, 100 mg PO b.i.d. ×10 days or tetracycline, 0.5 g PO q.i.d. *OR* Clindamycin, 900 mg IV q8h, plus gentamicin, 2.0 mg/kg IV, then 1.5 mg/kg t.i.d. ×4 days then clindamycin, 450 mg 5 ×1 day PO ×10–14 days total Supportive care Gynecologic consultation Close follow-up as outpatient	
Disseminated gonococcal infection	Ceftriaxone, 1.0 g IV q24h until asymptomatic ×48 hr, then complete 1 wk of therapy with cefuroxime 0.5 g b.i.d. or amoxicillin 0.5 g t.i.d with clavulinic acid Cefoxitin, 1.0 g IV q8h Cefotaxime, 1.0 g IV q8h	

(Data from Abramowicz M [ed]: Drugs for sexually transmitted diseases. Med Lett 33:119, 1991; and 1989 STD treatment guidelines, Centers for Disease Control. MMWR 38(Suppl 8):S_1–S_{43}, 1989.)

Trichomoniasis

Most, but not all, cases of trichomonas infection are sexually transmitted (see Table 7–21). Females have vaginitis and are more likely to be symptomatic than males. A thin, frothy vaginal discharge and cervical "strawberry hemorrhages" are characteristic. Diagnosis is made by visualization of motile, flagellated protozoans in the urine or in a saline wet mount. Single-dose treatment of both sexual partners with 2 g of metronidazole is effective. Trichomoniasis often is associated with other STDs, such as gonorrhea and chlamydia infection.

Nonspecific Bacterial Vaginosis

In postpubertal females who have a thin, gray, foul-smelling vaginal discharge and mild vaginitis, *G. vaginalis* often is found on culture of the discharge (see Table 7–21). In addition to *G. vaginalis*, anaerobic bacteria such as *Bacteroides*, *Mobiluncus*, and *Peptostreptococcus* are important in the pathogenesis. The pH of the discharge is greater than 4.5, and, on microscopic examination, the squamous epithelial cells are studded with rod-shaped organisms (clue cells). With the addition of potassium hydroxide to the discharge, there is a characteristic "fishy" odor because of the release of aromatic amines ("whiff" test). The clinical significance of this nonspecific bacterial vaginosis remains in doubt, but treatment with oral metronidazole, 500 mg twice a day, or oral ampicillin, 500 mg 4 times a day, for 1 wk is usually effective.

Vaginal discharge in prepubertal girls may be due to poor hygiene or irritants, such as bubble bath, deodorants, and detergents used to clean underwear. Nylon or rayon undergarments cause a moist environment to develop that may cause inflammation. Foreign bodies, pinworms, and sexual abuse also should be considered. *N. gonorrhoeae* also may cause vaginitis in the prepubertal female because of the thinner epithelial layer in this age group. When seen in prepubertal girls, gonorrhea almost invariably is due to sexual abuse.

Moniliasis

Genitourinary infection with *C. albicans* usually is not venereally acquired (see Table 7–20). It most commonly occurs after a course of systemic antibiotics that eliminates normal vaginal flora and allows for fungal overgrowth. Additional predisposing variables include obesity, pregnancy, birth control pills, and steroids. Vulvar symptoms of edema, pruritus, and inflammation predominate, but a vaginal discharge resembling cottage cheese characteristically is present as well. Gram stain of the discharge reveals thick, blue hyphae or budding yeast forms. Recurrent candidal infections suggest the possibility of diabetes mellitus. Treatment with miconazole or clotrimazole cream by vaginal applicator for 3–7 nights is effective in most cases.

Herpes

Primary genital *herpes simplex type 2* often is associated with headache, fever, malaise, myalgia, painful genital lesions, regional lymphadenopathy, discharge, and dysuria; some primary and many secondary lesions are asymptomatic (see Table 7–19). The multiple vesicles are red and painful. Secondary (recurrent or reactivation) eruptions are not as dramatic. Viral cultures are positive in 24 hr, but an immediate diagnosis can be made with a Tzanck test showing multinucleated giant cells. The PAP smear also will demonstrate these cells. Latency develops as the virus becomes dormant in the sacral nerve ganglion. In primary herpes simplex infection, viral shedding lasts 10–14 days and ulcer healing occurs in 16–20 days, whereas in recurrent disease virus is present for less than 7 days and the time of healing is 8–10 days. Many patients experience five to eight recurrences per year. Oral acyclovir is effective in reducing the severity and duration of symptoms in primary cases. Local hygiene and sitz baths may relieve some discomfort. Education of patients to use condoms and to avoid having sex with anyone who has genital ulcers can help prevent the spread of this disease.

Genital Warts

Warts can occur on the squamous epithelium or mucous membranes of the genital and perineal structures of both females and males (see Table 7–20). They are usually multiple firm gray to pink excrescences. They can become tender if macerated or secondarily infected. On cornified skin, cryotherapy with liquid nitrogen or cryoprobe is the recommended treatment, or topical 20% podophyllin in benzoin can be applied weekly until the lesions regress. Care should be taken to avoid allowing the tincture to come into contact with any normal skin; thorough washing with soap and water 4–6 hr after each application should be advised. Warts on mucous membranes, that are unresponsive to topical treatment or that occur during pregnancy can be treated with cryosurgery, laser ablation excision, or electrodesiccation, but should not be treated with podophyllin; recurrences after treatment are common. Human papillomavirus infection most commonly is asymptomatic but has been associated with carcinoma of the cervix.

References

Anonymous: Treatment of sexually transmitted diseases. Med Letter 32:5, 1990.

Behrman RE (ed): Nelson Textbook of Pediatrics. 14th ed. Philadephia, WB Saunders, 1992, Sec. 10.17.

Centers for Disease Control: 1989 STD treatment guidelines. Morbid Mortal Weekly Rep Surveill Semin 38(suppl):1–43, 1991.

Hammerschlag MR, Golden NH, Oh MK, et al: Single dose azithromycin for the treatment of genital chlamydial infections in adolescents. J Pediatr 122:961–965, 1993.

Shafer MA: Sexually transmitted disease syndromes. In McAnarney ER, Kreipe RE, Orr DP, Comerci GD (eds): Textbook of Adolescent Medicine. Philadelphia, WB Saunders, 1992, pp 696–710.

Schydlower M, Shafer MA (ed): AIDS and other sexually transmitted diseases. Adolescent Med State Art Rev 1: 409–642, 1990.

Rape

Rape is a legal, not a medical, term for unlawful, nonconsensual intercourse by force; almost one half of victims are adolescents. The attacker is known in 50% of cases. Although gathering historic and physical evidence that may be used in later criminal investigation is important, the physician's primary responsibility to an alleged rape victim is to provide medical examination and treatment in a supportive, nonjudgmental manner. The acute trauma of rape can result in physical injury and/or untoward psychologic responses, ranging from a state of panic to extreme withdrawal. The history is important and should include details of the sexual assault, whether the victim cleansed herself, the last menstrual period, and previous sexual activity, if any.

Specimens from body surfaces, the mouth, vagina, and anus, as well as any photographs taken to document the extent of injuries, should be labeled and handled as evidence in a manner that cannot be called into question in court. Specimens should be taken to identify sperm by microscopy, fluorescence in a Wood lamp, agglutination, and acid phosphatase content of posterior vaginal fornix and other locations. Attempts to identify gonorrhea, chlamydia and trichomonas also are helpful.

In addition to physical trauma, specific immediate medical issues include prevention of pregnancy and prophylaxis for STDs. Pregnancy may occur in 7–10% of victims and can be prevented reliably if treatment is instituted within 72 hr (e.g., 2 Ovral tablets [or the equivalent] at once and again in 12 hr). The risk of STDs is low, and the need for immediate treatment is controversial. Whether treatment is initiated or not, follow-up culture and VDRL and

HIV studies are indicated. The regimen for STDs with the broadest coverage and highest compliance is doxycycline, 100 mg PO twice a day for 7 days. Long-term sequelae are common; patients should be offered immediate and ongoing psychologic support, such as that offered at local rape crisis services.

Toxic Shock Syndrome

See Chapter 10.

SKIN CONDITIONS

Acne

Although it usually is not a serious medical problem, at least 85% of adolescents have some acne; it may have devastating effects on physical appearance, body image, and self-esteem. Effective treatment should be offered to any adolescent with acne, regardless of the extent of involvement, to avoid physical and psychologic scarring.

Many *pathogenic factors* cause acne. Androgenic stimulation of the sebaceous glands leads to an outpouring of lipid-rich sebum that lubricates the hair follicle. The epidermal cells lining the follicle canal obstruct the flow of sebum onto the surface of the skin. The retained material then acts as a medium for the growth of commensal bacteria, such as *Propionibacterium acnes* and coagulase-negative staphylococci. These bacteria produce lipases that hydrolyze the triglycerides contained in sebum, releasing free fatty acids. Inflammation occurs because neutrophils summoned by bacterial chemotactic factors produce hydrolases that disrupt the walls of the pilosebaceous unit. Because the adolescent may apply manual pressure to such lesions, the inflammatory products are released into the dermis rather than onto the surface of the skin. Open comedones are the earliest lesions and are due to dilation of the follicular canal from retained epidermal lining cells (blackheads). A whitehead, or closed comedo, is impaction of debris leading to inflammation and bacterial digestion of lipids, which results in the formation of papules, pustules, nodules, and cysts.

Treatment includes comedolytics (topical benzoyl peroxide, retinoic acid), topical bacteriostatics (benzoyl peroxide, erythromycin, clindamycin, tetracycline), oral bacteriostatics (tetracycline, erythromycin), oral contraceptives, and 13-*cis*-retinoic acid (Accutane). The latter drug causes congenital anomalies and should not be given to pregnant adolescents.

Crabs

Predominantly sexually transmitted, the pubic crab louse *(Phthirus pubis)* lives out its life cycle on pubic hair; therefore, the characteristic intense pruritus, erythematous papules, and egg cases (nits) of "crabs" are not seen before puberty (see Table 7–20). Treatment consists of education regarding personal and environmental hygiene and the application of an appropriate pediculocide, such as permethrin or 1% gamma benzene hexachloride (Kwell).

Jock Itch and Athlete's Foot

See Chapter 10.

EATING DISORDERS

See Chapters 1 and 2.

BEHAVIORAL PROBLEMS

Psychosocial Conditions
NORMAL VERSUS ABNORMAL BEHAVIOR

Normal adolescents may intermittently defy parents, provoke their teachers, and challenge physicians. They may refuse to participate in family events and argue incessantly with siblings. It is sometimes difficult to know whether these behaviors are a part of normal adolescent independence and individuality struggles or are pathologic. Differentiation between normal and abnormal behavior generally can be made by taking into account the degree of interference that a particular behavior produces with regard to schoolwork, family life, activities with friends, or work.

DEPRESSION

Younger depressed adolescents, whose cognitive development usually is concrete operational, may not be able to acknowledge their affective state, but the condition may be indicated by boredom, restlessness, difficulty concentrating or decreasing school performance, preoccupation with somatic complaints (fatigue, vague or localized pains), running away, fights with peers, flight to or from people, and other "acting-out" behaviors. Older adolescents who are formal operational in their thinking may be able to reflect on their feelings of depression and sadness. The mood disturbance in depression includes feeling sad or "blue" for more than 3 hr more than 3 times a week. Other symptoms include early morning awakening or hypersomnia, changes in appetite, loss of sexual interest, psychomotor retardation or fatigue, inability to concentrate, and feelings of excessive guilt, worthlessness, self-reproach, or hopelessness.

Biologic markers, such as an abnormal dexamethasone suppression test, blunted response to thyroid-releasing hormone, blunted growth hormone secretion on provocation, and abnormalities of sleep electroencephalogram, are not yet sufficiently specific to be used as diagnostic tests in adolescents. Antidepressant medication can be useful in adolescents who have a family history of depression or alcoholism (see suicide, under Violent Behaviors, below).

VIOLENT BEHAVIORS

Violence is a major and increasing health problem among contemporary adolescents. In 1987, the overall death rate for 10–14 yr olds was 26.9/100,000 and for 15–19 yr olds was 84.6/100,000. Accidents are the leading cause, followed by suicide and homicide. Homicide is a particular problem among urban black males.

Prevention of violent and destructive adolescent behavior is an important goal. Identifying high-risk antecedents of depression, attention deficit disorder, impulse control problems, risk-taking behavior, and substance abuse prior to accidents, homicides, or suicides is critical for prevention.

Accidents, particularly motor vehicle accidents, often result from risk-taking by adolescents; judgment impaired by alcohol or by drugs is frequently a contributing factor. Efforts have been made in several states to mandate seat belt use and to raise the drinking age to 21 yr. Data indicate a decrease in deaths from motor vehicle accidents following the use of such measures. Education programs do not appear to be as effective in changing behavior as legislation, but physicians should educate their young adolescent patients about the hazards of drinking, driving, or both.

Homicide is disturbingly common among young people of lower socioeconomic status living in crowded urban areas. A possible response to this situation may be to institute, at the local and national level, a combination of social programs providing perpetrators, potential perpetrators, and would-be victims with alternatives to violent behavior and destructive modes of thinking and relating to others. Gun control may lower the disturbing and premature deaths of young black males.

Suicide is the second leading cause of death among adolescents 15–24 yr of age in the United States. Suicide and attempted suicide may result from despair over the breakup with a boyfriend or girlfriend, grief over the death of a loved one, and a chronic depression. Data suggest that adolescents are more likely to try to harm themselves after viewing programs depicting suicide or after friends or classmates commit suicide, resulting in so-called "cluster suicides." Other risk factors include poor impulse control, psychosis, family history of suicide, or risk-taking by the adolescent. Attempts outnumber successful suicides by a ratio of at least 100:1, with females accounting for over 80% of attempts. Males outnumber females in successful suicide, however, because they are more likely to use violent means, such as guns or hanging, rather than poisoning.

References

Behrman RE (ed): Nelson Textbook of Pediatrics. 14th ed. Philadelphia, WB Saunders, 1992, Sec. 3.33–3.39, 10.1–10.3, 10.20.

Friedman SB, Sarles RM: "Out of control" behavior in adolescents. Pediatr Clin North Am 27:97–107, 1980.

Gourash L, Puig-Antich J: Medical and biologic aspects of adolescent depression. Semin Adolesc Med 2:299–310, 1986.

Hodgman CH, McAnarney ER: Adolescent depression and suicide: Rising problems. Hosp Pract 27:73–96, 1992.

Weiner IB: Normality during adolescence. In McAnarney ER, Kreipe RE, Orr DP, Comerci GD (eds): Textbook of Adolescent Medicine. Philadelphia, WB Saunders, 1992, pp 86–90.

Substance Abuse

With changing social norms and the wide availability of many psychoactive compounds, substance use and abuse are significant health problems of adolescents. This requires physicians to be aware of current problems in adolescent substance use and abuse in their own communities.

Exploratory drug use may be seen as part of normal psychosocial development for the contemporary adolescent. Many adolescents abandon or lessen their drug use as they develop into adults. However, it is hazardous to adopt an "everybody's doing it" attitude, especially with the more vulnerable younger adolescent, for several reasons (Table 7–23). The use of drugs is often purposive, goal directed, and psychologically adaptive. For example, drug use may allow the adolescent to attain independence from parental control and regula-

Table 7–23. Classification of Substance Use by Adolescents

Nonuse	Abstinence from psychoactive or addictive substances for personal, family, or religious reasons
Experimental use	Infrequent, episodic use of various drugs during contact with peers that does not interfere with activities at home, in school, or at work
Recreational use	Episodic use of tobacco, alcohol, or marijuana during social encounters with peers, intended to make one feel accepted or at ease
Circumstantial use	Repeated substance use because of a learned association between its use and decreased anxiety or stress, with drugs serving as a coping tool; depending on stressors, such use can quickly lead to physical or psychologic dependency
Habitual use	Substance(s) use involves most, if not all, areas of life, with the adolescent being psychologically and socially addicted; because everything in the adolescent's life revolves around obtaining and using substance(s), drug use becomes its own reward
Compulsive use	Physiologic addiction to substance(s) so that the adolescent is unable to help himself or herself stop using the drug; because habituation underlies such use, it is best treated in a conscientiously prescribed program of abstinence, change of friends, change of school, and change of all other patterns that were associated with the substance(s) use

(From Obermeier G, Henry P: Inpatient treatment of adolescent alcohol and polydrug abuses. Semin Adolesc Med 1:293–301, 1985.)

tion; to express opposition to social norms; to cope with anxiety, frustration, and depression; or to gain admission to a peer group. The adolescent may fail to develop healthy ways of dealing with these problems if drugs are used as a ready solution.

Furthermore, the use of substances by young people is linked systematically to a larger constellation of problem behaviors that are also considered inappropriate by society, such as prostitution and stealing. Compared with nonusing peers, adolescents who abuse drugs have lower grades, higher truancy rates, and fewer plans to attend college; they work less, have less of a religious commitment, have more radical political views, spend less time at home, and spend more time dating.

Finally, the average age at which young people first use substances is declining, and younger age at first use is correlated with a higher likelihood of continued use and abuse. In this context, alcohol and tobacco are often "gateway drugs." By providing a positive experience to a 7th grader, the experimental use of alcohol or tobacco can lead to experimentation with other psychoactive substances for which the risk of psychologic or physical addiction is great.

EPIDEMIOLOGY

Approximately two thirds of teenagers in the United States try some form of illicit drug before finishing high school; almost all have tried alcohol, and 40% have used some illicit drug other than marijuana. About 5% of high school seniors smoke cigarettes daily, drink alcohol daily, or both. In addition, there is an alarming increase in the use of nonprescription diet pills among females and cocaine and its derivatives among males and females. The clinician must determine the epidemiology of substance use for the individual adolescent as part of routine health care or whenever the adolescent is seen for any problem.

CLINICAL MANIFESTATIONS

Important factors in the history include types, frequency, timing, setting, circumstances, and outcomes of substance use. Although alcohol use may be considered statistically normative, adolescent alcohol abuse is characterized by consumption of large amounts over a short time, often to the point of intoxication. Even though an adolescent may drink "only" with friends at weekend parties, he or she can still be the victim of a fatal motor vehicle accident while driving home intoxicated after a party.

There are few physical findings associated with most chronic adolescent substance use, except in cases of intoxication or overdose (Tables 7–24 and 7–25). However, this does not mean that the commonly used substances are harmless. In the late 1970s, cocaine snorting and smokeless tobacco dipping became popular "recreational" activities among some adolescents, behaviors often modeled after those of some sports and rock music heroes. Devastating reports of sudden death from the cocaine derivative "crack" and oral cancers from snuff are now reported.

Table 7–24. Immediate Effects, Duration of Action, Toxicity, and Withdrawal Symptoms of Substance Abuse in Adolescents

Substance	Immediate Effects	Duration of Action	Toxicity	Signs and Symptoms of Withdrawal	Treatment of Overdose
Alcohol	Respiratory depression, central nervous system (CNS) depression, ataxia, slurred speech	Depends on amount ingested and adolescent's tolerance	Cirrhosis, gastrointestinal hemorrhage, thiamine and folate deficiency, CNS depression, impaired motor performance and mental function, stupor, deep anesthesia, death	Insomnia, restlessness, anxiety, tremulousness, hypertension, tachycardia, diaphoresis; auditory or visual hallucinations or both, seizures, delirium tremens are rare in adolescents	Supportive ventilation if needed
Amphetamine, other stimulants	↑ blood pressure (BP), activity, and alertness; tachycardia; insomnia, anorexia; ↓ fatigue; euphoria; excitation; aggression; hostility	2–8 hr	Agitation; ↑ heart rate, BP, and temperature; hallucinations; paranoia, psychosis; convulsions; death, arrhythmias	Apathy, hallucinations, irritability, excessive sleep, depression, psychosis, suicidal, sudden death	Paranoia with haloperidol; seizures with diazepam
Tobacco	↑ BP and heart rate; ↓ temperature, CNS stimulation, skeletal muscle relaxation	Minutes	CNS stimulation	Restlessness, anxiety, insomnia, agitation, nausea, headache, ↑ appetite, inability to concentrate	None
Cocaine, crack	↑ alertness, exultation, euphoria, insomnia; ↓ appetite; ↑ BP and heart rate, aphrodisiac, local anesthesia	15–30 min	Agitation; ↑ temperature, pulse, and BP; tremors; convulsions; tachyarrhythmias; paranoia, psychosis; myocardial infaction; death	Apathy, long periods of sleep, irritability, depression, suicidal, disorientation	Paranoia with haloperidol; seizures with diazepam; cooling for hyperthermia; nitroprusside, labetalol for hypertension
Inhalants (solvents, gasoline)	Respiratory depression, CNS depression, ataxia, slurred speech, bradycardia	5–30 min	Arrhythmias, hallucinations, seizures, encephalopathy, renal tubular acidosis, peripheral neuropathy, lead poisoning, death	Rare: chills, hallucinations, headache, abdominal pain, muscle cramps, delirium tremens	See Chapter 3
LSD, other hallucinogens	Dysphoria; hallucinations; anxiety; paranoia; psychosis; ↑ BP, heart rate, and temperature; dilated pupils; incoordination; ↑ creativity	2–12 hr; can produce exhaustion lasting for days	Long, intense "trips"; psychotic reactions not always reversible; flashbacks; suicide attempts; deaths with some drugs	None	Reassurance; haloperidol
Marijuana, hashish	Euphoria, ↓ reaction time, ↓ inhibitions, ↑ appetite	2–4 hr	Dysphoria, acute anxiety attacks, acute psychosis, fatigue, paranoia, lack of motivation	Insomnia, hyperactivity, ↓ appetite	
PCP and PCP analogues	Ataxia, nystagmus, ↑ BP, slurred speech, dysphoria, hallucinations, paranoia, confusion	Hours to days	Psychosis; convulsions, paranoia; flashbacks; deaths have resulted from suicide, accidents	None	Haloperidol, diazepam
Opioids	Euphoria, ataxia, slurred speech, miosis, stupor	Hours	Respiratory depression, hypothermia, hypotension, pulmonary edema, apnea, coma, death	Increased sympathetic nervous system activity, hunger, antisocial behavior, gooseflesh, diaphoresis, rhinorrhea (flu), yawning; treatment with clonidine	Naloxone; ventilation

LSD = lysergic acid diethylamide; PCP = phencyclidine.
(Data from Jones RL: Substance abuse. *In* Shearin RB [ed]: Handbook of Adolescent Medicine. Kalamazoo, MI, Upjohn Company, 1983, pp 133–152; and Abramowicz M [ed]: Treatment of acute drug abuse reactions. Med Lett 29:83, 1987.)

Table 7–25. Long-Term Effects, Tolerance, Dependence, Adulteration, and Methods of Administration of Substances Adolescents Abuse

Substance	Long-Term Effects	Tolerance	Dependence Psychologic	Dependence Physical	Adulteration or Substitution	Method of Administration
Alcohol	Blackouts; behavioral changes; ↑ accidents; homicide, suicide; gastritis; peptic ulcer; alcoholic hepatitis; fatty liver; pancreatitis	Yes	Yes	Yes	Methanol	Ingested
Amphetamine, other stimulants	Weight loss, insomnia, anxiety, paranoia, hallucinations; skin abscesses and amphetamine psychosis following injections	Yes	High	Yes	More than 90% of speed is adulterated with caffeine, asthma medications, PCP, LSD, strychnine, sugars	Ingested, injected
Tobacco	↑ risk of chronic bronchitis, heart disease, and cancer (oral cancer with smokeless tobacco)	Yes	Yes	Yes	No	Smoke inhaled, snuff dipping, chewed
Cocaine, crack	Nasal perforation with snorting, weight loss, insomnia, anxiety, paranoia, hallucinations, soft tissue abscesses with injections	Yes	High	Yes, especially following smoking or injection	Local anesthetics, sugars, PCP	Snorted, smoked, ingested, injected
Inhalants (solvents, gasoline, "white out," etc)	Liver damage with toluene, trichloroethylene, gasoline; anemia with tetraethyl lead; leukemia with benzene; kidney damage with trichloroethylene	Yes, especially with toluene	Yes	Yes	None	Sniffing rags soaked with the compound, inhaling fumes through the mouth
LSD, other hallucinogens	Flashbacks, pronounced personality changes, ↑ risk of chronic psychosis	Yes, cross-tolerance with mescaline, DMT, and psilocybin	Degree unknown	No	Sold as tablets, in liquids, in microdots in many colors; often adulterated with or substituted for other drugs	Ingested, injected, sniffed
Marijuana, hashish	Great variety involving several body systems; ↓ motivation	Yes	Degree unknown	No	With PCP	Smoke inhaled, ingested
PCP and PCP analogues	Personality disorders, flashbacks, catatonia, neuropsychologic disturbances, increased risk of schizophrenia	Yes	High	Degree unknown	Often added to other drugs or advertised as other drugs	Ingested, injected, smoked
Opioids	↓ motivation, antisocial behavior, crime to support habit, skin abscess, endocarditis, osteomyelitis, nephritis, hepatitis, HIV, amenorrhea	Yes	Yes	Yes	Quinine, sugar	Ingested, injected, subcutaneous (skin-popping), intravenous

LSD = lysergic acid diethylamide; PCP = phencyclidine.
(Modified from Jones RLK: Substance abuse. *In* Shearin RB [ed]: Handbook of Adolescent Medicine. Kalamazoo, MI, Upjohn Company, 1983, pp 133–152.)

Acute Overdose

Many drugs (most commonly alcohol, amphetamine, opiates, and cocaine) can result in a toxicologic emergency, which occurs most often the first time an adolescent uses a substance, sometimes being unaware of its nature; such an initial reaction makes identification of the offending agent difficult. Initial management should be directed at appropriate supportive medical treatment, with follow-up counseling after the toxic effects have diminished (Table 7–25).

Acute Illness

Heavy alcohol use can cause both acute gastritis and acute pancreatitis. Intravenous drug use can result in right-sided bacterial endocarditis, vertebral or sternoclavicular osteomyelitis, septic pulmonary embolism, hepatitis B infection, or acquired immunodeficiency syndrome. Chronic marijuana or tobacco use is associated with bronchoconstriction and bronchitis.

Chronic Use

Compulsive drug or alcohol use results in the adolescent's being unable to help himself or herself out of drug dependency and the psychosocial sequelae that attend such habituation (stealing, prostitution, drug dealing, unemployment, school failure, and social isolation).

TREATMENT

Specific management of substance use by adolescents depends on many individual patient factors. However, because of the highly addictive (physical or psychologic) nature of most substances, residential drug treatment facilities are becoming increasingly utilized, especially for younger adolescents.

References

Behrman RE (ed): Nelson Textbook of Pediatrics. 14th ed. Philadelphia, WB Saunders, 1992. Sec. 10.4–10.12.
Graham CJ: Emergency care of the substance-abusing adolescent. Adolescent Med: State Art Rev 4:167–180, 1993.

Functional (Psychosomatic) Disorders

Symptoms of pain or loss of function for which no physical cause is found are common during adolescence. Although the evidence for biologic disorders should be sought simultaneously with evidence for psychologic disorders, we must realize that our knowledge regarding the relationship between these two domains remains primitive. It is important that the adolescent not be led to believe that the physician, in finding no evidence of disease, judges the symptoms to be feigned or imaginary ("all in your head"). In such a situation, psychologic factors may indeed play a role, but rarely does the physician have the adolescent's trust and confidence required for the treatment to be effective. Even if the physician and adolescent can agree that psychologic factors are operating, this does not guarantee that there is not some organic pathology underlying the symptoms. Thus, rather than labeling symptoms for which no organic cause can be determined "psychosomatic," it is preferable to categorize them as "functional" (Table 7–26), which avoids the connotation that the symptoms are psychologic (they are somatic) and allows the difficulty to be recast in terms of disordered bodily functioning (rather than in terms of the imagination), triggered by previously unappreciated stressors.

A problem of increasing concern is the chronic fatigue syndrome. During adolescence it is often a postviral phenomenon, but its etiology is undetermined.

References

Behrman RE (ed): Nelson Textbook of Pediatrics. 14th ed. Philadelphia, WB Saunders, 1992, Sec. 3.24, 3.32.
Buchwald D, Smith MS: Chronic fatigue. In McAnarney ER, Kreipe RE, Orr DP, Comerci GD (eds): Textbook of Adolescent Medicine, Philadelphia, WB Saunders, 1992, pp 879–885.
Prazar G: Conversion reactions in adolescents. Pediatr Rev 8:279–286, 1987.

School Problems

School problems often indicate underlying psychologic or environmental difficulties. Common school problems include school phobia, truancy, and underachievement.

SCHOOL PHOBIA

Adolescents who avoid or refuse to go to school may have histories of separation anxiety and multiple vague somatic complaints, such as headaches, abdominal pain, and fatigue. They often have been seen by numerous specialists and undergo elaborate medical evaluations. Their absence from

Table 7–26. Features of Functional Disorders of Adolescents

Psychophysiologic Disorder
Presenting complaint is a physical symptom
Physical symptom caused by a known physiologic mechanism
Physical symptom is stress-induced
Patient may recognize association between symptom and stress
Symptom responds to medication, biofeedback, and stress reduction

Conversion Reaction (see also Chapter 1)
Presenting complaint is physical (loss of function, pain, or both)
Physical symptom not caused by a known physiologic mechanism
Physical symptom related to unconscious idea, fantasy, or conflict
Patient does not recognize association between symptom and the unconscious
Symptom responds slowly to resolution of unconscious factors

Somatization Disorder
Presenting complaint is >13 physical symptoms in females, >11 in males
Physical symptoms not caused by known physiologic or pathologic mechanism
Physical symptoms related to need to maintain the sick role
Patient convinced that symptoms unrelated to psychologic factors
Symptoms tend to either persist or change character despite treatment

Hypochondriasis
Presenting complaint is a physical sign or symptom
Physical sign or symptom is normal
Physical symptom is interpreted by patient to indicate disease
Conviction regarding illness may be related to depression or anxiety
Symptom does not respond to reassurance; medication directed at underlying psychologic problems often helpful

Malingering
Presenting complaint is a physical symptom
Physical symptom is under voluntary control
Physical symptom is used to gain reward (money, avoid military service, etc.)
Patient consciously recognizes symptom as factitious
Symptom may not lessen once reward is attained (need to retain reward)

Factitious Disorder (e.g., Munchausen syndrome)
Presenting complaint is symptom complex mimicking known syndrome
Symptom complex is under voluntary control
Symptom complex is used to attain medical treatment (including surgery)
Patient consciously recognizes symptom complex as factitious, but is often very psychologically disturbed so that unconscious factors also are operating
Symptom complex often results in multiple diagnoses and multiple operations

school often is mistaken as a consequence of their symptoms. In reality, the expression of their symptoms is a means of avoiding school and gaining the attention of a parent. These adolescents may have either a valid or an irrational concern about a parent and thus refuse to leave home, or they may have had an unpleasant experience in school. Rarely do they have a true phobia related to schoolwork. When challenged with the prospect of returning to school, these young people often become extremely anxious and incapacitated with escalating symptoms. School phobia that first becomes manifest during adolescence may be an expression of severe underlying psychopathology. If there is no medical contraindication for the young person to return to school and if he or she refuses to return, psychiatric consultation is indicated.

TRUANCY

Truancy is absenteeism from school without permission. It is often peer initiated. Truancy is more common in adolescents from lower socioeconomic status and low educational backgrounds. The truant adolescent leaves home ostensibly to attend school but either does not go to school or, once having arrived at school, leaves early. A review of the young person's curriculum for appropriateness and formal education testing are indicated, because truancy is often a sign of borderline intellectual abilities or learning disability. Young people who are truant often drop out of school when they become 16 yr of age.

ACADEMIC FAILURE

This is common during adolescence and often is a reflection of increasing demands of high school work and inability of adolescents to keep up with these demands for any number of reasons. Causes of academic failure should be sought. An initial history, physical examination, and laboratory evaluation by the pediatrician may define physical causes, such as visual or hearing impairment or neurologic dysfunction, or previously undiagnosed chronic illness, such as anemia. A careful behavioral assessment may identify undiagnosed depression. School records should be sought to compare academic capability measured by intelligence quotient (IQ) tests, teacher observations of the student's ability, and the student's actual performance reflected in school grades. Formal educational and psychologic evaluation may be indicated if there is not sufficient information in the school records to identify the cause of academic failure. Intervention involves developing a concerted plan to remedy the situation. The adolescent, the parents, the pediatrician, and the school authorities should participate in this planning.

References

Behrman RE (ed): Nelson Textbook of Pediatrics. 14th ed. Philadelphia, WB Saunders, 1992, Sec. 3.31–3.32, 3.39, 3.5.

Koplewicz HS, Gallagher R: School-related anxiety and related conditions. In McAnarney ER, Kreipe RE, Orr DP, Comerci GD (eds): Textbook of Adolescent Medicine. Philadelphia, WB Saunders, 1992, pp 994–1002.

Nader PR, Bullock D, Caldwell B: School phobia. Pediatr Clin North Am 22:605–617, 1975.

Sahler OJZ: The teenager with failing grades. Pediatr Rev 4:293–300, 1983.

SERIOUS PSYCHIATRIC ILLNESS

Psychoses related to drug ingestion, schizophrenia, or manic–depressive illness or as isolated episodes of decompensation during emotional stress often first occur during adolescence. It is unusual for an adult with psychosis to have had an uneventful adolescence. If there is any question about the possibility of psychosis, or impending psychosis, early psychiatric evaluation is indicated.

Schizophrenia generally presents before adulthood. It is characterized by loosening of associative thought patterns, inappropriate affect, ambivalent emotional state, and gradual but marked withdrawal from family, school, and peers. Perceptual disturbances are frequent. Health care providers frequently see adolescents in the early stage of their schizophrenic decompensation because of behavioral or somatic symptoms.

Manic–depressive psychosis often is mislabeled as schizophrenia during adolescence. The distinct periods of elevated, expansive, or irritable moods associated with hyperactivity and distractibility may alternate rapidly with periods of severe depression lasting for several days or weeks. The family history usually is positive for mental illness.

Acute confusional states can be related to numerous panic inducers, including drugs. The hallucinogens (most notably lysergic acid diethylamide [LSD] and phencyclidine [PCP]), amphetamines, and marijuana all have been associated with an acute toxic psychosis marked by confusion, disorientation, anxiety, agitation, and disturbances of perception, judgment, or reason. Major tranquiliz-

ers and a quiet, safe, nonthreatening environment are helpful in such cases (see Table 7–24).

References

Behrman RE (ed): Nelson Textbook of Pediatrics. 14th ed. Philadelphia, WB Saunders, 1992, Sec. 3.45–3.48.

McAnarney ER, Kreipe RE, Orr DP, Comerci GD (eds): Textbook of Adolescent Medicine. Philadelphia, WB Saunders, 1992, Sec. 24.

MISCELLANEOUS CONDITIONS

Runaway Behavior

Nearly 1 million young people run away from their families of origin during adolescence. Running away from home may indicate environmental stress, including abuse (over two thirds of female runaways report sexual abuse), or it may indicate intrapsychic problems of the adolescent. Psychologic evaluation of the adolescent includes seeking evidence for depression, characterologic personality disturbance, or a combination of these conditions. Runaway youths are at particularly high risk of being used by adults for illicit activities, such as drug-related crimes or prostitution. Hotlines are available for runaway youths to seek help.

Abuse

Abuse of adolescents may include physical, verbal, or sexual abuse. Adults often believe that adolescents are unlikely to be abused, because they have developed the capacity to ask for outside help or to leave the family to seek care. However, adolescents may be reluctant to report the abusive situation, because they may want to protect the abusing parent or may be too embarrassed to seek help. Evidence of physical abuse, including unexplained bruises and cuts, should be considered as evidence of abuse as in younger children. Sexual abuse and/or exploitation, either in incestuous relationships or for prostitution, may become evident when adolescents, particularly early adolescents, become pregnant. If a pregnant adolescent is unable to identify the father of the baby openly to the clinician, one should suspect either incest or prostitution.

References

Behrman RE (ed): Nelson Textbook of Pediatrics. 14th ed. Philadelphia, WB Saunders, 1992, Sec. 3.51–3.53, 5.5.

Daniel WA (ed): Adolescence II—psychosocial aspects. Pediatr Ann 15:759–814, 1986.

Immunology and Allergy

8

John W. Yunginger

THE IMMUNE SYSTEM

The immune system consists of all lymphatic tissue plus phagocytes, T and B lymphocytes, immunoglobulins, and the complement system. Together with physical barriers, such as the skin and motile cilia of the respiratory mucosa, the primary function of the immune system is the protection of the host against infection and malignancy. The pathologic costs of this protection are allergy, autoimmunity, and rejection of organ transplants.

Genetics

Genes of the major histocompatibility complex (MHC) encode cell-surface molecules that are strong transplantation antigens (i.e., they elicit a strong immunologic response in a recipient of a transplanted organ when the donor antigens differ from those of the recipient). Genes of the MHC also control immunologic responsiveness to foreign antigens; these genes are known as immune response (Ir) genes. In humans the MHC is termed human leukocyte antigen (HLA) and is located on the short arm of chromosome 6. The HLA-A, HLA-B, and HLA-C loci encode for Class I molecules that are expressed on all nucleated cells. The HLA-DP, HLA-DQ, and HLA-DR loci encode for Class II molecules that are expressed on macrophages, Langerhans cells, dendritic cells, B lymphocytes, and some activated T lymphocytes.

Cells

The cells of the immune system arise from totipotent stem cells in the fetal liver and bone marrow. Phagocytes include tissue macrophages, circulating monocytes, and polymorphonuclear leukocytes. Lymphoid stem cells differentiate into two major lines: T cells (which mature in the thymus gland between 8 and 12 wk gestation) and B cells (which mature in the bone marrow between 12 and 16 wk gestation). During maturation, both T and B cells acquire cell membrane molecules known as

cluster of differentiation (CD) antigens that are recognized by monoclonal antibodies. During maturation in the thymus, T cells acquire antigen receptors composed of two polypeptide chains (alpha and beta). T cells also acquire either CD8 or CD4 surface molecules that enable mature T cells to react with antigen combined with either Class I or Class II histocompatibility molecules, respectively. The thymus also monitors and destroys potentially damaging T cell clones. B cell receptors also are acquired during B cell differentiation. Mature T and B cells migrate to the spleen and peripheral lymph nodes; some lymphocytes continue to circulate through the lymphatic channels and vascular system.

Serum Proteins

Immunoglobulin (Ig) production for all classes is possible by the 20th wk of gestation. Most fetal IgG is transferred actively across the placenta after the 32nd wk of gestation. The complement system is composed of at least 25 distinct plasma proteins capable of interacting with each other, with antibody, and with cell membranes. Complement proteins comprise 10–15% of the plasma globulin fraction and normally circulate as inactive molecules.

Immune Response Events

Foreign antigens usually are ingested and partially digested by macrophages, then presented, along with Class I or Class II histocompatibility molecules located on the macrophage surface, to surface receptors on B or T cells. Occupation of the receptor site initiates a complex series of biochemical events that culminates in the activation and proliferation of a clone of antigen-reactive cells. This process may be amplified by the complement system or by soluble cytokines such as interleukins, interferons, and tumor necrosis factor.

Antibody-Mediated Immunity

When antigen combines with the B cell antigen receptor, the B cell differentiates into a plasma cell

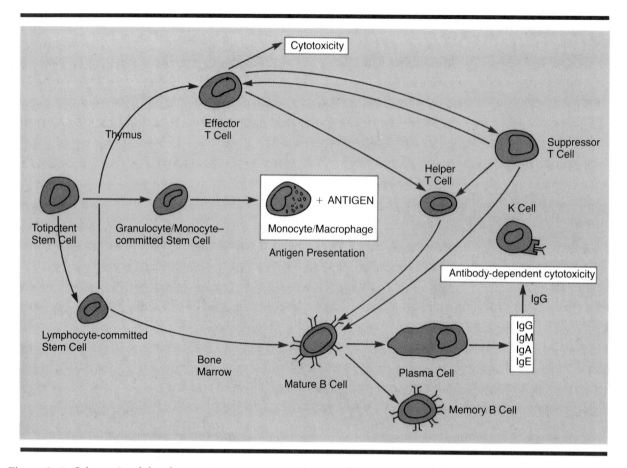

Figure 8–1. Schematic of development, response to antigen, and interactions of the cells involved in cell-mediated and antibody-dependent immunity.

clone that secretes identical antibody molecules of the IgG, IgA, IgM, IgD, or IgE isotype. A few plasma cells revert to long-lived lymphocytes that retain the capacity to increase antibody secretion on subsequent antigen exposure (Fig. 8–1). In fetal life and infancy, the initial antibody response is primarily of the IgM class, followed by a progression to IgG and then to IgA synthesis. This progression is reflected by the sequential acquisition of adult levels of IgM by 1 yr of age, of IgG at 5–7 yr of age, and of IgA at 10–14 yr of age.

IgM comprises 10% of all immunoglobulins and is confined to the intravascular pool. IgM forms rapidly following primary antigenic stimulation, binds complement efficiently, and assists the reticuloendothelial system in clearing circulating bacteria by opsonization and agglutination.

IgG is 70–75% of the total immunoglobulin pool and is the major antibody of secondary (rechal-

lenge) immune responses. It is distributed between the intra- and extravascular pools. IgG is the major antibody against bacteria, virus, and fungi and is considered the memory antibody because it persists after antigenic stimulation. IgG includes four subclasses (IgG1, IgG2, IgG3, and IgG4). Different subclasses respond preferentially to various antigens (e.g., polysaccharide antigens induce a preferential but not exclusive IgG2 subclass response). IgG4 cannot fix complement.

IgA constitutes 15–20% of the immunoglobulin pool and is the major protective antibody in saliva, lacrimal fluid, and colostrum. IgA is present in nasal, bronchial, and intestinal secretions and provides local immunity. It may also act to prevent systemic access of foreign proteins. Secretory IgA is distinguished from serum IgA by the presence of a component (called secretory piece) and by a short polypeptide J chain.

IgD accounts for less than 1% of the immunoglobulin pool and serves as an antigen receptor or receptor site on circulating B cells.

IgE is present in serum in very small amounts but is the principal mediator of immediate hypersensitivity reactions. It may play a role in parasite immunity. IgE is found on the surfaces of mast cells and basophils, and allergic individuals generally have high serum levels of this immunoglobulin.

Cell-Mediated Immunity

T lymphocytes comprise 65–80% of circulating small lymphocytes. Many of these T cells serve as "memory" cells, capable of enlisting the effector machinery of cell-mediated immunity when a familiar antigen is encountered. Subpopulations of T cells include helper cells, required for production of antigen-specific IgG and IgA, and suppressor cells to modulate ongoing immune responses. Subpopulations of T cells have been identified by specific cell surface antigen markers detected with monoclonal antibodies. All mature T cells have surface glycoproteins termed CD3 and CD2. CD8 positive (+) T cells react with antigens combined with Class I molecules, whereas CD4+ T cells react with antigens combined with Class II molecules. It was thought that all helper cells were CD4+ and that all suppressor/cytotoxic cells were CD8+, but these functions are now known not to be exclusively associated with these surface markers. Approximately 70% of circulating T cells are CD4+ and 30% of circulating T cells are CD8+.

Cell-mediated cytotoxicity is an important T cell function, producing lysis of target cells. Three cell types have roles in cytotoxicity. *Killer (K) cells* lyse cells that are coated with antibody in a process termed antibody-dependent cell-mediated cytotoxicity. *Natural killer (NK) cells* destroy target cells without antibody or prior antigenic stimulation. Both K and NK cells are called null cells because they lack T and B cell surface markers. *Cytotoxic T cells* respond to antigenic stimulation by lysing target cells without damaging nearby cells.

T lymphocytes are important in controlling fungal, viral, and protozoan infections. They are the cell type involved in contact dermatitis, allograft rejection, and graft-versus-host disease. Helper and suppressor T cells influence the regulation of antibody synthesis.

Complement

The complement system is composed of the two parallel but independent pathways (the classic and the alternative or properdin) that lead to the activation of factors resulting in the generation of various biologic activities, such as phagocytosis and antibody-dependent and -independent cell lysis (Fig. 8–2). Complement components have numbers in the classic pathway and letters in the alternative pathway. The third component of complement, C3, is most abundant and is the pivotal factor linking both pathways. Once C3 is activated, the remainder of the components are activated in a standard cascade. The endpoint is lysis of the target cell by a complex consisting of C5b,6,7,8,9. The classic pathway may be activated by antigen-antibody complexes (IgG and IgM complexes) and, nonimmunologically, by C-reactive protein and trypsin-like enzymes. The alternative pathway may be activated by C3b generated through classic complement activation and, nonimmunologically, by lipopolysaccharides, fungal substances, or bacterial polysaccharide (endotoxin).

The complement system performs several functions, including the lysis of target cells, such as enveloped viruses and gram-negative bacteria, the processing and clearance of immune complexes. the modification of opsonization and phagocytosis, and the recruitment and activation of immunologically active cells to sites of inflammation. The cleavage fragments of complement proteins have important functions, such as opsonization (C3b), mediator release from mast cells and leukocytes (C3a, C4a, C5a), neutralization of viruses (C1,4, C1,4,2,3), and chemotaxis of neutrophils, monocytes, and eosinophils (C5a). Complement also plays a role in resistance to *Neisseria* infections (C5, C6, C7, C8).

Phagocytic System

The phagocytic system is composed of monocytes and polymorphonuclear granulocytes. Blood monocytes represent the circulating pool and migrate into tissue to become *macrophages.* Macrophages are present in the liver, kidneys, lungs, spleen, brain, and lymph nodes and form a network called the reticuloendothelial system. Monocytes and macrophages have surface receptors for the Fc portion of IgG and for complement (C3b), which are important for adherence and phagocytosis of micro-organisms. Opsonization is the process that prepares bacteria for phagocytosis. Opsonins, such as IgG and complement, bind bacteria to phagocytes by membrane receptors on the monocytes. Monocytes contain several intracellular acid hydrolases and peroxidases that are important in the intracellular killing of microorganisms. Macro-

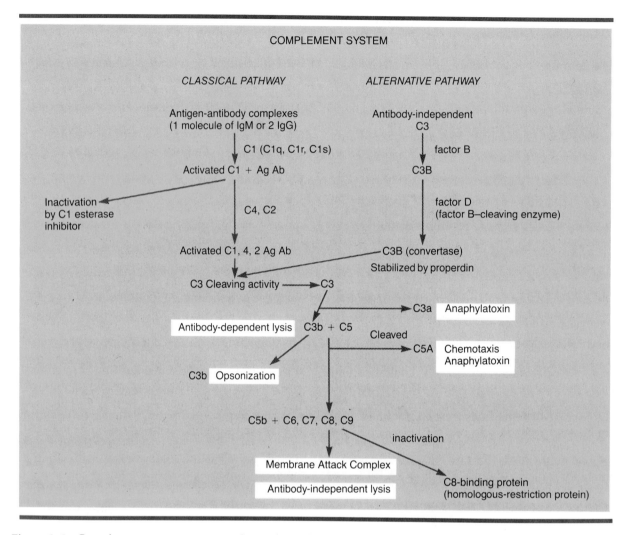

Figure 8–2. Complement component cascade involving the classical and the alternate, or properdin, pathways. The initiating events for both pathways differ but result in production of C3 cleaving enzyme activity, which is the pivotal step as the two pathways converge to the terminal activation sequences. Ag Ab = antigen–antibody complex.

phage function also can be enhanced by cytokines released from T lymphocytes and other cells, which can affect migration, chemotaxis, and bactericidal activity.

Macrophages function as antigen-presenting cells and as inflammatory, tumoricidal, and microbicidal cells in the effector limb of the inflammatory response. The function of both monocytes/macrophages and polymorphonuclear granulocytes can be enhanced by cytokines from T and B lymphocytes.

Polymorphonuclear granulocytes are classified as neutrophils, basophils, and eosinophils on the basis of staining reactions of their granules. Neutrophils represent over 90% of the circulating granulocytes and, like the monocyte/macrophage, have receptors for C3b and the Fc portion of the immunoglobulin molecule, which enhance phagocytosis if the bacteria are prepared for engulfment by opsonins (IgG, C3b). Ingested organisms are destroyed by both aerobic and anaerobic bactericidal systems.

Eosinophils comprise between 2% and 5% of blood leukocytes, and, although capable of phagocytizing and killing ingested micro-organisms, they do so less efficiently than neutrophils. Eosinophils may play a role in the immunity against parasitic infections by this mechanism; eosinophil proteins, major basic protein (MBP), eosinophil cationic protein (ECP), and eosinophil peroxidase (EPO) are in the granules and cause direct damage to parasites.

Eosinophils also may be capable of releasing these cellular materials that can adversely affect normal tissues in humans.

Basophils comprise 0.5–2% of circulating blood leukocytes and have a significant role in immediate-type hypersensitivity. Under appropriate stimulation when antigen crosslinks with surface-bound IgE, mediators of immediate-type hypersensitivity are released, including histamine, leukotrienes, and various chemotactic factors, all of which are responsible for the clinical manifestations of allergic disease.

References

Behrman RE (ed): Nelson Textbook of Pediatrics. 14th ed. Philadelphia, WB Saunders, 1992, Sec. 11.1–11.3.
Lockey RF, Bukantz SC: Fundamentals of Immunology and Allergy. Philadelphia, WB Saunders, 1987, p. 7.

IMMUNODEFICIENCY DISORDERS

The immunodeficiency disorders are a diverse group of conditions that share the common characteristic of an increased susceptibility of the host to infection. Primary immunodeficiencies are classified based on the location of the immune defect: B cell, T cell, phagocytic, and complement. Each system may act independently or together with one or more of the other immune systems. Immunodeficiencies may be congenital (e.g., X-linked agammaglobulinemia), acquired (e.g., common variable immunodeficiency acquired immunodeficiency syndrome [AIDS]), secondary to an embryologic abnormality (e.g., DiGeorge syndrome), or idiopathic.

Secondary immunodeficiencies result from non-immunologic diseases (prematurity, malnutrition, Hodgkin disease), injury (burns, splenectomy), or therapy (steroids, radiation, anticancer). The immunodeficiency may be permanent or transient, resolving with adequate treatment of the primary disease.

Clinical Manifestations

Primary immunodeficiency is uncommon; therefore, other conditions with increased susceptibility to infection should be considered first. These conditions include foreign bodies (e.g., central venous catheters, aspirated foreign bodies), obstructive disorders (e.g., eustachian tube dysfunction, cystic fibrosis), congenital cardiac defects, and unusual microbiologic factors (e.g., antibiotic-resistant organisms). Symptoms of allergic disease often are confused with those of immunodeficiency disorders and, in certain instances, may predispose the patient to infection in the upper respiratory tract. Symptoms of immunodeficiency relate to the degree of deficiency and the affected immune component. Certain characteristic clinical features are suggestive of specific immune abnormalities (Table 8–1). A family history of early infant death and

Table 8–1. Clinical Characteristics of Primary Immunodeficiencies

B Cell Defects
Recurrent pyogenic infections with extracellular encapsulated organisms, such as pneumococcus, *Haemophilus influenzae*, and streptococci
Otitis, sinusitis, recurrent pneumonia, bronchiectasis, conjunctivitis
Few problems with fungal or viral infections (except enterovirus encephalitis and poliomyelitis)
Decreased levels of immunoglobulins in serum and secretions
Diarrhea common, especially secondary to infection with *Giardia lamblia*
Growth retardation not striking
Compatible with survival to adulthood or for several years after onset unless complications occur

T Cell Defects
Recurrent infections with less virulent or opportunistic organisms such as fungi, mycobacteria, viruses, and protozoa
Growth retardation, malabsorption, diarrhea, and failure to thrive are common
Anergy
Susceptible to graft-versus-host reactions if given unirradiated blood
Fatal reactions may occur from live virus or BCG vaccination
High incidence of malignancy
Rarely survive beyond infancy or childhood

Phagocytic Defects
Recurrent dermatologic infections with bacteria and fungi, such as *Staphylococcus, Pseudomonas, Escherichia coli*, and *Aspergillus*
Subcutaneous, lymph node, lung and liver abscesses
Pulmonary infections common, including abscess and pneumatocele formation, contributing to chronic disease
Bone and joint infection common

Complement Defects
Recurrent bacterial infections with extracellular pyogenic organisms, such as pneumococcus, *H. influenzae*
Unusual susceptibility to recurrent *gonococcal* and *meningococcal* infections
Increased incidence of autoimmune disease (SLE)
Severe or recurrent skin and respiratory tract infection

BCG = bacillus Calmette-Guerin; SLE = systemic lupus erythematosus.

severe infection often is present because many primary immunodeficiency syndromes are inherited.

The *physical examination* of a child with immune deficiency may reveal a chronically ill, pale, and irritable child. Muscle and adipose tissue mass may be reduced and lymph node or tonsil size reduced or these organs absent. Eczema may be present in Wiskott-Aldrich syndrome; in hyperimmunoglobulin E syndrome; and in polymorphonuclear, B cell, and other immune defects. Seborrheic dermatitis may be seen in C5 deficiency (Leiner disease), AIDS, and combined immunodeficiency syndrome. Chronic mucocutaneous candidiasis (T cell defects), subcutaneous abscesses (leukocyte defects, hyperimmunoglobulin E), and draining ears (B and T cell defects) may be noted. Petechiae occur in the Wiskott-Aldrich syndrome, whereas telangiectasia is present in the ataxia–telangiectasia syndrome. Hypocalcemic tetany, mandibular hypoplasia, and congenital heart disease (aortic arch or conotruncal anomalies) may be noted in DiGeorge syndrome. Dental caries may occur in patients with B cell defects, whereas hepatomegaly often is noted in patients with chronic granulomatous disease (neutrophil defect). Congenital bone abnormalities are observed in adenosine deaminase (ADA) deficiency and cartilage–hair hypoplasia syndrome, whereas chronic osteomyelitis is noted with neutrophil defects.

B Cell Defects

The B cell disorders are due to abnormalities in the maturation of stem cells into plasma cells, which synthesize and secrete immunoglobulins. Abnormalities may be related to intrinsic defects in the B cell subpopulation or to regulatory defects in T cell subpopulations that lead to abnormalities in immune regulation (Fig. 8–1). Defects of antibody production may involve all antibody classes, selective antibody classes, selective deficiency of IgG subclasses, or an inability to respond to a specific antigen. Deficiencies of antibody production may be classified as congenital, late onset, transient, and secondary.

Congenital defects produce problems in the latter half of the 1st year of life when passively acquired immunoglobulins from the mother decline to their lowest level. The loss of transplacental immunoglobulin (IgG) also coincides with increased exposure to pathogens. The severity of symptoms depends on the degree of antibody deficiency. Major immunologic features of congenital (X-linked) agammaglobulinemia include absence of lymph nodes and B cells in peripheral blood, and serum concentrations of IgG, IgA, and IgM that usually are less than 200 mg/dL.

Late-onset or *common variable immunoglobulin deficiency* is similar to X-linked hypogammaglobulinemia, except that symptoms usually appear later in life. It is a heterogeneous group of disorders, with defects at different stages of B cell maturation in different individuals. B cells usually are normal in number, whereas total immunoglobulin levels usually are less than 300 mg/dL, with IgG usually less than 250 mg/dL. IgM and IgA may be present in significant amounts or may be absent. An increased incidence of autoimmune disease and a familial pattern have been noted.

Transient hypogammaglobulinemia of infancy is a temporary condition characterized by delayed immunoglobulin production of unknown cause coupled with the normal physiologic decline in immunoglobulin concentrations observed in the first 3–7 mo of life. B and T cells are present in these patients, and antibodies can be synthesized to antigens, such as diphtheria and tetanus toxoids. Immunoglobulin levels increase to normal age-appropriate levels, usually between 18 and 36 mo of age.

Secondary hypogammaglobulinemia may result from loss of immunoglobulins or lymphocytes into the gastrointestinal tract (e.g., protein-losing enteropathy) or the urinary tract (e.g., nephrotic syndrome). The abnormality will resolve if the primary disorder responsible for the condition is corrected.

Selective IgA deficiency is defined as serum IgA levels of less than 5 mg/dL accompanied by normal or increased levels of other immunoglobulins. It is the most common antibody deficiency, with a reported incidence of 1:700 to 1:328. Patients with this disorder may be asymptomatic but may have recurrent sinopulmonary infections, *Giardia* infection, and autoimmune disease.

Selective IgM deficiency also occurs, as does a rare and poorly understood *immunodeficiency with hyperIgM.* Immunodeficiency also may occur in *Epstein-Barr virus associated familial lymphoproliferative disease* (Duncan disease).

Selective deficiency of each of the four IgG subclasses has been described when total serum IgG levels were either normal or decreased. Depending on the subclass affected and levels present, some patients respond with normal antibody production following antigenic stimulation and others do not. These disorders are similar to other antibody deficiencies and cause recurrent pyogenic sinopulmonary infections.

T Cell Defects

Isolated T cell defects are rare, and, in most patients, defective T cell immunity is associated with defective B cell immunity, reflecting the interactions between T and B cells (see Fig. 8–1). Children with congenital abnormalities of cellular immunity are seen in early childhood with viral or fungal infections. Symptoms usually are more severe in patients with T cell abnormalities than in patients with B cell defects. The DiGeorge anomaly involves an embryologic developmental field defect that usually, but not always, affects the thymus and parathyroid glands. Affected infants may exhibit neonatal hypocalcemic tetany, conotruncal and aortic arch anomalies, micrognathia, and cellular immunodeficiency. A variable degree of thymic and parathyroid hypoplasia is due to poor development of the third and fourth pharyngeal pouches. The lymphocyte count is below 1200 cells/mm³ and T cells are markedly diminished. Episodes of recurrent infections, chronic candidiasis, and failure to thrive occur if these infants survive past the newborn period. Severely affected patients resemble patients with severe combined immunodeficiency disorder (see later).

Chronic mucocutaneous candidiasis is primarily a T cell disease characterized by localized chronic candidal infections of the skin, mucous membranes, and nails of the hands and feet. Endocrinopathies involving the parathyroid, thyroid, adrenal, and pancreatic glands occur in some patients; associated autoantibodies may be present. The cellular immune defect is limited to Candida, and immunity to other pathogens usually is normal.

Combined Defects

Severe combined immunodeficiency disease (SCID) is characterized by a profound lack of T and B cell function, although varying numbers of B and T cells may be present. Symptoms usually occur within the first few months of life, and failure to thrive is a striking feature. Clinical findings associated with poor T cell function predominate, although a variety of severe bacterial infections may occur. Chronic candidiasis, protozoan infections such as *Pneumocystis carinii*, low-grade opportunistic organisms, intractable diarrhea, and recurrent respiratory infections are common. Patients exhibit eczema, seborrhea, alopecia, neutropenia, anemia, thrombocytosis, and monocytosis. These patients also are susceptible to graft-versus-host disease if given fresh blood or immunocompetent foreign tissue. Two forms of inheritance have been distinguished in patients with SCID: autosomal recessive

and X-linked recessive. Combined defects also occur in *Nezelof syndrome* (cellular immunodeficiency with abnormal immunoglobulin synthesis), Duncan disease, and ADA and nucleoside phosphorylase (NP) deficiencies. The latter two are nonimmunologic diseases that cause immunodeficiency because metabolic products accumulated as a result of the inability to catabolize purines have a toxic effect on lymphocytes. ADA deficiency presents with severe diarrhea, pneumonia, and failure to thrive in the neonatal period; abnormalities of the ribs and scapulae may be seen on roentgenographs. NP deficiency presents later in childhood and may be associated with megaloblastic anemia, pure red cell aplasia, or spastic tetraparesis.

PARTIAL COMBINED DEFECTS

Several disorders have a combination of T cell and B cell defects but are less severe than those in SCID. The *Wiskott-Aldrich syndrome* is an X-linked disorder characterized by eczema, thrombocytopenia (small platelets), and susceptibility to infection. IgA and IgE are increased, IgM is decreased, and IgG is normal. There is an inability to respond to polysaccharide antigens, and cell-mediated immunity becomes progressively abnormal with aging, resulting in malignancy and opportunistic infections.

Ataxia–telangiectasia syndrome is an autosomal recessive condition characterized by progressive cerebellar ataxia, oculocutaneous telangiectasias, chronic sinopulmonary disease, malignancy, and a variable humoral and cellular immunodeficiency. There is a defect in DNA repair mechanisms, with a high incidence of chromosomal breaks. Immunologic attrition occurs with age, involving both humoral and cellular immunity. The most frequent abnormalities are deficiencies of IgA and IgE and the presence of low-molecular-weight IgM.

Phagocytic Defects

Phagocytic disorders may be classified as quantitative or qualitative. Granulocytopenia may be congenital or due to bone marrow dysfunction secondary to malignancy or drugs, or to increased destruction from antigranulocyte antibodies. Qualitative disorders can be either extrinsic, such as those that occur from deficiencies of opsonins secondary to antibody or complement abnormalities, or intrinsic, such as those that occur from enzyme deficiencies within the metabolic pathway necessary for killing bacteria. Disorders may result from a defect occurring in any stage of phagocytosis by

Table 8–2. Phagocytic Disorders

Name	Defect	Comment
Chronic granulomatous disease	Bactericidal	X-linked recessive (66%), autosomal recessive (33%); eczema, osteomyelitis, abscesses caused by *Staphylococcus aureus, Pseudomonas cepacia, Aspergillus fumigatus;* X-linked defect in cytochrome b produces negative nitroblue tetrazolium test
Chédiak-Higashi syndrome	Bactericidal plus chemotaxis	Autosomal recessive; oculocutaneous albinism, neuropathy, giant neutrophilic cytoplasmic inclusions; malignancy
Hyperimmunoglobulin E (Job syndrome)	Chemotaxis	Eczema, staphylococcal abscesses, red hair; granulocyte and monocyte chemotaxis affected; antistaphylococcal IgE
Myeloperoxidase deficiency	Bactericidal, fungicidal	Reduced chemiluminescence; autosomal recessive (1:4000); persistent candidiasis in diabetics
Glucose-6-phosphate dehydrogenase deficiency	Bactericidal	Phenotypically similar to chronic granulomatous disease
Burns, malnutrition	Bactericidal plus chemotaxis	Reversible defects
Lazy leukocyte syndrome	Chemotaxis	Normal bone marrow cells but poor migration; granulocytopenia
Leukocyte adhesion deficiency	Adherence, chemotaxis, phagocytosis; reduced lymphocyte cytotoxicity	Delayed separation or infection of umbilical cord; lethal bacterial infections; autosomal recessive; neutrophilia
Ciliary dysfunction	Locomotion, chemotaxis	Kartagener syndrome; immotile cilia syndrome; abnormal microtubule function
Schwachman syndrome	Chemotaxis	Pancreatic insufficiency, metaphyseal chondrodysplasia; autosomal recessive

polymorphonuclear neutrophils, including motility, recognition, adhesion, ingestion, degranulation, and intracellular killing. In these disorders, the number of cells may increase during an acute infection but the dysfunctional cells contribute little to host defenses. Signs and symptoms may be delayed because of the decreased numbers or the abnormal influx of granulocytes into infected sites. Representative phagocytic disorders are listed in Table 8–2.

Chronic granulomatous disease (CGD) is a model of a functional disorder leading to recurrent clinical infection. CGD is inherited most commonly as an X-linked but also as an autosomal recessive trait. It is characterized by defective intracellular killing of bacteria, leading to severe infections accompanied by generalized granulomatous processes and reactive hypergammaglobulinemia. Skin, lungs, and perianal tissue commonly are infected with *Staphylococcus aureus.* In addition, *Aspergillus* and *Candida* infections frequently are found. The defect is due to reduced white cell oxidative phosphorylation and free radical oxygen killing. Organisms that have catalase and detoxify H_2O_2 survive within the cell, producing granulomas and abscesses.

Complement Defects

Complement deficiencies may be hereditary or acquired. Complement is necessary for normal opsonization, bacterial killing, and neutrophil chemotaxis. Complement abnormalities have been associated with recurrent pyogenic infections, autoimmune disease, and *Neisseria* infection (Table 8–3). Acquired deficiency usually results from consumption of complement components because of immune complex deposition, as seen in systemic lupus erythematosus, bacterial endocarditis, and hepatitis. Sickle cell disease has been associated with a defect in alternative pathway function that is needed for opsonization of pneumococci.

Laboratory Evaluation of Suspected Immunodeficiency Syndromes

The competence of each limb of the immune response must be assessed, including both quantitative and qualitative tests of cell type or cell products. Screening tests should be employed initially, and the more specific tests should be reserved for when abnormalities are discovered or strongly suspected (Table 8–4). Results always should be com-

Table 8–3. Complement Deficiencies

Type	Associated Clinical Findings
Hereditary	
C2	SLE, MPGN, H-S purpura, septicemia
C3	Severe infections with extracellular organisms
C4	SLE
C5, C6, C7, C8	Disseminated gonococcal, meningococcal disease
C1 INH	Hereditary angioedema
Properdin	Fatal meningococcal disease
Acquired	
C3	MPGN, burns
C1, C4, C2, C3	SLE, SBE, hepatitis, Epstein-Barr virus
Alternate pathway function	Decreased in patients with sickle cell disease

H-S = Henoch-Schönlein; INH = inhibitor; MPGN = membranoproliferative glomerulonephritis; SBE = subacute bacterial endocarditis; SLE = systemic lupus erythematosus.

pared with appropriate age-related normals. Human immunodeficiency virus (HIV) infection should be excluded. Additional diagnostic tests are required if screening test results are abnormal or ambiguous (Table 8–5).

Table 8–4. Initial Screening Tests for Suspected Immune Deficiency

General
Complete blood count, including hemoglobin, differential white cell count and morphology, and platelet count
Roentgenograms to document infection in chest, sinus, mastoids, long bones, if indicated by clinical history
Cultures, if appropriate
Erythrocyte sedimentation rate

Antibody-Mediated Immunity
Quantitative immunoglobulin levels: IgG, IgA, IgM, IgE
Isohemagglutinin titers (anti-A, anti-B): measures IgM function
Pre-existing antibody levels: diphtheria, tetanus, polio, rubella, *Haemophilus influenzae*

Cell-Mediated Immunity
Lymphocyte count and morphology
Delayed hypersensitivity skin tests (*Candida*, tetanus toxoid, tuberculin, mumps): measures T cell and macrophage function

Phagocytosis
Neutrophil cell count and morphology
Nitroblue tetrazolium dye test

Complement
Total hemolytic complement (CH50): measures complement activity
C3, C4 levels: measure important pathway components

Table 8–5. Advanced Laboratory Tests for Suspected Immune Deficiency

Antibody
HIV antibody by ELISA; if positive, confirm with Western blot
B cell quantitation
Specific antibody response to immunization with pneumococcal or *Haemophilus influenzae* vaccine: monitor titers before and after immunization
IgG subclasses
Secretory antibody levels

Cell-Mediated
T cell subset quantitation
Mitogen stimulation tests with PHA, concanavalin A, and pokeweed mitogen
Cytokine assays
Cytotoxicity assays using target cells

Phagocyte
Rebuck skin window
Chemotaxis, adhesion, and aggregation assays
Enzyme assays—myeloperoxidase
Metabolic assays—chemiluminescence
Phagocytic and bactericidal assays

Complement
Individual components of classic pathway
Chemotactic factors
Opsonic assays
Alternative pathway activity assays
C1 esterase inhibitor—functional and antigenic assays
Complement receptors

ELISA = enzyme-linked immunosorbent assay; PHA = phytohemagglutinin.

Treatment

The treatment of patients with primary immunodeficiency disorders requires a combination of antibiotics, protective isolation, and replacement of missing humoral or cellular immunologic functions when possible. Antibiotics should be administered at the first indication of bacterial or fungal infections. Aggressive antibiotic treatment has become a standard part of management in the treatment of certain phagocytic disorders such as CGD and hyper-IgE syndrome. *Prevention* of infections may be accomplished with the administration of intravenous immunoglobulin to patients and bacterial capsular polysaccharide vaccines to family members and patients, if they are capable of immune response. Live vaccines should not be administered.

Treatment of antibody deficiency disorders includes the administration of intravenous immunoglobulin and the appropriate use of antibiotics. The treatment of T cell disorders varies depending on the defect, but, in general, the only adequate treatment is immunologic reconstitution by transplantation of immunocompetent tissue. Mature bone marrow, fetal liver, and fetal thymus all have been used successfully. A variety of immunomodulating agents that augment existing cellular immunity have been used, including levamisole, thymosin, and transfer factor, with variable results. ADA deficiency may be treated by enzyme replacement with infusions of polyethylene glycol–modified ADA or by gene therapy. Interferon gamma has improved phagocytic function in patients with CGD.

References

Behrman RE (ed): Nelson Textbook of Pediatrics. 14th ed. Philadelphia, WB Saunders, 1992, Sec. 11.4–11.33.

Gelfand EW: SCID continues to point the way. N Engl J Med 322:1741, 1990.

Greenberg F: What defines DiGeorge anomaly? J Pediatr 115:412, 1989.

The International Chronic Granulomatous Disease Cooperative Study Group: A controlled trial of interferon gamma to prevent infection in chronic granulomatous disease. N Engl J Med 324:509, 1991.

Pachman L, Lynch P, Silver R, et al: Primary immunodeficiency disease in children. An update. Curr Prob Pediatr 19:9, 1989.

Shyur S-D, Hill HR: Immunodeficiency in the 1990s. Pediatr Infect Dis J 10:595, 1991.

Yang KD, Hill HR: Neutrophil function disorders: Pathophysiology, prevention, and therapy. J Pediatr 119:343, 1991.

GRAFT-VERSUS-HOST DISEASE

Graft-versus-host disease (GVHD) results from the unopposed action of donor immunocompetent cells (T killer cells) against antigens expressed on host cells. The requirements for the development of GVHD are histocompatibility differences between the graft (donor) and host (recipient), immunodeficient host cells, and immunocompetent graft cells. GVHD may result from the infusion of a blood product containing viable lymphocytes. Immunoincompetent newborns may develop the disease after maternofetal blood transfusion, intrauterine transfusion, or exchange transfusion. Patients with primary or secondary immunodeficiency may develop GVHD as a result of bone marrow, liver, fetal thymus, or fetal liver transplantation. GVHD may appear in acute and chronic forms.

Acute GVHD. The acute form develops in 30–70% of bone marrow transplant patients, within the first 100 days and usually as early as 7–14 days

Table 8–6. Clinical Grading of GVHD

Grade	Clinical Criteria
1	Maculopapular rash involving less than 50% of body Bilirubin 2–3 mg/dL No alimentary tract disease No change in overall performance ability
2	Maculopapular rash involving 50–100% of body Bilirubin 3–6 mg/dL Diarrhea 500–1500 mL/24 hr in adolescents Mild decrease in overall performance ability Minimal fever
3	Generalized skin rash (erythroderma) Bilirubin 6–15 mg/dL Diarrhea greater than 1500 mL/24 hr in adolescents Moderate to markedly decreased overall performance Persistent and significant fever (>38.5°C)
4	Generalized erythroderma with bullous formation and desquamation Bilirubin greatern than 15 mg/dL Diarrhea greater than 1500 mL/24 hr in adolescents Extreme debility and fever

after transplantation. The primary tissues affected are the skin, the gastrointestinal tract, the liver, and the lymphohematologic system. The severity of acute GVHD can be assessed by the degree of individual organ or system involvement (Table 8–6). The skin rash of acute GVHD is a fine, diffuse, erythematous macular rash often mistaken for a viral or allergic rash. The rash may become generalized and, in severe cases, may progress to desquamation similar to that of toxic epidermal necrolysis. Gastrointestinal manifestations may include malabsorption, diarrhea, and hemorrhage. Hepatosplenomegaly, jaundice, cardiac irregularity, pulmonary infiltrates (cytomegalovirus pneumonia), and central nervous system irritability also may occur in severe cases.

Chronic GVHD. The chronic form of GVHD occurs more than 100 days after transplantation and may arise de novo or evolve from acute GVHD. Chronic GVHD is a generalized multisystem disease with features similar to those of lupus erythematosus and scleroderma. Dryness of the ocular and oropharyngeal mucosa is similar to that in Sjögren syndrome. Chronic diarrhea, failure to thrive, biliary cirrhosis, esophagitis, and malabsorption may occur. Chronic GVHD is associated with hypergammaglobulinemia, eosinophilia, autoantibody formation, and immune complexes. Specific antibody formation is poor, and these patients are susceptible to recurrent infections with encapsulated bacteria and opportunistic organisms.

Diagnosis.   The diagnosis is suggested in an immunodeficient patient who has the clinical manifestations of GVHD and has received a transfusion of immunocompetent cells in the preceding several weeks. Biopsy of active GVH lesions may demonstrate eosinophils, mononuclear cells, and phagocytic and histiocytic cells.

Prevention and Treatment.   Immunodeficient patients who must receive blood products should receive irradiated blood products to prevent donor lymphocyte proliferation. Mature bone marrow that is HLA-identical with that of the recipient is the tissue of choice for bone marrow transplantation. If unavailable, haploidentical (half-matched) bone marrow can be used after being depleted of T cells by various techniques, but the stem cells should be left intact for transplantation. *Therapy* of established **acute GVHD** includes high-dose prednisone, antithymocyte globulin, cyclosporine, OKT3 monoclonal antibodies, or combinations of these agents. Therapy of **chronic GVHD** includes prednisone alone or in combination with azathioprine: cyclosporine or thalidomide also may be effective. *Prophylaxis* is more effective than therapy of GVHD and includes methotrexate, prednisone, cyclosporine, purging of T cells from the donor's marrow (associated with graft failure), and combinations of these methods.

References

Behrman RE (ed): Nelson Textbook of Pediatrics. 14th ed. Philadelphia, WB Saunders, 1992, Sec. 6.38–6.40, 11.21.

Ferrara J, Deeg HJ: Graft-versus-host disease. N Engl J Med 324:667, 1991.

Hong R: Transplantation immunity: Basic principles and future projections. Adv Pediatr 37:285, 1990.

HYPERSENSITIVITY REACTIONS

Hypersensitivity is an immunologically mediated interaction between exogenous or endogenous antigens and specific antibodies or lymphocytes. It occurs following re-exposure to a particular antigen (allergen) and the development of tissue injury. Traditionally, hypersensitivity reactions have been divided into immediate- and delayed-type reactions. However, a more helpful system consists of three types of hypersensitivity that are antibody-mediated and a fourth that is mediated primarily by T lymphocytes and macrophages.

Type I (Anaphylactic) Reactions

Type I or immediate hypersensitivity is mediated primarily, if not exclusively, by IgE (reagin). Following initial antigen exposure, B cell stimulation results in IgE production. The antigen-specific IgE then binds to specific receptors on mast cell and basophil surfaces. On subsequent challenge by specific antigen, the antigen is bound by the mast cell–anchored IgE. The interaction between IgE and antigen provokes the release of mediators from granules inside the mast cell. This process, known as degranulation (Fig. 8–3), releases histamine, leukotrienes, and prostaglandins that cause the symptoms of type I hypersensitivity (see later). Examples include anaphylaxis to insect stings, foods (peanuts), or penicillin.

Type II (Cytotoxic) Reactions

Type II hypersensitivity involves antibody directed against cell surfaces or tissue antigens and an interaction with complement and a variety of effector cells that damages cells and surrounding tissues. Two subtypes of reactions may be distinguished. In the first, complement-fixing antibody (IgG, IgM) is directed against endogenous antigenic determinants of the cell membrane, leading to cell damage by complement-mediated lysis, phagocytosis, and K cell activity (e.g., hemolytic disease of the newborn, Goodpasture syndrome). In the second, an exogenous antigenic determinant acts as a hapten, combining with the cell membrane and eliciting the immune response (e.g., drug-induced hemolytic anemia). The binding of activated C3 to target cells or antigens opsonizes the target for mononuclear phagocytes and neutrophils, which have receptors for activated C3.

Type III (Immune-Complex or Arthus) Reactions

Type III hypersensitivity reactions involve formation of soluble immune complexes of antigen and antibody. Large immune complexes are removed by the reticuloendothelial system in the liver, spleen, and lungs, whereas smaller complexes persist in the circulation and can localize at the glomerular basement membrane or other target

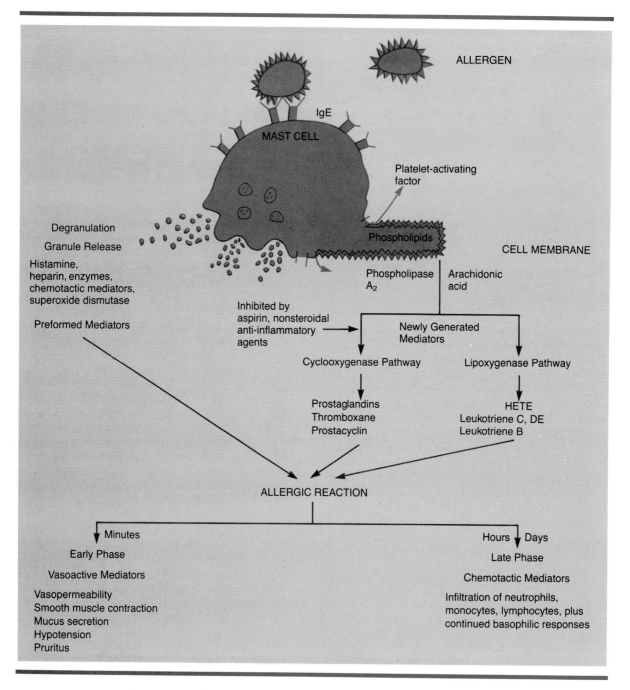

Figure 8–3. Mast cell mediators. HETE = hydroxyeicosatetraenoic acid.

organs. Tissue deposition occurs that may be facilitated by release of vasoactive amines from mast cells and basophils following the simultaneous interaction of IgE and antigen. Complement activation leads to the generation of C3a and C5a, which have anaphylactic and chemotactic properties. Immune complexes interact with Fc receptors on platelets, inducing platelet aggregation to form microthrombi that further increase vascular permeability. Complement activation induces leukocyte migration, phagocytosis, and release of permeability factors and proteases that cause tissue damage.

Polymorphonuclear leukocyte infiltration is necessary for the production of tissue injury in type III reactions. Clinical examples include autoimmune diseases, serum sickness, and local Arthus reactions.

Type IV (Cellular) Reactions

Type IV reactions, also known as delayed-type hypersensitivity, are mediated by antigen-specific T cells and macrophages. The reaction occurs 24–72 hr following antigen exposure. Several types of delayed-type hypersensitivity have been observed, including contact, tuberculin, and granulomatous-type reactions. Granulomatous reactions, which are identified morphologically by the presence of histiocytes, epithelioid cells, and giant cells, differ from the contact-type or tuberculin-type reactions in both morphology of the reaction and kinetics of granuloma formation, which occurs over several weeks rather than 48–72 hr. Following antigen exposure, T cells produce substances known as cytokines, which have numerous activities including macrophage activation, lymphocyte regulation, and induction of inflammation. Clinical examples include contact dermatitis, sarcoidosis, and GVHD.

Chemical Mediators of Immediate Hypersensitivity

Mast cells and basophils are the IgE-bearing, mediator-generating cells. Two types of mast cells are the connective tissue cells and the mucosal mast cells. There are 50,000–500,000 receptors for IgE on the surface of mast cells and basophils. The bridging of two or more IgE molecules by antigen causes mast cell degranulation, resulting in release of chemical mediators. Mediator release also can be caused by hypoxia, anaphylatoxins, and drugs. Different clinical effects in different organs may be related to the heterogeneous population of mast cells.

Mast cell mediators include preformed mediators, which are stored in and released from secretory granules, and newly generated mediators, which are synthesized de novo and secreted after IgE activation (Fig. 8–3). Histamine is a preformed bioactive amine that causes smooth muscle contractions of human bronchioles, increased permeability of capillaries, and increased secretion of nasal and bronchial mucous glands. High-molecular-weight neutrophil chemotactic factor and eosinophil chemotactic factor of anaphylaxis are two preformed mediators that attract neutrophils and eosinophils, respectively, into the area of allergic inflammation. Superoxide dismutase, lysomal hydrolases, kallikrein, Hageman factor cleaver, and myeloperoxidase are also preformed mediators.

Metabolites of arachidonic acid metabolism produced by mast cell activation are newly generated mediators responsible for bronchospasm, mucosal edema, and increased vascular permeability. Arachidonic acid, which is liberated from cell membrane phospholipid by phospholipase A2, subsequently is metabolized along two pathways (Fig. 8–3). Leukotrienes B_4, C_4, D_4, and E_4, formerly known as slow-reacting substances of anaphylaxis, are responsible for smooth muscle contraction and bronchoconstriction. Alternatively, prostaglandins (PGI_2, PGD_2, PGF_2, PGE_2) and thromboxanes (TXA_2) are produced. Adenosine, another newly formed mediator generated from the breakdown of adenosine triphosphate, is a potent vasodilator and causes bronchospasm. Platelet-activating factor is a generated mediator with biologic activities that include platelet aggregation, bronchoconstriction, and increased vascular permeability.

Heparin, tryptase, and chymase are granule-associated mediators. The latter two mediators play roles in proteolysis during the inflammatory process.

The consequences of mediator release may occur within minutes, which characterizes the "classic" early-phase allergic reaction, or may occur hours following the exposure, which characterizes the late-phase reaction. The mediators responsible for the late-phase reaction have not been conclusively determined.

References

Behrman RE (ed): Nelson Textbook of Pediatrics. 14th ed. Philadelphia, WB Saunders, 1992, Sec. 11.34–11.35.

Claman H: The biology of the immune response. JAMA 258: 2834, 1987.

Yunginger J: Anaphylaxis. Curr Prob Pediatr 22:130, 1992.

PRINCIPLES OF DIAGNOSIS AND TREATMENT OF ATOPIC DISEASE

Allergy History

A description of the onset and duration of symptoms, including severity, seasonal variation, environmental triggers, and response to medication, should be obtained. Associated allergic symptoms, such as rhinoconjunctivitis, asthma, drug or food allergy, urticaria, contact dermatitis, and eczema, frequently coexist in allergic individuals. A family history of allergy often is present.

The seasonal occurrence of mold spores and tree, grass, and weed pollens varies with geographic location. Perennial allergens, such as dust mites, animal dander, and indoor molds, may be responsible for chronic symptoms, especially when the house is sealed during the winter months. A detailed environmental history should include information on age of residence, heating and air-conditioning systems, carpeting, and pets. The bedroom is especially important because of the amount of time spent there. Pillows, mattresses, bookcases, curtains, rugs, and storage closets should be described. It is important to document symptoms after allergen exposure. It may be necessary to inquire about school or day care environments.

Physical Examination

Certain findings on physical examination may suggest the presence of allergic disease. Periorbital edema and bluish discoloration ("allergic shiners"), injected conjunctiva, watery rhinorrhea, pale nasal mucosa, transverse nasal crease, gaping facies, and mannerisms such as facial grimacing and frequent nose rubbing ("allergic salute") commonly are present. Wheezing and cough are present during exacerbations of asthma. Skin eruptions, such as urticaria, eczema, and angioedema, may be noted.

Laboratory Studies

Laboratory tests may be helpful in diagnosing the presence of allergic disease (Table 8–7). Eosinophilia ranging from 3% to 10% and a total eosinophil count greater than 250 cells/mm^3 are suggestive of atopy. Extreme elevations are not common

Table 8–7. Laboratory Evaluation of the Allergic Patient

General
Complete blood count with differential
Total eosinophil count
Nasal, sputum smears for eosinophils
Roetgenograms, if indicated—sinus, chest

IgE
Total serum IgE
Allergen-specific IgE—skin test or immunoassay

Provocation Tests
Bronchial
  Specific—pollen, dander, mites
  Nonspecific—methacholine, cold air, exercise
Ocular and nasal challenges
Oral challenges with foods or drugs

Table 8–8. Disorders Associated with Elevated Serum IgE

Allergic disease
Allergic bronchopulmonary aspergillosis
Hyperimmunoglobulin E syndrome
Wiskott-Aldrich syndrome
Hodgkin disease
Helminthic infections
Bullous pemphigoid
Atopic dermatitis
Idiopathic nephrotic syndrome

in allergic disease but may be associated with tissue-invading helminth parasites, drug reactions, immunodeficiency syndromes, and infiltrative lung disorders.

Elevated IgE levels are common in patients with allergic disease, but are not pathognomonic of atopy (Table 8–8).

Allergy skin tests produce a wheal and flare 15–20 min after an antigen is introduced into the skin by scratch, prick, puncture, or intradermal techniques. The positive skin test indicates the presence of antigen-specific IgE but does not necessarily indicate that clinical sensitivity is present. Results must be correlated with symptoms after allergen exposure.

Bronchial provocation tests are performed by having the patient inhale an aerosolized allergen and then recording changes of the patient's pulmonary function. Single- or double-blind food challenges under controlled circumstances may be helpful in diagnosing food hypersensitivity but can be difficult to interpret because of delayed reactions that occasionally occur hours after ingestion.

Treatment

The treatment of allergic disorders is based on environmental control measures, pharmacotherapy, and immunotherapy. Environmental measures, such as removal of a pet or feather pillow, may be easier to accomplish than the purchase of an expensive air filter or air-conditioning system. Complete elimination of certain allergens, such as pollen, dust mites, and molds, may not be possible. Environmental measures should be emphasized in the bedroom because of the greater time spent here.

Pharmacologic therapy interrupts the pathways of mediator release and tissue damage.

Antihistamines competitively inhibit histamine at receptor sites (H_1 and H_2) and are most effective prior to allergic exposure. *Adrenergics* stimulate specific alpha or beta receptors on cell surfaces to produce excitatory or inhibitory physiologic responses. *Methylxanthines* are bronchodilators. *Glucocorticoids* modify allergic reactions by a variety of mechanisms that inhibit the inflammatory response, and *cromolyn* reduces bronchial hyperactivity and bronchoconstriction by stabilizing mast cell membranes.

Immunotherapy consists of injections of increasing amounts of allergen in patients with type I immediate hypersensitivity. The mechanism of protection may be the production of blocking IgG, suppressor cell activation, or stabilization of mast cells. Immunotherapy is indicated for significant disease that cannot be controlled by pharmacotherapy and avoidance measures. Immunotherapy is effective in allergic rhinitis, Hymenoptera sensitivity, hay fever, and allergic asthma. Perennial therapy is recommended rather than preseasonal administration. A period of approximately 3–5 yr is considered adequate when high-dose immunotherapy is utilized. Small local reactions at the site of the injection are common, but anaphylaxis occasionally may occur (1–3% risk). The dose of allergen should be reduced during seasonal exposure to avoid severe reactions.

Prevention

Breast feeding and avoidance of allergens by the mother and infant may reduce the incidence of food allergies and eczema. Acaricide reduction in house dust mite exposure also may reduce allergic respiratory disorders.

References

Arshad SH, Matthews S, Gant C, et al: Effect of allergen avoidance on development of allergic disorders in infancy. Lancet 339:1493, 1992.

Behrman RE (ed): Nelson Textbook of Pediatrics. 14th ed. Philadelphia, WB Saunders, 1992, Sec. 11.36–11.39.

Dold S, Wjst M, von Mutius E, et al: Genetic risk for asthma, allergic rhinitis, and atopic dermatitis. Arch Dis Child 67:1018, 1992.

Eggleston PA: Immunotherapy for allergic respiratory disease. Pediatr Clin North Am 35:1103, 1988.

Ownby DR: Allergy testing: In vivo versus in vitro. Pediatr Clin North Am 35:995, 1988.

BRONCHIAL ASTHMA

Asthma is defined as reversible obstruction of large and small airways resulting from hyperresponsiveness to various immunologic and nonimmunologic stimuli. The disease is intermittent and characterized by recurrent episodes of cough, chest tightness, dyspnea, and wheezing. Between 5% and 10% of all children are affected at some time with asthma; 80–90% have the first episode of asthma by 4–5 yr of age. It is the most common chronic lung disease in children and is a leading cause of emergency room visits, hospital admissions, and school absenteeism. Its prevalance and mortality have increased in the last decade.

Pathophysiology. Three major pathologic events contribute to airway obstruction: mucosal edema with inflammation, smooth muscle contraction, and production of a thick, tenacious mucus. Obstruction occurs during expiration as the airway approaches the closing volume and results in distal airway gas trapping; more severe asthma may have diminished air flow during inspiration. A number of anatomic and physiologic characteristics predispose infants and young children to an increased risk (e.g., smaller airway size, lower elastic recoil of the lung, decreased smooth muscle support of the small airways, relative mucous gland hyperplasia, and decreased collateral channels of ventilation between alveoli).

Classification. Asthma may be classified into several categories based on the probable cause. *Allergic* or *extrinsic asthma* may be precipitated by pollens, foods, dust mites, mold spores, sulfites, and animal dander. It is associated with a history of eczema and is IgE mediated. An IgE response to respiratory syncytial virus (RSV) also occurs in infants and children with RSV-associated wheezing. *Intrinsic* or *nonallergic asthma* is non-IgE mediated; common triggers include temperature changes, cold air, odors, irritants, menses, and smoke. Viral infections such as RSV, parainfluenza virus, adenovirus, and rhinovirus also initiate these acute wheezing episodes. Psychologic factors have been overemphasized in childhood asthma but also play a role. *Combinations* of extrinsic and intrinsic triggering factors are more common in childhood. *Exercise-induced asthma* occurs in up to 95% of asthmatic children. Cold dry air is an important stimulus. *Aspirin-induced asthma* has been postulated to involve inhibition of the cyclooxygenase pathway of arachidonic acid metabolism, which increases production of leukotrienes by the alternate lipoxygenase pathway (Fig. 8–3). Other nonsteroidal anti-inflammatory agents and beta-adrenergic blocking agents may exacerbate asthma. Hyperplastic rhinitis and nasal polyps may be associated findings. Gastroesophageal reflux has been associated with asthma, probably as being secondary to cholinergic mechanisms or aspiration. Gastroesophageal reflux, sinusitis, pollutants (SO_2), and allergic bronchopulmonary aspergillosis have been implicated as causes of recalcitrant asthma.

Diagnosis. The history is most important in the diagnosis of asthma. Wheeze, cough, dyspnea, and chest pain are common during acute exacerbations. Wheezing may not always be present between episodes, but a history of persistent cough (cough-variant asthma), night cough, exercise-induced cough, post-tussive emesis from copious amounts of mucus, and cough following cold air exposure all are suggestive of asthma. Abdominal pain is common owing to the use of accessory muscles.

During acute episodes, the physical examination reveals a hyperinflated chest that is hyper-resonant to percussion. Tachypnea, tachycardia, cough, inspiratory and expiratory wheezing, a prolonged expiratory phase, and squeaky musical inspiratory rales are present. As the attack progresses, the following signs develop: cyanosis, use of accessory muscles of respiration, decreased breath sounds (tight "silent" chest) and diminished wheezing, agitation, inability to speak, tripod sitting position, diaphoresis, and pulsus paradoxus.

Differential Diagnosis. The causes of wheezing are listed in Table 8–9. Wheezing before 3 mo of age should suggest other conditions, such as pulmonary malformations, cardiac and gastrointestinal abnormalities, and cystic fibrosis (especially in the presence of clubbing, which is not seen in asthma). In infants and toddlers, bronchiolitis caused by RSV is a very common cause of wheezing. A foreign body in the airway or esophagus should be considered in patients over 1–2 yr of age who have sudden onset of wheezing and diminished breath sounds localized to one region on examination of the chest.

Laboratory studies (Table 8–10) can be helpful in determining the presence and type of asthma. Chest radiographs in both posteroanterior and lateral views should be obtained in all new patients to identify anatomic abnormalities, atelectasis, foreign bodies, or neoplasms. Pulmonary function testing can be helpful in assessing the severity of disease and response to therapy in the acute and chronic phases by measuring forced expired volume in 1 second (FEV_1), peak expiratory flow rate (PEFR), forced vital capacity (FVC), and average flow rate between 25% and 75% FVC (FEV_{25-75}).

During the onset of an asthma episode, hyperventilation due to mild airway obstruction produces hypocapnia accompanied by a respiratory alkalosis, with or without hypoxia. As airway

Table 8–9. Differential Diagnosis of Wheezing

Respiratory
Common
Bronchial asthma
Infection
Foreign body
Cystic fibrosis
Laryngotracheomalacia

Uncommon
Bronchopulmonary dysplasia
Alpha$_1$-antitrypsin deficiency
Allergic bronchopulmonary aspergillosis
Ciliary dyskinesia syndrome
Hypersensitivity pneumonitis
Bronchiectasis
Pulmonary hemosiderosis
Visceral larva migrans—hypereosinophilic disorders

Cardiovascular (Uncommon)
Congenital heart disease
Vascular rings/slings

Gastrointestinal (Uncommon)
Gastroesophageal reflux
H-type tracheoesophageal fistula
Foreign body

Miscellaneous (Uncommon)
Immunodeficiency disorder
Vasculitis, collagen vascular disease
Psychogenic cough

obstruction progresses, the arterial CO_2 level increases and hypoxia occurs. Thus, a normal CO_2 level is suggestive of moderately severe disease. With more severe airway obstruction, hypercapnia and a respiratory acidosis are present. If hypoxia persists, a mixed metabolic (lactic) and respiratory acidosis will develop. The severity can be assessed by a scoring system (Table 8–11).

Treatment. Counseling to determine the source of potential allergens in order to remove them from the patient's environment and to avoid or ameliorate the effects of other precipitating factors is the foundation of the long-term management of asthma. Pharmacologic treatment should complement this approach (see Allergic Rhinitis–Treatment).

Because of the central pathophysiologic role of inflammation and the risks of chronic beta$_2$-agonist therapy, anti-inflammatory agents are important therapies for acute symptomatic (oral or systemic glucocorticoids) or chronic (cromolyn; inhaled or oral glucocorticoids) asthma. Beta$_2$-adrenergic agonist inhalation therapy is best reserved for acute symptomatic episodes of wheezing rather than being used for routine chronic therapy during asymptomatic periods.

Theophylline preparations often are employed but are becoming less attractive because of a narrow therapeutic index and complex pharmacokinetics. A therapeutic level of 10–20 µg/mL is recommended, but significant cardiac, gastrointestinal, or neurologic toxicity may limit the dose. School performance and behavior may deteriorate, although other signs of toxicity may not be absent. The dose required to achieve therapeutic levels in children is extremely variable. Children metabolize theophylline more rapidly than adults and require relatively higher doses, except in infants under 6 mo of age, who require lower doses because of slower clearance rates. Theophylline clearance is decreased by hepatic disease, congestive heart failure, certain viral infections, and the administration

Table 8–10. Laboratory Studies in Asthma

Test	Comments
Complete blood count	Generally normal but eosinophils suggest allergic bronchopulmonary aspergillosis or atopic disease; leukocytosis suggests infection
Sputum examination	Tenacious and with eosinophils; purulent sputum suggests infection
Chest roentgenogram	Normal between episodes; hyperinflation atelectasis, increased lung markings appear acutely, pneumomediastinum or pneumothorax may occur
Pulmonary function testing	Assesses degree of obstruction and response to bronchodilators
Bronchial provocation	Demonstrates presence of nonspecific bronchial hyperreactivity by methacholine, exercise, and histamine
Serum IgE	Elevated levels may predict atopy; high levels with allergic bronchopulmonary aspergillosis
Allergy skin tests or immunoassay	Identifies potential environmental allergens
Arterial blood gases	Measures severity of acute obstruction and resultant ventilation–perfusion abnormalities

Table 8–11. Severity of Asthma Scoring System

Factor	Score*		
	0	1	2
PaO_2 (torr)	70–100	≤70 in room air	≤70 in 40% O_2
Cyanosis	None	In room air	In 40% O_2
$PaCO_2$ (torr)	<40	40–65	>65
Pulsus paradoxus (torr)	<10	10–40	>40
Accessory muscle use	None	Moderate	Marked
Air exchange	Good	Fair	Poor
Mental status	Normal	Agitated, depressed	Coma

* 0–4 = no immediate danger; 5–6 = impending respiratory failure, notify ICU and anesthesia; >7 = respiratory failure.
(Modified from Wood DW, Downes JJ, Lecks HI: Management of respiratory failure in childhood status asthmaticus. J Allergy Clin Immunol 42:261, 1968.)

of erythromycin and cimetidine (see Appendix 2). Theophylline clearance is increased by cigarette smoking; high-protein, low-carbohydrate diet; phenobarbital; and isoproterenol.

The selective *beta₂-adrenergic agents* are most useful for acute symptomatic exacerbations of asthma when given by inhalation (Table 8–12). Oral preparations of these agents may be employed in chronic stable asthma, whereas subcutaneous or intravenous routes are used less frequently for severe status asthmaticus. Beta₂-agonists are potent bronchodilators (even by aerosol with severe airway obstruction), enhance mucociliary clearance, and may attenuate the early phase of inflammation. Complications include tachycardia, palpitations, tremor, hypokalemia, agitation, excitability, and, if overused, tachyphylaxis or sudden death.

Inhaled *cromolyn sodium* stabilizes mast cells and is used to prevent bronchospasm. It is not a bronchodilator and is not helpful during acute episodes. Several weeks may be required to develop full clinical effectiveness. It is available as an inhaled powder (Spinhaler), an aqueous solution (air compressor required), and a metered-dose inhaler. It compares favorably with oral sustained-release theophylline preparations in the treatment of chronic asthma, often without the side effects produced by theophylline administration.

Glucocorticoids are recommended for severe asthma when bronchodilators do not control symp-

Table 8–12. Adrenergic Agents for Asthma Treatment

Drug	Dose	Form
Oral		
Albuterol*	0.4–0.6 mg/kg/24 hr, qid	2, 4-mg tablets (2 mg/5 mL)
Metaproterenol	1.2–2.0 mg/kg/24 hr, qid	10, 20-mg tablets (10 mg/5 mL)
Terbutaline	0.4–0.6 mg/kg/24 hr, qid	2.5, 5-mg tablets
Inhaled Beta₂-Agonists		
Albuterol*	2 puffs q 20 min × 3	90 µg/puff (metered dose inhaler)
	0.1–0.3 mg/kg/dose; up to 5 mg q 20 min for 1–2 hr (minimum dose 1.25 mg) in Emergency Department or 0.5 mg/kg/hr continuous inhalation (maximum 15 mg/hr) in Intensive Unit	5 mg/mL (nebulizer solution)
Metaproterenol	2 puffs	640 µg/puff (metered dose inhaler)
	5–15 mg (maximum 15 mg)	50 mg/mL (nebulizer solution)
Terbutaline	2 puffs q 20 min × 3	200 µg/puff (metered dose inhaler)
Systemic/Parenteral Beta-Agonists		
Epinephrine HCl	0.01 mg/kg (0.3 mg maximum) subcutaneously q 20 min × 3 doses	1:1000 (1 mg/mL)
Terbutaline	0.01 mg/kg (0.3 mg maximum) subcutaneously; 10-µg/kg bolus intravenous loading dose over 10 min, in hospital followed by 0.4–6.0-µg/kg/min intravenous maintenance infusion titrated to patient status in severe status asthmaticus	1 mg/mL

* Currently albuterol (oral, inhaled) is recommended. Inhalation is the preferred route in acute symptomatic exacerbations of asthma.

(Adapted from Executive Summary; Guidelines for the Diagnosis and Management of Asthma. US Department of Health and Human Services Publ #91-3042A. Washington, DC, U.S. Government Printing Office, 1991.

toms and for hospitalized patients with status asthmaticus. The benefit of steroid administration usually occurs 6–12 hr after administration. Alternate-day oral steroid administration or divided daily doses of inhaled glucocorticoids may be used in children who have chronic steroid-dependent asthma. The complications associated with chronic oral administration limit steroid usefulness, but topically active steroid aerosols have reduced systemic complications significantly.

Emergency treatment of asthma should include aerosolized beta₂-agonists to avoid the unpleasant side effects of subcutaneous epinephrine or terbutaline. The use of intravenous aminophylline is controversial. It may be administered in the appropriate loading dose (5–7 mg/kg), but, to avoid overdosage and toxicity, the previous 24-hr theophylline intake must have been determined first. If theophylline has been administered previously, the aminophylline dose should be reduced according to the serum level. If a response occurs, the patient can be discharged from the emergency room. Prednisone should be given to asthmatics who demonstrate exacerbations despite having received maximal bronchodilator therapy.

If respiratory distress continues without response to treatment, **status asthmaticus** is present and requires hospitalization. Aminophylline should be administered by continuous infusion (range: 0.7–1.2 mg/kg/hr). Hypoxia should be corrected by the administration of oxygen. Dehydration resulting from poor fluid intake and fluid loss secondary to a combination of hyperventilation, diaphoresis, and emesis should be corrected. Bicarbonate can be administered to correct a metabolic acidosis, if present. Intravenous methylprednisolone (1 mg/kg every 6 hr) is indicated in all cases until improvement occurs. Beta-agonist aerosols are continued; atropine aerosols may be beneficial. Continuous intravenous beta-agonists (terbutaline) also may be beneficial and avoid mechanical ventilation (Table 8–12). Mechanical ventilation may be needed when respiratory failure is present.

Prognosis. Asthma can be a fatal disease. Factors associated with poor prognosis of an acute exacerbation include delay in seeking medical attention; underestimation of the severity of the episode by patient, parents, and physician; disturbed family psychosocial relations; sedation; underutilization of glucocorticoids; onset during sleep; black race; male sex; a history of prior respiratory failure; and severe, rapidly progressive bronchospasm. Education can help avoid many of these problems. The long-term prognosis of childhood asthma is good. Many children with onset of asthma before age 5 yr "outgrow" it. Children with severe chronic asthma and those patients with onset during adolescence often continue to have recurrent asthma in adulthood. Asthma patients who are dependent on glucocorticoids may develop Cushing habitus, growth failure, acne, osteoporosis, cataracts, and opportunistic infections.

References

Behrman RE (ed): Nelson Textbook of Pediatrics. 14th ed. Philadelphia, WB Saunders, 1992, Sec. 11.41.

Hendeles L, Weinberger M, Szefler S, et al: Safety and efficacy of theophylline in children with asthma. J Pediatr 120:177, 1992.

Larsen GL: Asthma in children. N Engl J Med 326:1540, 1992.

Spitzer WO, Suissa S, Ernst P, et al: The use of β-agonists and the risk of death and near death from asthma. N Engl J Med 326:501, 1992.

Sporik R, Holgate ST, Cogswell JJ: Natural history of asthma in childhood—a birth cohort study. Arch Dis Child 66:1050, 1991.

Warner JO: Asthma: A follow up statement from an international paediatric asthma consensus group. Arch Dis Child 67:240, 1992.

ALLERGIC BRONCHOPULMONARY ASPERGILLOSIS

Allergic bronchopulmonary aspergillosis (ABPA) results from immunologic reactions in the lung to antigens of the mold *Aspergillus fumigatus*. ABPA is not due to fungal invasiveness. Aspergillosis antigens react with IgG, IgE, and sensitized T and B lymphocytes, causing bronchial wall damage and pulmonary eosinophilic consolidation. ABPA has been identified in corticosteroid-dependent asthma, in cystic fibrosis, and in bronchiectasis.

Clinical Manifestations.   The onset of ABPA may precede the clinical recognition of disease for many years. ABPA often is diagnosed initially as asthma with peripheral eosinophilia; irreversible lung damage may occur before the correct diagnosis is made. In addition to a history of bronchial asthma, patients often demonstrate marked immediate skin reactivity to *A. fumigatus*, other molds, and inhalant allergens. Acute exacerbations are char-

acterized by anorexia, headache, fever, fatigue, and increased sputum production. During acute exacerbations, rales, wheezing, and bronchial breathing may be present, resembling an acute exacerbation of asthma.

Laboratory Manifestations.   Peripheral blood eosinophils generally are greater than $1000/mm^3$. Large numbers of eosinophils and fungal mycelia may be present in sputum. Antigen-specific IgE and/or IgG may be elevated. A variety of transient roentgenographic changes may occur. Permanent changes are related to proximal bronchiectasis, but peripheral bronchi may be normal.

Treatment.   Prednisone is the drug of choice because it reduces the clinical symptoms and sputum production, decreases the incidence of positive sputum cultures, and clears roentgenographic lesions. The total serum IgE typically declines within 2 mo of initiating prednisone therapy, and failure to achieve this reduction suggests noncompliance or an exacerbation of the disease. Antifungal therapy is not helpful.

References

Behrman RE (ed): Nelson Textbook of Pediatrics. 14th ed. Philadelphia, WB Saunders, 1992, Sec. 12.108.

Slavin RG: Allergic bronchopulmonary aspergillosis. Clin Rev Allergy 3:167, 1985.

ALLERGIC RHINITIS

Allergic rhinitis occurs in 10% of children and accounts for 2 million school days lost yearly. Symptoms are rare before 4–5 yr of age and may be seasonal, perennial, or perennial with seasonal exacerbations.

Pathogenesis.   Allergic rhinitis is due to exposure to an antigen and a genetic predisposition to respond with IgE production. The binding of IgE and antigen to mast cells and basophils located on the nasal mucosal surface triggers the release of mediators (Fig. 8–3). Histamine release causes increased capillary permeability accompanied by edema formation and increased mucus secretion from stimulated goblet cells. Recurrent sneezing, pruritus, and glandular hypersecretion also occur by stimulation of H_1 receptors on sensory nerves, which triggers a parasympathetic response. Other mediators isolated from mucus include high-molecular-weight neutrophil chemotactic factor, kinins, prostaglandin D_2, and leukotrienes C, D, and

E. Seasonal allergens include pollens and outdoor molds, whereas perennial symptoms are due to allergens in the house, such as dust mites, animal dander, and house molds.

Clinical Manifestations.   The symptoms of allergic rhinitis consist of nasal congestion; watery rhinorrhea; sneezing; and pruritus of eyes, nose, ears, and throat. The mucus is thin and watery, and irritates the upper lip and nares. A transverse nasal crease may be present across the bridge of the nose. Allergic shiners (pale dark circles under the eyes), along with the allergic salute (nasal rubbing), often are present. Other findings may include snoring, abnormal facial development, and pale injected conjunctiva. Chronic serous otitis media, poor auditory function, and sinusitis also may be noted.

Examination reveals a boggy, edematous nasal mucosa with copious amounts of clear mucus. The mucous membranes are pale and blue and the turbinates are swollen, completely obstructing the nasal passages. The sclera and conjunctiva may be reddened; excessive lacrimation and chemosis (*allergic conjunctivitis*) also may be present. Purulent secretions indicate secondary infection either from sinusitis or, if unilateral, from a possible foreign body.

Laboratory Findings.   The presence of eosinophils on nasal smear usually indicates allergic rhinitis. Allergy skin tests or IgE immunoassays may confirm the presence of a specific offending allergen that correlates with the history.

Differential Diagnosis (Table 8–13).   Congenital abnormalities usually become apparent in the neonatal period. Foreign bodies, such as seeds and beads, typically cause a unilateral hemorrhagic or purulent discharge. Nasal polyps are uncommon in childhood and suggest cystic fibrosis, aspirin sensitivity, or primary ciliary dyskinesia. Topical decongestant abuse may lead to *rhinitis medicamentosa.*

Purulent rhinorrhea of several weeks' duration suggests the possibility of sinusitis, which can be confirmed by the presence of opacification or mucoperiosteal thickening in a computerized tomogram of the sinuses or in an erect Waters sinus roentgenogram. Other causes of chronic infection may be ciliary abnormalities or immunodeficiency.

Nonallergic rhinitis with eosinophilia syndrome differs from allergic rhinitis in several characteristics, including negative family history of atopy, negative skin tests, adult onset, and normal or low IgE levels. *Vasomotor rhinitis* also mimics allergic rhinitis and is thought to be caused by an autonomic nervous system imbalance.

Treatment

Environmental Control.   The easiest and most effective treatment is allergen avoidance. This includes dust control in the house, especially in the bedroom; elimination of animals; and avoidance of certain activities, such as mowing the grass during pollen season. Vacations can be planned to avoid the pollen season in a particular locale. Air conditioners and air filters may be helpful in creating a controlled environment.

Symptom Therapy.   Antihistamines, especially nonsedating antihistamines, are the treatment of choice. Decongestants may be used alone or in fixed combination with antihistamines to reduce

Table 8–13. Differential Diagnosis of Childhood Rhinitis

Congenital	Inflammatory	Neoplastic
Choanal atresia	Eosinophilic	Benign
Posterior choanal stenosis	Allergic	Angiofibroma
Encephalocele	Nonallergic (NARES)	Papilloma
Dermoid cyst	Neutrophilic (infection)	Hemangioma
Glioma	Nasopharyngitis	Malignant
Syphilis	Sinusitis	Lymphoma
	Nasal polyps	Rhabdomyosarcoma
Anatomic	Mastocytosis	Neuroblastoma
Septal anatomic deviation	Granulomatous (Wegener)	
Adenoidal hypertrophy		
Foreign body	**Noninflammatory**	
	Rhinitis medicamentosa	
	Vasomotor rhinitis	
	Hypothyroidism	
	Cerebrospinal fluid rhinorrhea	
	Encephalocele	

NARES = nonallergic rhinitis with eosinophilia syndrome.

mucous membrane edema. Topical decongestants have no role in chronic therapy.

Topical glucocorticoids and cromolyn also offer significant relief in more severe cases. Both require daily administration on a prophylactic basis to be effective. Adrenal suppression has not been reported with the glucocorticoid nasal sprays, although side effects such as stinging and occasional epistaxis occur.

Immunotherapy. The decision to immunize the patient should be based on multiple factors, including severity of disease, age, offending antigen, duration of symptoms, and adequacy of symptomatic measures in controlling symptoms. Injections should be administered only in settings where emergency therapy is available.

References

Behrman RE (ed): Nelson Textbook of Pediatrics. 14th ed. Philadelphia, WB Saunders, 1992, Sec. 11.40.
Simons FER: Allergic rhinitis: Recent advances. Pediatr Clin North Am 35:1053, 1988.

FOOD REACTIONS AND HYPERSENSITIVITY

Food allergy is a frequently misdiagnosed disorder because the majority of adverse food reactions cannot be shown to have an immunologic basis. Laboratory studies such as immunoassays for specific IgE and skin testing are not helpful in such instances. Nonimmunologic adverse food reactions include chemical sensitivities to foods such as wine and cheese with tyramine, hot dogs with nitrites, or Chinese food with monosodium glutamate (Table 8–14). The term "food allergy" should be reserved for immunologic reactions only.

Pathophysiology. The majority of allergic reactions to foods are IgE mediated and occur up to 2–4 hr after ingestion. Following ingestion, significant quantities of macromolecular food antigens can traverse the intestinal epithelium and provoke an immune response. Secretory IgA limits the absorption of intact molecules, preventing the adverse immune response. The frequent occurrence of food allergy in infancy may be related in part to the relative absence of secretory IgA. With maturation, the IgA barrier develops and prevents the absorption of allergens.

Clinical Manifestations. These may be classified by the underlying immunologic mechanism. *IgE-*

Table 8–14. Differential Diagnosis of Food Hypersensitivity

Classification	Examples
Food allergy	Anaphylaxis, urticaria, angioedema, asthma, eczema
Food additives	Dyes (tartrazine), flavorings (MSG), preservatives (metabisulfite, sorbitol)
Toxins	Staphylococcal food poisoning, botulism
Infections	*Salmonella, Giardia, Yersinia, Escherichia coli*
Accidental contaminants	Heavy metal (lead, mercury, iron), antibiotics (penicillin)
Endogenous pharmacologic agents	Caffeine, tyramine, alcohol, histamine
Gastrointestinal disease	Lactase deficiency, cystic fibrosis, gastroesophageal reflux, ulcer disease
Metabolic	Phenylketonuria, Wilson disease, hyperammonemia
Psychologic	School phobia

MSG = monosodium glutamate.

mediated reactions typically involve the respiratory, skin, and gastrointestinal systems. Respiratory involvement includes rhinoconjunctivitis, asthma, and laryngeal edema. Skin reactions include urticaria, angioedema, eczema, and maculopapular eruptions. Gastrointestinal tract symptoms may include vomiting, diarrhea, and abdominal pain. Generalized anaphylaxis can occur. Onset of these reactions is usually rapid, occurring within minutes to hours of the ingestion.

Non–IgE-mediated reactions may mimic reaginic reactions; in many of these reactions the immune pathogenesis is unclear. Several foods, including milk, gluten, and soy, have been demonstrated to induce both acute and chronic gastroenteropathies characterized by malabsorption, vomiting, diarrhea, and fecal blood loss. Protein loss in the stool can result in hypoalbuminemia.

Diagnosis. The clinical manifestations of food allergy and nonimmunologic adverse food reactions can be very similar. A careful and detailed history and a thorough physical examination are important tools used to distinguish among underlying organic disease, psychologic reactions, and the presence of food additives, contaminants, and endogenous pharmacologic agents (Table 8–14). The suspected food should reproduce symptoms on ingestion. Dietary manipulation does not establish an immunologic basis because symptoms caused by nonimmunologic mechanisms also subside when a causative food is excluded. Elimination diets for 7–14 days are useful in confirming an adverse reaction to a suspected food. Reintroduction of the food with resumption of symptoms is diagnostic. In children, the common food allergens include cow's milk, eggs, wheat, legumes (peanuts and soybeans), fish, and shellfish. Juices and fruits often cause rash and diarrhea in infancy without an immune basis. If no significant improvement occurs, it is unlikely that the food is responsible for symptoms. Double-blind food challenges with dried foods in gelatin capsules can be used to document food allergy. Challenges must be supervised and occasionally require hospitalization in cases of suspected severe food reactions.

Laboratory Findings. Skin tests can provide a guide for elimination diets and food challenges. However, there may be false positives and false negatives (nonimmune or non-IgE reactions). The diagnosis of food allergy requires the demonstration of symptoms following food challenges and positive skin tests (if IgE-mediated).

Treatment. The treatment of food hypersensitivity is the elimination of the offending food while continuing to meet nutritional requirements. Careful challenges under appropriate supervision should be performed periodically because sensitization and reactions to foods such as milk and egg often are transient. If complete avoidance is ineffective, pharmacologic management may be required. Antihistamines may be used to treat minor reactions, although, in severe cases, a subcutaneous epinephrine autoinjector should be provided for emergency use by the family. Oral cromolyn and ketotifen have been used experimentally for prophylaxis.

References

Behrman RE (ed): Nelson Textbook of Pediatrics. 14th ed. Philadelphia, WB Saunders, 1992, Sec. 11.49.

Bock SA: Prospective appraisal of complaints of adverse reactions to foods in children during the first 3 years of life. Pediatrics 79:683, 1987.

Sampson HA: Immunologic mechanisms in adverse reactions to foods. Immunol Allergy Clin North Am 11:701, 1991.

Sampson HA, Mendelson L, Rosen JP: Fatal and near-fatal anaphylactic reactions to food in children and adolescents. N Engl J Med 327:380, 1992.

Yunginger JW: Lethal food allergy in children. N Engl J Med 327:421, 1992.

URTICARIA AND ANGIOEDEMA

Urticaria

Urticaria (hives) affects up to 20% of the population at some time. It is characterized by raised, pruritic, erythematous lesions with well-circumscribed serpiginous borders and blanched centers. The lesions are evanescent and vary in size and pattern. Urticaria that persists for longer than 6 wk is chronic. Acute urticaria may occur in any age group but is most common in children and among atopic individuals. The cause of chronic urticaria in children frequently is undetermined. Angioedema is a similar process, occurring deeper in the dermis and subcutaneous tissues.

Pathogenesis. Urticaria may be initiated by IgE antigen reactions or activation of complement producing C3a and C5a (anaphylatoxins). The reactions cause basophil and mast cell mediators to be released, producing vasodilation and edema. An axonal reflex produces erythema. Direct mast cell activation also can occur with certain drugs such as morphine. Histamine, bradykinin, and kinins are primary mediators, but other substances, such as prostaglandins, leukotrienes, and plasmin, have been implicated. Factors that produce cutaneous vasodilation (e.g., exertion, heat, fever, and hyperthyroidism) exacerbate urticaria.

Etiology and Diagnosis. Both acute and chronic urticaria may be produced by a number of factors (Table 8–15). Acute urticaria is more likely to be IgE mediated, and in younger patients it is usually a benign condition.

A cause of acute urticaria may be evident from the history. Exposure to cold can induce immediate as well as delayed urticaria, which may occur on exposed areas or as a generalized condition. Swimming in cold water may be dangerous, resulting in symptoms of urticaria, angioedema, wheezing, and hypotension. Patients with infections (especially viral) or connective tissue disease also may develop cold-induced urticaria that is rarely associated with cryoglobulinemia, cryofibrinogenemia, or cold hemolysin.

Evaluation. In general, laboratory tests are not helpful except to determine the presence of systemic disease. In most instances of acute urticaria, extensive laboratory evaluation is not warranted. In specific instances, provocative challenges with a suspected antigen, elimination diets, and drug avoidance may be useful.

Table 8–15. Etiology of Urticaria

Drugs
Antibiotics (penicillin), aspirin, codeine, blood products

Foods and Food Additives
Eggs, peanuts, fish, tartrazine

Infectious Diseases
Streptococcal pharyngitis, sinusitis, hepatitis, mononucleosis, viral infection, *Mycoplasma*, parasites

Insect Bites and Stings
Bee stings, flea bites, mite bites

Collagen Vascular Diseases
Lupus erythematosus, vasculitis, polymyositis

Inhalant Allergens
Cat, horse

Idiopathic

Physical Agents
Dermatographism, cold, heat, solar, cholinergic, pressure, aquagenic, exercise, vibratory

Genetic Types
Familial cold, heat, and vibration

Contactants
Cat scratches, moth scales, caterpillars, nettle plants,
food processes

Neoplasms
Hodgkin disease, leukemia

Mastocytosis–Urticaria Pigmentosa

Endocrine System
Hyperthyroidism, hypothyroidism, pregnancy

Treatment. The preferred treatment is avoidance of the causative agent in cases of urticaria induced by drugs, food, inhalants, insects, and physical elements. If present, an underlying systemic
disease should be treated. Acute severe urticaria
can be treated with epinephrine 1:1000, at a dose
of 0.01 mL/kg (maximum 0.3 mL) subcutaneously
to provide temporary relief, and should then be
followed by oral administration of the H_1 class of
antihistamines. Hydroxyzine also has been very effective for acute and chronic urticaria. Cyproheptadine is the drug of choice for cold-induced urticaria.
Several long-acting, nonsedating antihistamines,
including terfenadine and astemizole, are promising in treatment of the disorder.

If antihistamines are unsuccessful, the addition
of a sympathomimetic agent, such as ephedrine or
terbutaline, may be a useful adjunct. Tricylic antidepressants such as doxepin, which has combined
H_1 and H_2 antihistaminic properties, have been
used in recalcitrant cases. Glucocorticoids should
be avoided except in refractory cases or to relieve
acute severe symptoms. Antihistamines should not
be discontinued when steroids are administered.
Drug desensitization may be needed (see Penicillin
Hypersensitivity).

Angioedema

Angioedema occurs in association with urticaria,
although it occurs alone in 10% of cases. Angioedema is colorless, asymmetric in distribution,
and variably pruritic. It affects the periorbital and
perioral areas, lips, tongue, scalp, scrotum, and
dorsum of hands and feet. Upper airway involvement produces stridor, hoarseness, dyspnea, and
airway obstruction that may be life threatening.
The pathogenesis, evaluation, and treatment of angioedema are similar to those of urticaria; however,
the inherited form known as *hereditary angioedema*
(HAE) is treated differently.

HAE is transmitted as a mendelian autosomal
dominant trait. It is caused by a partial deficiency
of an $alpha_2$-neuraminoglycoprotein that inhibits
the activation of the first component of complement. The C1 esterase inhibitor (C1 INH) inhibits
kinin formation in inflammation, inhibits factor XI
in clotting, and inhibits plasmin in the fibrinolytic
pathway for fibrinolysis. The functional absence of
this inhibitor allows activation of the complement
cascade and resultant symptoms. There are three
types of HAE: type 1 occurs in 85% of affected patients and is characterized by low levels of intact
C1 INH; type II occurs in 15% of patients and is
characterized by the presence of C1 INH in normal
amounts but with abnormal function; and an acquired form of C1 INH deficiency has been associated with underlying hematologic malignancy and
autoimmune disease caused by an antibody to C1
INH.

Clinical Manifestations. The symptoms of HAE
consist of recurrent episodes of angioedema affecting the extremities, face, airway, and intestine. Urticaria is not a feature. The angioedema is painless,
nonpitting, and nonpruritic. Laryngeal edema may
occur and is the major cause of death. Abdominal
symptoms may mimic an acute abdomen, with
nausea, emesis, and pain. Attacks may occur spontaneously or after trauma, emotional stress, or
change in environmental temperature.

Diagnosis. The diagnosis of HAE is established
by finding low levels of C4 and C1 INH. C4 levels
usually are low during both symptomatic and
asymptomatic periods. C2 levels are low during

symptomatic periods but may return to normal at other times. Functional assays of C1 INH also should be performed to detect the 15% of patients with normal C1 INH levels.

Treatment. Emergency management of an acute attack includes maintenance of the airway and tracheostomy, if necessary. The administration of epinephrine, H_1 antihistamines, glucocorticoids, and salicylates is generally ineffective. Antifibrinolytic agents such as epsilon-aminocaproic acid and tranexamic acid have been used, but significant side effects limit their long-term use. The treatment for HAE is the administration of either danazol or stanozolol, which corrects the defect and restores C4 levels toward normal. These androgens are not recommended for use in children. Purified C1 INH is not readily available but has been used with success for intermittent attacks and prophylactic administration.

References

Behrman RE (ed): Nelson Textbook of Pediatrics. 14th ed. Philadelphia, WB Saunders, 1992, Sec. 11.43.

Huston DP, Bressler RB: Urticaria and angioedema. Med Clin North Am 76:804, 1992.

Kaplan AP: Urticaria and angioedema. In Middleton E Jr, Reed CE, Ellis EF et al (eds): Allergy Principles and Practice. 4th ed. St. Louis, CV Mosby-Year Book, 1993, p 1553.

ATOPIC DERMATITIS/ECZEMA

Atopic dermatitis is a common skin disorder of infancy and childhood affecting 3–5% of children before 5 yr of age. Seventy percent of affected children have first degree relatives exhibiting some form of allergic disease; 30–50% of children with atopic dermatitis will go on to develop allergic rhinitis or asthma. Approximately 60% of affected children develop atopic dermatitis in the 1st yr of life and 90% within the first 5 yr of life.

Pathogenesis. The cause of atopic dermatitis is unknown. Antigen-specific IgE, demonstrated by either skin testing or immunoassay, has been detected in affected patients but does not always play a pathophysiologic role. The elevated IgE levels may be related to disordered control of IgE synthesis caused by a deficiency of suppressor T cell function. The skin of patients with atopic dermatitis reacts abnormally to light strokes (white dermographism) and histamine or acetylcholine (delayed

blanching). The skin also demonstrates abnormal rates of cooling and warming.

Clinical Manifestations. The hallmark of atopic dermatitis is severe pruritus, which is a constant feature and creates an "itch–scratch–itch cycle." Atopic dermatitis may be defined as an "itch that rashes, not a rash that itches." Pruritus leads to incessant scratching and rubbing.

Three distinct clinical phases have been described: infantile, childhood, and adult. The infantile stage begins between 2 and 6 mo of age and affects the cheeks, forehead, and extensor surfaces of the extremities. It is characterized by pruritus, erythema, papules, vesicles, oozing, and crusting. It frequently resolves between 3 and 5 yr of life. The childhood stage occurs between 4 and 10 yr of age, involving the popliteal and antecubital fossae, wrists, and ankles. Eruptions are dry and papular in appearance, extremely pruritic, and chronic. Flexor rather than extensor surfaces are involved, and skin thickening by lichenification is common. The adult stage begins at puberty and involves eyelids (loss of eyebrows because of rubbing), neck, flexor folds, upper arms, and dorsal aspects of hands, feet, fingers, and toes. In the adult stage, the lesions are most localized and often dry and thick, forming large, lichenified plaques. Weeping, crusting, and exudation may occur in both the childhood and adult stages, but these signs usually indicate secondary infection.

Atopic dermatitis tends to remit and exacerbate. It has been estimated that 75% of affected individuals outgrow the disorder by adolescence, and it is extremely rare over 40 yr of age. Typically, the eruption becomes milder with age, and longer remissions occur.

Diagnosis. The diagnostic criteria are based on a combination of signs, symptoms, and associated family history (Table 8–16). However, eczematous lesions are not exclusively due to atopic dermatitis, and a variety of metabolic, immunodeficiency, and congenital skin disorders should be considered (Table 8–17). In early infancy, seborrheic dermatitis (cradle cap) may be the most difficult to differentiate. *Seborrheic dermatitis* typically occurs earlier than atopic dermatitis and is minimally pruritic. The lesions begin on the scalp with characteristically yellow, greasy-appearing scales. Occasionally, a skin biopsy may be necessary to rule out other serious causes of eczematous eruptions, such as Letterer-Siwe disease.

Laboratory Findings. The eosinophil count and serum IgE level are often elevated. IgE levels wax

Table 8–16. Diagnostic Criteria for Atopic
Dermatitis—Absolute Features

The patient must have each of the following:

1. Pruritus
2. Typical morphology and distribution
   a. Flexural, lichenification in adults
   b. Facial and extensor involvement in infants and children
3. Tendency toward chronic or chronically relapsing dermatitis

plus

Two or more of the following features:

1. Personal or family history of atopic disease (asthma, allergic rhinitis, atopic dermatitis)
2. Immediate skin test reactivity
3. White dermatographism and/or delayed blanching to cholinergic agents
4. Anterior subcapsular cataracts

or

Four or more of the following features:

1. Xerosis (dry skin) ichthyosis/hyperlinear palms (increased palmar skin creases)
2. Pityriasis alba (dry, white patches on cheeks)
3. Keratosis pilaris (dry, thickened hair follicles on extensor surface of upper arm)
4. Facial pallor/infraorbital darkening
5. Dennie-Morgan infraorbital fold
6. Elevated serum IgE
7. Keratoconus
8. Tendency toward nonspecific hand dermatitis
9. Tendency toward repeated cutaneous infections

(From Hanifin JM, Lovits WC: Newer concepts of atopic dermatitis. Arch Dermatol 113:663, 1977.)

and wane with the activity of the disease. A more detailed immunologic evaluation may be necessary in the presence of failure to thrive and recurrent systemic infections. Skin tests may have a role in identifying offending allergens.

Table 8–17. Differential Diagnosis of Atopic
Dermatitis

Seborrheic dermatitis	Agammaglobulinemia
Diaper dermatitis	Ataxia–telangiectasia
Contact dermatitis	Hyper-IgE syndrome
Scabies	Leiner disease (C5 deficiency)
Psoriasis	Histiocytosis X (Letterer-Siwe
Fungal infections	disease)
Drug reactions	Acrodermatitis enteropathica
Hartnup syndrome	Phenylketonuria
Ichthyosis vulgaris	Pellagra
Wiskott-Aldrich	Biotinidase deficiency
syndrome	Erythrokeratoderma variabilis

Complications. The most common complication of atopic dermatitis is bacterial infection by *Staphylococcus aureus* (90%) and beta-hemolytic streptococci. A more serious complication is eczema herpeticum (Kaposi varicelliform eruption), which is caused by herpes simplex type I. It is clinically indistinguishable from eczema vaccinatum, which occurs as a complication of smallpox vaccination. Patients with atopic dermatitis also are more susceptible to molluscum contagiosum and verruca vulgaris wart viruses. The increased susceptibility to these viral infections may result from a combination of reduced cell-mediated immunity, depressed phagocytic function, and chronically excoriated skin. Other complications of atopic dermatitis include cataract formation, keratoconus, and otitis externa.

Treatment. Therapy is directed at controlling the dryness, inflammation, and pruritus. General measures include avoiding extremes of temperature and humidity, chemicals, soaps, certain allergy-triggering foods, wool, and synthetic materials. Scratching may be prevented by covering the lesions. Humidification of the house in winter may be helpful.

The treatment will depend on whether the patient presents in the acute or chronic phase. The acute phase is characterized by intense pruritus, marked erythema, and generalized crusty, weepy lesions. Removal of the crusts and exudate can be accomplished with cool, wet dressings consisting of Burow solution applied to the affected regions for 15–30 min, 4 times daily. Systemic antibiotics should be employed for secondary infection. Aveeno baths in combination with wet dressings reduce pruritus and inflammation. Antihistamines should be used to control the pruritus. Diphenhydramine (Benadryl), 5 mg/kg/day, or hydroxyzine (Atarax), 2 mg/kg/day, are quite effective. Topical steroids suppress inflammation and decrease pruritus. Initially, more potent fluorinated steroids should be applied topically to affected areas on the trunk and limbs until a clinical response occurs, after which less potent preparations can be substituted. Hydrocortisone cream (1%) should be used for affected areas of the head and neck.

Maintenance therapy of atopic dermatitis is more difficult. Management of chronic atopic dermatitis is directed at rehydration of the skin with emollients and appropriate bathing. The emollients are applied frequently throughout the day to reduce skin dryness and break the "itch–scratch–itch" cycle. A mild nonirritating soap (Neutrogena, Aveeno) may be used to wash. When the lubricant is applied, it is best administered over slightly moistened skin. In general, frequent bathing with irritant soap and water should be avoided because it will further dry the skin. Topical steroids should be applied frequently if flare-ups occur and, subsequently, should be tapered over a period of days. Topical steroids must be used cautiously in children because of potential systemic absorption and subsequent adrenal suppression. Local side effects also may occur, including skin atrophy, striae formation, and acneiform eruptions. Systemic steroids should be avoided whenever possible because of the potential for adrenal suppression and to avoid the rebound that occurs when the steroids are stopped.

Immunotherapy has no role in treatment and may exacerbate the dermatitis.

References

Behrman RE (ed): Nelson Textbook of Pediatrics. 14th ed. Philadelphia, WB Saunders, 1992, Sec. 11.42.

Bernhisel Broadbent J, Sampson HA: Food hypersensitivity and atopic dermatitis. Pediatr Clin North Am 35:1115, 1988.

Hanifin JM: Atopic dermatitis. In Middleton E Jr, Reed CE, Ellis EF, et al (eds): Allergy Principles and Practice. 4th ed. St. Louis, CV Mosby-Year Book, 1993, p 1581.

DRUG ALLERGY AND ADVERSE DRUG REACTIONS

An adverse drug reaction is any undesirable response to a drug occurring during or following a course of therapy. Adverse drug reactions may be divided into two major groups—predictable and unpredictable. Approximately 70–80% of adverse drug reactions are predictable, dose dependent, and related to the pharmacologic action of the drug. The latter include direct local or systemic *toxic effects* (e.g., morphine overdose); unavoidable, undesirable *side effects* (e.g., antihistamine drowsiness); indirect *secondary effects* (changed bacterial flora from antibiotics); and *drug interactions* (e.g., decrease of theophylline metabolism by cimetidine).

Unpredictable reactions usually are dose independent and related to the susceptible patient's immunologic response (allergy) or to genetic differences in susceptible patients (idiosyncrasy). Differences in drug metabolism also produce some idiosyncratic reactions. *Intolerance* is an expected adverse reaction that occurs at a lower than expected dosage. The classic example of a *coincidental* reaction is the appearance of a viral exanthem during a course of antibiotic therapy. *Psychogenic reactions* are the attribution of symptoms to a drug when the reaction actually is due to a psychologic reason. Drug teratogenicity and maternal–child drug transfer also must be considered as potential adverse drug reactions. As many as 5% of admissions to medical and pediatric services result from adverse drug reactions.

Pathophysiology. Most drugs are simple organic chemicals of low molecular weight and are not complete immunogens. They are haptens and require binding to a carrier molecule, such as a serum protein or a cell surface, to become immunogenic. The immune response may be directed at the hapten (which is generally a metabolic breakdown product of the drug) or the carrier protein (autoimmunity). A classification of the types of hypersensitivity–immune drug reactions is discussed under Hypersensitivity Reactions. Drugs also produce pseudoallergic reactions by nonspecific liberation of mast cell histamine, mimicking type I reactions (intravenous contrast dyes, vancomycin [red man syndrome], narcotics).

Clinical Manifestations. Clinical manifestations of hypersensitivity reactions are protean and may involve any organ system. Skin eruptions are the most common manifestations of drug allergy and include urticaria; angioedema; maculopapular, morbilliform, or erythematous eruptions; eczema; erythema nodosum; and fixed-drug eruptions. More serious non–IgE-mediated reactions, such as *Stevens-Johnson syndrome* (erythema multiforme) and toxic epidermal necrolysis or *Lyell syndrome* (sulfonamides, anticonvulsants, nonsteroidal antiinflammatory agents), may be potentially life threatening. Generalized nondermatologic reactions, such as anaphylaxis, serum sickness, vasculitis, and drug-induced autoimmunity, may occur independently. Fever can be the single sign of an adverse drug reaction in children. Drug reactions during anesthesia may be due to the malignant hyperthermia syndrome (halothane, succinylcholine), anaphylaxis to latex from the gloves of surgeons, or non–IgE-mediated histamine release (narcotics, d-tubocurare). A drug reaction always must be considered as potentially responsible for any unexplained finding or complication that occurs during the course of an illness.

Diagnosis. The history is most helpful in making the diagnosis. Allergic reactions typically do not resemble the known pharmacologic effects of the drug. An initial induction period of 7–10 days is necessary unless a drug possessing a cross-reacting structure has been introduced previously. A temporal relationship between drug administration and clinical manifestations should be established, although occasionally the interval can be prolonged. Discontinuation of the drug and subsequent recovery in several days is presumptive evidence of drug allergy.

Laboratory Findings. There is no single test to diagnose drug allergy. Immediate-type skin testing can be used to diagnose IgE-mediated reactions (e.g., antisera, hormones, penicillin). Skin testing is unreliable for other haptens. Delayed-type testing may be helpful in certain types of contact skin reactions. Patch testing may be predictive for contact dermatitis and photoallergic reactions. Skin testing does have significant risks and should not be performed without careful consideration.

In vitro laboratory tests are not very helpful, except in certain circumstances. Rarely, elevation of serum IgE and eosinophilia may occur during an acute reaction. The detection of drug-induced IgG and IgM antibodies may be helpful in hematologic reactions, such as drug-induced thrombocytopenia, hemolytic anemia, and agranulocytosis. Specific antipenicillin IgE, IgG, and IgM may be detected in penicillin hypersensitivity.

Prevention. Potential risks may be reduced by carefully considering prior history of drug reactions, availability of predictive tests prior to administration, alternative drugs when indicated, and pretreatment with antiallergy medications. The oral route is preferred because it is the least sensitizing.

If a known drug allergy does exist, it may be possible to "desensitize" a patient to the specific drug when it must be administered and no alternative treatment exists. This approach has been used successfully in patients with penicillin allergy and among those with positive skin tests to immunization materials (see Penicillin Hypersensitivy later).

Treatment. The initial treatment of a drug reaction is withdrawal of the offending drug. Symptomatic treatment is directed at controlling the clinical manifestations until the reaction subsides. Colloid baths, emollients, and topical steroids are helpful in treating cutaneous eruptions. Subcutaneous epinephrine, intravenous pressor agents, and volume expanders may be necessary to treat anaphylaxis. Non–life-threatening reactions can be treated with antihistamines such as diphenhydramine or hydroxyzine. Glucocorticoids will completely control most allergic reactions and are in-

dicated when symptoms are severe. Doses of prednisone at 1–2 mg/kg/day usually are sufficient.

Penicillin Hypersensitivity

Penicillin is the most common cause of serious allergic drug reactions in children (~3% of patients). Anaphylaxis has been reported to occur following parenteral, oral, topical, and inhalational routes, although parenteral administration is the most likely route to produce anaphylaxis (~0.02% of treatments). Nonetheless, because of inappropriate diagnosis, as many as 85% of patients who had some reaction to penicillin may be able to tolerate the drug on readministration.

Pathophysiology. Penicillin is a low-molecular-weight compound that is unable to elicit an immune response unless it combines with a carrier such as a protein, polysaccharide, or cell membrane. When penicillin G (benzylpenicillin) is degraded, the beta-lactam ring opens and reacts with tissue proteins to form the benzylpenicilloyl (BPO) group, which is referred to as the "major determinant" because approximately 95% of benzylpenicillin reacts in this manner. The remaining available haptens, "minor determinants," account for 5% of products responsible for immediate reactions.

Penicillin is capable of eliciting antibody responses of all major classes as well as producing delayed-type hypersensitivity. Immediate reactions occurring within 1 hr after administration are mediated by IgE directed against the minor determinants and, on rare occasions, the major determinants. Accelerated reactions, occurring between 1 and 72 hr, and delayed reactions, occurring later than 72 hr after administration, are mediated by BPO-specific IgE, which may be modified by the presence of BPO-specific IgG acting as a "blocking antibody." BPO-specific IgG and IgM have been associated with hemolytic anemia, maculopapular eruptions, and urticaria. Delayed-type hypersensitivity reactions have been associated with contact dermatitis.

Clinical Manifestations. Penicillin may produce a wide variety of hypersensitivity reactions. Reactions may be systemic (e.g., anaphylaxis, vasculitis), cutaneous (e.g., urticaria, angioedema, maculopapular eruptions), hematologic (e.g., Coombs-positive hemolytic anemia), and renal (e.g., interstitial nephritis). Occasionally, penicillin may be responsible for more severe cutaneous eruptions such as Stevens-Johnson syndrome, exfoliative dermatitis, and toxic epidermal necrolysis.

A maculopapular, non-urticarial rash during *ampicillin administration* occurs in 5–10% of patients. It is non-IgE mediated and does not correlate with prior history of penicillin therapy. The incidence of the rash is higher in certain viral infections, such as mononucleosis and cytomegalovirus. The maculopapular eruption is not necessarily an indication to discontinue the drug, and the rash may resolve despite continued therapy. To avoid falsely labeling patients as penicillin allergic, it is important to distinguish between penicillin hypersensitivity and the ampicillin rash.

Diagnosis. Penicillin hypersensitivity can be diagnosed by in vivo skin tests. Skin testing with both the major and minor determinants must be performed to detect the full spectrum of IgE activity. The major determinant is commercially available as a penicilloyl-polylysine (Pre-Pen). The minor determinants are not commercially available but some persons sensitized to minor determinants can be identified by skin tests with diluted penicillin G. Skin testing is performed using a combination of prick testing, and, if negative, intradermal testing with appropriate dilutions of the above antigens. Testing with both Pre-Pen and penicillin G will identify 95% of potential reactors. Skin tests are not predictive in non–IgE-mediated reactions.

Treatment. The treatment of a penicillin reaction is to discontinue the drug. If penicillin administration is mandatory in a penicillin-allergic patient, penicillin desensitization may be necessary. The desensitization procedure varies with the level of sensitivity and the route of drug administration. Desensitization has been successfully accomplished using the oral, subcutaneous, and intravenous routes. The desensitization process involves the administration of gradually increasing amounts of drug over a short period of time by personnel experienced in the procedure and capable of treating anaphylaxis. Once penicillin has been stopped for more than 48 hrs following a desensitization procedure, the patient is no longer considered "desensitized," and future administration would require similar precautions.

References

Behrman RE (ed): Nelson Textbook of Pediatrics. 14th ed. Philadelphia, WB Saunders, 1992, Sec. 11.46.

Blaiss MS, de Shazo RD: Drug allergy. Pediatr Clin North Am 35:1131, 1988.

International Rheumatic Fever Study Group: Allergic reactions to long-term benzathine penicillin prophylaxis for rheumatic fever. Lancet 337:1308, 1991.

Weiss M: Drug allergy. Med Clin North Am 76:789, 1992.

INSECT HYPERSENSITIVITY

Allergic reactions to insect stings result in significant morbidity in children. Stinging female insects of the order Hymenoptera include honeybees, wasps, yellow jackets, hornets, and fire ants. Although the majority of allergic reactions occur in individuals under 20 yr of age, children are at lower risk for subsequent serious systemic reactions than are adults.

Clinical Manifestations. Reactions are classified as immediate, occurring within minutes to several hours after the sting, or delayed, occurring from several hours to weeks following the sting (Table 8–18). Anaphylaxis, the most serious reaction, follows a sting and occurs in 0.4–0.8% of the population. Symptoms of anaphylaxis may involve the skin (e.g., generalized urticaria, flushing, angioedema), the cardiovascular system (e.g., circulatory collapse and hypotension), the respiratory tract (e.g., upper airway edema of the pharynx, epiglottis, trachea; bronchospasm), and gastrointestinal tract (e.g., diarrhea, cramps).

Pathophysiology. Venom-specific IgE antibodies are produced following an initial exposure to insect venom and become bound to tissue mast cells and circulating basophils. Local reactions are due to venom-associated histamine, formic acid,

Table 8–18. Classification of Sting Reactions

Immediate	
Normal	Localized swelling (less than 2 inches), transient pain, erythema all lasting less than 24 hr
Toxic	Follows multiple stings, produced by exogenous vasoactive amines in venom
Large local	Swelling contiguous to sting lasting more than 24 hr
Systemic	Generalized symptoms involving signs or symptoms remote from sting site; may be non–life threatening (distal urticaria, angioedema), or life threatening (laryngeal edema, bronchospasm, hypotension)
Delayed	
Systemic	May take several clinical forms, including serum sickness–like reactions, myocarditis, transverse myelitis, nephrosis

hyaluronidase, and kinins. Following a sting, degranulation and release of mediators may result in local signs and symptoms or in anaphylaxis.

Diagnosis.   A positive history of an immediate systemic reaction is necessary before venom testing and immunotherapy should be considered. The honeybee has a barbed stinger that remains embedded following a sting. The more aggressive yellow jacket and hornet may sting unprovoked and repeatedly. Nonetheless, identification of the offending insect is usually difficult.

Laboratory Findings.   Venom skin testing is the most sensitive means to detect venom-specific IgE. Five purified venoms are available: honeybee, yellow jacket, wasp, white hornet, and yellow hornet. No good correlation exists between the severity of the systemic reaction and the degree of skin test positivity. Venom-specific IgE antibodies may also be measured by immunoassay.

Treatment.   Avoiding bright clothing and exterminating infested areas will decrease the risk of accidental stings. Local reactions should be treated initially by removing the stinger if present, cleaning the site, applying cold compresses, and administering oral antihistamines and analgesics. In cases of severe, large local reactions, a short course of prednisone may be recommended.

Treatment of systemic reactions should be very aggressive. Epinephrine at a dose of 0.01 mL/kg of a 1:1000 solution (maximum 0.3 mL) is the drug of choice rather than an antihistamine, although both may be administered concurrently. Theophylline, pressor agents, and intravenous colloid solutions are necessary for more severe reactions. Glucocorticoids are not first-line drugs for the reaction because of their delayed onset of action, but they should be administered to prevent recurrent or prolonged symptoms.

Patients at risk should be instructed in the use of injectable epinephrine. Automatic injections, such as EpiPen (delivering 0.30 mg) and EpiPen Jr. (delivering 0.15 mg), are especially useful.

Patients with histories of normal, large local, toxic, or delayed systemic reactions are not candidates for *immunotherapy*. Venom immunotherapy is recommended for pediatric patients exhibiting a systemic reaction that involves the cardiovascular or respiratory tracts but not for patients having cutaneous reactions only. In childhood, cutaneous systemic reactions carry a 10% risk that a subsequent systemic reaction will occur on re-sting. The therapy is effective, with almost a 98% nonreaction rate on subsequent stings.

Biting Insects

Unusually large local reactions may develop to the salivary secretions of biting insects such as mosquitos, flies, and fleas in certain susceptible patients. The reaction appears urticarial (*papular urticaria*) and probably results from vasoactive or irritant substances present in the insect secretions. The immune mechanism is unknown. Treatment consists of avoidance, antihistamines for pruritus, topical corticosteroids, and treatment of secondary infection, if present.

References

Behrman RE (ed): Nelson Textbook of Pediatrics. 14th ed. Philadelphia, WB Saunders, 1992, Sec. 11.47.

Valentine M, Schuberth K, Kagey-Sobotka A, et al: The value of immunotherapy with venom in children with allergy to insect stings. N Engl J Med 323:1601, 1990.

ANAPHYLAXIS

Anaphylaxis is an acute, generalized allergic reaction in which signs and symptoms are immunologically mediated following exposure to an antigen. *Anaphylactoid reaction* refers to a reaction clinically similar or identical to anaphylaxis but not immunologically mediated because it occurred in the absence of an antigen-antibody interaction.

Etiology.   Antigen can be introduced by inhaled, oral, topical, and parenteral routes. Most cases of anaphylaxis are due to hypersensitivity to drugs, food, or insect stings. Penicillin causes anaphylaxis more frequently than any other drug. Any food can cause anaphylaxis, but certain foods have greater risk (e.g., nuts, fish, and egg white) (see Drug Allergy and Adverse Drug Reactions). Occasionally, in a condition termed *recurrent idiopathic anaphylaxis*, no etiologic agent is found. Exercise-induced anaphylaxis also occurs.

Pathophysiology.   Anaphylaxis is a type I hypersensitivity reaction mediated by IgE bound to mast cells and to basophils (Fig. 8–3), leading to the secretion and activation of vasoactive, chemotactic, and inflammatory mediators. Histamine levels are high during anaphylaxis. Non-IgE mechanisms also may cause anaphylaxis by activating mast cells via the anaphylatoxins C3a, C4a, and C5a. Certain drugs, such as opiates, radiocontrast media, and curare, can react with mast cells to release mediators nonimmunologically.

Clinical Manifestations.   The severity of the reaction is directly proportional to the rapidity of onset.

Symptoms usually occur within 30 min of challenge and may involve the skin (urticaria, flushing, angioedema, pruritus); respiratory tract (stridor, hoarseness, cough, wheezing, chest tightness, tachypnea, rhinitis); cardiovascular system (hypotension, tachycardia, shock, cardiac arrhythmias); and gastrointestinal tract (dysphagia, nausea, vomiting, diarrhea, abdominal pain). Early manifestations such as uneasiness, apprehension, and diaphoresis may herald the onset of more severe signs and symptoms. In fatal reactions, death may occur within moments after exposure to antigen.

Diagnosis. The diagnosis usually is apparent from the history and the physical examination. Anaphylaxis should be considered in any pediatric patient who presents with vascular collapse. Detection of IgE by skin testing or immunoassay to a specific antigen must correlate with the history, and a negative result does not rule out anaphylactic sensitivity. The *differential diagnosis* of anaphylactic shock includes cardiac failure, sepsis, endotoxic shock, hemorrhage, hereditary angioedema, serum sickness, pheochromocytoma, systemic mastocytosis, and vasovagal collapse. Vasovagal collapse is most often confused with anaphylaxis but is characterized by bradycardia, nausea, and the absence of respiratory and cutaneous symptoms.

Treatment. Prompt treatment is extremely important and should relate to the organ system involved and the severity of symptoms. After the airway is stabilized, epinephrine should be given by the intramuscular or the subcutaneous route. If an insect sting or desensitization injection caused the anaphylaxis, one half the dose of epinephrine should be injected at the site. Venous access for intravenous vasopressor medications and volume replacement (normal saline) must be obtained. Glucocorticoids have no role in treating the early stages of anaphylaxis but should be administered later for their anti-inflammatory actions. Diphenhydramine and cimetidine should be administered to block the systemic effects of histamine released during anaphylaxis and may be especially useful in treating urticaria and angioedema.

Prevention. Agents known to have precipitated anaphylaxis should be avoided, including structurally related cross-reacting allergens. In life-threatening situations that require the administration of a drug known to cause anaphylaxis (e.g., penicillin, insulin), desensitization may be performed in certain cases. In selected patients known to be sensitive to a particular drug, premedication with antihistamines and steroids may be beneficial. A Medic-Alert tag may be helpful in identifying the patient at risk. Epinephrine also should be available for the patient at risk.

References

Behrman RE (ed): Nelson Textbook of Pediatrics. 14th ed. Philadelphia, WB Saunders, 1992, Sec. 11.44.
Bochner B, Lichtenstein L: Anaphylaxis. N Engl J Med 324: 1785, 1991.
Yjunginger JW: Anaphylaxis. Curr Prob Pediatr 22:130, 1992.

SERUM SICKNESS

Serum sickness results from an immunologic response to injected foreign proteins mediated by the deposition of immune complexes. It is a type III hypersensitivity reaction and is relatively uncommon today because of the decreased use of heterologous animal antisera that had been administered in the past to treat infections such as rabies and diphtheria. IgE-mediated events also occur. Serum sickness–like reactions may occur following administration of nonprotein drugs, vaccines, insect venoms, allergy extracts, and hormones. Penicillin is the most common cause of these reactions. Nonetheless, the incidence is greater for cefaclor (0.14%), followed by trimethoprim–sulfamethoxazole (0.09%), penicillin (0.04%), and amoxicillin (0.007%). In contrast to other allergic reactions, serum sickness develops during or after the first exposure to antigen and needs no prior sensitization.

Pathogenesis. Following the introduction of antigen, immunoglobulins of all five classes may be formed after a latent period of 4–10 days. IgG and IgM are efficient complement activators and are most responsible for some of the manifestations of serum sickness. Circulating immune complexes deposit in small blood vessels, a process facilitated by release of vasoactive amines, such as histamine, that increase vascular permeability. Immune complex deposition activates the complement pathway by producing C3a, C5a, and C5,6,7 and by subsequently recruiting polymorphonuclear leukocytes. Vasoactive amines may be released either by antigen combining with specific IgE on basophils or by complement activation with IgG and IgM, resulting in anaphylatoxin production and subsequent mast cell and basophil degranulation. Proteolytic enzymes released from the lysosomal granules of the neutrophils mediate tissue damage and are responsible for the widespread vasculitis.

Clinical Manifestations. Serum sickness is characterized by pruritus, fever, polyarticular arthritis–arthralgia, lymphadenopathy, and urticaria–angioedema. It usually begins 7–14 days after antigen administration. An accelerated reaction may develop within 2–4 days if prior sensitization has occurred. Symptoms usually last 1–2 wk before spontaneously subsiding.

The onset of symptoms may be heralded by pruritus, pain, and swelling at the injection site. Skin eruptions occur in 90% of cases and may include urticaria (most common eruption), erythema multiforme, angioedema, and maculopapular and purpuric lesions. A characteristic serpiginous erythematous eruption on the hands and feet has been described. Arthritis or arthralgia is present in 10–50% of cases, affecting large and, occasionally, small joints. Lymphadenopathy occurs in 10–20% of patients and is usually regional, involving nodes draining the antigen injection site. Generalized lymphadenopathy associated with splenomegaly also may occur. Cardiovascular, pulmonary, and renal involvement is uncommon, but myocarditis, pericarditis, pleuritis, and nephritis do occur. Involvement of the nervous system, including cranial nerve palsies, optic neuritis, transient hemiplegia, and Guillain-Barré syndrome, rarely may occur.

Laboratory Findings. Laboratory studies usually are not helpful because no universal abnormality exists. Leukopenia and leukocytosis, with or without associated eosinophilia, are seen. The erythrocyte sedimentation rate often is elevated. Circulating immune complexes have been detected. Proteinuria, microscopic hematuria, and hyaline casts may be present on urinalysis. Serum complement levels (C3, C4, CH50) are not always decreased. Circulating plasma cells occasionally are seen on peripheral smear. Forssman antibodies may be detected.

Treatment. Treatment is usually symptomatic because the nature of the disease is self-limited. Antihistamines may relieve the urticaria and, if given prophylactically at the time of antigen exposure, potentially may decrease the incidence of serum sickness by inhibiting the actions of vasoactive amines. Aspirin is effective for symptoms of fever and joint pain. Severe cases should be treated with corticosteroids. Avoiding the offensive agent is the way to prevent the syndrome.

References

Behrman RE (ed): Nelson Textbook of Pediatrics. 14th ed. Philadelphia, WB Saunders, 1992, Sec. 11.45.

Bielory L, Gascon P, Lawley TJ, et al: Human serum sickness: A prospective analysis of 35 patients treated with equine anti-thymocyte globulin for bone marrow failure. Medicine 67:40, 1988.

Heckbert S, Stryker W, Coltin K, et al: Serum sickness in children after antibiotic exposure: Estimates of occurrence and morbidity in a health maintenance organization population. Am J Epidemiol 132:336, 1990.

Lawley TJ, Frank MM: Immune complexes and allergic disease. In Middleton E Jr, Reed CE, Ellis EF, et al (eds): Allergy Principles and Practice. 4th ed. St. Louis, CV Mosby-Year Book, 1993, p 990.

Rheumatic Diseases of Childhood   9

Deborah W. Kredich

The rheumatic diseases of childhood (autoimmune or collagen vascular diseases) are entities characterized by inflammatory changes that involve the connective tissues in the body. Common manifestations of rheumatic diseases include **synovitis** (arthritis), or inflammation of the joint synovium (Table 9–1); **enthesopathy**, or inflammation at the insertion of a ligament to a bone (sacroiliac joint arthritis, achilles tendinitis, plantar fasciitis); **serositis**, or inflammation of a serosal lining (Table 9–2); **myositis**, or muscle inflammation; **autoantibody** production (Table 9–3); and **vasculitis** (Table 9–4). Inflammation may be localized in one joint or tendon group or it may be generalized. Local inflammation is characterized by pain, swelling, erythema, limited range of motion, and warmth, whereas systemic inflammation is manifested by fever, malaise, anorexia, weight loss, and myalgias.

Currently, rheumatology is a descriptive subspecialty, and the pathophysiology of disorders included in this category is not precisely understood. Inflammation and tissue injury in rheumatic diseases are mediated by the immune response from the activation of monocytes, lymphocytes, polymorphonuclear leukocytes, complement, and antibodies. Specific autoantibodies may be produced, as are antiplatelet antibodies in systemic lupus erythematosus (SLE); or the injury may be mediated by deposition of non–tissue-specific antigen–antibody complexes in organs with large capillary beds, such as the glomerulus of the kidney. Furthermore, tissue damage may be mediated by local activation of macrophages and lymphocytes, as occurs in the synovium of patients with adult-type rheumatoid arthritis. In the latter condition, local inflammatory cells accumulate, as a result of immune complexes, and activate complement, which attracts more inflammatory cells. Cytokines, phospholipids, kinins, and other mediators of inflammation are released into the tissue, and hydrolytic enzymes (e.g., proteases and collagenases) are released, producing local damage. Synovitis produces synovial hypertrophy (pannus), which migrates into the articular cartilage. This hypertrophy, together with hydrolytic enzymes, further destroys, demineralizes, and enhances mechanical injury of the tissue. Although the description of each disorder is distinct, the individual patient often has overlapping signs and symptoms that may make a precise diagnosis difficult.

LABORATORY TESTS USED TO ASSESS RHEUMATIC DISEASES

Acute-Phase Reactants

The Westergren sedimentation rate (WSR), or erythrocyte sedimentation rate (ESR), is the most commonly used test to assess the activity of a rheumatic disease. It is nonspecifically increased in response to systemic inflammation (rheumatic disease, infection, malignancy). The sedimentation rate requires erythrocyte rouleaux formation and an interaction with fibrinogen or macroglobulins; afibrinogenemia, anemia, and sickle cell anemia may reduce the sedimentation rate. Other acute-phase reactants that are elevated in response to inflammation include the C-reactive protein, which is rapidly synthesized by the liver; platelet count; and total hemolytic complement (CH50). Any of the acute-phase reactants may be helpful in following the disease course in a given patient, but some patients will have active inflammatory disease with normal values for one or more acute-phase reactants.

Rheumatoid Factors

Rheumatoid factors are antibodies directed against the Fc portion of immunoglobulin (Ig) G. Most of the conventional tests for rheumatoid factor, such as the latex agglutination titer, detect rheumatoid factors that are IgM; IgG, IgA, and IgE rheumatoid factors can be measured by other techniques.

Table 9–1. Causes of Childhood Arthritis (Synovitis)

Common
Juvenile rheumatoid arthritis
Rheumatic fever
Systemic lupus erythematosus
Henoch-Schönlein purpura
Pyogenic infection (septic or immune complex)
Viral infection (parvovirus, rubella, mumps; possibly toxic synovitis)
Lyme disease
Serum sickness
Kawasaki disease

Less Common
Reflex sympathetic dystrophy
Diabetes mellitus
Leukemia
Reiter syndrome (enteric, genital)
Inflammatory bowel disease
Hypermobility syndrome
Dermatomyositis

Rare
Acneiform arthritis
Psoriatic
Wegener granulomatosis
Sarcoidosis
Scleroderma

A positive rheumatoid factor is not diagnostic. Most children with juvenile rheumatoid arthritis (JRA) are negative for conventional rheumatoid factors, whereas children with SLE and Henoch-Schönlein purpura may have rheumatoid factors. Rheumatoid factors also are present in viral infections, such as hepatitis B, and in other conditions including subacute bacterial endocarditis, sarcoidosis, tuberculosis, and congenital TORCH infections (toxoplasmosis, rubella, cytomegalovirus, and herpes simplex).

Table 9–2. Serositis

Manifestations
Pericarditis
Peritonitis
Pleuritis

Differential Diagnosis
Juvenile rheumatoid arthritis
Systemic lupus erythematosus
Tuberculosis
Viral (coxsackievirus)
Bacterial (meningococcus, gonococcus)
Malignancy

Table 9–3. Manifestations of Autoantibodies

Coombs-positive hemolytic anemia
Immune neutropenia
Immune thrombocytopenia
Thrombosis (anticardiolipin, antiphospholipid, lupus anticoagulant)
Immune lymphopenia

Antimitochondrial (primary biliary cirrhosis, SLE)
Antimicrosomal (chronic active hepatitis, SLE)
Antithyroid (thyroiditis, SLE)

Antinuclear Antibodies to Specific Nuclear Antigens and Associated Manifestations
Single-stranded DNA* (nonspecific, indicates inflammation)
Double-stranded DNA* (SLE, renal disease)
DNA-histone (drug-induced SLE)
Sm (Smith) (SLE, renal, central nervous system)
RNP (ribonucleoprotein) (SLE; Sjögren syndrome, scleroderma, polymyositis, MCTD)
Ro (Robert: SSA) (SLE; neonatal lupus–congenital heart block: Sjögren syndrome)
La (Lane: SSB) (SLE, Sjögren syndrome)
Jo-1 (polymyositis, dermatomysitis)
Sc1-70 (scleroderma)
Centromere (CREST syndrome, variant scleroderma)
PM-Sc1 (scleroderma, UCTD)

* Because antibodies to single-stranded DNA (ssDNA) are a nonspecific response to inflammatory diseases and because ssDNA may contaminate double-stranded DNA (dsDNA) preparations, the purer circular dsDNA of *Crithidia luciliae* (crithidia test) is preferred.
   CREST syndrome = calcinosis, Raynaud phenomenon, esophageal dysfunction, sclerodactyly, telangiectasia; SLE = systemic lupus erythematosus; UCTD = undifferentiated connective tissue disease; MCTD = mixed connective tissue disease.
   (Adapted from Condemi J: The autoimmune diseases. JAMA 268:2882, 1992.)

Antinuclear and Anticytoplasmic Antibodies (Table 9–3)

Autoantibodies against nuclear as well as cytoplasmic constituents often are found in the serum of patients with connective tissue diseases, but they also occur in individuals with nonrheumatic conditions (mononucleosis, endocarditis, chronic active hepatitis, malaria). Antinuclear antibodies (ANAs) are determined by indirect immunofluorescence techniques in which the patient's serum is incubated with a source of nuclei and a fluorescent-labeled immunoglobulin; the greatest dilution of serum at which a positive immunofluorescent pattern is observed then is recorded. Procedures differ in many laboratories, but frequently a 1:40 titer is the lowest dilution considered positive. The pattern of staining also is reported. The four major patterns are as follows:

Table 9–4. Vasculitis Syndrome

Type	Comment
Polyarteritis Nodosoa Group	
Polyarteritis nodosa (± hepatitis B antigenemia)	Multisystem—kidney, nerve, liver, skin; necrotizing vasculitis of small and medium muscular arteries
Churg-Strauss syndrome (allergic angiitis and granulomatosis)	Skin and pulmonary involvement; eosinophilia and asthma; granulomatous vasculitis of small and medium arteries
Polyangiitis overlap	Overlap of more than one of any type vasculitis with skin, lung, kidney, nerve involvement
Hypersensitivity Syndromes	
Henoch-Schönlein purpura	Palpable purpura, kidney, joint, intestine; inflammation of arteriole, capillary, and venule; leukocytoclastic vasculitis, IgA immune complexes
Serum sickness	Antigen–antibody hypocomplementemic, skin, joint, kidney
Vasculitis with infections	Meningococcemia, Rocky Mountain spotted fever
Connective tissue vasculitis (SLE, rheumatoid)	Cutaneous as SLE
Wegener Granulomatosis	Necrotizing granulomas; small and medium arteries; upper and lower respiratory tract, glomerulonephritis; positive anti-neutrophil cytoplasm antibodies
Giant Cell Arteritis	
Temporal/cranial	Medium-large arteries; retinal arteritis may cause blindness
Takayasu	Young women, inflammation of aortic arch
Others	
Behçet disease	Recurrent oral, gastrointestinal, and genital ulcers; uveitis; skin
Kawasaki disease	Arteritis, coronary artery aneurysm; immune complexes
Hypocomplementemic disease	Chronic urticaria

SLE = systemic lupus erythematosus.

1. *Speckled:* nonspecific for SLE and occurs in many connective tissue diseases (antigens include Sm, RNP, Ro, La, Jo-1, Scl-70, centromere; Table 9–3).
2. *Homogeneous:* also nonspecific and is the most common pattern seen in children with JRA who will develop uveitis.
3. *Rim (peripheral) pattern:* usually diagnostic of SLE (double-stranded DNA; Table 9–3) but is seen in a small proportion of SLE patients.
4. *Nucleolar:* most commonly seen in patients with scleroderma-like illnesses (PM-Scl; Table 9–3).

Complement

The various complement components (see Fig. 8–2), as well as the total hemolytic complement, may be elevated, as are the acute-phase reactants in rheumatic diseases. Decreased complement levels are noted in active SLE, particularly in SLE with nephritis; total hemolytic complement, an important screening test, is depressed in SLE and in various vasculitides. In addition, hereditary complement component deficiencies have been associated with familial cases of SLE and vasculitis.

Histocompatibility Antigens

Children with the human leukocyte antigen (HLA) B27 locus are at increased risk for ankylosing spondylitis, Reiter syndrome, psoriatic arthritis, and arthritis associated with inflammatory bowel disease. Seropositive polyarticular JRA is associated with the HLA-DR4 locus.

References

Behrman RE (ed): Nelson Textbook of Pediatrics. 14th ed. Philadelphia, WB Saunders, 1992, Sec. 11.50.
Condemi J: The autoimmune diseases. JAMA 268:2882, 1992.

JUVENILE RHEUMATOID ARTHRITIS

Arthritis occurring in an individual 16 yr of age or younger and persisting for at least 6 wk should suggest JRA when there is no other reason for the arthritis. JRA may be subdivided into three broad categories on the basis of the evolution of clinical manifestations over a 6-mo period. A child with JRA who exhibits initial temperature elevations greater than 39.4° C (103° F) for 2 wk, usually with a rash, is said to be in *systemic onset* (10%), regardless of how many joints are involved in the course of the illness. Patients who do not have fever or who have low-grade fever at presentation may be subdivided on the basis of the number of joints involved at the end of 6 mo; a child with four or fewer involved joints is termed *pauciarticular* (50%), and one with five or more involved joints is *polyarticular* (40%).

JRA is not a rare disease in childhood; it affects an estimated 100,000–250,000 children in the United States (incidence 1.4:10,000; prevalence 1:1000). The age of onset shows peaks at 1–3 yr and in the early teenage years.

Systemic-Onset JRA

Systemic-onset JRA is the most dramatic and least common form of the illness. It is the only type of JRA that affects males as frequently as females.

Clinical Manifestations.   The onset in children is usually 16 yr or younger, and the sexes are equally affected. These patients usually appear ill and often have high spiking fevers of at least 39.4° C (103° F) for many weeks. They usually have associated truncal erythematous macular rash, splenomegaly, hepatomegaly, and lymphadenopathy. Irritability and arthralgia/myalgia are prominent features, particularly during fever spikes. The characteristic rash consists of small, salmon-colored macules located on the trunk and extremities that come and go with the fever spikes; rarely, the rash is pruritic. Arthritis often is absent during the first weeks or even 6–8 mo of illness. Later in the course, chronic polyarticular arthritis may occur. Therefore, JRA becomes a suspected diagnosis and one of exclusion. The *differential diagnosis* includes occult infection (Epstein-Barr virus), malignancy (leukemia), and acute rheumatic fever (Table 9–5).

Other systemic features of the disease include serositis; asymptomatic pericarditis occurs with or without pleuritis, and abdominal serositis is less common. Myocarditis occasionally is seen. Growth retardation is a prominent feature of this type of illness. Chronic uveitis is an uncommon manifestation of systemic JRA.

Laboratory Findings.   There are no diagnostic laboratory features of systemic-onset JRA. The child typically has anemia that may be profound and is generally the normocytic/normochromic anemia of chronic disease. The white blood cell count frequently is elevated and may show a distinct shift to the left; often platelet counts are elevated, as are acute-phase reactants. Sedimentation rate usually is extremely high. The serum is uniformly negative for rheumatoid factors and ANAs.

Prognosis.   Some children have intermittent episodes of febrile illness for years after onset; others (25%) progress to severe chronic, destructive polyarticular joint disease without recurrent fevers. Death is uncommon in the course of JRA, but it is most likely to occur in the child in whom the condition had a systemic onset, in which case it usually is due to myocarditis or infection, especially if the child has been immunosuppressed.

Polyarticular JRA

Children in whom five or more joints have been involved in the first 6 mo of illness are further subcategorized into those who are seronegative (35%) and those who are seropositive (5%) for rheumatoid factor. Girls outnumber boys in both categories.

Invariably in *polyarticular disease* the small joints of the hands and, usually, the feet are involved. Large joint involvement also is common. The cervical spine, temporomandibular joint, sternoclavicular joint, and distal interphalangeal joints also may be affected. Systemic manifestations of disease are much less striking than in patients having disease with systemic onset; mild anemia, leukocytosis, fever, lymphadenopathy, and hepatosplenomegaly may occur.

Approximately one fourth of the *seronegative polyarticular JRA* patients have positive tests for ANAs; a few of these will have associated chronic uveitis. The onset of illness usually occurs when the child is 10 yr or younger. The course of the disease in this type of illness generally is favorable, with few extra-articular manifestations and 10–15% finally being categorized in functional class III or IV (Table 9–6). Seronegative JRA patients, in general, respond better to treatment with nonsteroidal anti-inflammatory drugs (NSAIDs) than do seropositive patients. The differential diagnosis includes Lyme disease, rheumatic fever, and SLE (Table 9–5).

Only about 5–8% of all children with chronic arthritis are *seropositive for rheumatoid factor*. The onset of illness usually occurs when the child is 9–16 yr of age. Most of these children have evidence of erosive, destructive arthritis on roentgenograms at the end of 1 yr of illness. Nodules over tendons

Table 9–5. Differential Diagnosis of Pediatric Arthritis Syndromes

Characteristic	Systemic Lupus Erythematosus	Juvenile Rheumatoid Arthritis	Rheumatic Fever	Lyme Disease	Leukemia	Gonococcemia	Kawasaki Disease
Sex	F > M	Type dependent	M = F	M = F	M = F	F > M	M = F
Age	10–20 yr	2–16 yr	5–15 yr	2–20 yr	2–10 yr	>12 yr	<4 yr
Arthralgia	Yes	Yes	Yes	Yes	Yes	Yes	Yes
Morning stiffness	Yes	Yes	No	No	No	No	No
Rash	Butterfly; discoid	Salmon-pink macules	Erythema marginatum	Erythema chronicum migrans	No	Palms/soles papulopustules	Diffuse maculopapular
Mono/pauciarticular	Yes	50%	No	Yes	Yes	Yes	Late onset
Polyarticular	Yes	Yes	Yes	Rare	Yes	No	Yes
Small joints	Yes	Yes	No	No	Yes	No	Yes
Temporomandibular joint	No	Rare	No	Rare	No	No	No
Eye disease	Uveitis/retinitis	Iridocyclitis	No	Keratitis	No	No	Conjunctivitis, uveitis
Total WBC count	Decreased	Increased	Normal to increased	Normal	Increased or neutropenia ± blasts	Increased	Increased
ANA	Positive	Positive (50%)	Negative	Negative	Negative	Negative	Negative
Rheumatoid factor	Positive	Positive (10%)	Negative	Negative	Negative	Negative	Negative
Other laboratory results	↓ Complement	—	↑ ASO	↑ Cryoglobulin, ↑ immune complexes	+ Bone marrow	+ Culture for GC	Thrombocytosis, ↑ immune complexes
Erosive arthritis	No, rare	Yes	No, rare	Rare	No	Yes	No
Other clinical manifestations	Proteinuria, serositis	Fever, serositis	Carditis, nodules, chorea	Carditis, neuropathy	Thrombocytopenia	Sexual activity, menses	Fever, lymphadenopathy; swollen hands/feet, mouth lesions
Pathogenesis	Autoimmune	Autoimmune	Group A streptococcus	Borrelia burgdorferi	Acute lymphoblastic leukemia	Neisseria gonorrhoeae	Unknown
Treatment	NSAIDs, steroids	NSAIDs	Penicillin prophylaxis, aspirin, steroids	Penicillin, tetracycline, ceftriaxone	Steroids, chemotherapy	Ceftriaxone, cefoxitin	Aspirin, intravenous immunoglobulins

ASO = antistreptolysin-O titer; GC = gonococcus; NSAID = nonsteroidal anti-inflammatory drug; WBC = white blood cell.

(elbows, knees, scalp) are seen more frequently in seropositive than seronegative polyarticular disease. Vasculitis (lung, skin) also may occur. Approximately half of these adolescents have severe unremitting disease with a functional outcome that puts them in class III or IV. Disease persists into adulthood, and the natural history is similar to that of adult-onset rheumatoid arthritis. About 50% of patients have positive ANA tests, and there is an association with HLA antigens DW4 and DR4.

Pauciarticular JRA

About half of all children with chronic arthritis of childhood have this form of disease. There are two prominent subgroups of pauciarticular JRA: (1) a younger group of patients, primarily female, who often have chronic insidious uveitis; and (2) older children with later onset of disease, more frequently male, who may have the subsequent disease course of spondyloarthropathy.

Clinical Manifestations. *Pauciarticular arthritis in the younger child* has a peak age of onset at about 2 yr. Large joints most commonly are involved, and systemic signs and symptoms of illness generally are absent. The knee is the most commonly involved joint, followed by ankles and elbows; the hip almost never is involved. The child occasionally

Table 9–6. American College of Rheumatology Revised Criteria for Classification of Functional Status in Rheumatoid Arthritis*

Class I	Completely able to perform usual activities of daily living (self-care, vocational, and avocational)
Class II	Able to perform usual self-care and vocational activities, but limited in avocational activities
Class III	Able to perform usual self-care activities, but limited in vocational and avocational activities
Class IV	Limited in ability to perform usual self-care, vocational, and avocational activities

* Usual self-care activities include dressing, feeding, bathing, grooming, and toileting. Avocational (recreational and/or leisure) and vocational (work, school, homemaking) activities are patient desired and age and sex specific.

(From Arthritis Rheum 35:498, 1992.)

may have small swollen joints in the hand or foot. Pain frequently is absent in these children, and the diagnosis may be made after months of asymptomatic swelling, leading to the slow development of contractures. The joint disease rarely is destructive, and, because it is not associated with systemic signs and symptoms, the child usually appears well otherwise. Localized growth disturbance may occur as a result of unilateral joint disease; this growth disturbance is particularly noticeable when arthritis is in the knee, because in this case it may lead to an overgrowth in the length of the affected leg. Signs and symptoms of uveitis are few (occasionally poor vision, red eye), and the diagnosis usually is made only with the aid of slit-lamp examination; therefore, there is a risk of blindness secondary to late diagnosis of eye disease. The differential diagnosis includes Lyme disease (Table 9–5).

Most *laboratory tests* are normal; these include hemoglobin level, sedimentation rate, and white blood cell count. Rheumatoid factor rarely is present, but many of the children have positive tests for ANAs (>50%). The presence of ANAs in the very young female patient with pauciarticular arthritis is closely associated with the development of chronic iridocyclitis. The disease is associated with HLA-DR5, -DR6, and -DR8.

Treatment of uveitis with local steroid eyedrops and dilating agents usually is successful. A minority of patients may require systemic steroids. Severe arthritis occurs in 10% of patients. If there is a *significant leg length discrepancy* from overgrowth of a leg, the child may experience a severe pelvic tilt, compensatory scoliosis, and a gait abnormality that is easily corrected by placing a lift on the shoe

of the normal (shorter) leg. The lift equalizes leg length and normalizes the gait.

Pauciarticular arthritis in older children usually occurs after 8 yr of age and has a propensity to involve the joints of the lower extremity in an asymmetric fashion; *enthesopathy* often occurs. Hips commonly are involved. The knee is the most commonly involved joint, and the ankle and the first metatarsophalangeal joint are the next. Some children have asymmetric upper extremity joint involvement. Many children have a positive family history of significant low back pain, immobility syndromes, psoriasis, inflammatory bowel disease, ankylosing spondylitis, or reactive (e.g., Reiter) arthritis.

The usual pattern is slowly diminishing motor performance and often attendant emotional depression. Commonly, the patient has a history of slowly decreasing exercise capacity, malaise, and nagging aches and pains. Occasionally, the child may have significant systemic signs accompanied by weight loss, fever, anorexia, and diffuse arthralgia/myalgia. In the first years of their illness, most children complain not of low back pain but rather of painful inflammation at points of insertion of tendons and ligaments (**entheses**). Therefore, a young boy may begin with pain in or about his Achilles tendon, around his knee, or in his plantar fascia. Much later, the actual joint effusion in the knee or the ankle may be detectable. Uveitis, when it occurs, tends to be acute in nature (decreased visual acuity, erythema), and is nondestructive; the symptoms are sufficient to lead the family to seek ophthalmologic assistance. Bowel disease and features of Reiter syndrome may occur.

Laboratory Tests. Older children with pauciarticular arthritis inevitably have normal findings on laboratory tests except, perhaps, children with constitutional symptoms, who may have markedly elevated sedimentation rates or depressed hemoglobin levels; these children frequently are positive for HLA-B27. Rheumatoid factor and ANA are negative.

General Characteristics of Arthritis in Childhood

Morning stiffness is characteristic of JRA as it is of adult rheumatoid arthritis, but children rarely complain specifically of stiffness as such; more often they responded "yes" to questions regarding "slowness in the morning." This morning stiffness may be ameliorated by setting an earlier time for arising, providing a warm morning bath, and using heating pads or electric blankets at night. Stiffness also occurs after periods of immobility, and teachers need to be reminded that children with arthritis need extra freedom to move about the classroom throughout the day.

Pain is variable in JRA. Many children experience little or no pain, but later in life this lack of pain often may conceal the presence of a long-standing arthritis, possibly accompanied by significant flexion contractures, before the joint disease finally is appreciated. Some children have significant pain or discomfort.

Generalized **growth retardation** may occur in the systemic form of the disease and in severe polyarticular disease and is accentuated if corticosteroids have been used in the treatment. If the systemic illness remits, some catch-up growth occurs, but many children have such prolonged disease that the height that is ultimately achieved is severely restricted.

Localized overgrowth and undergrowth occur in areas of asymmetric arthritis, particularly in the child not systemically ill with pauciarticular arthritis. In this case, there is generally marked overgrowth and acceleration of epiphyseal maturation in the affected joints so that, for example, the leg with the arthritic knee becomes much longer than the normal leg. If the cervical spine is involved, neck instability, stiffness, and torticollis may develop. Undergrowth of the mandible may result in a marked micrognathia and severe cosmetic and orthodontic deformity.

Roentgenographic changes in JRA usually are minimal. A child who has severe JRA for many years may have only osteopenia. Older children who are seropositive for rheumatoid factor may have evidence of erosive disease; these findings generally appear quite late in children who are seronegative for rheumatoid factor.

Prognosis of JRA

One of the most difficult concepts for parents to accept is that it is not possible to predict accurately the ultimate outcome for any particular child, although 60% of all children with JRA ultimately "outgrow" their disease. The prognosis is even more favorable in the young female with pauciarticular disease, but it is far less favorable in the child with seropositive polyarticular disease. However, a few children with pauciarticular JRA ultimately progress to a polyarticular involvement with severe destructive disease. Naturally, each time a child experiences a remission of disease, the family hopes that this is a permanent remission; relapse brings

profound disappointment. The physician caring for the child should maintain a positive attitude, because meticulous medical management, physical therapy, splinting, and psychologic support can improve the quality of life for the child with JRA.

Treatment

Most children respond to aspirin or NSAIDs with a lessening of arthritis or systemic signs such as fever. Because aspirin is associated with Reye syndrome following influenza or varicella, NSAIDs are preferred by some rheumatologists. Influenza virus vaccine also may reduce this risk when aspirin is used. Splinting, physical therapy, and, rarely, joint replacement (e.g., total hip replacement) may be needed. Steroids are indicated for serious complications, such as pericarditis or when the cricoarytenoid joint obstructs the airway.

Second-line agents for patients not responding to NSAIDs include low-dose oral methotrexate (10 mg/m²). Pulse methylprednisolone and cyclophosphamide in addition to methotrexate may benefit more refractory patients.

References

Behrman RE (ed): Nelson Textbook of Pediatrics. 14th ed. Philadelphia, WB Saunders, 1992, Sec. 11.51.

Giannini E, Brewer E, Kuzmina N, et al: Methotrexate in resistant juvenile rheumatoid arthritis. N Engl J Med 326: 1043, 1992.

Kredich DW: Chronic arthritis in childhood. Med Clin North Am 70:305, 1986.

Schneider R, Lang B, Reilly B, et al: Prognostic indicators of joint destruction in systemic-onset juvenile rheumatoid arthritis. J Pediatr 120:200, 1992.

SYSTEMIC LUPUS ERYTHEMATOSUS

This autoimmune disease may involve nearly every organ system in an inflammatory process. SLE occurs more frequently in females and has a higher incidence in the black population than in Caucasians. Peak ages of onset correlate roughly with menarche and menopause; the preponderance of females demonstrating onset of the disease during these ages and in the postpartum period is even more striking than that prior to puberty.

Clinical Manifestations. Arthritis or arthralgia is the most common complaint that brings a child with SLE to medical attention, although frequently weight loss, fever, malaise, or rash also are present at the onset of illness. The arthritis affects small more than large joints and is disproportionately painful relative to the physical findings. Many patients have a typical "butterfly" rash over the malar area of the face, sparing the nasolabial folds. Many other rashes are common with SLE and may vary from papular to bullous in character; some of these rashes exhibit photosensitivity. Any serosal surface also may be inflamed, resulting in pericarditis, pleuritis, or acute abdominal pain secondary to abdominal serositis.

Renal disease is universal in SLE, although in some patients it may be clinically inapparent. Renal biopsy demonstrates various lesions accompanied by deposition of complement and immunoglobulins within the glomerulus. At the onset of disease, some patients will have a diffuse proliferative nephritis with compromised renal function; others may have a mild mesangial involvement that may not be progressive.

Hematologic disorders are common and again reflect autoantibody formation. They include Coombs-positive hemolytic anemia, leukopenia secondary to antineutrophil antibodies, and thrombocytopenia associated with antiplatelet antibodies.

A broad spectrum of neurologic disorders may result from SLE, the most common being seizures or psychotic states. Low cerebral spinal fluid (CSF) complement, elevated CSF ANAs, mild CSF mononuclear pleocytosis, mild CSF protein elevation, and an abnormal magnetic resonance imaging study may occur. Other causes of central nervous system (CNS) symptoms, such as steroid psychosis, uremia, infection (toxoplasmosis, cryptococcosis, Nocardia, Listeria), or stroke (from the lupus anticoagulant) must be considered in the differential diagnosis. *Diagnostic criteria* for SLE and additional clinical manifestations are presented in Tables 9–7 and 9–8, respectively.

Laboratory Findings.   Nearly all patients have positive ANAs, although this is not a diagnostic test (Table 9–3). Most patients with SLE have antibodies to double-stranded DNA and decreased levels of total hemolytic complement. With effective therapy, complement levels may return to normal, except in rare patients with familial complement deficiencies. Other less specific tests, such as a false-positive test for syphilis (VDRL) or the presence of a rheumatoid factor, may help in the diagnosis of SLE. A usually reversible form of SLE also may be induced by various drugs (hydralazine, procainamide, isoniazid, chlorpromazine, pheny-

toin, carbamazepine, quinidine, propylthiouracil); in 95% of patients, this condition is associated with antihistone antibodies. When the drug is withdrawn, the lupus-like syndrome resolves.

Treatment.   Treatment varies with the disease manifestation. Arthritis and less serious manifestations usually are managed easily with aspirin or other NSAIDs. The skin manifestations of lupus respond to sunscreens, sun avoidance, and the use of hydroxychloroquine. Most patients have widespread organ system involvement that requires use of oral corticosteroids or, with very serious disease, intravenous pulses of steroids. Severe recalcitrant disease sometimes requires the use of cytotoxic agents (cyclophosphamide). Serologic parameters and complement levels are useful reflections of disease activity, thus allowing the physician to use the lowest possible doses of medication for the shortest possible period of time.

Hypertension is a frequent complication of renal disease and steroid therapy and may require ag-

---

Table 9–7. Clinical Diagnostic Criteria for SLE*

Physical Signs

Butterfly rash (malar)
Discoid lupus
Photosensitivity
Oral/nasopharyngeal ulcers
Nonerosive arthritis (≥2 joints with effusion, tenderness)
Pleuritis *or* pericarditis
Seizures *or* psychosis in absence of metabolic toxins or drugs

Laboratory Data

Renal Disease
Proteinuria (greater than 500 mg/24 hr) *or*
Cellular casts (RBC, granular, tubular)

Hematologic Disease
Hemolytic anemia with reticulocytosis *or*
Leukopenia (<4000 on 2 occasions) *or*
Lymphopenia (<1500 on 2 occasions) *or*
Thrombocytopenia (<100,000)

Serologic Data
Positive anti-dsDNA *or*
Positive anti-Sm *or*
Positive LE prep *or*
False-positive VDRL for >6 mo

Positive ANA in absence of drugs known to induce lupus

* Table shows the 1982 revised criteria for diagnosing SLE. A patient must have 4 of the 11 criteria in order to establish the diagnosis of SLE. These criteria may be present at the same or at different times during the patient's illness. Additional, less diagnostic manifestations are noted in Table 9–8.
LE = lupus erythematosus; RBC = red blood cell.

Table 9–8. Additional Manifestations of SLE

Systemic	Gastrointestinal
Fever	Pancreatitis
Malaise	Mesenteric arteritis
Weight loss	Serositis
Fatigue	Hepatomegaly
	Hepatitis (chronic–lupoid)
Musculoskeletal	Splenomegaly
Myositis, myalgia	
Arthralgia	**Renal**
	Nephritis
Cutaneous	Nephrosis
Raynaud phenomenon	Uremia
Alopecia	Hypertension
Urticaria	
Panniculitis	**Reproduction**
Livedo reticularis	Infertility
	Repeat abortions
Neuropsychiatric	Neonatal lupus
Personality disorders	Congenital heart block
Stroke	
Peripheral neuropathy	**Hematologic**
Chorea	Anticoagulants (factors
Transverse myelitis	VIII, IX, XII, others caus-
Migraine headaches	ing hemorrhage)
	Antiphospholipid
Cardiopulmonary	antibodies (lupus antico-
Endocarditis	agulant causing throm-
Myocarditis	bosis)
Pneumonitis	
	Treatment-Induced
Ocular	Steroid toxicity
Episcleritis	Immunosuppression
Sicca syndrome	Opportunistic infections
Retinal cytoid bodies	

gressive use of antihypertensive agents. End-stage renal disease may be managed with dialysis or transplantation. Children with CNS lupus and seizures require antiseizure medications in addition to the therapy for the lupus itself.

Prognosis. The outlook for long-term survival has improved in childhood lupus; most centers, using a variety of treatment regimens, report a better than 85% 5-yr survival rate. With earlier diagnosis and treatment, renal failure is less commonly a cause of death, but secondary infection with opportunistic organisms has become a leading cause of mortality. Cerebritis, vasculitis, and acute nephritis are less common causes of mortality.

As with any child with chronic disease, psychologic support is crucial to the long-term well-being of the lupus patient.

References

Behrman RE (ed): Nelson Textbook of Pediatrics. 14th ed. Philadelphia, WB Saunders, 1992, Sec. 11.54, 18.7.

Lockshin M: Therapy for systemic lupus erythematosus. N Engl J Med 324:189, 1991.
McCurdy D, Lehman T, Bernstein B, et al: Lupus nephritis: Prognostic factors in children. Pediatrics 89:240, 1992.

NEONATAL LUPUS SYNDROME

See Chapter 6.

DERMATOMYOSITIS

Dermatomyositis is a distinct clinical entity that produces vasculitis in children and involves primarily skin, striated muscle, and the gastrointestinal tract. The illness is more common in females and tends to peak in the 8–12 yr age range, although disease is seen from infancy to adulthood.

Clinical Manifestations. The clinical syndrome is associated with a characteristic rash, symmetric proximal muscle weakness, elevated muscle enzymes, an abnormal electromyogram, and a muscle biopsy that shows loss of muscle fibrils commensurate with damage to the blood supply of the affected muscle. The typical pattern of onset is insidious and, when the patient finally comes to medical attention, the history is one of very slowly diminishing capabilities, unnoticed by parents and teachers alike, until there is some major motor dysfunction (i.e., the child may no longer be able to climb stairs, step onto the school bus, comb his or her own hair, or get up out of a chair). In retrospect, the child may have had malaise or become apathetic, but usually there have been no specific complaints. The lassitude and nonspecific complaints may have caused the parents to seek medical attention; it is usual for the child to have been seen by numerous physicians before a diagnosis is made.

The rash is said to be pathognomonic, but similar rashes occur in other disease entities. However, the rash is exceedingly characteristic and often overlooked. It is primarily telangiectatic, but often the telangiectasias are small enough so that only discoloration is noticed. A "heliotrope" rash of purplish discoloration is present over the upper eyelids and is associated with a malar flush and often with periorbital edema. *Gottron papules* are areas of erythema, atrophy and/or hyperkeratosis over the metacarpophalangeal and proximal interphalangeal joints, without associated arthritis. Very commonly an associated nonspecific papular eruption covers the elbows and knees and, on occasion, occurs in the sun-exposed V-area of the neck as well. Calcifications over pressure points (knee, elbow)

Table 9–9. Dermatomyositis: Criteria for Diagnosis

Rash typical of dermatomyositis
Symmetrical proximal muscle weakness
Elevated muscle enzymes (SGOT, SGPT, LDH, CPK, aldolase)
EMG abnormalities typical of dermatomyositis
Positive muscle biopsy

CPK = creatine phosphokinase; LDH = lactic dehydrogenase; EMG = electromyographic; SGOT = serum glutamic oxaloacetic transaminase; SGPT = serum glutamic pyruvic transaminase.

or in soft tissue may occur. If the characteristic rash is present, only three of the other four criteria are necessary for diagnosis (Table 9–9).

Rarely, children may exhibit fulminant dermatomyositis/polymyositis with an acute course of proximal muscle weakness, often with dysphagia and/or respiratory muscle compromise. The rash may not be appreciated at onset and its course may be rapid enough to necessitate intensive care support. Cardiac involvement may be present but is uncommon. A history of regurgitating liquids through the nose and laboratory evidence of markedly diminished vital capacity require that such a child be placed immediately in an intensive care facility. Every child with the diagnosis of dermatomyositis needs to have both palatal function and voluntary respiratory muscle function (spirometry) adequately assessed after the initial diagnosis and at regular intervals during the course of the disease. Proximal muscle weakness also should be monitored and scored according to loss of function (Table 9–10). Hip (heel–toe walking) and shoulder (arm raising) weakness are evident in almost every patient.

Involvement of the gastrointestinal tract with vasculitis may result in massive gastrointestinal bleeding or intestinal perforation. Vasculitis occurs in other organ systems far less commonly than in the gastrointestinal system, the striated muscle, and the skin. Dilated capillaries are noted at the base of fingernails.

The *differential diagnosis* includes relatively uncommon disorders, such as trichinosis, tropical pyomyositis, hypereosinophilic syndromes, steroid myopathy, metabolic myopathies, SLE, overlap syndrome, emetine abuse, azidothymidine, and hyper- or hypothyroidism. Chronic myositis also may be due to persistent coxsackievirus infection. Acute viral (enterovirus, influenza) myositis is common and associated with rhabdomyolysis, myoglobinuria, elevated creatine phosphokinase, and tender muscles.

Treatment. Most pediatric rheumatologists recommend 2 mg/kg of prednisone equivalent per day as initial therapy unless the child is so severely affected that intravenous pulse steroids are indicated. Usually, a child responds within weeks with improved muscle function and markedly decreased muscle enzymes; the steroid dose then can be tapered slowly over the course of months. Most children do not tolerate alternate-day steroids until they are well into their illness. Under the usual treatment regimen, the steroid dose is reduced to 10–15 mg/day before switching to alternate-day steroids. The natural history of the active disease spans approximately 2–3 yr, so most physicians plan a treatment regimen that involves at least alternate-day low-dose steroids for a total duration of 2 yr.

Prognosis. Before the advent of steroids, one third of children died in the acute phase of illness, one third were severely compromised by disease, and one third recovered. Currently, the mortality rate from dermatomyositis is significantly less than 10%. Most children totally recover after their disease has run its course. Some children have a remitting and exacerbating course, and a few unfortunate children have severe and unremitting disease, which may require them to receive immunosuppression with drugs such as methotrexate.

A complication of dermatomyositis is *calcinosis*, which occurs in patients with a prolonged disease course (at least 1 yr in duration) and, therefore, is not seen in patients during the acute onset of disease. The calcium deposition may be minimal, sporadic, and unimportant or may be severe enough to significantly retard movement in all joints, thus resulting in a major disability. No effective treatment exists for the calcinosis of dermatomyositis; it may remit spontaneously or progress unremittingly and produce severe debilitation.

Table 9–10. Scoring System for Muscle Weakness

Score	Function
0	No movement or contraction
1	Contraction without extremity movement
2	No movement against gravity
3	Movement only against gravity
4	Movement against examiner resistance
5	Normal movement and strength

References

Behrman RE (ed): Nelson Textbook of Pediatrics. 14th ed. Philadelphia, WB Saunders, 1992, Sec 11.62.

Dalakas U: Polymyositis, dermatomyositis, and inclusion-body myositis. N Engl J Med 325:1487, 1991.

Pachman LM: Juvenile dermatomyositis. Pediatr Clin North Am 33:1097, 1986.

SCLERODERMA

In childhood, scleroderma (hardening of the skin) is a very rare condition that can be subdivided into localized and general disease entities. Girls are affected more than boys.

Clinical Manifestations. *Localized scleroderma* may appear as morphea or patch-like scleroderma on the trunk or as linear scleroderma that involves an extremity. The initial lesion may be inflammatory, exhibiting purplish discoloration and raised borders, some heat, and mild pain. Very rapidly progressing scleroderma lesions evolve into areas with hypopigmentation and atrophy. Even localized scleroderma can be a "full-thickness" entity in which not only skin and subcutaneous tissue but also muscle, supporting structures, and even bone are involved; in linear scleroderma this extensive involvement can lead to marked contractures and undergrowth of limbs, resulting in crippling. When linear scleroderma involves the scalp, extension to underlying structures can produce seizures, hypoplasia of the face, and severe cosmetic problems.

At times, what appears to be localized scleroderma can mask severe *progressive systemic sclerosis* (PSS), which involves organ systems that include the kidneys, resulting in severe hypertension and renal failure; the gastrointestinal tract, leading to esophageal and intestinal motility problems; the lungs, causing restrictive disease and pulmonary hypertension; and the joints, resulting in arthritis.

PSS also involves the skin, such that there is marked tightening of the skin in an acral distribution and an associated loss of secondary skin structures. Tightening of the skin becomes generalized, and facial creases disappear. Cutaneous lesions may be diffuse or limited. The former are characterized by the onset of Raynaud phenomenon after skin signs have been present for 1 yr, involvement of truncal and acral skin, tendon friction rubs, early visceral disease, and the absence of anticentromere antibodies. The latter are characterized by Raynaud phenomenon more than 1 yr before skin signs appear; involvement of the hands, face, feet, and skin; the late onset of pulmonary hypertension; and the presence of CREST syndrome and anticentromere antibodies.

Bone in the distal phalangeal tuft often disintegrates, resulting in tapering of the ends of the fingers, termed "sclerodactyly." Calcinosis is relatively common in patients with PSS.

The *CREST syndrome* represents a more benign pattern of illness that includes calcinosis, Raynaud phenomenon, esophageal hypomotility, sclerodactyly, and telangiectasia. **Raynaud phenomenon**, which may precede scleroderma for as many as 10 yr, is characterized by intense pallor (vasoconstriction) followed by cyanosis (partial recirculation) and then by marked erythema (recirculation of blood) of the fingers in response to cold or stress. Approximately 15–20% of patients with Raynaud phenomenon develop connective tissue disorders, which may be predicted by the presence of abnormal nail fold capillaries.

Systemic sclerosis may also occur without scleroderma, with only visceral disease.

Scleroderma-like conditions may occur secondary to drugs (bleomycin), toxins (polyvinyl chloride), and chronic graft-verus-host disease following bone marrow transplantation.

Differential Diagnosis. This includes idiopathic Raynaud disease (rather than phenomenon), toxin exposure (toxic oil, vinyl chloride), carcinoid syndrome, hereditary telangiectasia, porphyria, lichen sclerosis et atrophicus, idiopathic pulmonary hypertension, and *overlap syndrome*. The latter syndrome also is referred to as mixed connective tissue disease (MCTD) or undifferentiated syndrome. MCTD is an overlap syndrome with manifestations of rheumatoid arthritis, SLE, scleroderma, and myositis, including arthritis, polyserositis, myopathy, rash, and Raynaud phenomenon. Each disease manifestation may result from the pathophysiologic mechanisms commonly noted in SLE, dermatomyositis, and scleroderma: immune-inflammation, proliferative-erosive, or fibrotic-atrophic-insufficiency–mediated injury. Antibodies to extractable nuclear antigen and ribonucleoprotein are elevated in MCTD, but these antibodies are not specific for this syndrome.

Laboratory Findings. There is no pathognomonic test for scleroderma, although the presence of ANAs, anticentromere antibodies, and rheumatoid factor is common. Capillaroscopy may reveal nail fold capillary changes, such as enlarged capillary loops, disruption or loss of capillaries, tortuosity, and pseudoglomerular (bushy) capillaries. Vital capacity and carbon monoxide diffusion capacity are useful tests to evaluate pulmonary interstitial fibrosis and pulmonary endothelial damage, respectively.

Prognosis and Treatment. Scleroderma sometimes goes into remission, but it also can run an inexorable course in which complications of malignant hypertension, restrictive lung disease, cardiac failure, or inanition secondary to gastrointestinal disease result in death. The 5-yr mortality rate is 30–70% and depends on the severity of heart, lung, and kidney disease. Response to steroids is poor except in MCTD, which may have a better prognosis unless severe renal involvement is present. Penicillamine may be effective in some patients. Isolated Raynaud phenomenon may be managed by avoiding cold and, if pain is severe, by administering calcium channel blocking agents and utilizing biofeedback.

Eosinophilic Fasciitis

A subset of scleroderma patients have eosinophilic fasciitis. These are young adult and adolescent patients who may have engaged in strenuous physical activity and whose involved muscles subsequently have become swollen and edematous; they also exhibit marked skin changes characterized by an "orange peel" appearance without Raynaud phenomenon. Flexion contractures of the extremity are seen commonly and occur without active synovitis. Biopsy reveals evidence of eosinophilic infiltration into the fascia, peripheral eosinophilia, and an elevated ESR. Some patients develop local scleroderma lesions without sclerodactyly.

Therapeutic response to steroids usually is excellent, although the long-term outlook for children with eosinophilic fasciitis is unknown. Physical therapy may be used to avoid and treat contractures.

References

Allen RC, St-Cyr C, Maddison P, Ansell B. Overlap connective tissue syndromes. Arch Dis Child 61:284, 1986.

Behrman RE (ed): Nelson Textbook of Pediatrics. 14th ed. Philadelphia, WB Saunders, 1992, Sec. 11.63–11.65.

Miller J: The fasciitis-morphea complex in children. Am J Dis Child 146:733, 1992.

Silman A: Epidemiology of scleroderma. Ann Rheum Dis 50:846, 1991.

KAWASAKI DISEASE

This illness, first described in Japan by Dr. Kawasaki in 1967, was recognized in the United States in the early 1970s and now has been found throughout the world. There is a marked predilection for children of Japanese ancestry. It occurs in childhood, mostly in very young children, particularly under the age of 2 yr. The etiology of Kawasaki disease is unknown, although many believe it is viral in origin.

Clinical Manifestations. This illness is primarily a multisystem vasculitis; a significant number of these children (10–20%) have coronary artery aneurysms as sequelae to the disease. Criteria for diagnosing Kawasaki disease are listed in Table 9–11; five of the six criteria are required to make a diagnosis. Other disease manifestations are noted in Table 9–12. In addition, other disease processes must be excluded (Table 9–13).

The disease can be subdivided into three stages. The acute phase lasts about 10 days, during which all of the diagnostic criteria are most likely to be present. The children uniformly have high fever, conjunctivitis, changes in oral mucous membranes and in the extremities, and rash. A desquamating perineal rash may be present. Cervical lymphadenopathy is less frequent. Irritability is profound in children with Kawasaki disease, and aseptic meningitis frequently is found. Myocarditis and pericarditis may occur.

Table 9–11. Kawasaki Disease: Criteria for Diagnosis

Fever persisting for 5 days or more

Changes of peripheral extremities
Initial stage: reddening of palms and soles, indurative edema
Convalescent stage: membranous desquamation from fingertips

Polymorphous exanthem

Bilateral conjunctival congestion

Changes of lips and oral cavity: reddening of lips, strawberry tongue, diffuse injection of oral and pharyngeal mucosa

Acute nonpurulent cervical lymphadenopathy (>1.5 cm in diameter)

Table 9–12. Complications of Kawasaki Disease

Coronary artery aneurysms	Polyarticular arthritis (early)
Coronary artery thrombosis	Pauciarticular arthritis (late)
Myocardial infarction	Sterile pyuria (urethritis)
Myopericarditis	Thombocytosis (late)
Congestive heart failure	Peripheral artery aneurysm
Uveitis	Diarrhea
Hydrops of gallbladder	Pancreatitis
Aseptic meningitis	Peripheral gangrene

Table 9–13. Differential Diagnosis of Kawasaki Disease

Scarlet fever
Staphylococcal toxic shock syndrome
Stevens-Johnson syndrome (erythema multiforme)
Leptospirosis
Epstein-Barr virus
Juvenile rheumatoid arthritis
Measles
Acrodynia
Polyarteritis nodosa
Rocky Mountain spotted fever
Drug reaction
Scalded skin syndrome

The subacute phase of the disease (from days 11 through 21) usually is associated with a decrease in fever. Arthritis occurs in many children at this time, although in a few arthritis had already appeared in the acute phase of the disease. A dramatic skin desquamation occurs in virtually all children beginning on about day 14; usually this desquamation begins at the junction of the nail and the fingertip, is very thick in nature, and is not painful. It is most common on the hands and feet but may occur in other regions.

The third phase of the disease, the convalescent phase, begins about day 21. During this phase of the illness, coronary artery aneurysms are often detected by echocardiogram. Arthritis and thrombocytosis may persist, but generally the acute-phase reactants subside. Myocardial infarctions and rupture of aneurysms may occur in either the subacute or convalescent phases.

Treatment. High doses of aspirin generally are used in the acute phase (100 mg/kg/24 hr) and shorten the duration of fever; as the child improves, low doses of aspirin generally are employed for their effect in preventing platelet aggregation. Low-dose aspirin therapy (3–5 mg/kg/24 hr) generally is continued until both the thrombocytosis and the other acute-phase reactants have returned to normal (i.e., end of convalescent phase). Intravenous immunoglobulin therapy (2 g/kg × 1 dose) during the acute phase reduces coronary aneurysm formation.

The death rate from Kawasaki disease when it was first described was about 3%; this rate has dramatically decreased over the last 20 yr.

References

Behrman RE (ed): Nelson Textbook of Pediatrics. 14th ed. Philadelphia, WB Saunders, 1992, Sec. 11.58.

Burns J, Mason W, Glode M, et al: Clinical and epidemiologic characteristics of patients referred for evaluation of possible Kawasaki disease. J Pediatr 118:680, 1991.
Gersony W: Diagnosis and management of Kawasaki disease. JAMA 265:2699, 1991.

HENOCH-SCHÖNLEIN PURPURA

This is the most common vasculitis of childhood and is characterized by palpable nonthrombocytopenic purpura: periarticular, scrotal, and scalp swelling, edema, and inflammation; gastrointestinal bleeding (with or without intussusception); and nephritis (see Table 9–4). The cutaneous manifestations of Henoch-Schönlein purpura (HSP) are striking, with circular purpuric lesions 2–3 cm in size typically occurring over the buttocks and the posterior surfaces of the arms and legs. Skin lesions and the renal glomeruli contain IgA immune complexes.

Clinical Manifestations. The onset of the illness often follows a nonspecific upper respiratory tract infection in a 4–10 yr old child. The skin lesions are the hallmark of the disease, but cramping, intermittent abdominal pain, hematochezia, periarticular swelling, and tense scalp or scrotal edema may be present. Glomerulonephritis is common within 1–2 months of onset and becomes manifest as asymptomatic hematuria, with or without proteinuria. Five percent of patients have acute renal insufficiency, and another 5% have a slow progression, with renal failure developing months to years later. Initial manifestations of nephritis, nephrotic syndrome, or nephritic nephrosis increase the long-term risks of hypertension, renal impairment, or pre-eclampsia. Encephalopathy and pulmonary hemorrhage are rare manifestations of HSP. Most patients recover without therapy, but a small percentage relapse and another small group has a much slower rate of recovery accompanied by the persistence of hematuria for 1–2 yr.

Treatment. Therapy is symptomatic because 90% of patients have a self-limited illness. Corticosteroids may relieve abdominal pain and joint, scalp, or scrotal edema, but this has not been proved in controlled studies. Steroids do not have a beneficial effect on renal disease. Renal transplantation may be needed for the few patients with irreversible renal insufficiency; in some transplant patients HSP has recurred in the transplanted kidney.

References

Behrman RE (ed): Nelson Textbook of Pediatrics. 14th ed. Philadelphia, WB Saunders, 1992, Sec. 11.57.

Goldstein A, White R, Akuse R, et al: Long-term follow-up of childhood Henoch-Schönlein nephritis. Lancet 339: 280, 1992.

Mills J, Michel B, Bloch D, et al: The American College of Rheumatology 1990 criteria for the classification of Henoch-Schönlein purpura. Arthritis Rheum 33:1114, 1990.

WEGENER GRANULOMATOSIS

This is an uncommon vasculitis in childhood (see Table 9–4). The disease may resemble HSP, exhibiting renal, skin, joint, and gastrointestinal involvement, or it may resemble an adult-type vasculitis, with lung, renal, sinus/nasopharynx, eye, and joint disease. Necrotizing midline upper respiratory tract granulomas (sinus, subglottic stenosis, nose, otitis) accompanied by renal vasculitis and pulmonary lesions (cavitary or nodular infiltrates) are typical in both age groups. Sinus disease is an early manifestation, demonstrating inflammation of the paranasal sinuses and, rarely, nasal septum perforation. Secondary infection may produce pyogenic sinusitis. Renal involvement may occur late and becomes manifest by hematuria, proteinuria, renal failure, and hypertension. Other manifestations include rash, arthralgia, peripheral neuropathy, and dacrocystitis. Wegener granulomatosis can be differentiated from HSP by the presence of lung involvement, absence of IgA immune complexes in dermal capillaries, presence of antineutrophil cytoplasmic antibodies and granulomas. Treatment includes both cyclophosphamide and corticosteroids. The response is favorable in most patients.

References

Behrman RE (ed): Nelson Textbook of Pediatrics. 14th ed. Philadelphia, WB Saunders, 1992, Sec. 11.60.

Rottem M, Fauci A, Hallahan C, et al: Wegener granulomatosis in children and adolescents: Clinical presentation and outcome. J Pediatr 122:26, 1991.

ACUTE RHEUMATIC FEVER

See Chapter 13.

PAIN SYNDROMES IN CHILDHOOD

Growing Pains

Many children, most frequently between the ages of 5 and 12, complain of recurrent evening or nighttime limb pains. These pains usually are intermittent and occur around and behind the knee, in the calves and thigh areas, and sometimes in the shins; occasionally upper extremity pain occurs. Typical "growing pains" occur at the end of a day of strenuous activity and are resolved totally by the following morning. There is no associated limp, but the pain may be severe enough to interfere with normal sleep.

Growth and development are normal, as is the physical examination. No associated effusions or limitations of joint motion are present. Systemic signs are absent and roentgenograms and laboratory studies are normal.

Treatment consists mainly of reassurance that no organic disease is present. Stretching exercises for the Achilles tendons and hamstrings may be beneficial. Pain medication (e.g., acetaminophen) and the application of heat frequently are helpful. Growing pains may be episodic and may recur over the course of months or years. Ultimately, the child outgrows the propensity for having these pains.

Fibromyalgia

This benign, intermittent, noninflammatory musculoskeletal pain syndrome is seen in children as well as in adults, is more common in females (5:1), and tends to occur much more often in adolescents than in younger childhood. There is arthralgia but no synovitis. A number of characteristically tender "trigger points" exist: those on the anterior chest (costochondral); on the inner aspect of the scapula medially (supraspinatus muscle); around the knee but beyond the joint margin; over the greater trochanters; and near the gluteus medius, low cervical spine (C5–C7), and low lumbar ligaments (L4–S1). Some patients have associated mild swelling of the hands, which also is not articular. Many patients relate their symptoms to changes in the weather, and some often experience an associated depression, morning stiffness, and a disturbance in sleep pattern. Many of these children miss an extraordinary amount of school. Associated nonrheumatic illnesses include headache and irritable bowel syndrome.

Chronic, unilateral extremity pain may be due to reflex sympathetic dystrophy, which is characterized by local burning pain, hyperalgesia, allodynia (pain from usually nonpainful stimuli, such as light touch), cyanosis, sweating, mottling, coldness, excessive hair growth, swelling, and, if not treated, contractures, demineralization, and atrophy. A prior history of mild-moderate trauma may be present.

The approach to fibromyalgia is: (1) to reassure

the patient that it is not a deforming, crippling disease, (2) to administer NSAIDs for pain control, (3) to support the patient through counseling for the depressive manifestations of the disease, (4) to offer biofeedback for relaxation and pain control, and (5) to introduce a graduated program of aerobic physical therapy to increase activity.

References

Behrman RE (ed): Nelson Textbook of Pediatrics. 14th ed. Philadelphia, WB Saunders, 1992, Sec. 11.68.

Sigal L, Patella S: Lyme arthritis as the incorrect diagnosis in pediatric and adolescent fibromyalgia. Pediatrics 90: 523, 1992.

Wilder R, Berde C, Wolohan M, et al: Reflex sympathetic dystrophy in children. J Bone Joint Surg 74A:910, 1992.

SARCOIDOSIS

Sarcoidosis is a chronic disease of unknown cause. Multisystem (>5) involvement is common. The arthritis may mimic pauciarticular JRA. In pediatrics, the peak age is during adolescence, but it has occurred in children as young as 2 mo of age. Young children frequently exhibit skin, joint, and eye disease; children older than 4 yr of age have lung, lymph node, and eye involvement. Sarcoidosis is more common in blacks. The *clinical manifestations* of sarcoidosis include weight loss, cough, fatigue, bone or joint pain, lymphadenopathy, dyspnea, parotid enlargement, fever, uveitis, nodules, maculopapular rash or erythema nodosum, and hepatosplenomegaly. Hilar adenopathy with pulmonary nodules or interstitial infiltrates also is common. *Laboratory findings* are not specific, but hypercalcemia, polyclonal gammopathy, and elevated angiotensin-converting enzyme are common. Slit-lamp examination reveals granulomatous anterior uveitis, and tissue biopsy demonstrates noncaseating granulomas. Pulmonary function tests may show a restrictive pattern, and gallium scanning demonstrates increased pulmonary uptake. Renal disease becomes manifest as hematuria and proteinuria. Cutaneous anergy is common. *Treatment* includes corticosteroids. The *prognosis* is fair to good; only 40–50% of patients remain symptomatic for 5 yr after therapy.

References

Behrman RE (ed): Nelson Textbook of Pediatrics. 14th ed. Philadelphia, WB Saunders, 1992, Sec. 25.3.

Nocton J, Stork J, Jacobs G, et al: Sarcoidosis associated with nephrocalcinosis in young children. J Pediatr 121: 937, 1992.

Pattishal E, Strope G, Spinola S, et al: Childhood sarcoidosis. J Pediatr 108:169, 1986.

Infectious Diseases

10

Alice Prince

BASIC PRINCIPLES OF PEDIATRIC INFECTIOUS DISEASES

Epidemiology

The ability to diagnose and appropriately treat specific childhood infections depends on an understanding of the epidemiology and risk factors associated with each infectious agent as well as the population at risk for certain pathogens. Susceptibility to specific infectious agents is a direct consequence of the maturity of the immune system, exposure to potential infectious agents, and the presence of underlying diseases. The host response varies with age. Thus, neonates prior to the development of their own immunologic repertoire are at risk for different types of infections than school-age children or adolescents. To approach the diverse types of infections seen in pediatrics, the clinician must consider the following questions:

Who gets a specific disease?
Does this occur in a normal host, an immunocompromised patient, or a child with a specific immunologic defect?
What organisms are involved?
Is the presentation one of a benign viral illness or more suggestive of bacterial infection?
How can the etiologic agent be identified?
What antimicrobial agents are available for treatment?
What can be done to prevent this disease?

The likelihood of many infections can be estimated by historic factors and host evaluation. Sociologic factors are important; for infants the adequacy of prenatal care, gestational age, maternal risk-taking behavior, and appropriate screening tests for congenital infection are helpful clues. The immunization history and living conditions, including exposure to infected adults or to other infants in a closed setting such as day care or an informal baby sitting arrangement, may be factors in the transmission of common infections. Other environmental factors, such as travel, exposure to air conditioners, the season, construction sites, insects, and animals or exotic pets may help the clinician assess the possibility of specific etiologic agents.

A careful and complete physical examination is critical to the diagnosis of many infectious diseases. Although initial complaints, particularly in infants, may be nonspecific (irritability, poor feeding, or lethargy), certain physical findings such as specific rashes may be diagnostic. Particular care should be given to identifying the sites of infection (Table 10–1). Knowledge of these common sites permits identification of the infecting organism and guides appropriate treatment. Rashes are a common manifestation of infections; appropriate classification of the rash morphology can be diagnostic for many infections (Table 10–2).

Prevention

The prevention of many previously fatal childhood diseases has been a triumph of pediatrics and has been accomplished through the use of routine vaccination (Tables 10–3 and 10–4). Vaccines may be live attenuated viruses (measles, mumps, rubella, varicella, polio) or consist of inactivated immunogenic components of either viruses or bacteria (polio, hepatitis B, pertussis, influenza, diphtheria, tetanus, *Haemophilus influenzae* type b, pneumococcus). Vaccine efficacy is dependent on the age of the child, the immune status, appropriate administration, and booster immunizations.

In addition to those vaccines recommended for all children, various high-risk situations (e.g., repeated exposure to a pathogen, altered cardiopulmonary status, or increased susceptibility to various bacteria) warrant additional vaccinations (Table 10–5). When there are no specific effective vaccines and the patient is at increased risk for the infectious disease owing to repeated exposure or to increased host susceptibility, antimicrobial prophylaxis is administered for as long as the patient remains at risk (Table 10–6).

Clinical Use of the Microbiology Laboratory

Laboratory diagnosis of infection involves a variety of techniques ranging from the simple micro-

Table 10–1. Localizing Manifestations of Infection

Site	Symptoms	Signs
Upper respiratory	Rhinorrhea, sneezing, cough, sore throat, drooling, stridor, trismus, sinus pain, fever, ear pain or drainage	Nasal congestion; pharyngeal erythema; enlarged tonsils with exudate; swollen, red epiglottis; red, bulging tympanic membrane
Lower respiratory	Cough, fever, chest pain, dyspnea; sputum production	Rales, wheezing, localized diminished breath sounds, intercostal retractions, tachypnea
Gastrointestinal	Vomiting, diarrhea, abdominal pain, anorexia, fever	Hyperactive bowel sounds, abdominal tenderness, hematochezia
Hepatic	Anorexia, vomiting; dark urine, light stools	Jaundice, hepatomegaly, hepatic tenderness
Genitourinary	Dysuria, frequency, urgency, fever, flank or suprapubic pain, vaginal discharge	Costovertebral angle or suprapubic tenderness, cervical motion and adnexal tenderness
Skeletal	Limp, bone pain, fever, pseudoparalysis	Local swelling, erythema, warmth, limited range of motion, tenderness
Central nervous system	Fever, lethargy, irritability, headache, neck stiffness, seizures	Kernig or Brudzinski sign, bulging fontanel, focal neurologic deficits
Cardiovascular	Dyspnea, palpitations, exercise intolerance, chest pain, fever, shock	Tachycardia, hypotension, cardiomegaly, hepatomegaly, splenomegaly, rales, petechiae, Osler nodes, Janeway lesions, new murmur, distended neck veins, pericardial friction rub, muffled heart tones

scopic examination of bacterial morphology using the Gram stain to the more technical molecular microbiologic methods such as the polymerase chain reaction. Current practices include (1) routine culture methods for isolation of specific pathogens from infected sites, (2) bacterial antigen detection utilizing either latex agglutination or fluorescent antibody, (3) detection of genomic DNA (or RNA) sequences of pathogens using complementary probes, (4) demonstration of an antibody response to an infection by serologic testing and/or Western hybridization technique, and (5) tissue culture to identify viruses and intracellular pathogens.

The laboratory also can provide critical information to optimize therapy and avoid toxicity, such as antimicrobial susceptibility testing, mean inhibitory (MIC) or bactericidal (MBC) concentrations of antimicrobial agents, or peak and trough drug levels.

FEVER

Healthy individuals maintain their core body temperatures within 1–1.5°C. Normal body temperature is considered to be 98.6°F (range from 97° to 99.6°). Most individuals have a diurnal variation, with maximal levels achieved in the late afternoon. The normal body temperature is maintained by the anterior hypothalamus utilizing a complex regulatory system. Rectal temperatures greater than 38°C (100.4°F) generally are considered abnormal.

Pathogenesis of Fever

All infections can produce fever, which begins with the release of endogenous pyrogens into the circulation after an infectious or immunologically mediated event. The endogenous pyrogens reach the anterior hypothalamus via the arterial blood supply, liberating arachidonic acid, which is metabolized to prostaglandin (PG) E$_2$, resulting in an elevation of the hypothalamic thermostat. Antipyretics work by altering the synthesis of prostaglandins, reducing production of PGE$_2$. Endogenous pyrogens are cytokines (interleukin [IL]-1, IL-6, tumor necrosis factor [TNF], and the interferons), which are released by monocytes, macrophages, mesangial cells, glial cells, epithelial cells, and B lymphocytes.

Intense muscle contraction (cocaine overdose) or muscle metabolism altered by drugs (neuroleptic agents) or anesthetics produces *malignant hyperthermia* (see Chapter 18). Heat stroke, a potentially fatal febrile illness, is due to excessively high environmental temperatures and failure of physiologic body heat-losing mechanisms.

Table 10–2. Differential Diagnosis of Fever and Rash

Lesion	Pathogen or Associated Factor
Maculopapular or Macular Rash	*Viruses* Measles, rubella, roseola (human herpesvirus-6), fifth disease (parvovirus), Epstein-Barr virus, enteroviruses, hepatitis B virus (papular acrodermatitis or Gianotti-Crosti syndrome), human immunodeficiency virus *Bacteria* Rheumatic fever (group A streptococcus), scarlet fever, erysipelas, *Arcanobacterium haemolyticum*, secondary syphilis, leptospirosis, *Pseudomonas*, meningococcal infection (early), *Salmonella*, Lyme disease *Rickettsia* Early Rocky Mountain spotted fever, typhus (scrub, endemic), ehrlichiosis *Other* Kawasaki disease
Diffuse Erythroderma	*Bacteria* Scarlet fever (group A streptococcus), toxic shock syndrome *(Staphylococcus aureus)* *Fungi* *Candida albicans*
Urticarial Rash	*Viruses* Epstein-Barr virus, hepatitis B, human immunodeficiency virus *Bacteria* *Mycoplasma pneumoniae*, group A streptococci
Vesicular, Bullous, Pustular	*Viruses* Herpes simplex, varicella-zoster, coxsackievirus *Bacteria* Staphylococcal scalded skin syndrome, staphylococcal bullous impetigo, group A streptococcal crusted impetigo *Other* Toxic epidermal necrolysis, erythema multiforme (Stevens-Johnson syndrome), rickettsialpox
Petechial–Purpuric	*Viruses* Atypical measles, congenitial rubella, cytomegalovirus, enterovirus, human immunodeficiency virus, hemorrhagic fever viruses *Bacteria* Sepsis (meningococcal, gonococcal, pneumococcal, *Haemophilus influenzae*), endocarditis *Rickettsiae* Rocky Mountain spotted fever, epidemic typhus, ehrlichiosis *Other* Vasculitis, thrombocytopenia, Henoch-Schönlein purpura, malaria
Erythema Nodosum	*Viruses* Epstein-Barr, hepatitis B *Bacteria* Group A streptococcus, tuberculosis, *Yersinia*, cat-scratch disease *Fungi* Coccidioidomycosis, histoplasmosis *Other* Sarcoidosis, inflammatory bowel disease, estrogen-containing oral contraceptives, systemic lupus erythematosus, Behçet disease
Distinctive Rashes Ecthyma gangrenosum	*Pseudomonas aeruginosa*
Erythema chronicum migrans	Lyme disease
Necrotic eschar	Aspergillosis, mucormycosis
Erysipelas	Group A streptococcus
Koplik spots	Measles

Table 10–3. Schedule for the Routine Immunization of Healthy Infants and Children, Based on the Recommendations of the American Academy of Pediatrics and the CDCP*

Recommended Age†	Immunizations‡	Comments
At birth	HBV	Alternate schedule for HBV vaccination: 1–2 mo, 4 mo, and 6–18 mo
1–2 mo	HBV	—
2 mo	DTP,§ HbCV,‖ OPV	DTP and OPV can be initiated as early as 4 wk after birth in areas of high endemicity or during outbreaks
4 mo	DTP, HbCV,‖ OPV	A 2-mo interval (minimum of 6 wk) is desirable for OPV to avoid interference from the previous dose
6 mo	DTP (HbCV‖)	A third dose of OPV is not indicated in the United States but is desirable in other geographic areas where polio is endemic
6–18 mo	HBV	—
12 mo	(HbCV‖)	—
15 mo	MMR (HbCV‖)	MMR may be given at 12 mo of age in areas of recurrent measles transmission; if given at less than 12 mo, it should be given again at 15 mo
15–18 mo	DTaP or DTP, OPV¶	These vaccines may be given simultaneously with MMR at 15 mo
4–6 yr	DTaP or DTP, OPV	At or before school entry
11–12 yr	MMR#	At entry to middle school or junior high school unless the second dose was previously given
14–16 yr	Td	—

* As of August 1992. For all products, consult the manufacturer's package insert for instructions on storage, handling, dosage, and administration. Biologics prepared by different manufacturers may vary, and package inserts from the same manufacturer may change from time to time.

† Recommended ages should not be construed as absolute.

‡ HBV = hepatitis B vaccine; DTP = diphtheria, tetanus toxoid, and pertussis vaccine; HbCV = *Haemophilus influenzae* type b conjugate vaccine; OPV = trivalent oral live poliovirus types 1, 2, and 3 vaccine; MMR = measles, mumps, and rubella vaccine; DTap = diphtheria, tetanus toxoid, and acellular pertussis vaccine; Td = tetanus toxoid (full dose) and diphtheria toxoid (reduced dose) for use in adults. Live virus vaccines (OPV, MMR) are contraindicated in immunodeficient patients. MMR may be given to some patients who are HIV positive.

§ Contraindications for pertussis vaccine include allergy to components, encephalopathy within 7 days of prior dose, convulsion within 3 days of a dose, persistent unconsolable crying for 3 or more hr within 48 hr of dose, collapse and shock-like state within 48 hr or dose, and temperature greater than 40.5°C (104°F) with 48 hr of dose. The vaccine may be temporarily deferred in the presence of a progressive neurologic disorder or a recent personal history of convulsions. A family history of seizures is not a contraindication. Acetaminophen (15 mg/kg q4–6h) may be given to reduce fever and risk of possible febrile seizures.

‖ For all doses of HbCV given to children less than 15 mo old, the same conjugate product should be used for each dose. The third dose of HbCV is given either at 6 or at 12 mo of age, depending on the product, and a fourth dose is indicated at 15 mo in the schedule for one product.

¶ OPV may be given simultaneously with MMR and HbCV at 15 mo or at any time between 12 and 24 mo; priority should be given to administering MMR at the recommened age.

The Advisory Committee on Immunization Practices recommends the second dose at school entry.

(Adapted from Peter G: Childhood immunizations. N Engl J Med 327:1794, 1992.)

The *pattern of fever* in children may differ depending on the age of the child and the nature of the illness. Neonates may not have a febrile response or may be hypothermic despite a significant infection, whereas older infants and children under 5 yr may have an exaggerated febrile response with temperatures as high as 105°F in response to either a serious bacterial infection or a benign viral process. Fevers to this latter degree are unusual in older children and adolescents and suggest a significant pathologic process. Except in unusual circumstances, the fever pattern does not distinguish fever caused by bacterial, viral, fungal, or parasitic organisms from that resulting from malignancy, autoimmune diseases, or drugs.

Most febrile illness in children may be categorized as: (1) fever of short duration accompanied by localizing signs and symptoms in which a diagnosis can be established by clinical history and physical examination; (2) fever without localizing signs, usually occurring in a child under the age of 3 yr, in which a history and physical exam fail to

Table 10–4. Recommended Immunization Schedules for Children Not Immunized in First Year of Life*

Recommended Time/Age	Immunizations†	Comments
Younger Than 7 Years		
First visit	DTP, OPV, MMR	MMR if child ≥15 mo old; tuberculin testing may be done at same visit
	HbCV‡	For children age 15–59 mo, can be given simultaneously with DTP and other vaccines (at separate sites)§
Interval after first visit		
2 mo	DTP, OPV (HbCV)	Second dose of HbCV is indicated only in children whose first dose was received when younger than 15 mo
4 mo	DTP	Third dose of OPV is not indicated in the United States but is desirable in other geographic areas where polio is endemic
10–16 mo	DTP, OPV	OPV is not given if third dose was given earlier
4–6 yr (at or before school entry)	DTP, OPV	DTP is not necessary if the fourth dose was given after the fourth birthday; OPV is not necessary if third dose was given after the fourth birthday
11–12 yr	MMR	At entry to middle school or junior high
10 yr later	Td	Repeat every 10 yr throughout life
7 Years and Older‖,¶		
First visit	Td, OPV, MMR	
Interval after first visit		
2 mo	Td, OPV	
8–14 mo	Td, OPV	
11–12 yr	MMR	At entry to middle school or junior high
10 yr later	Td	Repeat every 10 yr throughout life

* High-risk groups who should receive hepatitis B immunization regardless of age: hemophiliac patients and other recipients of certain blood products; intravenous drug abusers; heterosexual persons who have had more than one sex partner in the previous 6 mo and/or those with a recent episode of a sexually transmitted disease; sexually active homosexual and bisexual males; household and sexual contacts of hepatitis B virus (HBV) carriers; members of households with adoptees from HBV-endemic, high-risk countries who are HBsAg-positive; children and other household contacts in populations of high HBV endemicity; staff and residents of institutions for the developmentally disabled; staff of nonresidential day care and school programs for developmentally disabled if attended by known HBV carrier, other attendees in certain circumstances; hemodialysis patients; health care workers and others with occupational risk; international travelers who will live for more than 6 mo in areas of high HBV endemicity and who otherwise will be at risk; and inmates of long-term correctional facilities. (Adapted from Committee on Infectious Diseases, American Academy of Pediatrics: Report of the Committee on Infectious Diseases. 22nd ed. AAP, 1991.)

† Abbreviations are explained in the footnote‡ to Table 10–3.

‡ If child is younger than 15 mo, only one HbCV (HbOC), as of October 1990, is approved for use.

§ The initial three doses of DTP can be given at 1- to 2-mo intervals; hence, for the child in whom immunization is initiated at age 15 mo or older, one visit could be eliminated by giving DTP, OPV, and MMR at the first visit; DTP and HbCV at the second visit (1 mo later); and DTP and OPV at the third visit (2 mo after the first visit). Subsequent doses of DTP and OPV 10–16 mo after the first visit still are indicated. HbCV, MMR, DTP, and OPV can be given simultaneously at separate sites if failure of the patient to return for future immunizations is a concern.

‖ If person is ≥18 years old, routine poliovirus vaccination is not indicated in the United States.

¶ Minimal interval between doses of MMR is 1 mo.

establish a cause but a diagnosis may be suggested by laboratory studies; and (3) fever of unknown origin (FUO), fever present for more than 14 days *(in a child)* that does not have an etiology despite history, physical exam, and routine laboratory tests. In older children and adolescents an FUO usually is defined as a fever over 38°F for more than 3 wk that remains undiagnosed despite in-hospital evaluation for 7 days.

Fever without a Source: Occult Bacteremia

A common clinical pediatric problem is the evaluation of the febrile but well-appearing child with no localizing signs of infection. Although most of these children have self-limited viral infections, some (usually under the age of 3 yr) will have bacteremia, and a few will develop severe and potentially life-threatening illnesses such as bacterial

Table 10–5. Additional Special Vaccines

Vaccine	Indication
Influenza virus (inactivated virus)	Patients with chronic cardiorespiratory disease (cystic fibrosis, bronchopulmonary dysplasia); patients with sickle cell anemia, those on chronic salicylate therapy, or those with chronic immunosuppressed conditions
Pneumococcal vaccine (23-valent polysaccharide)	Chronic pulmonary disease, sickle cell anemia, functional or anatomic asplenia, nephrotic syndrome
Meningococcal (polysaccharide A/C/Y/W135)	Functional or anatomic asplenia, travel to an endemic area, patients with terminal complement deficiency; type B meningococcus not covered
Bacille Calmette-Guérin (BCG) (live attenuated *M. bovis* vaccine)	Tuberculin-negative infant in household with active disease; high tuberculosis incidence areas
Inactivated poliovirus	May be equally effective as TOPV; should be used when TOPV is contraindicated; should be given to family members if close contact is immunodeficient, or if an unimmunized adult
Rabies (human diploid cell vaccine)	
Pre-exposure	High-risk groups (e.g., veterinarians, animal handlers, and laboratory workers)
Postexposure	Must include human rabies immune globulin passive immunization, plus vaccine on days 1, 3, 7, 14, and 28, following high-risk animal bites: dog, raccoon, skunk, fox, cat, coyote, and bat

TOPV = trivalent oral polio vaccine.

meningitis. Particularly in the early stages of such illness, it is difficult, even for experienced clinicians, to differentiate patients with bacteremia from those with benign illness (Table 10–7).

FEVER IN CHILDREN BETWEEN 3 MONTHS AND 2 YEARS OF AGE

Etiology. Children between 3 mo and 2 yr of age are at risk for infection resulting from organisms with polysaccharide capsules, such as *Streptococcus pneumonia, H. influenzae* type b, meningococci, and salmonella. Effective phagocytosis of these organisms requires opsonic antibody. Although neonates receive maternal immunoglobulin (Ig) G transplacentally, this protection is gradually lost (3–6 mo), leaving the infant at risk for infection caused by encapsulated organisms until their own IgM and IgG are produced.

Clinical Manifestations/Diagnosis. In children between 3 mo and 2 yr of age, most febrile episodes will demonstrate an obvious source of infection as elicited by history or physical examination (e.g., pharyngitis, otitis media, bronchitis, or upper respiratory tract infection). The evaluation of infants who are febrile, well appearing, but without a focus of infection depends on the clinical assessment, which may include a complete blood count with white blood cell (WBC) differential, erythrocyte sedimentation rate (ESR), blood culture, urinalysis with urine culture, and perhaps a chest radiograph to attempt to find an infectious focus. In occult bacteremia, positive blood cultures more often are obtained from children with fever greater than 104°F.

The WBC count does not always predict accurately whether a child is bacteremic. Nonetheless, it can be helpful in dividing the population into high- and low-risk (<15,000/µL) groups. This division may be helpful in selecting patients for further investigation or therapy. The ESR is no more useful than the WBC in predicting bacteremia in ambulatory febrile patients. Other hematologic findings that have been considered suggestive of bacteremia but are too inconsistent and nonspecific include thrombocytopenia, Dohle inclusion bodies, neutrophil toxic granulations, and vacuolization of neutrophils. With or without thrombocytopenia, the finding of petechiae in a febrile child is suggestive of bacteremia. Tests for rapidly detecting minute amounts of bacterial antigen in blood or urine (e.g., latex agglutination, and enzyme-linked immunosorbent assay [ELISA]) may become sufficiently accurate, reliable, and economical for routine use in the emergency room and office. Variables that may

Table 10–6. Antimicrobial Prophylaxis

	Pathogen	Preventive Therapy
Pertussis	*Bordetella pertussis*	Erythromycin
Diphtheria	*Corynebacterium diphtheriae*	Penicillin, erythromycin
Meningitis	*Haemophilus influenzae* type b	Rifampin
	Neisseria meningitidis	Rifampin
Tuberculosis	*Mycobacterium tuberculosis*	Isoniazid
Sepsis/asplenia*	*Streptococcus pneumoniae*	Penicillin
	Haemophilus influenzae type b	Amoxicillin
Rheumatic fever	Group A streptococci	Penicillin
Interstitial pneumonia	*Pneumocystis carinii*	Trimethoprim–sulfamethoxazole, pentamidine
Influenza	Influenza A virus	Amantadine
Neonatal conjunctivitis	*Chlamydia trachomatis*	0.5% erythromycin topically
	Neisseria gonorrhoeae	1% silver nitrate or 0.5% erythromycin topically
Bacterial endocarditis		
Dental procedure	Streptococci	Amoxicillin (PO), ampicillin and gentamicin (IV)
Genitourinary/ gastrointestinal procedure	Enterococcus	Amoxicillin (PO), ampicillin and gentamicin (IV)

* Including sickle cell disease.

help in differentiating viral from bacterial disease are noted in Table 10–7.

Occult bacteremia due to pneumococcus in otherwise healthy children between 3 and 24 mo may be transient, with a small percentage of infants developing serious infections. In contrast, bacteremias caused by *H. influenzae* type b and *Neisseria meningitidis* are less benign, and serious localizing infections such as meningitis, septic arthritis, and pericarditis are possible sequelae.

Children with *sickle cell anemia* have deficiencies of splenic function and properdin-dependent opsonization, placing them at high risk for bacteremia, especially during the first 5 yr of life. Pneumococcal sepsis that is accompanied by meningitis, and, less commonly, bacteremia and meningitis that are due to *H. influenzae* type b are potentially serious and fulminant infections in patients with

sickle cell disease. Salmonella sepsis may result in osteomyelitis.

Treatment. Because of the low incidence of occult bacteremia (4–5%) and because most episodes of occult bacteremia are due to pneumococci and usually are transient in healthy immunocompetent children, most physicians do not administer antibiotics to febrile infants whose infection has no focus or to those patients who do not appear to be septic. After obtaining a blood culture, some physicians administer ceftriaxone (IM) and discharge the well-appearing infant with follow-up within 24 hr.

Any ill-appearing infant should be considered seriously infected, admitted to the hospital, and treated with antibiotics. A well-appearing febrile infant between 3 and 24 mo of age should be carefully evaluated, a blood culture from the infant ob-

Table 10–7. Differentiating Viral from Bacterial Infections

Variable	Viral	Bacterial
Petechiae	Present	Present
Leukocytosis	Uncommon*	Common
Shift to left ($\uparrow$ bands)	Uncommon	Common
Neutropenia	Possible	Suggests overwhelming infection
$\uparrow$ ESR	Unusual*	Common
$\uparrow$ CRP	Unusual	Common
$\uparrow$ Elastase–alpha-1-protease	Uncommon	Common
$\uparrow$ TNF, IL-1, PAF	Uncommon	Common
Meningitis (pleocytosis)	Lymphocytic	Neutrophilic
Meningeal signs positive†	Present	Present

* Adenovirus and herpes simplex may cause leukocytosis and increased ESR; Epstein-Barr virus may cause petechiae and increased ESR.

† Nuchal rigidity, bulging fontanel, Kernig or Brudzinski sign.

CRP = C-reactive protein; ESR = erythrocyte sedimentation rate; PAF = platelet activating factor.

tained, and the child sent home with follow-up in 24 hr. If the blood culture becomes positive for pneumococci and the child is afebrile, appears well, and has no localizing signs, the child need not be treated; a repeat blood culture should be obtained. If the initial blood culture is positive for pneumococcus and the child remains febrile or has localizing signs suggestive of pneumonia or meningitis, the child should be treated with appropriate antibiotics in the hospital.

If the bacteremia is due to *H. influenzae* type b or *N. meningitidis*, the child should be hospitalized, a lumbar puncture performed, and intravenous antibiotics administered. Prior to the administration of antibiotics, a repeat blood culture should be obtained in all children to determine the persistence of the bacteremia. (Antibiotic dosages are noted in Appendix I.)

FEVER IN INFANTS LESS THAN 3 MONTHS OF AGE

This may be associated with a higher risk of serious bacterial infections than fever in older infants. These younger infants may not demonstrate localizing signs, and bacteremia, meningitis, urinary tract infection, and pneumonia may be present in the infant exhibiting nonspecific signs, such as poor feeding. Often fever is the only manifestation of serious bacterial infection in very young infants. Urinary tract infection (*Escherichia coli*), bacteremia (*Salmonella*, group B streptococci, pneumococcus, *H. influenzae*, meningococcus), pneumonia (*Staphylococcus aureus*, pneumococcus), meningitis (viral or group B streptococci, meningococcus, pneumococcus, *H. influenzae* type b), and osteomyelitis (*S. aureus*, group B streptococci) are common types of infection. Nonetheless, most febrile diseases in this age group are due to common viral pathogens. Differentiation between viral and bacterial infections often is difficult (Table 10–7). Therefore, infants less than 3 mo of age who appear sick and all infants less than 1 mo of age (especially with uncertain follow-up) usually are admitted to the hospital. After blood, urine, and cerebrospinal fluid are cultured, broad-spectrum antibiotics are administered to many of these infants. The choice of antibiotics depends on the possible pathogens involved and any localizing findings, such as pneumonia, septic arthritis/osteomyelitis, or meningitis. Well-appearing febrile infants without an infectious focus (otitis media, skin, soft tissue, bone, or joint) who are over 1 mo of age, with good follow-up, no history of prematurity or prior antimicrobial therapy, and a WBC count between 5,000 and 15,000, less than 1,500 bands, less than 10 WBC/high-power field (HPF) on examination of centrifuged urine (or negative leukocyte esterase), and less than 5 WBC/HPF on examination of stool in infants with diarrhea, may be discharged home without therapy. Some physicians administer ceftriaxone (IM) to these infants after obtaining a blood culture. In either case, careful outpatient management requires close phone contact for 48 hr and a return visit within 24 hr.

References

Baraff LJ, Bass J, Fleisher G, et al: Practice guidelines for management of infants and children 0 to 36 months of age with fever without source. Pediatrics 92:1, 1993.

Behrman RE (ed): Nelson Textbook of Pediatrics. 14th ed. Philadelphia, WB Saunders, 1992, Sec. 9.58–9.60, 12.1–12.9.

Lieu TA, Baskin MN, Schwartz S, et al: Clinical and cost-effectiveness of outpatient strategies for management of febrile infants. Pediatrics 89:1135, 1992.

Powell KR: Antimicrobial therapy for suspected sepsis in infants less than three months of age. Pediatr Infect Dis J 11:143, 1992.

Wald ER, Dashefsky B: Cautionary note on the use of empiric ceftriaxone for suspected bacteremia. Am J Dis Child 145:1359, 1991.

Fever of Unknown Origin

FUO (fever >100.4°F lasting for more than 14 days with no obvious cause despite a complete history, physical exam, and routine laboratory evaluation) historically was a difficult problem because most patients remained undiagnosed despite in-hospital evaluation for 1 wk. The differential diagnosis between occult infections and neoplasms often required invasive procedures. With the improved capability of diagnostic imaging techniques (combined with imaging-guided needle biopsy), including ultrasound, computerized tomography (CT), magnetic resonance imaging (MRI), and radionuclide scanning with gallium or technetium, the number of undiagnosed patients in this category has decreased substantially.

Etiology. In addition to carefully documenting several instances of an elevated temperature, a thorough *history* should be undertaken, including the impact the fever has had on the child's health; weight loss; presence of an associated disease such as diabetes mellitus or malignancy; involvement of vital organs such as liver, heart, or brain; use of drugs, medications, or immunosuppressive therapy; exposure to industrial or hobby-related chemicals; blood transfusions; domestic or foreign travel to endemic areas (malaria, histoplasmosis, coccidioidomycosis, *Cryptococcus neoformans,* Colorado tick fever); genetic background; recent surgical procedure or dental work; and sexual activity. Specific attention should be paid to the social history and exposure to pathogens (malaria, tuberculosis, day care) or animals (birds, livestock, bats, reptiles, pets) and insects (tick, mosquito).

Because the etiology of most occult infections is an unusual presentation of a common disease, an evaluation for diseases typical to a geographic locale should pursued. Thus, an adolescent from an urban area with a FUO requires a careful evaluation for bacterial diseases, including tuberculosis, salmonellae, and spirochetes, as well as viral entities, including Epstein-Barr virus (EBV), cytomegalovirus (CMV), human immunodeficiency virus (HIV), and hepatitis A, B, and C viruses. Inhabitants of or travelers to rural areas should be evaluated for zoonosis and insect or water-borne pathogens.

In the absence of localizing signs (heart murmur, abdominal pain, abnormal liver function), it may be difficult to focus the evaluation. Furthermore, entities such as sinusitis, endocarditis, intra-abdominal abscesses (perinephric, intrahepatic, subdiaphragmatic), and central nervous system (CNS) lesions (tuberculoma, cystercercosis, abscess, toxoplasmosis) may be relatively asymptomatic. A FUO also may be the presentation of an immunodeficiency disease.

Differential Diagnosis.   The three most common categories of FUO in children are infectious diseases, connective tissue or inflammatory diseases, and neoplasms. A diagnosis is not established in 10–20% of children with FUO.

The bacterial diseases most commonly implicated in children can be grouped into two categories—generalized infections caused by specific organisms and localized infections caused by a variety of organisms. In the United States, organisms and conditions most frequently associated with FUO in children that produce a generalized infection include *Brucella, Salmonella, Mycobacterium,* tularemia, spirochetes (leptospirosis, Lyme disease, rat-bite fever, syphilis), CMV, hepatitis viruses, and EBV. Localized infections include endocarditis, intra-abdominal or liver abscess, sinusitis, mastoiditis, osteomyelitis, pneumonia, and pyelonephritis or perinephric abscess.

The connective tissue (inflammatory) diseases that most commonly manifest as FUO are juvenile rheumatoid arthritis (JRA), systemic lupus erythematosus (SLE), polyarteritis nodosa, rheumatic fever, inflammatory bowel disease, and undefined vasculitis (see Chapter 9).

Malignancies are a less common cause of FUO in children than in adults, accounting for about 10% of all episodes. Malignancies that may be associated with FUO include Hodgkin and non-Hodgkin lymphoma, leukemia, Ewing sarcoma, and neuroblastoma.

Factitious fever is another important consideration: Fever should be documented in the hospital by a reliable individual who remains with the patient when the temperature is taken. Psychiatric disorders frequently are masked by the family's denial and desire to find an organic cause for their child's problems. Continuously observing the patient over a long period of time and repetitive evaluation are indicated.

Clinical Manifestations.   By definition, *physical findings* are minimal in children with FUO, but several important areas often are overlooked. Accurate weight measurements help document the impact of the FUO process on the nutritional status of the patient. Sweating should be noted; its absence suggests dehydration resulting from vomiting and diarrhea, central or nephrogenic diabetes insipidus, anhidrotic ectodermal dysplasia, familial dysautonomia, or exposure to atropine.

Red, weeping eyes may be a sign of systemic disease, particularly polyarteritis nodosa, sarcoidosis, inflammatory bowel disease, Kawasaki disease, or JRA. Palpebral conjunctivits may be a clue to measles, coxsackievirus, tuberculosis, infectious mononucleosis, lymphogranuloma venereum, cat-scratch disease, or Newcastle disease. In contrast, bulbar conjunctivitis in a child with FUO suggests leptospirosis, Kawasaki disease, or rheumatologic disorders.

FUO may be caused by hypothalamic dysfunction. A clue to this disorder is the failure of the pupils to constrict because of the absence of the sphincter constrictor muscle of the eye. This muscle develops embryologically when hypothalamic structure and function also are undergoing differentiation. Lack of tears, insensitivity to pain, a smooth tongue displaying an absence of fungiform papillae, an absent corneal reflex, failure to thrive and gastroesophageal reflux may suggest fever from **familial dysautonomia.**

Tenderness to tapping over the sinuses and teeth should be sought, and the sinuses should be transilluminated. Oral candidiasis may be a clue to various disorders of the immune system, especially acquired immunodeficiency syndrome (AIDS). Fever blisters are common findings in patients with pneumococcal, streptococcal, malarial, or rickettsial infection. Hyperemia of the pharynx, with or without exudate, may suggest infectious mononucleosis, CMV, toxoplasmosis, salmonellosis, tularemia, or leptospirosis.

Repetitive chills and temperature spikes are common in children with septicemia, regardless of cause, particularly when associated with renal, liver, or biliary tract disease; endocarditis; malaria; brucellosis; rat-bite fever; or loculated collections of pus. Careful ophthalmologic evaluation is helpful in establishing collagen vascular and granulomatous diseases, CMV, endocarditis, fungal infection, leukemia, sarcoidosis, syphilis, toxoplasmosis, and tuberculosis.

The muscles and bones should be palpated carefully. Point tenderness over a bone suggests osteomyelitis or neoplastic bone marrow invasion. Tenderness over the trapezius muscle may be a clue to a subdiaphragmatic abscess. Generalized muscle tenderness suggests dermatomyositis, trichinosis, polyarteritis, or mycoplasma, influenza, or arboviral infection.

Rectal or pelvic examination may reveal tenderness and suggest a deep pelvic abscess, iliac or mesenteric adenitis, or pelvic osteomyelitis. A guaiac test on stool should be performed because occult blood loss suggests inflammatory bowel disease. Hyperactive deep tendon reflexes suggest thyrotoxicosis.

Diagnosis. Children with unexplained fever should be evaluated in a logical sequence beginning with a meticulous history, comprehensive physical examination, and compilation of screening laboratory data. An organ system approach is helpful. The urgency of further testing will depend on the clinical status of the patient and the tempo of the disease processes. Not all patients with unexplained fever need be evaluated for all of the conditions associated with FUO. Young infants with unexplained fever frequently have undefined viral illnesses such as EBV infections. Other causes of FUO in infants include pyogenic bacterial infections, JRA, or Kawasaki disease. A more aggressive approach would be required to evaluate an infant with daily fever spikes to 105°F and significant toxicity.

The *immunologic competency* of the host may need to be evaluated, by monitoring T cell function by skin testing with an anergy panel as well as an intermediate-strength purified protein derivative, checking for lymphocytosis or leukocytosis with a WBC and differential count, doing T cell subsets, evaluating B cell function by immunoglobulin lev-

Table 10–8. FUO Evaluation: Additional Screening Tests

CBC with WBC differential and smear
ESR, CRP
Urinalysis
Blood electrolytes, glucose, calcium
Liver function tests—transaminase enzymes, bilirubin (direct and total)
CPK, albumin, globulin

Cultures
Blood (off all antimicrobial agents)
Urine
Stool—including examination for ova and parasites

Serologic Tests
VDRL/ART
Antinuclear antibodies
Rheumatoid factor
Complement
Immune complexes
Monospot—EBV titers

Roentgenographic Tests
Chest roentgenogram
Abdominal ultrasonography
CT scan
MR imaging

CBC = complete blood count; CPK = creatine phosphokinase; CRP = C-reactive protein; VDRL/ART = Venereal Disease Research Laboratory test/automated reagin test.

els, and measuring complement. Additional screening tests for the evaluation of an FUO are listed in Table 10–8. These additional tests should be used judiciously and should focus on areas suggested by the screening tests, physical findings, or historic data.

Central Nervous System. The child with headache, possible sinusitis, or other signs suggestive of CNS involvement should have a CT scan. Although acute bacterial meningitis is not a cause of FUO, a lumbar puncture and analysis of cerebral spinal fluid (CSF) may be informative and lead to diagnoses such as SLE, Lyme disease, or syphilis. A parameningeal focus may be suggested by CSF findings that could then be identified by CT scan with contrast or MRI. Silent CNS lesions, such as small brain abscesses, tuberculomas, toxoplasmosis, or cystercercosis may be identified.

Cardiovascular Disease. Bacterial endocarditis is an important cause of FUO but may be difficult to diagnose, because patients frequently are given oral antibiotics that sterilize blood cultures but are inadequate to sterilize intracardiac vegetations (see Chapter 13). The evaluation of myocarditis, endocarditis, or pericarditis includes echocardiography and both transthoracic and transesophageal echocardiography.

Pulmonary Disease. Even in the absence of respiratory manifestations, pulmonary disease may be a cause of FUO. Patients with significant parenchymal disease, pleural disease, mediastinal widening, or hilar adenopathy may be asymptomatic. The determination of arterial blood gases may be helpful to define alveolar disease. CT scan or MRI may assist in the assessment of the extent of disease and suggest a diagnosis. Hilar adenopathy may suggest lymphoma, sarcoidosis, histoplasmosis, or tuberculosis. The diagnosis of sarcoidosis requires a tissue biopsy via fiberoptic or rigid bronchoscopy. Interstitial infiltrates may be associated with histiocytosis, CMV, *Pneumocystis carinii* or HIV infection. Bronchoalveolar lavage and examination of fluid is indicated in such patients.

Gastrointestinal Disease. Many causes of FUO originate from the gastrointestinal tract, either as walled-off occult abscesses from clinically inapparent appendiceal perforations or hepatic, pelvic, and splenic abscesses, or as inflammatory bowel disease. CT with contrast or MRI may be helpful following screening ultrasonography. These tests are useful in ruling out mass lesions and evaluating the integrity of the gastrointestinal tract and bowel wall. Children suspected of inflammatory bowel disease may require contrast studies and endoscopy.

Weight loss and diarrhea may indicate parasitic infection, which may occur in a normal or immunodeficient child. In addition to the screening tests (above), careful evaluation for parasites also may include a total eosinophil count and a string test for *Giardia*. In HIV-infected patients, usually innocuous organisms such as *Blastocystis hominis* may be associated with significant symptoms.

Genitourinary Disease. The genitourinary tract may be the source of several causes of FUO, including tuberculosis, (heralded by sterile pyuria), perinephric abscess, and neuroblastoma. Ultrasound followed by CT is utilized in the evaluation of possible renal pathology, pelvic abscess, pelvic inflammatory disease, or other occult genitourinary infections.

Musculoskeletal Disease. The usual presentation of osteomyelitis or septic arthritis is that of an acute localized infection. However, vertebral or pelvic osteomyelitis that is not apparent may cause FUO. Similarly, a psoas abscess may present as vague back pain without localizing signs. Technetium pyrophosphate radionuclide imaging, which is highly sensitive for osteoclast and osteoblast activity, is extremely useful in detecting bony involvement. Similarly, a gallium scan, which indicates collections of polymorphonuclear leukocytes, may be useful to screen for abscesses. CT scan or MRI is helpful in demonstrating the presence of Ewing sarcoma, which often presents as bone pain with FUO.

The presence or history of arthritis, even if evanescent or migratory, may be very important in establishing the diagnosis of Lyme disease, autoimmune processes (see Chapter 9), or one of the postinfectious arthritides, such as Reiter's syndrome. Appropriate screening serologic tests may be helpful (Table 10–8). Myositis frequently is suggested by myalgias, muscle tenderness, and a high serum creatine phosphokinase (CPK) level.

Hematologic Disease. Children with FUO and/or chronic infection are frequently anemic. Examination of a peripheral blood smear may indicate findings suggestive of the "anemia of chronic disease" or the toxic granulations suggestive of bacterial infection. An examination of the bone marrow may be indicated to exclude hematologic malignancy or storage cells. Bone marrow aspirates should be examined and cultures for fungi (histoplasmosis) and mycobacteria (*Mycobacterium tuberculosis* and *M. avium-intracellulare*) as well as for other bacteria.

Treatment. By definition, a FUO is a chronic process. Every effort should be made to come to a specific diagnosis before initiating therapy, particularly with those modalities that may mask significant underlying diseases.

References

Behrman RE (ed): Nelson Textbook of Pediatrics. 14th ed. Philadelphia, WB Saunders, 1992, Sec. 12.3.

Hayani A, Mahoney DH, Fernbach DJ: Role of bone marrow examination in the child with prolonged fever. J Pediatr 118:919, 1990.

Knockaert DC, Vanneste LJ, Vanneste SB, et al: Fever of unknown origin in the 1980s: An update of the diagnostic spectrum. Arch Intern Med 152:51, 1992.

Steele RW, Jones SM, Lowe BA, et al: Usefulness of scanning procedures for diagnosis of fever of unknown origin in children. J Pediatr 119:526, 1991.

Fever in the Immunocompromised Host

The evaluation of fever in immunologically impaired patients is quite different than in normal hosts. Although a FUO may be the initial presentation of an immune deficiency, it is more common to be faced with a febrile patient with a known immunodeficiency. The types of infections and their management can be predicted by which part(s) of the immune system are abnormal.

FEVER AND NEUTROPENIA

Infection is the major cause of death in patients with hematologic malignancy or after transplantation. The use of antineoplastic agents that cause neutropenia (myelosuppression), as well as the regimens used for bone marrow transplantation, deplete bone marrow granulocyte precursor cells, resulting in a high frequency of bacterial sepsis. As the peripheral WBC count decreases below 500, patients are at risk for bacterial sepsis caused by their own endogenous flora (gastrointestinal aerobic gram-negative rods or cutaneous staphylococci). Febrile episodes in neutropenic patients routinely are treated with combinations of broad-spectrum antimicrobial agents (e.g., vancomycin or nafcillin–ceftazidine or antipseudomonas penicillin–aminogycoside) until the WBC count improves; some patients are placed on prophylactic antimicrobial agents to prevent sepsis. The use of recombinant granulocyte colony-stimulating factor or granulocyte-macrophage–stimulating factor stimulates neutrophil production by the bone marrow, reduces the duration and severity of neutropenia, and decreases the risk of infection.

Fungal infection (*Candida,* aspergillosis) also becomes a problem in persistently neutropenic patients. A febrile neutropenic patient, who remains febrile despite broad-spectrum antibacterial agents may require administration of amphotericin B. Fungal infections may produce fungemia, sinusitis, pneumonia, endophthalmitis and soft tissue, hepatic, splenic, or renal abscesses. Neutropenic patients may receive prophylactic antifungal agents (fluconazole).

In the absence of neutrophils to localize an infection, it often is difficult to determine the source of infection by physical examination. For example, the chest examination may be negative, despite significant infection, but abnormalities may be revealed by chest roentgenogram and arterial blood gases. Bronchoalveolar lavage is recommended to identify pulmonary pathogens. Many patients have indwelling central venous catheters to facilitate chemotherapy and blood drawing. Coagulase-negative staphylococci frequently colonize these catheters and are a source of infection in the absence of signs. Sinus infection (bacteria, *Aspergillus,*

Zygomycetes) is common in neutropenic hosts and may only be appreciated by CT scan. Perirectal abscess is another focus of infection in neutropenic hosts; tenderness and erythema may be the only clues to a significant local infection. In addition to antibiotics effective against gram negative and staphylococcal bacteria, metronidazole is indicated to treat anaerobic bacteria in perirectal abscesses.

FEVER IN THE TRANSPLANT PATIENT

The management of fever following an organ transplant is somewhat different than during leukemic or bone marrow transplantation. The use of cyclosporine and steroids decreases T cell function. The transplant patient is more likely to develop infection with herpes simplex, varicella zoster, CMV, *P. carinii,* or toxoplasmosis. The transplanted organ itself may be the source of CMV or toxoplasmosis. Most transplant protocols use prophylactic antimicrobial agents such as trimethoprim–sulfamethoxazole, acyclovir and/or gancyclovir, and fluconazole.

References

Behrman RE (ed): Nelson Textbook of Pediatrics, 14th ed. Philadelphia, WB Saunders, 1992, Sec. 12.13.
Kim JH, Perfect JR: Infection and cyclosporine. Rev Infect Dis 11:677, 1989.
Pizzo PA, Rubin M, Freifeld A, et al: The child with cancer and infection. I. Empiric therapy for fever and neutropenia, and preventive strategies. J Pediatr 119:679, 1991.

BACTEREMIA AND SEPTICEMIA

Bacteremia is bloodstream infection documented by positive blood cultures. This is distinguished from *sepsis,* which is the systemic response to infection and includes tachypnea, tachycardia, hyperthermia, hypothermia, and neutropenia or leukocytosis. The *sepsis syndrome* (also called the systemic inflammatory response syndrome, SIRS) includes the clinical diagnosis of sepsis with evidence of altered organ perfusion, including hypoxemia, oliguria, or elevated blood lactate level. In approximately 10% of patients having a sepsis syndrome the blood culture is negative. *Septic shock* includes the clinical diagnosis of the sepsis syndrome plus hypotension despite fluid resuscitation. See Chapter 3 for discussion of shock.

Etiology and Epidemiology.   The age and immunization status of the child are important factors in determining which organisms must be considered

Table 10–9. Risk Factors for Bacterial Sepsis

Age
Premature > full term > infant under 2 yr old

Immunodeficiency
AIDS
Sickle cell anemia plus other asplenic conditions
Neutropenia and immunosuppression (malignancy)
Neutrophil chemotactic defects
Complement deficiency
Malnutrition
Severe combined immunodeficiency syndrome
B cell defects (agammaglobulinemia)

Associated Disease States
Malignancy
Nephrotic syndrome
Galactosemia
Intravenous drug abuse
Paraplegia
Gonococcal genitourinary infection
Contact with *N. meningitidis* or *H. influenzae* (day care, etc.)

Medical Instrumentation/Procedures
Indwelling intravascular catheters
Indwelling urinary catheter
Endotracheal intubation (nasotracheal > orotracheal)
Ventriculoatrial shunts
Continuous peritoneal dialysis
Surgery
Prosthetic heart valves

(Table 10-9). In neonatal sepsis, the important micro-organisms are group B streptococci, *E. coli*, other streptococci, *S. aureus*, *Staphylococcus epidermidis* and *Listeria monocytogenes*. In the immunocompetent older febrile child with no localizing findings, the most common pathogens are *S. pneumoniae*, *H. influenzae* type b, *N. meningitidis*, *Salmonella*, *S. aureus*, and group A streptococci. Infants with galactosemia and children with pyelonephritis often have gram-negative bacteremia (e.g., *E. coli*).

Immunocompromised children (those with asplenia, sickle cell disease, neutropenia, malignancy, AIDS, or indwelling foreign bodies) are infected by a broader spectrum of organisms and are more prone to develop septicemia. Illness may be due to common organisms or may be associated with a wide variety of bacteria or fungi.

In some patients, bacteremia or septicemia may be associated with focal infections (e.g., pyelonephritis, pneumonia, cellulitis, osteomyelitis, endocarditis, meningitis). In such cases, when bacteremia or septicemia is strongly suspected, cultures should be obtained and intravenous broad-spectrum antibiotics administered.

Pathophysiology of Septic Shock. The pathophysiology of septic shock is based, in large part, on the body's response to microbial products. Lipid A (endotoxin) of gram-negative bacteria triggers a cascade of events, probably mediated by the resultant activation or production of inflammatory mediators (complement, prostaglandins, leukotrienes, kinins) and cytokines. Endotoxin stimulates the production of several cytokines from macrophages, including IL-1 and TNF, that produce fever, increased vascular permeability, and hypotension; increase the numbers of circulating neutrophils from the bone marrow; mobilize amino acids from skeletal muscle (catabolism); and amplify the immune response (see Chapter 3). Reactions in the lung lead to the development of the often fatal adult respiratory distress syndrome (ARDS) (see Chapter 12) and multiorgan system failure (see Chapter 3).

Clinical Manifestations. A clinical diagnosis of presumptive septicemia should be made when the child's fever and toxic appearance (tachycardia, hyperventilation, agitation, lethargy, poor perfusion) suggest serious illness. The history and physical examination may indicate the site of origin. The early features of septicemia are similar to those of many infections. The child usually is febrile; however, hypothermia may be an important sign of sepsis in the neonate, the neutropenic immunosuppressed patient, or the burn patient. Chills, hyperventilation, tachycardia, hypotension, and peripheral vasodilation are early signs. There may be petechiae and purpura. Apprehension, confusion, and agitation also are often early signs of septic shock, which often progresses to lethargy and coma. Profound hypotension with cold, clammy, mottled skin, cyanosis, poor capillary refill, a weak pulse, lethargy, and coma are observed later in the progression of shock.

Cutaneous lesions, such as purpura and petechiae, classically are seen in meningococcemia but may occur in infection with other organisms. *Pseudomonas aeruginosa* causes a characteristic skin lesion called *ecthyma gangrenosum*. These lesions are single round or oval lesions that look like a bull's eye, with a necrotic ulcer in the center surrounded by a rim of redness and induration. Disseminated intravascular coagulation (DIC) is common and becomes manifest as purpura and bleeding from puncture sites. Hypotension may result in peripheral gangrene, anuric renal failure, and lactic acidosis.

Diagnosis and Differential Diagnosis. In all patients, especially those immunocompromised by an underlying disease or by cancer therapy, the outcome of sepsis depends on early diagnosis and treatment. Several blood cultures should be obtained to identify the specific organism. All suspected sites of infection should be examined by culture and Gram stain for evidence of bacterial infection; these sites include cerebrospinal fluid, sputum, skin lesions, urine, and the buffy coat. The latter is the leukocyte-rich fraction of a centrifuged sample of blood and is located between the serum and erythrocyte interface. Gram-, methylene blue–, or acridine orange–stained leukocytes demonstrate bacteria in many patients with bacteremia. Latex agglutination may be helpful to identify certain bacteria, including *H. influenzae* type b, *S. pneumonia, N. meningitidis,* and group B streptococci in less than 2 hr. These tests are particularly helpful when previous antibiotics were given before obtaining cultures. A chest roentgenogram is indicated to identify pneumonia, pleural effusions, or ARDS.

Neutropenia is an important early laboratory finding caused by infection-mediated neutrophil storage pool depletion and margination of cells. Thrombocytopenia and reduced factor VIII concentration reflect DIC, whereas fibrin split products are the result of fibrinolysis. Thrombocytopenia also may be due to platelet antibodies produced during sepsis. Clotting factor abnormalities also may be a result of liver failure or antibiotic toxicity. Lactic acidosis is due to tissue hypoxia from shock or pulmonary insufficiency.

Many infectious and noninfectious diseases are associated with systemic symptoms similar to those of bacteremia or septicemia. Infectious diseases include rickettsial disease, such as Rocky Mountain spotted fever, staphylococcal toxic shock syndrome, leptospirosis, plague, Lyme disease, tuberculosis, tularemia, yersiniosis, viral sepsis (herpes simplex, enterovirus), malaria, and fungal diseases (Cryptococcosis, candidiasis). Noninfectious diseases include anaphylactic shock, toxic ingestions, hemorrhagic shock, midgut volvulus, vasculitis, and Kawasaki disease.

Treatment. Broad-spectrum antibiotics that are bactericidal against both gram-negative and gram-positive bacteria should be initiated before the causative bacteria are identified. Therapy of suspected gram-negative sepsis includes an aminoglycoside plus an antipseudomonas penicillin (ticarcillin or piperacillin) or a broad-spectrum third-generation cephalosporin (such as ceftazidime) (see Appendix I for dosages). Treatment of nosocomial infections may be aided by knowledge of the susceptibility patterns of bacteria prevalent in the hospital setting. When methicillin-resistant *S. aureus* and *S. epidermidis* are suspected, vancomycin should be added. Anaerobic bacteremia frequently complicates infections of the mouth, abdomen, rectum, or pelvis and requires therapy with either clindamycin or metronidazole in addition to antibiotics active against gram-negative enteric pathogens. Identifying the specific bacteria and performing antimicrobial susceptibility tests form the basis for administering antibiotics having a narrow spectrum, which avoids superinfection by yeast or resistant bacteria and reduces antibiotic toxicity.

Supportive care for shock is best performed in a pediatric intensive care unit where continuous monitoring of vital signs is possible (see Chapter 3). Venodilation, transcapillary fluid losses, and hemorrhage require the expansion of the circulating blood volume (with colloid of crystalloid solutions) to maintain the perfusion of vital organs. In addition to volume replacement, septic shock must be treated with sympathomimetic drugs, such as dopamine, dobutamine, or epinephrine. These drugs improve cardiac output and renal and systemic perfusion and may increase vascular tone. The mortality rate for patients having septic shock is 40–70%. When multiple organ systems fail (e.g., in ARDS or renal or hepatic failure), the mortality rate approaches 90–100%.

References

Behrman RE (ed): Nelson Textbook of Pediatrics. 14th ed. Philadelphia, WB Saunders, 1992, Sec. 12.14–12.15.

Bone RC, Balk RA, Cerra FB, et al: Definitions for sepsis and organ failure and guidelines for the use of innovative therapies in sepsis. Chest 101:644, 1992.

Cohen J, Glauser MP: Septic shock: Treatment. Lancet 338: 736, 1991.

Glauser MP, Zanetti G, Baumgartner J-D, et al: Septic shock: Pathogenesis. Lancet 338:732, 1992.

Martin MA, Silverman HJ: Gram-negative sepsis and the adult respiratory distress syndrome. Clin Infect Dis 14: 1213, 1992.

OSTEOMYELITIS AND SEPTIC ARTHRITIS

Infections of bones (osteomyelitis) and joints (septic arthritis) usually are due to bacterial pathogens and must be differentiated from cellulitis, trauma, inflammatory reactions, and malignancy.

Osteomyelitis

Osteomyelitis may occur at any age but is most common in children between the ages of 3 and 12 yr and affects boys twice as frequently as girls.

Pathogenesis. Infections of the bone may result from hematogenous dissemination or by direct spread from a contiguous focus of infection. Osteomyelitis in children is most often the consequence of bacteremia and involves rapidly growing bone, particularly the metaphyses of long bones (distal femur, proximal tibia, distal humerus, distal radius). Bacteria lodge in sharp loops of nutrient arteries supplying the growth plates of these bones. Blood in the large sinusoidal veins flows slowly and there are no phagocytic cells in this area. Obstruction to flow by bacterial microemboli produce small areas of avascular necrosis with a resultant metaphyseal abscess. Trauma often is noted prior to the onset of osteomyelitis and may result in local areas of bone injury that predispose to infection. This may mislead the clinician to think the bone symptoms are due to trauma. In infants less than 1 yr of age, the capillaries perforate the epiphyseal growth plate, permitting spread across the epiphysis, causing a septic arthritis (Fig. 10–1). In older children the infection is contained in the metaphyseal sinusoidal veins because the vessels no longer cross the epiphyseal plate (Fig. 10–2). Osteoarthritis also may be seen in joints where the capsule inserts on the metaphysis proximal to the epiphyseal plate. Pyoarthritis is common in these joints (hip, elbow,

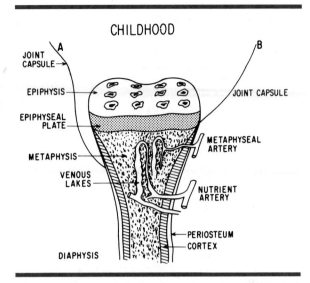

Figure 10–2. Major structures of the bone of a child. Joint capsule *A* inserts below the epiphyseal growth plate, as in the hip, elbow, ankle, and shoulder. Rupture of a metaphyseal abscess in these bones is likely to produce pyarthrosis. Joint capsule *B* inserts at the epiphyseal growth plate, as in other tubular bones. Rupture of a metaphyseal abscess in these bones is likely to lead to a subperiosteal abscess but seldom to an associated pyarthrosis. (From Gutman LT: Acute, subacute, and chronic osteomyelitis in children. Curr Probl Pediatr 15: 7, 1985.)

shoulder, knee) (Fig. 10–2). Infection spreads through the haversian system and Volkmann canals; as infection spreads laterally, the periosteum is lifted. In chronic osteomyelitis the infected periosteum may calcify into a shell of new bone around the infected portion of the shaft and is called an *involucrum*. The host defense mechanisms may wall off a metaphyseal abscess, producing a chronic infection with a sclerotic rim called a *Brodie abscess*. Dead bone within this space is called *sequestrum*.

Contiguous osteomyelitis is less common in children and usually occurs following spread of cellulitis, as a result of an infected wound such as a decubitus or sinus or periodontal disease, or following surgical procedures. Osteomyelitis also may result from direct inoculation from a penetrating wound, heel punctures, paronychia, open fracture, orthopedic surgery, and human or animal bites.

Etiology. *Staphylococcus aureus* is responsible for most infections. *H. influenzae* type b, group B (in neonates) or other streptococci, anaerobic microorganisms, gram-negative enteric bacteria, and *M.*

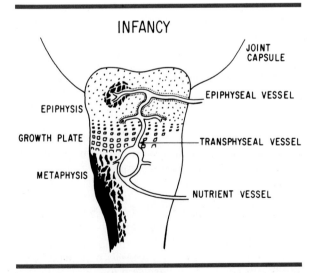

Figure 10–1. Major structures of the bone of an infant prior to maturation of the epiphyseal growth plate. Note the transphyseal vessel, which connects the vascular supply of the epiphysis and metaphysis, facilitating spread of infection between these two areas. (From Gutman LT: Acute, subacute, and chronic osteomyelitis and pyogenic arthritis in children. Curr Probl Pediatr 15:6, 1985.)

tuberculosis also cause osteomyelitis. Other factors that predispose the patient to osteomyelitis include furunculosis, infected lesions of varicella, infected burns, prolonged intravenous or central parenteral alimentation, intravenous drug abuse, and trauma. Sickle cell anemia and other hemoglobinopathies predispose the patient to osteomyelitis caused by *Salmonella* or *Staphylococcus* species, or, less commonly, *S. pneumoniae*. Osteomyelitis secondary to dog or cat bites may be caused by *Pasteurella multocida*. *Pseudomonas* osteomyelitis commonly follows puncture wounds of the foot (in sneaker wearers) or intravenous drug abuse.

Clinical Manifestations. Hematogenous osteomyelitis in children usually involves a single bone (after infancy) and occurs either as an acute illness with fever, focal bone pain, and sepsis or as a subacute illness with mild systemic signs but with local complaints at the site of involved bone. These complaints include severe pain, exquisite tenderness, warmth, erythema, and swelling. Weight bearing and spontaneous or requested motion are refused, which mimics paralysis (pseudoparalysis). Muscle spasm may make the extremity difficult to examine. Hematogenous osteomyelitis involving the vertebrae is notable for an insidious onset, vague symptomatology, backache, occasional spinal cord compression, and usually little associated fever or systemic toxicity. With osteomyelitis of the pelvis, presenting signs may include limp; abdominal, hip, groin, or thigh pain; and fever. Table 10–10 shows features of acute hematogenous osteomyelitis.

Diagnosis. Marked tenderness over the involved site identifies the infected bone. Leukocytosis may be present. The ESR usually is elevated and is of great help in monitoring the response to treatment. Blood cultures (positive in 60%), cultures of an aspirate of cellulitis, and a diagnostic aspirate of the periosteal space (or, if negative, of the bone itself) should be obtained prior to instituting antibiotic therapy. The evaluation of patients with chronic disease includes obtaining a tuberculin test and performing a chest roentgenogram. The tuberculin test may be especially helpful in establishing a diagnosis in vertebral osteomyelitis.

Roentgenograms of the affected areas should be obtained to allow observation of soft tissue swelling, periosteal elevation and calcification, and bone destruction, and to consider a possible alternative diagnosis, such as bone tumors, bone cysts, leukemia, or histiocytosis. Plain films of the bone generally are normal during the early phase (10–14 days); the radionuclide technetium-99 bone scan may be valuable if plain films are normal.

Treatment. Initial intravenous antibiotic therapy should be based on results of Gram stain of bone aspirate, blood culture reports, age, and associated diseases. Initial therapy should cover the penicillinase-producing staphylococci (oxacillin, nafcillin, methicillin, clindamycin) (see Appendix I for dosages) and the possibility of methicillin-resistant staphylococci should be considered. In patients with sickle cell anemia, *Salmonella* and *S. aureus* must both be covered (cefotaxime, ceftriaxone). Gram-negative organisms may be present if wound contamination or a history of intravenous drug abuse is discovered. *H. influenzae* should be suspected in young children and requires therapy with ceftriaxone, cefotaxime, or ampicillin/sulbactam. *Candida*, *Aspergillus*, and *Rhizopus* are potential pathogens in immunocompromised patients or those receiving long-term parenteral hyperalimentation and require appropriate antifungal therapy (amphoteracin B).

The response to appropriate intravenous antibiotics usually occurs within 48 hr, and lack of improvement in fever and pain after this time indicates that surgical drainage may be necessary or

Table 10–10. Clinical Manifestations of Acute Hematogenous Osteomyelitis by Age Groups

Age	Usual Site of Involvement	Symptoms and Signs	Expected Organism
Neonate	Varied; 40% may have multiple sites	Usually few systemic signs; local edema; reduced limb motion; joint effusion (60–70%)	Group B streptococci, *Escherichia coli*, *Staphylococcus aureus* or *Candida*
1–24 mo	Long bones; may involve joints	Pseudoparalysis, fever, limp	*S. aureus*, group B streptococci
2–20 yr	Metaphysis of long bones; rarely, vertebral bodies or pelvis	Focal pain with fever (90%) for days to weeks; focal tenderness (70%); focal swelling (70%) or joint effusion (20%)	*S. aureus* (60–90%), streptococci (10%), *Salmonella*; rarely, gram-negative bacilli, anaerobes, or fungi

that an unusual pathogen *(M. tuberculosis)* may be present. Surgical drainage may be appropriate at an earlier time if a sequestrum is present, if the disease is chronic or atypical, if the hip joint is involved, or if the disease occurs in the presence of spinal cord compression.

Standard therapy consists of administering antibiotics parenterally for 4–6 wk or longer. Oral antibiotics are effective after a good response to intravenous therapy (see Septic Arthritis). If oral antibiotics are administered, (1) patients may need to be hospitalized for the entire period of therapy, (2) intravenous antibiotics should be provided for an initial period of 5–7 days, (3) good clinical response to intravenous therapy should be documented, (4) satisfactory activity of the oral drug against the organism isolated from the patient should be demonstrated, and (5) oral absorption should be assessed by measuring the patient's serum bactericidal activity against the specific pathogen. Dosage should achieve a peak bactericidal titer of at least 1:8–1:16.

Inadequate or delayed antibiotic therapy of osteomyelitis often leads to chronic abscess formation, draining sinus tracts, pathologic fractures, orthopedic deformity, and amyloidosis.

Septic Arthritis

Septic or suppurative arthritis is a serious infection of the joint space occurring most commonly during the first 2 yr of life and during adolescence.

Pathogenesis. Septic arthritis results from (1) hematogenous dissemination of bacteria, (2) contiguous spread from surrounding soft tissues, and (3) spread of osteomyelitis through the epiphysis into the joint space in young children (Figs. 10–1 and 10–2). Septic arthritis must be differentiated from postinfectious joint effusions, which are sterile and often due to antigen–antibody complex deposition. Joint effusions developing after 7 days of a bacterial illness (bacteremia, meningitis, diarrhea, urethritis) more often are immunologically mediated, whereas those presenting in the first 3 days more often represent hematogenous spread of bacteria.

Etiology. *Staphylococcus aureus* is the most common agent, but *H. influenzae* type b is the most frequent cause in the 2 mo to 4 yr old child, followed by staphylococci, streptococci, pneumococci, and meningococci. Joint effusions may develop in patients with *H. influenzae* type b infection or with meningococcal sepsis and meningitis (see Patho-

genesis). Meningococcal arthritis may occur in the absence of sepsis or meningitis. Gonococcal arthritis associated with disseminated gonococcal infection is the most common cause of polyarthritis or monoarticular arthritis in adolescents. In endemic areas Lyme arthritis also must be considered.

Clinical Manifestations. The presentation has the typical features of infection: erythema, warmth, swelling, and tenderness over the affected joint, with a palpable effusion and decreased range of movement. The onset may be sudden, resulting in an ill-appearing child with fever and chills, or may be insidious, with symptoms only noted when the joint is moved, such as during a diaper change, or if parents become aware of decreased voluntary movement (pseudoparalysis) of a joint or limb. Toddlers may present with a limp. It is often difficult to assess septic arthritis of the hip, which may cause referred pain to the knee. The limb may be positioned in external rotation and flexion to minimize pain from pressure on the hip's joint capsule. Similarly, the knee and elbow joints usually are held in flexion. An acute septic arthritis most often involves a single joint (knee, hip, ankle, shoulder, elbow, wrist), with multiple joints affected in less than 10% of cases.

Diagnosis and Differential Diagnosis. Leukocytosis and an elevated ESR are common. Arthrocentesis is the test of choice for rapidly diagnosing suppurative arthritis (Table 10–11). During arthrocentesis, it is important to avoid crossing an overlying area of cellulitis to prevent the inoculation of bacteria and the conversion of a deep cellulitis into septic arthritis. Blood and/or joint cultures are positive in up to 85% of patients infected with *H. influenzae.* Joint fluid that exhibits the characteristics of pyogenic infection may not reveal bacterial pathogens in up to 30% of patients who have never received antibiotic therapy, because synovial fluid exerts a bacteriostatic effect. Antigen detection, KOH preparation for fungi (neonates, immunosuppressed patients), acid-fast stain, and Gram stain are helpful if no bacteria are covered. In chronic arthritis, synovial biopsy may distinguish between an infectious and a noninfectious process. Because septic arthritis may be present with osteomyelitis, roentgenograms or bone scans of the adjacent bone usually are indicated once therapy is initiated. Adolescents with acute septic arthritis should have urethral, cervical, rectal and pharyngeal cultures obtained for *N. gonorrhoea.*

The *differential diagnosis* of suppurative arthritis includes infections, postinfectious (Reiter syndrome rheumatic fever), and noninfectious (rheu-

Table 10–11. Synovial Fluid Findings in Various Joint Diseases

Condition	Appearance	White Blood Cell Count (/μL)*	Polymorphonuclear Cells (%)	Mucin Clot	Synovial Fluid–to-Blood Glucose Difference (mg/dL)	Comment
Normal	Clear, yellow	0–200 (200)*	<10	Good	No difference	—
Trauma	Clear, turbid, or hemorrhagic	50–4000 (600)	<30	Good	No difference	Common in hemophilia
Systemic lupus erythematosus	Clear or slightly turbid	0–9000 (3000)	<20	Good to fair	No difference	LE cell positive, complement decreased
Rheumatoid arthritis reactive arthritis (Reiter syndrome, inflammatory bowel disease)	Turbid	250–80,000 (19,000)	>70	Poor	30	Decreased complement
Infectious Pyogenic infection	Turbid	10,000–250,000 (80,000)	>t90	Poor	50–90	Positive culture, positive Gram stain
Tuberculosis	Turbid	2500–100,000 (20,000)	>60	Poor	40–70	Positive culture, PPD, and acid-fast stain
Lyme arthritis	Turbid	500–100,000 (20,000)	>60	Poor	70	History of tick bite or erythema chronicum migrans

* Average in parentheses.
LE = lupus erythematosus; PPD = purified protein derivative of tuberculin.

matoid arthritis, systemic lupus erythematosus and other collagen vascular diseases, serum sickness, and inflammatory bowel disease) diseases. Other entities that should be considered include Henoch-Schönlein purpura, leukemia, metabolic diseases involving joints, and traumatic arthritis. Viral infections may cause arthritis (rubella, rubella vaccine, parvovirus, hepatitis B). *Toxic tenosynovitis* of the hip is presumed to be viral in etiology and is a common condition of children ages 3–6 yr (see Chapter 19). This self-limited disorder is far more common than septic arthritis. Other bacterial infections causing arthritis including tuberculosis, syphilis, and Lyme disease. These must be considered in the child or adolescent with the signs of an acutely inflamed joint or joints but without typical findings of pyogenic infection.

Treatment. The therapy of septic arthritis is based on knowledge of the likely organism, the Gram stain of joint fluid, and the host's immunologic status. Parenteral antimicrobial agents are the mainstay of therapy, with surgical intervention reserved for specific situations. Pyogenic arthritis of the hip or shoulder caused by *S. aureus* usually requires prompt surgical drainage to prevent joint destruction and long-term sequelae. However, staphylococcal infection of the knee may be treated with repeated arthrocenteses to remove infected fluid, and continuation of appropriate parenteral antibiotics. Irrigation of the joints with antimicrobial agents is rarely if ever indicated. Infections due to gonococci or meningococci rarely require surgical intervention in a normal host.

There are a number of antimicrobial agents available which provide adequate antibiotic levels in joint spaces to eradicate the typical bacterial infections. For empiric therapy in the neonate a cephalosporin with activity against staphylococci, group B streptococci, and aerobic gram negative rods (ceftriaxone or cefotaxime) could be used depending upon the results of the joint fluid Gram stain. Infants ages 3 mo to 4 yr should receive antibiotics active against *S. aureus* and *H. influenzae* type b until culture results are known. These would include ceftriaxone or ampicillin/sulbactam. Intravenous methicillin (nafcillin, oxacillin) is the treatment of choice for *S. aureus;* methicillin resistant organisms are treated with vancomycin. The length of therapy depends upon clinical resolution (afebrile, less pain) and reduction of the ESR. Organisms such as *S. aureus* usually require more lengthy treatment (14–21 days or more), while gonococcal or meningococcal arthritis responds to 7 days of penicillin. Ceftriaxone is preferred for gonococcal arthritis due to the large number of penicillin resistant isolates. Treatment may be changed to oral antibiotics (see osteomyelitis) for staphylococcal and other infections if compliance can be assured. Oral agents with excellent activity against *S. aureus* include augmentin, cloxacillin, dicloxacillin, cephalexin, clindamycin, and ciprofloxacin (in older children); these are often used to complete therapy.

References

Behrman RE (ed): Nelston Textbook of Pediatrics. 14th ed. Philadelphia, WB Saunders, 1992, Sec. 12.16–12.17.

Nelson J: Skeletal infections in children. Adv Pediatr Infect Dis 6:59, 1991.

Rodriguez AF, Kaplan SL: Outpatient management of skeletal infections in children. Semin Pediatr Infect Dis 1:365, 1990

CENTRAL NERVOUS SYSTEM INFECTIONS

Acute Bacterial Meningitis beyond the Neonatal Period

Meningitis is an inflammation of the leptomeninges. Although this may be caused by bacteria, viruses, or rarely fungi, bacterial meningitis is a common complication of septicemia in children and must be treated as an emergency. A limited number of bacteria are associated with meningitis in normal hosts; thus the principles of supportive management and the initial choice of antibiotics can be generalized. Meningitis during the neonatal period is discussed in Chapter 6.

Etiology. Bacterial meningitis in children 2 mo to 12 yr of age usually is due to *S. pneumoniae*, or *N. meningitidis*, and *H. influenzae* type b. Infection with *H. influenzae* may occur at any age, but it is most common before 4 yr of age; the incidence of *H. influenzae* disease has decreased after the introduction of conjugated vaccine against the organism for infants (Table 10–3). Meningitis usually is due to *S. pneumoniae* or *N. meningitidis* in children over 5 yr of age. Meningitis associated with ventricular–peritoneal shunts generally is due to *S. epidermidis* or corynebacteria; meningitis in patients with an open neural tube defect may be due to *S. aureus* or enteric bacteria. Immunosuppressed patients with T cell defects are susceptible to cryptococcal and *L. monocytogenes* meningitis. Patients with CSF leaks due to sinus fractures frequently develop pneumococcal meningitis, whereas patients with penetrating head trauma or neurosurgical procedures often develop staphylococcal disease.

Epidemiology. Bacterial meningitis occurs more frequently in the winter and spring, in more males than females, and most often between 2 mo and 2 yr of age. Close contact with a nasopharyngeal carrier (day care) or a patient ill with *H. influenzae* type b infection or meningococcal infection has been associated with an increased risk of meningitis. Meningococcal disease often follows viral upper respiratory tract infections.

Pathogenesis. Bacterial meningitis is usually the result of hematogenous dissemination of micro-organisms from a distant site of infection; bacteremia precedes the condition or occurs at the same time. Acquisition is by aerosol or droplet and leads to nasopharyngeal colonization, replication, invasion, and bacteremia. Hosts often lack preformed antiphagocytic polysaccharide capsule antibodies. Alaskan Eskimos and Navajo Indians are at increased risk for invasive *H. influenzae* disease owing, in part, to their poor immune response. Meningitis rarely may be due to bacterial spread from a contiguous focus of infection, such as sinusitis, otitis media, or mastoiditis. More often brain, epidural, or subdural abscesses follow contiguous infections. Bacterial meningitis in children with otitis media generally follows bacteremia. Hematogenous spread to the meninges may occur with infective endocarditis, pneumonia, or thrombophlebitis. Because there is a direct communication between the skin and meninges, the meninges may be invaded from a dermoid sinus tract or meningomyelocele. Osteomyelitis of the skull or vertebral column also may produce meningitis.

Children with sickle cell anemia or asplenia have an increased incidence of meningitis caused by *S. pneumoniae*. Without antimicrobial prophylaxis, approximately 1:24 patients with sickle cell anemia develops pneumococcal meningitis prior to 4 yr of age. Terminal complement deficiency predisposes some children to *Neisseria* sepsis and meningitis.

Meningeal bacterial proliferation and endotoxin release activate macrophages with local production of cytokines (IL-1, TNF). The ensuing inflammatory response increases the blood–brain barrier permeability, producing cerebral edema and increased intracranial pressure and activation of the coagulation system, producing local thrombosis and infarction. Increased CSF protein is due to this inflammatory response, whereas the reduced CSF glucose is due to alterations of the blood–brain barrier and increased CNS glucose utilization.

Clinical Manifestations. Manifestations of bacterial meningitis may be preceded by several days of upper respiratory tract symptoms. Rapid onset (<1 day) is common with *S. pneumoniae* or *N. meningitides*, whereas the course may be subacute (2–3 days) with *H. influenzae*. In young infants, signs of meningeal inflammation may be minimal; only irritability, restlessness, and poor feeding may be noted. Fever usually is present. Inflammation of the meninges is associated with headache, irritability, nausea, vomiting, anorexia, nuchal rigidity, lethargy, and, occasionally, photophobia. The older child may be confused, may complain of back pain, and usually demonstrates the Kernig and Brudzinski signs. Seizures and coma may occur.

Increased intracranial pressure is common and may be reflected in complaints of headache and diplopia. There may be a bulging fontanel. Ptosis, sixth nerve palsy, anisocoria, bradycardia with hypertension, and apnea are common signs of increased intracranial pressure and brain herniation, whereas a bulging fontanel usually is not associated with herniation. Papilledema is uncommon, unless there are occlusions of the venous sinus, subdural empyema, or a brain abscess. Focal neurologic signs, arthralgia, myalgia, transient arthritis, anemia, petechial or purpuric lesions, and signs of DIC are additional manifestations.

Diagnosis and Differential Diagnosis. Lumbar puncture should be performed in every child when bacterial meningitis is suspected, except when signs (other than a bulging fontanel) of increased intracranial pressure are present. Infection at the lumbar puncture site, suspicion of a mass lesion, and extreme patient instability are other reasons to defer a spinal tap. Cerebrospinal fluid examination should include a white cell count, differential, protein and glucose levels, and Gram stain (Table 10–12). Cultures should be performed for bacteria and, when appropriate, for fungi, viruses, and mycobacteria. The Gram stain is helpful in 90% of patients with bacterial meningitis. Latex agglutination tests detect bacterial antigen and can establish the diagnosis of bacterial meningitis due to *H. in-*

Table 10–12. Cerebrospinal Fluid Findings in Various Central Nervous System Disorders

Condition	Pressure	Leukocytes (/μL)	Protein (mg/dL)	Glucose (mg/dL)	Comments
Normal	50–180 mm H_2O	<4; 60–70% lymphocytes, 30–40% monocytes, 1–3% neutrophils	20–45	>50 or 75% blood glucose	
Acute bacterial meningitis	Usually elevated	100–60,000 +; usually a few thousand; PMNs predominate	100–500	Depressed compared with blood glucose; usually <40	Organism may be seen on Gram stain and recovered by culture
Partially treated bacterial meningitis	Normal or elevated	1–10,000; PMNs usual but mononuclear cells may predominate if pretreated for extended period	100+	Depressed or normal	Organisms may be seen; in disease caused by *H. influenzae*, organism may grow; pretreatment may render CSF sterile in pneumococcal and meningococcal disease, but antigen may be detected
Tuberculous meningitis	Usually elevated; may be low because of block in advanced stages	10–500; PMNs early but lymphocytes predominate later	100–500; may be higher in presence of block	<50 usual; decreases with time if treatment not provided	Acid-fast organisms may be seen on smear; organism can be recovered in culture or antigen and DNA testing; PPD, chest x-ray positive
Fungal	Usually elevated	25–500; PMNs early; mononuclear cells predominate later	20–500	<50, decreases with time if treatment not provided	Budding yeast may be seen; organism may be recovered in culture; India ink preparation or antigen may be positive in cryptococcal disease
Viral meningitis or meningoencephalitis	Normal or slightly elevated	PMNs early; mononuclear cells predominate later; rarely more than 1000 cells except in eastern equine	20–100	Generally normal; may be depressed to 40 in some viral diseases (15–20% of mumps)	Enteroviruses may be recovered from CSF by appropriate viral cultures
Abscess (parameningeal infection)	Normal or elevated	0–100 PMNs unless rupture into CSF	20–200	Normal	Profile may be completely normal

PMN = polymorphonuclear leukocyte; PPD = purified protein derivative of tuberculin.

fluenzae type b, *S. pneumoniae*, and *N. meningitidis* groups A, C, D, X, Y, Z, and W 135 even if the patient was pretreated with antibiotics. Additional diagnostic tests include blood cultures (positive in 50–90% of patients), complete blood count, and sickle cell screening test.

Tuberculosis meningitis, fungal meningitis, aseptic meningitis, spirochete infection (syphilis, Lyme disease), brain abscess, encephalitis, Rocky Mountain spotted fever, intracranial or spinal epidural abscesses, bacterial endocarditis with embolism, subdural empyema (with or without thrombophlebitis), subarachnoid hemorrhage, and brain tumors may mimic bacterial meningitis. The differentiation of these disorders depends on careful examination of CSF and additional laboratory tests and roentgenographic studies (Table 10–12).

Treatment. Treatment of bacterial meningitis focuses on decreasing the CNS damage caused by the inflammatory response, use of appropriate antimicrobial agents that penetrate the CSF, and maintenance of systemic and cerebral perfusion. For patients suspected of having *H. influenzae* meningitis, dexamethasone (0.6 mg/kg/hr, q6h × 4 days) administration is recommended prior to antimicrobial therapy. Cefotaxime (200 mg/kg/24 hr, q6h) or ceftriaxone (100 mg/kg/24 hr, q12h) is appropriate for bacterial meningitis of unknown etiology. For sensitive *S. pneumoniae* or meningococcus, penicillin G (300,000 units/kg/24 h, q6h) is recommended. Cefotaxime, ceftriaxone, and vancomycin usually are active against penicillin-resistant pneumococci. For infants under the age of 2 mo, ampicillin (300 mg/kg/24 hr, q6h) is added to cefotaxime (or ceftriaxone) to cover the possibility of *L. monocytogenes*. Treatment for 7 days (meningococcus) or 10 days (*H. influenzae* type b and *S. pneumoniae*) is recommended.

Supportive therapy includes the treatment of shock, DIC, inappropriate antidiuretic hormone secretion, seizures, increased intracranial pressure, apnea, arrhythmias, and coma. Subdural effusions (detected by CT scan) are common in infection with *H. influenzae* type b. Most subdural effusions are asymptomatic and do not require drainage unless associated with increased intracranial pressure or focal neurologic signs. Persistent fever is common with *H. influenzae* type b infection but also may suggest a subdural effusion, pericardial or joint effusions, drug fever, thrombophlebitis, or nosocomial infection. Repeat lumbar puncture is not indicated for fever in the absence of other signs of persistent CNS infection. Prior to discharge, children with *H. influenzae* type b meningitis or meningococcal meningitis should be treated with rifampin to eliminate nasopharyngeal carrier status.

Prevention. Chemoprophylaxis with rifampin for family contacts of individuals with *H. influenzae* type b and *N. meningitis* infections is recommended. Vaccines or prophylactic antibiotics against *N. meningitidis* are recommended for at-risk individuals, and routine immunization against *H. influenzae* is recommended for all infants (see Tables 10–3 and 10–5).

Prognosis. Even with appropriate antibiotic therapy, the mortality rate for bacterial meningitis in children is significant (8%, *H. influenzae*; 15%, meningococcal; 25%, pneumococcal). As many as 35% of the survivors (particularly following pneumococcal infection) have some sequelae resulting from their disease, including, in order of frequency, deafness, seizures, learning disabilities, blindness, paresis, ataxia, or hydrocephalus. All patients with meningitis should have a hearing evaluation prior to discharge. Poor prognosis is associated with (1) young age, (2) long duration of illness prior to effective antibiotic therapy, (3) the presence of pneumococci or gram-negative enteric bacteria, (4) a high number of organisms and/or quantity of bacterial antigen present in the CSF, (5) late-onset seizures, (6) coma at presentation, (7) shock, (8) low or absent CSF WBC count in the presence of visible bacteria on Gram stain of the CSF, and (9) immunocompromised status. *Relapse* may occur 3–14 days after treatment and is due to the same pathogen, possibly from parameningeal foci; *recrudescence* occurs during inappropriate therapy; and *recurrence* occurs later and may be due to the same or another pathogen, suggesting an underlying immunologic or anatomic defect that predisposes the patient to infection of the CNS.

References

Behrman RE (ed): Nelson Textbook of Pediatrics, 14th ed. Philadelphia, WB Saunders, 1992, Sec. 12.15.

Bonadio WA, Smith DS, Goddard S, et al: Distinguishing cerebrospinal fluid abnormalities in children with bacterial meningitis and traumatic lumbar puncture. J Infect Dis 162:251, 1990.

Pomeroy SL, Holmes SJ, Dodge PR, et al: Seizures and other neurologic sequelae of bacterial meningitis in children. N Engl J Med 323:1651, 1990.

Saez-Llorens X, Ramilo O, Mustafa M, et al: Molecular pathophysiology of bacterial meningitis: Current concepts and therapeutic implications. J Pediatr 116:671, 1990.

Spanos A, Harrell FE, Durack DT: Differential diagnosis of

acute meningitis: An analysis of the predictive value of initial observations. JAMA 262:2700, 1989.

Acute Aseptic Meningitis

Aseptic meningitis, an acute inflammation of the meninges, is a common illness with many causes. The cerebrospinal fluid usually is characterized by lymphocytic pleocytosis, normal glucose, slightly elevated protein levels, and absence of bacterial micro-organisms on Gram stain or culture.

Etiology.   Although an etiologic agent is not always identified, viruses are usually the responsible agents. Enteroviruses cause approximately 85% of all cases of aseptic meningitis; coxsackievirus B5 and echoviruses 4, 6, 9, and 11 are the most common types. St. Louis and California encephalitis viruses are the most commonly implicated arboviruses in the United States, accounting for 5–7% of all cases of aseptic meningitis. Other etiologic viral agents include HIV, varicella, EBV, lymphocytic choriomeningitis, natural or vaccine-associated measles, mumps, rubella, or polio, rabies, influenza, and parainfluenza. Acute aseptic meningitis also may be caused by mycoplasma, chlamydia, various fungi and protozoa and other parasites, as well as by postinfectious reactions to various viruses.

The most common cause of nonviral aseptic meningitis is partially or inappropriately treated bacterial disease, tuberculosis, parameningeal infections, toxoplasmosis, and Kawasaki disease. Less common causes include leptospirosis, syphilis, cryptococcosis, Lyme disease, Rocky Mountain spotted fever, malignancy, intracranial hemorrhage, and reactions to nonsteroidal anti-inflammatory drugs, intravenous immunoglobulins, or trimethoprim–sulfamethoxazole.

Epidemiology.   Because 85% of cases are due to enteroviral infections, the epidemiologic pattern is typical of these agents. In temperate climates most cases occur in the summer and fall. The epidemiology of aseptic meningitis due to other agents also depends on season, geography, climatic conditions, exposures to animals or insects, and other factors related to the specific pathogens.

Clinical Manifestations.   The onset usually is acute, although it may be insidious or preceded by a nonspecific febrile illness. In older children, the initial manifestation is severe headache; in infants, irritability. Fever, nausea, and other neurologic complaints, such as vomiting, a stiff neck, photophobia, and retrobulbar pain, are frequent, but convulsions are uncommon. Examination often reveals nuchal rigidity without significant localizing neurologic signs. Exanthems that precede or accompany the infection may occur, especially in infections with echoviruses and coxsackieviruses. Parotitis or orchitis is noted with mumps, lymphadenopathy and hepatosplenomegaly with CMV, HIV, or EBV infections, and petechiae with Rocky Mountain spotted fever. The child with aseptic viral meningitis usually appears less ill than the child with bacterial meningitis; however, the two may be indistinguishable (Table 10–7).

The disease may become manifest in a meningeal or an encephalitic pattern, but the children exhibiting the latter pattern have a great incidence of headache, confusion, altered consciousness, and seizures.

Diagnosis.   The CSF contains a few to several thousand cells per microliter. Early in the disease the cells may be polymorphonuclear; later, lymphocytes or mononuclear cells predominate (Table 10–12). No organisms are seen on laboratory stain, and the protein level is normal to slightly elevated. The CSF glucose concentration is normal in most viral infections; glucose may be decreased with medulloblastoma, leukemia infiltration, *Mycoplasma pneumoniae* infection, inadequately treated bacterial meningitis, tuberculosis, and, rarely, certain viral infections. Specimens for viral culture include CSF, throat swabs, and stool. A serum specimen should be obtained early in the illness and again in 2–3 wk for serologic identification of the virus.

Treatment.   Aseptic viral meningitis is usually a benign, self-limited disease. Hospitalization usually is necessary in young infants or more acutely ill children because of the possibility of bacterial disease. Treatment is supportive for viral meningitis except for aseptic meningitis caused by herpes simplex. Meningoencephalitis resulting from herpes simplex or complicated herpes zoster should be treated with acyclovir. Lyme disease should be treated with high-dose parenteral ceftriaxone. Headache, which may be severe in all cases of aseptic meningitis, should be treated with nonsteroidal anti-inflammatory agents or mild narcotics, such as codeine.

References

Behrman RE (ed): Nelson Textbook of Pediatrics, 14th ed. Philadelphia, WB Saunders, 1992, Sec. 12.11.
Walsh-Kelly C, Nelson D, Smith D, et al: Clinical predictors

of bacterial versus aseptic meningitis in childhood. Ann Emerg Med 21:910, 1992.

Wildin S, Chonmaitree T: Importance of laboratory in the diagnosis and management of viral meningitis. Am J Dis Child 141:454, 1987.

Encephalitis

Encephalitis is an inflammatory process of the brain parenchyma that is usually an acute process but may be a postinfectious encephalomyelitis, a chronic degenerative disease, or a slow virus infection. The diagnosis is established with absolute certainty by brain biopsy, but it usually is made in the presence of neurologic signs, epidemiologic data, and laboratory (CSF, electroencephalography [EEG], and brain imaging techniques) evidence of infection. Encephalitis may be diffuse or localized (e.g., cerebellar ataxia, brain stem encephalitis, a meningoencephalitis, meningoencephalomyeloradiculitis). There is considerable overlap between viral aseptic meningitis and meningoencephalitis. Neurologic manifestations suggestive of encephalitis but occurring in the absence of inflammation (intoxication, Reye syndrome) indicate *encephalopathy*.

Etiology. Encephalitis usually is caused by direct viral infection of the brain via a hematogenous or neuronal (peripheral or cranial) route. During epidemic seasons (summer or fall) arboviruses and enteroviruses are common pathogens. Other causes of encephalitis include varicella, mumps, measles, EBV, rubella, lymphocytic choriomeningitis, influenza, parainfluenza, adenovirus, and respiratory syncytial virus. Herpes simplex, the most common cause of sporadic encephalitis (herpes simplex virus [HSV] type I), is a common encephalitis seen in neonates (HSV type II > type I). Cerebellar ataxia commonly is due to varicella virus. Postinfectious, allergic demyelinating encephalitis may follow either vaccination or a viral infection and is an autoimmune process. HIV is an increasingly common cause of encephalitis in children and may present as an acute febrile illness, but more commonly it is insidious in onset (see Human Immunodeficiency Virus Infection later).

Epidemiology. St. Louis encephalitis virus, which is spread from the bird reservoir, is the most common arboviral (arthropod-borne) agent and is present throughout the United States. California encephalitis virus, common in the Midwest, is carried by rodents and spread by mosquitoes. The eastern equine encephalitis virus is limited to the East coast (mosquitoes, birds), whereas the western equine encephalitis virus is present throughout the Midwest and West (mosquitoes, birds). The spread of disease depends on the geographic area, season, arthropod vector, and animal reservoir. Epizootics in horses often precede human cases of eastern equine encephalitis, but the horse is not a direct source of disease to humans.

HSV infections account for approximately 10% of non-neonatal cases. Sporadic encephalitis caused by HSV occurs in newborn infants born to mothers with an active primary infection, or in adults as a primary infection or reactivation of latent virus (see Herpes Simplex Virus Infection later).

Rabies is a rare but important cause of encephalitis in developing countries and is endemic in parts of the United States. In the northeast raccoons may be infected, whereas in the southeast foxes and bats are potential sources. The management after exposure to potentially infected animals is the aggressive postexposure use of vaccine plus hyperimmune globulin to prevent infection.

Slow viral diseases present months to years after infection with dementia, poor cognition, and personality changes; agents include HIV, natural or vaccine-related measles (subacute sclerosing panencephalitis), rubella, HSV (Mollaret meningitis), and JC papovavirus (progressive multifocal leukoencephalopathy). Slow CNS infection may be due to small proteinaceous particles *(prions)*; diseases include Kuru or Creutzfeldt-Jakob disease. Slow viral or prion diseases are progressive and fatal; treatment is available only for HIV encephalopathy.

Clinical Manifestations. Signs and symptoms are similar to those in aseptic meningitis, except that in encephalitis more abnormalities of mental function are noted. Headache and fever are associated with confusion, delirium, irritability, hallucinations, memory loss, combativeness, coma, seizures (may be focal), ataxia, and signs of increased intracranial pressure.

Diagnosis and Differential Diagnosis. A history should take into account possible exposures to persons and animals with illnesses, to mosquitoes, and to ticks; the history also should note any extent of travel. Encephalopathy due to toxins, hypoglycemia, hypervitaminosis A, Reye syndrome, inborn errors of metabolism, or trauma should be considered. A patient with concurrent or recent mumps, measles, or varicella is at risk for infectious or postinfectious encephalitis; neurologic involvement may precede the development of other manifestations of these diseases.

Bacterial diseases to be considered include mycoplasma, tuberculosis, syphilis, leptospirosis, rickettsia, Kawasaki disease, Lyme disease, cat-scratch disease, and borreliosis. Parasites associated with encephalitis include *Toxoplasma gondii*, trypanosomiasis, cystercercosis, and malaria. Cryptococcal disease presents as an encephalitis and is common in older children with HIV infection. Noninfectious causes of an encephalitic disease include malignancy, sarcoidosis, and primary CNS or systemic vasculitis.

Examination of the CSF in viral encephalitis rarely may reveal findings that are normal. The findings often resemble those in aseptic meningitis. Increased erythrocytes may be seen with HSV, whereas extreme elevations of protein and reductions of glucose should suggest tuberculosis or cryptococcal infection. Cryptococcal disease can be diagnosed by India Ink smear and determination of CSF cryptococcal antigen. The EEG, CT scan, and MRI may be nonspecific, but in HSV infection they often reveal a temporal lobe focus. There are many causes of temporal lobe disease, and when HSV is suspected on clinical grounds, biopsy confirms the diagnosis in only 40–50% of cases. Brain biopsy therefore may be necessary for definitive diagnosis, especially in patients with focal neurologic findings or at risk for CNS lymphoma or toxoplasmosis (both treatable). Viral cultures of the nasopharynx, rectum, and CSF for HSV occasionally are helpful. In many cases of viral encephalitis, paired serology of plasma is needed to determine a rise of specific antibodies.

Treatment. For HSV infections acyclovir is the treatment of choice (see Appendix I). HIV infections may be treated with zidovudine or other antiretroviral agents. *Mycoplasma pneumoniae* infections may be treated with doxycycline, erythromycin or one of the newer macrolides, such as azithromycin or clarithromycin. Supportive care is extremely important to decrease elevated intracranial pressure and maintain cardiopulmonary function.

Prognosis. Most children with encephalitis recover without major sequelae. Disease caused by HSV, rabies, or *M. pneumoniae* is associated with a poorer prognosis. Encephalitis may be severe in young children (<1 yr) and those presenting with coma. Although most patients with epidemic forms of encephalitis (St. Louis, California, and enteroviral infections) do well, eastern equine encephalitis has a poorer outcome.

References

Behrman RE (ed): Nelson Textbook of Pediatrics. 14th ed. Philadelphia, WB Saunders, 1992, Sec. 12.12.

Rautonen J, Koskiniemi M, Vaheri A: Prognostic factors in childhood acute encephalitis. Pediatr Infect Dis J 10: 441, 1991.

Whitley RJ: Viral encephalitis. N Engl J Med 323:242, 1990.

Whitely RJ, Arvin A, Prober C, et al: Predictors of morbidity and mortality in neonates with herpes simplex infection. N Engl J Med 324:450, 1991.

RESPIRATORY TRACT INFECTIONS

Upper Respiratory Tract Infections

EAR INFECTIONS

Otitis Externa ("Swimmers' Ear")

This is an acute infection of the external auditory canal. Trauma or prolonged exposure to moisture predisposes to infection. *Pseudomonas aeruginosa* is the leading cause, followed by *S. aureus* and other skin flora. The child has severe unilateral pain localized to the ear. There is exquisite tenderness on manipulation of the pinna or tragus, a finding not observed in patients with otitis media. In otitis externa, the tympanic membrane is normal, whereas the canal is erythematous. **Malignant otitis externa** is noted in diabetics and presents as a severe cellulitis due to *P. aeruginosa*. Rarely, herpes zoster may produce otitis externa. The *differential diagnosis* includes the presence of a foreign body, such as small toys or insects, trauma, and referred pain. *Treatment* of uncomplicated otitis externa includes irrigation and topical antibiotics. Abscess formation requires incision and drainage; severe cellulitis requires parenteral antistaphylococcal and antipseudomonas antibiotics.

Otitis Media

This is a suppurative infection of the middle ear cavity and is most common in healthy children between 6 mo and 2 yr of age; in certain high-risk populations, such as children with cleft palate and Down syndrome; and in Eskimos and American Indians. Otitis media is also more common in boys, in lower socioeconomic status patients, in formula-fed infants, and in the winter months.

Pathogenesis. Bacteria gain access to the middle ear when the normal patency of the eustachian tube is blocked by local infection, pharyngitis, or hypertrophied adenoids. Air trapped in the middle ear is reabsorbed, creating negative pressure in this cavity, which permits reflux of bacteria. This bacterial reflux, plus obstruction of the flow of secretions from the middle ear to the pharynx, results in a middle ear effusion that becomes infected by nasopharyngeal bacteria. The common bacterial pathogens include the pneumococci, nontypable *H. influenzae* (10% are type b), *Moraxella catarrhalis*, and group A streptococci. Bacteria recovered from the nasopharynx do not correlate with those isolated by tympanocentesis. Viruses (respiratory syncytial virus [RSV], CMV, rhinovirus) have been recovered as copathogens or alone in 20–25% of patients.

Clinical Manifestations. Patients with otitis media are febrile and irritable and often pull at their ears. The disease usually occurs 1–7 days following a nasopharyngitis. Vomiting, diarrhea, a bulging fontanel, vertigo, tinnitus, and a draining ear also may be seen. The normal eardrum moves freely when negative or positive pressure is generated by the otoscope; it appears pink and translucent, and a cone of reflected light usually is noted radiating from the center to the anteroinferior margin. In otitis media the otoscope examination reveals a bulging, immobile, erythematous tympanic membrane, with loss of identifiable landmarks such as the short process and handle of the malleus. Perforation of the tympanic membrane also may occur and usually is associated with acute relief of pain. Otitis media may be associated with an ipsilateral conjunctivitis; both usually are due to nontypable *H. influenzae.*

Treatment. Otitis media should be treated initially without determining the specific pathogen. Amoxicillin, trimethoprim-sulfamethoxazole, cefaclor, and erythromycin–sulfisoxazole are effective. The latter three choices and amoxicillin–clavulanic acid are used if beta-lactamase–producing bacteria are suspected (see Appendix I). Decongestants or antihistamines are not effective alone or when combined with antibiotics. *Complications* of otitis media include hearing loss, chronic effusion, cholesteatoma formation (keratinized epithelial growth), petrositis, and mastoiditis.

Acute mastoiditis is a suppurative complication of otitis media, with inflammation and potential destruction of the mastoid air spaces. The disease progresses from a periostitis to an osteitis with abscess formation and draining tracts (e.g., through the tympanic membrane or into the neck). Posterior auricular tenderness and swelling and erythema are present, in addition to the signs of otitis

media. The pinna is displaced downward and outward. Roentgenograms of the mastoid reveal clouding of the air cells, demineralization, or bone destruction. Bacteria that cause acute otitis media are also those responsible for acute mastoiditis. *S. aureus, P. aeruginosa,* and anaerobic bacteria may be recovered in chronic cases. Culturing swabs of the external ear is not as specific as obtaining fluid by tympanocentesis, aspiration of posterior auricular cellulitis or the mastoid at surgery, or, rarely, a blood culture. Treatment includes systemic antibiotics and incision and drainage, if the disease has progressed to abscess formation.

NASOPHARYNGITIS

Rhinorrhea (Nasal Discharge)

This is a common manifestation of infectious, allergic, or mechanical conditions. Infectious rhinitis is associated with a mucopurulent discharge that contains polymorphonuclear leukocytes and is due to rhinovirus and other respiratory viruses, such as RSV. Low-grade fever, nasal stuffiness, and sneezing may be present. Hypersensitivity to allergens is another common cause of rhinitis and is characterized by eosinophils in the discharge and by other allergic manifestations, such as allergic shiners; nasal polyps; a pale, edematous, nasal turbinate mucosa; and a transverse crease on the nasal bridge. Other less common causes of rhinorrhea include foreign body, choanal atresia, vasomotor rhinitis, CSF fistula, diphtheria, tumor, congenital syphilis, and Wegener granulomatosis. Persistent rhinorrhea following a cold should suggest sinusitis. The treatment of viral rhinorrhea is usually supportive, with normal saline nose drops, steam, and, occasionally, decongestants.

Sinusitis

This is a suppurative infection of the paranasal sinuses and often complicates the common cold and allergic rhinitis. In addition, patients with cyanotic heart disease, cystic fibrosis, immunoglobulin deficiency (total or subclass), HIV infection, nasotracheal intubation, immotile cilia syndrome, and dental infection have an increased incidence of sinusitis. The maxillary, ethmoid, and sphenoid sinuses are present at birth, whereas the frontal sinus develops at 1 yr of life. Pneumatization of the sinuses is delayed relative to sinus formation; the frontal sinuses may not appear as air-filled spaces until 10 yr of age.

Etiology. Obstruction to mucociliary flow (preceding viral rhinitis) predisposes to bacterial proliferation. The bacteria producing acute sinusitis include pneumococci, nontypable *H. influenzae, M. catarrhalis,* anaerobic bacteria, and, rarely, streptococci and staphylococci. Nosocomial sinusitis may be due to *Klebsiella* or *Pseudomonas.* Neutropenic immunosuppressed patients may develop sinusitis as a result of infection by *Aspergillus* species or Zygomycetes. Culture of the nasal mucosa is not helpful in identifying the responsible bacteria. If necessary, antral puncture (for maxillary sinusitis) is the diagnostic procedure of choice.

Clinical Manifestations. These include persistent mucopurulent rhinorrhea; cough (especially at night); nasal stuffiness; nasal quality to voice; facial swelling, tenderness, and pain; and headache. Transillumination of the sinuses and sinus roentgenograms or CT will reveal clouding or an air–fluid level. Sinus aspiration usually is not needed in patients with uncomplicated sinusitis.

Treatment. Amoxicillin, amoxicillin–clavulanic acid, trimethoprim–sulfamethoxazole, and cefaclor usually are effective oral medications for treating acute sinusitis (see Appendix I). *Complications* should be treated with drainage and, if indicated, broad-spectrum parenteral antibiotics; these complications include orbital cellulitis, epidural or subdural empyema, brain abscess, dural sinus thrombosis, osteomyelitis of the outer or inner table of the frontal sinus (Pott puffy tumor), and meningitis. Sinusitis also may exacerbate bronchoconstriction in asthmatic patients.

Orbital Cellulitis

This is a complication of sinusitis following spread of bacteria into the orbit through the wall of the infected sinus. Typically, ethmoid sinusitis spreads through the lamina papyracea, a thin bony plate that separates the orbit and the ethmoid sinus. Infection of the extraocular structures of the orbit progresses in stages from (1) an inflammatory edema to (2) orbital cellulitis (edema plus chemosis; mild proptosis; limited extraocular muscle motion, with or without reduced visual acuity), to (3) a subperiosteal abscess (down-and-out position of globe in proptosis, resulting from abscess formation in periosteum), to (4) an orbital abscess (involvement of the orbital fat, muscle, and posterior cone of the orbit; severe ophthalmoplegia; vision loss; proptosis), to (5) cavernous sinus thrombosis (headache; nuchal rigidity; involvement of cranial nerves III, IV, V, and VI). The patient often has a high fever, orbital pain, limited extraocular motion (ophthalmoplegia), decreased vision, and proptosis. Infection of the orbit must be differentiated from that of the preseptal space (anterior to palpebral fascia, separating the eyelids and the orbit) or periorbital space. *Periorbital cellulitis* usually occurs in younger children (<4 yr) who may, like those with orbital cellulitis, have fever and lid swelling and appear toxic, but they do not have decreased visual acuity, ophthalmoplegia, sinusitis, or proptosis. Periorbital cellulitis may be due to hematogenous infection (*H. influenzae* type b, pneumococcus) or trauma (*S. aureus,* group A streptococcus).

Diagnosis. Orbital cellulitis is confirmed by a CT scan of the orbit. This essential examination will determine the extent of orbital infection and the need for surgical drainage. Additional laboratory studies include blood cultures, ESR, and CBC. Disorders to be considered in the differential diagnosis include mucormycosis, orbital aspergillosis, rhabdomyosarcoma, neuroblastoma, Wegener granulomatosis, inflammatory pseudotumor of the orbit, and trichinosis.

Treatment. The therapy of orbital cellulitis includes broad-spectrum parenteral antibiotics, such as oxacillin and ceftriaxone (see Appendix I). Draining the infected sinus or orbital abscess also is indicated in complicated cases.

Pharyngitis or Pharyngotonsillitis

This disorder presents with cough, sore throat, dysphagia, and fever. It is one of the most common types of pediatric infection. Inflammation confined to the pharynx is unusual, but if the involvement of the tonsils is prominent, the term *tonsillitis* is used.

Etiology. Pharyngitis in children less than 2 yr of age is often viral; group A streptococci are more common over the age of 5 yr, and *Mycoplasma,* gonococcus, and *Arcanobacterium haemolyticum* are more common among adolescents. Viral pathogens include rhinovirus, coronavirus, adenovirus, enteroviruses, EBV, CMV, and HSV; the bacterial agent is predominantly group A streptococci, which may be recovered from only 10–20% of patients. Less common causes include group C or G streptococcus, *Cornyebacterium diphtheriae,* tularemia, toxoplasmosis, and gonorrhea.

Clinical Manifestations. Examining the throat reveals erythema, exudate, palatine petechiae, enlarged tonsils, and, occasionally, anterior cervical lymphadenopathy. This appearance does not differentiate bacterial pathogens from viral pathogens. Nonetheless, vesiculation and ulceration suggest HSV and coxsackieviruses (herpangina); concomitant conjunctivitis suggests adenovirus; a gray–white fibrinous pseudomembrane with marked cervical swelling (bull neck), with or without carditis or neuropathy, suggests the diphtheria pathogen; and a macular rash suggests group A beta-hemolytic streptococci (scarlet fever) or, less frequently, *A. haemolyticum*.

Diagnosis. Streptococcal pharyngitis is diagnosed by performing a throat culture or by using rapid streptococcal antigen detection kits. It is important to diagnose streptococcal pharyngitis in all children because treatment (1) reduces symptoms; (2) prevents the poststreptococcal sequela of acute rheumatic fever; (3) prevents local suppurative complications; and (4) identifies the possibility of, but does not prevent the development of, the poststreptococcal sequela of acute glomerulonephritis. CBC and heterophil testing may be used to diagnose infectious mononucleosis, whereas cold agglutinins may be useful for mycoplasma. Streptococcal pharyngitis may be present in 25% of patients with mononucleosis.

The *differential diagnosis* of infectious pharyngitis includes other local infections of the oral cavity, retropharyngeal abscesses (*S. aureus*, streptococci, anaerobes), peritonsillar abscess (quinsy sore throat; unilateral tonsil swelling; infections caused by streptococci, anaerobes, or, rarely, *S. aureus*), Ludwig angina (anaerobic bacterial cellulitis of the floor of the mouth, which may be due to an odontogenic source), and epiglottitis (see Chapter 12). In addition, neutropenic mucositis (leukemia, aplastic anemia), thrush (candidiasis secondary to T cell immune deficiency), autoimmune ulceration (SLE, Behçet disease), and Kawasaki disease may cause pharyngitis. Signs suggesting that the disease is not a simple pharyngitis include persistent clinical manifestations for more than 1 wk, stridor, trismus, poor clearance of secretions, difficulty in swallowing, pain in the absence of erythema, presence of a mass, and blood in the pharynx.

Treatment. Group A streptococcal pharyngitis is treated with penicillin or erythromycin (see Appendix I). The latter drug is effective if *Mycoplasma* or *A. haemolyticum* is present. Peritonsillar abscesses may be treated initially with high-dose penicillin and aspiration; following resolution of these abscesses, tonsillectomy may be indicated. Retropharyngeal abscesses require oxacillin and frequently need drainage. Ludwig angina and other odontogenic infections may be treated with high-dose penicillin.

Epiglottitis

See Chapter 12.

References

Behrman RE (ed): Nelson Textbook of Pediatrics. 14th ed. Philadelphia, WB Saunders, 1992, Sec. 14.19–14.33, 22.21–22.22.

Brook I: Microbiology of retropharyngeal abscesses in children. Am J Dis Child 141:202, 1987.

de Marie S, Tjon A Tham RTO, van der Mey AGL, et al: Clinical infections and nonsurgical treatment of parapharyngeal space infections complicating throat infection. Rev Infect Dis 11:975, 1989.

Ĝiebink GS, Canafax DM, Kempthorne J: Antimicrobial treatment of acute otitis media. J Pediatr 119:495, 1991.

Ginsberg C: Aerobic microbiology of upper respiratory infections in infants and children. Pediatr Infect Dis 6:843, 1987.

Gwaltney JM Jr: Combined antiviral and antimediator treatment of rhinovirus colds. J Infect Dis 166:776, 1992.

Israele V, Nelson J: Periorbital and orbital cellulitis. Pediatr Infect Dis 6:404, 1987.

Ogle J, Laver B: Acute mastoiditis. Am J Dis Child 140:1178, 1986.

Shoemaker M, Lampe R, Weir M: Peritonsillitis: Abscess or cellulitis? Pediatr Infect Dis 5:435, 1986.

Wald ER: Sinusitis in children. N Engl J Med 326:319, 1992.

Wald ER, Guerra N, Byers C: Upper respiratory tract infections in young children: Duration of and frequency of complications. Pediatrics 87:129, 1991.

Lower Respiratory Tract Infections

BRONCHIOLITIS

See Chapter 12.

PNEUMONIA

See Chapter 12.

URINARY TRACT INFECTIONS

See Chapter 16.

BACTERIAL INFECTIONS

Antibiotic Therapy

DOSAGES

See Appendix I.

PRINCIPLES

The chemotherapy of bacterial infections depends on the isolation of the offending agent, characterization of the agent's antibiotic susceptibility, and delivering the appropriate antibiotic to the site of infection in sufficient quantities to either kill the bacteria (bactericidal) or alter it to permit the body's immune response to eventually kill it. The two major strategies are (1) to use broad-spectrum, empiric antibiotics in high-risk situations, such as neonatal sepsis or bacteremia in an immunocompromised host; and (2) to tailor antibiotic treatment to the specific pathogen in lower risk, immunocompetent patients. This second principle minimizes drug toxicity, the development of resistant micro-organisms, superinfection by fungi and previously resistant bacteria, and cost to the family.

Antibiotic efficacy and toxicity may be modified by various host factors. The site of the infection is an important consideration, because many antibiotics do not penetrate into abscess spaces, the meninges, the lung, or the heart valves. Foreign bodies (ventriculoperitoneal shunts, central venous catheters, prosthetic cardiac valves) often impair microbial killing by acting as a nidus of infection removed from the circulation and hence from the antibiotic agents. Infected vegetations on heart valves, bone fragments (sequestra), cutaneous ulcers, and abscess centers also are sites of infection that are removed from the circulation, thus preventing adequate levels of antibiotics from reaching the pathogens. Indeed, when sequestrum formation has occurred, or when large abscesses are evident, antibiotics alone are unsuccessful in effectively treating the infection. Surgically draining pus and administering antibiotics is the standard care of such infections. Enteric absorption of antibiotics may be reduced by gastric acid (penicillin), *Giardia* infection, or various foods or drugs (tetracycline). Reduced renal excretion associated with immaturity or renal failure may result in drug accumulation and drug toxicity, whereas enhanced clearance of drugs, as in cystic fibrosis, may produce subtherapeutic drug levels.

Antibiotic efficacy may be altered by the type of infection the patient hosts. Intracellular pathogens, such as *Salmonella, Brucella, Listeria,* and *Mycobacteria,* require antibiotics that can penetrate the macrophage and the leukocyte. Abscess formation produces an anaerobic and acidic collection of debris in the center of the infection so that antibiotics, such as aminoglycosides, cannot enter the abscess and cannot function well because the oxygen is reduced and the pH environment of the abscess is low. Slow-growing bacteria frequently are not killed by antibiotics, which function best during the cell division phase of the cell cycle.

Antibiotic efficacy also may be modified by inter-action among administered drugs. Thus, for various bacteria, *synergism* results when the combined effect of two antibiotics is greater than the effects of each used individually. Continuing two antibiotics is helpful when broad-spectrum coverage is needed prior to identification of the pathogen. In addition, combining two synergistic antibiotics may be desirable for serious and hard-to-treat infections. Enterococcal endocarditis is best treated with ampicillin and the added synergistic killing effect of gentamicin. Synergism also occurs when two drugs act on a bacterium along different pathways; hence trimethoprim–sulfamethoxazole, which inhibits sequential steps of bacterial folate metabolism, is administered in combination because it is more effective than either drug used alone.

Antibiotic *antagonism,* the result of one drug's interference with the action of the other, may occur in the infusion apparatus, such as when chloramphenicol and erythromycin form insoluble precipitates if mixed. Antagonism also may result when bactericidal and bacteriostatic drugs are given together. Thus, chloramphenicol and aminoglycosides together are less effective against various gram-negative enteric bacilli.

Finally, antibiotic treatment of serious infections should include a bactericidal drug. The penicillins, cephalosporins, and aminoglycosides are bactericidal and appropriate for infections such as sepsis, osteomyelitis, and pyelonephritis. Erythromycin, rifampin, and tetracycline are bacteriostatic. Chloramphenicol is bactericidal for *H. influenzae,* pneumococcus, and *N. meningitidis* but is bacteriostatic for other susceptible bacteria.

SELECTION OF ANTIBIOTICS

The choice of antibiotics depends on the epidemiology of the condition, site of infection, localizing manifestations (see Table 10–1), host factors, the need for antibiotic prophylaxis (see Table 10–6), and the spectrum of bacterial pathogens susceptible to the antibiotic (Table 10–13). The treatment of specific bacterial infections is covered in the following sections.

Anaerobic Infections Other Than the Clostridial Type

Etiology. Anaerobic bacteria are ubiquitous and are usually harmless commensal members of the normal human flora of the oropharynx, gastrointestinal tract, vagina, and skin. The fecal flora con-

Table 10–13. Commonly Used Antibiotics for Bacterial Infection

Antibiotic	Mechanism of Action/ Activity	Sensitive Bacteria/ Indications	Comments
Penicillins	Bind to penicillin-binding proteins (1,2,3); inhibit transpeptidation reaction of cell wall, causing eventual cell lysis		No activity for *Staphylococcus epidermidis, Mycoplasma, Chlamydia*
Penicillin		*Pneumococcus, Meningococcus, Gonococcus,* streptococci, anaerobic bacteria (*Bacteroides melaninogenicus*), *Pasteurella multocida, Actinomyces* sp.	Penicillinase-producing *Gonococcus, Pneumococcus,* and some anaerobes are becoming resistant
Ampicillin/amoxicillin	Extended spectrum; beta-lactamase susceptible	*Haemophilus influenzae, Listeria monocytogenes, Escherichia coli, Salmonella, Shigella, Proteus mirabilis*	Many of these organisms produce beta-lactamases and are resistant
Carbenicillin/ticarcillin	Antipseudomonas	*E. coli, Pseudomonas aeruginosa, Proteus* sp.	Carboxypenicillins not β-lactamase stable
Mezlocillin or piperacillin	Antipseudomonas	*P. aeruginosa, Klebsiella, Citrobacter, Acinetobacter*	Ureidopenicillins
Oxacillin/methicillin or nafcillin	Antistaphylococcus	*Staphylococcus aureus, Pneumococcus, Streptococcus*	Penicillinase-resistant penicillins; *S. epidermidis* is usually resistant
Amoxicillin/clavulanic acid	Extended spectrum	As for ampicillin, plus *S. aureus, Enterococcus, Bacteroides fragilis, Moraxella catarrhalis*	Clavulanic acid inhibits beta-lactamases; PO prep
Ampicillin/sulbactam	Extended spectrum	As for amoxicillin/clavulanic acid, plus anaerobes	Sulbactam inhibits β-lactamase; IV prep
Ticarcillin/clavulanic acid	Extended spectrum	As above, plus broader gram-negative coverage	IV prep
Cephalosporins	Bind to penicillin-binding proteins; inhibit cell wall cross-linking; produce cell lysis		No activity against *Listeria* or *Enterococcus*
1st generation Cefazolin or cephalothin		*S. aureus, E. coli, Klebsiella*	Good for *S. aureus,* other gram-positive organisms; *H. influenzae* type b is resistant
2nd generation Cefuroxime or cefamandole	Beta-lactamase stable	*H. influenzae* type b, *S. aureus, Klebsiella, E. coli*	
Cephamycins Cefoxitin	Anaerobic coverage	*B. melaninogenicus, Bacteroides fragilis, E. coli, Gonococcus*	Abdominal and genital tract infections
3rd generation Cefotaxime or ceftriaxone	Extended spectrum	*E. coli, Klebsiella, Gonococcus, H. influenzae, Pneumococcus, Meningococcus, S. aureus*	Better gram-negative enteric coverage, good CSF penetration

Continued

Table 10–13. (*Continued*)

Antibiotic	Mechanism of Action/ Activity	Sensitive Bacteria/ Indications	Comments
Ceftazidime, cefoperazone	Broad spectrum	Same as above, gram-negative plus *Pseudomonas*; not good against *P. cepacia*	Resistance may be induced during therapy
Other Antibiotics			
Imipenem	Thienamycin drug: binds to penicillin-binding proteins; very broad spectrum	Most gram-positive and gram-negative bacteria, *Listeria, Bacillus* sp., *Pseudomonas, Acinetobacter*	*Pseudomonas maltophilia*, methicillin-resistant *S. aureus*, enterococci are resistant; requires cilastatin to inhibit renal degradation
Aztreonam	Monobactam drug: binds to penicillin-binding protein of Enterobacteriaceae only; narrow spectrum	Most gram-negative bacteria	No action against anaerobic or gram-positive bacteria; *P. cepacia* is resistant; does not induce beta-lactamase production
Aminoglycosides	Inhibition of bacterial protein synthesis at ribosomes		Ototoxicity and nephrotoxicity, must monitor peak and trough serum concentrations
Gentamicin, tobramycin, netilmicin		Gram-negative Enterobacteriaceae, including *Pseudomonas*	Broad spectrum, synergy with beta-lactams; enterococci are resistant
Amikacin		Same as above	Less susceptible to aminoglycoside-inactivating enzymes
Streptomycin		Plague, tularemia, brucellosis (plus tetracycline)	
Other Antibiotics			
Tetracyclines	Inhibition of protein synthesis	*Chlamydia, Mycoplasma, Gonococcus, Actinomyces,* Lyme disease; pelvic inflammatory disease, Rocky Mountain spotted fever, urethritis, *Brucella* sp., tularemia, plague	Stains teeth, contraindicated before 10 yrs of age
Chloramphenicol	Inhibition of protein synthesis	*Salmonella, H. influenzae, Meningococcus, Pneumococcus, Shigella, B. fragilis,* Rocky Mountain spotted fever, typhoid fever	Reversible bone marrow suppression, aplastic anemia, gray baby syndrome
Rifampin	Inhibition of DNA-dependent RNA polymerase	*S. aureus, Mycobacterium tuberculosis, H. influenzae, Meningococcus*	Red discoloration of secretions; increases metabolism of drugs (e.g., oral contraceptives); resistance develops if used alone

Continued

Table 10–13. (*Continued*)

Antibiotic	Mechanism of Action/ Activity	Sensitive Bacteria/ Indications	Comments
Metronidazole	Damage of DNA by free radicals	*Bacteroides* sp., *Clostridium difficile*, anaerobic bacteria, *Gardnerella vaginalis*, *Capnocytophaga*, *Giardia*, *Entamoeba histolytica*	Seizures, encephalopathy, disulfiram reaction, metallic taste
Erythromycin	Macrolide: inhibits protein synthesis	*Corynebacterium diphtheriae*, *Mycoplasma*, *Chlamydia*, *Bordetella pertussis*, *Haemophilus ducreyi*, *Legionella* sp., *Campylobacter*	Often used as an alternative to penicillin G; nausea, hepatoxicity (estolate ester); increases theophylline and carbamazepine blood levels
Azithromycin	Macrolide	Less active than erythromycin against *S. aureus, Pneumococcus*, streptococci, more active against *H. influenzae*, *Mycoplasma, Chlamydia*, gram-negative bacilli; active against *M. catarrhalis, C. pneumoniae, Legionella pneumophila, Borrelia burgdorferi, Neisseria gonorrhoeae*	Possible efficacy for *Mycobacterium avium*, toxoplasma encephalitis, cryptosporidiosis; long half-life: single-dose treatment for uncomplicated *Chlamydia* urethritis or cervicitis
Clarithromycin	Macrolide	More active than erythromycin for *S. aureus, Pneumococcus, Streptococcus*	Similar to azithromycin
Clindamycin	Similar to erythromycin	*S. aureus, Streptococcus*, most anaerobic bacteria, *Actinomyces* (penicillin-allergic patients)	Pseudomembranous colitis toxicity
Vancomycin	Inhibits cell wall synthesis	Methicillin-resistant *S. aureus, S. epidermidis*, JK diphtheroids, *C. difficile, Enterococcus*, anaerobic bacteria	Red man syndrome if injected too fast, nephrotoxic
Trimethoprim–sulfamethoxazole	Inhibition of bacterial folate synthesis at two separate sites of the folate pathway	*E. coli, Proteus mirabilis, Salmonella, Shigella, H. influenzae, Yersinia, Pneumococcus, S. aureus, Pneumocystis carinii, M. catarrhalis, Nocardia*	Group A streptococci may be resistant; *P. aeruginosa* and enterococci resistant, Stevens-Johnson syndrome—anemia, neutropenia, glucose-6-phosphate dehydrogenase hemolysis
Ciprofloxacin	Similar to nalidixic acid; inhibition of bacterial DNA gyrase; broad spectrum	*P. aeruginosa, Shigella, Salmonella, E. coli, Klebsiella, Proteus* sp., *S. aureus*, enterococci, *S. epidermidis, H. influenzae*, Gonococcus, *Chlamydia, Listeria monocytogenes*	May be given by mouth; toxicity to growing bone; arthritis; CNS toxicity; not approved for children <17 yr of age

(Data from Med Clin North Am 71:1051–1216, 1987; Med Lett 34:49, 1992.)

tains as many as 500 different species of anaerobes. Obligate anaerobes require special culture media to grow. Gram-negative nonsporulating rods include *Bacteroides* and *Fusobacterium* species; gram-positive nonsporulating rods include *Eubacterium* and *Propionibacterium*; cocci include *Peptostreptococcus*, *Peptococcus*, and *Veillonella*.

Epidemiology. Blood, peritoneum, oropharynx, lungs, and soft tissues are the main sites of anaerobic infection. Infection follows disruption of mucous membrane barriers. Several anaerobes, or both anaerobes and aerobes, may be recovered concomitantly from infected tissue. The major clinical settings for anaerobic infection are (1) in the neonate following prolonged rupture of the membranes, amnionitis, or obstetric difficulty, (2) peritonitis or septicemia associated with intestinal obstruction or perforation (appendicitis), (3) aspiration pneumonia with lung abscess, (4) salpingitis and tubo-ovarian abscess, (5) orofacial infections, and (6) brain abscess.

Clinical Manifestations. Anaerobic infections of the *upper respiratory tract* have many different clinical manifestations. Periodontal infection (trench mouth) often is due to poor dental hygiene. Periapical abscesses or anaerobic osteomyelitis of the mandible or maxilla may be present. Anaerobic micro-organisms may be present in chronic sinusitis, chronic otitis media, mastoiditis, peritonsillar and retropharyngeal abscesses, and cervical lymphadenitis. Fusobacteria are important in the development of **Vincent stomatitis**, an infection characterized by ulcers covered by a brown or gray, foul-smelling exudate. Extensive tissue destruction can result in perforation of the carotid artery. **Ludwig angina** is an acute cellulitis of the sublingual and submandibular spaces that tends to spread rapidly without lymph node involvement or abscess formation. Edema of the tongue and airway may cause respiratory obstruction and require tracheotomy.

Anaerobic infection of the *lower respiratory tract* produces necrotizing pneumonia, putrid empyema, or lung abscess. A history of aspiration usually can be elicited. Pneumonia is followed by abscess formation.

Anaerobic infection of the *CNS* produces brain abscess, subdural empyema, or septic thrombophlebitis of cortical veins and venous sinuses. These lesions originate by direct spread from a contiguous infection or by hematogenous spread. Purulent meningitis rarely is caused by anaerobes; identification of anaerobes from the CSF indicates another focus, such as a brain abscess or subdural empyema.

Peritoneal spillage of gastrointestinal contents, especially that of the colon, is associated with a high incidence of anaerobic *intra-abdominal infection*. Peritonitis and abscess formation (subdiaphragmatic, pelvic) are common after intestinal perforation.

Anaerobic *bacteremia* is clinically indistinguishable from aerobic bacteremia. Anaerobic bacteremia frequently is associated with disease of the gastrointestinal and genitourinary systems.

Diagnosis. The diagnosis of anaerobic infection requires an awareness of anaerobe-associated infections and appropriate collection of specimens for cultures, with the use of special media and techniques. Factors that should increase the suspicion of an anaerobic infection include:

1. Presence of a foul-smelling exudate or discharge
2. Evidence of necrotic tissue, gangrene, or fasciitis
3. Infection located in proximity to a mucosal surface
4. Gas in tissue
5. Gram stain of material that reveals multiple types of organisms
6. Infection associated with tissue destruction (trauma or malignancy)
7. Failure to respond to antibiotics, especially aminoglycosides
8. Septic thrombophlebitis
9. Abscess formation

Added clues that suggest anaerobes include no growth on routine cultures (sterile pus); failure to grow but presence of bacteria on Gram stain; growth in thioglycollate broth or on media containing kanamycin, neomycin, or paromomycin; production of gas and foul odor in culture; and development of characteristic colonies on agar plates incubated anaerobically.

Rapid diagnosis is possible with indirect immunofluorescence assay and gas–liquid chromatography identification of specific bacterial fermentation profiles from purulent material.

Treatment. The pathogen usually can be predicted from the site of infection (above or below the diaphragm), and most anaerobes have predictable susceptibilities to antibiotic agents. Penicillin G is useful against gram-positive and most gram-negative anaerobes (except *Bacteroides fragilis*) and can be used to treat orofacial and pulmonary infections, unless beta-lactamase–producing anaerobes are present. Cefoxitin, amoxicillin/clavulanate, clindamycin, or metronidazole may be used to treat anaerobic infections at other sites. Anaerobes also usually are susceptible to cefotetan, imipenem, or ticarcillin/clavulanate. Metronidazole is very effective in treating anaerobic brain abscesses, whereas clindamycin is excellent for lung abscesses (see Appendix I).

References

Behrman RE (ed): Nelson Textbook of Pediatrics. 14th ed. Philadelphia, WB Saunders, 1992, Sec. 12.38, 12.40.

Styrt B, Gorbach SL: Recent developments in the understanding of the pathogenesis and treatment of anaerobic infections (first of two parts). N Engl J Med 321:240, 1989.

Styrt B, Gorbach SL: Recent developments in the understanding of the pathogenesis and treatment of anaerobic infections (second of two parts). N Engl J Med 321:298, 1989.

Clostridial Infections

Clostridial organisms have been associated with tetanus, gas gangrene (clostridial myonecrosis), food poisoning, necrotizing enteritis, antimicrobial-associated colitis, and botulism. Most of these disorders are the result of toxin elaboration by vegetative organisms.

TETANUS (LOCKJAW)

Etiology. *Clostridium tetani* is an anaerobic, spore-forming, gram-positive bacillus. The spores are resistant to many injurious agents and processes, including boiling. The vegetative forms of *C. tetani* are susceptible to heat and many disinfectants. *C. tetani* survives in soil for years and may be found in house dust, salt and fresh water, the oral cavities of mammals, and feces of many animal species. Spores and vegetative organisms may be found in the intestinal contents of humans.

Tetanus bacilli are not invasive but produce two toxins, tetanospasmin and tetanolysin. Tetanospasmin is a neurotoxin responsible for clinical manifestations. Except for botulinum toxin, tetanospasmin, a diffusible protein, is the most potent poison known. It is produced at a site of injury by the vegetative forms of the organism and then is transported through the circulation or via peripheral nerves to the CNS.

Epidemiology. Tetanus occurs throughout the world and, in the United States, is most common in the South during the summer and in unimmunized or poorly immunized patients. In developing countries, it is an important cause of neonatal death because of poor hygiene and absent maternal, and hence neonatal, antitoxin. Contamination of the umbilical cord is the source of infection in the newborn infant. In older children, the risk is greatest from a deep puncture wound or from an injury associated with tissue necrosis, conditions that favor toxin elaboration. Contaminated medical needles or those used by intravenous drug users is another source. Morbidity and mortality rates in the United States have been decreasing since 1950; however, case fatality rates are still 50–65%. In the United States, tetanus is more common among 1–5 yr old boys and elderly patients with waning immunity. The incubation period is usually 3–14 days after injury but may be as short as 1 day with serious infection or as long as several months. Tetanus is not transmitted from person to person.

Clinical Manifestations. There are several clinical forms of tetanus: localized, generalized, cephalic, and tetanus neonatorum. In each, an examination of the actual wound does not reveal an appearance that is different from that of an uninfected wound.

Localized tetanus is uncommon in children but produces pain and continuous rigidity and spasm of muscles in proximity to the injury; symptoms may persist for weeks and resolve without sequelae. Occasionally, this pattern precedes the generalized disorder. The fatality rate of localized tetanus is about 1%.

Generalized tetanus is the most common form. The onset may be insidious, with gradually increasing muscle stiffness; trismus is the presenting symptom in over 50% of cases. Spasm of the masseter muscles may be associated with stiffness of neck muscles and difficulty in swallowing. Restlessness, irritability, and headache are early manifestations. Spasm of facial muscles immobilizes the jaw, producing a fixed sardonic grin (risus sardonicus). Tonic contractions of the somatic musculature become generalized. Voluntary movement or sensory stimulation (cutaneous, auditory, visual) may initiate spasms or convulsions. The lumbar and abdominal muscles may become rigid; persistent spasm of the back muscles results in opisthotonos. Tetanic seizures are characterized by sudden bursts of tonic contractions of various muscle groups. Spasm of the airway or respiratory muscles causes airway obstruction and respiratory insufficiency. Spasm may cause fractures and local hemorrhages. The patient is completely conscious during the clinical course and experiences intense pain. Signs and symptoms increase over 3–7 days, reach a plateau during the second week, and gradually abate. Recovery is complete in 2–6 weeks.

Cephalic tetanus is rare and may precede generalized tetanus. The incubation period is 1–2 days after otitis media, trauma to the head and face, and the presence of nasal foreign bodies. Involvement of cranial nerves III, IV, VII (most common), IX, X, and XI is the most prominent feature of the disease.

Tetanus neonatorum begins 3–10 days after birth and is generalized. Difficulty in sucking, excessive crying, difficulty in swallowing, rigidity, tonic contractions, and opisthotonos are common.

Diagnosis and Differential Diagnosis. The diagnosis of tetanus is made on clinical grounds. A history of a wound or bite, the characteristic facial appearance, and spasms aid in establishing the diagnosis. Most cases occur in unimmunized individuals or in their infants. Wound cultures are positive for *C. tetani* in one third of instances. Gram stains of the wound may show gram-positive rods with terminal, drumstick-like spores. Trismus may be associated with tooth, peritonsillar, or retropharyngeal abscesses. Spasms also may be seen in rabies, hypocalcemia, and strychnine or phenothiazine intoxication. Rabies and, rarely, tetanus may follow animal bites. Rabies causes pain and numbness at the bite, fever (not noted in tetanus), painful esophageal spasm on drinking, CSF pleocytosis, and, eventually, coma and paralysis.

Treatment. The objectives of therapy are to remove the source of tetanospasmin, to neutralize remaining circulating toxin before it reaches the CNS, and to provide supportive care until tetanospasmin, which is fixed to neural tissue, can be metabolized. Supportive care includes diazepam, chlorpromazine, and seconal for convulsions, meperidine for pain, and artificial ventilation and tracheostomy for respiratory insufficiency. Induction of paralysis with pancuronium may be helpful to control spasms and improve ventilation. Human tetanus immune globulin (antitoxin) (3000–6000 U × 1 dose) should be given. Wounds should be irrigated and débrided. Penicillin therapy is indicated to eradicate vegetative *C. tetani* organisms. There is no transmission to humans, but body substance isolation should be used until rabies is excluded.

Prevention. Immediate and thorough surgical treatment of wounds is mandatory. The indications for active and passive immunoprophylaxis depend on the prior immunization status and the severity of the wound (Table 10–14). *Tetanus toxoid* also should be given following tetanus, because the disease does not induce natural immunity.

Prognosis. Case fatality rates of tetanus are approximately 30–55% despite modern care; rates for

Table 10–14. Tetanus Prevention Following Wounds

Tetanus Immunization History	Clean Td†	Minor TIG‡	All Others* Td	All Others* TIG
Uncertain or incomplete (<3 doses)	Yes	No	Yes	Yes
Complete (>3 doses plus booster)	No§	No	No‖	No

* Other wounds include those contaminated with soil, dirt, feces, saliva; and punctures, avulsions, crush injuries, burns, frostbite, and wounds resulting from missiles. All wounds require appropriate irrigation and debridement.
† If less than 7 yr old, DT may be given.
‡ Tetanus immune globulin (human).
§ Yes, if longer than 10 yr since last immunization.
‖ Yes, if longer than 5 yr since last immunization.
¶ DT = diphtheria–tetanus vaccine; Td = tetanus–diphtheria toxoid (adult type); TIG = tetanus immune globulin.
(Modified from Report of Committee on Infectious Diseases, 1991 Red Book. 22nd ed. American Academy of Pediatrics, 1991.)

neonatal tetanus are 60% or greater. Patients with an incubation period of 8–10 days, those with progression longer than 60 hr, and those who survive for 10 days recover completely. Tetanus does not produce sequelae other than those due to anoxia.

References

Behrman RE (ed): Nelson Textbook of Pediatrics. 14th ed. Philadelphia, WB Saunders, 1992, Sec. 12.37.
Bleck TP: The pharmacology of tetanus. Clin Neuropharmacol 9:103, 1986.

BOTULISM

Etiology. *Clostridium botulinum* is an anaerobic, gram-positive bacillus that produces heat-resistant spores. When spores survive food processing, they germinate in the container and elaborate neurotoxins. Seven antigenically distinct toxins have been identified (A–G). All except D have been associated with human disease.

Epidemiology. The three forms of botulism are:

1. *Food-borne botulism*, an intoxication from preformed botulinum toxin present in improperly preserved food. Home-preserved foods are the most frequent cause of this type of botulism in the United States.
2. *Wound botulism*, a rare botulism resulting from local wound infection and toxin production by *C. botulinum*.
3. *Infant botulism*, the most common cause of botulism

in the United States, caused by germination of spores of *C. botulinum* in the gastrointestinal tract accompanied by toxin produced in vivo rather than by the ingestion of preformed toxin.

Infant botulism usually occurs in children under 6 mo of age, has a peak onset from 1–3 mo, and is caused by type A and B strains. Adults also have developed this type of botulism. Sources for spores include soil, house and vacuum cleaner dust, honey, and possibly corn syrup. The majority of patients have been reported from California, Pennsylvania, Hawaii, and Utah, clusters correlating with areas of high soil spore concentration of *C. botulinum*. Botulism toxin is the most potent toxin known to humans. It inhibits release of acetylcholine from the prejunction motor nerve terminals.

Clinical Manifestations.   The course of *infant botulism* varies from mild constipation and poor feeding to severe neurologic deterioration and sudden, at times unexplained, death. Typically, a previously healthy, afebrile infant has constipation, poor sucking and swallowing; develops a weak cry and smile; and has bilateral ptosis, hypotonia, and poor head control. Symmetric, descending paralysis progresses over hours to days, involving facial muscles, trunk, and limbs. Ileus, bladder atony, nonreactive dilated pupils, and decreased tearing and salivation may be present. Infants require ventilatory support for apnea or hypoventilation. Because the CNS is not affected, the child is awake and may even appear alert.

The incubation of *food-borne botulism* usually takes 12–36 hr but can range from several hours to a week. Nausea, vomiting, diplopia, dysphagia, dysarthria, and dry mouth are common during the course of disease. Weakness, postural hypotension, absent or diminished deep tendon reflexes, urinary retention, and constipation (not diarrhea) also may develop.

The course of *wound botulism* may be similar to that exhibited after ingestion of *C. botulinum* toxin but is usually milder and more prolonged. The incubation period is 4–14 days.

Diagnosis and Differential Diagnosis.   The diagnosis of botulism is established by identifying *C. botulinum* organisms and/or toxin in feces, blood, or food products. Wound botulism is diagnosed by demonstrating the organisms in the wound and/or the toxin in blood. An electromyogram with brief, small, abundant potentials suggests botulism.

Infant botulism should be differentiated from septicemia, myasthenia gravis, poliomyelitis, Werdnig-Hoffmann disease, spinal cord injury, near-miss sudden infant death syndrome, hypothyroidism, and inborn errors of metabolism.

Food-borne botulism must be differentiated from myasthenia gravis, poliomyelitis, Guillain-Barré syndrome, drug intoxication, trichinosis, diphtheria, and various forms of electrolyte or mineral imbalances.

Treatment.   Antitoxin is of uncertain value in *infant botulism*. Intensive care alone usually is sufficient. Antibiotics do not shorten the clinical course or decrease intestinal colonization. Aminoglycosides exacerbate or accelerate paralysis and produce respiratory failure as a result of synergistic inhibition of neurotransmission at the neuromuscular junction. A cleansing enema may eliminate the site of toxin production.

All children with *food-borne botulism* must be hospitalized. Vomiting should be induced and gastric lavage initiated. Cathartics may be placed in the stomach at the conclusion of lavage and an enema given to facilitate elimination of unabsorbed toxin. Equine antitoxin has been efficacious in treating food-borne disease. The polyvalent preparation is preferred until the toxin type has been identified. Skin sensitivity testing is mandatory prior to administration. Penicillin G is given to kill *C. botulinum*, which may continue to produce toxin.

Wound botulism requires débriding and draining the wound. Performing supportive intensive care measures and administering antitoxin and antibiotics also are indicated.

Supportive care includes monitoring cardiorespiratory functions in anticipation of apnea, hypotension, or aspiration resulting from the absence of the gag reflex; managing constipation; and treating urinary retention, inappropriate antidiuretic hormone secretion, and urinary tract infection. Nutritional support by gavage feeding may be indicated if the gag reflex is absent.

Prevention.   Boiling food for 10 min destroys the toxin. A pressure cooker is required to kill spores of *C. botulinum*; pressure requirements vary with the food being processed. Because 10% of retail honey in the United States may contain *C. botulinum* spores, it should not be fed to infants less than 6 mo of age. Breast feeding may lessen the severity of the illness.

Prognosis.   Most infants recover without sequelae, if adequate intensive care and supportive therapy prevent hypoxia. Severity of illness in food-borne botulism is directly related to the titer of toxin ingested and inversely related to the duration of the incubation period. Complete recovery is delayed for many months and requires regeneration of the previously destroyed presynaptic terminals. Because the toxin does not cross the blood–brain barrier, intelligence is normal in the absence of prior hypoxic episodes.

References

Behrman RE (ed): Nelson Textbook of Pediatrics. 14th ed. Philadelphia, WB Saunders, 1992, Sec. 12.39.

Hutchinson DN: Foodborne botulism: New techniques for preserving foods bring the need for greater awareness of the risks. BMJ 305:264, 1992.

Schreiner MS, Field E, Ruddy R: Infant botulism: A review of 12 years' experience at the Children's Hospital of Philadelphia. Pediatrics 87:159, 1991.

Infection Due to *Corynebacterium diphtheriae*

Etiology and Pathophysiology. *Corynebacterium diphtheriae* is a gram-positive, nonsporulating bacillus with three colony types (mitis, gravis, and intermedius). Infection of *C. diphtheriae* by a lysogenic bacteriophage containing the gene for the toxin is required to produce disease. Toxigenic and nontoxigenic strains of *C. diphtheriae* cause disease, but only strains that produce toxin are responsible for myocarditis and neuritis. Diphtheria is characterized by local inflammation and the production of a pseudomembrane composed of necrotic epithelium and coagulated inflammatory cells in the upper respiratory tract (nasal or oral pharynx), which may cause airway obstruction. In addition, toxin production causes injury to distant visceral tissues (nerve, heart, kidney). By cleaving NAD, the toxin inhibits protein synthesis.

Epidemiology. Humans are the only known reservoir of *C. diphtheriae*. The incidence peaks in the winter; 80% of cases occur in unimmunized individuals less than 15 yr of age. The incidence is highest among the poor who live in close, crowded conditions. Diphtheria is acquired by close contact with respiratory droplets from either an asymptomatic carrier or a person with the disease. Fomites and dust occasionally are vehicles of transmission. The incubation period is 2–4 days.

Clinical Manifestations. The manifestations of diphtheria depend on the location of infection, the immunization status of the host, and whether toxin enters the systemic circulation. Manifestations are classified by the location of the diphtheritic pseudomembrane: nasal, tonsillar, pharyngeal, laryngeal or laryngotracheal, conjunctival, cutaneous, and genital; more than one anatomic site may be involved.

Nasal diphtheria initially resembles a common cold. Gradually, the nasal discharge becomes mucopurulent and serosanguineous as the gray pseudomembrane excoriates the nasal mucosa and nares. Nasal diphtheria is uncommon, occurs most often in infants, and is characterized by a mild course.

Tonsillar and/or pharyngeal diphtheria is the most common type, beginning insidiously with malaise, low-grade fever, and a mild sore throat. Within 1–2 days a membrane forms; its size and extent vary according to the host's immune status. The membrane initially is thin, white, and localized; as the disease progresses, it coalesces and extends from the tonsil to the contiguous soft or hard palate, pharyngeal wall, larynx, and trachea. This pattern distinguishes diphtheria from other diseases producing membranous tonsillitis. The membrane becomes gray and the breath may have a foul, garlic odor. Removal of the exudate is followed by bleeding. Bilateral cervical lymphadenitis is variable. Ten percent of patients present with high fever, toxicity, rapid progression of the pseudomembrane, and edema of the soft tissues of the neck (bull neck). The edema is brawny, pitting, warm, and tender; it occurs in children over 6 yr of age and carries a more severe prognosis. In less severe cases, recovery may be complicated by myocarditis or neuritis caused by systemic absorption of toxin.

Laryngeal diphtheria usually results when the membrane extends downward from the pharynx. In 10% of cases, only the larynx is involved. Hoarseness and stridor produce acute and potentially fatal obstruction if the membrane occludes the airway. In severe cases, the membrane may extend downward, forming a cast over the entire tracheobronchial tree.

Cutaneous diphtheria, which is common in warmer climates, often is indistinguishable from other skin infections (e.g., impetigo). Skin lesions may be an important source of person-to-person transmission. *Conjunctival lesions* usually are limited to the palpebral conjunctiva, which appears red, edematous, and membranous; corneal erosion may occur. *Aural diphtheria* is characterized by otitis externa accompanied by a persistent, purulent, and frequently foul-smelling discharge.

The more extensive the primary lesion and the lower the antitoxin titer, the more severe the toxicity. Cardiac toxicity occurs in 10% of patients, appears between the 7th and 14th day of illness, and is characterized by heart failure, atrioventricular nodal block and arrhythmias. Isolated peripheral neuropathies involving the palate, pharynx, larynx, extraocular muscles, or diaphragm appear in 2–6 wk. Paralysis of the extremities and elevated CSF protein resembling Guillain-Barré syndrome may occur. Hepatitis, nephritis, and gastritis also may occur.

Diagnosis and Differential Diagnosis. Determining the diagnosis requires isolating *C. diphtheriae* from the membrane or the exudate beneath the membrane. The bacillus is readily recovered on selective media (tellurite) using inhibitors that retard the growth of other micro-organisms. Microscopic examination of diphtheritic lesions is unreliable. *C. diphtheriae* should be tested for toxigenicity.

Tonsillar and/or pharyngeal diphtheria must be differentiated from streptococcal pharyngitis, infectious mononucleosis, viral tonsillitis, primary herpetic tonsillitis, thrush, blood dyscrasias (such as agranulocytosis and leukemia), toxoplasmosis, cytomegalovirus, *Francisella tularensis*, and Vincent angina. Laryngeal diphtheria must be differentiated from viral croup, the presence of foreign bodies, retropharyngeal abscesses, and laryngeal tumors (papillomas, hemangiomas, lymphangiomas).

Treatment. Treatment of diphtheria requires neutralizing the circulating toxin and eradicating *C. diphtheriae* with antibiotics. Equine antitoxin must be given as soon as possible because, once toxin is bound to tissue, antitoxin has no effect. Antibiotics help stop the production of additional toxin. Penicillin and erythromycin are effective against most strains of *C. diphtheriae* but will not alter the evolution of the disease. The diphtheria carrier state can be treated with penicillin G benzathine, penicillin G, or oral erythromycin. The endpoint of antibiotic therapy and infectivity is indicated by three consecutive negative cultures. Supportive care may include endotracheal intubation for respiratory insufficiency due to airway obstruction or paralysis.

Prevention. Prevention requires isolation of the patient and treatment of close contacts who are likely to become ill (if nonimmune) or become carriers. Previously immunized carriers should be given a booster injection of diphtheria toxoid and should be treated with penicillin or erythromycin. Nonimmunized asymptomatic carriers should have samples taken for culture, should receive diphtheria toxoid and penicillin or erythromycin, and should be examined carefully for 7 days. Because diphtheria does not always produce persistent immunity, patients should receive toxoid after the illness.

Prognosis. Prior to the use of antitoxin and antibiotics, the mortality rate from diphtheria was 30–50%. Death was most common in younger children (<4 yr old) and often resulted from airway obstruction by the diphtheritic pseudomembrane. Today the mortality rate is less than 5%, and death is due to severe myocarditis. Nasopharyngeal persistence of *C. diphtheriae* may be noted in 5–10% of convalescing patients.

References

Behrman RE (ed): Nelson Textbook of Pediatrics. 14th ed. Philadelphia, WB Saunders, 1992, Sec. 12.23.

Kjeldsen K, Simonsen O, Heron I: Immunity against diphtheria 25–30 years after primary vaccination in childhood. Lancet 1:900, 1985.

Rappuoli R, Perugini M, Falsen E: Molecular epidemiology of the 1984–1986 outbreak of diphtheria in Sweden. N Engl J Med 318:12, 1988.

Infection Due to *Haemophilus influenzae*

Etiology. *Haemophilus influenzae* are small, fastidious, pleomorphic gram-negative coccobacilli that at times produce, especially if they are pretreated with antibiotics, a Gram stain that is variable, often causing diagnostic confusion. Encapsulated strains are classified according to their soluble capsular polysaccharides (polyribosyl ribitol phosphate [PRP]) and are designated as types a through f. Type b produces serious invasive infections (meningitis, septic arthritis, epiglottitis, pericarditis, facial cellulitis, pneumonia) in children. Infants lacking anti-PRP IgG have deficient phagocytosis of these encapsulated organisms. Nontypable unencapsulated strains are associated with sinusitis, conjunctivitis, otitis media, and bronchitis. *H. influenzae* organisms also contain endotoxin, IgA protease, and, for purposes of attachment, pili or fimbriae. Some strains produce beta-lactamase and thus are resistant to ampicillin.

Epidemiology. Asymptomatic colonization is common; most children have unencapsulated strains in their pharynx, and 2–5% carry type b organisms. The mode of transmission is by breathing respiratory droplets or by directly contacting toxic secretions. *H. influenzae* type b meningitis is more common in children less than 4 yr of age and in boys, blacks, American Indians, Alaskan Eskimos, and day care attenders; also, its occurrence is more common in urban settings. Children with asplenia (from congenital and surgical causes and sickle cell anemia), those with antibody deficiencies (e.g., IgG2), and patients receiving chemotherapy for malignancies are at an increased risk for infection. *H. influenzae* type b disease is usually endemic but may cause outbreaks in day care centers or chronic care facilities. For about 30 days after the onset of *H. influenzae* type b meningitis, the risk in household and day care contacts less than 4 yr of age is greater than the age-adjusted risk in the general population; the first 7 days after onset carry the highest risk for these household and day care contacts. The risk of secondary infection in day care centers is less than that for household contacts.

INFECTIONS CAUSED BY *HAEMOPHILUS INFLUENZAE* TYPE B

Clinical Manifestations

Meningitis. *H. influenzae* type b was a common cause of bacterial meningitis in children between ages 1 mo and 4 yr prior to the widespread use of HIB vaccine. Meningitis caused by *H. influenzae* cannot be distinguished from that due to *N. meningitidis* or *S. pneumoniae* on the basis of clinical presentation. The illness may be complicated at the time of presentation or later by other sites of infection with *H. influenzae*, including pneumonia, arthritis, osteomyelitis, pericarditis, cellulitis, and endophthalmitis.

Acute Epiglottitis. This potentially lethal condition, which may result in airway obstruction from an acutely inflamed epiglottis, usually occurs in children between 2 and 7 yr old (see Chapter 12).

Pneumonia. The incidence of *H. influenzae* pneumonia in children is unknown, but it is most common in children less than 6 yr of age. The signs and symptoms of pneumonia caused by *H. influenzae* cannot be distinguished from those caused by other micro-organisms. Pleural effusions and lobar and patchy infiltrates may be noted. Associated infections include otitis media, meningitis, and epiglottitis.

Septic Arthritis. *H. influenzae* type b is the most common agent producing septic arthritis in children less than 3 yr of age. Large joints, such as knees, hips, ankles, and elbows, commonly are affected, often in association with infections such as meningitis. Arthritis that appears late in the course of *H. influenzae* meningitis infection may be an antigen–antibody reaction and not a true joint space infection. Septic arthritis caused by *H. influenzae*

type b is indistinguishable from that caused by other bacterial pathogens.

Cellulitis. Over 85% of children with *H. influenzae* type b cellulitis are 2 yr of age or younger. Frequently, an upper respiratory tract infection precedes the acute onset of cellulitis. There are high fever, marked toxicity, bacteremia, and leukocytosis without a prior history of local trauma. The face and neck, particularly the cheek (buccal) and the periorbital area, are the most common sites. The lesion has indistinct margins, is tender and indurated, and may have a violaceous or bluish purple color. Meningitis with facial cellulitis may occur.

Pericarditis. *H. influenzae* type b causes up to 15% of bacterial pericarditis cases in children. Children are usually 2–4 yr of age and often have had an antecedent upper respiratory tract infection or adjacent pneumonia.

Bacteremia without an Associated Focus. Bacteremia caused by *H. influenzae* type b may occur without any apparent focus of infection other than signs of an upper respiratory tract infection or pharyngitis. Although affected children may appear only mildly ill at the initial visit, they are at substantial risk of developing pneumonia or meningitis, a finding that is in marked contrast to occult pneumococcal bacteremia, which has a much lower risk of metastatic foci or infection following bacteremia without a source.

Neonatal Disease. In the neonate, nontypable *H. influenzae* is more common than type b. Septicemia, pneumonia, meningitis, and respiratory distress syndrome produced by nontypable *H. influenzae* are indistinguishable from those due to other neonatal bacterial pathogens. Nontypable *H. influenzae* are acquired by the infant from the mother's genitourinary tract.

Diagnosis. CSF, blood, synovial fluid, cellulitis aspirate, or other material should be cultured on a selective medium, such as chocolate agar. Latex agglutination tests for detecting capsular antigen in CSF, blood, and urine aid in rapid diagnosis. Beta-lactamase production and antibiotic susceptibility tests should be performed on all isolates to determine resistance to ampicillin and chloramphenicol.

Treatment (see also Central Nervous System Infections). Invasive infections presumed to be due to *H. influenzae* initially should be treated with intravenous ceftriaxone or cefotaxime. If beta-lactamase production is present, the organism is resistant to ampicillin. Regionally, the prevalence of ampicillin-resistant strains varies from 10% to 40%. Strains of *H. influenzae* type b may be resistant to chloramphenicol because of their production of a plasmid-mediated acetyltransferase. Cefotaxime and ceftriaxone are useful for treating such resistant *H. influenzae* infections because they penetrate the CSF and they are active against ampicillin- and chloramphenicol-resistant strains (see Appendix I).

Prevention. Conjugate vaccines with PRP covalently linked to diphtheria toxoid or OMP (outer membrane protein of *N. meningitidis*) should be administered to infants at 2, 4, 6, and 15 mo and to unimmunized 24–60 mo old children (Tables 10–3 and 10–4). Because the risk for secondary infection caused by *H. influenzae* type b in close contacts is high, rifampin is recommended for all family contacts (adults, index case, plus young children) of individuals with *H. influenzae* disease when there are other children in the household who are less than 4 yr of age. Close contacts in day care centers also may be candidates for rifampin therapy.

References

Behrman RE (ed): Nelson Textbook of Pediatrics. 14th ed. Philadelphia, WB Saunders, 1992, Sec. 12.22.

Dagan R and the Israeli Pediatric Bacteremia and Meningitis Group: A two-year prospective, nationwide study to determine the epidemiology and impact of invasive childhood *Haemophilus influenzae* type b infection in Israel. Clin Infect Dis 15:720, 1992.

Korones DN, Marshall GS, Shapiro ED: Outcome of children with occult bacteremia caused by *Haemophilus influenzae* type b. Pediatr Infect Dis J 11:516, 1992.

Santosham M, Wolff M, Reid R, et al: The efficacy in Navajo infants of a conjugate vaccine consisting of *Haemophilus influenzae* type b polysaccharide and *Neisseria meningitidis* outer-membrane protein complex. N Engl J Med 324:1767, 1991.

Mycobacterial Infections

TUBERCULOSIS

Etiology. Tuberculosis is caused by *M. tuberculosis*, an aerobic, acid-fast–staining (resistant to acid decolorization) pleomorphic rod. It is a slow-growing organism (requiring 3–6 wk) that does not produce pigment. The cell wall contains complex lipids (hence its quality of acid fastness) and protein, which produces delayed sensitivity reactions to tuberculin.

Epidemiology. Tuberculosis currently is increasing in frequency and is a major cause of mortality throughout the world. Reservoirs of tuberculosis include the elderly, immigrants (Asian, African, Latin American), the homeless, and patients with AIDS. Tuberculosis is more common in crowded semi-industrialized societies and among the poor. Infection in children occurs following inhalation of contaminated respiratory droplets (coughing, sneezing) from heavily infected respiratory tract secretions. Infection in children typically is due to prolonged close contact with an individual having untreated, active, cavitary, sputum-positive disease. The incubation period from infection to development of a positive tuberculin skin test is 2–6 wk.

Immunity. Following inhalation into the alveolus, the tuberculosis bacillus is ingested but not killed by the pulmonary macrophage. The bacilli multiply, form pulmonary granulomas, spread to local lymph nodes, and disseminate to extrathoracic organs by lymphatic and hematogenous spread. The alveolar macrophage presents the antigenic material to T lymphocytes, producing delayed-type hypersensitivity, which, together with newly activated macrophages, causes intracellular killing of the bacilli and granuloma formation. Genetic factors, age (<3 yr, puberty), immunosuppression (AIDS, malnutrition, pertussis, measles, lymphoma, corticosteroids), pregnancy, and other factors predispose the patient to serious disease because they alter the immune response.

Clinical Manifestations. When a nonimmune host inhales organisms, that host develops a primary complex, which involves the lung parenchyma (usually lower or middle lobes) and its draining lymph node. The organism is then disseminated to other body sites (upper lobes, bone, meninges). Acquired immunity in the healthy host usually contains the infection in dormant foci in lungs, regional lymph nodes, and visceral organs. In the lung, this may be noted 1–2 yr after primary infection as calcified lesions or the **Ghon complex.** Lesions that apparently have healed may contain dormant but viable bacilli. In addition, disease progression may occur in the lungs or at distal sites of infection. Progression of the primary complex to pulmonary disease or miliary tuberculosis, or progression of CNS granulomas to meningitis, is most common in the 1st yr after primary infection and in children less than 5 yr. Pulmonary progression also is common during puberty. Skeletal lesions often are delayed 2–3 yr after the primary infection. In hosts with subsequent alteration of immunity, reactivation of the foci also can result in pulmonary or extrathoracic symptoms. Hilar adenopathy may compress the bronchus or trachea, producing airway obstruction and wheezing. Compression of the recurrent laryngeal nerve (hoarseness), phrenic nerve (diaphragm palsy), and vena cava (superior vena cava syndrome) causes additional problems.

Primary pulmonary tuberculosis in older infants and children is usually an asymptomatic illness. It is diagnosed only by a positive skin test, often with minimal abnormalities (infiltrate with hilar adenopathy) on the chest roentgenogram. Malaise, low-grade fever, erythema nodosum, phlyctenular keratoconjunctivitis, or symptoms resulting from lymph node enlargement may occur after the development of delayed hypersensitivity. In older children and adolescents, primary illness presents as an upper lobe infiltrate and cavitation without calcification. In children under 3 yr, primary pulmonary infection may be progressive and merge with miliary tuberculosis or progressive CNS disease to produce tuberculous meningitis.

Progressive pulmonary tuberculosis occurs when the primary infection is not contained and produces bronchopneumonia or lobar pneumonia (usually middle or lower) and cavitation with associated fever, weight loss, night sweats, malaise, hemoptysis, and productive cough. The tuberculin skin test is positive.

Reactivation pulmonary tuberculosis, uncommon in young children but more common in adolescents, usually is confined to apical segments of upper lobes or superior segments of lower lobes. There is usually little lymphadenopathy and no extrathoracic infection as a result of established hypersensitivity. This is a manifestation of a secondary expansion of infection at a site seeded years previously during primary infection. Cavitation and endobronchial spread of bacilli occur and are associated with fever, night sweats, malaise, and weight loss. A productive cough and hemoptysis often herald cavitation and bronchial erosion.

Upper respiratory tract tuberculosis, which involves the larynx (croupy cough, sore throat, hoarseness) or middle ear (hearing loss, otorrhea, thick perforated eardrum), is a complication of advanced pulmonary disease.

Pleural effusions are usually an allergic response to tuberculous antigens. Less often effusions may be secondary to discharge of tubercle bacilli into the pleural space from subpleural foci during postprimary tuberculosis. Pleural exudative effusions often are unilateral and may be associated with pericarditis and peritonitis. Biopsy of pleural tissue has a higher diagnostic yield than examination of fluid. The fluid is reabsorbed gradually during therapy.

Hilar *lymphadenopathy* is common in primary pulmonary disease. The most common extrathoracic sites of adenitis are the cervical, supraclavicular, and submandibular areas (scrofula). The illness usually is insidious, unilateral more often than bilateral, and associated with a history of exposure to an infected family member. The nodes are nontender and firm. Chest roentgenograms may reveal pulmonary tuberculosis as well. Suppuration of the nodes may lead to fluctuance and draining sinus tracts. Enlargement may cause compression of adjacent structures. Differential diagnosis includes infections caused by atypical mycobacteria, cat-scratch disease, fungal infection, viral or bacterial disease, toxoplasmosis, sarcoidosis, drug reactions, and malignancy. Diagnosis may be confirmed by fine-needle aspiration, but may necessitate excisional biopsy accompanied by appropriate histologic and microbiologic studies.

Miliary tuberculosis refers to widespread hematogenous dissemination with infection of multiple organs. The lesions are of roughly the same size as that of a millet seed, from which the name miliary is derived. Miliary tuberculosis is characterized by abrupt onset of fever, weakness, malaise, anorexia, weight loss, lymphadenopathy, night sweats, and hepatosplenomegaly. Diffuse bilateral pneumonitis always is present and meningitis is noted in 30% of patients. Anemia, monocytosis, thrombocytopenia, hyponatremia, hypokalemia, and abnormal liver function tests are common. The chest roentgenogram reveals bilateral miliary infiltrates demonstrating overwhelming infection. The tuberculin skin test may be nonreactive as a result of anergy. Liver or bone marrow biopsy may be needed for the diagnosis.

Tuberculous meningitis occurs in recently infected individuals. In developing countries, it usually occurs before age 5 yr and within 6 mo of the primary infection, whereas in developed countries, it has become an illness of adults. Rupture of CNS tubercles, which were seeded during primary infection, results in a severe inflammatory basilar meningitis (brain stem, basal cisterns, blood vessels). This insidious disease progresses through stages: the nonspecific influenza-like stage one, lasting 1–2 wk, which is manifested by low-grade fever and subtle personality changes; stage two, in which neurologic signs and symptoms develop that may include headache, stiff neck, positive Kernig or Brudzinski sign, and cranial nerve palsies (III, VI, VII, VIII), including aphasia, disorientation, ataxia, hemiplegia, and seizures; and stage three, which is demonstrated by increasing intracranial pressure (as a result of obstruction of basal cisterns), stupor, coma, decerebrate or decorticate posturing, and death. Without therapy, death is nearly inevitable within several weeks after the onset of symptoms.

There also may be evidence of concurrent pulmonary disease and hyponatremia caused by the syndrome of inappropriate antidiuretic hormone secretion. A CT scan may show periventricular lucencies, edema, infarctions, and hydrocephalus. Lumbar puncture usually reveals increased spinal fluid pressure. CSF studies reveal a modest increase in cells (50–500 cells/μL), mostly of lymphocytes, although polymorphonuclear leukocytes may predominate early. Glucose is low and protein is elevated. The tubercle bacilli are seen in less than 30% of patients; the culture requires weeks to grow organisms. The skin test is positive in about two thirds of cases, but in very ill individuals anergy may be present. In such children often a history of close contact with a person who has active tuberculosis will be revealed. Skin testing and chest roentgenograms of close contacts may facilitate diagnosis and recovery of the organism. An early diagnosis improves the outcome; however, sequelae such as deafness, paralysis, retardation, and hydrocephalus may occur.

In some children, an expanding mass presenting as a CNS infection with focal neurologic signs and low-grade fever may be due to a *tuberculoma of the CNS.* The CT scan may reveal a hypodense area surrounded by edema. As in tuberculous meningitis, children often have a history of contact with an infected adult, a positive skin test, and concurrent pulmonary disease.

Tuberculosis of the heart and pericardium rarely may result from rupture of mediastinal nodes into the pericardial space or from hematogenous dissemination. The signs and symptoms resemble those seen in pericarditis that is due to other etiologies, and the exudate resembles that of tuberculous pleuritis. The skin test is usually positive. The diagnosis can be confirmed by examining and culturing the pericardial membranes. Constrictive pericarditis is a late complication.

Abdominal tuberculosis occurs secondary to swallowing infected material, including contaminated milk or sputum. This is a relatively uncommon complication in developed nations where dairy herds are inspected for tuberculosis. Manifestations include dysphagia, pain, or signs of obstruction, perforation, hemorrhage, fistula formation, or colitis. Tuberculous peritonitis presents as fever, anorexia, and abdominal pain. Diagnosis depends on skin test results and on histology and culture of involved tissue and peritoneal fluid.

Urogenital tuberculosis is a late reactivation complication and is rare in children. Symptomatic illness presents as dysuria, frequency, urgency, hematuria, and "sterile" pyuria.

Tuberculosis of bone occurs following dissemination or erosion from adjacent caseating lymph nodes. The spine (Pott disease) is the most common site, followed by the hip and the fingers and toes (dactylitis). Roentgenograms demonstrate cortical destruction.

Diagnosis. The *skin test* response to tuberculin antigen is a manifestation of a T cell–mediated delayed hypersensitivity. It is usually positive 2–6 wk after onset of infection (occasionally 3 mo) and at the time of symptomatic illness. Multiple puncture tests (such as the tine test) are no longer recommended for screening high-risk populations. The Mantoux test, an intradermal injection, usually on the volar surface of the forearm, of 5 TU (units) (intermediate test strength) of Tween-stabilized purified tuberculous antigen (purified protein derivative, standard [PPD-S]) is the standard for screening high-risk populations and for diagnosis in all ill patients or contacts. A 10-mm induration reaction after 48 hr traditionally indicated infection, but erythemia has no significance; 5- to 10-mm induration indicates infection in high-risk populations (urban, contacts, HIV) but occasionally may be due to atypical mycobacteria or prior bacille Calmette-Guérin (BCG) vaccine vaccination. In northern states, where atypical bacilli are not endemic, 5–9 mm may be more significant. BCG immunization alone rarely can produce induration to PPD-S greater than 10 mm. A 15 mm induration may be positive for low risk patients. False-negative responses may occur early in the illness, with use of inactivated antigen (as a result of poor storage practice or inadequate administration), or as a result of immunosuppression (secondary to underlying illness, AIDS, malnutrition, or overwhelming tuberculosis). Tests with questionable results should be repeated after several weeks of therapy and adequate nutrition. An antigen panel should be included with the PPD-S to determine a more global state of anergy.

Although *histologic* demonstration of caseous granulomas is not a diagnostic finding, identifying the bacilli in tissue or secretions by acid-fast staining or nonspecific absorption of fluorescent dyes (fluorochrome stain) suggests the diagnosis.

The ultimate diagnostic confirmation relies on *culture* of the organism, a process that usually is more successful when tissue is utilized (e.g., pleural biopsy, pericardial membrane), rather than only the pleural or pericardial fluid. In young infants, gastric material (often mixed with swallowed sputum) may yield positive results when sputum is unobtainable. Large volumes of fluid (CSF, pericardial fluid) will yield a higher rate of recovery of organisms, but slow growth of the mycobacteria (3–6 wk) makes culture less helpful in very ill children. Rapid culture methods (^{14}C media) facilitate diagnosis and drug susceptibility testing. Once the organism is grown, the drug susceptibilities should be determined because of the increasing incidence of resistant organisms. Antigen detection and DNA probes have expedited diagnosis, especially in CNS disease.

Treatment. Hospitalization is not uniformly mandated but is necessary in several situations when the child needs specialized, continuous, or closely supervised care:

1. Therapy for severe or life-threatening disease
2. Initial evaluation and therapy of a young child (3 yr of age or less)
3. For acquisition of culture or biopsy by invasive techniques
4. Use of corticosteroid therapy or surgical intervention
5. Treatment of severe drug reaction
6. Treatment of severe coexisting disease
7. Initial evaluation and therapy when family or social disorganization would interfere with ambulatory management

Antituberculosis Drugs. In general, because of the emergence of drug resistance in vivo, most manifestations of tuberculosis, except those associated with the lowest level of replicating organisms (asymptomatic skin test conversions), are treated with at least two drugs to which the organisms are susceptible (Table 10–15). In life-threatening disease, such as meningitis or miliary tuberculosis, in patients with large numbers of organisms (cavitary lesions), or in regions where the incidence of primary drug resistance is high, four agents are initially utilized. Multiple drug therapy may shorten the duration of treatment and prevent emergence of drug resistance.

Isoniazid (INH) is the drug of choice for tuberculosis and is used in all regimens unless the organism is resistant. It is bactericidal, well absorbed orally, and appears in all body fluids, including CSF. The major side effects are hepatotoxicity (uncommon in children) and neuritis secondary to pyridoxine deficiency, which is rare in children but can be prevented in adolescents and adults by simultaneously administering pyridoxine. Mild elevations of serum glutamic oxaloacetic transaminase are common and are not a contraindication for continuing INH. However, if hyperbilirubinemia, he-

patomegaly, systemic "flu-like" illness, or a greater than 3-fold elevation of serum glutamic pyruvic transaminase occurs, INH should be discontinued.

Rifampin is the other drug of choice for tuberculosis therapy. It is also bactericidal (inhibits bacterial RNA polymerase), well absorbed orally, distributed into all body fluids, and accumulates in infected monocytes. Side effects include orange discoloration of body secretions (with permanent discoloration of soft contact lenses). The major side effect is hepatotoxicity, the risk of which is increased by simultaneously administering INH. Reducing the dosage decreases the risk. Thrombocytopenia, leukopenia, and an influenza-like syndrome are uncommon side effects. Rifampin interferes with metabolism of several drugs (see Appendix I). It is teratogenic in laboratory animals and contraindicated in the first trimester of pregnancy.

Ethambutol is a bacteriostatic oral agent that achieves low concentrations in CSF. It is highly active against tuberculosis. Its main limitation is ocular toxicity (blurred vision, color blindness, visual field constriction due to optic neuritis), which is

Table 10–15. Therapy for Children with Tuberculosis

Manifestation	Agent(s)*	Duration
Positive skin test	INH	9 mo†
Pulmonary (including hilar adenopathy)	*6-month regimen* INH, Rif, PZA (daily)‡	2 mo
	INH + Rif	4 mo
	or	
	INH, Rif, PZA (daily)	4 mo
	INH + Rif twice weekly	2 mo
	9-mo regimen INH + Rif (daily)	
	or	
	INH + Rif (daily)	1 mo
	INH + Rif twice weekly	8 mo
Extrapulmonary, disseminated (including meningitis)	INH, Rif, PZA, Sm	2 mo
	INH + Rif	10 mo§

* INH = isoniazid; PZA = pyrazinamide; Rif = rifampin; Sm = streptomycin.

† At least 6 consecutive mo of therapy should be given with good compliance. If daily therapy is not possible, twice-weekly therapy may be used for 9 mo.

‡ If possible drug resistance is a concern, a fourth drug should be added (ethambutol or streptomycin) until drug susceptibility has been determined.

§ Streptomycin is included in the initial regimen until susceptibility tests are available.

reversible. Because these toxicities are impossible to monitor in a young (< 6 yr) child, the use of ethambutol is precluded below this age unless drug resistance or severe disease is present.

Streptomycin is bactericidal, administered intramuscularly, and moderately ototoxic and nephrotoxic. It is utilized only in serious illness for a short period of time (up to 12 wk).

Pyrazinamide is a bactericidal oral agent distributed into CSF and an important drug used in multidrug short-course regimens. Side effects include hyperuricemia and polyarthralgias.

Ethionamide is a bacteriostatic oral agent utilized occasionally in therapy of drug-resistant organisms.

Corticosteroids are useful in the initial therapy of tuberculous meningitis to lower increased intracranial pressure, and in endobronchial tuberculosis and tuberculous pleuritis or pericarditis to speed the resolution of fluid and obstruction. Steroids should never be utilized in a patient with tuberculosis without concomitant antituberculosis therapy.

Prevention. Tuberculosis is prevented by (1) preventing contact with an actively infected person, (2) providing chemoprophylaxis with INH (see earlier), or (3) vaccinating using BCG vaccine. The use of BCG vaccine, a live attenuated mycobacterial vaccine, remains controversial, and studies of its efficacy are variable. It is advocated for use in:

1. Individuals with a negative skin test (especially infants) residing in a household with repeated exposure to untreated or ineffectively treated patients with positive sputum or exposure to INH- and rifampin-resistant organisms.
2. Groups at unusually high risk of new infections (>1%/ yr) in which routine chemoprophylactic and surveillance measures have failed (groups without regular health care or those exposed to resistant organisms).
3. As a public health measure in developing countries where skin test conversion rates exceed 1% annually.

It should not be used in patients with altered immunity. It also renders the skin test less useful, because it converts findings in the test to false positive. Nevertheless, in a recipient of BCG, over 10 mm of induration in response to a skin test performed 3 or more yr after BCG administration is probably an indication of active tuberculosis and not a response to BCG vaccine.

Tuberculosis during Pregnancy. Pregnancy does not interfere with a positive skin test, and the test is indicated in all pregnant women. Chest roentgenograms should be deferred in the asymptomatic woman until the end of the first trimester. Asymptomatic women with a positive skin test but normal chest roentgenograms should not receive INH until delivery because of the risk of hepatotoxicity. Women with active disease should receive INH, rifampin, ethambutol, and pyridoxine.

Infants Born to Mothers with Tuberculosis. Approximately one half of the infants born to mothers with active disease will develop tuberculosis in the 1st yr of life. If suspected of having congenital tuberculosis, the infant should be treated promptly with INH, pyrazinamide, streptomycin, plus rifampin. The skin test may not be positive for 6 mo. If the mother is asymptomatic (PPD positive) and no active disease is present in the family, the infant is tested (5 TU PPD) at 4–6 wk and 3–4 mo of age. If the family cannot be evaluated, INH (10 mg/kg/ 24 hr) may be started. If the mother has newly diagnosed but noncontagious disease at delivery, the asymptomatic infant should have a chest roentgenogram and 5 TU PPD (Mantoux) test at 4–6 wk, 3–4 mo, and 6 mo of age. INH is begun at birth and discontinued at 3–4 mo if the PPD is negative and there is no active disease in the family. With poor compliance, maternal positive sputum (culture or stain), and supervision unsure, BCG vaccination is indicated in the asymptomatic, PPD-negative infant. The latter measure may not prevent disease acquisition but may reduce severity and dissemination. If the mother is contagious, the mother and child are separated until she is noncontagious.

References

Bass JB Jr, Farer LS, Hopewell PC, et al: Diagnostic standards and classification of tuberculosis. Am Rev Respir Dis 142:725, 1990.

Behrman RE (ed): Nelson Textbook of Pediatrics. 14th ed. Philadelphia, WB Saunders, 1992, Sec. 12.47.

CDCP: Initial therapy for tuberculosis in the era of multidrug resistance. MMWR 42:(RR1)1, 1993.

Hussey G, Chisholm T, Kibel M: Miliary tuberculosis in children: A review of 94 cases. Pediatr Infect Dis J 10: 832, 1991.

Starke JR, Jacobs RF, Jereb J: Resurgence of tuberculosis in children. J Pediatr 120:839, 1992.

Waecker NJ Jr, Connor JD: Central nervous system tuberculosis in children: A review of 30 cases. Pediatr Infect Dis J 9:539, 1990.

NONTUBERCULOUS MYCOBACTERIAL INFECTION

Etiology. The staining and morphologic characteristics of nontuberculous *Mycobacterium* species (termed atypical mycobacteria) are similar to those of *M. tuberculosis*, but they differ in a variety of other characteristics, such as growth patterns and pigment production. The five species commonly associated with human disease include members of the Runyon Group I, the photochromogens, which form pigment on exposure to light (*M. kansasii, M. marinum*); Group II, the scotochromogens, which form pigment in the dark (*M. scrofulaceum*); Group III, the nonchromogens, which fail to produce pigment (*M. avium-intracellulare* complex); and Group IV, the rapid growers (*M. fortuitum-chelonei*). There are numerous other mycobacteria, but they rarely are associated with human disease.

Epidemiology. These agents are distributed worldwide and exist in soil, vegetation, dust, and water. They are pathogens in various animals. Infection occurs by inoculation of the skin or by inhalation. Atypical mycobacterial infections in immunocompetent patients are more common in warm, humid, rural environments, such as the southern states. No evidence exists for person-to-person spread. Nosocomial infection with *M. chelonei* and *M. fortuitum* have occurred, and opportunistic infection with *M. avium-intracellulare* organisms affects patients with advanced AIDS.

Clinical Manifestations. *Lymphadenitis* is the most frequent manifestation of infection in children, and is usually a unilateral cervical, submandibular, or preauricular (less commonly axillary and inguinal) swelling in a 1–5 yr old child with a normal chest roentgenogram and no history of exposure to tuberculosis. The node may suppurate and drain but usually is hard and painless. In the United States, lymphadenitis most often is due to *M. avium-intracellulare, M. scrofulaceum,* or, rarely, *M. kansasii*. Differential diagnosis should rule out infection due to *M. tuberculosis,* fungi, or bacteria as well as cat-scratch disease, toxoplasmosis, sarcoidosis, lymphoma, and drug reaction. The ratio of atypical mycobacterial infection to *M. tuberculosis* infection occurring in children under the age of 12 yr is 9:1. Diagnosis and therapy both are made by performing excisional biopsy; most species are resistant to antimicrobial drugs.

Cutaneous disease is usually the result of inoculation with *M. marinum* (swimming pool granuloma or fish tank granuloma) or with *M. fortuitum-chelonei*. The initial papule or nodule may enlarge and ulcerate. Infection in healthy children often is self-limited. *M. marinum* is treated for 3–4 mo with doxycycline, rifampin, and ethambutol, or trimethoprim–sulfamethoxazole. *M. fortuitum-chelonei* infection usually develops secondary to abrasions, puncture wounds, or foreign body placement during surgery and requires débridement, drainage, and often antibiotic therapy (amikacin, cefoxitin, erythromycin).

Pulmonary infection with these bacterial agents is uncommon in children and resembles tuberculosis. It may occur rarely with *M. kansasii* in adolescent patients, and treatment includes administration of rifampin, ethambutol, and INH.

Disseminated disease with bacteremia, pneumonia, diarrhea, and fever usually occurs in immunocompromised individuals and often is due to the *M. avium-intracellulare* complex, especially in patients with AIDS. Therapy includes the combinations of 3–4 drugs such as amikacin, ciprofloxacin, ansamycin, clofazamine, ethambutol, INH, rifampin, rifabutin, azithromycin or clarithromycin. Suppression of infection and symptoms is possible but bacteriologic cure is unusual.

Diagnosis. The diagnosis depends on staining and culture of secretions or tissue. The skin test reaction to PPD often is intermediately positive (5–10 mm of induration in the Mantoux test). Selective skin tests with specific nontuberculous antigens currently are being evaluated.

References

Behrman RE (ed): Nelson Textbook of Pediatrics. 14th ed. Philadelphia, WB Saunders, 1992, Sec. 12.48.

Huebner RE, Schein MF, Cauthen GM, et al: Usefulness of skin testing with mycobacterial antigens in children with cervical lymphadenopathy. Pediatr Infect Dis J 11:450, 1992.

Wolinsky E: Mycobacterial diseases other than tuberculosis. Clin Infect Dis 15:1, 1992.

Infections Caused by Neisseriae

Neisseriae are gram-negative, spherical or oval diplococci. The bacteria are observed within polymorphonuclear leukocytes obtained from diseased areas of the body. Neisseriae are aerobic and can be cultured on blood agar, but recovery is enhanced by use of appropriate media. Neisseriae normally are found in the nasal mucosa, pharynx, vagina, and lower intestinal tract. Human disease most commonly is due to infection with *N. meningitidis* and *N. gonorrhoeae* (see Chapter 7).

MENINGOCOCCAL INFECTIONS

Etiology. *N. meningitidis* colonizes the nasopharynx but may invade epithelial cells by receptor-mediated endocytosis and produce bacteremia.

Meningococcemia occurs when *N. meningitidis* (meningococcus) invades the blood stream and disseminates to other locations. Nine serogroups of *N. meningitidis* have been identified (A, B, C, D, X, Y, Z, 29E, and W135) on the basis of specific capsular polysaccharides. Groups B (45%), C (32%), Y (18%), and W135 are the common serogroups in the United States. Group B is noted in sporadic cases and groups A and C occur in epidemic cases. Each serogroup contains endotoxin.

Epidemiology. The rates of asymptomatic carriers of *N. meningitidis* vary from 2–5% in healthy children to as high as 90% in military personnel during epidemics. Meningococcal meningitis is a disease of young children who acquire *N. meningitidis* from an adult carrier, usually in the same family. Person-to-person transmission is through infected respiratory droplets. Age-specific attack rates are greatest for infants under 1 yr of age; 80% of cases of meningococcal disease occur in children under 10 yr of age. A second peak appears during adolescence. The estimated likelihood of meningococcal disease in family contacts, usually occurring within 1 wk of the first case (incubation period is 3–4 days), is 1%. This is 1000-fold greater than the risk in the community. Persons with deficiency of terminal complement component (C5–9) and IgG2 subclass are at high risk for recurrent disease. Properdin-deficient males may develop fatal meningococcemia. Meningococcal disease often follows viral upper respiratory tract infections.

Clinical Manifestations. Invasive meningococcal infections usually result in septicemic meningococcemia and/or meningitis. Acute meningococcemia initially occurs as an influenza-like illness but becomes fulminant within hours to days, accompanied by the occurrence of morbilliform, petechial, or purpuric lesions and hypotension; DIC; oliguria; renal failure; and coma. Acute meningococcemia may be associated with varying systemic severity. In meningitis, the signs and symptoms of meningeal irritation are similar to those of acute meningitis produced by *H. influenzae* and *S. pneumoniae*. Meningococcemia may be associated with acute endocarditis, myocarditis, pericarditis, and arthritis. Other, less common meningococcal diseases include pneumonia, endophthalmitis, vulvovaginitis, urethritis, pelvic inflammatory disease, adrenal hemorrhage (Waterhouse-Friderichsen syndrome), and chronic meningococcemia. The latter is characterized by intermittent fever, malaise, maculopapular rash, arthralgias, and arthritis.

Diagnosis and Differential Diagnosis. The diagnosis of meningococcal disease is established by stains and culture of blood, CSF, skin lesions, or other usually sterile sites. When meningitis is present, the laboratory characteristics of CSF reflect an acute bacterial meningitis. A poor prognostic sign is a normal CSF profile with no leukocytes but with sheets of gram-negative diplococci. Alternately, the Gram stain and culture may be negative if the patient was pretreated with antibiotics. Blood, cerebrospinal fluid, and urine can be tested by CIE or by latex agglutination, a technique that can allow the detection of capsular antigen from most *N. meningitidis* types.

The petechial or purpuric rash of meningococcemia is similar to that of diseases characterized by generalized vasculitis, including septicemia caused by gram-negative and gram-positive organisms; bacterial endocarditis; gonococcemia; Henoch-Schönlein purpura; Rocky Mountain spotted fever; endemic typhus; atypical measles; and infection with echoviruses, particularly types 6, 9, and 16, and coxsackieviruses, predominantly types A2, A4, A9, and A16. The morbilliform rash occasionally observed may be confused with any macular or maculopapular viral exanthem (Table 10–2).

Treatment. Intravenous penicillin is the drug of choice for patients with invasive disease. Ceftriaxone, cefotaxime, and chloramphenicol are alternative antibiotics (see Appendix I). Antibiotic treatment is given for a minimum of 7 days. Supportive measures include careful monitoring and treatment of shock, myocarditis, pericarditis, septic arthritis, ARDS, DIC, and necrotic cutaneous and/or extremity lesions.

Prevention. Meningococcal vaccine against serogroups A, C, Y, and W135 is available but is not routinely recommended for children. Vaccine should be administered to children over 2 yr of age who have functional or anatomic asplenia and to those with terminal complement component or properdin deficiencies. Household, day care, nursery school, and closely exposed medical contacts should receive rifampin chemoprophylaxis as soon as possible following diagnosis of the primary case. The patient should be placed in respiratory isolation for 24 hr after admission and receive rifampin prior to discharge.

Prognosis. The mortality rate of acute meningococcemia with septic shock may be as high as 20–50%. The mortality rate for patients with isolated meningococcal meningitis is less than 3%, if treated early. Poor prognostic signs include the development of hypotension, coma, rapidly progressive purpura (within 12 hr), DIC, absence of meningitis, absence of leukocytosis, thrombocytopenia, high antigen concentrations in serum and CSF, and a low sedimentation rate. Survival for 48 hr following initiation of therapy is a good prognostic sign. Sloughing of necrotic skin over purpuric areas usually heals uneventfully.

References

Begg N: Reducing mortality from meningococcal disease: Give antibiotics before admission. BMJ 305:133, 1992.

Behrman RE (ed): Nelson Textbook of Pediatrics. 14th ed. Philadelphia, WB Saunders, 1992, Sec. 12.23.

Hubert B, Watier L, Garnerin P, et al: Meningococcal disease and influenza-like syndrome: A new approach to an old question. J Infect Dis 166:542, 1992.

Welsby PD, Golledge CL: Meningococcal meningitis: A diagnosis not to be missed. BMJ 300:1150, 1990.

Pertussis (Whooping Cough)

Etiology. Pertussis, which means "intense cough," is predominantly caused by *Bordetella pertussis*, but a pertussis-like illness has been associated with infection by *B. parapertussis*, *B. bronchiseptica*, and adenovirus. *B. pertussis* organisms are gram-negative, pleomorphic bacilli with fastidious requirements for growth provided by Bordet-Gengou media.

Epidemiology. Pertussis is highly contagious, producing attack rates of over 90% in susceptible populations. Humans are the only known host of *B. pertussis*; transmission is by droplets released during intense coughing. The incubation period has a mean of 6 days and a range of 6–14 days. Patients are most contagious during the preparoxysmal stage. Risk of disease is highest in children under 5 yr of age; 30% of cases in the United States occur in infants less than 6 mo of age. Mortality is greatest in infants under 1 yr of age. There is little seasonal variation. *B. pertussis* rarely is isolated from asymptomatic individuals.

In the United States, the incidence has decreased dramatically since the pertussis vaccine has been used. Immunization reduces the incidence and mortality rate of pertussis, but immunity is neither complete nor permanent. As immunity wanes among adults, older patients can develop pertussis. In adults, the syndrome often is atypical, becoming manifest as a severe protracted cough without a whoop. Adults may serve as a reservoir of infection for very young children. Intrafamily spread is common. The younger the child, the more atypical the signs and symptoms of the disease; infants less than 6 mo of age may have apnea, cyanotic spells, and cough but no whoop. Pertussis is increasing in frequency in areas where immunization has declined.

Clinical Manifestations. Symptomatic illness lasts 6–8 wk and generally is divided into three states: *catarrhal* (prodromal, preparoxysmal), *paroxysmal* (spasmodic cough), and *convalescent*. The clinical manifestations depend on the specific pathogen, the patient's age, and the host's immunization status. Illness caused by *B. parapertussis* or *B. bronchiseptica* is less severe and of shorter duration than that caused by *B. pertussis*, an organism that adheres to and causes necrosis of the respiratory epithelium from the nasopharynx to the terminal bronchioles, resulting in bronchitis, atelectasis, and bronchopneumonia. The perihilar infiltrates produce the "shaggy" heart border on chest roentgenograms characteristic of pertussis.

Catarrhal Stage (1–2 wk). Rhinorrhea (clear to mucoid), conjunctival injection, lacrimation, mild cough, wheezing, and low-grade fever are noted. Unfortunately, a diagnosis of pertussis usually is not considered during this stage, even though at this time the organisms are present in the greatest concentration, because the manifestations are similar to those of most nonspecific viral upper respiratory tract infections.

Paroxysmal Stage (2–4 wk or longer). Episodes of coughing increase in severity and frequency. Multiple, repetitive series of 5–10 forceful coughs during an expiration are followed by a sudden massive inspiration, producing the whoop, as air is forcefully inhaled against a narrowed glottis. The whoop may be absent in children less than 6 mo of age or in adults. Facial petechiae and redness, venous engorgement, and cyanosis may be prominent during the attack. Post-tussive vomiting is sufficient evidence that the child should be suspected of having pertussis. Recurrent episodes are exhausting; patients appear apathetic and lose weight. Attacks may be initiated by yawning, sneezing, eating, drinking, and physical exertion. Paroxysms may produce anoxic brain damage; alternately, pertussis may produce encephalopathy.

Convalescent Stage (1–2 wk). Paroxysmal coughing and vomiting decrease in frequency and severity. During this phase chronic cough may persist for several months. Rarely, paroxysmal cough recurs accompanied by subsequent upper respiratory tract infections in the ensuing months.

Diagnosis and Differential Diagnosis. Pertussis is recognized readily during the typical paroxysmal stage. A history of incomplete immunization and of contact with a known case is helpful. Leukocytosis (counts of 20,000–100,000 cells/µL) with an absolute lymphocytosis is characteristic at the end of the catarrhal stage and during the paroxysmal stage of the disease. Lymphocytosis may not be evident in partially immunized or very young infants. Chest roentgenograms may show perihilar infiltrates, atelectasis, or emphysema.

The diagnosis depends on isolation of *B. pertussis,* usually accomplished during the early phases of illness by culture of nasopharyngeal swabs on glycerin-potato-blood agar medium (Bordet-Gengou) to which penicillin has been added to inhibit growth of other organisms. *B. parapertussis* and *B. bronchiseptica,* both morphologically similar to *B. pertussis,* can be differentiated by specific agglutination reactions. Fluorescent antibody staining of pharyngeal specimens provides a rapid specific diagnosis.

Attacks of coughing may be observed in bronchiolitis, pneumonia (due to *Chlamydia,* bacteria, CMV), cystic fibrosis, tuberculosis, asthma, and intrathoracic lymphadenopathy compressing the trachea and bronchi. A foreign body produces similar coughing and can be distinguished by sudden onset of symptoms and by roentgenography and endoscopy.

Complications. The most frequent complication is pneumonia caused by *B. pertussis* itself or resulting from secondary bacterial infection (pneumococcus, *H. influenzae, S. aureus*). Atelectasis may be secondary to mucus plugs. Otitis media and sinusitis are common and usually are due to *S. pneumoniae.* The force of the paroxysm may rupture alveoli and produce pneumomediastinum, pneumothorax, or interstitial or subcutaneous emphysema. Bronchiectasis may develop. Increased intrathoracic pressure and venous engorgement may cause epistaxis, retinal and subconjunctival hemorrhages, intraventricular and subarachnoid hemorrhage, rupture of the diaphragm, and inguinal hernia. Tetanic seizures may be associated with alkalosis related to persistent vomiting. Convulsions and encephalopathy occur in 2.5% and 0.5% of infants, respectively.

Treatment. Erythromycin aborts or eliminates pertussis when administered in the catarrhal stage of the disease but does not affect the duration of the paroxysmal stage. Erythromycin eliminates organisms from the nasopharynx within 3–4 days, thereby shortening the period of communicability (see Appendix I). Corticosteroids and salbutamol aerosols may be helpful in severe cases. Supportive care includes warm mist oxygen, nasopharyngeal suctioning, and parenteral fluids.

Prevention. Transplacental immunity to pertussis does not prevent disease. Active immunity induced by vaccine has an efficacy of 70–90%; the efficacy declines with fewer vaccinations. The risk of seizures (1:1750), encephalopathy (1:110,000), or permanent neurologic deficits (1:310,000) following pertussis immunization in the United States is lower than the risks from pertussis. Some of the reactions may be due to the method of vaccine preparation, which in the past has been from the "whole cell" of the bacterium. An acellular pertussis vaccine is now licensed for use (combined with tetanus and diphtheria toxoids [DPT]) at 15 mo and at 4–6 yr of age.

Prematurity is not believed to increase the risk of seizures following pertussis immunization. Erythromycin is effective in preventing disease in newborn infants and adults exposed to pertussis. Close contacts less than 7 yr of age who have received four doses of vaccine should receive a booster dose of DTP, unless a booster dose has been given within the preceding 3 yr. They also should be given erythromycin. Close contacts older than 7 yr of age should receive prophylactic erythromycin for 10–14 days but not the vaccine. For the primary immunization schedule and contraindications for DPT see Table 10–3. If pertussis exposure is probable, because of endemic or epidemic disease, the vaccine may be given at 2 wk of age. Patients who have pertussis do not require further pertussis vaccinations because the disease produces lifelong immunity.

Prognosis. The mortality rate is less than 1% but may reach 40% in infants under 5 mo of age. Most deaths are due to pneumonia or other pulmonary complications, asphyxia, or encephalopathy.

References

Behrman RE (ed): Nelson Textbook of Pediatrics. 14th ed. Philadelphia, WB Saunders, 1992, Sec. 12.26.

Blumberg D, Lewis K, Mink C, et al: Severe reactions associated with diphteria-tetanus-pertussis vaccine: Detailed study of children with seizures, hypotonic-hyporesponsive episodes, high fevers, and persistant crying. Pediatrics 91:1158, 1993.

Farizo KM, Cochi SL, Zell ER, et al: Epidemiological features of pertussis in the United States, 1980–1989. Clin Infect Dis 14:708, 1992.

Gan VN, Murphy TV: Pertussis in hospitalized children. Am J Dis Child 144:1130, 1990.

Hoppe JE and the Erythromycin Study Group: Comparison of erythromycin estolate and erythromycin ethylsuccinate for treatment of pertussis. Pediatr Infect Dis J 11: 189, 1992.

Infections Caused by *Streptococcus pneumoniae* (Pneumococcal Infections)

Streptococcus pneumoniae may colonize the upper respiratory tract but also can become an invasive pathogen.

Etiology. *S. pneumoniae* (formerly *Diplococcus pneumoniae*) is a gram-positive, encapsulated diplococcus. Eighty-three serotypes are identified by their type-specific capsular polysaccharide. The capsule impedes leukocytic phagocytosis and is an important virulence factor. Serotypes 6, 19, and 23 represent almost 50% of all isolates in children. These, plus types 1, 3, 4, 7, 9, 11, 14, 15, and 18, cause 80% of childhood pneumococcal infections. Carriage of a serotype does not induce local or systemic immunity sufficient to prevent later reacquisition of the same serotype. Colonization is greatest up to 2 yr of age and during the winter months.

Epidemiology. Males and blacks are more commonly affected than females and whites. Opsonophagocytosis depends on capsule-specific antibody and the reticuloendothelial system. Pneumococcal disease therefore has an increased frequency and severity in patients between 6 mo and 2 yr of age and patients with HIV, sickle cell disease, asplenia, Hodgkin disease, nephrotic syndrome, basal skull fractures through a sinus, deficiencies in humoral (B cell) immunity, and complement deficiencies. Transmission is through person-to-person contact by respiratory droplet.

Clinical Manifestations. *S. pneumoniae* is the most frequent bacterial cause of bacteremia, pneumonia, and otitis media; a common cause of sinusitis; and a common cause of meningitis in infants and children. The peak incidence of meningitis occurs among infants 3–5 mo of age, among children 6–12 mo of age who have otitis media, and among children 13–18 mo of age who are hospitalized for pneumonia. Pneumococcal meningitis is also a common cause of bacterial meningitis in older children and adults, and the pneumococcus is a common cause of bacterial pneumonia in all age groups, with or without the need for hospitalization. Local spread may cause empyema, pericarditis, mastoiditis, and epidural abscess. Bacteremia rarely is followed by meningitis, septic arthritis, osteomyelitis, and endocarditis. Pneumococcal bacteremia in young children having unexplained fever but no localizing signs or symptoms can occur without sequelae. Spontaneous pneumococcal peritonitis is common in patients with the nephrotic syndrome.

Diagnosis. The diagnosis is confirmed in older patients by performing a Gram stain and a culture of sputum and in all patients by recovering pneumococci from blood or CSF culture. Isolation of pneumococci from the nose or throat of patients with otitis media, sinusitis, pneumonia, septicemia, or meningitis is not proof of causation because the frequency of the carrier state is high. Latex agglutination of serum, CSF, and urine is very helpful in establishing the diagnosis of pneumococcal meningitis, pneumonia, and bacteremia. The total white blood cell count is elevated (20,000–30,000/μL), as is the ESR in serious pneumococcal disease. Paracentesis, Gram stain, and culture are required to differentiate pneumococcal from other pathogens (e.g., *E. coli*) in patients with peritonitis.

Treatment. Penicillin is the treatment of choice for pneumococcal disease. The dose and duration of treatment vary with the location of infection. Antimicrobial susceptibility (with an oxacillin disc) should be tested on all pneumococcal isolates from blood and CSF, because pneumococci that are relatively (MICs of 0.1–1 μg/mL) and absolutely resistant to penicillin have been isolated. If a pneumococcus is resistant to penicillin but susceptible to ceftriaxone or chloramphenicol, the latter drugs are the treatments of choice. High-level penicillin–resistant strains (MIC >1 μg/mL) often are resistant to multiple antibiotics and can be treated with intravenous vancomycin with or without rifampin. Erythromycin, cephalosporins, clindamycin, and chloramphenicol are good alternatives for penicillin-allergic patients (see Appendix I).

Prevention. A pneumococcal vaccine composed of purified capsular polysaccharide antigens of 23 pneumococcal serotypes has proved to be highly immunogenic and is associated with a low level of untoward reactions. However, responsiveness to pneumococcal polysaccharide vaccine is unpredictable in young children. This vaccine is recommended for children older than 2 yr of age with (1) asplenia, (2) nephrotic syndrome, (3) sickle cell disease, (4) other hemoglobinopathies, (5) HIV infection, (6) immunosuppression, and (7) about to undergo splenectomy for Hodgkin disease. Immunization does *not* prevent pneumococcal disease related to serotypes not found in the vaccine. Therefore, a history of immunization should not eliminate the need for antibiotics in high-risk situations, such as sickle cell anemia.

Administering gammaglobulin to children with hypogammaglobulinemia (IgG less than 200 mg/dL) will reduce the risk of pneumococcal bacteremia and meningitis but not necessarily pneumococcal respiratory infections. Oral penicillin (amoxicillin) should be given continuously to all infants with sickle cell anemia and to other patients who are anatomically or functionally asplenic to prevent sepsis.

References

Behrman RE (ed): Nelson Textbook of Pediatrics. 14th ed. Philadelphia, WB Saunders, 1992, Sec. 12.21.

Bruyn GAW, Zegers BJM, van Furth R: Mechanisms of host defense against infection with *Streptococcus pneumoniae*. Clin Infect Dis 14:251, 1992.

Chesney PJ: The escalating problem of antimicrobial resistance in *Streptococcus pneumoniae*. AJDC 146:912, 1992.

Friedland IR, Istre GR: Management of penicillin-resistant pneumococcal infections. Pediatr Infect Dis J 11:433, 1992.

Musher DM: Infections caused by *Streptococcus pneumoniae*: Clinical spectrum, pathogenesis, immunity, and treatment. Clin Infect Dis 14:801, 1992.

Infections Caused by Salmonellae

Salmonellae are important pathogens of animals and humans. Humans become infected by ingesting contaminated water or food, typically beef, poultry, milk, and eggs. Systemic infection with *Salmonella typhi* (typhoid fever) is uncommon in the United States but is endemic and epidemic in other parts of the world. Infections caused by other types of Salmonellae are common throughout the United States.

Etiology. Salmonellae are gram-negative, non-encapsulated bacilli. The principal antigens are the flagellum (H) antigens, the cell wall (O) antigens, and the envelope (Vi) heat-labile antigens. A typing scheme utilizing O and H antigens permits the differentiation of over 2200 salmonella serotypes. Salmonellae are classified into three groups: *S. enteritidis*, *S. typhi*, and *S. choleraesuis*. The first species contains all Salmonella serotypes except the latter two species, which have only one serotype. *S. typhimurium* (group B) is the most common type of salmonella isolated from people in the United States and belongs to *S. enteritides* (group D). An alternate classification includes 5 groups (A–E) based on somatic antigens.

SALMONELLOSIS (NONTYPHOIDAL)

Epidemiology.   More than two thirds of cases are in persons under 20 yr of age, with the higher attack rates among young infants (2–6 mo old) and males. Salmonella can infect many species of animals, but those particularly hazardous to human health are meat-producing animals, poultry (infection of tissues and eggs), and pets (dogs, cats, turtles). Animal infections usually are asymptomatic. Humans are important carriers of salmonella species and can cause localized epidemics of food poisoning by fecal–oral contamination of food at large gatherings, such as picnics. Intrafamilial transmission of salmonellosis is frequent. Contaminated human breast milk, marijuana, and carmine red dye have caused disease.

A large inoculum is needed because gastric acidity kills salmonella. Organisms subsequently bind to specific small bowel receptors as they invade the epithelial cell. The organism may survive and replicate in monocytes following phagocytosis. Dissemination, particularly with *S. choleraesuis* and in immunoincompetent patients, produces bacteremia and metastatic complications.

Seventy to 90% of individuals have a positive stool culture 2 wk following infection, about 50% at 4 wk, and 10–25% at 10 wk. The duration of salmonella excretion is longer in infants. Asymptomatic excretion is prolonged by antibiotic therapy. The incubation period for gastroenteritis is from 6 to 72 hr but usually is less than 24 hr.

Clinical Manifestations.   Salmonella gastroenteritis has a peak incidence in the late summer and early fall, correlating with food-borne outbreaks. Epidemics and disease found in small family clusters occur throughout the year. Onset is abrupt and is characterized by nausea, vomiting, and crampy abdominal pain followed by loose, watery stools that may contain mucus, leukocytes, and blood. Systemic signs of malaise, headache, and chills occasionally are noted. Fever of 38.3–38.9°C (101–102°F) is noted in 70% of patients and lasts for 48 hr. Symptoms subside within 2–5 days in healthy individuals. In patients who are compromised because of extremes of age, sickle cell disease, chronic granulomatous disease, AIDS, malignancy, antibiotic therapy, or corticosteroids, the illness may persist and become manifest as bacteremia with metastatic foci (meningitis, osteomyelitis). Septicemia accompanied by toxic appearance and high fever is much more common in the first 3 mo of life. Bacteremia in young infants and older children may clear spontaneously. Nonetheless, salmonella can localize and cause pneumonia, empyema, abscesses, osteomyelitis, septic arthritis, pyelonephritis, and meningitis. *S. choleraesuis* is one species that produces a greater incidence of septicemia and a higher mortality rate than those noted with other salmonella species. *S. choleraesuis* may cause bacteremia, with or without diarrhea.

Complications. Enteritis may produce significant dehydration, electrolyte disturbances, and hypovolemic shock. Other complications of nontyphoidal salmonellosis are unusual and are limited to the extraintestinal lesions noted above. In addition, children may develop reactive polyarticular arthritis about 2 wk after the diarrheal episode. There is a strong association with the presence of histocompatibility antigen human leukocyte antigen B27 and the reactive arthritis syndrome following salmonella infection. Full-blown Reiter disease (conjunctivitis, urethritis, and polyarthritis) also may be noted. The joint fluid is sterile.

Diagnosis. Culture of stool is indicated when there is fever and the presence of blood, mucus, or leukocytes in the stool. Blood should be cultured in young infants and immunocompromised patients. Cultures of stool, blood, urine, bone marrow aspirate, CSF, and foci of infection should be obtained in more complicated cases. Although three consecutive negative stool cultures suggest that infection has ceased, excretion may be intermittent. Salmonella gastroenteritis must be distinguished from other viral and bacterial causes of diarrhea (see Chapter 11). Rarely, the clinical course and roentgenographic findings suggest ulcerative colitis.

Treatment. Correction of shock, dehydration, and electrolyte imbalances are the most important aspects of the therapy of salmonella gastroenteritis. Uncomplicated enteritis in normal children usually is improving when stool culture results are known; these children require no antibiotics. Antibiotics are indicated for high-risk individuals because of the possibility of dissemination of disease (infants under 3 mo of age, children with immunologic deficiency, malnutrition, or malignancy).

Children with septicemia, enteric fever, or metastatic sites of infection initially should be treated with ceftriaxone or cefotaxime. Alternative antibiotics are determined on antimicrobial resistance patterns; useful agents for susceptible salmonella include amoxicillin, trimethoprim–sulfamethoxazole, chloramphenicol, or quinolones (for patients over 18 yr of age) (see Appendix I).

TYPHOID FEVER (ENTERIC FEVER)

Epidemiology. In the United States, 300–500 cases of typhoid fever occur each year. The majority of reported cases occur in persons under 20 yr of age and are imported from other countries (India, Mexico). The typhoid bacillus infects only humans, and chronic carriers therefore are responsible for new cases.

Pathogenesis. The upper small bowel is the predominant site of invasion. Monocytes phagocytize but do not kill the bacilli early in the disease, and carry the organisms from the blood to the mesenteric lymph nodes and other reticuloendothelial sites in which bacteria proliferate to produce inflammation in lymph nodes, liver, and spleen. Secondary septicemia is disseminated from these sites and usually is prolonged, seeding other organs. The gallbladder is particularly susceptible and is infected from the liver via the biliary system or from the blood. Micro-organisms that multiply in the gallbladder eventually are discharged into the intestine.

Clinical Manifestations. The pattern of typhoid fever in infants ranges from mild gastroenteritis to severe septicemia without diarrhea. Fever, hepatomegaly, jaundice, anorexia, lethargy, and weight loss can be marked.

In older children, the course is characterized by high fever, malaise, lethargy, myalgia, headache, rash, hepatosplenomegaly, and abdominal pain and tenderness. Diarrhea occurs in less than half of older children in the early stage, but constipation is noted in the later stages. The patient may become severely obtunded and exhibit delirium and confusion. At this stage of the disease, the spleen generally is enlarged and abdominal tenderness is present. A macular (rose spots) or maculopapular rash is observable on the skin of as many as 80% of patients. The paradoxic relationship of a high temperature and low pulse rate may be observed. Typically, for each degree rise above 38.3°C (101°F), the pulse should rise 10 bpm. Leukopenia is common.

Complications. Intestinal perforation at the site of inoculation, usually in the ileum, occurs in 0.5–3%, and severe gastrointestinal hemorrhage occurs in 1–10% of children with typhoid fever. Most complications occur during the second (dissemination) stage of disease and are preceded by a fall in temperature and blood pressure and a rise in pulse rate. Toxic encephalopathy, cerebral thrombosis, acute cerebellar ataxia, optic neuritis, aphasia, deafness, transverse myelitis, and acute cholecystitis may occur. Pneumonia is common during the second stage of illness but is caused by a superinfection. Pyelonephritis, endocarditis, meningitis, osteomyelitis, and septic arthritis are rare in the normal host. Septic arthritis and osteomyelitis are seen in individuals with hemoglobinopathies.

Diagnosis and Differential Diagnosis. Examination of stool reveals mononuclear leukocytes. Blood cultures are positive early in the disease, whereas urine and stool cultures become positive following the secondary septicemia. Bone marrow, lymph nodes, and reticuloendothelial tissues often contain organisms after the blood has been sterilized. In suspected cases with negative cultures, a culture of aspirated bone marrow or duodenal fluid (to evaluate possible biliary infection) may be helpful. A 4-fold rise in agglutinin titer in a nonimmunized individual usually is diagnostic.

During the initial stage of typhoid fever, the clinical diagnosis may be bronchitis, bronchopneumonia, gastroenteritis, or influenza. Subsequently, other infectious conditions caused by intracellular micro-organisms, may need to be considered. Concern about an acute abdomen may lead to unnecessary surgical intervention.

Treatment. Antibiotic resistance is common. Based on susceptibility, ceftriaxone, ampicillin, chloramphenicol, trimethoprim–sulfamethoxazole, and, in patients over 18 yr, ciprofloxacin are useful drugs (see Appendix I).

Corticosteroid therapy has been suggested for severe toxemia or prolonged symptoms. Third-generation cephalosporins may cure carriers, particularly drugs that are metabolized in the liver. Cholecystectomy may be indicated.

Prognosis. Antimicrobial therapy has reduced the mortality rate to less than 1% in most areas, but the presence of underlying debilitating disease, perforation of the gastrointestinal tract, severe hemorrhage, or coma increases the mortality rate. Meningitis or endocarditis may be associated with high morbidity and mortality rates. Relapse occurs in up to 10% of those who are not treated with antibiotics.

Individuals who excrete *S. typhi* for 3 or more mo are usually excreters at 1 yr and often for life. The risk of becoming a chronic carrier is low in children.

Prevention. Administering typhoid vaccine is indicated if a patient has had one of the following exposures: (1) intimate contact with a carrier, (2) an outbreak of typhoid fever in the community, and (3) travel to an endemic area. Typhoid vaccine can prevent disease that could be acquired via contaminated water. Typhoid carriers should be made aware of their potential contagiousness and of the importance of handwashing and personal hygiene in the prevention of transmission of the disease.

References

Behrman RE (ed): Nelson Textbook of Pediatrics. 14th ed. Philadelphia, WB Saunders, 1992, Sec. 12.28–12.29.
Baird-Parker AC: Foodborne salmonellosis. Lancet 336: 1231, 1990.
Butler T, Islam A, Kabir I, et al: Patterns of morbidity and mortality in typhoid fever dependent on age and gender: Review of 552 hospitalized patients with diarrhea. Rev Infect Dis 13:85, 1991.
St. Geme JW, Hodes HL, Marcy SM, et al: Consensus: Management of salmonella infection in the first year of life. Pediatr Infect Dis J 7:615, 1988.

Shigellosis (Bacillary Dysentery)
See also Chapter 11.

Etiology. Shigellae are non–lactose-fermenting, gram-negative bacilli. The genus *Shigella* is subdivided into four major groups (A, B, C, and D) on the basis of biochemical reactions and antigenic composition. Group A contains 10 serologic types, of which *S. dysenteriae* is the most important worldwide but is rarely encountered in the United States. *Shigella* group B contains six serologic groups, of which *S. flexneri* is commonly isolated in the United States; group C includes *S. boydii*; *S. sonnei* is the single serotype in group D and accounts for over half the *Shigella* isolates reported to the Centers for Disease Control.

Epidemiology. The highest incidence occurs in children under 2 yr of age. Humans are the major reservoir for *Shigella*. Animal reservoirs are not known; rarely, flies may be vectors. The organism is transmitted principally by the direct, person-to-person fecal–oral route, but outbreaks of waterborne and food-borne disease occur. Persons in close contact in unsanitary conditions are at high risk for outbreaks of shigellosis. Institutionalized children are at increased risk, as are children in day care centers, who transmit the disease to family members. Small numbers of bacteria are needed to produce infection. The incubation period varies from 1 to 7 days.

Clinical Manifestations. *Shigella* penetrates the epithelial cell, producing inflammation, edema, microabscess formation, and ulceration with bleeding. Toxin production contributes to but is not necessary for tissue invasion.

Mild *Shigella* infections result in watery diarrhea with minimal systemic symptoms. In severe cases, crampy abdominal pain, temperature greater than 40°C (104°F) lasting 1–3 days, and diarrhea containing blood and mucus can occur. The child may have nonlocalized lower abdominal tenderness. Shigellosis may mimic CNS diseases such as meningitis, particularly when high fever is associated with seizures. Seizures occur in 30% of children with *Shigella* gastroenteritis and are more common if the temperature exceeds 40°C (104°F).

Shigella infrequently may cause conjunctivitis and vaginitis from autoinoculation. Nonsuppurative arthritis and Reiter syndrome have been associated with *Shigella* infection. Hemolytic–uremic syndrome, possibly associated with toxin production, may coincide or follow enteritis caused by *S. dysenteriae* type 1.

Diagnosis.   Stool should reveal leukocytes and red blood cells. The complete blood count displays leukocytosis composed of immature forms. The diagnosis is established by isolating the organism from stool or rectal cultures. Shigellosis must be differentiated from other causes of dysentery, such as infection with invasive *E. coli*, amebae, *Campylobacter jejuni, Yersinia enterocolitica,* and salmonella, as well as from intussusception and acute appendicitis.

Treatment.   Antibiotic treatment decreases the duration of excretion of *Shigella* as well as the duration of diarrhea (see Chapter 11). Susceptibility patterns may vary among communities and among serotypes of *Shigella.* Trimethoprim–sulfamethoxazole is the drug of choice if susceptibility is unknown or if ampicillin resistance is present. Otherwise, ampicillin is the drug of choice for susceptible strains. Amoxicillin is less effective and should not be used (see Appendix I).

References

Behrman RE (ed): Nelson Textbook of Pediatrics. 14th ed. Philadelphia, WB Saunders, 1992, Sec. 12.30.

Bennish ML: Potentially lethal complications of shigellosis. Rev Infect Dis 13:S319, 1991.

Goren A, Freier S, Passwell JH: Lethal toxic encephalopathy due to childhood shigellosis in a developed country. Pediatrics 89:1189, 1992.

Lee LA, Shapiro CN, Hargrett-Bean N, et al: Hyperendemic shigellosis in the United States: A review of surveillance data for 1967–1988. J Infect Dis 164:894, 1991.

Staphylococcal Infections

Staphylococci are a common cause of pyogenic infections in infants and children. These organisms are gram-positive cocci that grow aerobically or as facultative anaerobes and appear in tetrads or grape-like clusters. Strains are classified as *S. aureus* (coagulase and mannitol positive), *S. epidermidis* species (coagulase and mannitol negative and novobiocin sensitive), and *S. saprophyticus* (coagulase negative, mannitol positive, novobiocin resistant).

INFECTIONS CAUSED BY *STAPHYLOCOCCUS AUREUS*

Etiology.   Disease may be the result of tissue inoculation or localization of bacteremia or result from a variety of bacterial toxins and enzymes. Strains of *S. aureus* can be classified by bacteriophage group typing. Exfoliative toxin, associated with phage group 2 and some non–group 2 staphylococci, is the cause of "scalded skin syndrome" (Ritter disease) and bullous impetigo. Staphylococcal enterotoxin (types A, B, C, D, E, and F) is elaborated by most strains of *S. aureus.* Ingestion of preformed enterotoxin A or D is associated with vomiting and diarrhea and, in some cases, with the development of profound hypotension. Staphylococcal enterotoxins B, C, and F as well as toxic shock syndrome toxin (TSST-1) have been associated with toxic shock syndrome (TSS).

Epidemiology.   *S. aureus* is part of normal human flora and is present in the anterior nares and moist areas of the body in about 30% of asymptomatic people. Transmission of *S. aureus* generally occurs via hands, nasal discharge, person-to-person contact, and, rarely, through air. Newborn infants are extremely susceptible to staphylococci; the nasopharynx, skin, and umbilical stump are the most common sites of colonization. Factors that increase the likelihood of infection include antibiotic therapy with a drug to which *S. aureus* is resistant, wounds, skin disease, intravenous drug abuse, intravenous or intrathecal catheterization, corticosteroid treatment, malnutrition, acidosis, and azotemia. The incubation period for bullous impetigo and scalded skin syndrome is 1–10 days; it is variable for other staphylococcal lesions.

Clinical Manifestations.   *S. aureus* causes a wide variety of suppurative lesions as well as septicemia and toxin-related diseases, including scalded skin syndrome, TSS, and food poisoning.

Skin.   Pyogenic skin infections may be primary or secondary to wounds or to a superinfection of other noninfectious skin disease (e.g., eczema) and include impetigo contagiosa, bullous impetigo, pustules, cellulitis, folliculitis, furuncles, and carbuncles. Toxin produces *staphylococcal scalded skin syndrome* (Ritter disease) and a rash resembling that in scarlet fever. In these conditions, staphylococci are not present in the lesions.

Respiratory Tract. Infections of the upper respiratory tract caused by *S. aureus* are rare, considering the rate of colonization of this area. Otitis media and sinusitis caused by *S. aureus* rarely may occur. Suppurative parotitis is a rare infection, but *S. aureus* is a common cause. *S. aureus* is a common cause of suppurative cervical adenitis. Tracheitis resembling viral croup but with high fever and toxicity may be caused by *S. aureus.* Pneumonia caused by *S. aureus* is noted in children under 1 yr of age and is associated with pneumatoceles, empyema, and sepsis.

Sepsis. Staphylococcal bacteremia and sepsis may be primary infections without an initiating focus or localized lesion. Later, organisms may localize in the lungs, heart valves, joints, bones, kidneys, and brain.

Muscle. Localized staphylococcal abscesses in muscle associated with elevation of muscle enzymes have been called *tropical pyomyositis.* Multiple abscesses occur in 30–40% of cases. Surgical drainage and appropriate antibiotic therapy are essential.

Bones and Joints. *S. aureus* is the most common cause of osteomyelitis and septic arthritis in children. These diseases are derived from hematogenous dissemination rather than direct extension of infection from an adjacent skin or soft tissue lesion.

Central Nervous System. Meningitis caused by *S. aureus* is rare but may follow bacteremia or may originate from direct extension of otitis media or osteomyelitis of the skull or vertebrae. Trauma or infection of meningomyelocele also may predispose the patient to *S. aureus* meningitis. Staphylococcal infection following neurosurgical procedures generally is due to *S. epidermidis. S. aureus* can be recovered from brain abscesses following CNS trauma and spinal epidural abscess.

Heart. Acute bacterial endocarditis in children may follow staphylococcal bacteremia and occur in the absence of valvular heart disease. Perforation of heart valves, myocardial abscesses, heart block, acute hemopericardium, purulent pericarditis, and sudden death may ensue.

Kidney. *S. aureus* is a common cause of renal and perinephric abscess. Uncomplicated urinary tract infection caused by *S. aureus* is unusual.

Intestinal Tract. Food poisoning may be caused by ingestion of preformed staphylococcal enterotoxins that contaminate foods. The short (1–7 hr) incubation period, lack of fever, short illness, and profuse emesis help differentiate it from other causes of food poisoning. Enterotoxins A and D are the most common causes in the United States.

Diagnosis. The diagnosis of staphylococcal infection follows the isolation of the organisms from skin lesions, abscess cavities, blood, CSF, or other usually sterile sites. Gram stains reveal gram-positive cocci in clusters. Following isolation, identification is made on the basis of Gram stain and coagulase and mannitol reactivity. Patterns of susceptibility to antibiotics should be assessed to guide therapy. Diagnosis of staphylococcal food poisoning is made on the basis of epidemiologic (e.g., unrefrigerated meats, mayonnaise, or creamed foods) and clinical findings. Food suspected of contamination should be examined by Gram stain culture and tested for enterotoxin.

Treatment. Loculated collections of purulent material must be incised and drained. Foreign bodies associated with infection may need to be removed. More than 90% of all staphylococci are resistant to penicillin; therefore, therapy should include a penicillinase-resistant antibiotic, such as methicillin, oxacillin, and nafcillin, or first-generation cephalosporins (cephalothin and cefazolin) and clindamycin. Vancomycin may be used to treat methicillin-resistant *S. aureus* or *S. epidermidis* (see Appendix I). Strains that hyper-produce beta-lactamase may be treated with amoxicillin/clavulanate, ticarcillin/clavulanate, ampicillin/sulbactam, imipenem, first-generation cephalosporins, fluoroquinolones, or vancomycin.

Prevention. Staphylococcal infection is transmitted by hand-to-hand contact. Observance of strict handwashing techniques is the most effective measure for preventing the spread of staphylococci. Local antibiotic ointment, antiseptic dyes, rifampin, or ciprofloxacin may be useful in reducing the carrier state.

Prognosis. Mortality rates have been reduced to 20% by appropriate antibiotic treatment. Staphylococcal pneumonia can be fatal and is more likely to produce morbidity and mortality in young infants. A total white blood cell count below 5000 cells/µL or a polymorphonuclear leukocyte response of less than 50% is a grave prognostic sign. Endocarditis may require prolonged treatment and eventual valve replacement.

References

Behrman RE (ed): Nelson Textbook of Pediatrics. 14th ed. Philadelphia, WB Saunders, 1992, Sec. 12.19.
Espersen F, Frimodt-Moller N, Rosdahl VT, et al: *Staphylococcus aureus* bacteraemia in children below the age of one year. Acta Paediatr Scand 78:56, 1989.
Hodes DS, Barzilai A: Invasive and toxin-mediated *Staphylococcus aureus* diseases in children. Adv Pediatr Infect Dis 5:35, 1990.
Marrack P, Kappler J: The staphylococcal enterotoxins and their relatives. Science 248:705, 1990.

TOXIC SHOCK SYNDROME

Toxic shock syndrome is an acute, multisystem disease characterized by high fever, hypotension, an erythematous rash, and other less specific manifestations.

Etiology and Epidemiology. Most cases occur in menstruating women using tampons in the presence of vaginal colonization and/or infection with toxin-producing *S. aureus*. Cases in children are associated with nasal packing, wounds, abscesses, infected insulin pump sites, staphylococcal tracheitis, and pneumonia. There is a high recurrence rate (30%) in menstruation-related cases. Secondary cases are milder and may occur with each menstrual cycle. The overall mortality rate is 3%.

A majority of responsible *S. aureus* strains are phage type 29/52, are noninvasive, and do not adhere to vaginal epithelial cells, but produce a number of extracellular toxins. TSST-1 is the responsible toxin in over 90% of menstrual associated cases. This toxin acts as a "superantigen" which can activate a large subset of T-cells.

Clinical Manifestations. The onset is abrupt, with high fever, vomiting, diarrhea, and myalgias, with or without sore throat, headache, and malaise. A diffuse erythematous sunburn-like macular rash appears within 24 hr and is associated with hyperemia of pharyngeal, conjunctival, and vaginal mucous membranes. Symptoms often include alterations in the level of consciousness, oliguria, and hypotension, which may progress to shock or may be postural in mild cases. Coagulopathy, hypocalcemia, hypoalbumenemia, leukocytosis, and elevated blood urea nitrogen, creatinine, and serum glutamic oxaloacetic transaminase, or CPK may be present. Recovery occurs within 7–10 days and is accompanied by desquamation of the palms and soles; hair and nail loss may be observed.

Differential Diagnosis. Kawasaki disease resembles TSS but many features of TSS are absent or rare in Kawasaki disease, including diffuse myalgia, vomiting, abdominal pain, diarrhea, azotemia, hypotension, ARDS, and shock. In addition, Kawasaki disease occurs in children under 5 yr of age who often have aneurysms of the coronary artery or other arteries. Scarlet fever, Rocky Mountain spotted fever, leptospirosis, toxic epidermal necrolysis, drug rash, and measles should be considered.

Treatment and Prevention. Fluid replacement should be aggressive to prevent or treat hypotension. Eradication of the source of toxin producing *S. aureus* (e.g., tampon, nasal packing, abscess) is necessary. Parenteral administration of a beta-lactamase–resistant antistaphylococcal antibiotic such as nafcillin, oxacillin, or methicillin is indicated in all cases for treatment and prevention of recurrences. The risk of acquiring TSS can be reduced by not using tampons or by using them intermittently during each menstrual period.

References

Behrman RE (ed): Nelson Textbook of Pediatrics. 14th ed. Philadelphia, WB Saunders, 1992, Sec. 12.20.
Resnick SD: Toxic shock syndrome: Recent developments in pathogenesis. J Pediatr 116:321, 1990.
Williams GR: The toxic shock syndrome: Many cases are not associated with menstruation. BMJ 300:960, 1990.

INFECTIONS CAUSED BY COAGULASE-NEGATIVE STAPHYLOCOCCI

Etiology. Coagulase-negative staphylococci (CONS) are common, usually nonpathogenic skin flora that, because of the use of indwelling catheters, are important causes of nosocomial infection. Infectivity is enhanced by their ability to adhere to plastic and their antimicrobial resistance.

Epidemiology. CONS readily colonize indwelling vascular catheters. CONS also cause infections in preterm neonates (with or without catheters) and in immunocompromised patients with intravascular central lines. CONS produce an extracellular polysaccharide slime that facilitates their attachment to foreign bodies.

Clinical Manifestations. In premature neonates infection caused by CONS presents as nosocomial sepsis (see Chapter 6). In older children bacteremia may be accompanied by intermittent fever; patients generally have few other signs of systemic infection. Persistent bacteremia may represent an infected thrombus or endocarditis in patients with prosthetic valves or Dacron grafts. Such infections often are more indolent than those caused by *S. aureus*, and may be difficult to diagnose. Often single positive blood cultures with *S. epidermidis* species are considered contaminants, when they may, in fact, represent a significant infection. CONS are common causes of infection in CNS ventriculoperitoneal shunts.

Staphylococcus saprophyticus is a cause of urinary tract infection, particularly in adolescent girls. Urine cultures that grow gram-positive cocci in symptomatic girls should not be dismissed as contaminants.

Treatment. CONS synthesize beta-lactamases and have altered penicillin-binding proteins, producing methicillin resistance. Treatment therefore requires vancomycin. Rifampin also may be added to treat CNS infections. Infected intravenous catheters may be treated without removal in many instances, but CNS shunts must be replaced.

References

Behrman RE (ed): Nelson Textbook of Pediatrics. 14th ed. Philadelphia, WB Saunders, 1992, Sec. 12.19.
Hall SL: Coagulase-negative staphylococcal infections in neonates. Pediatr Infect Dis J 10:57, 1991.
Patrick CC: Coagulase-negative staphylococci: Pathogens with increasing clinical significance. J Pediatr 116:497, 1990.

Group A Streptococcal Infections

Etiology. Streptococci are gram-positive cocci that grow in chains and that are classified by their ability to produce a zone of hemolysis on blood agar: those producing the enzyme hemolysin that causes partial hemolysis (alpha-hemolytic), those causing complete hemolysis (beta-hemolytic), and those with no hemolysis (gamma-hemolytic). Streptococci are further separated on the basis of differences in carbohydrate cell wall components; streptococcal Lancefield groups A–H and K–T have been identified. The cell walls of group A beta-hemolytic streptococci contain M protein, an important virulence factor, the presence of which inhibits phagocytosis by leukocytes. Most of the 75 immunologically distinct M protein bacterial types cause pharyngitis and potentially may cause rheumatic fever. Less than a dozen serotypes of group A streptococci are associated with acute glomerulonephritis. Most streptococci excrete toxins, enzymes, and hemolysins. Erythrogenic toxins cause the rash of scarlet fever. Exposure to streptolysin O is followed by systemic antibody production, which aids in diagnosing prior streptococcal infection.

Epidemiology. Group A streptococci are normal inhabitants of the nasopharynx; colonization occurs in 15–20% of the population throughout the year. The incidence of pharyngeal disease is highest in school-age children (5–15 yr of age), in the winter, in northern climates, and in settings of crowding and close contact. Person-to-person spread is by droplets from sneezing and coughing. Occasionally, a pet dog or contaminated food may be the source of infection. Streptococci are normal skin flora. Streptococcal infection of the skin is most common in children under 6 yr of age and during summer or in warmer climates in which skin abrasions or insect bites become infected.

Clinical Manifestations. The incubation period of streptococcal pharyngitis is 2–5 days.

Respiratory Tract Infection. Streptococcal pharyngitis is associated with an acute sore throat with fever, headache, and tender anterior cervical lymph nodes. Occasionally, vomiting, abdominal pain, and rash may be present. The tonsils are hyperemic, edematous, and covered with exudate. The pharynx is inflamed and covered by a membrane in severe cases. The tongue may be edematous and reddened.

Scarlet Fever. This disease is due to infection with group A streptococci, which elaborate an erythrogenic toxin that produces a characteristic rash appearing 24–48 hr after the onset of pharyngitis. The epidemiology, symptoms, sequelae, and treatment of scarlet fever are the same as those of streptococcal pharyngitis. The exanthem is red, punctate, or finely papular. In some patients, it may be palpated more readily than it is seen, having the texture of coarse sandpaper (goose flesh). The rash first appears in the axillae, groin, and neck but within 24 hr becomes generalized. Areas of more intense erythema are noted in the creases of the fingers and groin and the antecubital fossae (Pastia lines). The face appears flushed and there is circumoral pallor. The rash begins to fade 3–4 days after the onset; desquamation of fine flakes from the face and peeling of the palms and fingers may occur after 1 wk. The tongue has a white coat through which the red and edematous papillae project (white strawberry tongue). After several days the white coat desquamates; the red tongue with prominent papillae persists (red strawberry tongue). Scarlet fever rarely may follow infection of wounds (surgical scarlet fever), burns, or streptococcal skin infection. Scarlet fever must be distinguished from measles, rubella, erythema infectiosum, infectious mononucleosis, enteroviral infections, roseola, severe sunburn, TSS, drug reactions, and Kawasaki disease.

Skin Infections. The most common skin infection caused by group A beta-hemolytic streptococci is superficial pyoderma (*impetigo*), which begins as a single papulovesicular lesion surrounded by erythema that later becomes one or many golden yellow–crusted, weeping lesions. Fever and systemic signs other than regional lymphadenopathy are uncommon. Streptococcal *cellulitis* is a painful, erythematous, indurated infection of the skin and subcutaneous tissues. *Lymphangitis* and regional lymphadenitis are common. Streptococcal soft tissue *abscesses* are rare. Acute poststreptococcal glomerulonephritis may follow impetigo despite adequate treatment (see Chapter 16).

Erysipelas. This is an acute cellulitis and lymphangitis of the skin with rapid progression to contiguous skin. The lesion is very erythematous and indurated; the margins have a raised firm border. Erysipelas is associated with fever, vomiting, toxicity, and irritability; progression to bacteremia or abscesses is common. Cellulitis caused by *S. aureus* is characterized by diffuse brawny edema without discrete margins, whereas that caused by *H. influenzae* appears purple and is usually located on the face.

Bacteremia. Streptococcal bacteremia may follow streptococcal disease of the skin, respiratory tract, rectum, or vagina and has been noted without an obvious focus. DIC, shock, and peripheral gangrene can occur. Hematogenous dissemination may result in meningitis, osteomyelitis, arthritis, soft tissue abscesses, pneumonia, or endocarditis.

Streptococcal toxic shock–like syndrome manifests as hypotension, multisystem organ dysfunction, and musculoskeletal complaints, with or without an erythematous macular rash. It may occur after streptococcal superinfection of varicella lesions. Bacteremia resulting from a virulent pyrogenic exotoxin A–producing group A streptococcus is present in most cases.

Vaginitis. Group A streptococci are a common cause of vaginitis in prepubertal girls. There usually are a serous discharge, marked erythema, and irritation of the vulvar area, accompanied by discomfort on walking and on urination. Proctitis is rare but may be seen in either sex.

Diagnosis. The diagnosis of streptococcal infection is suggested by typical but not pathognomonic findings and should be established by isolating organisms from throat, skin, or blood. Rapid diagnostic tests based on identifying group A antigen from throat swabs are available but vary in their sensitivity and specificity. If such tests are positive, a throat culture is not necessary, but if they are negative, a throat culture should be obtained. The immunologic response to streptococcal antigen can be assessed by measuring titers to antistreptolysin O (ASO), antideoxyribonuclease B (the best serologic test for pyoderma), and antihyaluronidase (elevated with less regularity than ASO titers). Unfortunately they are of no value in diagnosing and managing acute streptococcal infection. Throat swabs incubated on blood agar demonstrate a zone of hemolysis, with growth inhibited by bacitracin, which typically inhibits only group A streptococci.

The *differential diagnosis* of acute pharyngitis includes infectious mononucleosis, infection due to cytomegalovirus, HSV, adenovirus, diphtheria, tularemia, toxoplasmosis, and, rarely, aplastic anemia. Pharyngitis and scarlatiniform rash in adolescents may be due to *A. haemolyticum*. Streptococcal pyoderma and cellulitis must be differentiated from staphylococcal skin disease. Bullous impetigo is usually staphylococcal, whereas the golden crusted lesions are caused by streptococci.

Complications. These are due to extension of streptococcal infection from the nasopharynx, which results in sinusitis, otitis media, mastoiditis, cervical adenitis, retropharyngeal and peritonsillar abscess, or bronchopneumonia. Hematogenous dissemination of streptococci may cause meningitis, osteomyelitis, or septic arthritis. Nonsuppurative complications include rheumatic fever (see Chapter 13) and acute glomerulonephritis (see Chapter 16).

Treatment. Penicillin is the treatment of choice for all streptococcal infections; if the patient is allergic to penicillin, erythromycin or clindamycin is used. Bacteremia, erysipelas, and bone or joint infection require intravenous therapy (see Appendix I). Impetigo also may be treated locally with mupirocin.

Prevention. Preventive therapy is indicated to avoid rheumatic fever. Administering daily oral or monthly intramuscular, long-acting penicillin in patients with an episode of rheumatic fever will prevent most cases of streptococcal disease and recurrent illness, if the drug is provided prior to the onset of symptoms. Treatment prevents the later occurrence of rheumatic fever, but not glomerulonephritis. Penicillin prevents rheumatic fever if initiated 7–14 days after the onset of the antecedent pharyngitis. Patients treated with penicillin for pharyngitis may be considered noncontagious within 48 hr of therapy.

References

Behrman RE (ed): Nelson Textbook of Pediatrics. 14th ed. Philadelphia, WB Saunders, 1992, Sec. 12.18.

Givner LB, Abramson JS, Wasilaukas B: Apparent increase in the incidence of invasive group A beta-homolytic streptococcal disease in children. J Pediatr 118:341, 1991.

Jackson MA, Burry VF, Olson LC: Multisystem group A β-hemolytic streptococcal disease in children. Rev Infect Dis 13:783, 1991.

Yersinia enterocolitica and *Yersinia pseudotuberculosis* Infections

Etiology.   *Y. enterocolitica* and *Y. pseudotuberculosis* are oxidase-negative, gram-negative bacilli. *Y. enterocolitica* has 35 serotypes and *Y. pseudotuberculosis* has 5.

Epidemiology.   The source of the organisms include wild and domestic animals, raw milk, chitterlings, oysters, and water supplies. Infection from dogs and human-to-human spread occurs. Infants and children appear most susceptible. The incubation period varies from 1 to 3 wk.

Clinical Manifestations.   *Y. enterocolitica* commonly is associated with enteritis and enterocolitis, which mimic inflammatory bowel disease and become manifest by fever and bloody diarrhea with mucus and abdominal pain. Young infants may have a nonspecific gastroenteritis or dysentery-like disease. Other manifestations include acute mesenteric adenitis, pharyngitis, hepatosplenic abscesses, arthritis, osteomyelitis, hepatitis, carditis, meningitis, Reiter syndrome, septicemia, and erythema nodosum. Septicemia has been associated with iron intoxication and has occurred after accidental overdose of oral iron in previously healthy children. Treatment with desferoxamine, an iron siderophore that chelates iron in hypertransfused patients having chronic anemia or iron intoxication, may present iron to the dormant organism,

which requires iron for growth. Septicemia is associated with a case fatality rate of nearly 50%, despite antibiotic treatment. Mesenteric adenitis typically affects older children and adolescents; the severe abdominal pain may simulate appendicitis. The duration of the illness generally is 2–3 wk without treatment, but occasionally diarrhea may persist for several months and simulate inflammatory bowel disease.

Y. pseudotuberculosis has been associated with mesenteric adenitis and terminal ileitis. Abdominal pain may be severe and may suggest acute appendicitis. Septicemia is unusual; other findings include diarrhea and erythema nodosum.

Diagnosis.   The diagnosis may be established by identifying the organism in stool, mesenteric lymph nodes, bowel mucosa at endoscopy, peritoneal fluid, or blood. Because identification requires special techniques, laboratory personnel should be notified. Passive hemagglutination tests also may confirm the diagnosis. Antibodies are detectable 8–10 days after the onset of illness and may persist for several months.

Treatment.   Most strains of *Y. enterocolitica* and *Y. pseudotuberculosis* are susceptible to aminoglycosides, tetracycline, chloramphenicol, and trimethoprim–sulfamethoxazole. Patients with septicemia or sites of infection outside the gastrointestinal tract should receive therapy. Trimethoprim–sulfamethoxazole and gentamicin are the drugs of choice for serious infection. The benefits of treating patients with enterocolitis or mesenteric adenitis are unknown (see Appendix I).

References

Behrman RE (ed): Nelson Textbook of Pediatrics. 14th ed. Philadelphia, WB Saunders, 1992, Sec. 12.34.

Lee LA, Taylor J, Carter GP, et al: *Yersinia enterocolitica* 0: 3: An emerging cause of pediatric gastroenteritis in the United States. J Infect Dis 163:660, 1991.

Ostroff SM, Kapperud G, Lassen J, et al: Clinical features of sporadic *Yersinia enterocolitica* infections in Norway. J Infect Dis 166:812, 1992.

Spirochetal Infections

SYPHILIS

Etiology.   Syphilis is caused by *Treponema pallidum,* a long, slender, coiled spirochete. It cannot routinely be cultivated in vitro, but can be seen by dark-field microscopy.

Epidemiology.   The disease is acquired through sexual contact, transplacentally from an infected mother to her fetus, and, less commonly, at birth, in the postpartum period, or by infected blood. Infants with congenital syphilis often are born to HIV-positive and crack cocaine–using women. Infection in males is 3 times more common than in females. Sexual abuse should be considered in young children who have acquired syphilis. The incubation period for primary syphilis is 10–90 days after exposure.

Clinical Manifestations

Congenital Syphilis.   Early manifestations occurring between birth and the 1st yr of life include fever, anemia, failure to thrive, irritability, local mucocutaneous lesions (maculopapular rash on trunk, palms, and soles; condylomata lata; bullous eruptions), persistent rhinitis (snuffles), hepatosplenomegaly, lymphadenopathy, dactylitis, and pseudoparalysis resulting from osteochondritis. Laboratory evaluation may show direct hyperbilirubinemia, elevated liver function tests, multiple sites of osteochondritis, thrombocytopenia, Coombs-negative hemolytic anemia, and leukocytosis. The moist secretions of early congenital syphilis are highly contagious. In an untreated pregnant woman, syphilis may be transmitted to the fetus at any time, but transmission to the fetus is more common during the 1st yr after syphilis has been acquired by the mother. Although some newborns demonstrate symptoms of the disease within the first 4–8 wk after birth, many infants are symptomatic at birth and exhibit nonimmune hydrops with anemia; thrombocytopenia; leukopenia; pneumonia; hepatitis, with or without nephrosis; and osteochondritis.

Late congenital syphilis appears many years after birth and becomes manifest as multiple bone signs (frontal bossing, saber shins), Hutchinson teeth (peg or screw-like), mulberry molars, a saddle-nose deformity, rhagades (perioral linear scars), juvenile paresis, juvenile tabes, interstitial keratitis, VIIIth nerve deafness, and Clutton joints (painless joint effusions). These manifestations are all rare in the modern era in which penicillin therapy is used to control congenital syphilis.

Acquired Primary Syphilis.   Three to 6 wk following inoculation, a single *painless* papule appears, becomes indurated, and progresses to a *painless* ulcer (chancre). This ulcer usually is found on the genitalia but may appear at any other site of inoculation.

Secondary Syphilis.   An influenza-like illness occurs 6–8 wk after the primary chancre, with generalized adenopathy and a generalized erythematous, maculopapular rash, which is present on the palms and soles. Plaque-like skin lesions (condylomata lata) and mucous membrane lesions also occur and are all infectious. Other manifestations of secondary syphilis may include meningitis, hepatitis, glomerulonephritis, bursitis, and periostitis.

Other Types of Syphilis.   *Latent syphilis* has no clinical manifestations, but a history of untreated syphilis and serologic evidence of infection may be discovered. *Late syphilis,* a slowly progressive disease typically involving the CNS and heart, is not seen in children.

Diagnosis.   Serologic tests for syphilis include the nontreponemal reagin antibody tests, which are directed against a poorly characterized lipoidal antigen. These tests include the Venereal Disease Research Laboratory (VDRL) test, a rapid plasma reagin (RPR) test, and an automated reagin test (ART). The specific tests include the *T. pallidum* immobilization test, which rarely is used; the fluorescent treponemal antibody–absorption (FTA-ABS) test; and the microhemagglutination test for *T. pallidum.* The specific tests are less likely to be falsely reactive in collagen vascular disease, pregnancy, drug addiction, malaria, infectious mononucleosis, and other infectious diseases ("biologic false-positive tests") than the nontreponemal tests. The serologic tests are uniformly positive in secondary and later stages of syphilis. The VDRL test becomes positive within 4–6 wk after infection. Treatment results in declining titers of the VDRL test, RPR test, and ART, but not the FTA-ABS test.

In diagnosing congenital syphilis, maternal transplacentally passed antibody often confuses the diagnosis. It is frequently difficult to determine if the infant only has passive acquisition of antibody. This is particularly true in HIV-infected patients, who may have absent or exaggerated antibody responses. Specific Western blot methods or polymerase chain reaction may improve the diagnosis of asymptomatic but infected patients. Positive CSF VDRL or RPR tests warrant therapy for CNS syphilis in congenital or acquired disease. Dark-field examination of chancres, mucous membranes, or cutaneous lesions may reveal motile organisms.

Treatment.   *T. pallidum* is extremely sensitive to penicillin, which remains the drug of choice for therapy of all forms of syphilis. Alternate therapy includes tetracycline or erythromycin. Dosage regimens vary according to stage of disease and the presence of neurologic involvement and congenital infection. Current regimens for therapy of gonorrhea also effectively treat incubating syphilis. Exposure to a documented case of syphilis warrants "prophylactic" therapy and serologic follow-up. A pregnant woman with documented or possible syphilis should be treated with penicillin to prevent illness in the mother and her offspring. Erythromycin does not treat the fetus. A systemic, febrile reaction, the Jarisch-Herxheimer reaction, occurs in 15–20% of syphilitic patients treated with penicillin. Patients with syphilis who also have AIDS may require prolonged therapy.

References

Behrman RE (ed): Nelson Textbook of Pediatrics. 14th ed. Philadelphia, WB Saunders, 1992, Sec. 12.50.

Brion LP, Manuli M, Rai B, et al: Long-bone radiographic abnormalities as a sign of active congenital syphilis in asymptomatic newborns. Pediatrics 88:1037, 1991.

Dorfman DH, Glaser JH: Congenital syphilis presenting in infants after the newborn period. N Engl J Med 323: 1299, 1990.

Hook EW III, Marra CM: Acquired syphilis in adults. N Engl J Med 326:1060, 1992.

Zenker PN, Berman SM: Congenital syphilis: Trends and recommendations for evaluation and management. Pediatr Infect Dis J 10:516, 1991.

BORRELIA BURGDORFERI INFECTION (LYME DISEASE)

Etiology. Lyme disease is a tick-borne illness caused by a fastidious spirochete, *Borrelia burgdorferi*. Ticks of the *Ixodes* genus and possibly other blood-sucking insects feed off animal reservoirs, such as the white-footed mouse, the deer, or the dog.

Epidemiology. Lyme disease has been reported in most states but is endemic to the coastal Northeast, Minnesota, Wisconsin, California, Texas, and Nevada; the predominant vector is *I. dammini* in the East and Midwest and *I. pacificus* in the West. In Europe, Lyme disease may be atypical relative to the clinical presentation in the United States and may be associated with other ticks. Because exposure to ticks is more common in the summer, Lyme disease is noted predominantly in this season.

Clinical Manifestations

Stage 1. Although not all patients recall a tick bite, the typical pattern of disease evolves from this bite. Three to 32 days (mean 7 days) after a tick bite, the site forms an erythematous papule that expands to form a red, raised border and a clear center. Multiple rings may form and new areas of this annular lesion may appear distal to the original site. The lesion, *erythema chronicum migrans,* may be 15 cm wide, may be pruritic or painful, and may contain *B. burgdorferi* organisms. This skin lesion is not present in all patients. The lesions fade within 1 mo. During this early stage, systemic manifestations include malaise, lethargy, fever, headache, arthralgias, stiff neck, myalgias, and lymphadenopathy. All of these early manifestations resolve without treatment in 1 mo.

Stage 2. *Cardiac manifestations* occur within 5 wk and include myocarditis, atrioventricular node block (occasionally requiring external pacemakers), ST depression, and T wave inversion. Cardiac disease is serious, present in approximately 10% of patients, and reversible. *Neurologic manifestations* occur within 4 wk and include lymphocytic "aseptic" meningitis, encephalitis, cranial neuritis (Bell palsy of the VIIth nerve), polyradiculitis, peripheral neuropathy, mononeuritis multiplex, or transverse myelitis. Neurologic manifestations resolve by 3 mo.

Stage 3. Arthritis may develop in 50–60% of patients within weeks to years of the tick bite. Intermittent arthritis also is noted in stage 2 and may be monoarticular, pauciarticular, or polyarticular, resembling JRA. The knee, shoulder, elbow, and, rarely, the small joints of the hands are involved. Chronic erosive arthritis may persist in 10% of patients, with involvement of the knee more than other joints. The male-to-female ratio is 7:1. Popliteal cysts may develop, and joint fluid is typically inflammatory, with leukocytic predominance and a total white count between 500 and 100,000 cells/μL (Table 10–10). These patients are rheumatoid factor negative and ANA negative.

Diagnosis. A history of a tick bite and the classic rash are helpful but not present in all cases. The ESR is elevated and complement may be reduced in patients with arthritis. The VDRL test may be falsely positive. Cryoglobulins and circulating immune complexes may precede or coincide with arthritis. CSF reveals a lymphocytic pleocytosis with normal glucose levels and slightly raised protein levels. The diagnosis is confirmed by serologic tests specific for *B. burgdorferi*. Because of high false-positive rates, the ELISA should be confirmed by a Western blot. The *differential diagnoses* are many and relate to the organ involved, as discussed under aseptic meningitis, arthritis, and myocarditis. In children, JRA must be considered (see Chapter 9).

Treatment.   Stage 1 disease, especially erythema chronicum migrans, may be treated with oral amoxicillin or, in older children, doxycycline for 2–3 wk. Early treatment may prevent carditis and meningitis. Stages 2 and 3 usually are treated with high-dose parenteral penicillin, tetracycline, or ceftriaxone if severe complications are present. Oral doxycycline or amoxicillin are effective for milder disease. Treatment is for 10–30 days for oral and 14–21 days for intravenous therapy (see Appendix I).

References

Behrman RE (ed): Nelson Textbook of Pediatrics. 14th ed. Philadelphia, WB Saunders, 1992, Sec. 12.57.

Committee on Infectious Diseases: Treatment of Lyme borreliosis. Pediatrics 88:176, 1991.

Cryan B, Wright DJM: Lyme disease in paediatrics. Arch Dis Child 66:1359, 1991.

Szer IS, Taylor E, Steere AC: The long term course of Lyme arthritis in children. N Engl J Med 325:159, 1991.

Chlamydial Infection

Etiology.   Chlamydiae are obligate intracellular parasites that contain DNA and RNA and do not stain with Gram stain. Infected cells contain cytoplasmic Giemsa stain–positive inclusions. There are two subgroups of the genus *Chlamydia.* Group A contains *C. trachomatis* and the agent of lymphogranuloma venereum (LGV). Group B contains the agent of psittacosis/ornithosis and Reiter syndrome, as well as several zoonoses.

CHLAMYDIA TRACHOMATIS INFECTION

C. trachomatis contains 15 serotypes that are divided into two groups—oculogenital (subtypes A–K) and LGV (subtypes L-1 and L-3). Trachoma is caused by subtypes A–C.

Epidemiology.   *C. trachomatis* is a common cause of sexually transmitted disease, causing about 40% of cases of nonspecific urethritis, as well as cervicitis, salpingitis, endometritis, epididymitis, and tubal infertility. Infection rates as high as 30% have been observed in certain adolescent groups (Chapter 7). About 12% of pregnant women are infected, the rates being higher in lower socioeconomic status groups. In infants born vaginally to infected mothers, about 50% are culture positive, 35% develop conjunctivitis, and 20% develop pneumoni-

tis. Approximately 20–30% of infants with the afebrile pneumonitis syndrome are infected with *Chlamydia.* The incubation period varies, depending on the type of infection.

Clinical Manifestations.   *Conjunctivitis* caused by *Chlamydia* in the neonate may appear from 3 days to 6 wk after delivery, but usually occurs in the 2nd wk of life. The eyes are inflamed, with purulent discharge issuing from one or both eyes. Recurrences can occur even with appropriate therapy, but residual eye damage is rare. **Trachoma** is a chronic follicular keratoconjunctivitis resulting from repeated infection and may result in blindness in older children or adults because of extensive local scarring and inflammation.

Pneumonitis develops at 3–10 wk of age. The child generally appears well, is afebrile, but has tachypnea and a cough. Apnea also may occur. One half of affected patients have concomitant conjunctivitis. Examination reveals rales and wheezing. Roentgenograms of the chest reveal hyperinflation and diffuse interstitial or patchy infiltrates. Mild eosinophilia (about 400/μL), hypergammaglobulinemia, and mild hypoxemia are common. The illness is self-limiting but may last for weeks.

Beyond infancy, urethritis in both sexes and cervicitis in females may occur. These infections may be protracted and recurrent, and, in females, may result in chronic pelvic inflammatory disease and infertility.

Diagnosis.   *Chlamydia* can be grown in treated tissue culture cells, which is the standard method of isolation. Monoclonal antibody detection tests have been useful in the evaluation of genital secretions and in pneumonitis or conjunctivitis of infants. If conjunctivitis is present, scraping the eyelid and staining the exfoliated cells to demonstrate cytoplasmic inclusion bodies may be diagnostic.

Conjunctivitis must be differentiated from inflammation (red eye) caused by silver nitrate (chemical), gonococcal infection, or viral infection (Table 10–16). The pneumonitis must be differentiated from that caused by viruses (especially cytomegalovirus and RSV), *Ureaplasma, P. carinii,* and, less commonly, other bacteria and mycobacteria.

The adenopathy of LGV must be differentiated from that caused by cat-scratch disease, pyogenic bacteria, chancroid, granuloma inguinale, syphilis, HSV, and neoplasms. Examining the node may reveal inclusions using Giemsa stain. Chlamydial cultures may be positive. Serology usually is diagnostic.

Table 10–16. The Red Eye

Condition	Etiology	Signs/Symptoms	Treatment
Bacterial conjunctivitis	*H. influenzae, H. aegyptius, S. pneumoniae* *Neisseria gonorrhoeae*	Mucopurulent unilateral or bilateral discharge, normal vision, photophobia Conjunctival injection and edema (chemosis); gritty sensation	Topical antibiotics, ceftriaxone for *Gonococcus, H. influenzae*
Viral conjunctivitis	Adenovirus, ECHO virus, coxsackievirus	As above; may be hemorrhagic, unilateral	Self-limited
Neonatal conjunctivitis	*Chlamydia trachomatis, Gonococcus*, chemical (silver nitrate), *S. aureus*	Palpebral conjunctival follicle or papillae; as above	Ceftriaxone for *Gonococcus* and erythromycin for *C. trachomatis*
Allergic conjunctivitis	Seasonal pollens or allergen exposure	Itching, incidence of bilateral chemosis (edema) greater than that of erythema, tarsal papillae	Antihistamines, steroids, cromolyn
Keratitis	Herpes simplex, adenovirus, *S. pneumoniae, S. aureus, Pseudomonas, Acanthamoeba*, chemicals	Severe pain, corneal swelling, clouding, limbus erythema, hypopyon, cataracts; contact lens history with amebic infection	Specific antibiotics for bacterial/fungal infections; keratoplasty, acyclovir for herpes
Endophthalmitis	*S. aureus, S. pneumoniae, Candida albicans*, associated surgery or trauma	Acute onset, pain, loss of vision, swelling, chemosis, redness; hypopyon and vitreous haze	Antibiotics
Anterior uveitis (iridocyclitis)	JRA, Reiter syndrome, sarcoidosis, Behçet disease, Kawasaki disease, inflammatory bowel disease	Unilateral/bilateral; erythema, ciliary flush, irregular pupil, iris adhesions; pain, photophobia, small pupil, poor vision	Topical steroids, plus therapy for primary disease
Posterior uveitis (choroiditis)	Toxoplasmosis, histoplasmosis, *Toxocara canis*	No signs of erythema, decreased vision	Specific therapy for pathogen
Episcleritis/scleritis	Idiopathic autoimmune disease (e.g., SLE, Henoch-Schönlein purpura)	Localized pain, intense erythema, unilateral; blood vessels bigger than in conjunctivitis; scleritis may cause globe perforation	Episcleritis is self-limiting; topical steroids for fast relief
Foreign body	Occupational exposure	Unilateral, red, gritty feeling; visible or microscopic size	Irrigation, removal; check for ulceration
Blepharitis	*S. aureus, S. epidermidis*, seborrheic, blocked lacrimal duct; rarely molluscum contagiosum, *Phthirus pubis, Pediculus capitis*	Bilateral, irritation, itching, hyperemia, crusting, affecting lid margins	Topical antibiotics, warm compresses

Continued

Table 10–16. (Continued)

Condition	Etiology	Signs/Symptoms	Treatment
Dacryocystitis	Obstructed lacrimal sac: *S. aureus, H. influenzae, Pneumococcus*	Pain, tenderness, erythema and exudate in area of lacrimal sac (inferiomedial to inner canthus); tearing (epiphora); possible orbital cellulitis	Systemic, topical antibiotics; surgical drainage
Dacryoadenitis	*S. aureus, Streptococcus,* CMV, measles, EBV, enteroviruses; trauma, sarcoidosis, leukemia	Pain, tenderness, edema, erythema over gland area (upper temporal lid); fever, leukocytosis	Systemic antibiotics; drainage of orbital abscesses
Orbital cellulitis (postseptal cellulitis)	Paranasal sinusitis; *H. influenzae, S. aureus, S. pneumoniae, Streptococcus;* Trauma: *S. aureus;* Fungi: *Aspergillus, Mucor* sp. if immunodeficient	Rhinorrhea, chemosis, vision loss, painful extraocular motion, proptosis, ophthalmoplegia, fever, lid edema, leukocytosis	Systemic antibiotics, drainage of orbital abscesses
Periorbital cellulitis (preseptal cellulitis)	Trauma: *S. aureus,* streptococcus; Bacteremia: *H. influenzae,* pneumococcus, streptococcus	Cutaneous erythema, warmth, normal vision, minimal involvement of orbit; fever, leukocytosis, toxic appearance	Systemic antibiotics

(Data from Am J Med 79:545, 1985; BMJ 296:1720, 1988; Infect Dis Clin North Am 2:99, 1988; Lancet 338:1498, 1991; Ped Ann 22: 353, 1993.)

Treatment. Although topical therapy of conjunctivitis using sulfonamides is effective, oral erythromycin or sulfisoxazole also should be administered to treat either conjunctivitis (to eradicate the nasopharyngeal colonization and risk of subsequent pneumonitis) or pneumonitis. Prophylactic therapy of the infected mother and her sexual partner can decrease the rate of infection in the newborn. For uncomplicated genital tract infection caused by *C. trachomatis* in adolescents and adults, tetracycline, doxycycline, or azithomycin is recommended. LGV is treated with tetracycline or sulfonamides (see Appendix I).

References

Behrman RE (ed): Nelson Textbook of Pediatrics. 14th ed. Philadelphia, WB Saunders, 1992, Sec. 12.58–12.62.

Bell TA, Stamm WE, Pin Wang S, et al: Chronic *Chlamydia trachomatis* infections in infants. JAMA 267:400, 1992.

Brasfield DM, Stagno S, Whitley RJ, et al: Infant pneumonitis associated with cytomegalovirus, *Chlamydia, Pneumocystis,* and *Ureaplasma:* Follow up. Pediatrics 79:76, 1987.

Martin DH, Mroczkowski TF, Dalu ZA, et al: A controlled trial of a single dose of azithromycin for the treatment of chlamydial urethritis and cervicitis. N Engl J Med 327: 921, 1992.

Rettig PJ: Infection due to *Chlamydia trachomatis* from infancy to adolescence. Pediatr Infect Dis 5:449, 1986.

Mycoplasmal Infection

Etiology. Mycoplasmas are the smallest free-living organisms. They lack a cell wall and are distinct from bacteria but grow on artificial media and are not viruses. Pathogenic species of mycoplasmas include *M. pneumoniae* (pneumonia, systemic infection), *M. hominis* (genitourinary tract infection), and *Ureaplasma urealyticum* (genitourinary tract, neonatal pneumonia).

Epidemiology. *M. pneumoniae* is a major cause of illness in school-age children and young adults. Clinical illness is unusual before 4 yr of age, and the peak attack rate occurs at 6–15 yr of age. *M. pneumoniae* is estimated to cause one-half million cases of pneumonia and over 11 million cases of tracheobronchitis in the United States annually. Illness occurs at irregular intervals, tending to begin in the fall with smoldering epidemics. Transmission is presumed to be by droplet spread from symptomatic patients. The incubation period is 2–3 wk.

Clinical Manifestations.   Onset of illness (*atypical pneumonia*) is gradual, with headache, malaise, fever, sore throat, and cough. Sputum production, rales, and pleural effusions are frequent. Severe pulmonary disease has been reported in children with sickle cell anemia. Other manifestations include skin eruptions (maculopapular rashes, erythema nodosum, Stevens-Johnson syndrome) and, less commonly, meningoencephalitis, Guillain-Barré syndrome, hemolytic anemia, thrombocytopenia, myocarditis, and pericarditis. The nonrespiratory tract illnesses are less firmly established as being due to *M. pneumoniae*.

Diagnosis.   Cold agglutinin titers tend to reflect the severity of illness and are likely to be positive in the school-age child with pulmonary infection due to *Mycoplasma*. Confirmation of the diagnosis is achieved by demonstrating an increase of specific antibodies.

Treatment.   Erythromycin or tetracycline (in children over 10 yr of age) is the drug of choice (see Appendix I).

References

Behrman RE (ed): Nelson Textbook of Pediatrics. 14th ed. Philadelphia, WB Saunders, 1992, Sec. 12.63.
Broughton RA: Infections due to *Mycoplasma pneumoniae* in childhood. Pediatr Infect Dis 5:71, 1986.
Editorial: *Mycoplasma pneumoniae* Lancet 337:651, 1991.

Cat-Scratch Disease

Etiology.   The cat-scratch disease agent *Rochalimaea henselae* is a small, pleomorphic, gram-negative bacillus that stains with Warthin-Starry silver impregnation of material from aspirated lymph nodes. It also causes bacillary angiomatosis and peliosis hepatis.

Epidemiology.   The disease has a worldwide distribution, is more common in males, and occurs in temperate climates in the fall and winter months. In over 90% of cases, the disease follows the scratch (rarely, a lick) of a kitten (less often, of an older cat). The cats are not sick. Rare cases have occurred in association with dogs, thorns, or wood splinters.

Clinical Manifestations.   A primary cutaneous papule or conjunctival granuloma develops 3–10 days after the initial contact. Lymphadenopathy localized to the draining regional nodes develops 2 wk (range) (1–7 wk) later, usually on the head, neck, and axilla. The nodes enlarge to 1–8 cm, may suppurate, and are painful in the early stage of the illness. There is no lymphangitis and usually few systemic signs, although fever and malaise may be noted in 30% of patients. Lymphadenopathy lasts 1–4 mo. Additional, but rare, features include erythema nodosum, osteolytic lesions, encephalitis, septic-like appearance, oculoglandular (Parinaud) syndrome, polyneuritis, transverse myelitis, hepatic or splenic granulomas, thrombocytopenia, and pneumonia.

Diagnosis.   Usually, the disease is suspected by a history of exposure to cats, the primary lesion localized at the site of the scratch or bite, and a single enlarged node. The cat-scratch skin test is prepared from exudative material pooled from excised lymph nodes but currently is not used for diagnosis. Aspiration of the node with subsequent microscopic evidence of the bacillus by Warthin-Starry silver stain is diagnostic and may be curative.

Treatment.   Usually no treatment is required, because the lymphadenopathy resolves in 2–4 mo without sequelae. Aspiration is indicated for large, painful, and uncomfortable lesions. Rifampin ciprofloxacin, gentamicin, or trimethoprim–sulfamethoxazole may enhance resolution of more severe disease. After an illness, immunity is lifelong. The disease is not contagious; therefore, the patient does not need to be isolated.

References

Behrman RE (ed): Nelson Textbook of Pediatrics. 14th ed. Philadelphia, WB Saunders, 1992, Sec. 12.102.
Margileth AM: Antibiotic therapy for cat-scratch disease: Clinical study of therapeutic outcome in 268 patients and a review of the literature. Pediatr Infect Dis J 11: 474, 1992.
Zangwill K, Hamilton D, Perkins B, et al: Cat scratch disease in Connecticut. Epidemiology, risk factors and evaluation of a new diagnostic test. N Eng J Med 329:8, 1993.

VIRAL DISEASES

Antiviral Chemotherapy

Therapy against viral disease must take into consideration the intracellular nature of viral replication and, to avoid toxicity to the host's cells, must be directed at viral specific proteins. Viral enzymes (e.g., HIV and reverse transcriptase) or enzymes with different substrate specificity compared with

Table 10–17. Antiviral Chemotherapy

Drugs	Mechanism of Action	Indication	Comments
Acyclovir	Requires viral thymidine kinase to produce acyclovir monophosphate, which inhibits DNA polymerase	Herpes simplex 1 and 2, varicella-zoster (systemic, mucocutaneous)	Oral, intravenous, topical; varicella requires higher drug levels; toxic encephalopathy, renal dysfunction
Amantadine/rimantadine	Inhibits viral replication	Influenza A	Prophylaxis and therapy; CNS toxicity with poor concentration, confusion
Ganciclovir	As acyclovir	CMV, herpes viruses	Neutropenia, recurrence when discontinued
Foscarnet	Inhibits viral DNA polymerase	CMV retinitis, ganciclovir-resistant CMV; acyclovir-resistant HSV and varicella-zoster virus	Nonmyelosuppressive; nephrotoxic, $\downarrow \uparrow$ CA^{2+}, Mg^{2+}
Ribavirin	Inhibits RNA synthesis and reverse transcriptase	Aerosol for RSV, parenteral for influenza, Lassa virus	Aerosol has few side effects; indicated for complicated RSV infection
Zidovudine (azidothymidine [AZT])	Inhibits reverse transcriptase	HIV-AIDS	Bone marrow depression
Didanosine (DDI) and dideoxycytosine (DDC)	Inhibits reverse transcriptase	Advanced AIDS if intolerant of or deteriorating on AZT	Painful peripheral neuropathy, pancreatitis

(Data from Med Lett 34:31, 1992; Infect Dis Clinic North Am 1:311, 1987.)

the host's enzyme (thymidine kinase, DNA polymerase of herpes viruses) are targets for antiviral chemotherapy. In addition, recombinant human factors that naturally reduce virus replication and kill viruses, such as interferon and high dose intravenous immunoglobulin, have been used. To date, the most successful antiviral agents are those nucleotide analogs that interfere with viral DNA or RNA synthesis (Table 10–17).

Adenoviral Infection

Etiology. Adenoviruses are DNA viruses. More than 40 distinct types have been associated with human illness.

Epidemiology. Adenoviruses produce respiratory tract disease year-round, with a higher incidence in the spring, early summer, and mid-winter. Infection occurs early in childhood by respiratory, fecal, oral, and, possibly, conjunctival inoculation. Transmission occurs from person to person, usually by respiratory spread. Asymptomatic infections are common. Enteric strains of ade-

novirus may be transmitted by the fecal–oral route. The period of communicability is highest during the first several days of illness. The incubation period ranges from 2–14 days.

Clinical Manifestations
Pharyngoconjunctival Fever (Types 1, 2, 3, and 5). Manifestations of this type of infection are high fever, pharyngitis, conjunctivitis, cervical adenopathy, and rhinitis, all of which last 4–5 days and are accompanied by malaise, lethargy, weakness, and headache of longer duration. Epidemics that may spread from contaminated swimming pools have been reported in summer camps. Pharyngitis, one of the most common manifestations of adenovirus, is a typical symptom in young infants.

Other Manifestations. Adenovirus may cause epidemic keratoconjunctivitis (primary in adults), as well as acute follicular conjunctivitis. Conjunctivitis in children often occurs with pharyngitis (Table 10–16). Seven to 10% of hospitalized children with pneumonia are infected with adenovirus. This infection may be particularly severe or fatal and is associated with high fever, leukocytosis, elevated ESR, or the development of bronchiolitis obliterans. Noncultivatable "enteric" adenoviruses have been associated with a small proportion of the episodes of diarrhea in infants. Adenovirus also has been recovered from lymph nodes of children who have intussusception, mesenteric adenitis, and lymphadenitis, but in these settings it is not clear whether the virus is the etiologic agent. The sudden onset of hematuria, dysuria, and urinary frequency, accompanied by bacteriologically sterile urine, has been associated with adenovirus types 11 and 21. Hemorrhagic cystitis lasts 1–2 wk.

Disseminated Adenoviral Disease.   This condition commonly occurs in immunocompromised patients, particularly those with T cell defects and those who have undergone bone marrow transplantation. Clinical manifestations include hepatosplenomegaly, liver failure, DIC, shock, and, ultimately, death. Several other manifestations of severe adenoviral infection, including conjunctivitis, pneumonitis, and pharyngitis, may be variably present.

Diagnosis.   A striking rise in the polymorphonuclear leukocyte count may occur that is unlike that usually seen in viral infection. Most adenoviruses are culturable in tissue culture, whereas a group of "enteric adenoviruses" thought to be responsible for diarrhea in infants are diagnosed by antigen detection methods or tissue culture techniques available only in research laboratories. Enteric adenoviruses may be identified by electron microscopy of stool specimens.

Treatment and Prevention.   There are no currently approved antiviral drugs for therapy or prevention of adenoviral infection. Vaccination is recommended for epidemics, such as those occurring in military recruits.

References

Behrman RE (ed): Nelson Textbook of Pediatrics. 14th ed. Philadelphia, WB Saunders, 1992, Sec. 12.77.

Edwards KM, Thompson J, Paolini J, et al: Adenovirus infections in young children. Pediatrics 76:420, 1985.

Ruuskanen O, Meurman O, Sarkkinen H: Adenoviral diseases in children: A study of 105 hospital cases. Pediatrics 76:79, 1985.

Enteroviruses

Enteroviruses, a group of RNA viruses, include 23 group A coxsackieviruses (types A1–A24, except type A23), six group B coxsackieviruses (B1–B6), three polioviruses, and 31 echoviruses (types 1–33, except types 10 and 28). More recent isolates are designated enteroviruses (types 68–71).

Epidemiology.   These hardy viruses maintain activity for days at room temperature. They are spread from person to person, primarily by the fecal–oral route and possibly by the respiratory route, especially among susceptible children in lower socioeconomic status groups and in tropical areas where poor hygiene may exist. There is a peak incidence in summer and fall in temperate climates that is less evident in the tropics. Males and females are equally affected by the disease, although males are more likely to become symptomatically ill. Young children frequently are infected; the disease in neonates may be fulminant, whereas older children have more benign illness unless paralysis or significant myocarditis is present. The incubation period is 3–6 days.

Pathogenesis.   After initial upper respiratory tract viral implantation, viral replication occurs in regional lymph nodes, followed several days later by a low-grade (minor) viremia. This viremia may involve many secondary sites (heart, skin, pericardium, pleura, lung, liver, brain, spinal cord). Viral replication in these sites coincides with clinical illness and the second (major) viremia. Viral replication is halted by the appearance of antibody on approximately the 7th day of infection. Gastrointestinal tract viral replication and shedding are generally of longer duration but do not necessarily produce gastrointestinal symptoms.

Pathology and Pathophysiology.   Each of the groups of enteroviruses has a predilection for specific organ systems. The pathognomonic finding in *poliomyelitis* is viral multiplication in motor neurons, a process that occurs predominantly in the spinal cord (especially anterior horn cells), but the medulla, mid-brain, thalamus, hypothalamus, pallidum, and motor cortex also may be involved. Typical organ involvement by *coxsackieviruses* includes pharyngitis (herpangina); skin (hand–foot–mouth disease); myocarditis; meningoencephalitis; and involvement of adrenals, pancreas, liver, pleura, pericardium, and, at times, the lung. Hepatic necrosis has been observed in some severe *echovirus* infections. Myositis, pneumonia, and adrenal involvement may also occur.

Clinical Manifestations
Polioviruses.   The major forms and clinical manifestations of poliomyelitis are outlined in Table

Table 10–18. Clinical Manifestations of Polio Virus Infection (Poliomyelitis)

Asymptomatic infection	95% of infected persons are asymptomatic
Abortive form (nonspecific febrile illness)	Fever, malaise, anorexia, nausea, vomiting, headache, pharyngitis, abdominal pain
Nonparalytic form (aseptic meningitis)	Similar to the abortive form plus stiff neck and signs of meningeal inflammation, soreness of back muscles, tripod sign, positive Kernig and Brudzinski signs, and bulging fontanel; decrease in both superficial (cremasteric, abdominal) and deep tendon reflexes heralds paralysis
Paralytic form	Similar to the nonparalytic form, plus weakness of skeletal or cranial muscle groups; with deeper brain involvement the signs and symptoms may be pain, spasticity, hypertonia, respiratory and cardiac arrhythmias, blood pressure and vasomotor changes, and bladder and bowel dysfunction; hallmark is asymmetric, flaccid paralysis in spinal, bulbar, and encephalitic forms
Spinal form	Axial and extremity muscle weakness that may involve intercostal muscles and diaphragm
Bulbar form	Cranial nerve weakness and respiratory and circulatory disturbances
Encephalitic form	Irritability, disorientation, drowsiness, and tremors

10–18. The clinician must be vigilant regarding respiratory insufficiency resulting from both respiratory muscle and/or central respiratory center involvement. Such involvement may result in anxiety; jerky, breathless speaking; tachypnea; signs of respiratory distress (nasal flaring, use of accessory muscles of respiration); decreased cough; paradoxic abdominal movement; and immobility of intercostal spaces. Arm and deltoid weakness is a clue to impending respiratory paralysis.

In *bulbar poliomyelitis,* a nasal twang in the voice indicates palatal and pharyngeal weakness, as do pooling of saliva; poor cough; nasal regurgitation of saliva and other fluids; deviation of palate, uvula, or tongue; hoarseness; or aphonia. Changes in respiratory and cardiac function or vasomotor function (blood pressure changes, flushing and mottling of the skin) point toward central involvement of the key regulatory nuclei of the brain stem. The differential diagnosis includes Guillain-Barré syndrome, other types of viral encephalitis, botulism, tetanus, demyelinating encephalomyelitis, tick paralysis, CNS tumor, and trauma. In the United States, most cases of paralytic poliomyelitis are due to the vaccine virus in normal or immunoincompetent hosts.

Nonpolio Enteroviral Infection. Unlike the rare or declining occurrence of polio in most developed countries resulting from successful vaccination, the nonpolio enteroviruses remain common. Their manifestations may be biphasic, in which the patient experiences several days of well being that occur between periods of 1–4 days of illness. Less than 50% of cases of enteroviral infection are *asymptomatic.*

The most common manifestation of all types of enteroviral infection is *nonspecific febrile illness.* It generally lasts 3 days and is associated with fever, malaise, headache, pharyngitis, and myalgia. In neonates, gastrointestinal tract symptoms may occur.

The enteroviruses have been associated with a variety of *respiratory tract illnesses,* including conjunctivitis, pharyngitis, herpangina, stomatitis, parotitis, croup, bronchitis, pneumonia, and pleurodynia. Pharyngitis is associated with pharyngeal erythema and, at times, with exudate. **Herpangina** (coxsackievirus A) is associated with fever, oral ulcers, and vesicles surrounded by erythema, usually in the posterior pharynx but also the anterior tonsillar pillars, palate, uvula, and posterior buccal surfaces. The duration is 3–6 days. **Pleurodynia** (Bornholm disease, devil's grip), an acute febrile illness, typically is associated with intense pleuritic chest and upper abdominal muscular pain that occurs in spasms and is intensified by breathing or coughing. The pain may mimic acute pulmonary or abdominal surgical processes and is due to intercostal muscle infection. This illness, often caused by a member of the coxsackie B group, generally occurs in outbreaks and may be associated with the other manifestations of enteroviral infection. Chest roentgenograms usually are normal, and the WBC count may be normal or elevated, with an increased percentage of myeloid cells.

Gastrointestinal manifestations commonly are associated with outbreaks of enteroviral infection. They include vomiting (in about 50% of cases), diarrhea (without blood), abdominal pain, mesenteric adenitis, and pseudoappendicitis.

Acute hemorrhagic conjunctivitis, particularly that associated with coxsackievirus A24 and enterovirus 70, may become manifest as eye pain, photophobia, blurred vision, lacrimation, erythema, congestion of the eye as a result of edema, chemotic eyelids, and eye discharge. Subconjunctival hemorrhages, conjunctivitis, keratitis, and preauricular adenopathy are present. Outbreaks have occurred in tropical and temperate climates.

Pericarditis and myocarditis commonly are caused by enteroviruses, especially coxsackieviruses B1–B5, and must be distinguished from acute rheumatic fever and acute bacterial endocarditis. Myocarditis has a significant mortality rate from acute disease, especially in neonates and young infants. Older patients may develop chronic congestive heart failure and dilated cardiomyopathy after coxsackievirus myocarditis.

Genitourinary tract manifestations of the group B coxsackieviruses include orchitis and epididymitis. Rare manifestations include glomerulonephritis, pyuria, hematuria, cystitis, and vaginal ulcerative lesions.

Myositis, arthritis, and a dermatomyositis-like syndrome occurring in immunodeficient patients (usually with B cell defects) have been linked to chronic enteroviral infection.

Hand–foot–mouth syndrome, often associated with coxsackievirus A16 or enterovirus 7, is an illness characterized by small intraoral ulcers on the tongue and buccal mucosa associated with vesicular or erythematous macular lesions on the hands, feet, and, occasionally, the buttocks. Nonspecific maculopapular and even petechial rashes also are common during enteroviral infection.

The enteroviruses are the most common cause of seasonal *aseptic meningitis syndrome,* occurring in summer and fall in temperate climates. This syndrome may be associated with other manifestations of enteroviral infection or may be the sole manifestation of the condition. Rash (erythematous, maculopapular, or petechial), sore throat, muscle pain, and signs of meningeal irritation are common, except in infants under 12 mo of age who commonly are infected. CSF usually reveals an early polymorphonuclear cell predominance, shifting to a lymphocytic predominance in 12–24 hr. The median number of cells is 100–150/μL, but occasionally thousands of cells per microliter are seen. CSF protein is mildly elevated, and glucose is normal. The duration of illness is generally 4–6 days of fever and 7–14 days of neurologic signs or symptoms.

The enteroviruses also are probably the most common cause of seasonal *encephalitis* in locales with low arthropod-mediated arboviral activity.

As with poliovirus, the other enteroviruses uncommonly can cause an acute anterior horn cell infection resulting in *paralysis.* Peripheral neuritis and acute hemiplegia also have been associated with enteroviral infection.

Neonatal nonspecific febrile illness may be acquired transplacentally from a mildly ill mother or, more usually, at birth from the sick mother, another sick family member, or a nursery contact. The illness is characterized by fever, irritability, anorexia, mild vomiting, or diarrhea and often is indistinguishable from bacterial sepsis. The duration of the illness is 3–4 days. The peripheral WBC count often is elevated, accompanied by a predominance of polymorphonuclear leukocytes. This illness must be differentiated from neonatal bacterial sepsis and usually requires hospitalization for diagnostic evaluation and empiric antimicrobial therapy. Echovirus 11 has been associated with fulminating neonatal hepatic necrosis.

Myocarditis in the neonate often is due to coxsackieviruses B1–B5. Illness begins abruptly with fever, tachycardia, cardiomegaly, electrocardiographic changes, transient systolic murmurs, shock, and respiratory distress. In the newborn, fulminant *encephalomyocarditis* can occur.

Diagnosis.   Although the season, location, age of the patient, exposure, and clinical manifestations may suggest enteroviral infection, it often is difficult to differentiate this infection from bacterial infection or other viral infections. Definitive diagnosis may be made by culturing enterovirus from a normally sterile site or from biopsy material. Recovering virus from stool or pharyngeal secretions suggests but does not prove that infection exists, because a significant number of infants may be asymptomatically shedding enterovirus during an epidemic or continue to shed vaccine strains after polio immunization. Viral growth requires 3–7 days in tissue culture. If polio virus is isolated, it should be sent to the Centers for Disease Control to distinguish wild polio from vaccine strains. Many of the group A coxsackieviruses require suckling mouse inoculation for recovery. While a 4-fold or greater rise in specific antibody titers in serum is diagnostic, most laboratories will not perform serologic tests in the absence of an isolate because there are a multitude of enteroviruses. However, serum collected at the initial presentation of the patient with the illness and 2–4 wks later may confirm or refute infection, especially in the infant with fecal shedding of virus or in one who has an unusual illness. RNA hybridization with cDNA probes may identify the viral genome in infected tissues.

Treatment. Currently, there are no available specific antiviral therapies for enteroviral infections. In immunocompetent patients, therapy is aimed at anticipating and preventing complications and preparing for the more prolonged phases of rehabilitation, when necessary. Corticosteroid therapy is of no value in any form of enteroviral infection and has worsened experimental murine coxsackievirus myocarditis. Supportive therapy of myocarditis and meningitis is essential and includes providing cardiorespiratory care and controlling increased intracranial pressure, respectively.

Prevention. Poliovirus infection can be prevented almost entirely by vaccination (live oral or inactivated injected preparations) (see Tables 10–3, 10–4, and 10–5). Vaccination is not available for other enteroviruses. Immunocompromised individuals who are exposed to vaccine virus, either by receiving live oral polio vaccine themselves or by being exposed to siblings given polio vaccines, are at increased risk of acquiring paralytic disease. These patients should receive inactivated polio vaccine. In enteroviral epidemics in nurseries, human immunoglobulin may offer some protection to uninfected infants and may benefit immunocompromised patients having antibody deficiency (Bruton's agammaglobulinemia). Enteric precautions are indicated for hospitalized patients for 7 days after the onset of each of these illnesses.

Prognosis. In developed countries, the rate of early mortality from poliovirus infection is 5–7%. Residual disability is influenced by acute management and the extent of appropriate rehabilitation. The major sequelae of nonpolio enteroviral infections are related to myocardial and CNS damage. Young infants, especially those with seizures, may be at higher risk for neurologic sequelae.

References

Behrman RE (ed): Nelson Textbook of Pediatrics. 14th ed. Philadelphia, WB Saunders, 1992, Sec. 12.80.
Bergman I, Painter MJ, Wald ER, et al: Outcome in children with enteroviral meningitis during the first year of life. J Pediatr 110:705, 1987.
de Quadros C, Andrus JK, Olive J-M, et al: Eradication of poliomyelitis: Progress in the Americas. Pediatr Infect Dis J 10:222, 1991.
McKinney RE, Katz SL, Wilfert CM: Chronic enteroviral meningoencephalitis in agammaglobulinemic patients. Rev Infect Dis 9:334, 1987.
Sabin AB: Paralytic poliomyelitis: Old dogmas and new perspectives. Rev Infect Dis 3:543, 1987.
Sutter RW, Patriarca PA, Brogan S, et al: Outbreak of paralytic poliomyelitis in Oman: Evidence for widespread transmission among fully vaccinated children. Lancet 338:715, 1991.

Erythema Infectiosum (Fifth Disease)

Etiology. Erythema infectiosum is caused by human parvovirus B19, which, when following transplacental infection, also may cause hydrops fetalis and/or fetal anemia. Parvovirus is also the most common cause of aplastic crisis in children and adults with chronic hemolytic anemia (sickle cell anemia, spherocytosis, sickle cell–thalassemia). Because the virus reduces erythropoiesis, diseases with a shortened red blood cell half-life demonstrate increasing anemia, whereas patients with normal red cell life span (120 day) may demonstrate reduced reticulocytes but do not develop anemia.

Epidemiology. Community epidemics may occur, usually in the spring. The highest attack rate occurs in school-age children. The mode of transmission is from person to person, and the period of communicability is unknown. The incubation period is generally 12–14 days but may range from 4 to 14 days.

Clinical Manifestations. This illness becomes manifest by rash, low-grade or no fever, and, occasionally, by pharyngitis and mild conjunctivitis. The rash appears in three stages. The initial stage of the rash typically is demonstrated by erythematous cheeks, which gives a "slapped cheek" appearance to the patient as a result of intense facial erythema. One to 4 days later, an erythematous symmetric, maculopapular, truncal rash appears, but later fades as central clearing takes place, giving a distinctive lacy-reticulated rash that lasts 2–40 days (mean 11 days). This rash often is pruritic; does not desquamate; and may recur with exercise, bath, rubbing, or stress. Adolescents may experience myalgia, significant arthralgia or arthritis, headache, pharyngitis, coryza, and gastrointestinal upset. Parvovirus may produce pancytopenia in immunosuppressed patients.

Diagnosis and Differential Diagnosis. Serologic tests demonstrating antibody response to parvovirus and the presence of specific IgM antibody to parvovirus are diagnostic. In serum specimens taken during the acute stage, the virus has been detected by immune electron microscopy and DNA hybridization. A mild leukopenia, thrombocytopenia, and reticulocytopenia may be present. This illness is characteristic, although atypical cases may be confused with other viral exanthems, such as measles, rubella, and enterovirus, as well as with drug rashes or SLE.

Treatment. There is no specific therapy. Respiratory isolation is advisable for 7 days after the onset of illness. Patients with sickle cell anemia may require transfusion until reticulocytosis begins.

References

Behrman RE (ed): Nelson Textbook of Pediatrics. 14th ed. Philadelphia, WB Saunders, 1992, Sec. 9.72.

Bell LM, Naides SJ, Stoffman P, et al: Human parvovirus B19 infection among hospital staff members after contact with infected patients. N Engl J Med 321:485, 1989.

Chorba T, Coccia P, Holman RC, et al: The role of parvovirus B19 in aplastic crisis and erythema infectiosum (fifth disease). J Infect Dis 154:383, 1986.

Committee on Infectious Diseases: Parvovirus, erythema infectiosum, and pregnancy. Pediatrics 85:131, 1990.

Hepatitis

See Chapter 11.

Herpes Virus Infections

The human herpes virus family consists of cytomegalovirus, Epstein-Barr virus, herpes simplex virus, varicella-zoster virus, and human herpesvirus-6 (HHV6). The herpes viruses cause acute primary infection, maintain a state of latency in lymphoid and perhaps in other tissues (neural), may reactivate, and occasionally induce a clinical recurrence, especially in immunocompromised individuals.

CYTOMEGALOVIRUS INFECTION

Etiology. CMV is an enveloped DNA virus that exclusively infects humans.

Epidemiology. CMV is a ubiquitous virus. It is the most commonly known human virus that is transmitted vertically to the fetus (transplacentally, during birth, and by breast milk), but transmission also occurs horizontally from person to person (blood, urine, secretions). In addition, CMV persists in a latent form after a primary infection and reactivation may occur, particularly during immunosuppression. Infection rates are inversely correlated with socioeconomic status. Twenty to 50% of childbearing-age women in the United States are infected, whereas in developing countries the infection rate approaches 100%. Four to 10% of pregnant women excrete virus in cervical secretions or in their urine, and 5–25% shed it in milk during lactation. From 1–3% of children are infected prior to birth, and 10–20% acquire infection in the neonatal period. Day care centers are important areas of CMV transmission in infants and young children. These infected infants act as a source of infection for their seronegative parents.

The transmission of CMV infection requires close contact. Epidemic outbreaks have not been reported, although transmission is common in families, in day care centers, and among sexual partners. CMV can be isolated from saliva, urine, nasopharyngeal secretions, milk, semen, blood, and donor organs (kidneys, bone marrow). The incidence of CMV excretion in day care centers may reach 50–70% in 1–2 yr olds. Although infection of the fetus can result from either primary or recurrent disease in the mother, it is the primary form in the mother that results in symptomatic neonatal illness, which is estimated to occur in 5–10% of infants of mothers with primary infection. Horizontal transmission probably occurs most commonly via saliva, but urine also may be an important medium, especially in day care centers. Blood transfusion with CMV-infected blood cells may induce a mononucleosis-like syndrome in susceptible individuals, an effect that often is noted in massively transfused patients after cardiopulmonary bypass. Blood transfusions from CMV-seropositive donors to seronegative recipients are another source of infection in premature infants, in immunosuppressed patients, and following transplantation. Immunocompromised patients often experience severe primary infection and, usually, less severe recurrent syndromes. Sexually active individuals have a high rate of CMV infection.

The incubation period in horizontal transmission is unknown. Following transplantation of infected tissue, CMV disease occurs between 6 wk and 4 mo later; following blood transfusion, infection occurs in 3–12 wk.

Clinical Manifestations. These vary according to age and immune status of the host.

Neonatal Infection. Over 90% of congenitally infected infants are asymptomatic. A significant number (15%) of infants born to women with asymptomatic or symptomatic primary infection occurring early in pregnancy will have a "TORCH syndrome" (see Chapter 6). Infants infected during maternal reactivation have less severe disease. Premature neonates who are CMV seronegative and who receive blood from CMV-positive donors may develop a syndrome characterized by respiratory distress, pallor, sepsis-like signs, hepatosplenomegaly, neutropenia, thrombocytopenia, and lymphocytosis. A small percent of term infants with perinatally acquired disease develop CMV pneumonitis, petechial rash, intracranial calcifications, and hepatosplenomegaly. Some congenitally infected infants who appear to be asymptomatic at birth will have hearing loss or learning disability in infancy or childhood.

Older Children. Asymptomatic infections are the most common type in older children. A characteristic syndrome caused by CMV in healthy children is a heterophil-negative, mononucleosis-like syndrome and hepatitis. The former often includes fever, malaise, myalgia, headache, anorexia, abdominal pain, and hepatosplenomegaly. Atypical lymphocytosis and reversal of the T cell helper to suppressor cell ratio is characteristic. The degree of pharyngitis and lymphadenopathy generally is less striking than that seen in the EBV-induced mononucleosis syndrome. As occurs in patients with infectious mononucleosis, an ampicillin-induced rash and abnormal serologic reactions, including the presence of cold agglutinins, antinuclear antibodies, rheumatoid factor, and cryoglobulins, may occur in this CMV syndrome. A CMV hepatitis syndrome without other manifestations of the mononucleosis syndrome may occur.

Immunocompromised Hosts. CMV commonly causes serious infection in immunocompromised hosts: In HIV-infected patients, CMV causes retinitis, pneumonia, gastrointestinal ulcers, and encephalitis. The spectrum of disease is different in organ or bone marrow transplant recipients in whom CMV pneumonitis and neutropenia are major problems. Transplanting CMV-negative tissue into CMV-negative patients is recommended. CMV-positive patients may reactivate their endogenous infection or acquire new strains from CMV-positive donors. Active CMV infection may be associated with organ rejection.

Diagnosis. The diagnosis may be difficult to establish because of the high rate of asymptomatic excretion, the frequency of reactivation infections, and the presence of IgM antibody in some episodes of reactivation.

Neonatal Infection. The diagnosis of congenital disease relies on demonstrating CMV in urine, in pharyngeal secretions, or in peripheral blood leukocytes during the 1st wk of life, or on demonstrating a positive CMV-IgM serologic test. The serologic diagnosis is complicated by maternal transplacental IgG antibody and the common occurrence of perinatally acquired disease, making studies after the first few weeks of life inconclusive in establishing the diagnosis of congenital CMV. Negative serologic studies of the infant generally exclude the latter diagnosis, as do negative maternal serologic studies.

The *differential diagnosis* of congenital CMV includes infection with *Toxoplasma*, syphilis, rubella, HSV, HIV, *Listeria monocytogenes*, varicella, and enterovirus.

Acquired Infection. Diagnosis of CMV depends on viral isolation and seroconversion. Diagnosis is especially complicated in immunosuppressed patients, who may not mount an immune response and in whom the finding of CMV in the urine is so common as to be nondiagnostic. Thus, diagnosis of CMV hepatitis or pneumonitis may rest on isolation of CMV from the specific site by biopsy, bronchoscopy (bronchoalveolar lavage), or other invasive tests. The isolation of CMV from blood or buffy coat cells has been associated with the presence of invasive CMV disease. Appropriate serologic tests should exclude infection caused by hepatitis A and B viruses and EBV. New antigen detection tests by nucleic acid hybridization or ELISA may simplify the diagnosis of CMV, if appropriate tissue specimens are available.

Treatment. Serious CMV infections in immunocompromised patients can be treated with ganciclovir or foscarnet (Table 10–17). CMV pneumonitis has been treated with ganciclovir and intravenous immunoglobulin. Minimally symptomatic immunocompetent patients require no treatment.

Prevention. In several patient populations, including immunocompromised individuals, seronegative premature neonates, or individuals about to receive a renal transplant, use of blood or kidneys from CMV-seronegative donors or glycerol frozen blood can prevent potentially serious primary infection. Seronegative premature infants should not receive fresh human milk from nonmaternal sources because the rate of CMV excretion in milk is high. Prophylactic ganciclovir may reduce infection in transplant recipients.

Prognosis. Symptomatic congenital infection carries a guarded outlook regarding neurologic sequelae, especially in the child with microcephaly or intracranial calcifications. Hearing loss is a common complication of congenital CMV infection. Acquired infection in the healthy host usually is self-limited, whereas it may be fatal in the immunocompromised host as a result of pneumonitis, encephalitis, or secondary opportunistic infections.

References

Behrman RE (ed): Nelson Textbook of Pediatrics. 14th ed. Philadelphia, WB Saunders, 1992, Sec. 12.71.

Boppana SB, Pass RF, Britt WJ, et al: Symptomatic congenital cytomegalovirus infection: Neonatal morbidity and mortality. Pediatr Infect Dis J 11:93, 1992.

Horwitz CV, Henle W, Henle G, et al: Clinical and laboratory evaluation of cytomegalovirus-induced mononucleosis in previously healthy individuals. Medicine 65:124, 1986.

Ljungman P, Engelhard D, Link H, et al: Treatment of interstitial pneumonitis due to cytomegalovirus with ganciclovir and intravenous immune globulin: Experience of European bone marrow transplant group. Clin Infect Dis 14:831, 1992.

Murph JR, Baron JC, Brown CK, et al: The occupational risk of cytomegalovirus infection among day-care providers. JAMA 265:603, 1991.

Ramsay MEB, Miller E, Peckham CS: Outcome of confirmed symptomatic congenital cytomegalovirus infection. Arch Dis Child 66:1068, 1991.

EPSTEIN-BARR VIRUS INFECTION (INFECTIOUS MONONUCLEOSIS)

Etiology. EBV, a DNA virus, is a human herpes virus that causes infectious mononucleosis in children.

Epidemiology. EBV infection occurs at an early age in persons in developing countries; most children are seropositive by 3 yr of age. In developed countries, age of infection is inversely related to socioeconomic level; 60–80% of adolescents from lower socioeconomic levels are seropositive. In higher socioeconomic levels, infection typically occurs during high school or college attendance. Susceptible Yale University students demonstrated a 15% seroconversion rate per year. Endemic disease in group settings of adolescents is common.

EBV is transmitted by salivary exchange, contact with contaminated objects, or, less commonly, blood transfusions. It is spread by intimate contact, and EBV is shed in the saliva before and during clinically apparent infection. In addition, 10–20% of healthy seropositive individuals and 60% of seropositive immunosuppressed individuals shed virus intermittently; therefore, the period of communicability is not known. The incubation period is 30–50 days.

Pharyngeal epithelial cells are probably the initial target of viral infection and replication. Circulating B lymphocytes then are infected and widely disseminate the virus until the immune system (particularly natural killer cells and T cells) limits infection. The B cells remain latently infected and immortalized in vitro when cultured.

Clinical Manifestations. The clinical manifestations of EBV are age related and range from asymptomatic to fatal infections. Infants and young children infected with EBV usually are asymptomatic or experience mild disease that may include tonsillitis, fever, or upper respiratory tract disease. In older children and young adults, a typical infectious mononucleosis syndrome (pharyngitis, fever, lymphadenopathy, hepatosplenomegaly, lymphocytosis) may develop after EBV infection.

The prodromal period of infectious mononucleosis includes malaise, fatigue, headache, nausea, and abdominal pain lasting 1–2 wk. The typical symptoms and signs of mononucleosis include pharyngitis (with enlarged tonsils and exudate), an enanthema (pharyngeal petechiae), fever, lymphadenopathy (posterior cervical; epitrochlear; less commonly, generalized), splenomegaly (up to 50% of patients), and hepatomegaly (10–20%). Eyelid edema and maculopapular or urticarial rash occur in 5–15% of cases. Group A streptococci may be recovered from the pharynx in 30% of children. Approximately 80% of patients treated with ampicillin will develop a diffuse erythematous rash. The symptoms last 2–4 wk, then slowly abate.

Oncogenicity of EBV. EBV is probably the initiator of African Burkitt lymphoma in children and of adult nasopharyngeal carcinoma in the Orient. Polyclonal B cell lymphoma in immunocompromised patients and X-linked lymphoproliferative disease (see under Complications) have been shown to be EBV associated.

Complications. As a result of rapid swelling, splenic rupture may occur. The pharyngeal tonsillar hypertrophy may cause airway obstruction. Neurologic complications include seizures, ataxia, aseptic meningitis syndrome, Bell palsy, transverse myelitis, encephalitis, and Guillain-Barré syndrome. Other complications include hepatitis (85% of cases); myocarditis; interstitial pneumonia; Coombs-positive hemolytic anemia; antibody-mediated thrombocytopenia; hemophagocytic syndrome; and, rarely, aplastic anemia, pancreatitis, parotitis, orchitis, and Reye syndrome.

In several kindreds, a rare syndrome of *X-linked lymphoproliferative disease* (Duncan syndrome) following EBV infection has occurred. The affected males may die of overwhelming infection; may survive and develop B cell lymphoproliferative disease; or may develop hypoplastic syndromes, such as aplastic anemia or hypogammaglobulinemia. Rarely, immunocompromised patients (transplantation, AIDS, ataxia-telangiectasia, severe combined immunodeficiency disorders) and apparently healthy patients may have the same fate.

Diagnosis.   Nonspecific findings often include a leukocytosis of 10,000–20,000 cells/μL, with at least 20–40% being atypical lymphocytes. These lymphocytes are T cells responding to EBV-infected B cells. Children under 5 yr of age have less striking atypical lymphocytosis. Mild thrombocytopenia occurs in 50% of individuals and elevated liver enzymes occur in approximately 85%.

Nonspecific tests for the heterophil antibody include the Paul-Bunnell test and the slide agglutination reaction, both of which are based on the appearance of IgM antibody against sheep, horse, or oxen red blood cells not absorbable by guinea pig kidney cells. These are present in the serum for up to 6 mo after EBV infection. This antibody response generally is absent in children under 5 yr of age, but will identify about 90% of cases in older children and adults. Specific diagnosis of EBV infection involves analysis for several types of antibodies against specific EBV antigens.

Serologic Response to EBV Infection.   The most commonly performed test is that for detecting antibodies to viral capsid antigen (VCA). At the time of the onset of symptoms, most patients have high IgG anti-VCA and IgM anti-VCA antibodies, as well as antibodies to early antigen (EA). The absence or low level of antibody to Epstein-Barr nuclear antigen (EBNA) and the presence of the anti-VCA antibody indicates acute infection. High levels of IgG anti-VCA and anti-EBNA and absence of IgM anti-VCA and anti-EA indicate previous (not acute) infection. Absence of all anti-EBV antibodies indicates a susceptible, uninfected individual. These serologic tests are particularly useful for evaluating young patients who have heterophil-negative infectious mononucleosis or for those with isolated organ manifestations, such as myocarditis, FUO, or encephalitis.

EBV DNA also can be demonstrated in infected cells by DNA hybridization.

Differential Diagnosis.   The differential diagnosis includes cytomegalovirus infection, toxoplasmosis, hepatitis A, lymphoma, and leukemia. Less commonly confused conditions are rubella, leptospirosis, Kawasaki syndrome, HIV infection, human herpesvirus-6, and streptococcal infection.

Treatment.   The typical patient with mononucleosis requires no antiviral therapy. Bed rest is indicated by the patient's needs and does not improve the course. Acyclovir may have some beneficial effects in life-threatening EBV infection. Corticosteroids have been utilized for respiratory distress resulting from tonsillar hypertrophy, thrombocytopenia, hemolytic anemia, and neurologic complications. Although steroids have been shown to shorten the course of the acute illness, they should not be used in uncomplicated cases.

Prevention.   There are no measures to prevent EBV infection. Patients with recent EBV infection should not donate blood. Splenic trauma should be avoided by limiting athletics and repeated examinations.

References

Alpert G, Fleisher GR: Complications of infection with Epstein-Barr virus during childhood: A study of children admitted to the hospital. Pediatr Infect Dis 3:304, 1984.

Behrman RE (ed): Nelson Textbook of Pediatrics. 14th ed. Philadelphia, WB Saunders, 1992, Sec. 12.72.

Grierson H, Purtillo DT: Epstein-Barr infections in males with the X-linked lymphoproliferative syndrome. Ann Intern Med 106:538, 1987.

Sumaya CV: Epstein-Barr virus infection: The expanded spectrum. In Aronoff SC, Hughes WT Jr, Kohl S, et al (eds): Advances in Pediatric Infectious Diseases. Chicago, Year Book Medical Publishers, 1986, p 75.

HERPES SIMPLEX VIRUS INFECTION

Etiology.   HSVs are large DNA viruses of two types exhibiting major antigenic and genomic differences. Although either virus can be found in any site, nongenital type 1 (HSV-1) usually occurs above the waist (CNS, eyes, mouth), and genital type 2 (HSV-2) generally involves the genitalia and skin below the waist; HSV type 2 generally occurs in the neonate at any site. *Primary infection* occurs in nonimmune individuals who have never been previously infected. This infection often is asymptomatic but may cause a typical clinical syndrome. In the majority of infected individuals, the virus attains a state of *latency* in neural tissue. *Reactivation* of latent virus may result in a characteristic clinical syndrome of herpetic *recurrence*. In addition, another exposure to a second type or even a second strain of the same type can result in exogenous *reinfection*.

Epidemiology.   The incubation period is 2–12 days, with a mean of 6–7 days. Approximately 85% of infections are asymptomatic. Institutional and family outbreaks have occurred. Close body contact (saliva, kissing, wrestling, sexual) and inoculation of mucous membranes or disrupted skin are required for infection. After the loss of transplacental antibodies, infants and young children begin to be infected with HSV-1. At the onset of sexual activity, HSV-2 infection becomes more common. HSV infection occurs more frequently in individuals from lower socioeconomic status groups. Approximately 2–5% of healthy individuals will shed HSV in oral secretions at any time.

Pathology.   The classic findings are intranuclear inclusion bodies and multinucleated giant cells. Immunity requires T cell–mediated activity and anti-HSV antibodies.

Clinical Manifestations

Skin and Mucous Membranes.   Primary infection of the skin in neonates is common. Autoinoculation from another site may cause a localized vesicular eruption on an erythematous base. Healing is complete in 7–14 days. Recurrences occur at the same site. Infection of a digit causes a viral paronychia, referred to as a **herpetic whitlow**, which is painful, erythematous, and occasionally presents with a vesicular eruption. It is found in children who suck their thumbs and bite their nails. In older children it may be found concomitantly with genital herpes, whereas in health care professionals it usually is nosocomially acquired. Abraded or burned skin is quite susceptible to HSV infection. In this setting, the lesions often are atypical, with ulcers predominating. Wrestlers and rugby players acquire cutaneous herpes from close body contact with the cutaneous infections of other players (herpes gladiatorum and herpes rugbiaforum). Erythema multiforme also is associated with HSV.

Acute Herpetic Gingivostomatitis.   This is the most common clinical manifestation of primary HSV infection in infants and children beyond the neonatal period. It generally occurs in 1–3 yr olds, although it may occur at any age. The onset is abrupt, with mouth pain, salivation, fetor oris, dysphagia, anorexia, and fever. The vesicles usually rupture, and the typical lesion is ulcerative. The anterior and, less commonly, the posterior oropharynx are involved, with lesions in the gingiva, buccal mucosa, tongue, and lips and, following autoinoculation, on the skin of neck and nose. Regional lymphadenopathy is common. The illness lasts 7–14 days. **Herpangina**, an enteroviral infection, may be differentiated by its vesicles and ulcers, which occur predominantly in the posterior pharynx. In adolescents, a severe exudative pharyngitis may be the manifestation of primary oral HSV infection.

Recurrent stomatitis is the typical fever blister that occurs on the mucocutaneous junction. These lesions are a recurrence of oral HSV infection and are not associated with systemic signs or symptoms.

Eczema Herpeticum (Kaposi Varicelliform Eruption).   This is a serious, usually primary HSV infection that occurs in individuals with eczema. It may be generalized and involve many areas of skin, producing vesicles, ulcers, and hemorrhagic crusts. High temperature (40.0–40.5°C [104–105°F]) for 7–10 days and recurrent attacks are common. In severe cases, the widespread infection acts as a burn, causing fluid loss and hyponatremia. Dissemination to visceral organs or the brain may occur. In previous times, this infection had to be differentiated from vaccinia, variola, and varicella.

Ocular Lesions.   Conjunctivitis and keratoconjunctivitis may be manifestations of primary or recurrent infection at any age. The conjunctiva is erythematous and swollen, without purulence. Corneal lesions may occur as dendritic or ameboid ulcers or more commonly, in recurrent infection, as a deep keratitis. Vesicular lid lesions, if present, should suggest the diagnosis. HSV, along with bacteria and other viruses, always should be included in the differential diagnosis of conjunctivitis (Table 10–15). Steroids, which worsen HSV ocular infection, should not be used in patients with herpes conjunctivitis. Ocular manifestations of neonates infected with HSV may include cataracts, uveitis, and chorioretinitis, in addition to conjunctivitis and keratoconjunctivitis.

Encephalitis.   HSV is the most common cause of fatal, sporadic viral encephalitis. Beyond the neonatal period, it is predominantly caused by HSV-1. It may be a manifestation of primary or recurrent disease. The mortality rate is over 75% if the infection is not treated. Although it resembles other forms of encephalitis with alterations of mentation, fever, and seizures, the characteristic features of HSV encephalitis are clinical signs of *focal* CNS disease, as evidenced by EEG or neuroradiologic signs of focality, especially in the temporal lobe. The spinal fluid usually reveals lymphocytosis, elevated protein, normal glucose, and red blood cells. The CSF culture is negative for bacteria or HSV (HSV may be recovered in neonatal disease). Detection of HSV antigen or DNA may aid the diagnosis.

Genital Herpes. This condition occurs most commonly in adolescents or young adults. It may be a sign of early sexual activity or child abuse in younger children. About 75% of cases are due to HSV-2. Primary symptomatic infection becomes manifest by vesicular, ulcerative, and crusted lesions in the genital areas of males or females. In females, the cervix is involved as well. Systemic symptoms of fever, adenopathy, paresthesia, and dysuria are common. The course of illness lasts 10–20 days. In patients practicing rectal intercourse, a similar syndrome involving the perirectal area occurs.

Recurrent genital tract disease is characterized by localized vesicles, ulcers, and crusts that last for several days without systemic symptoms. Recurrences occur in 50–80% of patients with primary symptomatic genital tract disease.

Complications of primary genital tract herpes infection include a self-limited aseptic meningitis syndrome. HSV infection of the genital tract of pregnant women can result in the transmission of infection to their offspring.

Disseminated (Systemic) Infection of the Neonate. The majority of neonatal HSV is caused by HSV-2 and is acquired when the infant passes through an infected birth canal. Infants also can be infected by nongenital maternal or nosocomial sources. The majority of infected mothers are asymptomatic, and usually no history of maternal or paternal genital HSV infection is discovered. The incidence of premature birth is higher than expected. Initial symptoms of disseminated neonatal disease generally occur within 1 wk of birth; diseases localized to the CNS or to the skin, eyes, and mouth more often occur 2–3 wk following birth.

Clinical manifestations in the neonate include (1) a vesicular or pustular eruption; (2) a nonfocal meningoencephalitis syndrome; (3) a respiratory distress pneumonic syndrome; and (4) a generalized, systemic infection involving several internal organs, including the CNS and liver. The systemic infection progresses to acidosis, coagulopathy, shock, and death in the majority of untreated cases. Unfortunately, the telltale vesicular eruption often is late in appearing or does not appear at all (20–30%) prior to the infant's demise. Of all infants who present with only local signs, such as vesicles, conjunctivitis, and mouth lesions, 70% will have infection that will disseminate to other organs. Thus, *any* manifestation of HSV infection in the neonate should be treated with antiviral chemotherapy. If left untreated, the mortality of neonatal HSV infection is 50%, with 50% of survivors having significant sequelae. Even localized disease of the skin, eyes, and mouth is associated with sequelae in 10–15% of infants.

Immunocompromised Patients. Patients with T cell disorders, severe combined immunodeficiency, AIDS, lymphoma, leukemia, or severe malnutrition and those undergoing chemotherapy or transplantation procedures have a significant increase in susceptibility to serious HSV infection. This becomes manifest rarely as disseminated disease but frequently as severe recurrences, which are typically focal, necrotic, painful lesions that heal slowly. Rarely, these lesions disseminate to other areas of skin or visceral organs. In immunosuppressed patients, HSV commonly causes mucositis and esophagitis as a result of local spread from oral infection. Less commonly, pneumonitis, hepatitis, and, rarely, chronic encephalitis occur.

Diagnosis. Cytologic examination (Tzanck stain, Papanicolaou stain) may reveal cells with characteristic intranuclear inclusions or giant cells. These indicate either HSV or varicella-zoster virus infection. Antigen detection tests, such as fluorescent antibody and enzyme-linked immunoassays, are rapid and specific but are only 50–80% sensitive. The test of choice is tissue culture for viral cytopathic effects, which is rapid (2–5 days), specific, and sensitive.

Acute and convalescent antibody testing may be diagnostic in primary infection but is not helpful for making clinically useful decisions. Most neonates have transplacental anti-HSV antibody, patients with recurrences have high and stable levels of antibody, and severely immunosuppressed children may fail to produce any antibody.

Treatment. Therapy of HSV infection depends on the type of the disease (primary, recurrent), the anatomic sites involved, and, most importantly, the immune status of the host. No treatment is needed for mild, self-limited infection in immunocompetent children (gingivostomatitis, "cold sores"). Acyclovir is used either orally for uncomplicated infections (primary genital lesions) or intravenously for more serious (encephalitis) or disseminated (immunocompromised host, neonate) infections. Topical therapy with trifluridine, vidarabine, or iododeoxyuridine is indicated for ocular infection.

Prevention. The acquisition in neonates is greatest when mothers have a primary genital infection at the time of delivery; operative delivery is suggested to prevent neonatal disease. Prepartum HSV cultures do not predict the presence of the virus at the time of delivery. Chronic acyclovir occasionally is used in patients with frequent or severe recurrences of genital herpes infections. The use of condoms provides some protection against sexual transmission of herpes simplex.

References

Behrman RE (ed): Nelson Textbook of Pediatrics. 14th ed. Philadelphia, WB Saunders, 1992, Sec. 12.68.

Belongia EA, Goodman JL, Holland EJ: An outbreak of herpes gladiatorum at a high-school wrestling camp. N Engl J Med 325:906, 1991.

Gibbs RS, Mead PB: Preventing neonatal herpes—current strategies. N Engl J Med 326:946, 1992.

Mertz GJ, Benedetti J, Ashley R, et al: Risk factors for the sexual transmission of genital herpes. Ann Intern Med 116:197, 1992.

Whitley R, Arvin A, Prober C, et al: A controlled trial comparing vidarabine with acyclovir in neonatal herpes simplex virus infection. N Engl J Med 324:444, 1991.

Whitley R, Arvin A, Prober C, et al: Predictors of morbidity and mortality in neonates with herpes simplex virus infections. N Engl J Med 324:450, 1991.

VARICELLA-ZOSTER VIRUS INFECTION

Etiology. Varicella-zoster virus (VZV) causes a primary infection (varicella or chickenpox) or an endogenously reactivated recurrent infection (herpes zoster or shingles). In primary infection VZV enters the conjuctivae or the upper respiratory tract. VZV replicates in the regional lymphatic tissues and disseminates via a primary viremia. Replication then occurs in the liver, spleen, and elsewhere and is followed by a secondary viremia, resulting in cutaneous infection with the characteristic vesicular rash. There is one antigenic type of varicella; humans are the only source of infection.

Varicella (Chickenpox)

Epidemiology. Varicella is a highly contagious infection of childhood. The peak age of occurrence is 5–10 yr; 90% of children in temperate climates are infected by age 10. The secondary household attack rates in susceptible individuals is 90%. The peak seasonal infection rate is late winter and spring. Transmission is by direct contact, droplet, and air. The incubation period is generally 14–16 days, with a range of 11–20 days after contact. The period of communicability ranges from 2 days before to 7 days after the onset of the rash when all lesions are crusted. Patients with zoster may initiate varicella in seronegative contacts.

Clinical Manifestations. Primary infection with VZV results in chickenpox. Prodromal symptoms (fever, malaise, anorexia) may precede the rash by 1 day. The characteristic rash appears initially as small red papules that rapidly progress to nonumbilicated, oval, "teardrop" vesicles on an erythematous base. The fluid progresses from clear to cloudy, and the vesicles ulcerate, crust, and heal. New crops appear for 3–4 days, usually beginning on the trunk and then the head, the face, and, less commonly, the extremities. In total, there may be 100–300 lesions, with all forms of lesions being present at the same time. Pruritus is almost universal. Lesions may be present on all mucous membranes. Lymphadenopathy may be generalized. The severity of the rash varies, as do systemic signs and fever, which generally abate after 3–4 days.

Congenital Varicella. Varicella in the pregnant woman may result in fetal varicella infection, characterized by low birth weight, cortical atrophy, seizures, mental retardation, chorioretinitis, cataracts, microcephaly, intracranial calcifications, and diagnostic cicatricial scarring of the body or extremities.

In mothers with varicella (not shingles) occurring 5 days before or 2 days after delivery, a severe varicella syndrome develops that is thought to be due to the lack of transplacental antibody in these neonates. These infants should be treated as soon as possible with zoster immune globulin (ZIG) to attempt to prevent or ameliorate their infection. Children who were exposed in utero to VZV may develop zoster early in life without ever exhibiting varicella.

Complications. Although VZV infection is generally a mild disease, complications are common. Varicella is a more severe disease for neonates, adults, and immunosuppressed individuals. Secondary infection of skin lesions by streptococci or staphylococci is the most common complication. Thrombocytopenia and hemorrhagic lesions or bleeding also may occur (purpura fulminans, varicella gangrenosa). Pneumonia is uncommon in healthy children but occurs in 15–20% of healthy adults and immunosuppressed patients. Myocarditis, pericarditis, orchitis, hepatitis, ulcerative gastritis, glomerulonephritis, and arthritis complicate VZV. Reye syndrome may be preceded by varicella and, therefore, aspirin should be avoided during varicella infection.

Neurologic complications include postinfectious encephalitis, cerebellar ataxia, nystagmus, and tremor. Guillain-Barré syndrome, transverse myelitis, cranial nerve palsies, optic neuritis, and hypothalamic syndrome have been associated with varicella.

In immunodeficient or immunosuppressed children, primary varicella can be a fatal disease as a result of visceral dissemination, encephalitis, and pneumonitis. In children with leukemia who have not received prophylaxis or therapy for varicella, the mortality rate approaches 10%.

Diagnosis.   Vesicles contain polymorphonuclear leukocytes. Cytology and electron microscopy of vesicular fluid or scrapings may reveal intranuclear inclusions, giant cells, and virus particles. VZV is fastidious and difficult to culture. If the cytology is consistent with either HSV or VZV but is culture negative, it may indicate VZV. Infection can be confirmed by detection of varicella specific antigen in vesicular fluid with immunofluorescence of monoclonal antibodies or by testing acute and convalescent antibody for VZV antibody.

Treatment.   Symptomatic therapy of varicella includes nonaspirin antipyretics, cool baths, and careful hygiene. Intravenous acyclovir is effective in treating varicella in immunocompromised patients. Early therapy prevents severe complications, including pneumonia, encephalitis, and death. Oral acyclovir shortens the duration of illness in normal children; however, it is uncertain if acyclovir's cost justifies its use in otherwise healthy children. ZIG is not effective therapy once the disease has been contracted.

Prevention.   A live attenuated vaccine is licensed in several countries and is undergoing clinical trials in the United States. It appears safe for all individuals, including some immunocompromised children.

Passive immunity can be induced by use of ZIG, which is indicated within 96 hr of exposure for susceptible individuals at risk for severe illness. Candidates for ZIG include immunocompromised or immunosuppressed individuals, neonates of infected mothers who had onset of chickenpox within 5 days before delivery or 48 hr after delivery, premature infants of less than 28 wk or those born to mothers lacking a prior history of chickenpox, and possibly children older than 15 yr or adults with a close exposure to varicella. Children should not return to school until all vesicles have crusted. The hospitalized child with varicella should be isolated in a room that will prevent the air-circulation system from transmitting the virus.

Herpes Zoster (Shingles)

Epidemiology.   This condition is a recurrence of VZV in individuals previously infected. After the episode of chickenpox, VZV remains latent in nerve ganglion cells, but for unknown reasons (other than immunosuppression) a local recurrence occurs. Herpes zoster is unusual in children under 10 yr of age. Infants and young children with herpes zoster often will have a history of early or presumed in utero varicella. Immunocompromised or immunosuppressed children have an increased incidence of herpes zoster.

Clinical Manifestations.   The pre-eruption phase of shingles includes intense localized pain and tenderness along a dermatome, accompanied by malaise and fever. In several days, the eruption of papules, which quickly vesiculate, occurs in the dermatome or in two adjacent dermatomes. Groups of lesions occur for 1–7 days, then progress to crusts and healing. The typical areas involved are dorsal and lumbar, although cephalic and sacral lesions may develop. Lesions generally are unilateral and are accompanied by regional lymphadenopathy. In one third of patients, a few vesicles occur outside the primary dermatome.

Any branch of the Vth cranial nerve may be involved, which also may cause corneal and intraoral lesions. Involvement of the VIIth cranial nerve may result in facial paralysis and ear canal vesicles (Ramsay Hunt syndrome). Ophthalmic zoster may be associated with ipsilateral cerebral angiitis and stroke. Immunocompromised patients may have unusually severe, painful herpes zoster that involves cutaneous and, rarely, visceral dissemination (to liver, lungs, and CNS). Skin lesions may be chronic and hemorrhagic. Postherpetic neuralgia and ocular complications are rare in normal children. Secondary bacterial infections may occur.

Diagnosis.   The differentiation between VZV and HSV infections is difficult because HSV may cause infection in a dermatome distribution. The previously healthy patient with more than one recurrence probably has HSV infection, which can be confirmed by culture.

Treatment.   VZV infection in immunocompromised patients is treated with acyclovir, either orally or parenterally depending on the severity of the infection. Acyclovir therapy decreases pain, shortens the duration of viral shedding, and decreases visceral dissemination.

Prevention. There is no clinically useful way to prevent herpes zoster. Patients with herpes zoster are infectious to VZV-susceptible individuals.

References

Behrman RE (ed): Nelson Textbook of Pediatrics. 14th ed. Philadelphia, WB Saunders, 1992, Sec. 12.69.

Brunell PA: Varicella in pregnancy, the fetus, and the newborn: Problems in management. J Infect Dis 166(Suppl 1):S42, 1992.

Dunkle LM, Arvin AM, Whitley RJ, et al: A controlled trial of acyclovir for chickenpox in normal children. N Engl J Med 325:1539, 1991.

Gershon AA, Steinberg S, NIAID Collaborative Varicella Vaccine Study Group: Live attenuated varicella vaccine: Protection in healthy adults in comparison to leukemic children. J Infect Dis 161:661, 1990.

Jackson MA, Burry VF, Olson LC: Complications of varicella requiring hospitalization in previously healthy children. Pediatr Infect Dis J 11:441, 1992.

Whitley RJ, Gnann JW, Hinthorn D, et al: Disseminated herpes zoster in the immunocompromised host: A comparative trial of acyclovir and vidarabine. J Infect Dis 165:450, 1992.

Human Herpesvirus-6 (Exanthem Subitum, Roseola Infantum)

Etiology. Roseola infection also is referred to as exanthem subitum or sixth disease and is caused by primary infection with human herpesvirus-6. This virus also commonly causes an acute illness characterized by high fever and otitis media in young children but without the roseola rash.

Epidemiology. Illness predominates in the spring and fall. The incubation period is 7–17 days. It is a sporadic disease of infants 6–18 mo of age but occasionally occurs in small outbreaks or epidemics in older age groups. Blood and throat washings from acutely infected patients have transmitted infection to infants and monkeys. Reactivation and salivary secretion may be another source of infection from asymptomatic adults.

Clinical Manifestations. The onset of high fever (temperature rising to 41.1°C [106°F]), occasionally with a seizure, is typical. Physical findings are minimal and the child generally appears well. The WBC count is often 16,000–20,000 cells/μL, and an increase in neutrophils occurs during the first 24–36 hr. By the 2nd day, leukopenia is evident,

accompanied by lymphocytosis. By the 3rd or 4th day, the fever rapidly declines, at which point a macular or maculopapular eruption appears. The rash begins on the trunk, spreads to the arms and neck, and may involve the face and legs. The rash fades in 24 hr.

Immunosuppressed patients may develop hepatitis, interstitial pneumonia, or asymptomatic reactivation.

Differential Diagnosis. The characteristic timing of the onset of rash immediately following defervescence of fever is not typical of other viral exanthems (rubella, rubeola, enteroviral infection). The differential diagnosis of the infant with high fever and granulocytosis must include local infections (otitis media, pneumonia, pyelonephritis, meningitis) and nonlocalized bacteremia (especially pneumococcal). No specific diagnostic tests are known.

Treatment and Prevention. No prophylaxis or specific therapy is available for this condition.

References

Behrman RE (ed): Nelson Textbook of Pediatrics. 14th ed. Philadelphia, WB Saunders, 1992, Sec. 12.66.

Leach CT, Sumaya CV, Brown NA: Human herpesvirus-6: Clinical implications of a recently discovered, ubiquitous agent. J Pediatr 121:173, 1992.

Pruksananonda P, Hall CB, Insel RA, et al: Primary human herpesvirus 6 infection in young children. N Engl J Med 326:1445, 1992.

Human Immunodeficiency Virus Infection (Acquired Immunodeficiency Syndrome)

Etiology. The cause of AIDS in infants, children, and adults is HIV. HIV is one of several retroviruses that are RNA viruses possessing the unique enzyme reverse transcriptase that allows viral RNA to act as a template for DNA transcription and incorporation into the host genome.

Pathogenesis. HIV selectively infects human helper T cells (CD4 cells, OKT4 or Leu3 +) via the CD4 surface receptor, which results in the lytic destruction of T helper cells, thereby reducing their number. Because helper T cells are important for delayed hypersensitivity, for T cell–dependent B cell antibody production, and for T cell–mediated lymphokine activation of macrophages, their destruction produces a profound combined (B and T cell) immunodeficiency. Lack of T cell regulation and unrestrained antigenic stimulation results in a nonspecific and ineffective polyclonal hypergammaglobulinemia. Infection of macrophages disseminates the virus throughout the body. Infection of brain tissue accounts for the encephalopathy and cerebral atrophy associated with the condition.

Epidemiology. HIV is transmitted by contaminated blood and blood products, body secretions (semen, breast milk), infected organs, and, in the pregnant woman, vertically to the fetus. Thus, lifestyles (homosexual or heterosexual promiscuity, intravenous drug use, prostitution), conditions requiring multiple or frequent use of blood products (hemophilia, sick neonates), or birth to an infected mother leads to a high risk of HIV infection. As the rate of infected women increases as a result of heterosexual or parenteral drug abuse transmission, so will the incidence of infant AIDS. In the pediatric population, the mode of acquisition depends on the age of the individual. The neonate and infant (<15 mo old) acquire HIV from vertical transmission as a result of birth to an infected mother (with an estimated 20–40% transmission rate, accounting for 80% of pediatric AIDS) or from receipt of infected blood products. As adolescents become sexually active and experiment with intra-

Table 10–19. Indicator Diseases for Presumptive Diagnosis of AIDS in Children*

Pneumocystis carinii pneumonia
Multiple severe bacterial infections
Kaposi sarcoma
Lymphoid interstitial pneumonia
Candidiasis (esophagus, trachea, lung)
Extrapulmonary cryptococcosis, coccidioidomycosis, or histoplasmosis
Persistent cryptosporidiosis or isosporiasis (diarrhea >1 mo)
CMV (retinitis, colitis, pneumonia)
HSV (pneumonitis, esophagitis, cutaneous ulcer)
CNS lymphoma
CNS toxoplasmosis
HIV encephalopathy
Progressive multifocal leukoencephalopathy (papovavirus)
Mycobacterium avium-intracellulare infection (nonpulmonary)
Mycobacterium tuberculosis infection
Recurrent pyogenic bacteremia (*Pneumococcus, Salmonella*)
Lymphoma (atypical)
HIV wasting syndrome

* Other causes of immunodeficiency or immunosuppression should be excluded.
(Modified from JAMA 258:1143, 1987.)

Table 10–20. Manifestations of AIDS

Infant
Failure to thrive
Lymphoid interstitial pneumonia
Opportunistic infection
Chronic otitis media
Recurrent bacterial sepsis
Persistent diarrhea
Hepatosplenomegaly
Lymphadenopathy
Salivary gland enlargement
Encephalopathy
Thrombocytopenia
Hypergammaglobulinemia
Heart failure
Nephropathy

Older Child and Adolescent
Fever
Lymphadenopathy
Opportunistic infection
Thrombocytopenia
Failure to thrive (wasting syndrome)
Encephalopathy
Malignancy
Syphilis (refractory to therapy)
Bacillary angiomatosis

venous drugs, their modes of acquisition are similar to those of adults.

Currently pediatric AIDS is predominantly an illness of blacks (58%) and hispanics (23%) because of the risk factors of maternal drug addiction and heterosexual activity with high-risk males. In Africa, AIDS is transmitted by heterosexual activity and by receiving infected blood.

Clinical Manifestations. The incubation period may be as long as 7–10 yr, but it is 1–24 mo with a mean of 5 mo after vertical transmission, a much shorter period than seen in adults. The major clinical manifestations of AIDS are related to immunodeficiency, resulting in frequent and often unusual infections (Table 10–19). In adults and adolescents, a prodromal period of weight loss, fever, malaise, lymphadenopathy, and diarrhea occurs. The manifestations in infants and children are noted in Table 10–20. Pulmonary manifestations are common and include *P. carinii* pneumonia, which must be differentiated from **lymphoid interstitial pneumonia.** The latter is characterized by cough, digital clubbing, lymphadenopathy, and a nodular chest roentgenographic pattern, whereas *P. carinii* pneumonia becomes manifest as tachypnea, retractions, reduced breath sounds, rales, and fever. *P. carinii* infection often is related to CD4 cell counts and occurs when CD4 cell counts are less than 750 in children under 2 yr of age or less than 500 in older children.

The mortality rate in symptomatic pediatric AIDS is approximately 65%, with an increasing rate as the period of follow-up lengthens.

Diagnosis. HIV infection results in a decrease in helper T cells, decreased T helper–T suppressor ratio (normal 1.5:1–2:1; AIDS, <1:1), polyclonal hypergammaglobulemia, and decreased or absent response of lymphocytes to mitogens and antigens. These characteristic findings also usually are associated with the presence of anti-HIV antibody and HIV antigen (p24) in serum and of HIV virus and RNA in blood.

The early destruction of the immune system in infants may result in hypogammaglobulinemia and absent antibody to HIV. In children born to mothers who are HIV seropositive, the diagnosis of HIV infection can be established prior to onset of symptoms by demonstrating persistent or rising HIV antibody titers, by demonstrating the presence of IgM or IgA to HIV, or by detecting antigen or RNA (by polymerase chain reaction) or virus. Initial infection is associated with viremia (antigenemia), which may be followed by clearance of virus and the appearance of antibody as determined by ELISA. The isolation of specific antibody is confirmed by Western blot (antibody to specific viral protein). Decline of these antibodies may herald the reappearance of virus (antigen) and the onset of AIDS.

The diagnosis of AIDS is made by serologic evidence of HIV infection and the presence of an indicator disease (Table 10–19). The definition of AIDS in children differs from that for adults in two ways. First, multiple or recurrent serious bacterial infections and lymphoid interstitial pneumonia/pulmonary lymphoid hyperplasia are accepted as indicative of AIDS among children but not among adults. Second, for children less than 15 mo of age whose mothers are thought to have had HIV infection during the child's perinatal period, the laboratory criteria for establishing HIV infection are more stringent because the presence of IgG HIV antibody in the child is insufficient evidence for HIV infection because passively acquired maternal antibodies persist for up to 15 mo after birth.

The *differential diagnosis* includes primary immunodeficiency syndromes (usually found in HIV-negative children whose parents have no risk factors for HIV infection) and intrauterine infection caused by other agents.

Treatment. Azidothymidine (zidovudine; AZT) is the standard treatment for AIDS (Table 10–17).

Didanosine and dideoxycytosine are potential therapies for children who do not respond to AZT. Intravenous immunoglobulin prevents bacterial infection in children with CD4 counts greater than 400 but does not affect survival. Opportunistic infections should be treated aggressively, as with any infection in an immunodeficient host. Prevention of *P. carinii* pneumonia is possible with low-dose trimethoprim–sulfamethoxazole or aerosolized pentamidine. Although routine immunizations may result in suboptimal antibody concentrations, they remain indicated except for the use of most live vaccines in symptomatically infected children. Because of the risk of fatal measles in children with AIDS, live measles vaccine is indicated in presymptomatic, HIV-seropositive patients. Children exposed to varicella or measles should receive ZIG or serum immune globulin, respectively. Household contacts of children with AIDS should receive inactivated, not live, poliovirus vaccine.

Prevention. Preventing AIDS or HIV infection in adults will decrease the incidence of infection in children. Adult prevention may result from behavior changes ("safe sex," decrease in intravenous drug use), abortion, or avoidance of pregnancy and breast feeding (in developed countries) in high-risk women. Screening of blood donors already has markedly reduced the risk of transmission from blood products, including those used to treat hemophilia. HIV infection almost never is transmitted in a casual or nonsexual household setting. Currently, no vaccine exists.

References

Behrman RE (ed): Nelson Textbook of Pediatrics. 14th ed. Philadelphia, WB Saunders, 1992, Sec. 12.83.

Borkowsky W, Krasinski K, Pollack H, et al: Early diagnosis of human immunodeficiency virus infection in children <6 months of age: Comparison of polymerase chain reaction, culture, and plasma antigen capture techniques. J Infect Dis 166:616, 1992.

Bryant ML, Ratner L: Biology and molecular biology of human immunodeficiency virus. Pediatr Infect Dis J 11: 390, 1992.

Centers for Disease Control: Revision of the CDC surveillance case definition for acquired immunodeficiency syndrome. MMWR 36:S1, 1987.

Duliege AM, Messiah A, Blanche S, et al: Natural history of human immunodeficiency virus type 1 infection in children: Prognostic value of laboratory tests on the bimodal progression of the disease. Pediatr Infect Dis J 11: 630, 1992.

Glatt A, Chirgwin K, Landesman S: Treatment of infections associated with human immunodeficiency virus. N Engl J Med 318:1439, 1988.

Hauger SB, Nicholas SW, Caspe WB: Guidelines for the care of children and adolescents with HIV infection. J Pediatr 119S:1, 1991.

Mofenson LM, Moye J, Bethel J, et al: Prophylactic intravenous immunoglobulin in HIV-infected children with CD4+ counts of 0.20 × 10^9/L or more: Effect on viral, opportunistic, and bacterial infections. JAMA 268:483, 1992.

Rubinstein A, Moracki R, Silverman B, et al: Pulmonary disease in children with acquired immune deficiency syndrome and AIDS-related complex. J Pediatr 1008:498, 1986.

Ruff AJ, Halsey NA, Coberly J, et al: Breast-feeding and maternal-infant transmission of human immunodeficiency virus type 1. J Pediatr 121:325, 1992.

Tovo PA, deMartino M, Gabiano C: Prognostic factors and survival in children with perinatal HIV-1 infection. Lancet 339:1249, 1992.

Influenza Viral Infection

Etiology. Influenza viruses are RNA orthomyxoviruses. Three antigenic types—A, B, and C—exist. Epidemics are caused by types A and B. Influenza A viruses are subclassed by two antigens: neuraminidases (N), of which there are 9; and hemagglutinins (H), of which there are 12. An example of classification is A/Hong Kong/68 (H3N2). Minor variations within the same subtype (*drift*) and major changes (*shift*) in either the H or N antigens result in antigenic fluctuations. Antigenic shift has occurred only in influenza A, whereas drift occurs in both influenza A and B. The variants cause cycles of disease, usually one at a time, although several strains may circulate at once. Three hemagglutinin subtypes (H1, H2, and H3) and two neuraminidases (N1 and N2) have been associated with human infection. Specific antibodies to these antigens are important determinants of immunity.

Epidemiology. Influenza A shifts result in major antigenic change and severe pandemic disease every 10–40 yr. Antigenic drift is probably the cause of less intense epidemics every 2–3 yr worldwide. Influenza B, which does not undergo shifts, causes an outbreak every 4–7 yr. In large urban areas, influenza activity takes place each year, with infection occurring during cooler or rainy seasons. A new strain results in the highest rate of infection in children. Spread is by airborne infected respiratory secretions transmitted from person to person or by articles contaminated with nasopharyngeal secretions. The period of communicability begins 24 hr before symptoms and continues until resolution. The incubation period is 1–3 days.

Pathogenesis. During the incubation period, virus is present in the respiratory tract but rarely in blood and other organs. Virus binds to respiratory epithelial cells, replicates, and causes cell death, desquamation, and decreased mucociliary clearance of bacteria. Immunity correlates better with secretory antibody than with serum antibody, although the latter is associated with protection.

Clinical Manifestations

Older Children and Adolescents. In this group, the manifestations are similar to those seen in adults. There is an abrupt onset of high fever, flushed face, headache, myalgia, cough, and chills. Pharyngitis occurs in 50% of patients and ocular symptoms (tearing, photophobia, burning, pain on eye motion) and nasal stuffiness are common. These symptoms last 2–5 days. As the systemic signs and symptoms resolve, the cough and nasal congestion become more prominent and last 4–10 days. Leukopenia occurs in 25% of patients, and 10% have clinical and roentgenographic evidence of bronchopneumonia.

Younger Children. The classic influenza illness is less common in younger children, who manifest laryngotracheitis, bronchiolitis, bronchitis, pneumonia, and/or a mild upper respiratory tract syndrome. Influenza B has been associated with myositis. Parotitis has been reported in influenza A infection. Fever tends to be higher in younger children than in older children. In neonates, the sudden fever and nonspecific signs simulate sepsis, although a nasal discharge may suggest the diagnosis of a viral respiratory tract infection. Influenza C infection has been associated with an upper respiratory tract syndrome.

Complications. The most important complication is secondary bacterial infection of the respiratory tract, including otitis media, sinusitis, and pneumonia. These complications should be treated with antibiotics effective against *Haemophilus*, pneumococcus, and staphylococcus. Viral-related complications include pneumonia, rarely neurologic syndromes, myocarditis, myoglobinemia, and Reye syndrome. Salicylates should be avoided in children and adolescents with influenza.

Diagnosis. In community-wide outbreaks of winter respiratory tract disease involving all age groups, influenza is the most likely agent. Virus may be isolated in 2–6 days from nasopharyngeal secretions in tissue culture. Rapid diagnosis may be made by immunofluorescent techniques or ELISA. Serologic responses are helpful for retrospective diagnosis.

Treatment. Amantadine has been proved efficacious in early therapy of influenza A infection in adults. Ribavirin aerosol, a licensed therapy for RSV infection, also has been shown effective in therapy of influenza A or B infection. These agents should not be utilized routinely but may be necessary in unusually severe infection. Antibiotics should be avoided unless a bacterial superinfection is suspected. Non–aspirin-containing antipyretics increase the patient's comfort and do not carry the risk of the development of Reye syndrome.

Prevention. Inactivated vaccine, given on a yearly basis, is indicated for children at risk for complications and, probably, for other children and adults who live in a household with high-risk children. The latter include children with cardiovascular, pulmonary (cystic fibrosis, bronchopulmonary dysplasia), metabolic, renal, or neurologic disorders and those who are immunosuppressed or have a hemoglobinopathy, including sickle cell disease.

Amantadine is effective as prophylaxis against influenza A and should be used in unimmunized high-risk children during an outbreak.

References

Behrman RE (ed): Nelson Textbook of Pediatrics. 14th ed. Philadelphia, WB Saunders, 1992, Sec. 12.74.

Douglas RG Jr: Prophylaxis and treatment of influenza. N Engl J Med 322:443, 1990.

Groothuis JR, Levin MJ, Rabalais GP, et al: Immunization of high-risk infants younger than 18 months of age with split-product influenza vaccine. Pediatrics 87:823, 1991.

Troendle JF, Demmler GJ, Glezen WP, et al: Fatal influenza B virus pneumonia in pediatric patients. Pediatr Infect Dis J 11:117, 1992.

Measles (Rubeola)

Etiology. Measles virus is an RNA paramyxovirus with one antigenic type. It is stable at room temperature for 1–2 days and can be cultivated in human or monkey cells, with cytopathic changes visible in 5–10 days.

Epidemiology. Measles virus is present in blood, urine, and nasopharyngeal secretions of infected individuals. Maximum contagiousness occurs during the prodromal (catarrhal) stage by droplet spray. The infected person is contagious from 1 to 2 days before until 5 days after onset of the characteristic rash. Measles is extremely contagious, with few subclinical cases. In areas of low vaccine use, measles occurs primarily in 5–10 yr old children. In areas of high vaccine use, it occurs primarily in unvaccinated teenagers or adults or in infants too young to be vaccinated. Outbreaks often are due to cases imported from other areas. Measles is a major cause of mortality in malnourished infants and of morbidity in immunosuppressed patients, including those who have AIDS.

Most neonates and young infants are protected from measles by transplacental maternal antibody. They become susceptible toward the middle and end of the 1st yr. Passive immunity may interfere with vaccination until 12–15 mo of life. The incubation period is 8–12 days from exposure to onset of symptoms and 14 days from exposure to onset of rash.

Clinical Manifestations. The manifestations of the prodromal period include cough, coryza, conjunctivitis, and the pathognomonic Koplik spots (gray–white, sand grain–sized dots on the buccal mucosa opposite the lower molars), which last 12–24 hr. The conjunctiva may reveal a characteristic transverse line of inflammation along the eyelid margin (Stimson line). The rash phase often is accompanied by high fever (40.0–40.5°C [104–105°F]). The macular rash begins on the head and spreads over most of the body in 24 hr in a descending fashion. It fades in the same manner. The severity of the illness is related to the extent of the rash. It may be petechial or hemorrhagic (black measles). As the rash fades, it undergoes desquamation and brownish discoloration.

Cervical lymphadenitis, splenomegaly, and mesenteric lymphadenopathy (with abdominal pain) may be noted. Otitis media, pneumonia, and gastrointestinal tract symptoms are more common in infants. Liver involvement is more common in adults. Leukopenia is characteristic. In patients with acute encephalitis, the CSF reveals an increased protein, a lymphocytic pleocytosis, and normal glucose levels.

Complications. Measles frequently is complicated by otitis media. Interstitial pneumonia may be caused by measles or, more commonly, may be due to a secondary bacterial infection. The anergy associated with measles may activate latent tuberculosis. Myocarditis and mesenteric adenitis are infrequent complications. Encephalomyelitis occurs in 1–2:1000 cases and usually occurs 2–5 days after the onset of the rash. Early encephalitis probably is due to viral activity in the brain, whereas later onset encephalitis is a demyelinating and probably an immunopathologic phenomenon. *Subacute sclerosing panencephalitis* is a late complication of slow measles infection, occurring years after the acute illness.

Diagnosis. The clinical presentation is characteristic. Confirmation includes (1) multinucleated giant cells in nasal mucosal smears, (2) virus isolation in culture, and (3) diagnostic antibody rises in convalescent serum.

The rash must be differentiated from exanthem subitum, rubella, enteroviral or adenoviral infection, infectious mononucleosis, toxoplasmosis, meningococcemia, scarlet fever, rickettsial disease, Kawasaki syndrome, serum sickness, and drug rash. The constellation of cough and conjunctivitis is fairly diagnostic for measles. Measles modified by transplacental or administered antibody may be less characteristic. Koplik spots usually are pathognomonic but are not always present at the time of the most pronounced rash.

Treatment. Therapy is supportive. Photophobia is intensified by strong light, which should be avoided. Immunoglobulin and steroids are of no proven value in established disease. Vitamin A (200,000 U × 1, PO) improves outcome in infected malnourished infants. Intravenous ribavirin also may be of benefit in severe infections.

Prevention

Active Immunization. Live measles vaccine prevents infection and should be administered to children at 12–15 mo and at 4–5 or 11–12 yr of age. The effects of vaccination are obstructed by transplacental antibody or passive immunization with immunoglobulin (for ~12 mo in the former case and for 3 mo in the latter case). A skin test for tuberculosis prior to or concomitant with vaccination is advised, because vaccination may induce a state of anergy for 1 mo. The live vaccine is contraindicated in pregnant women, immunodeficient or immunosuppressed children (see Human Immunodeficiency Virus Infection) during a febrile illness, or if immunoglobulin has been administered within 3 mo. If inadvertently vaccinated, immunocompromised patients should receive immunoglobulin. Vaccination shortly after exposure to measles may prevent illness.

Passive Immunization. Immune serum globulin may prevent or ameliorate measles if given within 5 days of exposure. A large dose (0.25 mL/kg) is protective, whereas a smaller dose (0.05 mL/kg) attenuates the illness. Protection is indicated for chronically ill, immunosuppressed, or immunodeficient children, who should receive 0.5 mL/kg (maximum 15 mL).

References

Behrman RE (ed): Nelson Textbook of Pediatrics. 14th ed. Philadelphia, WB Saunders, 1992, Sec. 12.64.
Gindler JS, Atkinson WL, Markowitz LE, et al: Epidemiology of measles in the United States in 1989 and 1990. Pediatr Infect Dis J 11:841, 1992.
Hussey GD, Klein M: A randomized, controlled trial of vitamin A in children with severe measles. N Engl J Med 323:160, 1990.
Kaplan LJ, Daum RS, Smaron M, et al: Severe measles in immunocompromised patients. JAMA 267:1237, 1992.

Mumps

Etiology. Mumps is caused by a paramyxovirus. Humans are the only known natural host.

Epidemiology. Mumps occurs worldwide and spreads by direct contact, aerosolization of respiratory secretions, and fomites. It affects both sexes, and 85% of infections occur in persons under 15 yr of age. Epidemics are most frequent in late winter and spring. The incidence of natural infection in developed countries has decreased as a result of immunization.

Although the virus may be isolated from saliva 6 days before and 9 days after the onset of parotid swelling, the illness can be transmitted 1 day before until 3 days after swelling. Transplacental antibody protects infants from infection in the first 6 mo of life. Infection is associated with lifelong immunity. The incubation period is usually 16–18 days but may range from 12 to 25 days after exposure.

Clinical Manifestations. Thirty to 40% of the cases of infection are subclinical, but when symptoms occur, the onset is characterized by fever, muscle pain, headache, malaise, and pain and swelling in the parotid glands lasting 3–7 days. The swelling obscures the angle of the mandible and pushes the earlobe upward and outward. Pain is elicited by palpation of the gland and also by agents, such as citrus juice, that stimulate salivary flow. Swelling and erythema also surround the Stensen duct. Swelling also may be present in the pharynx and larynx and over the manubrium and upper chest (probably as a result of lymphatic obstruction). Swelling of the submandibular glands may accompany parotid swelling, and in 10–15% of cases they may be the only glands involved. The sublingual glands are involved less commonly.

Meningoencephalomyelitis. Sixty-five percent of patients with parotitis will have CSF pleocytosis, and over 10% will have clinical manifestations of meningoencephalitis. In the preimmunization era, mumps was one of the most common causes of aseptic meningitis. Early-onset meningitis probably is due to direct viral infection of the brain, whereas meningoencephalitis that occurs 10 days or more after the onset of illness is a postinfectious, demyelinating syndrome.

Orchitis, Epididymitis. These complications occur in 15–35% of adolescents and adults and rarely occur before puberty. They become manifest at the end of the 1st wk of illness. Bilateral illness occurs in 3% of affected patients. The testes are red, swollen, and tender. Atrophy is common as a sequela but infertility is rare.

Pancreatitis. Mild pancreatitis is common and may become manifest as epigastric pain, tenderness, and vomiting. An elevated serum amylase value usually is present in mumps, with or without clinical pancreatitis. It may indicate pancreatic or salivary gland involvement.

Rare Complications. Examples of rare complications include nephritis (viruria is common but nephritis is rare), thyroiditis, myocarditis, mastitis, deafness, ocular complications, arthritis, and thrombocytopenia. No firm evidence for a fetal mumps syndrome has been discovered.

Diagnosis. The diagnosis is made clinically. Elevated serum amylase is typical and its onset parallels parotid swelling. Specific diagnosis can be confirmed by isolation of the virus from saliva, urine, CSF, or blood by routine viral culture. A rise in serum antibody to mumps also is diagnostic.

Parotitis also may be caused by other viruses, such as enterovirus, lymphocytic choriomeningitis virus, and influenza A virus. Cytomegalovirus may cause parotitis in immunocompromised children, and infants with AIDS may present with parotitis. Suppurative parotitis, which usually is due to *S. aureus,* can be diagnosed by expression of purulent material containing bacteria through the Stensen duct. Other causes of swelling in the parotid area include salivary calculus, recurrent parotitis (etiology unknown), salivary gland tumors, lymphomas, and cervical adenitis, which may mimic parotitis.

Treatment. No therapy is available except for supportive care.

Prevention. Live attenuated mumps vaccine has markedly diminished the incidence of mumps and should be administered to 15 mo old children as part of their measles, mumps, and rubella (MMR) vaccine (Table 10–3). Parotitis and meningoencephalitis are rare complications of the highly protective mumps vaccination.

References

Behrman RE (ed): Nelson Textbook of Pediatrics. 14th ed. Philadelphia, WB Saunders, 1992, Sec. 12.73.

McDonald JC, Moore DL, Quennec P: Clinical and epidemiologic features of mumps meningoencephalitis and possible vaccine-related disease. Pediatr Infect Dis J 8: 751, 1989.

Sullivan KM, Halpin TF, Kim-Farley R, et al: Mumps disease and its health impact: An outbreak-based report. Pediatrics 76:533, 1985.

Parainfluenza Viral Infection

Etiology. Parainfluenza viruses are RNA paramyxoviruses. Five antigenically distinct types (1, 2, 3, 4A, and 4B) cause illness in humans.

Epidemiology. By age 3 yr, most children have been symptomatically infected with parainfluenza types 1–3. Type 4 infection also is common but usually asymptomatic. Symptomatic reinfection is common. Infection occurs worldwide, with epidemics occurring in the fall and endemic activity occurring throughout the year. Transmission is from person to person by direct contact, aerosolization of respiratory secretions, and articles contaminated by respiratory tract secretions. The period of contagiousness generally is 4–9 days but may last for up to 2–3 wk. The incubation period is 2–4 days. Infection does not provide complete immunity, but reinfections are usually mild.

Clinical Manifestations. The major manifestations include laryngotracheitis (croup), bronchitis, bronchiolitis, and, less commonly, pneumonia, particularly in immunodeficient children. Illness lasts approximately 5 days. Less common manifestations include parotitis, Guillain-Barré syndrome, and Reye syndrome. Secondary bacterial infections, including otitis media, tracheitis, and pneumonia, may occur. In the immunocompromised host, progressive pneumonia may occur.

Diagnosis. Tissue culture may be used to provide specific diagnosis within 1 wk. Serologic diagnosis is possible, but results may be confused by cross-reactivity with other paramyxoviruses. Rapid identification of viral antigen in nasopharyngeal secretions through immunofluorescent techniques or ELISA may be used to establish the diagnosis. Differential diagnosis includes infection caused by other respiratory viruses (influenza virus, RSV, adenovirus, rhinovirus) and mycoplasma. In addition, bacterial infection (acute epiglottitis), aspirated foreign bodies, and angioneurotic edema must be differentiated from viral laryngotracheobronchitis.

Treatment.   No specific antiviral therapy is available for parainfluenza infection. Secondary bacterial infections must be treated.

Prevention.   No chemotherapeutic or vaccine modalities are available for prevention.

Reference

Behrman RE (ed): Nelson Textbook of Pediatrics. 14th ed. Philadelphia, WB Saunders, 1992, Sec. 12.75.

Respiratory Syncytial Virus Infection

Etiology.   RSV is an RNA virus of the paramyxovirus family. Humans are the only source of infection.

Epidemiology.   Worldwide outbreaks of respiratory illness caused by RSV occur among infants each winter or early spring. These outbreaks lead to predictable, yearly increases in infant hospitalization for bronchiolitis and pneumonia. The partially protective effect of transplacental antibody probably accounts for the relative lack of severe infection before 4–6 wk of life. Infection is universal by age 2 yr. Reinfections are common and tend to be mild. RSV is responsible for 55–85% of cases of bronchiolitis, 15–25% of cases of childhood pneumonia, and 6–8% of cases of croup. Illness generally is introduced into families by an older sibling, parents with "colds," and infants exhibiting the more severe syndromes. Nosocomial infection is extremely common among infants during RSV epidemics. The virus is spread by large droplets delivered, either airborne or via the hands, to nose or eyes. The period of viral shedding is 3–8 days but may last for up to 4 wk in young infants. The incubation period is 5–8 days.

Clinical Manifestations.   RSV causes acute respiratory tract disease in all ages, but in infants and young children it is the most important cause of bronchiolitis and pneumonia (Chapter 12). The initial manifestations of RSV infection include rhinorrhea, pharyngitis, cough, tachypnea, and low-grade fever. If the illness progresses, the cough worsens, wheezing ensues, and signs of respiratory distress appear. Chest roentgenograms usually reveal hyperexpansion and, at times, pneumonitis. In young infants, pneumonia may occur alone or concomitantly with bronchiolitis, a combination that often is associated with a paroxysmal cough resembling that of pertussis. In the very young infant, the premature infant, or the child with underlying respiratory or cardiac illness, only apnea and periodic breathing may occur. Long-term abnormalities in pulmonary function and subsequent wheezing that accompany respiratory infections have been reported in children with RSV bronchiolitis or pneumonia. RSV infection is very severe and life-threatening in patients with pulmonary hypertension (congenital heart disease, bronchopulmonary dysplasia), immunosuppression, or immunodeficiency.

Diagnosis.   The season of the year, the occurrence of community outbreaks, and the presence of a sibling with an upper respiratory tract infection should alert the physician to the likelihood of RSV infection in an infant with bronchiolitis or pneumonia. Routine laboratory tests are of little use in specific diagnosis. Tests of blood gases often reveal a higher level of hypoxemia than expected and, as the infant's condition worsens, hypercapnia ensues. Specific diagnosis can be made by virus isolation from nasopharyngeal secretions (2–5 days) or tests for rapid detection of RSV antigen.

The differential diagnosis of RSV pneumonia in young infants must include infection caused by *Chlamydia*, which often is accompanied by conjunctivitis and eosinophilia; infection caused by pertussis, which usually occurs in an unimmunized child with lymphocytosis; or infection caused by other viral or bacterial agents.

Treatment.   Symptomatic therapy is usually all that is necessary for most children with RSV infection. Oxygen is indicated for hypoxia. In the severely ill child or in high-risk patients as noted above, the use of aerosolized ribavirin and beta-sympathomimetic agents in the hospital have been shown to be efficacious.

Prevention.   No vaccines are available to prevent RSV infection. Breast feeding has been linked to less severe illness in infants. In the hospital setting, meticulous hand washing and the use of gown, gloves, and eye and nose protection has been shown to decrease the occurrence of infection in staff and to decrease the nosocomial spread of RSV.

References

Behrman RE (ed): Nelson Textbook of Pediatrics. 14th ed. Philadelphia, WB Saunders, 1992, Sec. 12.75.

Hall CB, Walsh EE, Schnabel KC, et al: Occurrence of groups A and B of respiratory syncytial virus over 15 years: Associated epidemiologic and clinical characteristics in hospitalized and ambulatory children. J Infect Dis 162:1283, 1990.

Klassen TP, Rowe PC, Sutcliffe T, et al: Randomized trial of salbutamol in acute bronchiolitis. J Pediatr 118:807, 1991.

Shaw KN, Bell LM, Sherman NH: Outpatient assessment of infants with bronchiolitis. Am J Dis Child 145:151, 1991.

Smith DW, Frankel LR, Mathers LH, et al: A controlled trial of aerosolized ribavirin in infants receiving mechanical ventilation for severe respiratory syncytial virus infection. N Engl J Med 325:24, 1991.

Rubella (German or Three-Day Measles)

Etiology.   Rubella is caused by an RNA virus that can be isolated in tissue culture.

Epidemiology.   Humans are the only hosts. Viral spread occurs by oral droplets from nasopharyngeal secretions or via the transplacental route. In unvaccinated populations, the illness occurs in 5–14 yr olds. In vaccinated populations, it occurs more commonly in teenagers and young adults (especially in large institutions, such as colleges and hospitals). Health care personnel should be screened for rubella antibody and immunized if seronegative. Maximum communicability of postnatal rubella appears to be 2 days before and 5–7 days after onset of the characteristic rash. The incubation period for postnatal rubella ranges from 14 to 21 days but most commonly is 16–18 days. Infants with congenital rubella may shed virus in nasopharyngeal secretions and urine for more than 1 yr after birth and may transmit the virus to susceptible contacts.

Transplacental antibody is protective during the first 6 mo of life. In closed populations, the infection rate approaches 100%, whereas it is 50–60% among susceptible family members. Subclinical cases outnumber clinically apparent cases by a ratio of 2:1. Rubella generally occurs in the spring, with epidemics occurring in cycles of every 6–9 yr in unvaccinated populations. Infection confers lifelong immunity. Surveys indicate that 10–20% of young adults are susceptible to rubella.

Clinical Manifestations.   The prodromal phase of rubella (mild catarrhal symptoms) may go unnoticed. The characteristic signs of rubella are retroauricular, posterior cervical, and posterior occipital lymphadenopathy accompanied by an erythematous, maculopapular, discrete rash. The rash begins on the face and spreads to the body; it lasts for 3 days. An enanthem consisting of rose-colored spots on the soft palate may appear before the rash. Other signs include mild pharyngitis, conjunctivitis, anorexia, headache, malaise, and low-grade fever. Polyarthritis (usually of the hands) may occur, especially among older females, but it usually resolves without sequelae. Paresthesia and tendonitis may occur. The WBC count usually is normal or low, and thrombocytopenia rarely occurs.

Diagnosis.   Rubella has a relatively nonspecific appearance. The clinical diagnosis can be made with confidence only during a rubella epidemic. The *differential diagnosis* includes scarlet fever, mild rubeola, enteroviral infection, infectious mononucleosis, and drug eruptions. Specific diagnosis can be established by viral isolation from nasopharyngeal secretions or by a 4-fold antibody rise from acute to convalescent serum. Blood, urine, and CSF also may yield the virus, especially in infants with congenital infection.

Treatment.   No antiviral therapy is available for rubella.

Prevention.   Immunoglobulin should be used in pregnant, nonimmune women exposed to rubella who refuse to have an abortion, even if documented infection has occurred. Serology will determine the immune status of a pregnant, exposed woman.

Active immunization with a live attenuated vaccine prevents rubella. Following vaccination, virus is shed from the nasopharynx for several weeks, but it is not readily communicable. In the United States, vaccination is indicated for all children (given at 15–18 mo of age), for all nonimmune prepubescent children, and for all postpubescent females who are nonimmune and will not become pregnant within 3 mo. This regimen has reduced the incidence of rubella and of the congenital rubella syndrome, primarily by preventing epidemics of rubella. Other countries immunize only pubescent girls. This does not prevent rubella outbreaks but may decrease the percentage of nonimmune pregnant women.

Although highly attenuated and not associated with fetal damage, the vaccine virus has been recovered from fetuses. Therefore, rubella vaccination is contraindicated in pregnant women. Inadvertently using the vaccine in this setting is not an indication for abortion. Vaccination is contraindicated in a patient with an immunodeficiency state, immunosuppressed condition, vaccine hypersensitivity, or acute febrile illness, as well as in a patient who has received immunoglobulin within the last 3 mo. Fever, lymphadenopathy, rash, arthralgia, and arthritis (the latter two especially in older girls and women) may follow vaccination.

References

Behrman RE (ed): Nelson Textbook of Pediatrics. 14th ed. Philadelphia, WB Saunders, 1992, Sec. 12.65.

Lee SH, Ewert DP, Frederick PD, et al: Resurgence of congenital rubella syndrome in the 1990s. JAMA 267:2616, 1992.

McIntosh EDG, Menser MA: A fifty-year follow-up of congenital rubella. Lancet 340:414, 1992.

MYCOTIC INFECTIONS

Diseases caused by fungi frequently cause cutaneous (candidiasis, "ringworm," tinea) or mucocutaneous (candidal thrush, vulvovaginitis) infections in immunocompetent patients or systemic illnesses in immunoincompetent and immunosuppressed patients. Localized pulmonary diseases (histoplasmosis, cryptococcosis) are common among immunocompetent patients, whereas unusual or disseminated disease is more common among neutropenic, lymphopenic, or immunosuppressed patients. These latter infections include invasive mucormycosis or aspergillosis, disseminated candidiasis, and CNS cryptococcosis.

Treatment depends on the presence of underlying immunologic disease, the site of infection, and the specific fungus involved. Treatment of systemic fungal infections usually requires prolonged antifungal therapy using empiric antifungal agents because most laboratories do not routinely perform antifungal susceptibility testing (Table 10–21).

Coccidioidomycosis

Etiology. Coccidioidomycosis (San Joaquin fever, desert rheumatism) is caused by *Coccidioides imitis*, a dimorphic fungus.

Epidemiology. This fungus is present in soil in the southwestern states, including western Texas, Arizona, New Mexico, and California. It also occurs in Mexico and certain areas of Central and South America. The infection is usually a childhood illness and, once contracted, confers permanent immunity. The spores are spread by inhalation or, less commonly, by implantation. Person-to-person spread does not occur. Hot summers, dry soil, and rodent burrows are an ideal environment for preserving infectious spores. The incubation period is 10–16 days, with a range of 1 wk to 1 mo.

Table 10–21. Antifungal Agents

Drug	Mechanism of Action	Indications	Comments/Toxicity
Amphotericin B	Polyene component of drug combines with fungal membrane sterols	Blastomycosis, candidiasis, histoplasmosis, cryptococcosis, aspergillosis, mucormycosis, coccidioidomycosis, sporotrichosis (extracutaneous)	Fever, chills, azotemia, hypokalemia, toxicity; may be combined with flucytosine
Nystatin	As above	Candidiasis	Topical/oral use only
Flucytosine	Conversion to 5-fluorouracil, which interferes with DNA synthesis	Combined with amphotericin B; candidiasis, cryptococcosis, aspergillosis, mucormycosis	Not used as a single drug; neutropenia, thrombocytopenia, hepatitis
Ketoconazole	Interferes with membrane sterol formation	Candidiasis (mucosal), nonmeningeal blastomycosis, or histoplasmosis; ringworm, tinea versicolor	Oral drug; gastrointestinal toxicity; inhibits testosterone synthesis; multiple drug interaction (see Appendix I)
Fluconazole	As ketoconazole	Candidiasis (oral, esophagitis), cryptococcosis	Intravenous or oral drug; gastrointestinal toxicity; drug interactions
Itraconazole	As ketoconazole	As ketoconazole; higher tissue levels, Aspergillus	Oral drug; headache, hypertension, edema; drug interactions
Griseofulvin	Disrupts mitotic spindle formation	Ringworm	Headache, gastrointestinal toxicity

(Data from Med Lett 28:41, 1986; 30:30, 1988; 32:57, 1990.)

Clinical Manifestations

Primary Coccidioidomycosis. The primary pulmonary infection is asymptomatic in 60% of patients. Symptomatic disease may resemble an influenza syndrome. Skin manifestations may include a diffuse maculopapular rash; urticaria; and, frequently, erythema nodosum or, less commonly, erythema multiforme. Skin infection can occur following trauma or with dissemination of the fungus and often occurs with arthralgias. Pleural effusions as well as pneumonitis may be present. The chest roentgenograms often are more impressive than the findings on physical examination.

Residual Pulmonary Coccidioidomycosis. Infrequently a cavity or chronic progressive fibrocavitary syndrome occurs.

Disseminated or Progressive Coccidioidomycosis. The fungus may occasionally disseminate to the skin, bones, and meninges of normal individuals or in immunocompromised patients. The mortality rate of meningitis without therapy is 100%. Hydrocephalus is a common complication of CNS disease.

Diagnosis. Histologic examination of pulmonary or other involved tissue reveals double-contoured spherules accompanied by endospores without budding. Culture on appropriate media should be performed cautiously because the fungus is highly contagious. A positive skin test indicates either recent or previous infection. A negative skin test does not exclude infection and typically may be negative in an individual with disseminated disease. In general, the higher the level of antibody in the serum complement fixation test the more severe the illness. In meningitis, the CSF almost always contains specific antibody. The level and persistence of complement fixation titers in serum and CSF are useful for determining the prognosis and for guiding therapy.

Treatment. Primary coccidioidal infection is self-limiting and requires no specific therapy. Persistent cavitary disease may require surgical excision, usually combined with amphotericin B treatment. Amphotericin B is the agent of choice for treatment of disseminated coccidioidomycosis (see Appendix I). Fluconazole also has been used with success. For meningitis, intrathecal administration usually is utilized in addition to systemic therapy. Therapy of meningitis is continued for 3 mo after normal protein and cells and a negative antibody titer in the CSF are demonstrated. Relapse, which is heralded by headache or by abnormal CSF chemistries, may occur years after therapy has ceased. Surgical débridement may be indicated for localized, symptomatic, or progressive lesions.

References

Behrman RE (ed): Nelson Textbook of Pediatrics. 14th ed. Philadelphia, WB Saunders, 1992, Sec. 12.109.

Kafka JA, Catanazaro A: Disseminated coccidioidomycosis in children. J Pediatr 98:355, 1981.

Tucker RM, Galgiani JN, Denning DW, et al: Treatment of coccidioidal meningitis with fluconazole. Rev Infect Dis 12:S380, 1990.

Histoplasmosis

Etiology. Histoplasmosis is caused by a dimorphic fungus, *Histoplasma capsulatum.*

Epidemiology. The organism grows particularly well in soil containing bird or bat droppings. In the United States, it is endemic in the Mississippi, Missouri, and Ohio river valleys. Infection is acquired by inhalation of airborne spores. Outbreaks have occurred following exploration and dust-raising activities in heavily contaminated areas. It is not transmitted from person to person. The incubation period is variable but is usually a few weeks from the time of exposure.

Pathogenesis. This infection is much like tuberculosis. Inhalation of spores results in primary infection of the lung, with seeding of multiple organs. An effective immune response results in granulomatous containment of the organism, occasionally associated with calcification.

Clinical Manifestations. Asymptomatic infection is most common and may be recognized by serologic and skin test conversion.

Acute Pulmonary Histoplasmosis. This condition is an influenza-like illness with hilar adenopathy. Splenomegaly and erythema nodosum or erythema multiforme may be present. Chest roentgenograms reveal patchy infiltrates and hilar adenopathy in about 25% of patients. Involved areas eventually may calcify, resulting in the characteristic "buckshot" areas of healed histoplasmosis. This self-limiting illness persists for 3–4 wk.

Secondary (Reinfection) Pulmonary Histoplasmosis. This condition occurs within 3 days of exposure. Signs and symptoms are the same as those that occur in mild primary disease, with chest roentgenograms revealing a miliary pattern.

Disseminated Histoplasmosis. This condition is typically an acute illness of infants, young children, and immunocompromised patients. If left untreated, it is fatal. Beginning as primary pulmonary histoplasmosis, it progresses to involve the reticuloendothelial system, with diffuse adenopathy, hepatosplenomegaly, pneumonitis, and bone marrow involvement, resulting in anemia, leukopenia, and thrombocytopenia. Death is due to respiratory failure, gastrointestinal tract bleeding, or bacterial sepsis.

Diagnosis. Diagnosis of acute histoplasmosis generally is made by demonstration of a serologic response. Sputum cultures usually are negative. In disseminated disease, the organism may be recovered and cultured from bone marrow, lymph nodes, or biopsy material. In patients with disseminated disease, the skin test may be nonreactive. Application of skin test antigen may induce a serologic response and, thus, it usually is not utilized for diagnostic purposes or is placed after blood for serologic studies has been drawn.

Treatment. Acute histoplasmosis in older children and adults is a self-limited disease and does not require therapy. Other forms of histoplasmosis, including symptomatic pulmonary disease in the infant and young child and disseminated disease, are treated with amphotericin B. Ketoconazole has been used in a small number of children with milder forms of histoplasmosis (see Appendix I).

References

Behrman RE (ed): Nelson Textbook of Pediatrics. 14th ed. Philadelphia, WB Saunders, 1992, Sec. 12.103.

Weinberg GA, Kleiman MB, Grosfeld JL, et al: Unusual manifestations of histoplasmosis in children. Pediatrics 72:99, 1983.

Wheat LJ, Kohler RB, Tewar RP: Diagnosis of disseminated histoplasmosis by detection of *Histoplasma capsulatum* antigen in serum and urine specimens. N Engl J Med 314:83, 1986.

Superficial Fungal Infections

Cutaneous manifestations of infection by relatively nonvirulent fungi are quite common (Table 10–22).

RICKETTSIAL DISEASE

Etiology. Rickettsiae are gram-negative coccobacillary organisms that resemble bacteria but have incomplete cell walls and have lost enzymes, and thus require an intracellular site for replication.

Epidemiology. Rickettsiae infect arthropod vectors and, with the exception of louse-borne epidemic typhus, are transmitted to humans only incidentally. Table 10–23 summarizes the agents, epidemiology, and serologic response to the more common rickettsial infections of humans. Rocky Mountain spotted fever (RSMF) is the most common human rickettsial illness in the United States. Rickettsiae have a limited geographic and seasonal occurrence related to arthropod life cycles, activity, and distribution.

Pathogenesis. The fundamental characteristic of the condition is infection of the blood vessels of skin, brain, and subcutaneous tissue resulting in vasculitis, increased vascular permeability, edema, and, eventually, decreased vascular volume, altered tissue perfusion, and widespread organ failure.

Clinical Manifestations. Local primary lesions are present in many rickettsial infections. Prominent features include fever, rash, headache, myalgias, and respiratory tract signs and symptoms. Patients with Q fever do not exhibit rash but may have pneumonia and hepatitis as part of their clinical presentation.

Diagnosis. Organisms can be detected in biopsy specimens (usually of skin) and by staining (usually by immunofluorescence). Staining procedures are specific but only moderately sensitive and not widely available. Serologic diagnosis may be accomplished by detection of specific antirickettsial antibodies or by the use of cross-reacting antibodies to *Proteus vulgaris* (Weil-Felix reaction). The specific antibody response is slow and may not be diagnostic until the illness has been present for several weeks. Although it is useful for etiologic confirmation, serologic response may not be helpful regarding therapeutic decisions. The Weil-Felix reaction is frequently unreliable because of its false-positive and false-negative results. Culturing of rickettsiae is possible in animals or tissue culture; it is hazardous and generally not available.

Treatment. Therapy with chloramphenicol or tetracycline is curative when begun early (see Appendix I). Other antimicrobial agents are of no value or may even enhance rickettsial replication (sulfonamides). In the child with renal failure, chloramphenicol is the agent of choice. Its use in patients with both renal and liver failure requires

Table 10–22. Superficial Fungal Infections

Name	Etiology	Manifestations	Diagnosis	Therapy
Tinea capitis (ringworm)	*Microsporum audouinii, Trichophyton tonsurans, M. canis*	Prepubertal infection of scalp, hairshafts; "black dot" alopecia; *T. tonsurans* common in blacks	*M. audouinii* fluorescence—blue–green with Wood lamp*; +KOH, culture	Griseofulvin; selenium sulfide shampoo
Kerion	Inflammatory reaction to tinea capitis	Swollen, boggy, crusted, purulent, tender mass with lymphadenopathy; secondary distal "id" reaction common	As above	As above, plus steroids for "id" reactions
Tinea corporis (ringworm)	*M. canis, T. rubrum,* others	Slightly pruritic ringlike, erythematous papules, plaques with scaling and slow outward expansion of the border; check cat or dog for *M. canis*	+KOH, culture; *M. canis* fluorescence—blug–green with Wood lamp; *differential diagnosis:* granuloma annulare, pityriasis rosea, nummular eczema, psoriasis	Local miconazole or clotrimazole
Tinea cruris (jock itch)	*Epidermophyton floccosum, T. mentagrophytes, T. rubrum*	Symmetric, pruritic, scrotal sparing, scaling plaques	+KOH, culture; *differential diagnosis:* erythrasma (*Corynebacterium minutissimum*)	Local miconazole, clotrimazole, undecylenic acid, or tolnaftate; wear loose cotton underwear
Tinea pedis (athlete's foot)	*T. rubrum, T. mentagrophytes*	Moccasin or interdigital distribution, dry scales, interdigital maceration with secondary bacterial infection	+KOH, culture; *differential diagnosis: C. minutissimum* erythrasma	Medications as above; wear cotton socks
Tinea unguium (onychomycosis)	*T. mentagrophytes, T. rubrum, Candida albicans*	Uncommon before puberty; peeling of distal nailplate; thickening, splitting of nails	+KOH, culture	Oral ketoconazole or griseofulvin
Tinea versicolor	*Malassezia furfur*	Tropical climates, steroids or immunosuppressive drugs; uncommon before puberty; chest, back, arms; oval hypo- or hyperpigmented in blacks, red-brown in whites; scaling patches	+KOH; orange–gold fluorescence with Wood lamp; *differential diagnosis:* pityriasis alba	Selenium sulfide shampoo, topical sodium hyposulfite, oral ketoconazole
Candidiasis	*C. albicans*	Diaper area, intense erythematous plaques or pustules, isolated or confluent	+KOH, culture	Topical nystatin; oral nystatin treats concomitant oral thrush

* Wood lamp examination uses an ultraviolet source in a completely darkened room. Trichophyton usually has no fluorescence.

careful attention to serum antibiotic concentrations, which may mandate dosage adjustments. In more advanced cases, usually as a result of delayed therapy where multisystem disease is present, intensive care is critical. Although corticosteroids are of unproven efficacy, they often are advocated in the patient who has vasculitis.

Immunity. Prolonged immunity and some degree of cross-immunity to other rickettsial infections is conferred by infection. Recurrent or recrudescent activation of rickettsial infection years after the first attack (as in Brill disease or scrub typhus) is common. Humoral antibodies are produced during infections, but cell-mediated immunity is probably of greater importance.

Prognosis. Mortality is lower in children than in adults. Early diagnosis and therapy markedly reduce the mortality rate. In the United States, the mortality rate is 5–10% in individuals younger than 30 yr of age with RMSF, the most serious form of rickettsiosis. Mortality rates are consistently higher in nonwhites, presumably because of the difficulty in appreciating the characteristic rash. When death occurs, it is usually in the 2nd wk of illness.

Rocky Mountain Spotted Fever

Epidemiology. This is the most common rickettsial illness in the United States, occurring primarily in the Eastern coastal, the Southeast, and the Western states, especially among 5–9 yr old children. Although the illness is transmitted by various ticks, 15–20% of infected individuals will not be able to describe tick bites or contacts. Most cases occur from April to September following outdoor activity in wooded areas.

Table 10–23. Rickettsial Diseases of Humans: Summary of Pertinent Features

Group Disease	Causative Agent	Arthropod Vector	Hosts	Incubation Period	Confirmatory Tests*	Geographic Distribution
Spotted Fever						
Rocky Mountain spotted fever	*R. rickettsii*	Tick	Dogs, rodents	1–8 days	IFA, DFA	Western hemisphere
Boutonneuse fever (Mediterranean spotted fever)	*R. conorii*	Tick	Dogs, rodents	3–15 days	IFA, DFA	Africa, Mediterranean region, India, Middle East
Rickettsialpox	*R. akari*	Mite	Mice	10–24 days	IFA	North America, Russia, Korea, South Africa
Ehrlichiosis	*E. canis*	Tick	Dogs	7–28 days	IFA	Southeast, south central United States
Typhus						
Epidemic typhus/Brill-Zinsser disease	*R. prowazekii*	Body louse	Humans	—	IFA	Highlands of Africa, Asia, Central and South America
Flying squirrel–associated typhus fever	*R. prowazekii*	Lice, fleas	Flying squirrels	10–14 days	IFA	Eastern United States (including Texas)
Murine (endemic) typhus	*R. typhi*	Cat or rat flea, rat louse	Rats	8 days	IFA	Worldwide
Scrub typhus						
Scrub typhus	*R. tsutsugamushi*	Mite	Rodents	8–10 days	IFA, IP	Pacific Islands, Australia, and central, eastern, and southeast Asia
Others						
Q fever	*Coxiella burnetii*	Ticks?	Cattle, sheep, goats, cats	18–20 days	IFA, CF	Worldwide

* Although not widely available or highly sensitive, a direct fluorescent antibody (DFA) test can be used to detect rickettsiae in skin biopsies or tissue samples. Preferred confirmatory serologic tests include indirect fluorescent antibody or microimmunofluorescent assay (IFA), complement fixation (CF), and immunoperoxidase (IP) assays. Cross-absorption of the patient's serum with specific rickettsial antigens can be done to distinguish the following infections: *R. rickettsii* versus *R. conorii* or *R. akari;* and *R. prowazekii* versus *R. typhi.*

(Adapted from Behrman RE (ed): Nelson Textbook of Pediatrics. 14th ed. Philadelphia, WB Saunders, 1992, p 858.)

Clinical Manifestations. The onset is nonspecific, with headache, malaise, and fever. In a few days, a pale, rose-red macular or maculopapular rash appears in 90% of cases. It begins peripherally and spreads to involve the entire body, including palms and soles. The early rash blanches on pressure and is accentuated by warmth. In several days, it progresses to a petechial and purpuric eruption. Fever, headache, myalgia, malaise, splenomegaly (33%), and facial edema become evident. In severe cases, symptoms of CNS inflammation, myocarditis, renal impairment, pneumonitis, and shock occur.

Thrombocytopenia and hyponatremia are common findings and may be important clues to the etiology of this syndrome. DIC is an ominous finding. The fatality rate in untreated patients is 10–40% compared with 5–7% in appropriately treated patients and nearly zero in those treated early.

Diagnosis. The epidemiologic data (locale, time of year, evidence of a tick bite) and clinical manifestations (especially the rash) should facilitate diagnosis. Absence of or failure to obtain appropriate information will greatly hinder diagnosis and increase the risk of a fatal outcome. Fever, headache, and myalgias lasting longer than 1 wk are more indicative of RMSF in endemic areas than of the typical influenza that usually has resolved or begins resolving after 1 wk of duration. The differential diagnosis includes a broad spectrum of illnesses, such as measles, collagen vascular diseases, viral infections, Henoch-Schönlein purpura, idiopathic thrombocytopenic purpura, infectious mononucleosis, ehrlichiosis (Table 10–23), and meningococcemia.

Treatment. Parenteral chloramphenicol or tetracycline plus supportive care constitutes the treatment of choice (see Appendix I).

Prevention. Protection from tick bites and rapid removal of ticks can prevent RMSF. Ticks are best removed by gentle upward traction with forceps to avoid infecting the patient or oneself with material from the crushed tick.

References

Abramson JS, Givner LB: Should tetracycline be contraindicated for therapy of presumed Rocky Mountain spotted fever in children less than 9 years of age? Pediatrics 86: 123, 1990.

Behrman RE (ed): Nelson Textbook of Pediatrics. 14th ed. Philadelphia, WB Saunders, 1992, Sec. 12.94–12.101.

Dumler JS, Taylor JP, Walker DH: Clinical and laboratory features of murine typhus in south Texas, 1980 through 1987. JAMA 266:1365, 1991.

Eng TR, Harkess JR, Fishbein DB, et al: Epidemiologic, clinical, and laboratory findings of human ehrlichiosis in the United States, 1988. JAMA 264:2251, 1990.

Kirk JL, Fine DP, Sexton DJ, et al: Rocky Mount spotted fever: A clinical review based on 48 confirmed cases, 1943–1986. Medicine 69:35, 1990.

PARASITIC INFECTIONS

Although much attention is focused on bacterial and viral infections, protozoal and helminthic infections are a more significant health problem in most parts of the world. Malaria is estimated to kill over 1 million individuals a year, mostly children.

Protozoal Disease

Protozoa are the simplest organisms of the animal kingdom. They are unicellular and most are free living, but some have a commensalistic or parasitic existence. Protozoal disease is considered under the groupings of intestinal and systemic protozoal infections.

INTESTINAL PROTOZOAL INFECTIONS

Amebiasis

Etiology. Amebiasis is caused by *Entamoeba histolytica*, a protozoan that exists as a resistant infectious cyst (10–18 μm, with 4 nuclei) or as a motile, invasive trophozoite.

Epidemiology. Humans are the natural host and reservoir of *E. histolytica*. It is transmitted via contaminated food or water and by person-to-person contact.

Pathogenesis. Once ingested, a cyst becomes a trophozoite that can cause invasive disease and produce a characteristic flask-shaped ulcer in the intestinal mucosa. The amebas may disseminate to the liver or, less commonly, to other areas, such as the pleura, skin, brain, and lungs. The disease is distributed worldwide, although it is more prevalent in areas of poor sanitation. A patient is intermittently infectious if not treated.

Clinical Manifestations. Most infected individuals are asymptomatic, but some present with acute, cramping diarrhea. In 2–8% of infected persons, intestinal amebiasis may be associated with diarrhea that contains blood and mucus and that is associated with fever, abdominal pain, headache, and chills. Symptoms last for days to weeks and recur without therapy. *Ameboma* (a mass due to amebas), extraintestinal lesions, or intestinal perforation and hemorrhage may occur. Twenty-five percent of patients have ulcerative lesions that can be visualized by sigmoidoscopy. These lesions may lead to perforation of the colon and subsequent peritonitis.

Hepatic amebiasis is the most common manifestation of disseminated infection. Amebic liver abscess with fever, abdominal pain, distention, and a tender liver occurs in 1% of infected individuals. These patients often do not have a history of intestinal amebiasis, and their stool is negative for amebas.

Diagnosis. The diagnosis of intestinal illness relies on demonstration of the organism in stool or biopsy of ulcers or liver abscess tissue. In invasive intestinal amebiasis and in cases of liver abscess, antibody to ameba is present in over 90% of cases. Ultrasound or CT will delineate the liver abscess, which is usually singular and located in the right lobe.

Treatment. Therapy of amebiasis depends on the type of illness. Metronidazole or tinidazole is recommended for forms that invade tissue, followed by iodoquinol for intraluminal organisms.

References

Ahmed L, El Rooby A, Kassem MI, et al: Ultrasonography in the diagnosis and management of 52 patients with amebic liver abscess in Cairo. Rev Infect Dis 12:330, 1990.

Behrman RE (ed): Nelson Textbook of Pediatrics. 14th ed. Philadelphia, WB Saunders, 1992, Sec. 12.111.

Fuchs G, Pickering LK: Amebiasis in the pediatric population. In Ravdin JI (ed): Amebiasis: Human Infection by

Entamoeba histolytica. New York, John Wiley & Sons, 1988, pp 594–613.

Cryptosporidiosis

Etiology. *Cryptosporidium* is a coccidian protozoan that can produce an acute illness in immunocompetent and immunocompromised hosts (particularly those with AIDS).

Epidemiology. Person-to-person transmission occurs; outbreaks have been reported in day care centers and with contaminated water. Prevalence of infection may be as high as 4–7% in sporadic epidemics of enteritis. The incubation period is unknown.

Clinical Manifestations. This condition can appear as an acute and self-limited enteritis in normal individuals who exhibit watery diarrhea, nausea, and cramps lasting 12–14 days or as a chronic severe enteritis in immunocompromised individuals, who have profuse, watery diarrhea, and profound weight loss.

Treatment. No specific therapy is available. In the immunocompromised patient, fluid replacement often is necessary because of the voluminous fluid loss.

References

Behrman RE (ed): Nelson Textbook of Pediatrics. 14th ed. Philadelphia, WB Saunders, 1992, Sec. 12.113.
Miron D, Kenes J, Dagan R: Calves as a source of an outbreak of cryptosporidiosis among young children in an agricultural closed community. Pediatr Infect Dis J 10:438, 1991.
Soave R, Armstrong D: Cryptosporidium and cryptosporidiosis. Rev Infect Dis 6:1012, 1986.
Sorvillo FJ, Fujoka K, Nahlen B, et al: Swimming-associated cryptosporidiosis. Am J Publ Health 82:742, 1992.

Giardiasis

Etiology. Giardiasis is due to *Giardia lamblia,* a flagellated protozoan. The hardy cysts are ingested (often in water) and are the infectious form. The trophozoites are liberated after ingestion and are responsible for symptoms. Giardiae live in the duodenum.

Epidemiology. Giardia has a worldwide distribution and infects humans, dogs, and wild animals (beavers). Transmission occurs from person to person by fecal–oral spread or by drinking or eating contaminated water or food. Outbreaks occur in day care centers, in institutions for the mentally retarded, and in travelers to the Soviet Union and the Rocky Mountains.

Clinical Manifestations. Individuals vary in their response to infection and have the following clinical manifestations: (1) asymptomatic; (2) an acute illness with a sudden onset of explosive, watery, foul-smelling stools, flatulence, abdominal distention, nausea, and anorexia; and (3) chronic diarrhea and malabsorption (including that of antibiotics), with flatulence, abdominal distention, and abdominal pain, often lasting for months.

Diagnosis. Examination of several stool specimens is necessary for visualizing the organism, because intermittent excretion occurs. Examining duodenal contents obtained by direct aspiration or by use of a string test (Enterotest) is more sensitive. Rarely, duodenal intubation with fluid aspiration or biopsy may be required for diagnosis. ELISA can be used to detect *Giardia* antigen in stool specimens.

Treatment. Several drugs, including metronidazole, furazolidone, and quinacrine, are effective in the treatment of giardiasis.

References

Addiss DG, Juranek DD, Spencer HC: Treatment of children with asymptomatic and nondiarrheal *Giardia* infection. Pediatr Infect Dis J 10:843, 1991.
Behrman RE (ed): Nelson Textbook of Pediatrics. 14th ed. Philadelphia, WB Saunders, 1992, Sec. 12.112.
Gunasekaran TS, Hassall E: Giardiasis mimicking inflammatory bowel disease. J Pediatr 120:424, 1992.
Quick R, Paugh K, Addiss D, et al: Restaurant-associated outbreak of giardiasis. J Infect Dis 166:673, 1992.

SYSTEMIC PROTOZOAL INFECTIONS

American Trypanosomiasis (Chagas Disease)

Etiology. American trypanosomiasis is a zoonosis caused by *Trypanosoma cruzi,* a protozoan hemoflagellate.

Epidemiology. *T. cruzi* is transmitted to humans by blood-sucking insects called reduviid bugs. The trypomastigotes are released as the insect defecates near its bite. The trypanosome gains entry and amastigotes (intracellular forms) and trypomastigotes (vascular forms) are produced. The infected reduviid bugs have adapted to adobe, mud, and cane housing in most of South and Central America. It is estimated that 24 million South Americans are infected with *T. cruzi*. Several endogenous cases have occurred in Texas. Animal reservoirs, including rats, opossums, and raccoons, may be important. Although it is common to encounter infected reduviid bugs in the southwestern United States, infection in humans appears to be rare, possibly because of better housing, low adaptability of North American reduviids to domestic housing, or difference in *Trypanosoma* virulence. *T. cruzi* also may be transmitted congenitally or by infected blood. The incubation period is 1–2 wk.

Clinical Manifestations

Acute Infection.   Illness generally is asymptomatic or mild in young children in endemic areas. There may be local inflammation at the site of entry of the parasite. Half of infected children have unilateral eye swelling (Romaña sign), which is the first indication of disease. Some patients will develop a nodular skin lesion (chagoma) at the site of the original inoculation. Hematogenous dissemination results in malaise, fever, muscle pain, adenopathy, rash, hepatosplenomegaly, and, less often, meningoencephalitis. Myocardial involvement is noted in nearly one half of symptomatic patients, accompanied by tachycardia and arrhythmias. Most cases evolve into an asymptomatic chronic stage. The mortality rate is 10%. Congenital disease is characterized by low birth weight, hepatomegaly, and meningoencephalitis.

Chronic Trypanosomiasis.   In the symptomatic chronic stage, inflammation and fibrosis result in myocarditis, cardiac failure, or enlargement of a hollow viscus, especially of the esophagus (megaesophagus) or the colon (megacolon). This occurs in 10–15% of cases.

Diagnosis.   In acute disease, *T. cruzi* can be demonstrated in blood smears. It also can be isolated from blood by use of special media or can be identified by xenodiagnosis (i.e., infection of sterile reduviid bugs). Serodiagnosis is more useful in chronic disease.

Treatment.   Nifurtimox has been used successfully to treat acute trypanosomiasis.

Prevention.   Insect control and adequately protected housing are keys to breaking the bug–human cycle. Blood donors in endemic areas must be screened by serology.

References

Behrman RE (ed): Nelson Textbook of Pediatrics. 14th ed. Philadelphia, WB Saunders, 1992, Sec. 12.115.

Grant IH, Gold JWM, Wittner M, et al: Transfusion-associated acute Chagas disease acquired in the United States. Ann Intern Med 111:849, 1989.

Schiffler RJ, Mansur GP, Navin TR, et al: Indigenous Chagas disease (American trypanosomiasis) in California. JAMA 251:2983, 1984.

Malaria

Etiology.   Malaria is caused by one or more of four *Plasmodium* species: *P. falciparum, P. vivax, P. ovale,* and *P. malariae.*

Epidemiology.   Malaria usually is acquired from the bite of an infected female *Anopheles* mosquito. Less commonly, it is acquired transplacentally or via an infected blood transfusion. Infection transmitted through blood transfusion or the transplacental route occurs without the pre-erythrocytic hepatic phase. In children with no pre-existing immunity to malaria, the incubation period varies from 6 to 16 days depending on the *Plasmodium* species involved.

Pathology.   Infected red cells rupture, causing hemolytic anemia and pigment deposition in reticuloendothelial cells. The infected red blood cells also may sludge and stick in organs, interfering with circulation and inducing pneumonia, encephalitis, or enteritis. *P. falciparum* is associated with the heaviest degree of parasitemia and is the most lethal. Serum antibody production seems to be correlated with clearance of the erythrocyte (but not the hepatic) stage of parasites. Sickle cell anemia and glucose-6-phosphate dehydrogenase (G6PD) deficiency are associated with some protection against lethal malaria.

Clinical Manifestations.   Malaria is most severe in children lacking antibody and is milder in children having survived initial attacks. The illness is characterized by a nonspecific prodrome prior to the onset of sudden high fevers with chills. An abrupt return to normal temperature occurs after 2–12 hr. Fever is associated with headache, abdominal and back pain, nausea, and, often, splenomegaly. In established *P. vivax* or *P. malariae* infection, fever may occur every 2 or 3 days, respectively. *P. falciparum* infection also may produce encephalitis, pneumonitis, enteritis, and nephritis. The most serious form of malaria is due to severe and sudden intravascular hemolysis (blackwater fever), associated with heavy *P. falciparum* infection as well as with the use of drugs that induce hemolysis in G6PD-deficient individuals.

Diagnosis. Malaria and the species of *Plasmodium* may be diagnosed by examining thick and thin blood smears. These smears should be examined at 12-hr intervals because the level of parasitemia fluctuates. In convalescence, there is an antibody response to the parasite.

Treatment. Specific therapy for malaria depends on the species acquired, the mode of acquisition, and the locale of acquisition. Chloroquine is the therapy for malaria acquired in locales that do not have chloroquine-resistant malaria. In areas with *P. falciparum* known to be chloroquine resistant, including much of Africa, Oceania, Southeast Asia, the Indian subcontinent, and South America, therapy consists of mefloquin or quinine plus pyrimethamine–sulfadoxine or quinine plus tetracycline. Severe illness may necessitate the intravenous use of quinine or quinidine. To prevent relapse of mosquito-transmitted *P. ovale* and *P. vivax* infection, primaquine is utilized to eradicate the hepatic phase of the parasite cycle. Because a hepatic phase does not occur with congenital or transfusion-acquired *P. malariae* or *P. falciparum* infection, primaquine is not indicated in these situations. Primaquine induces hemolysis in patients with G6PD deficiency. In severe disease, multisystem support, transfusion, and possibly exchange transfusion are necessary.

Prevention. Malaria can be prevented by administering chemoprophylaxis, which includes the use of weekly dosages of chloroquine (which must also be taken for 6 wk after leaving the endemic area) and possibly the use of primaquine for terminal prophylaxis in order to eradicate hepatic forms. In areas in which Plasmodium species are chloroquine resistant, mefloquine or doxycycline may be used. Control of malaria relies on the prevention of mosquito bites by using special clothing, repellents, night netting, and mosquito eradication programs.

References

Behrman RE, Kliegman RM: Nelson Textbook of Pediatrics. 14th ed. Philadelphia, WB Saunders, 1992, Sec. 12.114.
Cook G: Prevention and treatment of malaria. Lancet 1: 132, 1988.
Freedman DO: Imported malaria—here to stay. Am J Med 93:239, 1992.
Subramanian D, Moise KJ Jr, White AC Jr: Imported malaria in pregnancy: Report of four cases and review of management. Clin Infect Dis 15:408, 1992.

Toxoplasmosis

Etiology. *Toxoplasma gondii,* an intracellular protozoan parasite, causes toxoplasmosis.

Epidemiology. Newly infected cats excrete the infectious oocysts in their feces. The oocysts and tissue cysts are infectious when ingested. High frequency of human infection occurs in warm, humid climates. Infection also occurs from ingesting undercooked meat containing cysts. Less commonly, transmission occurs by blood transfusion or organ transplant, or transplacentally during acute infection of pregnant women. In the United States the incidence of congenital infection is 1–2:1000 live births. The incubation period for acquired infection is about 7 days.

Clinical Manifestations
Congenital Toxoplasmosis. Most maternal infection is asymptomatic. Among women infected during pregnancy, 40–60% will give birth to an infected infant. The later in pregnancy that infection occurs, the more likely it is that the fetus will be infected, but the less severe the illness. Severely affected fetuses will be stillborn. In infants born live, illness may occur at birth and become manifest by poor feeding, fever, rash, petechiae, lymphadenopathy, hepatomegaly, splenomegaly, jaundice, hydrocephalus or microcephaly, microphthalmia, seizures, cerebral calcifications, and chorioretinitis. This illness must be differentiated from other congenital infections included in the TORCH syndrome (rubella, CMV, HSV, syphilis, hepatitis, and VZV). In 67–75% of infants who are asymptomatic at birth, subsequent defects, such as chorioretinitis, retardation, and neurologic disability, will develop years after birth.

Acquired Toxoplasmosis. This condition usually is an asymptomatic infection. Symptomatic infection is characterized as a heterophil-negative mononucleosis syndrome that includes lymphadenopathy, fever, and hepatosplenomegaly. Disseminated infection, including myocarditis, pneumonia, and encephalitis, is more common in immunosuppressed patients, especially those with AIDS. Localized lymphadenopathy that is difficult to differentiate from Hodgkin disease is one of the more common manifestations of toxoplasmosis.

Diagnosis. In toxoplasmosis involving the CNS, the parasites may be visualized in CSF by cytocentrifuge preparations or by growth in inoculated infant mice. Typical histopathology or cysts may be identified in biopsy specimens of involved lung, brain, or lymph node.

Serologic diagnosis can be established by performing several different antibody tests. A 4-fold rise in antibody titer or seroconversion from negative to positive indicates the presence of infection. In congenital infection, diagnosis is complicated by the presence of maternally derived transplacental antibody. If the maternal antibody status is negative, the diagnosis of congenital toxoplasmosis is excluded; if the maternal and neonate levels are positive, serial studies for several months are necessary to distinguish transplacental antibody (levels will fall) from congenital infection (levels will remain stable or rise). Several research laboratories can perform an IgM–anti-*Toxoplasma* antibody study on the serum from newborns; a positive result indicates infection.

Treatment. Treatment includes both pyrimethamine and sulfadiazine, which act synergistically against *Toxoplasma* organisms. Because these compounds are folic acid inhibitors, they are used in conjunction with folinic acid. Spiramycin, which currently is not licensed in the United States, also is utilized in therapy of toxoplasmosis. Corticosteroids are reserved for patients with acute CNS or ocular infection.

Prevention. Ingesting only well-cooked meat and avoiding cats or soil in areas where cats defecate is prudent in pregnant or immunocompromised patients. Cat litter should be disposed of daily, because oocysts are not infectious during the first 48 hr after passage. Administering spiramycin to infected pregnant women has been associated with lower risks of congenital infection in their babies.

References

Behrman RE (ed): Nelson Textbook of Pediatrics. 14th ed. Philadelphia, WB Saunders, 1992, Sec. 12.117.
Cohn JA, McMeeking A, Cohen W, et al: Evaluation of the policy of empiric treatment of suspected toxoplasma encephalitis in patients with the acquired immunodeficiency syndrome. Am J Med 86:521, 1989.
Mitchell CD, Erlich SS, Mastrucci MT, et al: Congenital toxoplasmosis occurring in infants perinatally infected with human immunodeficiency virus 1. Pediatr Infect Dis J 9:512, 1990.

Helminthiases

The helminths are divided into three groups: one group of round worms, the nematodes, and two groups of flat worms, the trematodes (flukes) and the cestodes (tapeworms).

INFECTIONS CAUSED BY INTESTINAL NEMATODES

Infections normally are acquired by inadvertently ingesting eggs or by larval forms from soil penetrating the skin.

Ascariasis

Etiology. Ascariasis is the most prevalent type of helminthiasis, involving 1 billion people. It is caused by *Ascaris lumbricoides*, a large nematode.

Epidemiology. After humans ingest the eggs, larvae are released and then penetrate the intestine, migrate to the lungs, ascend the trachea, and are reswallowed. On entering the intestines again, they mature and produce eggs that are excreted in the stool and are deposited in the soil, where they survive for prolonged periods. This is a ubiquitous parasite that generally occurs in warm areas. Human fecal soilage, use of human manure for agriculture, and hand-to-mouth spread are the major sources of ascariasis.

Clinical Manifestations. Manifestations may be due to migration of the larvae to other sites of the body or due to the presence of adult worms in the intestine. Pulmonary ascariasis occurs as the larvae migrate through the lung. The manifestations of the condition include cough, blood-stained sputum, eosinophilia, and transient infiltrates on chest roentgenograms. Adult larvae in the small intestine may cause abdominal pain and distention. It is rare that intestinal obstruction from adult worms occurs. Migration of worms into the bile duct may result in the rare occurrence of acute biliary obstruction. Steatorrhea and decreased vitamin A absorption may occur in heavily infected children. Asymptomatic infections are common.

Diagnosis. Results from examination of stool for characteristic eggs are diagnostic.

Treatment. Mebendazole currently is considered the drug of choice; pyrantel pamoate or albendazole are alternatives.

Prevention. Effective control of this worldwide parasite depends on adequate sanitary treatment and disposal of infected human feces, especially before it is used as fertilizer.

Enterobiasis (Pinworm)

Etiology. Pinworm is caused by *Enterobius vermicularis*, a nematode that is distributed worldwide.

Epidemiology. Enterobiasis affects individuals at all socioeconomic levels, especially children. Crowded living conditions predispose individuals to infection. Humans ingest the eggs carried on hands or present in house dust or on bedclothes. They hatch in the stomach, and the larvae migrate to the cecum and mature. At night the females migrate to the perianal area to lay their eggs, which are viable for 2 days.

Clinical Manifestations. The most common symptoms are nocturnal anal pruritus and sleeplessness, presumably resulting from the migratory female worms. Vaginitis and salpingitis can occur secondary to aberrant worm migration. *Enterobius* has been recovered from the appendix in several cases, although its role in appendicitis is doubtful.

Diagnosis. The eggs are detected by microscopically examining adhesive cellophane tape pressed against the anus in the morning to collect eggs. Less commonly, a worm may be seen in the perianal region.

Treatment. The drug of choice is pyrantel pamoate or mebendazole given as a single dose and repeated in 2 wk. Alternatives include piperazine and pyruvium pamoate. Repeated therapy may be necessary due to reinfection. Therapy of all family members at once also is often used.

Hookworm Infections

Etiology. Hookworm infection is caused by several species of hookworms; *Ancylostoma duodenale* and *Necator americanus* are the most important. *A. duodenale* is the predominant species in Europe, the Mediterranean region, northern Asia, and the west coast of South America. *N. americanus* predominates in the Western hemisphere, sub-Saharan Africa, Southeast Asia, and several Pacific islands.

Epidemiology. More than 9 million humans are infected with hookworms. Optimal soil conditions and fecal contamination are found in many agrarian tropical countries and in the southeastern United States. Infection typically occurs in young children, especially during the first decade of life. The larvae are found in warm, damp soil and infect humans by penetrating the skin. They migrate to the lungs, ascend the trachea, are swallowed, and reside in the intestine. The worms then mature and attach to the intestinal wall, where they suck blood and shed eggs.

Clinical Manifestations. Infections usually are asymptomatic. Intense pruritus ("ground itch"), which may include papules and vesicles, can occur at the site of larval penetration, usually the soles of the feet or between the toes. Migration of larvae through the lungs usually is asymptomatic. Symptoms of abdominal pain, anorexia, indigestion, fullness, and diarrhea occur with hookworm infestation. The major manifestation of infection is subsequent anemia. Chronic infection causes hypoalbuminemia and edema, which may lead to heart failure.

Diagnosis. Examination of fresh stool will reveal hookworm eggs.

Treatment. Pyrantel pamoate or mebendazole will eradicate hookworm infection. Therapy for anemia may necessitate iron therapy or, in severe cases, transfusion.

Prevention. Eradication depends on sanitation of the patient's environment and chemotherapy. Eradication essentially has been achieved in the southeastern United States.

SYSTEMIC NEMATODES

Visceral Larva Migrans (Toxocariasis)

Etiology. Visceral larva migrans (VLM) is caused by ingestion of the eggs of the dog or cat tapeworms *Toxocara canis*, *Toxocara catii*, and *Toxascaris leonina*.

Epidemiology. VLM is most common in young children with pica who have dogs or cats as pets. Ocular toxocariasis occurs in older children. Approximately 2% of dogs in the United States excrete *Toxocara* eggs, and up to 25% of soil samples in public parks contain the eggs. The eggs of these roundworms are produced by adult worms residing in the dog and cat intestine. Ingested eggs hatch into larvae that penetrate the gastrointestinal tract and migrate to the liver, lung, eye, CNS, and heart, where they die and calcify.

Clinical Manifestations. Symptoms are due to the number of migrating worms and the immune response they elicit. Most persons who are lightly infected are asymptomatic. Symptoms include fever, cough, wheezing, and seizures. Physical findings may include hepatomegaly, rales, rash, and adenopathy. Visual symptoms may include decreased acuity, strabismus, periorbital edema, or blindness. Eye examination may reveal granulomatous lesions near the macula or disc. These must be differentiated from retinoblastoma and other granulomatous infections.

Diagnosis. Eosinophilia and hypergammaglobulinemia associated with elevated isohemagglutinin levels suggest the diagnosis, which may be confirmed by serology (ELISA) or, less commonly, by biopsy.

Treatment. This is a self-limiting illness. In severe disease, steroids and thiabendazole or diethylcarbamazine may be useful.

Prevention. Avoiding pica and washing the hands after animal contact may help control the illness. Deworming puppies and kittens, the major excretors of eggs, will decrease the risk of infection.

INFECTIONS CAUSED BY TREMATODES (FLUKES)

Trematodes include flukes, which infect the intestine, liver, lung, and blood. Eosinophilia is a prominent clinical sign of trematode infection. These infections are uncommon in the United States.

Schistosomiasis

Etiology. The trematodes (flukes) include *Schistosoma haematobium, S. mansoni, S. japonicum,* and, rarely, *S. intercalatum* and *S. mekongi.*

Epidemiology. Schistosomiasis affects over 2 million people, mainly children and young adults. (The maximum incidence of infection is between the ages of 10 and 20 yr.) Humans are infected in contaminated water by cercariae that emerge in an infectious form from snails. They penetrate intact skin. Each adult worm migrates to specific sites: *S. haematobium* to the bladder plexus, and *S. intercalatum* and *S. mekongi* to the mesenteric vessels. The eggs are deposited by the adult flukes in urine (*S. haematobium*) or stool (*S. mansoni* and *S. japonicum*). Intermediate hosts for these complex parasites are freshwater snails that are infected by miracidia, which hatch from eggs in freshwater. *S. haematobium* is prevalent in Africa and the Middle East; *S.* *mansoni* in Africa, the Middle East, the Caribbean, and South America; *S. japonicum* in China, the Phillipines, and Indonesia; *S. mekongi* in the Far East; and *S. intercalatum* in West Africa.

Clinical Manifestations. The pathogenesis of schistosomiasis is due to eggs that are trapped at the site of depository or at metastatic locations. Within 3–12 wk of infection, while the worms are maturing, a syndrome of fever, malaise, cough, abdominal pain, and rash can occur. This is followed by a resultant inflammatory response that leads to further symptoms. In infection with *S. haematobium*, bladder granulomas may lead to renal failure and cancer of the bladder. In the other schistosomal infections, intestinal and hepatic egg deposition and inflammation lead to ulceration of the intestine, colic, abdominal pain, and bloody diarrhea. Parasinusoidal liver obstruction causes hepatosplenomegaly, portal hypertension, ascites, and hematemesis. *Katayama fever* is an acute condition, with fever, weight loss, hepatosplenomegaly, and eosinophilia.

Diagnosis. Eggs may be found in the stool or urine (*S. haematobium*) of infected individuals. Biopsy of the bladder or rectal mucosa may be helpful but usually is not necessary.

Treatment. Praziquantel is the drug of choice for therapy of schistosomiasis in children.

Prevention. Sanitary measures, molluscicides, and therapy for infected individuals may help control the illness.

TISSUE TAPEWORMS

Etiology. Canines become infected with tapeworms by eating infected sheep or cattle viscera. The larval stage of the canine tapeworm *Echinococcus granulosus* (hydatid disease) infects humans when *Echinococcus* eggs from dog feces or dog feces–contaminated material are ingested. Humans then become an intermediate host. The embryos pass through the intestine to the liver and other visceral organs, forming cysts up to 2 cm in diameter.

The cysticercus stage of *Taenia solium* (pork tapeworm) is responsible for *neurocysticercosis.* Humans are infected after consuming raw or undercooked larva-containing pork from pigs that were fed raw sewage contaminated with human feces containing *T. solium.*

Epidemiology. *E. granulosa* has a worldwide distribution but is endemic in sheep- and cattle-raising areas of Australia, South America, South Africa, the Soviet Union, and the Mediterranean region. The prevalence is highest in children. *T. solium* is endemic in Asia, Africa, and Latin and South America.

Clinical Manifestations. Symptoms due to *E. granulosa* result from space-occupying cysts and are most typical in adults. Pulmonary cysts may cause hemoptysis, cough, dyspnea, and respiratory distress. Brain cysts appear as tumors; liver cysts cause problems as they compress and obstruct blood flow.

Neurocysticercosis presents with generalized or focal seizures, variable eosinophilia, and calcification of cerebral cysts.

Diagnosis. Radiologic diagnosis is possible in endemic areas. Ultrasound will confirm the cystic nature of the granulosa mass. Neurocysticercosis demonstrates CT findings of calcified cysts. Serologic tests also are helpful.

Treatment. Large or asymptomatic granulosa cysts are removed surgically. Treatment with mebendazole has shown some benefit. Neurocysticercosis is treated with praziquantel, steroids and anticonvulsant drugs.

References

Behrman RE (ed): Nelson Textbook of Pediatrics. 14th ed. Philadelphia, WB Saunders, 1992, Sec. 12.120–12.138.

Despommier DD: Tapeworm infection—the long and the short of it. N Engl J Med 327:727, 1992.

Hall A, Anwar KS, Tomkins AM: Intensity of reinfection with *Ascaris lumbricoides* and its implications for parasite control. Lancet 140:1253, 1992.

The Medical Letter: Drugs for parasitic infections. Med Lett 34:17, 1992.

The Gastrointestinal Tract

11

Barbara S. Kirschner
Dennis D. Black

Gastrointestinal complaints are common pediatric problems. A careful history and physical examination are necessary to determine whether the symptoms are due to a primary gastrointestinal illness or to systemic disease states that may produce abdominal complaints. For example, abdominal pain in patients with sickle cell anemia may represent sickle cell pain crisis, transfusion-associated hepatitis, hemolysis-associated bilirubin stones and cholecystitis, renal papillary necrosis, or the usual causes of abdominal pain not associated with sickle cell anemia, such as gastroenteritis, appendicitis, and lactose malabsorption. Knowledge of the family history and questions that determine the relationship of symptoms to feeding, the color of emesis, the number and character of stools, the nature of defecation and the location of maximum pain will help formulate a differential diagnosis and select laboratory tests or diagnostic (roentgenographic, endoscopic) procedures.

It is important to recognize diseases and their manifestations that are associated with particular age groups. Hence, most patients with intestinal obstruction resulting from congenital anomalies of the esophagus, small intestine, and large bowel will have symptoms in the 1st wk of life, whereas the age of onset of inflammatory bowel disease is usually during adolescence. Common manifestations of many gastrointestinal illnesses, both benign and serious, include pain, diarrhea, emesis, constipation, and gastrointestinal hemorrhage.

CLINICAL MANIFESTATIONS OF GASTROINTESTINAL DISEASE

Abdominal Pain

This is the most frequent gastrointestinal complaint bringing children and adolescents to the physician. Abdominal pain is classified as visceral, somatic, or referred. The sensation of pain from the abdominal viscera is produced in response to: (1) stretching or distending of the wall of a hollow organ or the capsule of a solid organ, (2) inflammation, or (3) ischemia. Visceral pain usually is dull or crampy and is poorly localized along the dermatomes that innervate the organ. Pain originating from the liver, pancreas, biliary tree, stomach, or proximal small intestine is felt in the epigastrium; pain from the distal small intestine, right colon, and appendix is felt in the periumbilical region; and pain from the left colon, urinary tract, or genital organs usually is felt in the suprapubic area. Parietal or somatic pain represents peritoneal inflammation and is localized to the area of the involved viscera. Peritoneal pain is steady and sharp and associated with voluntary guarding or involuntary rigidity of the overlying abdominal muscles, with or without rebound pain. Referred pain is due to local irritation, with referral along the pathway of innervation of the organ. Pain that begins as dull and poorly localized but that becomes more diffuse and severe suggests that a hollow viscus has ruptured and has progressed to peritonitis.

Critical to the evaluation of abdominal pain is both "how ill" the child appears and whether the onset of the complaint is new or recent (acute), or recurrent (chronic). As part of the history, it is necessary to determine: (1) the age of onset, the location of the pain, its relation to feeding, its severity, time and frequency of occurrence, and duration and nature; (2) the presence or absence of associated symptoms, such as weight loss, fever, vomiting, bloating, diarrhea, hematochezia, or urinary symptoms; and (3) whether any intercurrent illness or recent trauma has occurred (Table 11–1).

ACUTE ABDOMINAL PAIN

In children, acute gastroenteritis is one of the most common causes of acute abdominal pain. In infants less than 2 yr of age, trauma, intussuscep-

Table 11–1. Distinguishing Features of Abdominal Pain in Children

Disease	Onset	Location	Referral	Quality	Comments
Functional: irritable bowel syndrome	Recurrent	Periumbilical	None	Dull, crampy, intermittent, duration 2 hr	Family stress, school phobia, diarrhea/constipation
Esophageal reflux	Recurrent, after meals, bedtime	Substernal	Chest	Burning	Sour taste in mouth. Sandifer syndrome
Duodenal ulcer	Recurrent, before meals, at night	Epigastric	Back	Severe burning, gnawing	Relieved by food, milk, antacids, family history
Pancreatitis	Acute	Epigastric/hypogastric	Back	Constant, sharp, boring	Nausea, emesis, marked tenderness
Intestinal obstruction	Acute or gradual	Periumbilical—lower abdomen	Back	Alternating cramping (colic) and painless periods	Distention, obstipation, bilious emesis, increased bowel sounds
Appendicitis	Acute	Periumbilical or epigastric, localized to right lower quadrant	Back or pelvis if retrocecal	Sharp, steady	Nausea, emesis, local tenderness, ± fever
Meckel diverticulum	Recurrent	Periumbilical—lower abdomen	None	Sharp	Hematochezia; painless unless intussusception or perforation
Inflammatory bowel disease	Recurrent	Depends on site of involvement		Dull cramping, tenesmus	Fever, weight loss, ± hematochezia
Intussusception	Acute	Periumbilical—lower abdomen	None	Cramping, with painless periods	Guarded position with knees pulled up, "currant jelly" stools
Lactose intolerance	Recurrent with milk products	Lower abdomen	None	Cramping	Distention, gaseousness, diarrhea
Urolithiasis	Acute, sudden	Back	Groin	Severe colicky pain	Hematuria
Pyelonephritis	Acute, sudden	Back	None	Dull to sharp	Fever, costochondral tenderness, dysuria, urinary frequency
Cholecystitis/cholelithiasis	Acute	Right upper quadrant	Right shoulder	Severe colicky pain	Hemolysis ± jaundice

(Adapted from Andreoli TE, Carpenter CJ, Plum F, et al: Cecil Essentials of Medicine. Philadelphia, WB Saunders, 1986, p 261.)

tion, incarcerated hernias, urinary tract infections, intestinal malrotation, and volvulus also must be considered. Between 2 and 5 yr of age, sickle cell anemia, lower lobe pneumonia, and urinary tract infections also should be considered. In the older child and adolescent, appendicitis is more common and may be difficult to distinguish from gastroenteritis. In the adolescent girl, mittelschmerz, ectopic pregnancy, ovarian cysts, and pelvic inflammatory disease are important considerations. Less common causes of acute pain include pancreatitis, Henoch-Schönlein purpura, mesenteric adenitis, lead poisoning, diabetic ketoacidosis, renal stones, and cholecystitis. Sudden acute, excruciating pain suggests obstruction (stones), perforation, or ischemia. Complete blood count (CBC) with differential, urinalysis, pregnancy test, bacterial cultures, serum amylase or lipase, ultrasonography, and abdominal plain films support the findings of a careful history and physical examination. Re-examination several hours later may be necessary to help establish the diagnosis.

Reference

Siegel M, Carel C, Surratt S: Ultrasonography of acute abdominal pain in childhood. JAMA 226:1987, 1991.

CHRONIC ABDOMINAL PAIN

Ten to 15% of all children between the ages of 5 and 15 yr experience chronic abdominal pain. *Chronic recurrent abdominal* pain is defined as three or more episodes of pain, severe enough to affect activities, occurring over a period of 3 mo.

In a large percentage no specific underlying organic cause is found; the pain may be due to dysfunctional bowel with altered motility. The term *irritable bowel syndrome* frequently is applied to this condition. Associated symptoms include pallor, nausea, headaches, vomiting, lethargy, and diarrhea. Disorders such as nocturnal enuresis, fears, or sleep disturbances are seen in 30% of those with this syndrome. The mother, the father, or other siblings often suffer from abdominal pain. Social factors such as a new school, new teacher, examinations, peer group conflict, moving, family illness or death, sibling rivalry, or parental pressure for achievement frequently precipitate or are associated with attacks of pain.

An unknown proportion of patients with chronic pain have lactose intolerance, also manifested by bloating, gaseousness, or diarrhea. In infants, chronic abdominal pain also may be due to colic, gastroesophageal reflux and esophagitis, celiac disease, malrotation, and intra-abdominal tumors. Older children may have pain resulting from acid peptic disease (esophagitis, gastritis, gastric or duodenal ulcer), giardiasis, inflammatory bowel disease, sickle cell anemia, and, rarely, porphyria, hereditary angioedema, systemic lupus erythematosus (vasculitis, serositis), and familial Mediterranean fever. Menstrual-related pain is common in adolescence.

Diagnostic evaluation includes CBC, sedimentation rate, urinalysis, stools for occult blood and ova and parasites, abdominal ultrasound, and upper gastrointestinal series with small bowel follow-through. Breath hydrogen testing after a lactose challenge will identify lactose intolerance. A barium enema is indicated when malrotation or intussusception are suggested.

Treatment of the irritable bowel syndrome should be directed at: (1) explaining the functional and benign nature of this syndrome, (2) identifying sources of stress and providing guidance on how to relieve them, and (3) offering sympathetic reassurance. In some patients, short-term antispasmodic anticholinergic agents may relieve pain, and a high-fiber diet may be beneficial, especially when constipation is present. Formal psychiatric intervention occasionally may be necessary. Specific therapy for other conditions is discussed later in this chapter.

Diarrhea and Malabsorption

The small intestinal mucosa is composed of villous epithelium, crypt epithelium, lamina propria, and muscularis mucosa (Fig. 11-1).

PATHOPHYSIOLOGY OF DIARRHEA

Five mechanisms explain the pathophysiology of diarrhea (Table 11–2). More than one of these may

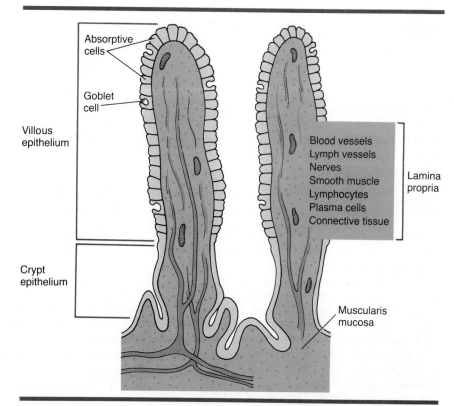

Figure 11–1. Anatomy of the mucosa of the small intestine.

Table 11–2. Mechanisms of Diarrhea

Primary Mechanism	Defect	Stool Examination	Examples	Comment
Secretory	Decreased absorption, increased secretion	Watery, normal osmolality; osmols = 2 × (Na$^+$ + K$^+$)	Cholera, toxigenic E. coli, carcinoid, VIP, neuroblastoma, congenital chloride diarrhea, *Clostridium difficile*, *cryptosporidiosis* (AIDS)	Persists during fasting; bile salt malabsorption also may increase intestinal water secretion; no stool leukocytes
Osmotic	Maldigestion, transport defects, ingestion of unabsorbable solute	Watery, acidic, + reducing substances; increased osmolality; osmols > 2 × (Na$^+$ + K$^+$)	Lactase deficiency, glucose–galactose malabsorption, lactulose, laxative abuse	Stops with fasting, increased breath hydrogen with carbohydrate malabsorption, no stool leukocytes
Increased motility	Decreased transit time or stasis (bacterial overgrowth)	Fecal-like, stimulated by gastrocolic reflex	Irritable bowel syndrome, thyrotoxicosis, postvagotomy dumping syndrome	Infection also may contribute to increased motility
Decreased surface area	Decreased functional capacity	Watery	Short bowel syndrome, celiac disease, rotavirus enteritis	May require elemental diet plus parenteral alimentation
Mucosal invasion (motile or secretory)	Inflammation, decreased colonic reabsorption, increased motility	Blood and increased WBCs in stool	*Salmonella, Shigella,* amebiasis, *Yersinia, Campylobacter*	Dysentery = blood mucus, and WBCs

AIDS = acquired immunodeficiency syndrome; VIP = vasoactive intestinal peptide; WBC = white blood cell.

be present at the same time. A number of disease processes directly affect the secretory and absorptive function of the enterocyte. Some of these processes act by increasing cyclic adenosine monophosphate (cAMP) levels (*Vibrio cholerae, Escherichia coli,* heat-labile toxin, vasoactive intestinal peptide–producing tumors); other processes cause secretory diarrhea by unknown mechanisms (*Shigella* toxin, congenital chloridorrhea). Activation of intestinal production of cAMP produces secretory diarrhea by inhibiting free mucosal sodium chloride absorption and stimulating mucosal chloride secretion. Stimulation of cyclic guanosine monophosphate by *E. coli* heat-stable toxin produces the same effect. Virulence factors for various enteropathogens are noted in Table 11–3. Intestinal resection, inflammation, and infection reduce mucosal surface area, which impairs both digestion and absorption. Abnormal intestinal motility reduces mucosal contact time, decreasing both digestion and absorption.

ACUTE DIARRHEA

A differential diagnosis of acute diarrhea in children is presented in Table 11–4. In addition to a complete history, which includes epidemiologic data (day care, travel), antibiotic exposure, and a physical examination, the stool should be tested for occult blood and white blood cells (with methylene blue smear). If the stool is negative for both blood and white blood cells, and there is no history to

Table 11–3. Virulence Characteristics of Enteropathogens

Organisms	Virulence Properties
Campylobacter jejuni	Invasion; enterotoxin
Clostridium difficile	Cytotoxin; enterotoxin
Cryptosporidium	Adherence
Cyclospora	Inflammation
Entamoeba histolytica	Cyst resistant to physical destruction; invasion; enzyme and cytotoxin production
Enteric adenovirus	Mucosal lesion
Escherichia coli	
Enteropathogenic	Unknown, possibly cytotoxin or adherence
Enterotoxigenic	Enterotoxins (heat stable or labile)
Invasive	Invasion
Enterohemorrhagic (0157:H7)	Cytotoxin
Giardia lamblia	Cyst resistant to physical destruction; adheres to mucosa
Norwalk-like viruses	Mucosal lesion
Rotavirus	Damage to microvilli
Shigella	Invasion; enterotoxin; cytotoxin
Salmonella	Invasion; enterotoxin
Vibrio cholerae	Enterotoxin
Vibrio parahaemolyticus	Invasion; cytotoxin
Yersinia enterocolitica	Invasion; enterotoxin

Table 11–4. Differential Diagnosis of Diarrhea

Infant	Child	Adolescent
Acute		
Common		
Gastroenteritis	Gastroenteritis	Gastroenteritis
Systemic infection	Food poisoning	Food poisoning
Antibiotic associated	Systemic infection	Antibiotic associated
Overfeeding	Antibiotic associated	
Rare		
Primary disaccharidase deficiency	Toxic ingestion	Hyperthyroidism
Hirschsprung toxic colitis		
Adrenogenital syndrome		
Chronic		
Common		
Postinfectious secondary lactase deficiency	Postinfectious secondary lactase deficiency	Irritable bowel syndrome
Cow's milk/soy protein intolerance	Irritable bowel syndrome	Inflammatory bowel disease
Chronic nonspecific diarrhea of infancy	Celiac disease	Lactose intolerance
Celiac disease	Lactose intolerance	Giardiasis
Cystic fibrosis	Giardiasis	Laxative abuse (anorexia nervosa)
AIDS enteropathy	Inflammatory bowel disease	
	AIDS enteropathy	
Rare		
Primary immune defects	Acquired immune defects	Secretory tumor
Familial villous atrophy	Secretory tumors	Primary bowel tumor
Secretory tumors	Pseudo-obstruction	Gay bowel disease
Acrodermatitis enteropathica		
Lymphangiectasia		
Abetalipoproteinemia		
Eosinophilic gastroenteritis		
Short bowel syndrome		
Intractable diarrhea syndrome		
Autoimmune enteropathy		

AIDS = acquired immunodeficiency syndrome.

suggest contaminated food ingestion, the cause most likely is viral. Parasitic infestations other than giardiasis, cryptosporidiosis, and, where endemic, amebiasis are not common causes of acute diarrhea. Stool examinations for parasites usually are not helpful unless the diarrhea persists. If the stool is positive for blood and white blood cells, bacterial causes must be excluded first. The absence of bacterial pathogens and toxins suggests the diagnosis of inflammatory bowel disease, particularly in the adolescent patient who demonstrates weight loss, fever, and abdominal pain (see Table 11–4).

Specific Causes of Infectious Diarrhea

Viral Causes. Viruses associated with gastroenteritis in infants include the *rotavirus, calicivirus, enteric adenovirus, astrovirus,* and members of the *Norwalk agent* group. **Rotavirus** is the most frequent cause of diarrhea during the winter months. Primary infection with rotavirus in infancy may cause moderate to severe disease, whereas reinfection in adolescence leads to mild illness. Rotavirus invades the epithelium of upper small intestine and, in se-

vere cases, may extend throughout the small bowel and colon, resulting in villus damage, secondary transient disaccharidase deficiency, and inflammation in the lamina propria. Vomiting may last for 3–4 days and diarrhea for 7–10 days; dehydration is noted in younger patients. The *diagnosis* may be confirmed on Rotazyme (enzyme-linked immunosorbent assay) testing of the stool. *Treatment* is supportive and consists of supplying fluid and electrolytes to prevent dehydration.

Bacterial Causes. Only certain strains of *Escherichia coli* produce diarrhea. *E. coli* is classified by the mechanism of diarrhea: enteropathogenic (EPEC), enterotoxigenic (ETEC), enteroinvasive (EIEC), enteroadherent (EAEC), and enterohemorrhagic (EHEC) (Table 11–3). EPEC and ETEC adhere to the epithelial cells in the upper small intestine and produce disease by liberating toxins that induce intestinal secretion and limit absorption. EIEC invades the colonic mucosa, producing widespread mucosal damage with acute inflammation. EPEC is responsible for many of the epidemics of diarrhea in nurseries for neonates and day care cen-

Table 11–5. Antibiotic Therapy of Diarrhea

Organism	Treatment*	Comment
Salmonella typhi	Ampicillin§, chloramphenicol§, trimethoprim–sulfamethoxazole, cefotaxime	Invasive, bacteremic disease
Other *Salmonella*	Usually none; amoxicillin, ampicillin, trimethoprim–sulfamethoxazole	Treatment indicated if less than 3 mo of age, or if malignancy, sickle cell anemia, AIDS, evidence of nongastrointestinal foci of infection are present
Shigella	Trimethoprim–sulfamethoxazole, ampicillin	Amoxicillin is not recommended; treatment reduces infectivity and improves outcome
E. coli Toxigenic	Usually none if endemic; trimethoprim–sulfamethoxazole or ciprofloxacin for traveler's diarrhea	Prevention of traveler's diarrhea with bismuth subsalicylate, doxycycline, or ciprofloxacin†
Invasive or pathogenic	Trimethoprim–sulfamethoxazole, neomycin	
Campylobacter	Mild disease needs no treatment; erythromycin for diarrhea, gentamicin for systemic illness	If started early (days 1–3), treatment reduces symptoms and fecal organisms
Yersinia	None for diarrhea; gentamicin, chloramphenicol, trimethoprim–sulfamethoxazole for systemic illness	Value of treatment of mesenteric adenitis with antibiotics is not established
Vibrio cholerae	Tetracycline, trimethoprim–sulfamethoxazole	Fluid maintenance is critical
Clostridium difficile	Oral vancomycin, metronidazole‡	*C. difficile* is an agent of antibiotic-associated diarrhea and pseudomembranous colitis
Giardia lamblia	Quinacrine, furazolidone, metronidazole‡	Furazolidone only preparation available in liquid form
Cryptosporidium	None; azithromycin or paromomycin + octreotide in AIDS	A serious infection in immunocompromised patients (AIDS)
Entamoeba histolytica	Metronidazole‡, tinidazole followed by iodoquinol	

* All treatment is predicated on knowledge of antimicrobial sensitivities.
† Ciprofloxacin is not indicated for children with growing bones (less than 17 yr).
‡ The safety of metronidazole in children is unknown.
§ Often resistant.
AIDS = acquired immunodeficiency syndrome.

ters. ETEC plays a major role in *traveler's diarrhea.* EHEC is responsible for a hemorrhagic colitis and some cases of the *hemolytic–uremic syndrome,* especially the *E. coli* 0157:H7 strain. *Treatment* is indicated for infants under 3 mo of age with EPEC and for those patients who remain symptomatic (Table 11–5).

Salmonella is transmitted through contact with infected animals or from contaminated food products, such as milk, eggs, and poultry. The organism produces disease by invading the intestinal mucosa. *Treatment* of mild illness does not shorten the clinical course, but does prolong bacterial excretion. Antibiotic therapy is necessary only for high-risk patients who have symptoms of toxicity, de-

velop metastatic foci, or have *S. typhi* infection (Table 11–5).

Shigella may cause disease by producing toxin either alone or in combination with tissue invasion. Infection is spread by person-to-person contact or by the ingestion of contaminated food. The colon is selectively affected. Antibiotic *treatment* will produce a bacteriologic cure in 80% of patients after 48 hr, thus reducing the spread of the disease. Many *S. sonnei,* the predominant strain affecting children, are ampicillin resistant. Treatment with trimethoprim–sulfamethoxazole generally is effective (Table 11–5).

Campylobacter jejuni may account for 15% of episodes of bacterial diarrhea. The infection is spread by person-to-person contact and by contaminated water and food. The organism invades the mucosa of the jejunum, ileum, and colon, producing enterocolitis. Most patients recover spontaneously before the diagnosis is established. *Treatment* speeds recovery and reduces the duration of the carrier state (Table 11–5).

Yersinia enterocolitica is transmitted by pets and by contaminated food (e.g., chitterlings). Infants and young children characteristically have a diarrheal disease, whereas older children usually develop acute lesions of the terminal ileum or acute mesenteric lymphadenitis resembling appendicitis or Crohn disease. Arthritis, rash, and

spondylopathy may develop. The course usually is self-limited, lasting 3 days to 3 wk. The efficacy of antibiotic *treatment* is questionable, but children with septicemia or infection in sites other than the gastrointestinal tract should be treated (Table 11–5).

Clostridium difficile is a common cause of antibiotic-associated diarrhea. *Treatment* includes discontinuation of the prior antibiotic and, if diarrhea is severe, oral vancomycin or metronidazole.

Many bacterial agents may be food contaminants and cause food poisoning. Sudden onset, a common source, epidemic vomiting, and diarrhea should suggest food poisoning (Table 11–6).

Table 11–6. Common Causes of Food Poisoning

Agent	Mechanism	Source	Time of Onset	Signs
*Salmonella**	Tissue invasion	Dairy/meat products	16–48 hr	Fever, cramps, vomiting, bloody diarrhea
*S. aureus**	Preformed toxin	Meat, egg salad, pastries	1–6 hr	Vomiting, diarrhea
*C. perfringens**	In vivo toxin production	Meat, gravy	8–16 hr	Cramps, diarrhea
*C. botulinum**	Preformed toxin	Canned food, honey, fish	18–36 hr	Nausea, vomiting, diarrhea, constipation, paralysis
B. cereus				
Short incubation	Preformed toxin	Fried rice	1–6 hr	Nausea, vomiting
Long incubation	Toxin produced in vivo	Vegetables	8–16 hr	Vomiting, diarrhea, cramps
Norwalk agent	Invasion	Waterborne, shellfish	16–48 hr	Watery diarrhea
Heavy metals†	Direct toxicity	Acidic juices in metal containers, lemonade, fruit punch	1–4 hr	Vomiting, cramps, diarrhea
Scombroid	Histamine	Tuna	Minutes	Flushing, dizziness, headache, vomiting, diarrhea
Ciguatera	Toxin	Mackerel	1–6 hr	Paresthesia of lips, tooth pain, cramps, vomiting, diarrhea
Paralytic shellfish	Neurotoxin	Dinoflagellates of mollusks	1–3 hr	Paresthesia of lips and extremities, dysphagia, ataxia

* *Salmonella* (23%), *Staphylococcus aureus* (18%), *Clostridium perfringens* (8%), and *C. botulinum* (8%) are the most common causes of food poisoning.

† Includes copper, zinc, tin, and cadmium.

Parasitic Causes. *Entamoeba histolytica* and *Giardia lamblia* are important parasites found in North America that produce disease. Amebiasis occurs in warmer climates, whereas giardiasis is endemic throughout the United States and is common among infants in day care centers.

The site of infection with **Entamoeba histolytica** is the colon, although amebae may pass through the bowel wall and invade the liver, lung, and brain. Diarrhea is of acute onset, is bloody, and contains white blood cells. *Diagnosis* depends on identification of the organism in the stool and may be confirmed serologically. The drug of choice for *treatment* is metronidazole.

Giardia lamblia is transmitted through ingestion of cysts either from contact with an infected individual or from food or fresh or well water contaminated with infected feces. The organism adheres to the microvilli of the duodenal and jejunal epithelium. The onset of the illness usually is insidious but may be acute. *Clinical manifestations* include anorexia, nausea, gaseousness, abdominal distention, watery diarrhea, secondary lactose intolerance, and weight loss. The *diagnosis* may be made by identifying the organism in the stool, in duodenal aspirate, or in the mucosa of a small bowel biopsy. See Table 11–5 for *treatment*.

Cryptosporidium causes mild diarrhea in immunocompetent infants attending day care centers. In contrast to the severe diarrhea it produces in patients with acquired immunodeficiency syndrome (AIDS), cryptosporidiosis in normal infants is a self-limited disease (Table 11–5).

Management of Diarrhea

Therapy must be directed to cure the initiating event, to correct dehydration and ongoing fluid and electrolyte deficits, and to manage secondary complications resulting from mucosal injury. Antibiotic treatment is noted in Table 11–5. *Traveler's* diarrhea may be prevented by avoiding uncooked food and untreated drinking water; preventive medication with Pepto-Bismol, tetracycline (8 yr of age or older), or trimethoprim–sulfamethoxazole is controversial. In the near future, *rotavirus* diarrhea may be prevented by vaccination.

Treatment of fluid deficits requires an estimation of the degree of dehydration and the determination of any electrolyte imbalances, such as hypernatremia, hyponatremia, or metabolic acidosis (see Chapter 16). Acidosis is due to stool bicarbonate losses, lactic acidosis resulting from fermentation of malabsorbed carbohydrate or shock, and phosphate retention resulting from transient prerenal renal insufficiency. Therapy of severe fluid and electrolyte losses requires intravenous alimentation, whereas less severe degrees of dehydration (<10%) in infants without excessive vomiting may be managed with oral rehydration solutions containing glucose and electrolytes. Jejunal and ileal glucose absorption will carry sodium into the enterocyte, thus also drawing in water. Oral rehydration solutions contain 2% glucose, 75–90 mEq/L Na$^+$, 20 mEq/L K$^+$, 45–80 mEq/L Cl$^-$, and 30 mEq/L bicarbonate or citrate.

Severe infections may damage the mucosa, producing a secondary lactase deficiency that causes osmotic diarrhea if a lactose-containing formula is given to an infant. Therefore, a non–lactose-containing formula may be needed during the immediate rehabilitation phase following episodes of *severe* diarrhea. Drugs such as loperamide, paregoric, and diphenoxylate are potentially dangerous and have no place in the management of acute infectious diarrhea in children.

References

Ashkenazi S, Cleary TG: Antibiotic treatment of bacterial gastroenteritis. Pediatr Infect Dis J 10:140, 1991.

Behrman RE (ed): Nelson Textbook of Pediatrics. 14th ed. Philadelphia, WB Saunders, 1992, Sec. 12.10, 12.27–12.30, 12.34, 12.38 and 12.41–12.42.

Blacklow NR, Greenberg HB: Viral gastroenteritis. N Engl J Med 4:252, 1991.

Guerrant RL, Bobak DA: Bacterial and protozoal gastroenteritis. N Engl J Med 5:327, 1991.

Pickering LK: Therapy for acute infectious diarrhea in children. J Pediatr 118:118, 1991.

Snyder JD: Use and misuse of oral therapy for diarrhea: Comparison of US practices with American Academy of Pediatrics recommendations. Pediatrics 87:28, 1991.

Staat MA, Morrow AL, Reves RR, et al: Diarrhea in children newly enrolled in day-care centers in Houston. Pediatr Infect Dis J 10:282, 1991.

CHRONIC DIARRHEA (SEE TABLE 11–4)

During infancy, chronic diarrhea may be a manifestation of specific genetic diseases, such as disaccharidase deficiencies, cystic fibrosis, or immunologically mediated diseases. *Milk and/or soy protein intolerance* should be considered in infants less than 1 yr of age when the stool contains erythrocytes, with or without eosinophils. This can occur even in breast-fed infants if cow's milk proteins enter maternal milk. The mechanism by which milk proteins result in mucosal injury is poorly understood. Immune-mediated disease against gluten **(celiac disease)** begins once the infant is exposed to solid foods containing this protein. Cereals composed of wheat, barley, rye, and oats produce the disease, which may necessitate a lifelong withdrawal from these foods.

Chronic diarrhea also may be the only manifestation of **cystic fibrosis** or may occur in association with meconium ileus, rectal prolapse, hypoalbuminemia, hyponatremic dehydration, and hypoprothrombinemia. The diagnosis of cystic fibrosis is confirmed by documenting an elevated sweat chloride content. Primary metabolic disorders of absorption, such as *glucose–galactose malabsorption* and *congenital chloridorrhea*, will appear in the neonatal period.

The most common cause of chronic diarrhea during infancy is **chronic nonspecific diarrhea of infancy** or **toddler's diarrhea**. The onset is between 6 mo and 3 yr of age and is rarely accompanied by pain. Often the first stool in the morning is formed, but stools (4–6/24 hr) progress during the day to greater liquidity, sometimes containing mucus and food. The infants do not demonstrate fluid and electrolyte abnormalities, dehydration, or failure to thrive. There is often a family history of similar intestinal problems in siblings or in parents. Symptoms may be precipitated by teething or common infectious illnesses. In this same age group, a **lactase deficiency** following viral gastroenteritides also is common and may result in secondary lactose malabsorption that may persist for months. Increased breath hydrogen excretion following a standard oral lactose challenge, resulting from colonic bacterial fermentation of malabsorbed lactose, is diagnostic. Bloating, cramping, borborygmus, and flatus also are noted in lactose-intolerant patients during the lactose challenge. A non–lactose-containing formula may be needed until lactase activity regenerates. *Congenital sucrose deficiency* is rare and occurs after sucrose-containing foods (fruits, juices, vegetables) are added to the diet in sufficient quantities to exceed the digestive capacity of the brush border sucrase; treatment consists of avoiding sucrose sugar–containing foods.

Beyond infancy, lactase deficiency and parasitic infection, usually giardiasis, are important common causes of chronic diarrhea (Table 11–4). Diarrhea as the only manifestation of irritable bowel syndrome is unusual in older children and adolescents. During this older age period, *inflammatory bowel disease* should be considered, especially when diarrhea is associated with fever, hematochezia, abdominal pain, weight loss, rash, arthralgias or arthritis, and uveitis or episcleritis.

When chronic diarrhea persists and is associated with weight loss and global or specific nutritional deficiencies, a **malabsorption syndrome** exists. The usual early manifestations of malabsorption are frequent, bulky–oily, foul-smelling stools (steatorrhea), weight loss, and a ravenous appetite. Late manifestations include failure to thrive, muscle wasting, protuberant abdomen, secondary immune deficiency, and nutritional disorders. Malabsorption of specific nutrients—such as vitamin D, which results in rickets; vitamin K, which results in hemorrhage; vitamin B_{12}, folate, and iron, which result in anemia; and calcium, which results in hypocalcemic tetany—may develop. Mechanisms of malabsorption include impaired digestion, reduced absorption, decreased surface area, lymphatic obstruction, drugs, infection, collagen vascular disease, and endocrine abnormalities (Table 11–7). Cystic fibrosis, celiac sprue, short bowel syndrome, and giardiasis are common causes of malabsorption. Immune deficiencies usually associated with enteritis include Wiskott-Aldrich syndrome, common variable hypogammaglobulinemia, and AIDS. Certain AIDS related opportunistic intestinal infections (*Isospora belli, Cryptosporidium, Entamoeba,* and cytomegalovirus) also cause malabsorption and failure to thrive.

The **diagnosis** of a patient with chronic diarrhea begins with a careful history, including a family and dietary history as it relates to the onset of symptoms. It is important to remember that neither stool odor, which is usually unpleasant, nor stool color, unless blood is seen, has any consistent relationship to the presence of gastrointestinal disease. Physical examination should include a careful assessment of the patient's nutritional status (see Chapter 2) and a check for signs of infection.

Stool should be tested for blood, white blood cells, fat content, and carbohydrate malabsorption. The latter is assessed by identifying an acid stool pH and reducing substances. Fecal fat should not exceed 15% of intake in infants and 10% in older children. To exclude parasitic infection, three fresh stool specimens should be collected for examination. Barium studies should not be done within several days of the stool collection because parasites adhere to the barium. Roentgenographic findings may be diagnostic for inflammatory bowel disease, but for many of the small intestinal mucosal disorders only a nonspecific "malabsorption pattern," characterized by thickened mucosal folds, edema of the bowel wall, and flocculation of the barium, is present.

A number of studies are available to assess specific types of malabsorption. The D-xylose test provides an index of mucosal carbohydrate absorption. Lactose and sucrose malabsorption can be

Table 11–7. Malabsorption Syndromes

Reduced Digestion	
Pancreatic exocrine deficiency	Cystic fibrosis, pancreatitis, Schwachman syndrome
Bile salt deficiency	Cholestasis, biliary atresia, hepatitis, cirrhosis, bacterial deconjugation
Enzyme defects	Lactase, sucrase, enterokinase, lipase deficiencies
Reduced Absorption	
Primary absorption defects	Glucose–galactose malabsorption, abetalipoproteinemia, cystinuria, Hartnup disease
Decreased mucosal surface area	Crohn disease, malnutrition, short bowel syndrome, antimetabolite chemotherapy, familial villous atrophy
Small intestinal disease	Celiac disease, tropical sprue, giardiasis, immune/allergic enteritis, Crohn disease, lymphoma, AIDS
Lymphatic Obstruction	
	Lymphangiectasia, Whipple disease, lymphoma, chylous ascites
Others	
Drugs	Antibiotics, antimetabolites, neomycin, laxatives
Collagen vascular	Scleroderma
Infestations	Hookworms, tapeworm, giardiasis, immune defects

measured using the breath hydrogen technique. A Sudan stain of the stool may be used as a qualitative assessment of fecal fat, but steatorrhea is best quantitated by a 72-hr fecal fat study. Measurement of the fecal alpha-1-antitrypsin level is a screening study for documenting enteric protein loss. Quantitative measurements of protein loss can be made by assessing alpha-1-antitrypsin clearance with simultaneous serum and 24-hr stool concentrations. Serum calcium, prothrombin time, and vitamin A and E levels may be determined to assess fat-soluble vitamin deficiencies.

Peroral, **transpyloric biopsy** during gastroduodenoscopy of the small intestinal mucosa may be needed to document diseases such as celiac sprue, lymphangiectasia, giardiasis, abetalipoproteinemia, and tropical sprue.

Treatment must be directed at the primary disease and at the correction of associated deficiency states, such as rickets and hypoprothrombinemia. Primary treatment of cystic fibrosis requires lifelong pancreatic enzyme replacement, whereas therapy of celiac disease requires strict adherence to a gluten-free diet. Hyperalimentation may be needed for familial enteropathies, short bowel syndrome or refractory cases of chronic intractable diarrhea.

References

Behrman RE (ed): Nelson Textbook of Pediatrics. 14th ed. Philadelphia, WB Saunders, 1992, Sec. 13.14, 6.20, 12.10, 13.58–13.61, 13.65.

Camilleri M, Prather CM: The irritable bowel syndrome: Mechanisms and a practical approach to management. Ann Int Med 116:1001, 1992.

Phillips AD, Schmitz J: Familial microvillous atrophy: A clinicopathological survey of 23 cases. J Pediatr Gastroenterol Nutr 14:380, 1992.

Constipation/Encopresis

Constipation is defined as infrequent passage of hard, dry stools. Obstipation is the absence of bowel movements. The causes of constipation are noted in Table 11–8. Beyond the neonatal period, the most common cause (90–95%) of constipation is voluntary withholding or **functional constipation** (Table 11–9), a problem often beginning with the attempt to toilet train the infant. A family history of similar problems often is obtained. Stool retention may be due to conflicts in toilet training but usually is caused by pain on defecation, which creates a fear of defecation, and further retention. Voluntary withholding of stool increases distention of the rectum, which decreases rectal sensation, necessitating an even greater fecal mass to initiate the urge to defecate. Complications of stool retention include impaction, abdominal pain, overflow diarrhea resulting from leakage around the fecal mass, anal fissure, rectal bleeding and urinary tract infection caused by extrinsic pressure on the urethra.

Encopresis, which is daytime or nighttime soiling by formed stools beyond the age of expected toilet training (4–5 yr), is another complication of

Table 11–8. Causes of Constipation

Nonorganic (Functional)

Organic
  Intestinal
  Hirschsprung disease
  Neuronal dysgenesis
  Anal stenosis
  Anal stricture
  Anterior dislocation of the anus
  Pseudo-obstruction
  Collagen vascular diseases
  Rectal abscess/fissure
  Stricture post-NEC

  Drugs
  Lead
  Narcotics
  Antidepressants
  Psychoactive drugs (chlorpromazine [Thorazine])
  Chemotherapeutic agents (vincristine)

  Metabolic
  Dehydration
  Cystic fibrosis (meconium ileus equivalent)
  Hypothyroidism
  Hypokalemia
  Hypercalcemia

  Neuromuscular
  Infant botulism
  Absent abdominal muscle
  Myotonic dystrophy
  Spinal cord lesions (tumors or spina bifida)
  Chagas disease

NEC = necrotizing enterocolitis.

constipation (see Chapter 1). In older children it is important to ask specifically about soiling, because such information may not be expressed because of embarrassment. These children frequently are unable to sense the need to defecate because of stretching of the internal sphincter by the retained fecal mass.

In term infants, meconium should be passed within the first 24 hr of life, and failure to pass meconium suggests an underlying disorder. The consistency and frequency of bowel movements vary greatly both in the individual child and among different children. Breast-fed infants usually produce stool with every feeding but may produce stool only 1–2 times a day. Formula-fed infants usually produce stool daily but may produce stool once every 2 or 3 days. In general, the range of normal for infants is from 5 stools/day to as few as 1 every 3rd day.

Stool is produced as the fecal fluid is moved through the colon by three to four mass propulsive movements per day. Water and electrolytes are reabsorbed (95%) in the colon and rectosigmoid, resulting in formed stool. Stool is stored in the rectum until sufficient distention produces the urge to defecate. The internal anal sphincter then relaxes and stool enters the anal canal. The external anal sphincter is a voluntary muscle controlling fecal continence. Failure to defecate may be due to decreased peristalsis (aganglionic segment, spinal cord defect), decreased expulsion (weakened abdominal muscle), and anatomic malformations (anterior dislocation of the anus, neuronal dysgenesis, aganglionic Hirschsprung disease, stenosis). The exclusion of **Hirschsprung disease** is critical in the *differential diagnosis* of constipation, especially in infants because of the risk of bacterial overgrowth, enterocolitis, and intestinal perforation (Table 11–9).

Functional constipation may be self-perpetuating, often becoming more severe with time; symptomatic treatment is indicated. In infants, increases in the intake of juices and fruits, malt extract, or lactulose is effective. For older children, mineral oil, 1–3 oz/24 hr given either in divided doses or as a single dose 2 hr after meals, and increased dietary fiber content usually are successful. If there is marked fecal retention, the rectum must be cleared of impacted stool with enemas and/or cathartics. Once stools are softened, the oil and fiber supplements must be continued on a regular basis for several months, during which time the dose gradually is reduced. Psychologic problems leading to or resulting from the constipation may need special attention (see Chapter 1).

Vomiting

Vomiting occurs in both gastrointestinal and nongastrointestinal diseases in childhood. The forceful ejection of gastric contents, often is preceded by nausea and is due to the coordination of gastric atony (except in pyloric stenosis), relaxation of the gastroesophageal junction, and increased intragastric (abdominal) pressure from abdominal wall contractions. Vomiting is mediated by the medullary emesis center in the floor of the 4th ventricle, which is influenced by gastrointestinal (visceral afferent) or nongastrointestinal (chemoreceptive trigger zone) stimuli. The latter elements are affected by various stimuli, including drugs and motion sickness. **Regurgitation** is not vomiting but rather a passive, nonforceful ejection of gastric contents resulting from reflux through a relaxed lower esophageal sphincter. Most infants less than 3 mo

Table 11–9. Distinguishing Features of Hirschsprung Disease and Functional (Acquired) Constipation

	Functional Constipation	Hirschsprung Disease*
History		
Onset of constipation	After 2 yr of age	At birth
Encopresis	Common	Very rare
Forced bowel training	Usual	None
Stool size	Very large	Small, ribbon-like
Enterocolitis	None	Possible
Abdominal pain	Common	Common
Failure to thrive	Uncommon	Common
Examination		
Abdominal distention	Rare	Common
Poor growth	Rare	Common
Anal tone	Patulous	Tight
Rectal examination	Stool in ampulla	Ampulla empty
Malnutrition	Absent	Possible
Laboratory		
Barium enema	Massive amounts of stool, no transition zone	Transition zone, delayed evacuation (greater than 24 hr)
Rectal biopsy	Normal	No ganglion cells; ↑ acetylcholinesterase staining
Anorectal manometry	Distension of the rectum causes relaxation of the internal sphincter	No sphincter relaxation

* Note that ultrashort-segment Hirschsprung disease may have clinical features of functional (acquired) megacolon (e.g., constipation).

(From Behrman RE (ed): Nelson Textbook of Pediatrics. 14th ed. Philadelphia, WB Saunders, 1992, p 955.)

of age regurgitate formula with no apparent ill effects.

The *differential diagnosis* of vomiting should be approached by considering age-specific diseases. During the neonatal period, gastrointestinal obstruction often is due to congenital malformations (Table 11–10). In infants, gastroenteritis, overfeeding, and gastroesophageal reflux are the most common causes of emesis and regurgitation. Food allergy and milk protein intolerance also are common. Nongastrointestinal diseases that produce emesis in the infant include systemic infections, hyperammonemia, associated inborn errors of metabolism, adrenogenital syndrome, rumination, increased intracranial pressure and subdural hemorrhage.

In children and adolescents, vomiting commonly is caused by gastroenteritis, systemic infection, toxic ingestions, and appendicitis. Less common causes are Reye syndrome, hepatitis, ulcers, pancreatitis, malrotation, brain tumor, increased intracranial pressure, cyclic vomiting or abdominal migraine, middle ear infection, and chemotherapy.

Children also may have vomiting associated with pertussis syndrome and achalasia. Vomiting also may occur in adolescence as a result of bulimia and inflammatory bowel disease.

A careful history and physical examination are necessary to determine whether the source of vomiting is gastrointestinal or some other systemic disturbance. Neonates with polyhydramnios, drooling, a large amount of gastric aspirate (10–20 mL), persistent emesis, abdominal distention, bile- or blood-stained vomitus may be obstructed and should have a contrast study to determine the site of the obstruction. Bile-stained emesis suggests obstruction distal to the ampulla of Vater. Persistent emesis in older children may require endoscopic evaluation, especially in the presence of dysphagia, gastrointestinal hemorrhage, or a foreign body. *Laboratory investigation* to determine the presence of infection (culture), reflux (prolonged esophageal pH testing), metabolic disorders (testing for acidosis, hyperammonemia), pancreatitis (testing for amylase and lipase), pyloric stenosis (testing for alkalosis, ultrasound, contrast radiograph) and inflammatory bowel disease (erythrocyte sedimentation rate, mucosal biopsy, roentgenographic contrast study) should be directed by the information obtained from the history and physical examination.

Treatment of emesis is directed toward the underlying disorders and toward correction of dehydration and electrolyte disturbances. Short periods of small frequent feedings of clear fluids may be all that is needed to stop emesis. Rarely, drugs such as promethazine, chlorpromazine, or prochlorperazine by rectal suppository may be useful,

but extrapyramidal side effects may ensue. Ondansetron, a serotonin antagonist, is effective treatment for chemotherapy-induced emesis and other causes of refractory vomiting.

References

Behrman RE (ed): Nelson Textbook of Pediatrics. 14th ed. Philadelphia, WB Saunders, 1992, Sec. 3.26, 3.29, 13.14, 13.32.
Hatch TF: Encopresis and constipation in children. Pediatr Clin North Am 35:257, 1988.
Partin JC, Hamill SK, Fischel JE, et al: Painful defecation and fecal soiling in children. Pediatrics 89:1007, 1992.
Madoff RD, Williams JG, Caushaj PF: Fecal incontinence. N Engl J Med 15:1002, 1992.
Rollins MD, Shields MD, Quinn RJM, et al: Value of ultrasound in differentiating causes of persistent vomiting in infants. Gut 32:612, 1991.

Gastrointestinal Hemorrhage

Hemorrhage may occur at any location in the gastrointestinal tract, and the differential diagnosis depends to a large extent on the patient's age. **Hematemesis**, blood-stained emesis, results from bleeding proximal to the ligament of Treitz. Less severe upper gastrointestinal bleeding results in a coffee grounds appearance of the emesis. **Melena** refers to soft, usually black or dark-colored stool of a tarry consistency; it usually is suggestive of bleeding from the oropharynx into the proximal small intestine. With stasis of blood in the right colon, bleeding lesions in that area also may appear as melena. **Hematochezia** refers to bright red or maroon-colored stools. While typically the lesion is colonic, massive upper gastrointestinal bleeding may cause bright red blood per rectum because blood is a cathartic and decreases transit time. *Bright red streaks* of blood coating the surface of a stool suggest a rectal or anal lesion. **Occult gastrointestinal bleeding** is defined as significant, ongoing blood loss in the absence of a discernible change in the color or texture of stools; such loss may produce iron-deficiency anemia if it persists.

Before proceeding with an evaluation, it is important to be sure that the stool does indeed contain blood and that the blood is from the gastrointestinal tract. A number of commonly ingested substances may simulate hematochezia: noncarbonated drinks (Kool-Aid, Hawaiian Punch), colored gelatins, beets, fruit bars, clingstone peaches, and antibiotics. Similarly, melena is simulated by the ingestion of compounds containing bismuth (Pepto-Bismol), therapeutic iron supplements, charcoal, and spinach. Swallowed blood from a

Small Intestine

Table 11–10. Causes of Gastrointestinal Obstruction

Esophagus
Congenital	Tracheoesophageal fistula
	Isolated esophageal atresia
Acquired	Caustic agent esophageal stricture
	Peptic stricture
	Chagas disease
	Collagen vascular disease

Stomach
Congenital	Antral webs
	Pyloric stenosis
Acquired	Bezoars/foreign body
	Pyloric stricture (ulcer)
	Crohn disease
	Eosinophilic gastroenteropathy
	Prostaglandin induced
	Chronic granulomatous disease

Small Intestine
Congenital	Duodenal atresia
	Annular pancreas
	Malrotation/volvulus
	Malrotation/Ladd bands
	Ileal atresia
	Meconium ileus
	Inguinal hernia
Acquired	Postsurgical adhesions
	Crohn disease
	Intussusception
	Meconium ileus equivalent

Colon
Congenital	Meconium plug
	Hirschsprung disease
	Colonic atresia, stenosis
	Imperforate rectum
	Rectal stenosis
	Malrotation/volvulus
Acquired	Ulcerative colitis (toxic megacolon)
	Crohn disease
	Chagas disease
	Stricture post-NEC

NEC = necrotizing enterocolitis.

Table 11–11. Differential Diagnosis of Gastrointestinal Bleeding in Childhood

	Infant	Child	Adolescent
Common	Swallowed maternal blood Anal fissure Milk protein allergy Necrotizing enterocolitis Intussusception Bacterial gastroenteritis	Anal fissure Bacterial gastroenteritis Intussusception Ulcer/gastritis Swallowed epistaxis Juvenile polyp Mallory-Weiss syndrome	Bacterial gastroenteritis Inflammatory bowel disease Ulcer/gastritis Mallory-Weiss syndrome Polyps Hemorrhoids
Rare	Volvulus Hemorrhagic disease of newborn Meckel diverticulum	Esophageal varices Esophagitis Coagulopathy Meckel diverticulum Lymphonodular hyperplasia Foreign body Hemangioma Sexual abuse Hemolytic–uremic syndrome Henoch-Schönlein purpura	Esophageal varices Esophagitis Coagulopathy Telangiectasia (angiodysplasia) Gay bowel disease

briskly bleeding nasopharyngeal or oral lesion, which is subsequently regurgitated, also may be misinterpreted as upper gastrointestinal bleeding. Rarely, hemoptysis may be confused with hematemesis. Vaginal bleeding and hematuria have been mistakenly interpreted as hematochezia.

The *differential diagnosis* of gastrointestinal hemorrhage is based primarily on a careful history and a physical examination of the child (Table 11–11) and on the site of bleeding (Table 11–12). Abdominal pain that awakens the patient at night, is relieved by food and is accompanied by hematemesis is highly suggestive of peptic ulcer disease. Substernal pain suggests esophagitis. Infants and older children with chronic hepatic disease and cirrhosis who exhibit hematemesis probably have bleeding esophageal varices. A history of neonatal omphalitis and subsequent portal vein thrombophlebitis also suggests variceal bleeding secondary to portal vein obstruction. However, for many children who have acute gastrointestinal hemorrhage, no obvious diagnosis is evident at the time of the first episode of bleeding.

The goals of *management of acute gastrointestinal hemorrhage*, in order of importance, are (1) to correct hypovolemia, (2) to correct anemia, (3) to stop the bleeding, (4) to prevent recurrence, (5) to diagnose the cause, and (6) to apply specific therapy. The immediate approach to the patient includes (1) assessing pulse and blood pressure (both supine and orthostatic changes), (2) establishing intravenous access for administering fluids, (3) expanding the intravascular volume in the presence of hypovolemia by providing crystalloid or colloid fluids, (4) determining blood hemoglobin content, and (5) typing and cross-matching whole blood or packed cells for continued replacement of whole blood or erythrocyte losses. If hepatic disease is present, co-

Table 11–12. Sites and Causes of Gastrointestinal (GI) Bleeding

Upper GI	Upper and Lower GI	Lower GI
Epistaxis Esophagitis Gastritis Gastric ulcer Duodenal ulcer Esophageal varices Mallory-Weiss syndrome Foreign body Caustic ingestion	Hemorrhagic disease of newborn Hemangioma Osler-Weber-Rendu syndrome Arteriovenous malformation Tumor	Milk/soy protein colitis Eosinophilic colitis Gastroenteritis Intussusception Henoch-Schönlein purpura Polyps Inflammatory bowel disease Volvulus Meckel diverticulum Lymphonodular hyperplasia Pseudomembranous colitis Hemolytic–uremic syndrome

agulation studies should be determined; if coagulopathy is present, therapy is initiated with parenteral vitamin K and fresh frozen plasma. In newborn infants with bright red bloody emesis or bright red blood passed per rectum, an Apt test should be performed to determine whether the blood is fetal or maternal. Swallowed maternal blood at the time of delivery or from a ruptured lacteal during breast feeding is a common cause of hematemesis or hematochezia in the newborn (see Chapter 6).

During the initial evaluation, an appropriately sized nasogastric tube should be placed in the stomach to determine whether the bleeding site is above the ligament of Treitz and to monitor the rate of upper gastrointestinal system hemorrhage. If the pylorus is closed, duodenal bleeding may not be detected with a nasogastric tube. If the gastric fluid return is clear, the source of the bleeding probably is below the ligament of Treitz. A small amount of hematemesis or melena may be misleading, because a source of major blood loss may be concealed within the intestines. Furthermore, an initial normal hemoglobin and hematocrit may give a false sense of security, since re-equilibration may take 2–4 hr to demonstrate blood losses.

To diagnose the specific cause of upper gastrointestinal bleeding, **endoscopy** should be performed after the hemorrhaging has decreased or stopped. An upper gastrointestinal tract contrast roentgenographic study also may be helpful. Lower intestinal bleeding may be evaluated with proctosigmoidoscopy, colonoscopy, arteriography, or specific scans. The technetium-99m (^{99m}Tc) pertechnetate scan, preceded by pentagastrin stimulation, or a histamine H_2-receptor antagonist (cimetidine), will identify the ectopic acid–secreting cells creating the hemorrhage in **Meckel diverticulum**.

When the site of bleeding is unclear, arteriography, ^{99m}Tc sulfur colloid, or ^{99m}Tc-labeled autologous red blood cells can be infused intravenously. Arteriography and ^{99m}Tc sulfur colloid detect rapid bleeding, whereas intermittent bleeding is more reliably identified by ^{99m}Tc-labeled red blood cells.

The *treatment* of gastrointestinal hemorrhage should be specific for the underlying disorder. H_2-receptor–blocking drugs and antacids are useful agents for gastritis, esophagitis, and peptic ulcer disease, whereas the Mallory-Weiss syndrome requires the above plus close inpatient observation. Acute abdominal crises, such as volvulus or intussusception, require immediate contrast studies, which may be therapeutic for intussusception. Bleeding esophageal varices may be managed with intravenous vasopressin or sclerotherapy. Rarely, emergency portosystemic shunts are r... stop variceal hemorrhage in children. ... massive hemorrhage that is unresponsiv... apy may require surgical exploration, whether or not a lesion has been identified. New techniques that may avoid emergency surgery include direct intra-arterial infusion of vasopressin, selective embolization of an arteriovenous malformation or isolated bleeding site, and electrocoagulation and laser photocoagulation for a bleeding ulcer or bleeding from angiodysplastic lesions.

Jaundice

Jaundice (icterus) is the yellow discoloration of the skin, mucous membranes, and sclera caused by increased serum bilirubin concentrations that are deposited in tissue. Although indirect hyperbilirubinemia appears on the skin as yellow–brown coloration and direct hyperbilirubinemia gives the skin a yellow–green appearance, laboratory evaluation is needed to diagnose and classify the jaundice. Hyperbilirubinemia may be due to overproduction, decreased hepatic uptake or metabolism, and decreased hepatic excretion of bilirubin. Jaundice is the most common physical finding of hepatic dysfunction in children of all ages. Jaundice may be due to a benign process (as in physiologic jaundice of the newborn) or may be a sign of serious underlying disease such as hepatitis. The production and excretion of bilirubin is discussed in Chapter 6.

Jaundice in the neonatal patient is discussed elsewhere (Chapter 6). In older patients, jaundice always is a sign of significant disease. Icterus in the young infant may not be visible until the bilirubin level is 10 mg/dL, whereas older children and adolescents demonstrate jaundice when the bilirubin is 2.5 mg/dL. Additional signs of underlying hepatic disease include protuberant abdomen, ascites, edema, pruritus/excoriations, dark urine, and acholic whitish-gray stools. The differential diagnosis and laboratory evaluation of a jaundiced infant depend on whether there is indirect or direct hyperbilirubinemia (Figure 11–2). Patients with indirect hyperbilirubinemia should be evaluated further for evidence of immune- or nonimmune-mediated hemolysis by a CBC, peripheral blood smear, and Coombs test. Nonhemolytic indirect hyperbilirubinemia is common in newborn infants and older children with Gilbert syndrome. The remaining patients with indirect hyperbilirubinemia should have an appropriate laboratory assessment based on the history and physical examination

JAUNDICE

Unconjugated Hyperbilirubinemia			Conjugated Hyperbilirubinemia					
Hemolysis and Positive Coombs test	*Reticulocytosis Negative Coombs test*	*No Hemolysis*	*Obstructive*	*Infectious*	*Metabolic*	*Toxic*	*Idiopathic*	*Autoimmune*
ABO and Rh incompatibility	RBC enzyme defect (G6PD deficiency)	Gilbert syndrome	Biliary atresia	Hepatitis A, B, C, D, E	Wilson Disease	Total parenteral nutrition	Idiopathic neonatal hepatitis	Autoimmune chronic hepatitis
Autoimmune, systemic lupus erythematosus	Hemoglobinopathy (Sickle cell anemia)	Physiologic jaundice of the newborn	Choledochal cyst	Cytomegalovirus	Alpha-1-antitrypsin deficiency	Acetaminophen	Alagille syndrome	Sclerosing cholangitis
Drug induced and idiopathic acquired hemolytic anemia	RBC membrane defect (Hereditary spherocytosis)	Breast milk jaundice	Cholelithiasis	Herpes simplex-1,2,6	Galactosemia	Ethanol	Nonsyndromic paucity of intrahepatic bile ducts	Graft vs host disease
	Hemolytic-uremic syndrome	Crigler-Najjar syndrome	Tumor/neoplasia	Epstein-Barr virus	Tyrosinemia	Salicylates	Progressive familial intrahepatic cholestasis	
	Wilson disease	Hypothyroidism	Bile duct stenosis	Coxsackievirus	Fructosemia	Iron	Familial benign recurrent cholestasis	
		Pyloric stenosis	Spontaneous bile duct perforation	ECHO virus	Niemann-Pick Disease	Halothane	Cholestasis with lymphedema (Aagenaes syndrome)	
		Internal hemorrhage	Bile-mucus plus	Measles	Gaucher Disease	Isoniazid	Cholestasis with hypopituitarism	
				Varicella	Zellweger syndrome	Valproic acid	Familial erythrophagocytic lymphohistiocytosis	
				Syncytial giant cell (paramyxovirus)	Wolman disease	Veno-occlusive disease		
				Toxoplasmosis	Cystic fibrosis			
				Syphilis	Neonatal iron storage disease			
				Leptospirosis	Indian childhood cirrhosis			
				Bacterial sepsis/ urinary tract infection (especially gram negative)	Trihydroxycoprostanic acidemia			
				Cholecystitis				
				Curtis-Fitzhugh syndrome				

Figure 11–2. Differential diagnosis of jaundice in childhood. G6PD = glucose-6-phosphate dehydrogenase; RBC = red blood cell.

(e.g., constipation and a large anterior fontanel should suggest hypothyroidism).

All patients with direct-reacting hyperbilirubinemia (direct bilirubin >1 mg/dL or 20% of total bilirubin), regardless of age, should have a comprehensive diagnostic evaluation to determine potentially serious causes of hepatic dysfunction. The laboratory studies should be based on family history (metabolic or hepatic disease), exposure history (toxins, drugs, infectious agents), age-related diseases (biliary atresia in infancy), physical examination (unusual facies, splenomegaly, psychomotor retardation), and screening liver function tests. The latter tests include tests of hepatic synthetic function (i.e., serum albumin, prothrombin time); tests of biliary obstruction (i.e., direct bilirubin, serum alkaline phosphatase, 5'-nucleotidase, gammaglutamyl transpeptidase); and tests of hepatocellular injury (i.e., aspartate aminotransferase, alanine aminotransferase). In many infants, hepatic imaging with ultrasonography, radionucleotide or CT scans, and/or liver biopsy also may be necessary.

References

Behrman RE (ed): Nelson Textbook of Pediatrics. 14th ed. Philadelphia, WB Saunders, 1992, Sec. 13.22–13.24, 13.39–13.42, 13.82–13.83.

Caulfield M, Wyllie R, Sivak M, et al: Upper gastrointestinal tract endoscopy in the pediatric patient. J Pediatr 115: 339, 1989.

Doig C: Paediatric problems. II. Rectal bleeding. BMJ 305: 511, 1992.

Jones D: Lower gastrointestinal haemorrhage. BMJ 305: 107, 1992.

Steffen R, Wyllie R, Sivak M, et al: Colonoscopy in the pediatric patient. J Pediatr 115:507, 1989.

GASTROINTESTINAL DISORDERS BY ORGAN

Oral Cavity

Mastication, the primary function of the oral cavity, requires healthy teeth with proper approximation. Two sets of teeth include 20 *primary* or *deciduous* and the 32 *secondary* or *permanent* teeth. The schedule of dental eruption is indicated in Table 11–13. Disorders of tooth development include **enamel hypoplasia**, which appears as enamel fissures, pits, or grooves and which may be due to rickets, serious illness, or the intake of tetracycline. Because enamel formation of permanent teeth is complete between 8 and 10 yr of age, tetracycline

Table 11–13. Time of Eruption of the Primary and Permanent Teeth

Tooth Type	Primary Age (mo)		Permanent Age (yr)	
	Upper	Lower	Upper	Lower
Central incisor	6 ± 2	7 ± 2	7–8	6–7
Lateral incisor	9 ± 2	7 ± 2	8–9	7–8
Cuspids	18 ± 2	16 ± 2	11–12	9–10
First bicuspids	—	—	10–11	10–12
Second bicuspids	—	—	10–12	11–12
First molars	14 ± 4	12 ± 4	6–7	6–7
Second molars	24 ± 4	20 ± 4	12–13	11–13
Third molars	—	—	17–21	17–21

given after this age will not be incorporated and thus will not stain the teeth. Abnormally shaped teeth are seen in congenital syphilis. Natal, congenital, or prematurely erupted teeth are uncommon and usually not a clinical problem. **Delayed eruption** of all teeth indicates endocrine or nutritional disturbances, such as hypopituitarism, hypothyroidism, or rickets. Discoloration of the teeth may occur as a consequence of excessive fluoride (>5 ppm), prolonged neonatal hyperbilirubinemia, or the intake of tetracycline.

DENTAL CARIES

The development of dental caries depends on the interaction of dietary carbohydrate and oral bacteria, specifically *Streptococcus mutans*, on the tooth surface. Organic acids produced by the bacterial fermentation of carbohydrate demineralize the tooth surface, leading to pit formation that progresses to cavity formation. If unchecked, the process erodes through the tooth, permitting a bacterial invasion of the pulp that becomes painful (toothache). Further spread of the inflammatory process to the alveolar bone results in a dental abscess. Caries in primary teeth may disrupt the development of the permanent teeth.

The best *treatment* for caries is *prevention*, and the most effective preventive measure is fluoridation of the water supply to 1 ppm. In fluoride-deficient areas, supplementation may be necessary. Reducing dietary carbohydrate intake also is important.

To prevent the damaging effects of continuous bottle feeding (nursing bottle caries), bedtime bottles, if necessary, should contain only water. Brushing and flossing of teeth should begin by age 3, although most children under 10 yr of age do not have the eye-to-hand coordination to perform either properly. The parents must assume this responsibility according to the child's ability. Regular dental visits should begin by age 3.

Early dental *treatment* can salvage most carious teeth. Dental infection confined to the tooth itself may be managed with filling or extraction. When the infection extends to the adjacent alveolar bone, oral antibiotics (penicillin) should be initiated. More serious spread of infection to the submandibular space (**Ludwig angina**) and to the buccal or orbital spaces, both of which may produce cellulitis, should be managed with intravenous penicillin. The diseased tooth can be identified by localized pain and requires local treatment (filling or extraction) after the infection is treated.

OROPHARYNGEAL CANDIDIASIS (THRUSH)

Oral candidiasis is common in young infants. The diagnosis is made by visual inspection of white plaques covering the oropharyngeal mucosa. Initial treatment consists of the topical application of nystatin. All toys and nipples must be boiled daily to prevent reinfection. Refractory cases may require clotrimazole troches or, rarely, intravenous amphotericin. Persistent candidiasis resistant to therapy or the presence of this lesion in older infants who are not on broad-spectrum antibiotics suggests an immune disorder such as AIDS.

References

Behrman RE (ed): Nelson Textbook of Pediatrics. 14th ed. Philadelphia, WB Saunders, 1992, Sec. 13.1, 13.6.
Greene J, Louie R, Wycoff S: Preventive dentistry I. Dental caries. JAMA 262:3459, 1989.

Cleft Lip and Palate

CLEFT LIP

Cleft lip, with or without cleft palate, occurs in 1:1000 births and is more common in males. Unilateral cleft lip is due to failure of the ipsilateral maxillary prominence to fuse with the medial nasal prominence, a process that produces a persistent labial groove. Failure of bilateral fusion produces bilateral cleft lip. Multiple genetic as well as environmental factors appear to play a role in the etiology of cleft lip. The recurrence risk in siblings is 3–4%; the risk for a child of a mother with cleft lip is 14%. Associated malformations include hypertelorism and heart, foot, and hand anomalies. Most cleft lips are repaired shortly after birth or once the infant demonstrates steady weight gain. In general, feeding is not a problem with isolated cleft lip deformities.

CLEFT PALATE

Development of the palate proper, which includes the hard palate, soft palate, uvula, and maxillary teeth, is completed by the 9th wk of gestation. This region develops from the maxillary bone plates that are initially separated by the tongue. As the tongue descends in the floor of the mouth and moves forward, the two plates fuse. Failure of the tongue to descend produces the midline palatal clefts. The incidence of cleft palate is 1:2500 births. Genetic factors are important in its etiology. The recurrence risks are the same as those for cleft lip. Cleft palates are common in patients with chromosomal syndromes. Surgical repair usually is undertaken between 12 and 24 mo of age. In the immediate newborn period, respiratory and feeding problems may occur. Repositioning the tongue and feeding the baby on his or her side should resolve respiratory difficulties. Most patients do well with a long, soft nipple that has a hole that is larger than usual. Patients with sucking or swallowing difficulty will require gavage or gastrostomy feedings. The main problems after cleft palate repair are speech and tooth disturbances and recurrent otitis media. Although two thirds demonstrate acceptable speech, their speech may have a nasal quality or a muffled tone.

Pierre Robin syndrome is an identifiable sporadic or familial condition characterized by high arched or cleft palate, micrognathia, and glossoptosis. The latter is due to the smallness of the mandible and results in airway obstruction and feeding problems during infancy. As the mandible grows, respiratory and feeding disturbances resolve.

Esophagus

DEVELOPMENT

The esophagus develops as an elongation of the superior portion of the primitive foregut very early in the embryonic process. When the septation be-

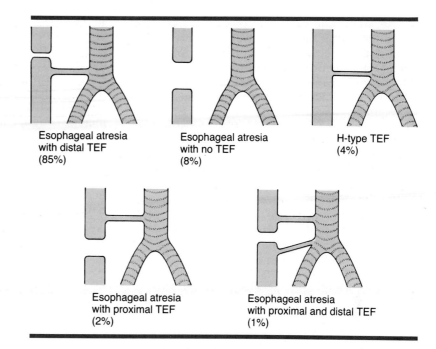

Esophageal atresia
with distal TEF
(85%)

Esophageal atresia
with no TEF
(8%)

H-type TEF
(4%)

Esophageal atresia
with proximal TEF
(2%)

Esophageal atresia
with proximal and distal TEF
(1%)

Figure 11–3. Various types of tracheoesophageal fistulas (TEF) with relative frequency (%).

tween the ventral tube and the dorsal esophagus develops abnormally, **esophageal atresia** results, a condition usually associated with **tracheoesophageal fistula** (TEF) (Fig. 11–3).

Forty percent of patients with TEF have associated anomalies; cardiovascular anomalies (patent ductus arteriosus, vascular ring, coarctation of the aorta) are the most frequent. The incidence of imperforate anus, malrotation, and duodenal anomalies also is increased. **VATER** syndrome describes the association between *v*ertebral defects (hemivertebra), *a*nal atresia, *T*EF, and *r*adial limb dysplasia.

Polyhydramnios and excessive salivation are early *clinical manifestations* of TEF, followed by choking, coughing, and cyanosis after the first feeding. The *diagnosis* may be made by passing a radiopaque catheter and observing coiling in the esophageal pouch on a chest roentgenogram or a pool of contrast dye collected in the atretic esophagus. Infants with TEF without esophageal atresia (H type) may have nonspecific symptoms for several months but usually exhibit chronic cough with feeding and recurrent pneumonia.

Primary surgical repair is the *treatment* of choice when the infant's condition is stable. Postoperative anastomotic leak occurs in 5–10% and requires parenteral or duodenal feedings. Strictures at the anastomotic site require dilating bougienage. Patients with TEF have a persistent derangement of esophageal motility. Abnormal lower esophageal sphincter (LES) function results in gastroesophageal reflux, which may lead to esophagitis, stricture formation, wheezing, and recurrent pneumonia. The survival rate for this lesion in term infants without other anomalies or complications is over 90%.

Clinical manifestations of esophageal diseases include a sensation that food is stuck in the esophagus (dysphagia), which may be due to motility disorders or obstruction. Pain on swallowing (odynophagia) may be due to reflux of acidic stomach contents. **Regurgitation**, rather than forceful emesis, is the most common manifestation of esophageal disease in children.

GASTROESOPHAGEAL REFLUX (CHALASIA)

Gastroesophageal reflux (GER) is a common problem during the 1st yr of life. A number of factors alone or in combination may be responsible. These include reduced LES pressure, inappropriate LES relaxation, large hiatal hernia, and delayed gastric emptying. The latter may suggest distal intestinal obstruction. In infants, regurgitation, vomiting, and irritability are the most frequent complaints, which, if severe, may result in failure to thrive, aspiration pneumonia, wheezing, or esophagitis with bleeding and anemia. On rare occasions, especially in premature infants, GER may be associated with apnea or bradycardia. **Sandifer syndrome** is GER associated with lateral head tilt and back arching resulting from esophagitis. GER in the older child or adolescent may present with regurgitation, retrosternal burning (esophagitis), dysphagia (stricture), or severe asthma.

The *diagnostic* evaluation of GER often includes a barium swallow with fluoroscopy, but at least 30% of infants have normal esophagrams as a result of the intermittent nature of GER. The study excludes anatomic causes, such as an antral web, duodenal web, pyloric stenosis, or annular pancreas. In patients with recurrent pneumonia, swallowing function should be assessed as part of the upper gastrointestinal series. The definitive test for establishing the presence of GER is the 24-hr esophageal pH probe study. This test documents the percent of time that the esophageal pH is less than 4.0, as well as duration of reflux episodes. Formula or food containing ^{99m}Tc can be used to assess gastric emptying. Esophageal manometry, which directly measures LES pressure, also may help determine the cause of GER. Finally, when blood loss, anemia, retrosternal burning, or dysphagia is present, endoscopy and esophageal biopsy will detect the presence of peptic esophagitis, infection, or stricture formation.

Patients with mild to moderate reflux can be managed with medical *treatment,* which may include feeding cereal-thickened formula and careful burping. Position therapy consisting of a 30-degree prone upright position after feeding has been recommended in the past but is now controversial. Most young infants outgrow reflux by 18 mo of age. In cases complicated by esophagitis, antacids, H_2-blocking agents, or sucralfate suspension may be beneficial in reducing acid reflux. Bethanechol, a parasympathomimetic drug, increases esophageal peristalsis and LES tone, whereas metoclopramide, a dopamine antagonist and cholinergic agonist, increases gastric emptying (reducing nausea) and LES tone. Both medications are associated with side effects, the most important being a dystonic type of extrapyramidal reaction with metoclopramide. Infants should receive medications other than theophylline for wheezing because this drug lowers LES pressure. Repeated episodes of pneumonia, failure to thrive, recurrent esophagitis with stricture, severe apnea, and failure to respond to 4–6 wk of medical management are indications for surgery. The most common antireflux operation is the Nissen fundoplication, in which the fundus of the stomach is wrapped 270–360 degrees around the distal esophagus. Gastric distention after a feeding will increase pressure around the wrap, thus preventing acid reflux.

FOREIGN BODIES

Coins, marbles, disc batteries, and pins frequently are swallowed and become lodged in the esophagus at one of three sites of narrowing (i.e., the cricopharyngeal muscle, the level of the aortic arch, and the LES at the diaphragm). Symptoms include cough, choking, stridor, odynophagia, retrosternal pain, and excessive salivation. However, many children are asymptomatic. If the foreign body is left in place, ulceration accompanied by bleeding and perforation may occur. Perforation is heralded by pain, fever, and shock. In experienced hands, smooth objects such as coins, buttons, or marbles may be removed by passing a Foley catheter (8–12 Fr) into the distal esophagus, inflating the balloon, and, by using fluoroscopic guidance, slowly pulling back with the object obtained. Others would favor removing these objects endoscopically or pushing them into the stomach to prevent aspiration. Resistant smooth objects and sharp objects that might penetrate the mucosa require general anesthesia and removal through an esophagoscope or bronchoscope.

CORROSIVE BURNS

Corrosive burns are a common cause of esophageal stricture. The most common chemicals producing esophageal damage are the tasteless alkali caustics found in drain cleaners. Household bleaches and ammonia-containing cleaners are much weaker and produce less damage. Alkali agents cause full-thickness–penetrating coagulation necrosis, whereas acid burns produce an eschar that coats the mucosa, preventing deeper penetration. Burns in the mouth suggest that the esophagus also is burned. However, the absence of burns on the oral mucosa does not preclude esophageal involvement.

Following a lye ingestion, vomiting should not be induced. Water or milk should be given to dilute the corrosive. Hospitalization, intravenous fluids, and endoscopy are recommended, even if there is a doubt about the ingestion. The presence of a burn warrants follow-up with a barium swallow 3–4 wk after the initial injury to check for stricture formation. Strictures will need bougienage dilation. Steroids are of no benefit.

References

Behrman RE (ed): Nelson Textbook of Pediatrics. 14th ed. Philadelphia, WB Saunders, 1992, Sec. 13.15–13.25.
Grill BB: Twenty-four-hour esophageal pH monitoring:

What's the score? J Pediatr Gastroenterol Nutr 14:249, 1992.
Lovejoy FJ: Corrosive injury of the esophagus in children: Failure of corticosteroid treatment reemphasizes prevention. N Engl J Med 323:668, 1990.
Orenstein SR: Controversies in pediatric gastroesophageal reflux. J Pediatr Gastroenterol Nutr 14:338, 1992.

Stomach

PYLORIC STENOSIS

After inguinal hernia, congenital hypertrophic pyloric stenosis is the most common condition requiring surgery during the first 2 mo of life. The incidence is 1:150 in males and 1:750 in females. The condition occurs in 5% of siblings and 25% of offspring if the mother was affected. Pylorospasm, secondary to reduced tissue nitric oxide levels (a mediator of relaxation) may lead to hypertrophic pyloric stenosis.

The typical *clinical manifestation* is nonbilious vomiting beginning between the 2nd and 4th wk of life. Emesis increases in frequency and eventually becomes projectile. Clear liquids and/or frequent feedings may lessen the severity of the vomiting temporarily, but weight loss becomes apparent as the obstruction becomes more complete. *Laboratory* abnormalities include hypokalemic metabolic alkalosis with paradoxic aciduria and dehydration. Indirect hyperbilirubinemia also may be present.

The *diagnosis* may be made by palpating an olive-shaped mass to the right of the umbilicus and witnessing marked peristaltic waves progressing from the left upper quadrant to the epigastrium. The diagnosis is confirmed by ultrasound demonstration of the thick hypoechoic ring in the region of the pylorus. Contrast roentgenographic studies rarely are necessary.

Pyloromyotomy is the *treatment of choice* once dehydration and electrolyte abnormalities are corrected. Within 1–2 days, most infants can tolerate formula feeding.

ACID-PEPTIC DISEASE

This designation refers to a variety of disorders of the proximal gastrointestinal tract resulting from the action of gastric secretions. Local mucosal infection with the urea-splitting bacteria *Helicobacter pylori* also may play an etiologic role. Included under "acid-peptic disease" are gastritis, gastric ulcer, duodenitis, and duodenal ulcer. Strictly speaking, gastritis and duodenitis refer to inflammatory processes in the mucosa, whereas ulcer implies a sharply circumscribed lesion.

Gastritis

Acute gastritis may be localized or diffuse. Necrosis of the superficial mucosal cells and damage to the blood vessels of the lamina propria may cause extravasation of blood (acute hemorrhagic gastritis). If erosions form (erosive gastritis) and extend to the submucosa and muscularis, an ulcer may form. Acute gastritis may follow viral infections, the ingestion of aspirin or nonsteroidal anti-inflammatory drugs, cancer chemotherapy, and the ingestion of corrosive agents, such as strong acids. Gastritis also may occur following severe trauma, major surgery, or septic shock. Hematemesis is the major *clinical manifestation*. Other symptoms include abdominal pain, nausea, and vomiting. Endoscopy is the diagnostic method of choice; barium studies usually are not helpful. Treatment is similar to that for peptic ulcer disease.

Gastric Ulcer/Duodenal Ulcer

Ulcers no longer are considered rare in children because increased rates have been detected by endoscopy. Primary ulcers occur in previously healthy individuals with no history of medication use. They are more duodenal than gastric and tend to have an insidious onset. Gastric ulcers occur in the antrum, whereas primary duodenal ulcers are found in the bulb and usually are solitary. The finding of multiple ulcers either in the 3rd or 4th portion of the duodenum or in the jejunum should raise suspicion of the **Zollinger-Ellison syndrome**. Secondary ulcers are seen in association with underlying systemic disorders (sepsis, burns, raised intracranial pressure) or occur as a consequence of drug therapy. They may hemorrhage or perforate without a prior history of pain, are more common in the stomach and frequently are multiple.

The *etiology* of ulcer disease is unknown. Genetics, personality traits, stress, alcohol abuse, *H. pylori* infection, and smoking are contributing factors. Excessive acid secretion or breaks in the mucous protective layer (defects in cytoprotection) are important pathophysiologic factors.

Epigastric burning or gnawing abdominal pain relieved by food or antacids and recurring 1–3 hr after eating is the most common *clinical manifestation*. Nocturnal pain that awakens a child from sleep is typical of peptic ulcer disease and occurs in 30% of children with primary peptic ulcers but is rare in children with psychophysiologic disorders.

Vomiting and nausea are other frequent symptoms. Documentation of an ulcer crater by an upper gastrointestinal roentgenographic series is sufficient to establish the *diagnosis* of peptic ulcer, but the ulcer may be undetected in up to 25% of cases. Endoscopy may be required to identify the lesion.

The goal of *treatment* is to reduce gastric acidity. Antacids are used but have a short duration of action. H_2-receptor–blocking agents, such as cimetidine and ranitidine, are effective for 6–12 hr and thus provide sustained relief. Drug interactions are common (see Appendix I). Sucralfate has a local coating action and is not absorbed. Therapy should be continued for 6–8 wk. Combination antimicrobial therapy (bismuth salts, amoxicillin, metronidazole) may be needed in refractory or recurrent disease to eradicate *H. pylori*. Indications for surgical vagotomy with pyloroplasty include perforation, obstruction, uncontrolled bleeding, rebleeding in the hospital, and intractable pain.

FOREIGN BODIES/BEZOARS

Most foreign bodies that reach the stomach will pass through to the intestine and should be managed conservatively. Objects without sharp edges should be removed endoscopically if serial roentgenograms show no progress after 3–4 wk. Objects with sharp points, such as safety pins, nails, and needles, should be monitored roentgenographically and be removed endoscopically if they do not move from the stomach after several days.

Three types of stomach bezoars occur in children: *trichobezoars* (composed primarily of hair), *phytobezoars* (composed of vegetable material), and *lactobezoars* (occurring from milk). Symptoms include abdominal pain, anorexia, vomiting, and weight loss. Children with trichobezoars may be retarded and may have alopecia. Lactobezoars, which may cause gastric outlet obstruction, usually are seen in neonates receiving high-caloric-density formulas by continuous drip.

References

Behrman RE (ed): Nelson Textbook of Pediatrics. 14th edition. Philadelphia, WB Saunders, 1992, Sec. 13.26–13.27, 13.39.

Drumm B, Rhoads JM, Stringer DA, et al: Peptic ulcer disease in children: Etiology, clinical findings, and clinical course. Pediatrics 82:410, 1988.

Prieto G, Polanco I, Larrauri J, et al: *Helicobacter pylori* infection in children: Clinical endoscopic and histologic correlations. J Pediatr Gastroenterol Nutr 14:420, 1992.

Disorders of the Intestine and Colon

CONGENITAL MALFORMATIONS

Abdominal Wall Defects

Omphalocele.   When the abdominal viscera herniate through the umbilical and supraumbilical portions of the abdominal wall into a sac covered by peritoneum and amniotic membrane, the defect is called an omphalocele. It results from a failure of migration of the bowel from the umbilical coelom, and its incidence is 1:6000 births. Large defects may contain the liver and spleen, as well as most of the gastrointestinal tract. The sac covering the defect is thin and may rupture in utero or during delivery. Ten percent of infants with omphaloceles are born prematurely; the incidence of associated malformations is high. Thirty-five percent have other gastrointestinal defects; 20%, congenital heart defects; and 10%, the **Beckwith-Wiedemann syndrome** (exophthalmos – macroglossia – gigantism–hyperinsulinemia–hypoglycemia).   Primary closure of small defects often is possible. Larger defects require staged repairs that involve covering the sac with a prosthetic material. Survival rates vary and depend on the severity of associated anomalies.

Umbilical Hernia.   Umbilical hernia results from the incomplete closure of the fascia of the umbilical ring. Herniated omentum or bowel is covered by skin. Umbilical hernia is more common in premature infants and blacks; it is found in up to 40% of black children less than 1 yr of age. Fascial defects with a diameter of less than 0.5 cm heal spontaneously before age 2 yr. With a ring between 0.5 and 1.5 cm, healing usually is complete by age 4 yr. Surgical closure is advisable if the defect exceeds 1.5 cm at 2 yr of age or if incarceration or symptoms such as abdominal pain have occurred. The practice of manually reducing the hernia and taping some device (such as a coin) over the ring does not accelerate the healing process.

Gastroschisis

Gastroschisis is the herniation, without a covering sac, of a variable length of small intestine and, occasionally, of portions of the liver, through an abdominal wall defect located to the right of the umbilical cord. The eviscerated uncovered mass of bowel is adherent, edematous, dark in color, and covered by a gelatinous matrix of greenish material. Sixty percent of these infants are born premature; 14% have associated jejunoileal malformations, usually stenosis or atresias; and 4% have nongastrointestinal malformations. Little evidence supports the notion that genetic factors play a role, and the risk of congenital anomalies in future pregnancies is small. Gastroschisis is a surgical emergency, and a single-stage primary closure is possible in only 10% of patients.

Intestinal Atresia

Duodenum.   Duodenal obstruction may be complete (atresia), owing to the failure of the lumen to recannalize, or partial (stenosis), owing to a web, band, or annular pancreas. Intrinsic duodenal lesions result from a failure of the lumen to recannalize during the 8th–10th week of gestation. Duodenal atresia is associated with other anomalies (30%), prematurity (25%), and trisomy 21 (20%).

With complete obstruction, bile-stained vomiting begins within a few hours after the first feeding. In utero polyhydramnios may be present. Abdominal roentgenograms usually show gastric and duodenal gaseous distention, which also is called the "double bubble" sign, proximal to the atretic site. The presence of gas in the distal bowel suggests partial obstruction, and a contrast roentgenographic study should be performed. Management is surgical. Mortality is related to prematurity and associated congenital anomalies.

Jejunum and Ileum.   Jejunoileal atresias occur more frequently (2:1) than duodenal atresias and probably are caused by infarction. Two thirds of cases involve complete obstruction of either the distal ileum or proximal jejunum, with multiple atresias accounting for only 10–20%. **Meconium ileus** with atresia is due to thick intestinal secretions from cystic fibrosis.

Polyhydramnios is present in 25% of cases. Vomiting of bile-stained material usually begins within 24–48 hr after birth. The abdomen becomes distended, and plain films show dilated loops of small bowel and an absence of colonic gas. Peritoneal calcifications signify **meconium peritonitis**, the result of intrauterine bowel perforation. A barium enema will show a narrowed unused colon (**microcolon**). Surgery is mandatory.

Malrotation/Volvulus

Anomalies of intestinal rotation result from failure of the midgut to appropriately re-enter the fetal abdomen. The severity of the malrotation depends on the extent of the rotational arrest. Volvulus occurs when the small intestine is not fixed in the abdomen and becomes suspended by a stalk containing the superior mesenteric artery. Twisting of bowel leads to arterial obstruction, midgut ischemia, and infarction. Further complicating the malrotation is the presence of peritoneal fixation bands (Ladd bands), which may result in partial duodenal obstruction.

Eighty percent of children with this anomaly experience symptoms within the 1st mo of life. Abdominal distention and bilious vomiting suggest obstruction. If volvulus occurs, bloody stools may be followed by perforation and peritonitis. Children who are brought to the physician's attention after the neonatal period have intermittent cramping, abdominal pain, vomiting, and diarrhea (often with hypoalbuminemia and secondary hypogammaglobulinemia) or constipation. The diagnosis of malrotation can be made by demonstrating an abnormal position of the duodenum in an upper gastrointestinal roentgenographic series with small bowel follow-through. Midgut volvulus is a surgical emergency.

Meckel Diverticulum

Meckel diverticulum, the vestigial remnant of the omphalomesenteric duct, is the most frequent anomaly of the gastrointestinal tract, is present in 2–3% of the population, and is located within 100 cm of the ileocecal valve along the antimesenteric border of the small intestine. The peak incidence is 2 yr of age. Heterotopic tissue, usually gastric, is 10 times more common in symptomatic cases because of acid secretion and ulceration.

The clinical signs of Meckel diverticulum include painless rectal bleeding (melena, 84%), intestinal obstruction (intussusception or volvulus, 10%), and painful diverticulitis mimicking appendicitis (6%). Diagnosis is discussed in the section on Gastrointestinal Hemorrhage. The definitive treatment is surgical resection.

Congenital Aganglionic Megacolon (Hirschsprung Disease)

The failure of retrograde migration of neural crest–derived ganglion cells in the developing colon results in an aganglionic segment of variable length. This disorder is 3 times more common among males and accounts for 20% of neonatal intestinal obstruction. In 75% of cases, the aganglionic segment is limited to the rectosigmoid colon; 15% extend beyond the splenic flexure. **Neuronal intestinal dysplasia** (hyperganglionosis) demonstrates hyperplasia of the intramural plexus and clinically resembles Hirschsprung disease.

The **diagnosis** should be suspected in any infant who fails to pass meconium within the first 24 hr and who requires repeated rectal stimulation to induce bowel movements. Failure to thrive and abdominal distention may occur. Fever and diarrhea are ominous signs that suggest the presence of coexisting enterocolitis. In some cases, particularly those with short segment (<5 cm) involvement, the diagnosis goes undetected into childhood. These children often are poorly nourished and suffer from massive abdominal distention and anemia. The presence of stool palpable throughout the abdomen and an empty rectum on digital examination are most suggestive of the disease (see Table 11–9).

The *treatment* of Hirschsprung disease is surgical and is performed in two stages. The first stage involves the creation of a colostomy through a section of bowel containing ganglion cells, thus permitting decompression of the dilated colon. In the second stage, the aganglionic segment is removed by pulling the ganglionic segment through the rectum. This procedure is postponed until the infant is 12–14 mo old or for 3–6 mo when the disease has been diagnosed in an older child. Mortality for this disorder is low in the absence of enterocolitis, and the major complications include anal stenosis (5–10%) and incontinence (1–3%).

Anorectal Malformation/Imperforate Anus

Anorectal anomalies arise either because of a failure of the urorectal septum to divide the cloaca completely or because of incomplete convergence of the anal tubercles around the termination of the hindgut. The incidence is 1:5000, and 50% of cases demonstrate associated vertebral or genitourinary malformations.

The recognition of anorectal malformations depends on careful inspection of the perianal area at birth. Figure 11–4 illustrates the various types of anomalies. Fistulization between the rectum and surrounding structures may occur. Rectourethral fistulas in males and rectovaginal fistulas in females are associated with "high" lesions, whereas fistulas through to the perineum are associated with "low" lesions. Contrast roentgenograms of a fistula or tube instillation of contrast into the rectum should allow delineation of the anatomy. Anal stenosis may be treated with simple dilation. Other lesions require surgery. Bowel control is achieved in 90% of children with low lesions but in only 50% of those with high lesions.

Inguinal Hernia

During development, a peritoneal sac precedes the testicle as it descends from the genital ridge into the scrotum. The lower portion of this sac (processus vaginalis) envelopes the testes and forms the tunica vaginalis, whereas the remainder of the sac atrophies. In 50% of patients, the processus vaginalis remains patent. If abdominal contents become trapped in the processus vaginalis, an *indirect hernia* exists. Indirect inguinal hernias are more common in males (4:1), in premature infants, and following increased intra-abdominal pressure (ascites). The hernia becomes manifest as a painless swelling in the inguinal area. Contents of the hernia sac usually can be reduced with gentle pressure. When the contents of the sac cannot be reduced, the hernia is said to be **incarcerated**, necessitating immediate surgery to avoid bowel necrosis and testicular infarction. Repair of an asymptomatic reducible hernia should be carried out as

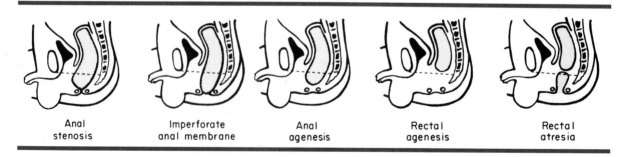

| Anal stenosis | Imperforate anal membrane | Anal agenesis | Rectal agenesis | Rectal atresia |

Figure 11–4. Various types of anorectal anomalies. The stippled line is a projection of the puborectalis sling. On a roentgenogram, it is drawn from the lower part of the pubis to the sacrococcygeal junction. (Modified from Silverman A, Roy CE [eds]: Pediatric Clinical Gastroenterology. St. Louis, CV Mosby, 1983.)

soon as possible unless other conditions preclude surgery.

References

Behrman RE (ed): Nelson Textbook of Pediatrics. 14th ed. Philadelphia, WB Saunders, 1992, Sec. 13.26, 13.28–13.36.
Ford EG, Senac MO, Srikanth MS, et al: Malrotation of the intestine in children. Ann Surg 215:172, 1992.
Martin LW, Torres AM: Hirschsprung's disease. Surg Clin North Am 65:1171, 1985.
St-Vil D, Brandt ML, Panic S, et al: Meckel's diverticulum in children: A 20-year review. J Pediatr Surg 26:1289, 1991.

DISACCHARIDASE DEFICIENCIES

Primary congenital disaccharidase deficiencies are rare. **Sucrase–isomaltase deficiency** is the most common form occurring in infancy and is inherited as an autosomal recessive trait. Osmotic diarrhea begins with the introduction of sucrose-containing foods or drinks, and may be associated with vomiting, dehydration, abdominal cramping, bloating, and growth failure. The diagnosis may be confirmed on breath hydrogen testing and quantitative determination of sucrase–isomaltase activity in jejunal mucosal biopsy. The treatment consists of excluding from the diet foods that contain more than 2% sucrose.

Congenital *lactase deficiency* is rare, but late-onset lactase deficiency is common. This inherited form has a striking ethnic variation, being present in 5–10% of whites compared to 70% of blacks. The absence of brush border lactase activity causes lactose malabsorption and osmotic diarrhea within hours of lactose ingestion. Symptoms begin between 8 and 15 yr of age and include crampy abdominal pain, bloating, and acidic diarrhea (containing reducing substances). The diagnosis may be made on breath hydrogen or lactose tolerance testing. Because the deficiency is relative rather than absolute, some lactose restriction from the diet usually is sufficient to prevent symptoms. Transient secondary lactase deficiency often occurs as a consequence of damage to the small intestinal mucosa following severe viral gastroenteritis. Mucosal recovery occurs in 4–6 wk. Treatment is with a non–lactose-containing formula.

PROTEIN INTOLERANCE/SENSITIVITY SYNDROMES

Cow/Soy Milk Protein Intolerance

The proteins in cow's milk and soy milk may cause an immune-mediated inflammatory injury of the small bowel, with villous atrophy, or an injury of the large bowel, producing colitis (inflammation with or without ulceration). The precise immune mechanisms are undetermined. Systemic signs, such as anaphylaxis, wheezing, rhinitis, pulmonary hemosiderosis, and urticaria, may be mediated by immunoglobulin (Ig) E antibody. Approximately 4% of all infants are intolerant to cow's milk proteins, and 20–50% of them also will be intolerant to soy protein. Milk protein intolerance syndrome usually has an onset within the 1st mo of life. When it causes **enterocolitis** there is vomiting, diarrhea, enteric blood loss, and anema. Rectal biopsy findings include inflammation, eosinophilic infiltration of the lamina propria and mucosa, ulceration, and crypt abscesses. Another syndrome of **enteropathy** begins at 2–3 mo of age, and clinical manifestations include prolonged diarrhea, protein-losing enteropathy (edema, hypoproteinemia), malabsorption, and failure to thrive. Small intestinal villous atrophy, at times associated with inflammatory colitis, is present. The *diagnosis* of cow or soy milk protein intolerance is made by history and mucosal biopsy. Improvement with protein-free casein hydrolysate formula and recurrence of symptoms when milk proteins are reintroduced confirm the diagnosis. Most infants eventually tolerate bovine or soy proteins by 2–3 yr of age. Infants with severe reactions (anaphylaxis) should not undergo challenge. Breast-fed infants may manifest similar symptoms because of the presence of dietary bovine proteins in human breast milk. Treatment requires elimination of dairy products by the mother and supplementing her with calcium and vitamin D.

Eosinophilic gastroenteropathy is not usually associated with cow's milk sensitivity and is characterized by eosinophilic infiltration of the intestinal mucosa, muscularis, or serosal layers and elevated IgE levels and peripheral eosinophilia. Protein-losing enteropathy, pyloric obstruction (muscular involvement), gastrointestinal bleeding with anemia (mucosal involvement), and ascites (serosal involvement) also may be present. The cause is unknown, but it is a chronic condition that responds poorly to therapy with corticosteroids. The differential diagnosis includes intestinal parasite infestation.

GLUTEN-SENSITIVE ENTEROPATHY (CELIAC DISEASE)

Celiac disease, an immunologically mediated intolerance to gluten-containing grains (wheat, rye, barley, oats), results in small intestinal villous atrophy with lymphocytic and plasma cell infiltration. The incidence in the United States is 1:3000 births. There is a genetic predisposition: 98% have human leukocyte antigen (HLA)-DQW2 and 80% are HLA-B8 positive.

Clinical manifestations usually begin between 6 and 18 mo, and include apathy, irritability, pain, vomiting, chronic diarrhea, steatorrhea, abdominal distention, and failure to thrive; some infants are asymptomatic. A wasted skeletal muscle mass, finger clubbing, and peripheral edema also may occur. Older children may present with unexplained growth failure or may be asymptomatic. The *diagnosis* is confirmed by an initially abnormal small bowel biopsy showing partial or subtotal villous atrophy, improvement of a second biopsy on a gluten-free diet, and then evidence on subsequent biopsy of disease reappearance following gluten challenge. The presence of serum IgG or IgA against gliadin, reticulin, or endomysial antibodies and a low D-zylose absorption are useful screening tests. *Treatment* consists of permanent elimination of gluten-containing foods. Older patients may not develop signs when rechallenged with cereals, but they will develop mucosal atrophy, which may place them at increased risk for intestinal lymphoma.

INFLAMMATORY BOWEL DISEASE

Inflammatory bowel disease (IBD) includes ulcerative colitis and Crohn disease. Both conditions result from an unknown cause, are more common among whites, Jews, and family members, and occur equally in males and females. Most pediatric patients are adolescents, but both diseases have been reported in infancy. Crohn disease may involve any part of the gastrointestinal tract (mouth to anus), whereas ulcerative colitis produces only colonic disease (Table 11–14). Both may have common extraintestinal manifestations, including arthralgias, polyarticular arthritis, primary sclerosing cholangitis, chronic active hepatitis, sacroiliitis, pyoderma gangrenosum, erythema nodosum, nephrolithiasis, and uveitis or episcleritis. The pathology of Crohn disease involves transmural inflammation in a discontinuous pattern (skipped lesions): granulomas are present in some specimens. Ulcerative colitis produces superficial diffuse colonic ulceration and crypt abscesses. It involves the rectum in 95% of patients, with or without contiguous extension higher in the colon.

Clinical Manifestations (Table 11–14). Most children with ulcerative colitis exhibit blood in the

Table 11–14. Comparison of Crohn Disease and Ulcerative Colitis

Feature	Crohn Disease	Ulcerative Colitis
Malaise, fever, weight loss	Common	Common
Rectal bleeding	Sometimes	Usual
Abdominal mass	Common	Rare
Abdominal pain	Common	Common
Perianal disease	Common	Rare
Ileal involvement	Common	None (backwash ileitis)
Strictures	Common	Unusual
Fistula	Common	Unusual
Skip lesions	Common	Not present
Transmural involvement	Usual	Not present
Crypt abscesses	Unusual	Usual
Granulomas	Common	Not present
Risk of cancer	Slightly increased	Greatly increased

(Modified from Andreoli TE, Carpenter CJ, Plum F, et al: Cecil Essentials of Medicine. Philadelphia, WB Saunders, 1986, p 746.)

stool (100%), abdominal pain (95%), and tenesmus (75%). Ninety percent of patients exhibit mild (<6 stools/day, no fever, anemia, or hypoalbuminemia) to moderate (>6 stools/day, fever, anemia, and hypoalbuminemia) disease. Severe disease may be a fulminant illness accompanied by high fever, abdominal tenderness, distention, tachycardia, leukocytosis, hemorrhage, more than 8 stools/day, and severe anemia. Toxic megacolon and subsequent intestinal perforation are rare complications.

The onset of Crohn disease often is subtle. Cramping abdominal pain, fever of unknown origin, weight loss, and diarrhea are common manifestations. Arthritis may precede gastrointestinal or other extraintestinal manifestations. Perianal disease may produce skin tags, fissures, fistulas, or abscesses.

Diagnosis. The differential diagnosis of IBD includes chronic bacterial or parasitic causes of diarrhea, such as *Clostridium difficile, Campylobacter jejuni, Yersinia enterocolitica,* amebiasis, and giardiasis. Because ulcerative colitis involves the rectum in 90% of patients, proctosigmoidoscopy and biopsy are indicated. Visualization of the mucosa in ulcerative colitis reveals diffuse superficial ulceration and easy bleeding. In Crohn disease, direct visualization and biopsy of the ileocecal area are not always possible. Roentgenographic examination with a double (air)-contrast barium enema will demonstrate diffuse colonic lesions and pseudopolyp formation in ulcerative colitis. This examination should be delayed in patients with severely active disease to avoid precipitating toxic megacolon. Crohn disease often reveals ileal and/or colonic involvement with skipped lesions, rectal sparing, segmental narrowing (string sign), and longitudinal ulcers.

Treatment. General management includes drug therapy combined with nutritional support (enteral or parenteral); dietary modifications as needed for control of diarrhea, presence of fistula, stenotic segments, or lactose intolerance; and transfusion for anemia.

Therapy for ulcerative colitis depends on the severity of the illness. Mild disease may be treated with oral sulfasalazine, which is poorly absorbed and is split by colonic bacteria into sulfapyridine and the active 5-aminosalicylate. Sulfasalazine is active against lipoxygenase and may reduce the elevated mucosal prostaglandin levels. Sulfapyridine may cause headache, hemolytic anemia, and gastrointestinal discomfort. Topical 5-aminosalicylate or hydrocortisone enemas also may be used in mild left-sided disease. They hasten healing but may be refused by children and adolescents. Oral mesalamine (5-aminosalicylate) may be used for colonic disease in patients who do not tolerate sulfasalazine. Moderate ulcerative colitis is managed with the addition of 1–2 mg/kg/day of prednisone (maximum 60 mg/day) to the above regimen. Sulfasalazine helps to maintain remission. Severe disease requires intravenous alimentation, systemic corticosteroids, and close monitoring for hypokalemia, acidosis, anemia, and intestinal perforation. Cyclosporine may be efficacious in severe refractory disease. Emergency colectomy is indicated for refractory toxic megacolon or severe, persistent hemorrhage. Colectomy also is indicated for chronic refractory disease, persistent growth failure, and the presence of moderate or severe dysplasia on biopsy. The risk of colon carcinoma is increased in patients with extensive disease of greater than 10 yr duration. Colonoscopic surveillance is mandatory to determine the presence of dysplasia.

Prednisone is the treatment of choice for Crohn disease of the small bowel. Colonic involvement also may benefit from the addition of sulfasalazine, whereas perianal disease and fistula may respond to metronidazole. Azathioprine and 6-mercaptopurine may permit reduction of corticosteroid dose in those children who are dependent on or refractory to prednisone. Surgery eventually is needed in approximately 25% of children with ulcerative colitis and 70% of children with Crohn disease because of failure of medical management, intestinal fistula or obstruction, and growth failure.

POLYPS

Most polyps in children are of the juvenile type, although some may occur in association with familial syndromes. These latter include **Peutz-Jeghers syndrome** (mucocutaneous pigmentation; autosomal dominant), **Gardner syndrome** (soft tissue–bone tumor, rectal cancer; autosomal dominant), and **familial polyposis coli** (carcinoma; autosomal dominant). Juvenile polyps are pedunculated harmartomas, which have a peak incidence between 3 and 5 yr. Seventy percent occur in the rectum or sigmoid colon, and the majority are solitary. The usual presenting symptom is painless rectal bleeding. If the polyp is in the rectum, the diagnosis may be made on digital examination. Otherwise, the diagnosis depends on a carefully performed air-contrast enema or colonoscopy. The latter affords the opportunity for removal of the polyp at the time of the procedure.

APPENDICITIS

This is the most common cause of an acute abdomen in older children and adolescents (4:1000 children <16 yr). The cause may be obstruction of the appendiceal lumen by a fecalith or by inflammatory edema produced by lymphatic hyperplasia from a nonspecific infection. Meconium ileus equivalent or ileus-producing drugs (vincristine) are rarer causes of obstruction.

Clinical manifestations include a 1–2 day history of periumbilical dull or crampy pain, *followed by* anorexia and nausea, with or without vomiting. The pain remains constant but then localizes in the right lower quadrant (McBurney point) as a result of irritation of the parietal peritoneum. With rupture, the pain initially may subside but then is followed by signs of peritonitis, such as high fever, abdominal wall muscle rigidity resulting from voluntary guarding, and involuntary spasm. Unfortunately, atypical presentations are common among children or patients with retrocecal (less peritoneal irritation: positive psoas sign) or pelvic (less peritoneal irritation: tender rectal exam) appendices. Fever is often 38–38.5° C (100–102° F), and the peripheral white blood cell count usually is normal unless perforation has occurred or peritonitis is present. Urinalysis occasionally may reveal proteinuria and mild pyuria. Abdominal roentgenograms often demonstrate a fecalith or acute scoliosis toward the right as a result of psoas muscle spasm. Ultrasonography reveals a noncompressable enlarged appendix surrounded by fluid (donut or target sign) but also excludes ovarian or pelvic disease, mesenteric adenitis, and calculi. The differential diagnosis includes those age- and sex-related diseases listed in Table 11–1. **Mesenteric adenitis** caused by *Yersinia* species also may mimic appendicitis, whereas **primary peritonitis** may be confused with a ruptured appendix. The latter is noted in patients with ascites, nephrotic syndrome, or, rarely, no underlying illness and is due to *Streptococcus pneumoniae* or *E. coli*.

Treatment is surgical excision of the acutely inflamed appendix. Peritoneal drainage and broad-spectrum antibiotics effective against anaerobic and gram-negative enteric organisms are added if perforation is present.

INTUSSUSCEPTION

Intussusception occurs when one segment of bowel telescopes into a distal segment. Idiopathic intussusception usually occurs between 6 and 18 mo of life, with only 10% of cases occurring after 3 yr of age. The cause is unknown, but lymphoid hyperplasia (Peyer patches) may form a lead point of the proximal intussusception segment. A lead point is seen in 5% of cases. In older children, Meckel diverticulum, lymphosarcoma, and polyps may form lead points. Intussusception also is seen in cystic fibrosis and in Henoch-Schönlein purpura. The ileocolic form is the most frequent, followed by ilioileal and colocolic. Intussusception causes an acute onset of colicky intermittent abdominal pain. During the episodes of pain the infant will cry, draw up the knees, and perhaps vomit. Lethargy and fever are late findings, as is the passage of currant jelly–colored stools. On physical examination, a sausage shaped mass may be found in the upper abdomen. Barium enema not only confirms the diagnosis but, with appropriate hydrostatic pressure, may reduce the intussusception in 75% of patients. Surgical reduction should be done if (1) there are clinical signs of peritonitis or shock, (2) medical reduction is unsuccessful, or (3) there is a high likelihood of finding a pathologic lead point.

References

Behrman RE (ed): Nelson Textbook of Pediatrics. 14th ed. Philadelphia, WB Saunders, 1992, Sec. 12.38, 13.40–13.47, 13.56–13.66.

Bhisitkul DM, Listernick R, Shkolnik A, et al: Clinical application of ultrasonography in the diagnosis of intussusception. J Pediatr 121:182, 1992.
The European Society for Paediatric Gastroenterology and Nutrition Working Group for the Diagnostic Criteria for Food Allergy: Diagnostic criteria for food allergy with predominantly intestinal symptoms. J Pediatr Gastroenterol Nutr 14:108, 1992.
Geier DL, Miner PB: New therapeutic agents in the treatment of inflammatory bowel disease. Am J Med 93:199, 1992.
Jones DJ: Appendicitis. BMJ 305:44, 1992.
Kirschner BS: Inflammatory bowel disease in children. Pediatr Clin North Am 35:189, 1988.
Neilson IR, Laberge J-M, Nguyen LT, et al: Appendicitis in children: Current therapeutic recommendations. J Pediatr Surg 25:1113, 1990.
Trier JS: Celiac sprue. N Engl J Med 325:1709, 1991.

Liver

Manifestations of hepatic disease may include abnormalities of any or all of the specific liver functions. The most common manifestations include jaundice (Figure 11–1), hepatomegaly, metabolic disturbances (hypoglycemia, hyperammonemia, encephalopathy, metabolic acidosis, hyperaminoacidemia), portal hypertension (cirrhosis, ascites, varices), and hemorrhage (varices).

Laboratory tests of hepatic function (Table 11–15) can be divided into two categories, those that suggest the presence of hepatobiliary disease and those that assess "liver function." "Liver function" tests do not quantitatively measure function but instead provide clinical information about the course or severity of disease. In interpreting these tests, it is important to remember that the liver has a large reserve capacity with the capability for regeneration.

ACUTE VIRAL HEPATITIS

A number of agents cause acute hepatic injury (Table 11–16). Characteristics of hepatitis A virus (HAV), hepatitis B virus (HBV), and hepatitis C virus (HCV) infection are shown in Table 11–17. The delta agent produces disease only in those patients with hepatitis B infection.

The *clinical course* for HAV and HBV is shown in Figure 11–5. A prodromal phase, which lasts approximately 1 wk, is characterized by headaches, anorexia, malaise, nausea, and vomiting and usually precedes the onset of clinically detectable disease. Infants with HBV may have immune complexes accompanied by urticaria and arthritis prior to icterus. Jaundice and a large tender liver are the

Table 11–15. Liver Evaluation Tests

Test	Mechanism	Significance
Hepatic Function		
Albumin	Decreased protein synthesis	Decreased synthesis, increased losses (ascites)
Prothrombin time	Decreased synthesis of factors 2, 7, 9, 10	Severe hepatic dysfunction is unresponsive to vitamin K; malabsorption responds to vitamin K
Ammonia	Decreased ureagenesis, increased portosystemic shunts	Increased ammonia associated with hepatic encephalopathy
Glucose	Decreased glycogenolysis; decreased gluconeogenesis	Hypoglycemia and central nervous system risk
Cellular Injury		
Aspartate aminotransferase (AST/SGOT)	Released from necrotic cells	Also released from heart and muscle
Alanine aminotransferase (ALT/SGPT)	Released from necrotic cells	More specific for liver injury
Biliary Obstruction		
Alkaline phosphatase	Bile duct cell proliferation	Must be fractionated to determine bone component
Gamma-glutamyltranspeptidase	Bile duct cell proliferation	More specific for biliary disease
5′-Nucleotidase	Bile duct cell release	Biliary disease
Direct bilirubin	Decreased excretion	Also noted with hepatocellular injury
Bile acids	Decreased extraction from blood, decreased excretion	Cholestasis, portosystemic shunt
Other		
Alpha-fetoprotein	Derepressed fetal gene	Hepatic tumor
Antismooth muscle, antimitochondrial, antinuclear antibodies	Autoimmunity	Chronic active hepatitis
Imaging		
Ultrasound	Gross anomalies	Cholelithiasis and choledochal cysts
Technetium-99m sulfur colloid	Kupffer cell uptake	Focal lesions >2–3 cm
Technetium-99m iminodiacetic acid (PIPIDA, HIDA)	Hepatocyte uptake and biliary excretion	Biliary atresia, obstruction
Gallium	Inflammatory, neoplastic cell uptake	Abscess, tumor

most common physical findings. However, infants and young children with HAV or HBV may not become icteric and mistakenly may be diagnosed as having the "flu." Liver enzymes may increase 15–20-fold. Resolution of the hyperbilirubinemia and normalization of the transaminases may take 6–8 wk.

A number of *serologic markers* are available to detect the presence of hepatitis A or B. Their appearance and time course also are shown in Figure 11–4. The presence of high-titer IgM-specific anti-body to HAV and a low or absent IgG antibody titer to the same virus is presumptive evidence for hepatitis A infection. The presence of hepatitis B virus surface antigen (HB$_s$Ag) signifies infection with HBV. Antigenemia may appear early in illness and may be transient. The presence of HB$_s$Ag also is diagnostic of the carrier state, and maternal HB$_s$Ag status always should be determined when infants less than 1 yr of age are diagnosed with hepatitis B infection. Hepatitis B "e" antigen (HB$_e$Ag) appears in the serum with HB$_s$Ag. The

Table 11–16. Causes of Acute Liver Disease in Childhood

Viral

Hepatitis A	Herpes simplex 1, 2
Hepatitis B	Lassa fever virus
Hepatitis C	Dengue
Hepatitis D (with B)	Yellow fever
Hepatitis E	Ebola virus
Epstein-Barr virus	Measles
Cytomegalovirus	Varicella-zoster virus
Enterovirus	Undefined paramyxovirus
Human herpesvirus-6	(syncytial giant cells)

Bacterial

Syphilis	Miliary tuberculosis
Leptospirosis	Gonococcus (perihepatitis)
Bacterial sepsis	*Chlamydia trachomatis*
Coxiella burnetii	(perihepatitis)

Toxic

Isoniazid	Iron
Oral contraceptives	Erythromycin estolate
Androgens	Alcohol
Carbon tetrachloride	Mushroom poisoning
Chlorpromazine	(*Amanita phalloides*)
Allopurinol	Valproic acid
Acetaminophen	Phenytoin
Salicylates	Carbamazepine
Hydralazine	Methotrexate
Halothane	6-Mercaptopurine

Other

Wilson disease	Veno-occlusive disease
Inborn errors of	Tumor
metabolism	Infarction
(galactosemia,	Shock
tyrosinemia)	Heart failure
Chronic active hepatitis	Anoxia

(From Behrman RE (ed): Nelson Textbook of Pediatrics. 14th ed. Philadelphia, WB Saunders, 1992, p 1018.)

continued presence of HB$_s$Ag and HB$_e$Ag in the absence of antibody to e antigen (anti-HB$_e$) is predictive of a high risk of transmission. Clearance of HB$_s$Ag from the serum precedes a variable "window" period followed by the emergence of the antibody to surface antigen (anti-HB$_s$), which confers lifelong immunity. Antibody to core antigen (anti-HB$_c$) is a useful marker for recognizing HBV infection during the window phase (i.e., when HB$_s$Ag has disappeared but before the appearance of anti-HB$_s$). Anti-HB$_e$ is useful in predicting a low degree of infectivity during the carrier state. Seroconversion following HCV may occur up to 6 mo after illness.

Recovery is the rule in most cases of acute viral hepatitis. Less than 1:1000 cases progress to fulminant hepatic necrosis, encephalopathy, and death

(see Fulminant Hepatic Failure). The virus-specific risks for chronic hepatitis, carrier state, and hepatocellular carcinoma are noted in Table 11–17.

The *treatment* of hepatitis is largely supportive and includes rest, hydration, and adequate dietary intake. Hospitalization is indicated for patients with severe vomiting and dehydration, a prolonged prothrombin time, or evidence of early hepatic encephalopathy. Once the diagnosis of viral hepatitis is made, attention should be directed toward preventing its spread. For HAV, careful hygienic measures include handwashing and the careful disposal of excreta, contaminated diapers or clothing, needles, and other blood-contaminated items. As soon as the diagnosis is established, immune serum globulin should be given to all immediate family contacts and, in the case of infants and toddlers, to all close playmates and

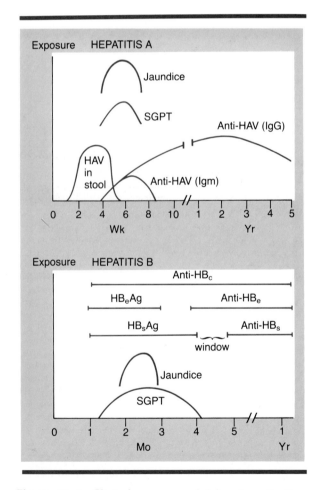

Figure 11–5. Clinical course and laboratory findings with hepatitis A and B. SGPT = serum glutamic pyruvic transaminase.

Table 11–17. Characteristics of the Agents Causing Acute Viral Hepatitis

	Hepatitis A Virus (HAV; enterovirus 72)	Hepatitis B* Virus (HBV)	Hepatitis C† Virus (HCV; formerly post-transfusion non-A, non-B virus)	Hepatitis D Virus (HDV)	Hepatitis E Virus (HEV; formerly enteral non-A, non-B virus)
Agent	27-nm RNA virus	42-nm DNA virus	30–60-nm RNA virus; similar to flaviviruses	36-nm circular RNA hybrid particle with HB$_s$Ag coat	27–34-nm RNA virus; similar to Norwalk-type viruses
Transmission	Fecal–oral, Food–water	Transfusion, sexual, inoculation, vertical	Parenteral, transfusion, vertical (sexual?)	Similar to HBV	Enteral: endemic and epidemic
Incubation period	30 days	60–180 days	30–60 days	Similar to HBV	35–60 days
Serum markers	Anti-HAV	Antigens*, anti-HB$_s$, anti-HB$_c$	Anti-HCV (IgG, IgM)	Anti-HDV, RNA	Anti-HEV
Fulminant liver failure	Rare	Uncommon unless with δ agent‡	Uncommon	Yes	Yes in pregnancy
Chronic liver disease	No	Yes	Yes	Yes	Uncommon
Carrier state	No	Yes§	Yes	Yes	No
Risk of hepatocellular cancer	No	Yes	Yes	No	No
Prophylaxis against	Immune serum globulin; hygiene	Hepatitis B immune globulin, vaccine Screen blood products for HB$_s$Ag	Screen blood for antibody appearing 4 mo postinfection (6 mo post-transfusion)	Screen blood for HBV markers	Screen blood for IgM, IgG antibody

* Hepatitis B whole virus particle is the Dane particle, which consists of a surface antigen HB$_s$Ag, a core antigen HB$_c$Ag, an e antigen HB$_e$Ag, and DNA with a DNA polymerase. Mutant HBV also may produce severe hepatitis.

† An unknown number of posttransfusion hepatitis cases are due to viruses other than HBV, HCV or cytomegalovirus, Epstein-Barr virus, human herpesvirus-6, or known agents and remain designated as caused by a non-A, non-B hepatitis agent.

‡ δ Agent or hepatitis D virus requires hepatitis B virus coinfection or superinfection of a chronic HBV carrier for replication.

§ Chronic carrier state common in Afro-Asian, Haitian, Eskimo, and South Pacific immigrants, drug abusers, Down syndrome, multiply transfused patients, homosexuals, patients on hemodialysis, and dental workers.

(From Behrman RE (ed): Nelson Textbook of Pediatrics. 14th ed. Philadelphia, WB Saunders, 1992, p 1017.)

children at day care centers. Similar hygienic measures are necessary for hepatitis B and C.

The *prevention* of hepatitis may be accomplished by immunization and isolation (Table 11–18). Immune globulin is recommended following exposure to hepatitis. High-risk groups should receive immunization against HBV (e.g., parenteral drug abusers; male homosexuals; prisoners; sexual partners of HBV-infected individuals; infants born to HB$_s$Ag-positive mothers; patients and staff in hemodialysis and oncology units; patients requiring frequent blood or clotting factor concentrates and health care personnel who handle these products; physicians, dentists, and morticians; household contacts of HB$_s$Ag carriers; and patients with Down syndrome). It currently is recommended to immunize all neonates and infants to HBV regardless of risk (see Chapter 10).

FULMINANT HEPATIC FAILURE

Fulminant hepatic failure may occur in patients who have had no pre-existing liver pathology. Massive hepatic necrosis is due either to a viral agent or to hepatotoxins. Impending acute liver failure should be suspected when transaminase values that initially were elevated 15–20-fold fall rapidly as prothrombin time becomes prolonged and unresponsive to parenteral vitamin K. The direct bilirubin level continues to rise. In severe liver failure the total bilirubin level continues to rise as the direct fraction decreases as a result of loss of conjugating function. Hepatic encephalopathy is the most dramatic sign of fulminant hepatic failure and improves with liver regeneration. Other complications include hypoglycemia, gastrointestinal hemorrhage, hyponatremia, renal insufficiency (hepatorenal syndrome), sepsis, and cerebral edema.

Treatment is supportive and includes (1) the discontinuation of oral feedings and the administration of lactulose by nasogastric tube to decrease enteric ammonia production; (2) central venous alimentation with quantities of glucose and fluid sufficient to prevent hypoglycemia and hypovolemia; (3) central venous pressure monitoring; (4) intracranial pressure monitoring and, in selected patients with elevated intracranial pressure, administration of mannitol, and hyperventilation; (5) the administration of antacids or cimetidine to keep the gastric pH above 4; and (6) the administration of intravenous vitamin K or fresh frozen plasma to

Table 11–18. Prevention of Hepatitis

Etiology	Clinical Situation	Treatment
HAV	Before and 1 wk following jaundice	Enteric isolation
	Household contacts	IG within 2 wk of exposure
	School outbreak	IG only in day care or custodial institutions with high risk of fecal–oral spread
HBV	Perinatal exposure	Vaccination + HBIG
	Sexual—acute infection	HBIG ± vaccination
	Sexual—chronic carrier	Vaccination
	Household contact—chronic carrier	Vaccination
	Household contact—acute case	None unless known exposure
	Household contact—acute case, known exposure	HBIG ± vaccination
	Infant (<12 mo)—acute case in primary caregiver	HBIG + vaccination
	Inadvertent—percutaneous or permucosal exposure	HBIG ± vaccination
HCV	Inadvertent—percutaneous exposure	IG*

* Efficacy in this situation not conclusively proven.
IG = immune serum globulin; HBIG = hepatitis B immune globulin.

improve or maintain clotting status. Liver transplantation is an effective therapy.

The short-term *prognosis* is poor, with mortality rates of 80–90%. However, for those who survive, the long-term prognosis is excellent, with full recovery of normal liver function following hepatic regeneration.

CHRONIC LIVER DISEASE

Chronic hepatitis is an inflammatory process that lasts more than 6 mo and may become manifest as hepatic failure or chronic liver disease. The *cause* of most cases is unknown. Viral infections with HBV and HCV are the most frequently identifiable causes. Other causes include drugs (such as alphamethyldopa, isoniazid, and methotrexate), Wilson disease, alpha-1-antitrypsin deficiency, cystic fibrosis, and inflammatory bowel disease.

Chronic hepatitis may be classified as either persistent or active based on the histologic appearance of the liver. In patients with **chronic persistent hepatitis**, the liver architecture is normal and the inflammatory process is confined to the portal area without extension into the periportal region. Patients may be asymptomatic or have fatigue, abdominal pain, slight hepatomegaly, mild jaundice, and anorexia. Laboratory studies demonstrate fluctuating transaminase levels, mild hyperbilirubinemia, normal prothrombin time, and HBV or HCV seropositivity in most patients. Chronic persistent hepatitis is the most common cause of chronic hepatitis and is a self-limited condition that requires reassurance of the child and family but no specific treatment. Recovery is the rule, but the pathologic lesion and mild biochemical abnormalities may persist for years.

Chronic active hepatitis is a more serious form of the disease because the inflammatory process of lymphocytes and plasma cells not only involves the portal area but also extends into the adjacent lobule (periportal hepatitis, piecemeal necrosis). Fibrosis may extend between portal areas (bridging fibrosis). Chronic active hepatitis may progress to cirrhosis and hepatic failure. The diagnosis should be considered in any child with persistent or relapsing jaundice 6 mo following an episode of HBV or HCV hepatitis. However, the majority of patients have no evidence of antecedent acute hepatitis. The most common form of chronic active hepatitis in children is the **autoimmune** form, which may have an indolent course. Many patients already have cirrhosis when the diagnosis is made.

Clinical manifestations include hepatosplenomegaly, jaundice, malaise, anorexia, and right upper quadrant pain. In addition to the aforementioned features of liver disease, patients with autoimmune chronic active hepatitis also may have extrahepatic manifestations, such as amenorrhea, arthritis, arthralgia, low-grade fever, and thyroiditis. Patients with autoimmune hepatitis have circulating markers, such as antismooth muscle (66%) and antimitochondrial (33%) and antinuclear (50%) antibodies. In chronic active hepatitis, the serum transaminase test shows a 5-fold or greater elevation and usually is accompanied by hypergammaglobulinemia. The *diagnosis* is made by liver biopsy, which is a prerequisite for treatment with immunosuppressive agents.

In cases of autoimmune hepatitis, *treatment* with prednisone may lead to a dramatic improvement in the clinical, laboratory, and histologic features of the disease, as well as a decrease in the mortality rate. Azathioprine is of value because of its steroid-sparing effect. Corticosteroids are contraindicated in patients with viral chronic active hepatitis. In children with autoimmune chronic active hepatitis, 75% respond to therapy but 50% will relapse with discontinuation of prednisone. Progression to cirrhosis may occur despite a good response to initial immunosuppression. Treatment of HCV chronic active hepatitis with interferon shows promise, but relapse may occur when therapy is discontinued.

CIRRHOSIS

Cirrhosis is the end result of destructive processes producing irreversible fibrosis, scarring, and hepatocellular regeneration, which leads to the formation of nodules. The nodules cause irreversible distortion of the hepatic vasculature and biliary system. Nodules may be small (<3 mm in micronodular cirrhosis) or large (>3 mm in macronodular cirrhosis). This distortion of the vascular bed leads to portal hypertension and portosystemic shunting. In childhood, the *causes* of cirrhosis include biliary malformations, alpha-1-antitrypsin deficiency, Wilson disease, galactosemia, tyrosinemia, chronic active hepatitis, and hemochromatosis. *Clinical manifestations* include palmar erythema, spider angiomata, gynecomastia, splenomegaly, ascites, hemorrhoids, cutaneous excoriations from pruritus, and jaundice. The liver may be large and hard (biliary cirrhosis) or small, scarred, and shrunken (postnecrotic cirrhosis). *Laboratory findings* depend on the cause and severity of the process. The major *complications* of cirrhosis in children include portal hypertension with variceal bleeding and hypersplenism, ascites, liver failure with encephalopathy, hepatorenal syndrome, and, rarely, hepatocellular carcinoma.

PORTAL HYPERTENSION

Although cirrhosis is an important cause of portal hypertension, any process leading to an increased resistance to portal blood flow into the liver (prehepatic or presinusoidal; e.g., portal vein thrombosis, omphalitis, schistosomiasis), through the liver (intrahepatic or sinusoidal), or from above the liver (suprahepatic or postsinusoidal; e.g., Budd-Chiari syndrome, veno-occlusive disease, pericarditis) will result in portal hypertension. Prehepatic and suprahepatic causes are more likely in children less than 5 yr of age with no prior history of liver disease. Although rare, lesions such as an arteriovenous malformation, which increases hepatic blood flow, also will result in portal hypertension. Portal hypertension leads to the formation of collaterals between the portal and systemic circulation. The most important of these connections is that between the portal vein and the azygos vein via submucosal veins (varices) in the stomach and esophagus.

Hemorrhage from *esophageal varices* is associated with hematemesis or melena (see Gastrointestinal Hemorrhage). In children, the bleeding often stops spontaneously, but rebleeding may occur. Impaired synthesis of clotting factors, resulting from severe hepatocellular dysfunction or hypersplenism induced thrombocytopenia, can result in uncontrollable hemorrhage. Management consists of replacing losses and intravenous infusion of vasopressin, which causes constriction of the splanchnic arterioles and a reduction of portal pressure and flow. Endoscopic sclerotherapy can be used to arrest acute bleeding and to prevent rebleeding. Repeated sclerosing injections lead to variceal obliteration. Portosystemic shunt surgery may decompress the entire portal system (portocaval anastomosis) or only the varices (distal splenorenal shunt). Portal hypertension also produces *hypersplenism* that becomes manifest by anemia, neutropenia, and thrombocytopenia.

ASCITES

Ascites is the accumulation of abnormal amounts of fluid in the peritoneal cavity. It results from hypoalbuminemia, portal hypertension, increased hepatic and splanchnic lymph production accompanied by impaired renal sodium and water excretion secondary to hyperaldosteronism and increased levels of antidiuretic hormone. Ascites is clinically detectable as a shifting dullness to percussion when at least 300 mL of fluid is present. Ascites caused by liver disease has the characteristics of a transudate (<3 g protein/dL). *Treatment* consists of the administration of spironolactone and the restriction of sodium intake. The administration of furosemide may be necessary in refractory cases. Diuresis usually should be accomplished slowly over several days, but aggressive diuresis with abdominal paracentesis or intravenous albumin followed by furosemide is indicated when respiratory function is compromised. The latter approach may lead to plasma volume depletion, hypokalemia, hepatorenal syndrome, and encephalopathy. Spontaneous bacterial peritonitis may be a complication of ascites and should be considered if fever and abdominal pain are present (see Peritoneal Cavity).

HEPATIC ENCEPHALOPATHY

Progressive deterioration of liver function results in impaired detoxification of metabolic products. This process, along with portosystemic shunting, results in hepatic encephalopathy. Encephalopathy may be acute, as seen in fulminant hepatic failure, or chronic, as seen in slowly progressive liver disease. The *cause* is unknown but may be related to disturbances in neuronal function resulting from the presence of a false neurotransmitter in the central nervous system. Ammonia and bacterial products, such as octopamine, mercaptan (fetor hepaticus), or endogenous benzodiazepines and gamma-aminobutyrate, may play important roles. However, serum ammonia levels correlate poorly with the degree of encephalopathy.

The *clinical manifestations* of hepatic encephalopathy are described by four stages: (1) impaired mentation; (2) lethargy, disorientation, and asterixis; (3) arousable stupor; and (4) coma. *Treatment* of chronic encephalopathy should focus on identification of the precipitating causes, such as intestinal bleeding, infection, central nervous system–depressing drugs, and complications of diuretic therapy. Therapy includes maintaining adequate nutrition and reducing ammonia production. Some protein restriction may be needed, but at least 1.0 g/kg/24 hr must be provided to meet metabolic requirements and to prevent endogenous protein breakdown. During acute encephalopathy, no protein should be given, but glucose infusions are needed to prevent hypoglycemia and proteolysis. Neomycin (oral) will reduce the number of bacteria in the intestine available for producing ammonia. Lactulose also should be given to reduce ammonia production; it lowers stool pH, trapping ammonia in the form of the nondiffusible ammonium ion, and is a cathartic, reducing intestinal stasis. Flumazenil, a benzodiazepine antagonist, may reverse hepatic encephalopathy.

NEONATAL CHOLESTASIS

Direct hyperbilirubinemia during the 1st mo of life signifies significant pathology resulting from hepatobiliary structural anomalies, infections, metabolic and genetic disease, drug and nutritional toxicity, and disorders of unknown cause (Fig. 11–1 and Chapter 6). Except for parenteral alimentation–induced cholestasis in premature infants, the most common disorders in full-term infants that are associated with neonatal cholestasis are extrahepatic biliary atresia and giant cell hepatitis. The usual manifestations of cholestatic diseases during infancy are jaundice, hepatomegaly, dark urine, and acholic stools.

After specific diagnostic tests are performed, the supportive management of these patients depends on the extent of the hepatocellular dysfunction and the severity of the cholestasis. Hepatocellular dysfunction predisposes the patient to complications, such as bleeding, encephalopathy, and hepatorenal syndrome, whereas bile salt deficiency may result in fat-soluble vitamin deficiencies, rickets, hypocalcemia (vitamin D deficiency), hemorrhage (vitamin K deficiency), and peripheral neuropathy (vitamin E deficiency). Retention of bile salts may produce pruritus. *Supportive therapy* includes fat-soluble vitamin supplementation; the administration of cholestyramine, to decrease reabsorption of bile salts from the gut; and phenobarbital, to increase the hepatic excretion of bile. The administration of oral ursodeoxycholic acid has improved bile secretion. *Definitive treatment* depends on the underlying process and may include an exclusion diet (lactose in galactosemia), surgery (in extrahepatic biliary atresia, choledochal cyst), or liver transplantation.

BILIARY ATRESIA

Biliary atresia is seen in 1 : 10,000 births and typically involves the extrahepatic bile ducts. In some patients, however, both intra- and extrahepatic biliary structures are involved as a result of an inflammatory process beginning in the perinatal period. It is more common in females, and the etiology is unknown.

Clinical manifestations usually present in a full-term infant in whom jaundice develops during the 2nd or 3rd wk of life. The stools often are acholic, although the shedding of bilirubin-laden intestinal mucosal cells may color the stool. The liver enlarges and becomes quite hard. Splenomegaly usually is detectable by 8 wk. Other than these physical findings, the infants usually appear healthy. There is an association with the polysplenia syndrome and with trisomy 13 and 18.

Laboratory tests demonstrate conjugated hyperbilirubinemia and elevated serum alkaline phosphatase, gamma-glutamyl transferase, and transaminases. Ultrasound examination is helpful in excluding a choledochal cyst. A biliary scan following 5 days of phenobarbital administration (5 mg/kg/day) demonstrates a normal hepatocyte uptake but a failure to excrete the isotope into the intestine after 24 hr. This test is less reliable in infants with serum bilirubin levels above 10 mg/dL. Percutaneous liver biopsy shows bile duct proliferation and confirms the diagnosis in 95% of patients.

Ultimately, patients with suspected biliary atresia require exploratory laparotomy. If biliary atresia is found, a **Kasai procedure** (hepatoportoenterostomy) is used to connect the bowel lumen and the porta hepatis. Without surgery, patients usually die from cirrhosis before 2 yr of age. Surgical success is judged by improvement in bile drainage; the earlier the operation (<2 mo of age), the greater the chance of establishing bile flow. Twenty-five to 50% of patients survive 5 yr after the Kasai procedure, but complications of the procedure include progressive biliary cirrhosis and ascending cholangitis. Another treatment for most infants is liver transplantation, which has an 80–90% survival rate.

BILIARY HYPOPLASIA

Patients with intrahepatic biliary hypoplasia may be classified as either "syndromic" (Alagille syndrome, arteriohepatic dysplasia) or "nonsyndromic." In addition to intrahepatic biliary hypoplasia, infants with Alagille syndrome have facial, cardiac (valvular or peripheral pulmonic stenosis), vertebral (butterfly vertebra), ocular (posterior embryotoxon), and renal (dysplastic kidneys) anomalies. Patients have hypercholesterolemia and associated cutaneous xanthomata. Many of the children have growth failure, and some are mildly mentally retarded. *Treatment* is directed at controlling hypercholesterolemia with diet and cholestyramine and at preventing manifestations of vitamin E deficiency (ataxia, areflexia, loss of vibratory and position sensation, and ophthalmoplegia) with aggressive vitamin E supplementation. Phenobarbital and ursodeoxycholic acid therapy also may help lower serum bilirubin and bile acid levels. The *prognosis* for hepatic disease of the "syndromic" form is better than that for the nonsyndromic form. Cirrhosis and liver failure usually occur in the nonsyndromic form before adolescence.

NEONATAL (GIANT CELL) HEPATITIS

Idiopathic neonatal hepatitis is responsible for most of the cases of intrahepatic cholestasis in infants who are not receiving parenteral nutrition. It usually presents at birth, is more common in males, and often is characterized by growth retardation. Idiopathic neonatal hepatitis represents more than

one disease resulting from infectious or familial causes. It is unusual to have acholic stools and a very high alkaline phosphatase level. Patency of bile ducts may be documented by a biliary scan, although severe cholestasis may cause a false-positive scan. Liver biopsy shows numerous giant cells, lobular disorganization, necrosis, and inflammation without the neoductular proliferation and fibrosis characteristic of extrahepatic atresia. The *differential diagnosis* includes TORCH infections, biliary atresia (which may be difficult to exclude without biopsy) and other causes of conjugated hyperbilirubinemia (Fig. 11–1). *Treatment* is as described for Alagille syndrome, and most patients recover within 6–8 mo.

PROGRESSIVE FAMILIAL INTRAHEPATIC CHOLESTASIS (BYLER DISEASE)

Progressive familial intrahepatic cholestasis (PFIC), inherited in an autosomal recessive manner, was first described in an Amish kindred (Byler), and usually presents in the 1st yr of life with progressive cholestasis and pruritis, out of proportion to the level of jaundice. PFIC progresses to cirrhosis, end-stage liver disease, and death by 3 yr without transplantation. PFIC is characterized by low serum gamma-glutamyl transpeptidase and normal cholesterol concentrations, in contrast to other childhood cholestatic disorders. Other than liver transplantation, chronic biliary diversion and ursodeoxycholic acid therapy may reduce pruritis and improve liver function in some patients.

REYE SYNDROME

Reye syndrome is characterized by encephalopathy and the noninflammatory fatty infiltration of the liver and kidney. It has been associated with epidemics of influenza A or B virus and varicella. The administration of aspirin predisposes the patient to this condition. The peak incidence is in children of 6 yr of age, with most cases occurring between 4 and 12 yrs of age.

The *clinical manifestations* of Reye syndrome begin with intractable vomiting during or immediately following recovery from an upper respiratory tract infection. Over a period of 2–24 hr, the child becomes confused, combative, agitated, stuporous, and, finally, comatose. In addition to the altered level of consciousness, physical findings include dilated pupils, hyperactive deep tendon reflexes, and Kussmaul respirations. Jaundice and fever are absent, and the liver may be normal to moderately enlarged in size. The serum transaminase and ammonia levels are elevated and the prothrombin time may be prolonged. Hypoglycemia and acidosis also may be present. Spinal fluid examination is normal and toxicology of the blood and urine are negative.

The *diagnosis* is made by liver biopsy. Histologic findings include a diffuse microvesicular steatosis, without necrosis or inflammation. The mitochondria are swollen. Infants under 2 yr of age should be evaluated for underlying inborn errors of metabolism, such as medium-chain acyl-coenzyme A dehydrogenase deficiency.

Treatment is supportive and similar to that outlined for fulminant hepatic failure. Careful monitoring and treatment of increased intracranial pressure are mandatory.

The *prognosis* correlates best with the depth of coma. Death from Reye syndrome usually is due to increased intracranial pressure, because liver regeneration is often present at the time of autopsy.

Prevention may be possible by avoiding salicylates during viral respiratory illnesses.

ALPHA-1-ANTITRYPSIN DEFICIENCY

The glycoprotein alpha-1-antitrypsin is produced by hepatocytes under the influence of two autosomally inherited, codominant alleles and makes up 80% of the serum alpha-1-globulin fraction. It functions as an inhibitor of trypsin, pancreatic elastase, neutral proteases of leukocytes, and acid proteases of alveolar macrophages. Uninhibited proteolytic activity by these enzymes may cause hepatic or pulmonary injury. There are 26 different alleles of this protease-inhibitor (Pi) system. The normal phenotype is MM; Pi ZZ is associated with liver or lung disease, whereas the MS, MZ, and SZ phenotypes may be associated with hepatic disease. The incidence of the ZZ phenotype is 1:2000–4000, but only 20% of patients with the ZZ phenotype have neonatal cholestasis. The pathogenesis of the liver disease is unknown; it appears that the hepatocytes are unable to excrete the protein that accumulates in the cell.

Cholestatic jaundice that is indistinguishable from neonatal hepatitis during the first 1–3 mo of life may be the initial presenting sign. Hepatosplenomegaly also may be present. Cirrhosis develops in 30–50% of patients, resulting in hepatic failure; progression may be extremely variable (months to years). Older patients may develop pulmonary emphysema, and hepatocellular cancer has developed following cirrhosis. Pancreatitis also may develop. The *diagnosis* is made by quantifying levels of circulating alpha-1-antitrypsin and phenotyping. Liver biopsy reveals the presence of eosinophilic cytoplasmic granules that stain intensely with periodic acid–Schiff stain.

There is no specific *treatment* for alpha-1-antitrypsin deficiency. Plasma or recombinant alpha-1-antitrypsin infusions restore plasma levels but have not yet been demonstrated to cure the hepatic complications. Therapy for cholestasis and the complications of cirrhosis are similar to those previously outlined. Severe cases may be treated with liver transplantation.

WILSON DISEASE (HEPATOLENTICULAR DEGENERATION)

This autosomal recessive disorder is caused by the accumulation of copper in the liver, brain, eyes, kidney, and bone. *Clinical manifestations* are unusual before 5 yr of age and include hepatosplenomegaly and jaundice resembling chronic active hepatitis, hemolytic anemia, deterioration of neurologic function (worsening school performance and handwriting, intention tremor, clumsiness, personality changes), renal tubular acidosis, and the appearance of corneal Kayser-Fleischer rings. Hepatitis is common in younger patients; neuropsychiatric problems are noted in older patients.

Low serum copper and low serum ceruloplasmin levels suggest the *diagnosis*, but normal copper values may be found early in the course of the disease. Quantitation of urinary copper output, with or without penicillamine administration or quantitation of hepatic copper levels, confirms the diagnosis.

The goal of *treatment* is to lower tissue copper levels. This has been successfully accomplished with the copper chelating agent D-penicillamine. Foods high in copper, such as chocolate, nuts, and dried fruits, should be avoided. *Prognosis* depends on early diagnosis and successful chelation of the copper.

References

Balistreri W: Mechanisms and management of pediatric hepatobiliary disease. J Pediatr Gastroenterol Nutr 10:138, 1990.

Behrman RE (ed): Nelson Textbook of Pediatrics. 14th ed. Philadelphia, WB Saunders, 1992, Sec. 13.81–13.102.

Editorial: The A to F of viral hepatitis. Lancet 336:1158, 1990.

Hassall E, Berquist W, Ament M, et al: Sclerotherapy for extrahepatic portal hypertension in childhood. J Pediatr 115:69, 1989.

Hussein M, Howard E, Mieli-Vergani G, et al: Jaundice at

14 days of life: Exclude biliary atresia. Arch Dis Child 66:1177, 1991.

Laker M: Liver function tests. BMJ 301:250, 1990.

Mortimer EA Jr: Reye's syndrome, salicylates, epidemiology, and public health policy. JAMA 257:1941, 1987.

Mullen K: Benzodiazepine compounds and hepatic encephalopathy. N Engl J Med 325:509, 1991.

Suruga K, Tsunoda S, Deguchi E, et al: The future role of hepatic portoenterostomy as treatment of biliary atresia. J Pediatr Surg 27:707, 1992.

Pancreas

Isolated disease of the exocrine pancreas is uncommon in children. Pancreatic exocrine insufficiency often is part of a genetic or systemic illness. Cystic fibrosis (Chapter 12) and severe malnutrition are the leading causes of pancreatic disease. Schwachman's syndrome (neutropenia, dysostosis), an autosomal recessive disorder, accounts for 3–5% of pancreatic insufficiency in childhood.

Pancreatic function tests include determination of the levels of serum amylase and lipase (which are increased when pancreatitis is present), and trypsinogen (which is increased in cystic fibrosis); examination of stool for fat droplets or meat fibers (indicating fat and protein maldigestion); and analysis of urine for reduced *para*-aminobenzoic acid (PABA) excretion (which is due to deficient pancreatic chymotrypsin) following ingestion of N-benzoyl-L-tyrosyl-PABA. Cannulation of the pancreatic duct and collection of fluid for enzyme analysis, with and without secretagogue stimulation (endoscopic retrograde cholangiopancreatoduodenoscopy), also may be helpful in evaluating pancreatic insufficiency.

ANNULAR PANCREAS

This rare malformation is due to a failure of rotation and fusion of the ventral and dorsal pancreatic buds. A complete pancreatic ring may obstruct the duodenum. **Pancreas divisum** is due to failure of fusion of the dorsal and ventral embryonic pancreas that drains through an accessory papilla. Pancreas divisum is a cause of recurrent pancreatitis.

PANCREATITIS

Pancreatic duct obstruction or nonspecific parenchymal inflammation results in tissue injury from digestive enzymes, which leads to autodigestion and further inflammation and edema. Fat necrosis and hemorrhage are additional complications of acute pancreatitis. The *etiology* is idiopathic in as many as 25% of cases. Other causes include infectious agents (mumps; coxsackievirus, hepatitis virus, influenza virus, mycoplasma), drugs (alcohol, thiazide diuretics, valproic acid, L-asparaginase, acetaminophen, corticosteroids, sulfonamides), cystic fibrosis, alpha-1-antitrypsin deficiency, gallstones, biliary "sludge," shock, pancreas divisum, hypertriglyceridemia, hypercalcemia, trauma, renal failure, familial disease, and vasculitis.

The *clinical manifestations* of pancreatitis include intense epigastric pain (occasionally radiating to the back), nausea, and vomiting. The abdomen may be tender and rigid, and a mass may be palpable if a pseudocyst has formed. Hemorrhagic pancreatitis may cause shock and produce a blue discoloration around the umbilicus (Cullen sign) or around the flank (Grey Turner sign). Left-sided pleural effusion and ascites are less common manifestations. Poor prognostic features include hyperglycemia (>200 mg/dL), leukocytosis (>16,000), elevated lactic dehydrogenase (>700 IU) and serum glutamic oxaloacetic transaminase (>250 U), and the development of anemia, hypocalcemia, azotemia (blood urea nitrogen >50 mg/dL), metabolic acidosis, hypoxia, and the need for continuous fluid resuscitation.

Laboratory findings include elevated serum amylase and lipase levels. Diabetic ketoacidosis, renal failure, parotid gland disease, perforated gastric ulcer, or acidosis may produce false elevations of serum amylase. Pleural or ascitic fluid amylase levels will be elevated. Hyperglycemia and hypocalcemia may be present. Abdominal roentgenograms may demonstrate a sentinel loop, pancreatic calcification, or a mass. Ultrasonography will demonstrate a swollen pancreas and/or pseudocyst.

Treatment includes fluid replacement for hypovolemic shock, bowel rest, nasogastric decompression, and pain medication. The treatment also is directed toward the relief of complications, such as anemia and hypocalcemia. Pseudocysts that persist beyond 6 wk may require surgery. Endoscopic retrograde cholangiopancreoduodenoscopy may have a role in the management of severe pancreatitis.

References

Behrman RE (ed): Nelson Textbook of Pediatrics. 14th ed. Philadelphia, WB Saunders, 1992, Sec. 13.70–13.80.

Dugernier T: Severe acute pancreatitis. The therapeutic dilemma: Medical or surgical intensive care. Intensive Crit Care Digest 10:47, 1991.

Schroder T, Sainio V, Kivisaari L, et al: Pancreatic resection versus peritoneal lavage in acute necrotizing pancreatitis. Ann Surg 214:663, 1991.

Weizman Z, Durie P: Acute pancreatitis in childhood. J Pediatr 113:24, 1988.

Peritoneal Cavity

Primary peritonitis is an acute inflammatory process in the peritoneal cavity attributable to a perforated viscus. It usually occurs in children after splenectomy or in those having chronic ascites, such as that seen in nephrotic syndrome or cirrhosis. *Clinical manifestations* include the acute onset of fever, severe abdominal pain, and vomiting. The *diagnosis* may be made on abdominal paracentesis. The fluid is an exudate, Gram stain reveals organisms, and many polymorphonucleated leukocytes are present. The responsible bacteria are *Pneumococcus* and gram-negative enteric pathogens. Peritonitis in patients receiving chronic ambulatory peritoneal dialysis includes that caused by *Staphylococcus epidermidis*.

Secondary peritonitis is an inflammatory response to bacteria, bile, or pancreatic enzymes in the abdominal cavity resulting from a ruptured viscus. Necrotizing enterocolitis, appendicitis, and penetrating wounds are common causes. *E. coli, Klebsiella, Proteus, Enterobacter,* and *Bacteroides fragilis* are frequently found pathogens. Combined therapy for anaerobic and gram-negative organisms and appropriate surgery are the treatment of choice.

Reference

Behrman RE (ed): Nelson Textbook of Pediatrics. 14th ed. Philadelphia, WB Saunders, 1992, Sec. 13.103.

The Respiratory System

12

Carolyn M. Kercsmar

Disorders of the respiratory system—for example, viral upper respiratory infections, otitis media, pneumonia, asthma, and cystic fibrosis—constitute a substantial part of the pediatrician's clinical practice. Respiratory disease may be insidious, because normally a large lung reserve capacity exists and more than half the total lung tissue (or function) may be lost before an individual complains of dyspnea. In addition, the typical symptoms (dyspnea, cough, chest pain) or signs (tachypnea, rales, wheezing) may be overlooked or may be subtle in young children. Fever may be the only symptom of pneumonia, tachypnea the only manifestation of asthma, and cough the only symptom of foreign body aspiration. During a child's development, the pediatrician also must consider genetic (cystic fibrosis), anatomic (congenital anomalies), iatrogenic (oxygen toxicity), immunologic (immunosuppression, immunodeficiency), and extrapulmonary (heart failure) conditions as etiologic variables contributing to pulmonary pathology.

DEVELOPMENT OF THE RESPIRATORY SYSTEM

At about 24 days' gestation in the developing human embryo, primordial lungs are detectable as a bud from the gut. Within another 4 days, the major bronchi are discernible. They then undergo rapid growth and repeated dichotomous branching. By 12 wk, lobes of lung tissue can be distinguished. This first stage of development, known as the "glandular" stage, is completed by 16 wk. During the "canalicular" phase of lung growth, which takes place between 16 and 24 wk, the airway epithelium and submucosal glands develop, and alveoli begin to appear late in this phase. The rapid proliferation of the alveoli constitutes the "alveolar phase," which begins at about 24 wk and continues into postnatal life.

The capillary network first develops during the 20th wk of gestation, but these capillaries are not closely associated with the alveolar surfaces until the 26th to the 28th wk, when the alveolar walls become much thinner. Without the presence of both alveolar surface and closely adjacent capillaries, extrauterine life is not possible.

The alveolar surfaces are lined by two types of cells: type I cells have a very thin cytoplasm and form the major tissue barrier between the air spaces and the capillaries across which gas diffuses; type II cells synthesize and secrete surfactant, a substance that reduces alveolar surface tension, thus reducing the pressure required to maintain alveolar volume. Surfactant is essential for normal respiration (see Chapter 6).

During early postnatal life, the lung continues to develop, primarily by increasing the number of alveoli and terminal airways. At birth, the normal full-term infant has approximately 25 million alveoli; this number increases to nearly 300 million in adulthood. Almost all of this alveolar growth takes place in the first 8 yr, the greatest amount in the first 3–4 yr.

References

Behrman RE (ed): Nelson Textbook of Pediatrics. 14th ed. Philadelphia, WB Saunders, 1992, Sec. 14.1.
Chernick V, Mellins RB: Developmental anatomy of the lung. Sec. II, Chapters 2–4. In Chernick V, Mellins RB (eds): Basic Mechanisms of Pediatric Respiratory Disease. Philadelphia, BC Decker, 1991, pp 11–54.

ANATOMY OF THE RESPIRATORY SYSTEM

Air enters the nostrils and passes over three turbinates (bony protrusions into the nasal cavity), which are covered by ciliated respiratory epithelium and which increase the total surface area within the nostril. This large surface area and the convoluted patterns the airflow takes as it passes over the turbinates create a high resistance but serve to warm, humidify, and filter the inspired air. Secretions draining from the paranasal sinuses are carried from the nasal cavity to the pharynx by the mucociliary action of the epithelium. The eustachian tubes open from the middle ear into the posterior aspect of the nasopharynx. Lymphoid tissue at this location (the adenoids) may obstruct the orifice of the eustachian tubes.

The epiglottis helps to protect the larynx during swallowing by deflecting swallowed material toward the esophagus. The epiglottis of children has a contour somewhat like the Greek letter omega and usually is shaped differently from that of adults. The arytenoid cartilages, which assist in opening and closing the glottis, usually are not very prominent in children. The vocal cords form a V-shaped opening (the glottis), with the apex of the V being anterior, at the base of the epiglottis. Beneath the cords, the walls of the subglottic space converge toward the cricoid ring, a complete ring of cartilage. In children less than 2 or 3 yr of age, the cricoid ring (in effect, the first tracheal ring) is the narrowest portion of the airway, whereas in older children and adults the glottis is the smallest part of the airway.

The trachea and main bronchi are supported by rings of cartilage, which extend about 320 degrees around the airway circumference; the posterior wall is membranous. Beyond the lobar bronchi, the cartilaginous support for the airways becomes discontinuous. The more peripheral airways are supported entirely by elastic forces within the lung parenchyma.

The right lung normally has three lobes (upper, middle, and lower) and occupies about 55% of the total lung volume. The left lung normally has two lobes. The left upper lobe has an inferior division (the lingula) that is analogous to the middle lobe on the right.

PULMONARY PHYSIOLOGY

Pulmonary Mechanics

The major function of the lungs is to exchange oxygen and carbon dioxide between the atmosphere and the blood. Factors that influence this function include the anatomy and mechanics of the airways, the mechanics of the respiratory muscles and rib cage, the structure of the blood–gas interface (the alveolar surface), the pulmonary circulation, and the central mechanisms for neuromuscular control of ventilation.

Air enters the lungs via the upper airway whenever the pressure in the thorax is less than that of the surrounding atmosphere. During inspiration at rest, the negative intrathoracic pressure is caused by contraction (and lowering) of the diaphragm. Accessory muscles of respiration may be recruited during labored breathing. The external intercostal, scalene, and sternocleidomastoid muscles lift the rib cage and thus function as muscles of inspiration. During quiet breathing, most exhalation is passive, but during forced exhalation, intrathoracic pressure is increased by the abdominal muscles and by the internal intercostal muscles, which pull the ribs together.

Airway resistance is determined by the diameter of the conducting airway, its length, the viscosity of the gas, and the nature of the airflow. During quiet breathing, air flow (especially in the smaller airways) may be laminar, in which case the resistance is inversely proportional to the 4th power of the radius of the airway. At higher flow rates (as during exercise), the flow becomes turbulent, and the resistance increases even more. Thus relatively small changes in airway diameter (e.g., increases with normal growth or decreases resulting from mucosal edema or bronchoconstriction) may produce very large changes in airway resistance, a phenomenon more dramatically demonstrated in infants because the same degree of airway narrowing in the smaller airways of an infant will produce proportionately greater physiologic effects than it will in the airways of an older child or an adult.

When all mechanical forces acting on the lung are at equilibrium (e.g., at the end of a normal relaxed breath), the lung contains a volume of gas known as the functional residual capacity (FRC) (Fig. 12–1). This gas volume is important in maintaining exchange of oxygen across the alveolar surface during exhalation. Alterations in pulmonary homeostasis that result in decreased FRC include surfactant deficiency, adult respiratory distress syndrome (ARDS), and restrictive lung diseases. Obstructive lung disease, such as cystic fibrosis, increases FRC.

Normal tidal breathing utilizes the middle range of lung volumes, reaching neither residual volume nor total lung capacity (Fig. 12–1). Residual volume (RV) is the volume of gas in the lungs at the end of a maximal exhalation, whereas total lung capacity (TLC) is the volume of gas in the lungs at the end of a maximal inhalation. Vital capacity (VC) is the difference between TLC and RV.

With *partial airway obstruction*, airways collapse during exhalation, preventing normal emptying and thus increasing RV while also decreasing VC. Increased degrees of obstruction eventually increase FRC as well. Another manifestation of obstruction is decreased expiratory flow rates. A useful technique to clinically define airway obstruction

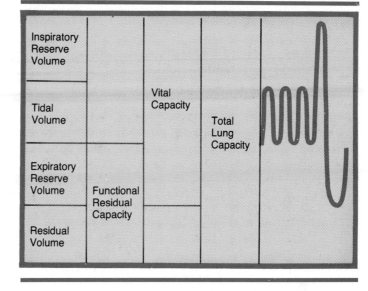

Figure 12–1. Lung volumes and capacities. Although vital capacity and its subdivisions can be measured by spirometry, calculation of residual volume requires measurement of functional residual capacity by body plethysmography, helium dilution technique, or nitrogen washout. (From Andreoli TE, Carpenter CJ, Plum F, et al [eds]: Cecil Essentials of Medicine. Philadelphia, WB Saunders, 1986, p 137.)

is measuring the volume of air exhaled during the 1st sec of a forced vital capacity maneuver (forced expiratory volume in 1 sec, FEV_1). The maximal midexpiratory flow rate (MMEF) is the volume of air exhaled per second during the forced expiratory maneuver between 25% and 75% of forced vital capacity. It is more sensitive to obstruction in peripheral airways than is FEV_1. VC, FEV_1, and MMEF are clinically useful measures and can be determined with a simple spirometer. Peak expiratory flow rate (PEFR) measures the most rapid rate of airflow (in liters/second or minute) during a forced expiratory maneuver, is largely a measure of airflow in central airways, and is highly dependent on patient effort. PEFR is best measured with a peak flowmeter, a simple hand-held device readily available in the office or emergency room setting.

Not all the air inspired during each breath reaches the alveoli. Normally, about 30% of each tidal breath fills the anatomic dead space (non–gas-exchanging parts of the respiratory system). The efficiency of ventilation therefore can be enhanced by increasing the tidal volume (because dead space is relatively constant). If tidal volume is decreased (as with central depression of respiratory drive or neuromuscular disease), the ratio of dead space to tidal volume will increase and alveolar ventilation will decrease.

The most common forms of lung disease in children result in airway obstruction. Excess secretions, bronchospasm, mucosal edema, stenosis, and airway compression all may produce symptomatic airway obstruction. *Restrictive disease* is less common and is characterized by normal to low FRC and RV, low total lung capacity and VC, decreased lung compliance, and relatively normal flow rates.

Respiratory Gas Exchange

Gas exchange depends on alveolar ventilation and pulmonary capillary blood flow, as well as on the ability of the gases to diffuse across the alveolar/capillary surfaces. Carbon dioxide diffuses 20 times more readily than oxygen. Thus, hypercapnia is a relatively late manifestation of disordered gas exchange, whereas hypoxemia occurs earlier. Under normal circumstances, physiologic matching of ventilation ($\dot{V}_A$) and blood flow ($\dot{Q}$) is maintained by anatomic mechanisms and local constriction of the pulmonary vessels in areas that are hypoventilated. The flow to the pulmonary circulation is capable of increasing at least 5-fold. A significant percentage of the capillary bed is not open under normal resting conditions, and blood normally is shunted away from underventilated areas of the lung. However, if hypoxic pulmonary vasoconstriction fails for any reason, the underventilated lung will continue to be perfused and the blood returning from that area will be unoxygenated, thus producing an intrapulmonary shunt with hypoxemia. Under normal circumstances, the hypoxemia would lead to an increased minute volume and a fall in the arterial carbon dioxide partial pressure (Pa_{CO_2}) as the shunt increases. Additionally, disorders of unequal ventilation–perfusion matching are much more common causes of hypoxemia than are ab-

Table 12–1. Differentiation of Mechanisms of Hypoxia

Etiology	Example	PaO₂	PaCO₂	A-aDO₂ (gradient)*		Q̇s/Q̇T (shunt)†	
		Pa_{O_2}	Pa_{CO_2}	*Room Air*	*100% O₂*	*Room Air*	*100% O₂*
Hypoventilation	Narcotic overdose, neuromuscular disease	↓	↑	N	N	N	N
Altitude	Mountain climbing	↓	↓	N	N	N	N
Intrapulmonary shunt	Atelectasis	↓	N or ↓	↑	↑	↑	↑
Cyanotic heart disease	Tetralogy of Fallot	↓	N or ↓	↑	↑	↑	↑
Pulmonary edema	Cardiomyopathy	↓	↓ N ↑	↑	N or ↑	↑	N or ↑
Adult respiratory distress syndrome	Sepsis, shock	↓	N to ↑	↑	N or ↑	↑	↑
Pneumonia	Lobar pneumococcal pneumonia	N or ↓	↓ or N	N or ↑	N	↑	↑
Pure V̇ₐ/Q̇ mismatch	Bronchopulmonary dysplasia, cystic fibrosis	↓	N or ↑	↑	N	↑	N
Diffusion defect	Scleroderma	↓	N	↑	N or ↑	↑	N

* A-aDO₂ = alveolar–arterial O₂ gradient, which is not influenced by changes in minute ventilation and is a measure of gas exchange. The A-aDO₂ can be determined by the *alveolar gas equation:* $A\text{-}aDO_2 = (P_B - pH_2O) \times FiO_2 - Pa_{CO_2}/R$, where P_B = atmospheric pressure (usually 760 mm Hg); pH_2O = partial pressure of H_2O (47 mm Hg); R = respiratory exchange ratio (.8); FiO_2 = inspired O₂ (21% for room air). Normal value of A-aDO₂ = 30–50 mm Hg (while breathing 100% O₂). Under normal conditions, alveolar or inspired O₂ should be close to arterial O₂.

† Q̇s/Q̇T = the calculation of venous admixture or shunt. Q̇s = flow through the shunt (area of perfusion but no ventilation). Q̇T = total cardiac output to well-ventilated and poorly ventilated (shunt) areas of the lung. An increased Q̇s/Q̇T is due to shunting or ventilation–perfusion inequality (V̇ₐ/V̇Q). With 100% O₂, V̇ₐ/V̇Q is eliminated and the Q̇s/Q̇T represents shunting.

N = normal; Pa_{CO_2} = arterial carbon dioxide partial pressure; Pa_{O_2} = arterial oxygen partial pressure.

normalities of diffusion, especially in children (Table 12–1).

Control of Ventilation

Ventilation is controlled by central chemoreceptors in the medulla, which respond to the intracellular pH (and, therefore, to the partial pressure of carbon dioxide [P_{CO_2}]) (Fig. 12–2). To a lesser extent, ventilation also is controlled by peripheral receptors in the carotid and aortic bodies, which respond predominantly to the partial pressure of oxygen (P_{O_2}). The central receptors are very sensitive; small changes in Pa_{CO_2} normally result in significant changes in minute ventilation. If Pa_{CO_2} is elevated for some time, however, equilibration of the cerebral intracellular space to a higher bicarbonate level may result in relative hypoventilation for the degree of carbon dioxide elevation. The peripheral receptors do not affect ventilation until the arterial oxygen partial pressure (Pa_{O_2}) falls to approximately 50 torr. These receptors may become very important when lung disease results in chronic elevation of Pa_{CO_2}.

The output of the central respiratory center also is modulated by reflex mechanisms. Full lung inflation inhibits inspiratory effort (the Hering-Breuer reflex) through vagal afferent fibers. Other reflexes from the airways and intercostal muscles may influence the depth and frequency of respiratory efforts (Fig. 12–2).

Lung Defense Mechanisms

The airways are a direct connection between the lungs and the atmosphere, which is not typically clean or sterile. Large particles are filtered primarily by the nose. The paranasal sinuses and the nasal turbinates are lined with ciliated epithelium, which carries these filtered particles to the pharynx. Particles smaller than 10 μ in diameter may reach the trachea and bronchi, where they are deposited on the mucosa. Particles smaller than 1 μ may reach the alveoli, where they either remain or are exhaled

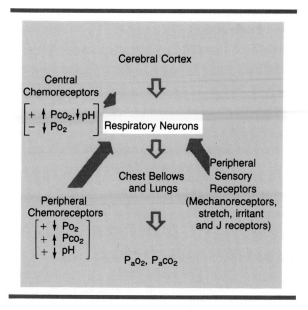

Figure 12–2. Schematic representation of the respiratory control system. The respiratory neurons in the brain stem receive information from the chemoreceptors, peripheral sensory receptors, and cerebral cortex. This information is integrated, and the resulting neural output is transmitted to the chest bellows and lungs. + = Stimulation, − = inhibition. (From Andreoli TE, Carpenter CJ, Plum F, et al [eds]: Cecil Essentials of Medicine. Philadelphia, WB Saunders, 1986, p 171.)

without being deposited. Ciliated cells line the airways from the larynx to the bronchioles; the cilia continuously move a thin layer of mucus toward the mouth, carrying inhaled particulates. Normally, mucociliary transport in the larger airways is fast, with rates averaging 10 mm/min. Alveolar macrophages and polymorphonuclear cells can engulf particles or pathogens opsonized by locally secreted immunoglobulin IgA antibodies or transudated serum antibodies.

Reflex mechanisms also protect the lungs. The most important of these mechanisms is cough, a forceful expiration that removes foreign or infected material from the airways. A cough may be voluntary or generated by reflex irritation of the nose, sinus, pharynx, larynx, trachea, bronchi, and bronchioles. During a cough, one inspires deeply, the glottis closes, the expiratory muscles contract to increase intrathoracic pressure, and the glottis opens suddenly, forcefully releasing air from the system. Loss of the cough reflex leads to aspiration and pneumonia. In young infants, secretions may be swallowed rather than expectorated. Nasal irritation may produce reflex bronchoconstriction to limit the penetration of noxious vapors.

References

Behrman RE (ed): Nelson Textbook of Pediatrics. 14th ed. Philadelphia, WB Saunders, 1992, Sec. 14.2–14.3.

Chernick V, Mellins RB: Developmental physiology of the lung. Chapters 5–11. In Chernick V, Mellins RB (eds): Basic Mechanisms of Pediatric Respiratory Disease. Philadelphia, BC Decker, 1991, pp 55–145.

West JB: Respiratory Physiology. The Essentials. 3rd ed. Baltimore, Williams and Wilkins, 1985.

Wilson AF (ed): Pulmonary Function Testing Indications and Interpretations. Orlando, FL, Grune & Stratton, 1985.

DIAGNOSTIC MEASURES

Evaluating the Patient, Taking the History, and Performing the Physical Examination

The diagnostic evaluation begins with a careful and complete history and physical examination. Much can be learned by seemingly casual observation of the child during the formal history taking with the parents. The physician should question the child, too, because children as young as 3–4 yr of age often know things their parents do not ("last week I choked on a peanut"). The signs or symptoms in children with airway disease often appear quite different during sleep, and, therefore, the physician should inquire specifically about observations of the sleeping child.

To avoid producing anxiety in the child, it often helps to have the mother hold the child in her lap during the physical examination. For the observation of the respiratory pattern, rate, depth, and retractions, the child should be quiet and not crying. Clothing should be removed from the upper half of the body so that the thorax may be clearly inspected. The observations made during auscultation of the chest may be misleading in young children, because they may not take a breath deep enough to produce audible crackles (rales) or rhonchi despite the presence of fluid in the alveoli and small airways. With patience, however, most infants can be observed during at least one deep inspiration, whereas older children may be induced to take a deep breath by asking them to pretend to blow out a candle.

The *respiratory rate* is an important indicator of respiratory status. Any factor that impairs respiratory mechanics is likely to result in more rapid breathing. Because anxiety or excitement will also increase respiratory rates, the sleeping respiratory rate is most reliable. Infants less than 1 yr old have sleeping rates ranging from 25 to 35 breaths/min; while awake, the same infants may take from 40

Table 12–2. Breathing Patterns

Pattern	Features
Normal rate (breaths/min)	*Preterm:* 40–60 *Term:* 30–40 *5 yr:* 25 *10 yr:* 20 *15 yr:* 16 *Adult:* 12
Obstructed Mild	Reduced rate, increased tidal volume
Severe	Increased rate, increased retraction of accessory muscles, anxiety, cyanosis
Restrictive	Rapid rate, decreased tidal volume
Kussmaul respiration	Increased rate, increased tidal volume, regular deep respiration; consider metabolic acidosis or diabetes mellitus
Cheyne-Stokes respiration	Gradually increasing tidal volume followed sequentially by gradually decreasing tidal volume and apnea; consider CNS injury, depressant drugs, heart failure, uremia, or prematurity
Biot respiration	Ataxic or periodic breathing with a respiratory effort followed by apnea; consider brain stem injury or posterior fossa mass
Gasping	Slow rate, variable tidal volume; consider hypoxia, shock, sepsis, or asphyxia

to 80 breaths each min. With increasing maturity sleeping rates gradually decline toward the adult range of 10–15/min (Table 12–2).

In addition to the rate of respiration, its *pattern* or depth and the degree of effort required for its maintenance are important points to note. Hyperpnea (increased depth of respiration) may occur with fever, acidosis, salicylism, pulmonary disease, or extreme anxiety (hyperventilation syndrome, panic attack). Hyperpnea without signs of respiratory distress should suggest a nonpulmonary etiology (acidosis, fever, salicylism). When the degree of effort is increased because of airway obstruction or decreased pulmonary compliance, the intrathoracic pressure may be more negative than usual and intercostal retractions can be observed (Table 12–2). Use of accessory muscles such as the sternocleidomastoids should be apparent on

physical examination and should alert the physician to the presence of pulmonary pathology. In children, increased inspiratory effort also will result in flaring of the alae nasi, which is a relatively reliable sign of dyspnea. **Grunting** (forced expiration against a partially closed glottis) should suggest hypoxia, atelectasis, pneumonia, or pulmonary edema.

The *sounds of breathing* deserve careful documentation. **Stridor**, usually heard on inspiration, is a harsh sound that emanates from the upper airway and is due to a partially obstructed extrathoracic airway. If accompanied by signs of respiratory distress or if present at rest, stridor requires immediate investigation and intervention. Stridor also may be chronic or congenital in nature, in which case it may be of less importance physiologically unless infection further compromises the airway. A

Table 12–3. Physical Signs of Pulmonary Disease

Disease Process	Mediastinal Deviation	Chest Motion	Fremitus
Consolidation	No	Reduced over area	Increased
Bronchospasm	No	Hyperexpansion with limited motion	Normal or decreased
Atelectasis	Shift toward lesion	Reduced over area	Decreased
Pneumothorax	Tension deviates trachea and PMI to opposite side	Reduced over area	None
Pleural effusion	Deviation to opposite side	Reduced over area	None
Interstitial process	No	Reduced	Normal to increased

wheeze is produced by partial obstruction of the lower airway and is heard on exhalation. Wheezes may be harsh and low pitched (usually from large, central airways) or high pitched and almost musical (from small, peripheral airways). Secretions in the intrathoracic airways may result in wheezing, but more commonly they result in irregular sounds called **rhonchi**. Fluid or secretions in the alveolar spaces or terminal airways may produce a sound that is characteristic of crumpling cellophane, variously termed **rales** or **crackles**. This sound may disappear after a few deep inspirations or a cough, but its persistence suggests pneumonitis or pulmonary edema. The quality of breath sounds may be **bronchial**, normally heard over the trachea, with inspiration and expiration clearly auscultated. More peripheral breath sounds are **vesicular**, with a greater proportion of inspiration heard as the expiratory component lessens. Bronchial breath sounds in the lung periphery suggest consolidation or the interface of a pleural effusion.

These physical findings, when combined with inspection for tracheal or cardiac deviation, chest wall motion, percussion, fremitus, voice signs, and the presence or absence of breath sounds, help identify the intrathoracic pathology (Table 12–3). **Digital clubbing** is a sign of chronic pulmonary disease, but it also may be noted in other chronic diseases (cyanotic congenital heart disease, endocarditis, celiac disease, inflammatory bowel disease, chronic active hepatitis, biliary cirrhosis, thalassemia, and Hodgkin disease).

Imaging Techniques

Chest roentgenograms are extremely useful in diagnosing respiratory disease in children, but they must be performed in a technically correct manner and be properly interpreted. Failure to obtain satisfactory inspiration, the most common problem, may lead to the erroneous impression of cardiomegaly or the presence of infiltrates. External skinfolds, rotation or other improper position of the chest, or motion also may produce a distorted or unclear image. Whenever possible, chest roentgenograms should be obtained in both the posteroanterior and the lateral projections. Lesions may be apparent on only one of the two views. Expiratory views or fluoroscopy is helpful in detecting the presence of partial bronchial obstruction; a lung or lobe that does not empty on expiration will appear hyperinflated.

A *barium esophagram* frequently is of great value in diagnosing chest disease in children. Disorders of swallowing or esophageal motility, tracheoesophageal fistulas, or gastroesophageal reflux may lead to aspiration and recurrent or persistent pulmonary disease. When the esophagram reveals that abnormal vascular structures are compressing the esophagus, it may be a major clue that those same vessels are compressing the airways. When searching for an H-type tracheoesophageal fistula, the contrast material should be injected into the esophagus under pressure through a catheter while the injection sites are observed in the lateral projection. Simple barium swallows are much less likely to demonstrate the often small connection between the trachea and esophagus.

Computerized tomography (CT) is very useful in diagnosing chest disease in children, especially in evaluating lesions in the mediastinum or hilum. Rapid, fine-cut CT provides information about the lumenal size or presence of masses within the central intrathoracic airways; bronchiectasis also may

Percussion	Breath Sounds	Adventitious Sounds	Voice Signs
Dull	Bronchial or reduced	Rales	Egophony,* whispering, pectoriloquy increased†
Hyperresonant	Normal to decreased	Wheezes, rales	Normal to decreased
Dull	Reduced	None or rales	None
Resonant	None	None	None
Dull	None	Friction, rub; splash if hemopneumothorax	None
Normal	Normal	Rales	None

* Egophony is present when *e* sounds like *a*.
† Whispering pectoriloquy produces clearer sounding whispered words.
PMI = pneumomediastinal interstitium.
(Adapted from Dantzker D, Tobin M, Whatley R: Respiratory diseases. In Andreoli TE, Carpenter CJ, Plum F, et al (eds): Cecil Essentials of Medicine. Philadelphia, WB Saunders, 1986, pp 126–180.)

be detected. *Magnetic resonance imaging* (MRI) can identify pathology in the trachea and large central airways. MRI also may visualize the relationships between the great vessels and central airways. *Ultrasonography* can determine the nature of some intrathoracic masses and the presence of pleural fluid.

Measures of Respiratory Gas Exchange

A properly performed *arterial blood gas analysis* is one of the most useful measures of lung function, but it is nonspecific in terms of the etiology of dysfunction. Because of the shape of the oxyhemoglobin dissociation curve, oxygen saturation does not fall appreciably until the Pa_{O_2} reaches approximately 60 torr.

The arterial pH and P_{CO_2} also are important measures of respiratory function; P_{CO_2} is regulated almost entirely by ventilation (given a constant CO_2 production). Bicarbonate concentration is regulated chiefly by the kidneys. It is important to distinguish between metabolic and respiratory causes of acidosis or alkalosis. At the normal pH of 7.4, the Pa_{CO_2} should be about 40 torr, and the bicarbonate about 25 mEq/L. This relationship is governed by the Henderson-Hasselbalch equation:

$$pH = 6.1 + \log [(HCO_3)/0.03\ P_{CO_2}]$$

Thus it is the ratio of bicarbonate to P_{CO_2} that governs pH. Metabolic acidosis, which exhibits low bicarbonate, can be compensated by hyperventilation, which lowers the P_{CO_2}, whereas respiratory acidosis, which is due to elevated P_{CO_2}, can be compensated by renal retention of bicarbonate. Respiratory compensation is a much faster process than renal compensation, which generally requires several days to reach equilibrium.

Noninvasive methods of assessing oxygenation and ventilation are available, although the information provided, while useful, has more limited value than arterial blood gas measurement. *Pulse oximetry* (measurement of oxygen saturation using light absorption) provides a painless, relatively easy and reliable means of measuring oxygenation. A small probe consisting of a light source and sensor is clipped to a finger or toe, and either continuous or single oxygen saturation measurements are obtained. *Capnography* (measurement of CO_2 by gas analysis) permits a measure of ventilation. Monitoring the content of CO_2 in expired air (sampled at end-expiration or averaged over the respiratory cycle) provides an approximate measure of alveolar P_{CO_2}. Although most commonly used in intubated and mechanically ventilated patients, capnography

units that monitor CO_2 content in expired air at the nares are now available. Similarly, transcutaneous electrodes may be used to monitor P_{O_2} and P_{CO_2} at the skin surface, but these techniques are best suited for continuous monitoring in an intensive care unit and for detecting trends rather than for providing absolute numbers.

Pulmonary Function Testing

The simplest clinically useful measures of ventilatory function are *vital capacity* and *expiratory flow rates*, which can be measured with a spirometer. Simple spirometry can be performed in most children 6 yr of age or older. Even an older child cannot be expected to perform reproducibly without training and experience with the technique, and great care must be taken in interpreting the results. Predicted values for lung functions are based on the height of the patient. Airway resistance, FRC, and RV (among other measures) require the use of a plethysmograph as well as a spirometer, and thus are even more difficult to obtain in young children. An expiratory flow–volume curve can be very informative; flow rates at lower lung volumes are relatively independent of effort and reflect the function of more peripheral airways.

Pulmonary function studies may be useful in evaluating an older child's functional status, although they rarely yield an etiologic diagnosis. Abnormal results may be described in terms of *obstructive disease* (low flow rates, increased RV or FRC) or *restrictive disease* (low VC and TLC, with relative preservation of flow rates and FRC); in addition, the extent of functional impairment often can be estimated.

Pulmonary function testing also can be used to detect reversible airway obstruction characteristic of asthma. In patients with pulmonary function tests consistent with obstructive disease, a significant increase in pulmonary function after the inhalation of a bronchodilator indicates reactive airway disease. These tests are useful not only for determining diagnosis but also for managing therapy. Inhalational *challenge testing* with methacholine, allergens, or histamine is another useful test for diagnosing reactive airways disease, but such tests are difficult to establish and interpret.

Endoscopic Evaluation of the Airways

Diagnostic *bronchoscopy* is indicated whenever necessary information about the lungs or airways can be most definitively, safely, or rapidly obtained by this method. Airway structure can be examined, the dynamics of the airways during breathing can be documented, and specimens can be obtained for a variety of diagnostic purposes. For patients of any age, no absolute contraindications to bronchoscopy exist, given that the proper equipment is available and the physician's skill is adequate. Flexible instruments are advantageous for most diagnostic purposes, whereas rigid instruments must be used for foreign body extraction and for most operative procedures. Bronchoscopy accompanied by bronchoalveolar lavage assists in diagnosing pulmonary infection in the immunocompromised patient.

Laryngoscopy often is useful in diagnosing stridor and should be performed carefully under appropriate conditions and with the use of sedation and/or anesthesia. The common technique of direct laryngoscopy at the bedside or in the treatment room in an unsedated infant or young child is traumatic to the child, and the results often are misleading. Mirror (indirect) laryngoscopy usually can be performed on children 4–5 yr of age or older, but in infants and younger children direct laryngoscopy, or preferably transnasal laryngoscopy using a flexible bronchoscope or nasopharyngoscope, will yield much better diagnostic information.

Examination of Sputum

Sputum specimens are important in evaluating inflammatory processes in the lower airways, although in young children they often are difficult to obtain. An expectorated specimen may not provide a representative sample of the lower airway secretions, but microscopic examination will help determine the source of a putative sputum specimen. Sputum should contain macrophages; often ciliated cells also are seen. Material containing large numbers of squamous epithelial cells either most likely is not from the lower airways or is heavily contaminated, so that diagnostic tests performed on such a specimen may yield misleading results. Infected sputum should have many polymorphonucleated leukocytes and one predominant organism in large numbers present on Gram stain. If sputum cannot be obtained, obtaining lung washings by bronchoscopy for microbiologic and/or cytologic diagnosis may be useful in selected situations (bronchoalveolar lavage).

Lung Biopsy

When less invasive methods have failed, lung biopsy may be required for the diagnosis of lung disease. Although transbronchial lung biopsy through a bronchoscope is useful in adults, a thoracotomy and open biopsy has major advantages in most pediatric patients: thoracotomy allows the surgeon to inspect and palpate the lung and, thus, initially to choose the best site for performing the biopsy; and open biopsy provides sufficient material for a variety of diagnostic tests. The site of biopsy should be chosen after inspecting the involved lobe on roentgenogram. In most cases, infants and children tolerate open lung biopsy well.

References

Behrman RE (ed): Nelson Textbook of Pediatrics. 14th ed. Philadelphia, WB Saunders, 1992, Sec. 14.6–14.15.

Effman EL: Basic concepts of lung imaging. In Chernik V, Mellins RB (eds): Basic Mechanisms of Pediatric Respiratory Disease. Philadelphia, BC Decker, 1991, pp 383–396.

Fisher MR: Magnetic resonance for evaluation of the thorax. Chest 95:166, 1989.

Paton J, Bautisa D, Stable W, et al: Digital clubbing and pulmonary function abnormalities in children with lung disease. Pediatr Pulmonol 10:25, 1991.

Schapp LM, Cohen NH: Pulse oximetry. Uses and abuses. Chest 98:1244, 1990.

Wood RE: Spelunking in the pediatric airways: Explorations with the flexible fiberoptic bronchoscope. Pediatr Clin North Am 31:785–799, 1984.

THERAPEUTIC MEASURES

Oxygen Administration

Any child in respiratory distress should be given supplemental oxygen as soon as feasible. Although depressing the respiratory drive is possible if the patient's central chemoreceptors are blunted by chronic hypercapnia, patients in such a state are rare in pediatric practice and should be readily recognized as having chronic, severe respiratory disease (e.g., cystic fibrosis, bronchopulmonary dysplasia). Even in these patients, oxygen therapy may be life saving without producing apnea.

In the acute situation, an appropriately sized mask is often the most useful technique for administering oxygen, although some children may become frightened. For a frightened child, a high-flow oxygen source may be held near the child's face until a more satisfactory method can be arranged. For chronic administration of oxygen, a nasal cannula may be helpful, because it frees the face and mouth, allowing the patient to eat and speak unhindered by the oxygen delivery system.

The concentration of oxygen administered should be high enough to relieve hypoxemia yet

442 The Respiratory System

as low as feasible to prevent oxygen toxicity. In general, inspired oxygen concentrations below 40% are safe for long-term use. Determining the concentration of inspired oxygen is more difficult in patients receiving oxygen by nasal cannula; titrating the delivery (in liters/minute) according to measurements of PaO_2 or by pulse oximetry is best. The optimal range of oxygen saturation is 92–94%. It is unnecessary to achieve 100% saturation, especially because this may require potentially toxic levels of inspired oxygen. Oxygen as obtained from tanks or wall sources is dry, and must be humidified to avoid dehydration of the mucosa of the upper respiratory tract.

Aerosol Therapy

Delivering therapeutic agents to the lower respiratory tract often is accomplished by having the patient inhale the agents in aerosol form. Employing aerosol generators that deliver relatively small particles (2–5 μ) is necessary to achieve optimum deposition in the lower airways. The pattern of the patient's breathing will greatly influence deposition of the particles. Slow, deep inspirations are needed for maximal effect, but most children, especially infants, cannot perform in this fashion. Therefore, inhaling aerosols from a face mask or mouthpiece for a period of several minutes during quiet tidal breathing is necessary. Metered dose inhalers produce a high-pressure stream of particles and deposit more of the aerosol on the teeth and oral mucosa than in the lungs. Infants and children should use spacer devices that trap the aerosol particles issuing from the inhaler into a chamber, from which the patient then breathes more slowly.

The drugs most often given by aerosol are bronchodilators. In certain situations, antibiotics may be given by aerosol.

Physical Therapy

When disease processes impair clearance of pulmonary secretions, physical therapy may help maintain airway patency. Percussion of the thorax over the pulmonary segments while the patient is positioned so that the airways of the percussed segments are directed downward may move secretions toward the central airways, from which they can be expectorated. A typical therapy session may require 15–30 min; most children with lung disease requiring chest physiotherapy need one to four such sessions daily. In older children, sustained (for 5–15 min) exercise that produces hyperpnea also can be helpful. Chest physiotherapy is most

beneficial for children with cystic fibrosis but also may be useful for individuals with neuromuscular disease and atelectasis. It generally is not beneficial for pneumonia.

Intubation

When the natural upper airway is obstructed because of disease or when assisted ventilation is needed because of disease or anesthesia, it may be necessary to provide an artificial airway for the patient. Intubation alters the physiology of the respiratory tract in a number of ways, not all of which are beneficial: it interferes with humidification, warming, and filtration of inspired air; with phonation; and with transport of secretions by mucocilia and through cough. Intubation also stimulates increased production of secretions. Depending on the reason for the intubation, the airway resistance may be increased or decreased, and the physiologic dead space may be increased.

Techniques for intubation are beyond the scope of this chapter, but it should be noted that endotracheal tubes can easily damage the larynx and the airways if they are of improper size or are not carefully maintained. Because the cricoid ring is the smallest portion of the airway in children and is completely surrounded by cartilage, it is vulnerable to damage, which results in subglottic stenosis. Pressure of the tube that exceeds capillary filling pressure (roughly 35 cm H_2O) against the airway mucosa produces mucosal ischemia and, within hours, mucosal necrosis. An endotracheal tube should allow a small air leak at the larynx.

Artificial airways of all types must be kept clear of secretions. Mucus plugs in artificial airways can be fatal. Providing adequate humidification of the inspired air and suctioning the tube will help reduce the probability of occlusion by secretions.

Tracheostomy

Tracheostomy is the surgical placement of an artificial airway into the trachea below the larynx. If prolonged intubation is anticipated, elective tracheostomy should be considered to prevent laryngeal trauma and subsequent subglottic stenosis and to increase the patient's comfort and the ease of nursing care. Unfortunately, no clear guidelines are available as to how long a given patient is likely to tolerate an endotracheal tube or when a tracheostomy is necessary. Once laryngeal damage has occurred, the probability of subglottic stenosis is much higher.

Children with *subglottic stenosis* may require a tracheostomy for a prolonged period. Because the tracheostomy tube typically prevents the child from effectively phonating, and thus from communicating distress, special attention must be given to ensure that the child is monitored carefully at all times. As with endotracheal tubes, tracheostomy tubes must be kept clear and clean, and vigilant care must be taken to reduce complications. Occlusion of the tube with secretions or accidental dislodgment of the tube can be fatal. Children with tracheostomies may be successfully cared for at home, if the caretakers are well trained and adequately equipped.

Mechanical Ventilation

Patients who are unable to maintain an adequate gas exchange because of airway obstruction, intrapulmonary pathology, neuromuscular disease, or other factors are candidates for mechanical ventilation. Techniques for mechanical ventilation involve inflation of the lungs with compressed gas. Exhalation is always passive. No method accurately mimics the natural breathing mechanisms, and all methods have their drawbacks and complications.

Positive pressure ventilation requires intubation or tracheostomy. Positive pressure is transmitted to the entire thorax and may impede venous return to the heart during inspiration (venous return increases during spontaneous inspiration). The airways and lung parenchyma may be damaged by high inflation pressures (as well as by high inspired oxygen concentrations). In general, inflation pressures should be limited to those necessary to provide sufficient lung expansion for adequate ventilation and prevention of atelectasis. Newer modes of ventilation include high-frequency jet ventilation and very-high-frequency oscillation; these techniques are used to reduce mean airway pressure and thus the probability of barotrauma (see Chapter 6).

Pressure-cycled ventilators frequently are used in infants and deliver an indefinite volume of gas at a fixed inflation pressure. A major disadvantage of this system is that the pressure is sensed in the ventilator circuit rather than in the lung, and increasing degrees of airway resistance (e.g., occlusion of the endotracheal tube) will result in decreasing delivered volumes. *Volume-cycled ventilators* deliver a fixed volume of gas at whatever inflation pressure is necessary (up to a preset maximum). These instruments are more often used in children and adolescents. In either case, the response of the patient must be assessed carefully and frequently. Regardless of the method chosen for ventilation,

alveolar ventilation (assessed by breath sounds, chest wall excursion, and arterial blood gas measurements) and oxygenation (assessed by arterial blood gas measurements or oximetry) must be adequate.

The normal tidal volume is 5–7 mL/kg body weight; values less than this will usually result in hypoventilation and hypercapnia. Patients with lung disease and uneven distribution of ventilation often require larger tidal volumes; most volume-cycled ventilators are operated at tidal volumes of 10–15 mL/kg body weight. Continuous ventilation at smaller volumes results in redistribution of surfactant and atelectasis. An occasional full lung inflation may be provided by a "sigh" on some ventilators or by inflation with an Ambu bag to prevent atelectasis.

References

Behrman RE (ed): Nelson Textbook of Pediatrics. 14th ed. Philadelphia, WB Saunders, 1992, Sec. 6.33–6.34, 14.3, 14.17.

Lough M: Respiratory treatment and equipment. In Blumer JL (ed): A Practical Guide to Pediatric Intensive Care. St. Louis, Mosby-Year Book, 1990, pp 926–996.

MAJOR PEDIATRIC PULMONARY SYMPTOM COMPLEXES

Upper Airway Obstruction

This condition is defined as obstruction of the portion of the airways located above the thoracic inlet, and it is manifested during inspiration because the pressure within the upper airway is negative relative to the atmosphere. This negative pressure tends to collapse the upper airway, producing the characteristic sounds associated with upper airway obstruction. Upper airway obstruction ranges from nasal obstruction associated with the common cold to life-threatening obstruction of the larynx or upper trachea. Nasal obstruction is usually more of a nuisance than a danger, because the mouth can be used as an airway. However, nasal obstruction may be a serious problem for neonates, who breathe predominantly through the nose. The etiologies of airway obstruction vary with the age of the child (Table 12–4), and diagnosis requires a careful history and physical examination.

The *clinical manifestation* most commonly associated with upper airway obstruction is inspiratory **stridor**, a harsh sound produced usually at or near the larynx by the vibration of upper airway structures. Less commonly, stridor also may be an expi-

Table 12–4. Age-Related Differential Diagnosis of Airway Obstruction

Newborn
Foreign material (meconium, amniotic fluid)
Congenital subglottic stenosis (uncommon)
Choanal atresia
Micrognathia (Pierre Robin syndrome, Teacher Collins syndrome, DiGeorge syndrome)
Macroglossia (Beckwith-Wiedemann syndrome, hypothyroidism, Pompe disease, trisomy 21, hemangioma)
Laryngeal web, clefts, atresia
Laryngospasm (intubation, aspiration, transient)
Vocal cord paralysis (weak cry; unilateral or bilateral, with or without increased intracranial pressure from Arnold-Chiari malformation or other CNS pathology)
Tracheal web, stenosis, malacia, atresia
Pharyngeal collapse (cause of apnea in preterm infant)

Infancy
Laryngomalacia (most common etiology)
Subglottic stenosis (congenital, acquired after intubation)
Hemangioma
Tongue tumor (dermoid, teratoma, ectopic thyroid)
Laryngeal papillomatosis
Vascular rings

Toddlers
Viral croup (most common etiology in children 3 mo–4 yr of age)
Bacterial tracheitis (toxic, high fever)
Foreign body (sudden cough; airway or esophageal)
Spasmodic (recurrent) croup
Laryngeal papillomatosis
Retropharyngeal abscess
Diphtheria (uncommon)

Over 2–3 Yr Old
Epiglottitis (epiglottis, aryepiglottic folds)
Inhalation injury (burns, toxic gas, hydrocarbons)
Foreign bodies
Angioedema (familial history, cutaneous angioedema)
Anaphylaxis (allergic history, wheezing, hypotension)
Trauma (tracheal or larynx fracture)
Peritonsillar abscess (adolescents)
Ludwig angina
Diphtheria

CNS = central nervous system.

Table 12–5. Differentiating Supraglottic from Subglottic Causes of Airway Obstruction

	Supraglottic	Subglottic
Example	Epiglottitis, peritonsillar and retropharyngeal abscess	Croup, angioedema, foreign body, tracheitis
Stridor	Quiet	Loud
Voice	Muffled	Hoarse
Dysphagia	Yes	No
Sitting-up or arching posture	Yes	No
Barking cough	No	Yes
Fever	High (40°C [104°F])	Low grade (38–39°C [100.4–102.2°F])
Toxic	Yes	No, unless tracheitis is present
Trismus	Yes	No
Drooling	Yes	No
Facial edema	No	No, unless angioedema is present

(Adapted from Davis H, et al: Acute upper airway obstruction: Croup and epiglottis. Pediatr Clin North Am 28:859, 1981.)

ratory noise. Hoarseness suggests involvement of the vocal cords, whereas stridor that changes with position of the child's head or neck suggests a supraglottic etiology. Children with laryngomalacia or pharyngeal hypotonia may exhibit much less stridor while crying because their muscle tone increases. In contrast, an obstructing lesion below the glottis usually will produce more stridor during crying because the inspiratory flow rates increase. In many children, stridor will decrease during sleep because inspiratory flow rates are lowest at that time. Positional stridor suggests an anatomic problem.

A child with upper airway obstruction usually will have some degree of suprasternal retraction as a result of the pressure gradient between the trachea and the atmosphere. Obstruction below the thoracic inlet seldom will result in suprasternal retraction because the major pressure drop will occur below the sternal notch.

Radiographic evaluation of the child with stridor should include views of the lateral neck and nasopharynx and an anteroposterior (AP) view of the neck taken with the head in extension. The subglottic space on the AP view should be symmetric, and the lateral walls of the airway should fall away steeply. Asymmetry suggests subglottic stenosis or a mass lesion, whereas narrow tapering suggests subglottic edema. An important differential diagnosis is that between supraglottic and subglottic obstruction (Table 12–5).

Lower Airway Obstruction

In contrast to upper airway obstruction, obstruction of the airways below the thoracic inlet produces more expiratory symptoms than inspiratory symptoms. During inspiration, intrathoracic pressure becomes negative relative to the atmosphere. Therefore, the airways tend to increase their diameter during inspiration, and unless substantial, relatively fixed, obstruction (or increased airway secretion) is present, few or no abnormal noises may be generated during inspiration. Intrathoracic pressure is increased relative to atmospheric pressure during exhalation, thus tending to collapse the intrathoracic airways and produce wheezing. A **wheeze** is a relatively continuous expiratory sound, generally with a more musical quality than stridor, that is produced by turbulent airflow. Partial airway obstruction may produce wheezing only during the later phase of exhalation.

There are many *etiologies* of wheezing (Table 12–6), the most common of which is diffuse bronchial obstruction resulting from constriction of bronchial smooth muscle, airway inflammation, or excessive secretions. However, the importance of the aphorism "All that wheezes is not asthma" cannot be overemphasized. Although it often is useful to administer a bronchodilator to determine whether the wheezing is acutely reversible, mere reversibility does not establish a diagnosis of asthma, nor does it eliminate anatomic causes of wheezing. Conversely, the most common cause of wheezing in childhood is reactive airway disease. Wheezing that begins in the first weeks or months of life or that is persistent despite maximal bronchodilator therapy is more likely to be due to some other cause, and more extensive diagnostic evaluation may be warranted. Because of their small airways, children less than 2–3 yr old are more likely to wheeze in response to viral infections. Wheezing that is localized to one area of the chest deserves especially close diagnostic attention (e.g., foreign body, compressing lymph node).

Although a child known to have reactive airway disease certainly does not need *roentgenographic evaluation* on each episode of wheezing, other children with significant respiratory distress, fever, history of aspiration, localizing signs, or persistent wheezing should have chest films included as part of their diagnostic evaluation. Both posterioanterior and lateral views should be obtained. Generalized hyperinflation, with flattening of the diaphragm and an increased AP diameter of the chest, suggests diffuse obstruction of small airways. Localized hyperinflation, especially on expiratory films, suggests localized bronchial obstruction, such as with a foreign body or anatomic anomalies.

Table 12–6. Causes of Wheezing in Childhood

Acute
Reactive Airway Disease
 Asthma
 Exercise-induced asthma
 Hypersensitivity reactions

Bronchial Edema
 Infection
 Inhalation of irritant gases or particulates
 Increased pulmonary venous pressure

Bronchial Hypersecretion
 Infection
 Inhalation of irritant gases or particulates
 Cholinergic drugs

Aspiration
 Foreign body
 Aspiration of gastric contents

Chronic or Recurrent
Reactive Airway Disease (see above)

Hypersensitivity Reactions, Allergic Aspergillosis

Dynamic Airway Collapse
 Bronchomalacia
 Tracheomalacia
 Vocal cord adduction

Airway Compression by Mass or Blood Vessel
 Vascular ring
 Anomalous innominate artery
 Pulmonary artery dilation (absent pulmonary valve)
 Bronchial or pulmonary cysts
 Lymph nodes or tumors

Aspiration
 Foreign body
 Gastroesophageal reflux
 Tracheoesophageal fistula

Bronchial Hypersecretion or Failure to Clear Secretions
 Bronchitis, bronchiectasis
 Cystic fibrosis
 Immotile cilia syndrome

Intrinsic Airway Lesions
 Endobronchial tumors
 Endobronchial granulation tissue
 Bronchial or tracheal stenosis
 Bronchiolitis obliterans
 Sequelae of bronchopulmonary dysplasia

Congestive Heart Failure

Cough

This is one of the most common (and sometimes most vexing) respiratory symptoms at all ages. Cough results from stimulation of irritant receptors in the airway mucosa or in other locations, including the ear. It may have many different characteristics, depending on anatomic factors and the cause of the irritation, and significant diagnostic information usually may be derived from the history and physical examination. Most cases of *acute cough* are associated with respiratory infections (pneumonia, tracheobronchitis, bronchitis, sinusitis, pertussis), and the cough subsides with resolution of the infection. A history of the sudden onset of choking and coughing is often described after aspiration of a foreign body. Other causes include pulmonary edema, thermal or chemical inhalation injury (smoke), and pulmonary embolism or hemorrhage. *Chronic cough* (daily cough for greater than 6 wk), however, has a more diverse etiology, including allergy (asthma, hypersensitivity pneumonitis), anatomic abnormalities (tracheoesophageal fistula, cysts, gastroesophageal reflux), chronic infection (cystic fibrosis, sinusitis, recurrent aspiration pneumonia, abscess, tuberculosis, fungal pneumonia, histoplasmosis, acquired immunodeficiency syndrome [AIDS]-related infection), environmental exposure to irritants (smoking, drug abuse), foreign body aspiration, psychogenic (habit), and neurologic dysfunction.

Children in the first several years of life often have frequent viral respiratory infections, especially if they are exposed to many other children, as in day care centers. Cough that resolves promptly and clearly is associated with a viral infection does not require further diagnostic evaluation. However, cough that persists and is not associated with classic viral upper respiratory tract infection symptoms may require investigation.

The circumstances under which *chronic cough* occurs are important to consider in diagnosis. Nocturnal cough suggests allergy (especially to antigens in the child's bedroom) or drainage from sinuses. Cough associated with exercise suggests reactive airway disease or bronchitis/bronchiectasis. Cough on first arising in the morning frequently is associated with excessive production of tracheobronchial secretions, such as occurs in asthma, bronchitis, bronchiectasis, or cystic fibrosis. Paroxysmal cough should suggest pertussis syndrome, foreign body aspiration, or cystic fibrosis. Chlamydial infections characteristically produce a repetitive, staccato cough. Children with a harsh, brassy cough often have an anatomic problem such as subglottic edema (croup), tracheomalacia, or tracheal compression but also may have habit cough. Habit cough disappears with sleep. Cough that arouses a child from sleep is usually the result of a pathologic process. Tumors, mediastinal or parabronchial lymphadenopathy, and pul-

monary vasculitis are uncommon causes of chronic cough.

The *diagnostic evaluation* of the child with chronic cough should include a chest roentgenogram and, if possible, an examination of sputum. In children too young to expectorate, a specimen often may be obtained with a throat swab placed deep into the posterior pharynx during coughing. Children with allergies most often will produce clear mucoid sputum, although microscopic examination should be performed (see Diagnostic Measures, earlier in this chapter). Some children with allergies may produce apparently purulent sputum that contains numerous eosinophils. Purulent sputum (containing many white blood cells) suggests infection and should be cultured. A variety of rapid diagnostic tests (immunofluorescence, enzyme-linked immunosorbent assay utilizing nasal washings or serum) are available to help reach a diagnosis of certain pulmonary infections.

References

Arnold J: Airway obstruction. In Blumer JL (ed): A Practical Guide to Pediatric Intensive Care. St. Louis, Mosby-Year Book, 1990, pp 91–94.

Behrman RE (ed): Nelson Textbook of Pediatrics. 14th ed. Philadelphia, WB Saunders, 1992, Sec. 14.2, 14.19–14.22, 14.76.

Fernald GW, Denny FW, Fairclough DL, et al: Chronic lung disease in children referred to a teaching hospital. Pediatr Pulmonol 2:27, 1986.

Irwin R, Curley F, French C: Chronic cough—the spectrum and frequency of causes, key components of the diagnostic evaluation and outcome of specific therapy. Am Rev Respir Dis 141:640, 1990.

Morgan WJ, Taussig LM: The chronic bronchitis complex in children. Pediatr Clin North Am 31:851, 1984.

STRUCTURAL AND DYNAMIC ABNORMALITIES

Many disorders of the pediatric respiratory system involve abnormalities either of structure or of the dynamic functions of otherwise normal structures.

The Upper Airway

The major abnormalities of the upper airway involve obstructive lesions. The most common is **adenoidal tonsillar hypertrophy**. The adenoids consist of lymphoid tissue arising from the posterior and superior wall of the nasopharynx in the region of the choanae. Lymphoid hyperplasia may result from recurrent infection, allergy, or nonspecific stimuli and may cause partial or total obstruction of the nasopharynx. The signs of adenoidal hypertrophy include persistent mouth breathing, snoring, and in some patients, obstructive sleep apnea. The eustachian tube enters the nasopharynx at the choanae and may be obstructed by enlarged adenoids, thus promoting recurrent or persistent otitis media. The diagnosis of adenoidal hypertrophy is confirmed by a lateral roentgenogram of the nasopharynx or by nasopharyngoscopy; treatment is by surgical excision. Because the adenoids are not a discrete organ but consist merely of lymphoid tissue, regrowth following adenoidectomy is not uncommon. Tonsils also may enlarge to the point of producing airway obstruction. Obstruction sufficient to produce sleep apnea, retractions, or cor pulmonale may require tonsillectomy.

Choanal stenosis or **atresia** may be bilateral or unilateral and is a relatively rare cause of respiratory distress in the newborn. The neonate is generally an obligate nose breather; thus, nasal obstruction may be fatal. Crying relieves the obstruction, which is worse during quiet activity. Failure to pass a small catheter through the nostrils easily should raise the suspicion of choanal atresia. An oral airway may be life saving. The diagnosis is confirmed by CT or roentgenographically by instilling a small amount of contrast material or by inspecting the area directly with a nasopharyngoscope or bronchoscope.

Stridor beginning at birth or shortly thereafter should raise the suspicion of the presence of **laryngomalacia** (see Table 12–4). This relatively common condition involves the collapse of the epiglottis and/or arytenoid cartilages during inspiration and usually is benign and self-limiting. In some infants the epiglottis alone is involved; these patients tend to become asymptomatic during the 1st yr of life. Other infants have very large arytenoid cartilages that prolapse into the glottis during inspiration; in these patients, stridor tends to last longer, sometimes for several years. Establishing a definitive diagnosis in suspected laryngomalacia is important both for its appropriate management and to exclude other, more serious lesions. The differential diagnosis should include vocal cord paralysis, laryngeal cysts or other mass lesions (especially when the stridor begins several weeks after birth), congenital subglottic stenosis, tracheomalacia, and compression of the upper trachea by an anomalous innominate artery (see Table 12–4). The child with laryngomalacia will have *inspiratory stridor* but should have no evidence of significant expiratory obstruction. The stridor typically is loudest when the child is feeding or quietly relaxing, or in a supine or neck flexion position, and usually will diminish during sleep or when the child is crying (when increased muscle tone may hold the supraglottic structures out of the air stream). Viral infections may exacerbate laryngomalacia. No treatment is needed unless the infant has hypoxia resulting from the airway obstruction; tracheostomy then may be required. Symptoms usually disappear by 18–24 mo of age.

Subglottic stenosis is a common problem that may be congenital or iatrogenic. Aggressive management of premature infants with intubation and mechanical ventilation may produce residual damage to the larynx. Infants with Down syndrome appear to have a smaller larynx than normal and are more susceptible to subglottic stenosis. Subglottic obstruction will produce stridor, and evidence of obstruction will be present on expiration as well as on inspiration. With increasing degrees of respiratory effort, the stridor will worsen (in contrast to laryngomalacia, in which the stridor may lessen with increasing respiratory efforts). Viral infection may exacerbate subglottic stenosis. Definitive diagnosis requires endoscopic evaluation. Treatment may necessitate tracheostomy; however, milder congenital cases improve with age as the larynx grows.

A number of *mass lesions* affect the larynx, but the most common laryngeal tumor in childhood is the **hemangioma** that usually is found in the subglottic space. Infants with stridor should be examined head to toe for cutaneous hemangiomas because the presence of such lesions greatly increases the likelihood that the stridor is due to a subglottic hemangioma and mandates endoscopic evaluation. Most patients who have subglottic hemangioma come to the physician's attention prior to 6 mo of age. Subglottic lesions produce asymmetric narrowing of the subglottic space and may be detected on AP roentgenograms of the larynx. The airway obstruction, which usually worsens with crying, may eventually produce pulmonary hypertension and cor pulmonale. Treatment is controversial, but in many patients, tracheostomy will be required. Laser therapy, interferon, and steroids have been used with moderate success. As with cutaneous hemangiomas, spontaneous regression is the rule, but this may require many months to several years. **Juvenile laryngeal papillomatosis**, benign tumors caused by human papillomavirus acquired at birth from maternal genital warts, occurs in infants less than 2 yr of age. Treatment includes laser therapy and interferon.

The Lower Airway

The most common anomaly of tracheal structure and dynamics, although a less common cause of upper airway obstruction, is **tracheomalacia**. The tracheal cartilage rings normally extend through an arc of approximately 300 degrees, thus maintaining rigidity of the trachea during changes in intrathoracic pressure. In tracheomalacia, the cartilage rings do not extend nearly so far around the circumference, and thus a larger portion of the tracheal wall is membranous. Therefore, the lumen of the intrathoracic portion of the trachea tends to collapse during expiration. This collapse may be apparent in most patients only during forced exhalation or with cough, but coarse, persistent wheezing may be a prominent symptom in other patients. The voice is normal, as is inspiratory effort. Tracheomalacia localized to the cervical trachea may result in inspiratory obstruction. Tracheomalacia almost invariably is present in children who have had esophageal atresia and a tracheoesophageal fistula. Tracheomalacia must be differentiated from extrinsic compressing lesions. In some patients, localized tracheomalacia may result after the trachea has been relieved of compression by a mass lesion or by an abnormal blood vessel. Viral infections may exacerbate the airway obstruction of tracheomalacia. Treatment usually is not necessary, but some patients may require long-term tracheostomy and ventilatory support.

Tracheoesophageal fistula is another relatively common anomaly of the trachea, occurring in 1:3000–4500 live births (see Chapter 11).

Compression of the trachea by abnormal vessels may produce persistent wheezing and/or stridor. The most common of these lesions is anterior compression resulting from an **anomalous innominate artery**, which arises more distally along the arch of the aorta than it normally does. Surgical treatment generally is required only for the most severe cases. A more serious lesion involves complete encirclement of the trachea at and just above the carina by a vascular ring. This anomaly may be caused by a double aortic arch or by a right aortic arch with a persisting ligamentum arteriosum. In addition to respiratory symptoms, emesis on dysphagia may be present as a result of esophageal compression. Definitive diagnosis often can be made by barium swallow, although vascular dye contrast study or magnetic resonance angiography may be required prior to surgical repair. Less common causes of extrinsic tracheal compression include mediastinal masses and cystic hygromas.

Endobronchial mass lesions are relatively uncommon in children, but when they occur, they most commonly consist of granulation tissue and they result from localized inflammatory lesions. Partial obstruction of an airway by either an intrinsic or an extrinsic mass may result in wheezing and/or obstructive emphysema if there is more obstruction during exhalation than during inspiration. If the airways become totally obstructed, atelectasis results. Chest roentgenograms, CT scans, bronchoscopy, or vascular contrast studies may be required for diagnosis. Primary tumors of the lungs and airways are rare in children and include nonsecreting carcinoid tumor and congenital bronchial cysts. Metastatic tumors, such as osteogenic sarcoma, may spread to the endobronchial airways from other areas of the body.

Bronchial stenosis may be congenital or acquired and may result in localized wheezing, air trapping, atelectasis, or infection. Acquired stenosis is usually the result of a chronic inflammatory process or localized trauma. Diagnosis usually requires bronchoscopy or bronchography.

Emphysema, a condition that results when alveolar septa are disrupted or destroyed, is relatively uncommon in children, but generalized or localized overinflation is common and is due to airway obstruction from a variety of causes. Although the term "emphysema" often is used somewhat inaccurately to refer to overinflation or to leakage of air into the interstitial tissues of the lung or into the subcutaneous tissue, this use of the term has become accepted. *Congenital lobar emphysema* consists of overinflation of one lobe, most often the left upper lobe, which may produce respiratory distress because the surrounding lung tissue has become compressed, shifting the mediastinum. Lobectomy may be required if respiratory distress is severe and progressive. True emphysema develops in the absence of antiproteases (alpha-1-antitrypsin deficiency) but rarely appears before the 3rd decade of life.

Chest Wall and Pleura

Scoliosis, when severe, may result in respiratory dysfunction (Chapter 19). Marked curvature of the thoracic spine is associated with chest wall deformity and limitation of chest wall movement, which decreases lung volumes (restrictive lung disease). In advanced scoliosis, bronchial obstruction may develop when the bronchi become kinked or compressed by the great vessels that shift to abnormal positions in relation to the airways. Significant loss of inspiratory capacity often leads to pulmonary hypertension, recurrent infection, atelectasis, and respiratory insufficiency.

Pneumothorax is the accumulation of air in the pleural space that may result from external trauma or from leakage of air from the lungs or airways. It may occur spontaneously in teenagers and young adults. Predisposing conditions include mechanical ventilation, asthma, cystic fibrosis, disorders of collagen (Marfan syndrome), and exertion with a Valsalva maneuver. The symptoms of pneumothorax include pain, dyspnea, and cyanosis; if the air leak communicates with the mediastinum, subcutaneous emphysema may become apparent. Physical findings may include decreased breath sounds, a tympanitic percussion note, signs of mediastinal shift, and subcutaneous crepitance (Table 12–3). Few or no physical signs of pneumothorax may be present if the amount of air collection is small, but symptoms may progress rapidly if the air in the pleural space is under pressure ("tension pneumothorax"), with death resulting if the tension is not relieved. The *diagnosis* is confirmed by chest roentgenogram. In infants, transillumination of the chest wall may help in the rapid diagnosis of pneumothorax.

Treatment depends on the amount of air collected and the nature of the underlying disease. Small pneumothoraces often do not need treatment and resolve spontaneously. Larger pneumothoraces (and certainly tension pneumothoraces) require immediate drainage of the air. In an emergency situation, a simple needle aspiration may suffice, but placement of a chest tube may be required for resolution. Sclerosing the pleural surfaces to obliterate the pleural space may benefit patients with recurrent pneumothoraces.

Pneumomediastinum results from the dissection of air from a leak in the pulmonary parenchyma into the mediastinum. The most common cause in children is acute asthma. Symptoms include pain and dyspnea. Physical findings may be absent or may include a crunching noise over the sternum on auscultation. Frequently, subcutaneous emphysema is present in the neck. The diagnosis is confirmed by roentgenogram. Treatment is directed toward the underlying lung disease.

Pleural effusion commonly accompanies inflammatory processes in the lungs and may be heralded by pain, dyspnea, and signs of respiratory insufficiency resulting from compression of the underlying lung (Chapter 10). Physical findings include dullness to percussion, decreased breath sounds, mediastinal shift, and decreased tactile fremitus (Table 12–3). The diagnosis is confirmed roentgenographically; decubitus views may be helpful to distinguish fluid collections from other densities in the thorax.

Fluid accumulates in the pleural space whenever the local hydrostatic forces pushing fluid out of the vascular space exceed osmotic forces pulling fluid back into the vascular space. The underlying causes of pleural effusion include congestive heart failure, hypoproteinemia, obstruction of lymphatic drainage, malignancy, collagen vascular disease, and inflammation or infection of the pleura. Infection may produce a reactive parapneumonic effusion or a more serious purulent **empyema**. The latter often is due to *Streptococcus pneumoniae*, *Haemophilus influenzae*, or streptococci (rarely *Mycobacterium tuberculosis*), whereas anaerobic bacteria produce empyema associated with aspiration pneumonia and dental, lung, or subdiaphragmatic abscesses. **Diagnostic thoracentesis** may be necessary to establish the cause of the effusion and to exclude infection. Most patients with effusions should undergo diagnostic thoracentesis unless the underlying causes for the effusion are clearly evident (e.g., systemic lupus erythematosus [SLE]), the patient does not have significant respiratory distress, and infection is not suspected. In the absence of inflammation, the fluid should have a low specific gravity (<1.015) and protein content (<2.5 g/dL), low lactic dehydrogenase activity (<200 IU/L), and a low cell count with few polymorphonuclear cells. In contrast, exudative pleural effusions resulting from inflammation have high specific gravity, high protein (>3.0 g/dL) and lactic dehydrogenase (>250) content, low pH (<7.0) and glucose (<40 mg/dL), and a high cell count with many polymorphonuclear leukocytes.

Treatment of pleural effusion is directed at the underlying condition that caused the effusion and at relief of the mechanical consequences of the fluid collection. Small effusions, especially if they are transudative, usually require no therapy. Large effusions may require drainage with a chest tube, especially if the fluid is purulent (empyema). In this latter case, the fluid often will be very thick and may be loculated, making simple drainage difficult. All patients with empyema require tube drainage.

If the underlying condition is treated successfully, the prognosis for patients with pleural effusions, including empyema, is excellent.

References

Behrman RE (ed): Nelson Textbook of Pediatrics. 14th ed. Philadelphia, WB Saunders, 1992, Sec. 14.19–14.49, 14.90–14.103.

Freij BJ, Kusjiesz H, Nelson J, et al: Parapneumonic effusions and emphysema in hospitalized children: A retrospective review of 227 cases. Pediatr Infect Dis 3:578, 1984.

Jay SJ: Diagnostic procedures for pleural disease. Clin Chest Med 6:33, 1985.

Landing BH: State of the art: Congenital malformations and genetic disorders of the respiratory tract. Am Rev Respir Dis 120:151, 1979.

Montgomery WW: Chronic subglottic stenosis. Otolaryngol Clin North Am 17:107, 1984.

Pagtakhan RD, Chernick V: Liquid and air in the pleural space. In Chernick V, Kendig EL (eds): Disorders of the Respiratory Tract in Children. 5th ed. Philadelphia, WB Saunders, 1990, pp 545–556.

Richardson MA, Cotton RT: Anatomic abnormalities of the pediatric airway. Pediatr Clin North Am 31:821, 1984.

GENETIC DISORDERS

Cystic Fibrosis

Cystic fibrosis (CF), a complex autosomal recessive disorder, is the most common lethal genetic disease affecting Caucasians (1:2500 live births). The gene for cystic fibrosis has been localized to the long arm of chromosome 7 and has been characterized as a large gene (over 250 kb of genomic DNA) that encodes a polypeptide of 1480 amino acids, termed *cystic fibrosis transmembrane regulator* (CFTR). The most common mutation, which occurs in approximately 70% of the CF chromosomes, is a specific deletion of three base pairs resulting in a deletion of phenylalanine at position ΔF 508. However, over 100 other different mutations also have been reported to result in the CF phenotype. Heterozygote detection and prenatal diagnosis of individuals with ΔF 508 deletion is readily accomplished.

Etiology.   The major organs involved in CF are epithelial; the secretory and absorptive characteristics of these tissues are affected. The CFTR protein appears to be involved in Cl^- conductance, consistent with the observation that 99% of patients with CF have elevated levels of sweat Cl^-. Although the CFTR currently is believed to be a chloride channel, it is possible that CFTR is a transporter molecule or indirectly modulates Cl^- channels. How the abnormal Cl^- conductance accounts for the clinical manifestations of CF is as yet uncertain.

Clinical Manifestations.   The respiratory epithelium of patients with CF exhibits marked impermeability to chloride and an excessive reabsorption of sodium. These alterations in the bioelectric properties of the epithelium lead to a relative dehydration of the airway secretions, resulting in impaired mucociliary transport and airway obstruction. *Chronic bronchial infection* then develops. Most patients are colonized with *H. influenzae, Staphylococcus aureus,* and/or *Pseudomonas aeruginosa* (which predominates in older patients with advanced disease). Chronic bronchial infection leads to cough, which is the most common initial pulmonary manifestation; sputum production; hyperinflation; bronchiectasis; and, eventually, pulmonary insufficiency and death. Digital clubbing is nearly universal in patients with significant lung disease.

Most patients with CF (90%) develop exocrine *pancreatic insufficiency* early in life (if not at birth) as a result of inspissation of mucus in the pancreatic ducts and consequent autodigestion of the pancreas. The original name for the disease, "cystic fibrosis of the pancreas," reflects this pancreatic involvement. Maldigestion with secondary malabsorption results in steatorrhea (large, fatty, floating, foul-smelling stools), azotorrhea, and a number of secondary deficiency states (vitamins K, D, A, and E) in the untreated patient. Nutrient malabsorption also results in failure to thrive despite a ravenous appetite. Approximately 10% of patients are born with intestinal obstruction resulting from inspissated meconium ("meconium ileus"). In older patients intestinal obstruction may occur because of maldigestion and thick mucus in the intestinal lumen ("meconium ileus equivalent"). Such events may occur after dietary indiscretions or with inadequate pancreatic enzyme replacement. In adolescent or adult patients, relative insulin deficiency may develop, and *hyperglycemia* may become symptomatic, although ketoacidosis is rare.

As in the respiratory and gastrointestinal tracts, inspissation of mucus in the *reproductive tract* leads to dysfunction. Female fertility is low and the cervical mucus is abnormal, but a number of patients have given birth to children. Secondary amenorrhea often is present as a result of chronic illness and markedly reduced body weight. Males almost universally are azoospermic, with atrophy or absence of the vas deferens.

The failure of the *sweat ducts* to conserve salt may lead to heat exhaustion or to unexplained hypochloremic alkalosis in infants but has relatively little clinical consequence otherwise.

CF is a chronic, insidiously progressive disease exhibiting multiple *complications* related to viscous mucus, malabsorption, and infection (Table 12–7).

Diagnosis.   The diagnosis of CF should be seriously considered in any patient with chronic or recurring respiratory or gastrointestinal symptoms.

Table 12–7. Complications of Cystic Fibrosis

Pulmonary Complications
Bronchiectasis, bronchitis, bronchiolitis, pneumonia
Atelectasis
Hemoptysis
Pneumothorax
Nasal polyps
Sinusitis
Reactive airway disease
Cor pulmonale
Respiratory failure
Mucoid impaction of the bronchi
Allergic bronchopulmonary aspergillosis

Gastrointestinal Complications
Meconium ileus
Meconium peritonitis
Meconium ileus equivalent (non-neonatal obstruction)
Rectal prolapse
Intussusception
Volvulus
Appendicitis
Intestinal atresia
Pancreatitis
Biliary cirrhosis (portal hypertension: esophageal varices, hypersplenism)
Neonatal obstructive jaundice
Hepatic steatosis
Gastroesophageal reflux
Cholelithiasis
Inguinal hernia
Growth failure
Vitamin deficiency states (vitamins A, K, E, D)
Insulin deficiency, symptomatic hyperglycemia

Other Complications
Infertility
Edema–hypoproteinemia
Dehydration–heat exhaustion
Hypertrophic osteoarthropathy–arthritis
Delayed puberty
Amyloidosis

Indications for sweat testing are shown in Table 12–8. To establish the diagnosis, the sweat chloride concentration must exceed 60 mEq/L on two separate sweat tests with adequate sweat volume (at least 50 mg of sweat, and preferably more than 100 mg, must be collected for accurate analysis). In addition to a positive sweat test, the patient must have (1) chronic obstructive lung disease, (2) exocrine pancreatic insufficiency, or (3) a confirmed family history of classic CF in a sibling or first cousin. Although highly specific for CF, the sweat test is subject to numerous technical problems and is reliable only in laboratories that perform the test frequently and with scrupulous quality control. False-positive and false-negative sweat test results

occur in a few well-defined clinical states (Table 12–9). A few patients may have typical, but mild symptoms and borderline or even normal sweat Cl^- levels. Other supportive tests, such as measurement of bioelectrical potential differences across respiratory epithelium, low levels of stool trypsin, or detection of the ΔF 508 genotype (or other known mutation) by DNA analysis may be useful. Prenatal detection of a known CF genotype may be accomplished by amniotic fluid or chorionic villus sampling.

Treatment. The complex management of CF is best coordinated by a tertiary referral center. As in the treatment of any chronic disease, the patient–physician relationship is of utmost importance. Physicians, patients, families, and other caretakers must work together to maintain an optimistic, aggressive approach to life and to treatment. Efforts to prevent the occurrence of compli-

Table 12–8. Indications for Sweat Testing

Pulmonary Indications
Chronic or recurrent cough
Chronic or recurrent pneumonia
Recurrent bronchiolitis
Atelectasis
Hemoptysis
Staphylococcal pneumonia
Pseudomonas aeruginosa in the respiratory tract (in the absence of such circumstances as tracheostomy or prolonged intubation)
Mucoid *P. aeruginosa* in the respiratory tract
Right upper lobe pneumonia

Gastrointestinal Indications
Meconium ileus
Neonatal intestinal obstruction (meconium plug, atresia)
Steatorrhea, malabsorption
Hepatic cirrhosis in childhood (including any manifestations such as esophageal varices or portal hypertension)
Pancreatitis
Rectal prolapse
Vitamin K deficiency states (hypoprothrombinemia)

Miscellaneous Indications
Digital clubbing
Failure to thrive
Family history of cystic fibrosis (sibling or cousin)
Salty taste when kissed; salt crystals on skin after evaporation of sweat
Heat prostration, especially under seemingly inappropriate circumstances
Hyponatremic hypochloremic alkalosis in infants
Nasal polyps
Pansinusitis
Aspermia

Table 12–9. Causes of False-Positive and -Negative Sweat Tests

False Positive	False Negative
Adult age	Edema
Adrenal insufficiency	Poor technique
Ectodermal dysplasia	Atypical cystic fibrosis
Nephrogenic diabetes insipidus	(uncommon)
Hypothyroidism	
Fucosidosis	
Mucopolysaccharidosis	
Malnutrition	
Poor technique	
Type I glycogen storage disease	
Panhypopituitarism	

cations and the progression of lung disease are vital, and immunization to influenza virus and other diseases should be kept up to date. Unfortunately, no universally accepted protocol for treatment exists, and many measures are controversial.

The *electrolyte loss* resulting from the sweat defect is treated by adding more salt to the patient's diet.

Lung disease is treated by combining physical measures to help remove mucus from the airways (chest physiotherapy, exercise), pharmacologic measures to clear mucus and improve airway patency (bronchodilators and other aerosols), and antibiotic therapy to control chronic infection. Monitoring pulmonary bacterial flora and providing aggressive therapy with appropriate antibiotics in full therapeutic doses (oral, aerosolized, and/or parenteral) help to slow the progression of the lung disease. Patients are hospitalized for high-dose intravenous antibiotic therapy whenever necessary, especially when they are infected with organisms resistant to oral agents (e.g., *Pseudomonas*). Under normal circumstances, therapy should last for at least 2 wk; even when using the most aggressive therapy, it is difficult to sterilize the lungs. Infection with *Pseudomonas cepacia* is particularly difficult to treat and may be associated with an accelerated clinical deterioration. **Allergic bronchopulmonary aspergillosis** also may complicate CF and require treatment with steroids. Pulmonary complications, such as pneumothorax, hemoptysis (check vitamin K status) or atelectasis, are treated as they are in other patients.

Pancreatic insufficiency is treated by replacing pancreatic enzymes, preferably in enteric-coated form, and by encouraging higher caloric intake than normal. Even with the best enzyme replacement, stool losses of fat and protein may be relatively high. Fat is not withheld from the diet, even when signifi-

cant steatorrhea exists. Instead, enzyme doses are increased to normalize the stools as much as possible. Fat-soluble vitamins are given in twice-normal doses, preferably in water-miscible form. Meconium ileus often requires surgical intervention but may respond to enemas of hyperosmolar roentgenographic contrast material. Intestinal obstruction in older patients is treated similarly or with oral laxatives.

Therapies under investigation are directed toward thinning mucus with inhaled DNAse, antiinflammatory medications (antiproteases, nonsteroidal anti-inflammatory agents), lung transplantation, and ultimately gene therapy.

Prognosis. Pulmonary disease is the major cause of morbidity in CF and is influenced by the inherent severity of disease and by therapy. Patients with meconium ileus have the same prognosis as others with CF if they survive the 1st yr of life. Current data from the Patient Registry of the Cystic Fibrosis Foundation indicate that the median survival age for patients with CF is approximately 27 yr, but patients vary greatly in the severity of their disease.

Immotile (Dysmotile) Cilia Syndrome

This syndrome is an inherited disorder in which ultrastructural abnormalities in the cilia result in absent or disordered movement. The most classic form of the syndrome, *Kartagener syndrome*, is an autosomal recessive disorder characterized by situs inversus, pansinusitis, and bronchiectasis. Otitis media also is common, and male infertility is universal (as a result of immotile sperm). The cilia lack dynein arms, an ultrastructural feature that represents an ATPase necessary for ciliary motility. Many other variants of the syndrome exist that have a variety of ultrastructural abnormalities of the cilia. In some patients, cilia may move but their beat is abnormal, usually uncoordinated, and ineffective.

Because respiratory tract cilia fail to beat normally, secretions accumulate in the airways and bacterial infection occurs. Chronic infection leads to bronchiectasis by early adulthood. The diagnosis should be suspected in individuals with early-onset chronic bronchitis or bronchiectasis; in patients with chronic, recurrent, or persistent pneumonia; and especially in patients with pansinusitis and/or chronic otitis media. Cystic fibrosis should be excluded by sweat testing. The *diagnosis* is confirmed by electron microscopy of respiratory cilia; the cilia may be obtained from nasal scrapings. Because chronic infection and inflammation may result in ultrastructural abnormalities in nasal cilia, care must be taken in confirming the diagnosis.

Treatment is similar to the pulmonary therapy in cystic fibrosis and is directed toward improving clearance of respiratory secretions and controlling infection. Chest physiotherapy, immunoprophylaxis of viral infections (e.g., influenza), and prompt treatment of bacterial infection are helpful, but the course of the disease tends to be slowly progressive, with most patients expiring in the 4th–5th decades.

Alpha-1-Antitrypsin Deficiency

Alpha-1-antitrypsin deficiency is an inherited absence (relative or absolute) of antiprotease activity. In the respiratory tract, the proteases (especially elastase) released by the normal turnover of phagocytic cells therefore are not inhibited, and, over a period of time (usually 2 or more decades), emphysema develops. In some forms of the disorder, liver disease appears early in life, but in most children with alpha-1-antitrypsin deficiency little evidence for lung disease exists in the 1st decade.

In children or adolescents, dyspnea is the first manifestation. Chest roentgenograms may reveal hyperinflation; often the disease may be confused with late-onset asthma. Progressive emphysema or pulmonary cyst formation may be associated with previous pulmonary infection or with exposure to cigarette smoke.

The *diagnosis* is confirmed by demonstrating reduced total alpha-1-antitrypsin levels and a ZZ phenotype. Recombinant alpha-1-antitrypsin is now available and has some efficacy in *treatment* and *prevention* of the lung disease.

References

Behrman RE (ed): Nelson Textbook of Pediatrics. 14th ed. Philadelphia, WB Saunders, 1992, Sec. 14.89, 14.53, 14.77.

Hubbard RC, Brantly ML, Sellers SE, et al: Anti-neutrophil-elastase defenses of the lower respiratory tract in α-1-antitrypsin deficiency directly augmented with an aerosol of α-1-antitrypsin. Ann Intern Med 111:206, 1989.

Tizzano EF, Buchwald M: Cystic fibrosis: Beyond the gene to therapy. J Pediatr 120:337, 1992.

INFECTIOUS DISORDERS

The Upper Airway

OTITIS MEDIA

See Chapter 10.

SINUSITIS

See Chapter 10.

CROUP

The most common syndrome of infectious upper airway obstruction is croup, or acute infectious laryngotracheobronchitis (see also Chapter 10). Croup is predominantly of viral etiology; parainfluenza types 1 and 2 viruses are the most common agents.

Clinical Manifestations. The typical episode begins in a child between 6 mo and 3 yr of age having symptoms of an upper respiratory infection (the common cold) and lasts less than 5 days. A brassy cough (typically characterized as sounding like the barking of a seal), inspiratory stridor, and respiratory distress may develop slowly or acutely. Signs of upper airway obstruction, such as labored breathing and marked suprasternal, intercostal, and subcostal retractions, are evident on examination. Associated lower airway disease accompanied by wheezing and a productive cough may be present. Although the majority of such children are not seriously ill, the airway obstruction may become severe, necessitating placement of an artifical airway. The subglottic space is the major site of obstruction, which is caused by edema resulting from the viral inflammation (see Table 12–5). Roentgenogram reveals the "steeple" sign of a narrowed subglottic space.

Treatment. Administering aerosolized racemic epinephrine may reduce the edema temporarily, producing marked clinical improvement, but the edema and obstruction soon return and the disease runs its course over several days. Epinephrine aerosol treatment may need to be repeated as often as every 20 min in severe cases. During inspiration, the walls of the subglottic space are drawn together, aggravating the obstruction (and probably also the edema), so that children should be kept as calm as possible to reduce their respiratory efforts. The best calming method for a child with croup is to sit in the mother's lap. Sedatives should be used very cautiously. Cool mist administered by tent or face mask may help to prevent drying of the secretions around the larynx.

Children with severe croup requiring hospitalization should be monitored carefully. When symptoms subside, it may indicate that the patient either is improving or is becoming fatigued and is in respiratory failure. Because aerosolized epinephrine has a short duration of action, most authorities believe that children requiring such therapy should be hospitalized for observation, even if their obstructive signs clear completely with the first aerosol treatment. Systemically administered corticosteroids is beneficial in treating croup but generally is reserved for seriously ill patients. If the patient is very young (less than 4 mo of age) or if symptoms continue for more than 1 wk, the patient should undergo careful laryngoscopy because there is an increased probability that another lesion exists (subglottic stenosis or hemangioma). Sudden worsening (fever, respiratory distress, leukocytosis) suggests a complicating bacterial tracheitis.

Some children have acute episodes of croup-like symptoms without having evidence of a viral infection. These episodes may be severe but usually are of short duration. This acute *"spasmodic croup"* is not well understood but may involve allergic mechanisms in some patients. It tends to recur and to respond to relatively simple therapies, such as exposure to cool or moist air.

EPIGLOTTITIS

Acute epiglottitis, another syndrome of upper airway obstruction, typically occurs in older children (2–7 yr old). The causative agent is predominantly bacterial (*H. influenzae* type b).

Clinical Manifestations. Epiglottitis is characterized by sudden onset, high fever, respiratory distress, fulminant progression, severe dysphagia, and a muffled voice (Table 12–5). Patients usually find it easier to breathe sitting erect, and they drool because of the dysphagia. Acute epiglottitis is a true pediatric emergency because the inflamed airway suddenly may become totally obstructed, leading to death. Examination of the pharynx should be discouraged.

Diagnosis. In typical cases, epiglottitis should be suspected on observing the patient's clinical presentation. The *differential diagnosis* includes severe croup, bacterial tracheitis, foreign body aspiration, Ludwig angina, and retropharyngeal and peritonsillar abscess. Confirmation of the diagnosis is based on direct observation of the inflamed and swollen supraglottic structures and cherry-red enlarged epiglottis, but this procedure should be performed only in the operating room with a competent surgeon and anesthesiologist prepared to place a nasotracheal tube or to perform a tracheostomy. *H. influenzae* may be recovered from the surface of the epiglottis or from blood culture. Epiglottitis may be distinguished from severe croup on the basis of a lateral neck film if there is doubt as to the clinical diagnosis ("thumb sign" of swollen epiglottis). A physician should accompany the patient to the radiology department and be prepared to perform an emergency intubation (which will be much more difficult than under normal circumstances) or tracheostomy.

Treatment. Nasotracheal intubation is currently the preferred method of treatment, but the intubated patient requires constant supervision and restraint to decrease the probability of accidental extubation. Tracheostomy is an acceptable alternative. Antibiotics (ceftriaxone) suitable for *H. influenzae* should be given at once. With effective therapy, clinical recovery is rapid, and most patients can be safely extubated within 48–72 hr. The severity of airway obstruction is directly correlated with the rapidity of onset; almost no deaths occur in patients presenting for medical attention more than 24 hr after onset of symptoms. *Prevention* is possible with the *H. influenzae* vaccine.

The Lower Airway

BRONCHIOLITIS

Bronchiolitis is an acute respiratory illness of young children resulting from inflammation of small airways and characterized by wheezing. Respiratory syncytial virus (RSV) is the principal agent, although other viruses, such as parainfluenza, adenovirus, influenza, rhinovirus, and, infrequently, *M. pneumoniae*, have been associated with the illness.

Epidemiology. Bronchiolitis is a common illness of young children; approximately 15% of children experience this illness during the first 2 yr of life. Children generally acquire the infection when exposed to family members who typically have symptoms of an upper respiratory tract infection or from infected children in a day care setting. The majority of cases occur during the winter and early spring, when the associated viral agents are most prevalent in the community.

Clinical Manifestations. Affected infants usually develop rhinorrhea, sneezing, cough, and low-grade fever, followed in several days by the onset of rapid breathing and wheezing. The child may feed poorly. *Physical examination* is notable for signs of acute respiratory distress, including nasal flaring, tachypnea, intermittent cyanosis, retractions, a prolonged expiratory phase, and wheezes and crackles in the chest. The white blood cell count usually is normal. Chest roentgenograms typically reveal air trapping and may show peribronchial thickening, atelectasis, and infiltrates. The principal physiologic abnormality is hypoxemia secondary to mismatching of ventilation and perfusion. It is unusual for hypercapnia to develop, but it can occur in the severely affected infant who becomes fatigued.

Pathology. The major pathologic findings are necrosis of small airway epithelium, peribronchiolar inflammation, airway edema, and plugging of small airways with mucus and debris. Patchy areas of atelectasis are common, and interstitial pneumonitis may occur.

Diagnosis. The diagnosis of bronchiolitis is based on clinical findings and on knowledge of the epidemiology of viral illnesses prevalent in the community. RSV may be identified on nasopharyngeal secretions by culture or antigen assay. Many other diagnoses should be considered in the young child who presents with an acute *wheezing-associated respiratory illness*. Asthma typically has a recurrent pattern and is responsive to bronchodilators. Pneumonia usually is associated with an infiltrate demonstrated on a chest roentgenogram and, if bacterial infection is present, with a high white blood cell count. In congestive heart failure, an enlarged heart usually is seen on the chest roentgenogram, and either related structural cardiac abnormalities or viral myocarditis may be present. Children with foreign body aspiration often have a history of having aspirated an object and may exhibit localized wheezing or air trapping. Wheezing associated with gastroesophageal reflux is likely to be chronic or recurrent, and the patient may have a history of frequent emesis. Cystic fibrosis may be associated with poor growth, chronic diarrhea, or a family history of the disease.

Treatment. The management of the child with bronchiolitis depends on the severity of the illness. Most children have mild symptoms and can be managed with supportive measures at home. Approximately 5% of children with bronchiolitis will require hospitalization. *Indications for hospitalization* include young age (<6 mo), moderate to marked respiratory distress (sleeping respiratory rates of 50–60 or higher), hypoxemia (Po_2 <60 mm Hg or oxygen saturation <92% on room air), the occurrence of apnea, inability to tolerate oral feeding, and lack of appropriate care available at home. Children with chronic lung disease, such as bronchopulmonary dysplasia, congenital heart disease (particularly with associated pulmonary hypertension), neuromuscular weakness, and immunodeficiency, are at increased risk of having severe, potentially fatal disease. Consideration should be given to the hospitalization of all of these high-risk children.

Supportive measures appropriate to the care of the child with bronchiolitis include administering adequate oral or (in the hospitalized child) parenteral fluids to ensure maintenance of normal hydration in the presence of increased insensible water losses associated with tachypnea. Fever, if high or associated with increased respiratory distress, may be treated with antipyretic agents. Supplemental humidified oxygen should be provided for the hospitalized child in a sufficient concentration to maintain a Pao_2 of 70–90 mm Hg (oxygen saturation ≥93%). The use of *bronchodilators*, such as aerosolized beta-2-agonists or theophylline, may be beneficial in selected patients and should be tried in severely affected children.

Administering *ribavirin aerosol*, a specific antiviral agent, to children with RSV infection has been demonstrated to be moderately efficacious in clinical trials. This should be considered in severely affected infants and in those at high risk of developing severe, protracted disease (e.g., chronic lung disease, congenital heart disease). Antibacterial therapy is not indicated unless evidence suggests the existence of a concomitant bacterial infection. *Intubation and mechanical ventilation* are required to treat respiratory failure or severe apnea.

Prognosis. Complications of bronchiolitis include apnea, respiratory failure, atelectasis, secondary bacterial infection, and pneumothorax or pneumomediastinum (in the child requiring mechanical ventilation). However, the immediate prognosis of most children with bronchiolitis is excellent, with symptoms resolving in 7–10 days. Several studies suggest that some children who experience an episode of bronchiolitis, particularly if they needed to be hospitalized, may be prone to experience further episodes of wheezing, may manifest allergic symptoms, have lower average levels of lung function, and have a modestly higher prevalence of increased airway reactivity later in life. Factors other than the occurrence of bronchiolitis, such as underlying increased bronchial reactivity or exposure to environmental pollutants like cigarette smoke, may contribute to the apparent sequelae of bronchiolitis.

BRONCHIOLITIS OBLITERANS

This condition is an uncommon form of chronic bronchiolitis in which there is endobronchiolar granulation tissue and peribronchiolar fibrosis. Most reported cases in children (particularly neonates and young infants) have been related to the occurrence of severe viral infection, most commonly adenovirus. Association with influenza, pertussis, measles, and *M. pneumoniae* has been reported. In adults, bronchiolitis obliterans also has been associated with toxic inhalational exposures, connective tissue disorders, and drug administration (such as penicillamine). The characteristic *pathologic lesion* is the partial or complete obliteration of small airways by granulation tissue and surrounding fibrosis. An interstitial pneumonia may be present. These abnormalities may be diffuse or localized.

Clinical Manifestations.   Much like acute bronchiolitis, the typical illness begins with fever, cough, tachypnea, and wheezing. Notable physical findings include retractions, wheezes, and rales. Chest roentgenograms typically show a nonspecific diffuse infiltrate exhibiting areas of atelectasis, but the roentgenograms may reveal a more miliary pattern. The course of the illness differs from that of acute, uncomplicated bronchiolitis in that the symptoms progress, often after a brief period of improvement, and are accompanied by an increasing shortness of breath, the development of productive cough, hypoxia, and persistent wheezing. Clinically, there is fixed airway obstruction that is poorly responsive to bronchodilators. Increased symptoms can occur as acute exacerbations or more insidiously over a prolonged period. Bronchography reveals obstruction of small airways; arteriography reveals a reduction of the pulmonary bed.

Complications include progressive respiratory failure, atelectasis, secondary bacterial infection, and the development of the unilateral hyperlucent lung syndrome in those in whom the pathology appears to be confined to one lung. Some patients die early in the course of the disease, whereas others experience a more chronic course.

Diagnosis.   Bronchiolitis obliterans should be considered in the child who has significant recurrent or persistent respiratory symptoms and evidence of fixed airway obstruction following a severe viral lung infection. Typical bronchographic findings support the diagnosis; confirmation requires lung biopsy. Other diagnoses to consider in a child with recurrent/persistent cough and wheezing with an infiltrate or atelectasis on chest roentgenogram include cystic fibrosis, asthma, gastroesophageal reflux, and foreign body aspiration.

Treatment.   No specific therapy is available, although corticosteroids often are used in an attempt to mitigate the progressive fibrosis. Appropriate supportive measures include supplemental oxygen, chest physiotherapy, a trial of bronchodilator therapy, and early, aggressive treatment of further lung infections.

PNEUMONIA

Pneumonia refers to the inflammation of pulmonary tissue and is associated with consolidation of the alveolar spaces. Pneumonitis is a general term for lung inflammation that may or may not be associated with consolidation. *Lobar pneumonia* describes pneumonia localized to one or more lobes of the lung in which the affected lobe or lobes are completely consolidated. *Bronchopneumonia* refers to inflammation of the lung that is centered in the bronchioles, resulting in the production of a mucopurulent exudate that obstructs some of these small airways and causes patchy consolidation of the adjacent lobules. Bronchopneumonia is usually a generalized process involving multiple lobes of the lung. The distinction between bronchopneumonia and bronchiolitis can be somewhat arbitrary. *Interstitial pneumonitis* refers to inflammation of the interstitium, which is composed of the walls of the alveoli, the alveolar sacs and ducts, and the bronchioles. Interstitial pneumonitis may be seen acutely with viral infections, but also may be a chronic process.

Anatomic respiratory system malformations, altered systemic or local immunity, and exposure to cigarette smoke predisposes the patient to infectious pneumonia. The cause of pneumonia depends on the age, immune status, presence of CF or other chronic lung disease, exposure history, and nosocomial versus community acquisition.

Etiology.   Pneumonia may be caused by a variety of infectious agents (bacterial, viral, fungal, rickettsial, and parasitic organisms), and inflammatory processes (SLE, sarcoidosis, histiocytosis), as well as by toxic substances (hydrocarbons, smoke, molds, dusts, chemicals, gases, gastric contents) that are inhaled and/or aspirated. The most common cause of pneumonia in children is viral infections; bacterial infections account for only 10–30% of all pediatric pneumonias. Certain infectious pneumonias are more common at a particular age (Table 12–10).

Table 12–10. Common Causes of Pneumonia at Different Ages*

Age	Bacterial	Viral	Others
Neonate	Group B streptococci, coliform bacteria	CMV, herpes virus	*Mycoplasma hominis, Ureaplasma urealyticum*
4–16 wk old	*S. aureus, H. influenzae, S. pneumoniae*	CMV, RSV, influenza virus, parainfluenza virus	*Chlamydia trachomatis, U. urealyticum*
Up to 5 yr old	*S. pneumoniae, S. aureus, H. influenzae*	RSV, adenovirus, influenza virus	
Over 5 yr old	*S. pneumoniae, H. influenzae*	Influenza virus	*Mycoplasma pneumoniae, Chlamydia pneumoniae, Legionella pneumophila*

* An increasingly important consideration is *Mycobacterium tuberculosis.*
CMV = cytomegalovirus; RSV = respiratory syncytial virus.

Micro-organisms gain access to the lung by hematogenous dissemination or local spread descending through the respiratory bronchial tree. Although aspiration pneumonia may be seen following seizures in patients with altered mental status, neuromuscular disease, and gastroesophageal reflux, most cases of pediatric pneumonia are not due to these causes. *H. influenzae* type b pneumonia often is associated with bacteremia, meningitis, and other sites of infection (arthritis, pleural effusion, cellulitis). *S. aureus* is a rare cause of pneumonia in infants; when present, the child is acutely ill with empyema, pneumatoceles, and respiratory failure. Staphylococcal skin infection may precede bacteremia and pneumonia. RSV, influenza viruses, and parainfluenza virus are common causes of viral pneumonia. Viral respiratory infections often precede bacterial pneumonias. Infants between 1 and 3 mo of age often have an *afebrile* pneumonia, which typically is due to congenitally or environmentally acquired agents such as *Ureaplasma urealyticum, Chlamydia trachomatis* (preceding by conjunctivitis), cytomegalovirus (CMV), *Pneumocystis carinii,* or RSV. Pneumonia in immunocompromised patients may be due to *P. carinii,* gramnegative enteric bacteria, fungi (aspergillosis, histoplasmosis), mycobacteria (*M. tuberculosis, M. avium*), or CMV, whereas disease in patients with CF usually is due to *S. aureus* (in infancy), *P. aeruginosa,* or *P. cepacia* (in older patients).

Children with immune system dysfunction, malnutrition, or defects in the normal defense mechanisms of the lung are very susceptible to pulmonary infections. The causative agents often are unusual, opportunistic organisms, including gramnegative enteric bacteria, anaerobes, CMV, measles, varicella, *P. carinii,* or fungi.

Clinical Manifestations. The typical clinical patterns of viral and bacterial pneumonias usually differ, although the distinction is not always clear for a given patient. Tachypnea, cough, malaise, pleuritic chest pain, and retractions are common to both. Viral pneumonias more often are associated with cough, wheezing, or stridor; fever is less prominent than in bacterial pneumonia. The chest roentgenogram in viral pneumonia shows diffuse, streaky infiltrates of bronchopneumonia, and the white blood count often is not elevated (lymphocytes are the predominant cell type). Bacterial pneumonias typically are associated with cough, high fever, chills, dyspnea, and auscultatory findings of lung consolidation (decreased or tubular breath sounds, dullness to percussion, and egophony in a localized region) (Table 12–3). The chest roentgenogram in bacterial pneumonia often shows lobar consolidation and pleural effusion (10–30%), and the white blood cell count is elevated (>15,000–20,000/mm), with a predominance of neutrophils. Many cases of pneumonia have characteristics that fall between these two typical patterns of viral and bacterial pneumonia. Lower lobe pneumonia may present with abdominal pain.

Diagnosis. Definitive diagnosis of pneumonia requires identification of the causative organism. Sputum (for culture) is not easily obtained from children. Certain viral agents (RSV, influenza, parainfluenza, adenovirus) may be identified by culture or by immunofluorescent staining of infected epithelial cells washed from the nasopharynx. CMV and enterovirus can be cultured from the nasopharynx, urine, or bronchoalveolar lavage fluid. *M. pneumoniae* may be suspected if cold agglutinins are present in peripheral blood samples and confirmed by detecting presence of *Mycoplasma*-specific immunoglobulin (Ig) G or IgM in serum. Bacterial agents may be cultured or identified by antigen detection (*Pneumococcus, H. influenzae*) from blood or from an associated pleural effusion. *M. tuberculosis* may be diagnosed by tuberculin skin tests and analysis of sputum or gastric aspirates.

Invasive procedures, such as bronchoscopy and bronchoalveolar lavage, lung aspiration, or lung biopsy, may be necessary to obtain culture specimens. These invasive procedures are not used in typical pneumonias, but they may be employed in special instances, such as pneumonia in the immunocompromised host or when the clinical picture is unusual.

Treatment. The management of pneumonia depends on the age of the patient and the clinical presentation (whether more consistent with viral or with bacterial pneumonia). Neonatal or congenital pneumonia is life threatening; therefore, infants less than 2 mo of age with pneumonia should be hospitalized and treated with intravenous antibiotics. If bacterial pneumonia is suspected at birth, antibiotics effective against group B streptococcus and coliform bacteria should be used (see Appendix 1). After the 1st wk of life, antibiotic coverage for *S. aureus* should be included if the roentgenogram demonstrates effusions or pneumatoceles. In older children, drugs effective against *H. influenzae* and *S. pneumoniae* should be used. Appropriate antibiotic choices in older children include amoxicillin, ceftriaxone, erythromycin–sulfadiazine, or trimethoprim–sulfamethoxazole for 10 days. Pneumonia in children 5–10 yr of age frequently is caused by *M. pneumoniae* or *S. pneumoniae* and may be treated with erythromycin. Outbreaks of penicillin-resistant *Pneumococcus* have occurred recently. These organisms often are resistant to multiple antibiotics and require therapy with ceftriaxone or vancomycin. A small percentage of children with pneumonia require hospitalization. Most children beyond early infancy may be managed as outpatients. Indications for hospitalization include (1) moderate to severe respiratory distress, (2) failure to respond to oral antibiotics, (3) inability to take oral antibiotics at home because of vomiting or poor compliance, (4) lobar consolidation in more than one lobe, (5) immunosuppression, (6) empyema, (7) abscess or pneumatocele, and (8) underlying cardiopulmonary disease (e.g., bronchopulmonary dysplasia or pulmonary hypertension).

Prognosis. Most children recover from pneumonia rapidly and completely, and the roentgenographic findings should return to normal within 6–8 wk. In a few children, pneumonia may persist longer than 1 mo or may be *recurrent*. In such cases, the possibility of underlying disease must be inves-

Table 12–11. Differential Diagnosis of Recurrent Pneumonia

Hereditary Disorders
Cystic fibrosis
Sickle cell disease

Disorders of Immunity
AIDS
Bruton agammaglobulinemia
Selective IgG subclass deficiencies
Common variable immunodeficiency syndrome
Severe combined immunodeficiency syndrome

Disorders of Leukocytes
Chronic granulomatous disease
Hyperimmunoglobulin E syndrome (Job syndrome)
Leukocyte adhesion defect

Disorders of Cilia
Immotile cilia syndrome
Kartagener syndrome

Anatomic Disorders
Sequestration
Lobar emphysema
Esophageal reflux
Foreign body
Tracheoesophageal fistula (H type)
Gastroesophageal reflux
Bronchiectasis

tigated further (Table 12–11). Evaluation then may include the tuberculin skin test, sweat chloride determination, serum immunoglobulin determinations, bronchoscopy, and barium swallow.

BRONCHIECTASIS

Bronchiectasis, or the dilation of bronchi, may be either *congenital* or *acquired* but most often results from long-standing localized bronchial infection.

Etiology. Cystic fibrosis, immotile cilia syndrome, foreign body aspiration, immunodeficiency states, and certain postinfectious conditions (adenovirus, pertussis, measles, tuberculosis) are the most common causes of bronchiectasis. Chronic sinusitis, allergic bronchopulmonary aspergillosis, and, rarely, asthma are other etiologic factors. Chronic infection and inflammation result in destruction of the bronchial wall, with dilation, loss of mucociliary transport, and chronic mucus hypersecretion with obstruction. In its early stages, bronchiectasis may be reversible, if the underlying problem can be corrected and the infection controlled.

Clinical Manifestations. The presentation of bronchiectasis may be subtle, but often includes productive cough, fever, hemoptysis, digital clubbing, and persistent moist rales over the affected area. Bronchiectasis results in the development of a rich bronchial blood supply to the affected area; thus, **hemoptysis** is a frequent *complication*. Atelectasis is common and is due to obstruction of the affected bronchus. Wheezing is infrequent.

Diagnosis. Chest roentgenograms may show dilated airways that usually are manifested as parallel densities ("tram tracks"), and CT scans may show dilated airways appearing as ring shadows. Although bronchography was used to characterize bronchiectasis, it has been replaced by rapid, fine-cut CT. Fusiform dilation ("cylindrical bronchiectasis") may be reversible when the disease is managed aggressively, but saccular dilation usually is irreversible.

Treatment. Therapy for bronchiectasis includes antibiotics and chest physiotherapy. Underlying conditions should be treated, if possible. When there is evidence of localized, irreversible bronchiectasis, pulmonary resection should be considered, because a focus of infection may spread to other uninvolved areas of the lung. Additional indications for surgery include hemorrhage and resectable disease accompanied by failure to thrive that does not respond to medical therapy.

LUNG ABSCESS

Lung abscess is an uncommon but serious problem in children and usually is due to aspiration of foreign material into the lung or to infection behind an obstructed bronchus. Occasionally, an abscess will develop from hematogenous spread of infection. The most commonly involved sites are the posterior segments of the upper lobes and the superior segments of the lower lobes (into which material will drain when the child is recumbent). A lung abscess results when there is localized infection that destroys lung tissue, leaving a cavity containing pus and debris. Anaerobic bacteria most often are isolated from abscess cavities, but other organisms also may cause abscesses, including *S. aureus*, *Klebsiella pneumoniae*, fungi, and mycobacteria. The clinical manifestations initially include fever and other systemic symptoms, but cough usually develops later in the course of the disease. Symptoms may be like those of typical pneumonia (from which abscesses sometimes evolve). Chest roentgenograms reveal a cavitary lesion, often with an air–fluid level, surrounded by parenchymal inflammation. If the cavity communicates with the bronchi, organisms may be isolated from sputum.

Diagnostic bronchoscopy may be indicated to rule out a foreign body and to obtain microbiologic specimens (especially if the patient does not produce sputum). In almost all cases the lesion will regress when appropriate antimicrobial therapy is administered. Antibiotics should be chosen to cover the most likely organisms (penicillin or clindamycin will cover the majority of anaerobic flora) and should be continued for several weeks until all signs of infection have cleared. In most patients, clinical and roentgenographic resolution is complete within several months. Occasionally, a patient with previously undiagnosed diaphragmatic hernia is suspected of having a lung abscess because air–fluid levels are present on a chest film. If the patient's symptoms do not correspond to the roentgenographic picture, an upper gastrointestinal series may help diagnose the condition.

PULMONARY TUBERCULOSIS

See Chapter 10.

PERTUSSIS

See Chapter 10.

References

Asher MI, Beaudry PH: Lung abscess. In Chernick V, Kendig EL (eds): Disorders of the Respiratory Tract in Children. Philadelphia, WB Saunders, 1990, pp 429–435.

Behrman RE (ed): Nelson Textbook of Pediatrics. 14th ed. Philadelphia, WB Saunders, 1992, Sec. 14.43–14.52, 14.54–14.69, 14.81–14.83.

Cohen GJ: Management of infections of the lower respiratory tract in children. Pediatr Infect Dis 6:317, 1987.

Denny FW, Murphy TF, Clyde WA, Jr, et al: Croup: An 11-year study in a pediatric practice. Pediatrics 71:871, 1983.

Epler GR, Colby TV, McLoud TC, et al: Bronchiolitis obliterans organizing pneumonia. N Engl J Med 312:152, 1985.

Lewiston NJ: Bronchiectasis in childhood. Pediatr Clin North Am 31:864, 1984.

Mauro R, Poole S, Lockhart C: Differentiation of epiglottitis from laryngotracheitis in the child with stridor. Am J Dis Child 142:679, 1988.

Nohynek H, Eskola J, Laine E, et al: The causes of hospital-treated acute lower respiratory tract infection in children. Am J Dis Child 145:618, 1991.

Super DM, Cartelli NA, Brooks LJ, et al: A prospective randomized double-blind study to evaluate the effect of dexamethasone in acute laryngotracheitis. J Pediatr 115: 323, 1989.

HYPERSENSITIVITY DISEASES

Asthma
See Chapter 8.

Hypersensitivity Pneumonitis

Nonasthmatic allergic pulmonary disease, also known as *extrinsic allergic alveolitis*, is due to inhalation of a variety of organic antigens found in dust and may occur as an acute syndrome or as a chronic, progressive disease. The most common antigens are from fungal organisms (such as thermophilic actinomycetes) and avian danders. They often are associated with occupational or agricultural exposure and include thermophilic bacteria found in moldy hay, grain, mushrooms, sugar cane, home or automobile air conditioners, heated humidifiers, *Bacillus subtilis* and ameba found in water, and animal proteins derived from feathers, serum, or excrement.

Clinical Manifestations.   *Acute symptoms*, which usually begin within 4–8 hr after exposure, include dyspnea, coughing, malaise, fever, and chills. Physical examination reveals tachypnea and diffuse rales without wheezing. There is often marked leukocytosis and elevation of serum immunoglobulins other than IgE. The immune mechanism is similar to a type III or Arthus-like immune response because antigen–antibody complexes are present and the polymorphonuclear leukocytes become activated (see Chapter 8). Chest roentgenograms reveal a diffuse interstitial infiltrate without hyperinflation.

The *chronic form* of the disease is characterized by persistent and progressive respiratory symptoms (dyspnea, exercise intolerance) without the fever and chills of the acute form. Anorexia and weight loss may be prominent. Fine basilar crackles are heard on physical examination, and the roentgenogram reveals diffuse interstitial fibrosis. Type III and type IV immune responses may be activated in chronic allergic alveolitis.

Pulmonary function testing reveals decreased vital capacity, which may be reversible in the acute form but becomes irreversible in the chronic form. Pao_2 is decreased as a result of reduced diffusion of oxygen; $Paco_2$ usually is decreased because of hyperventilation. Precipitating IgG antibodies to the inciting antigen usually are found in the serum but also may be seen in asymptomatic patients.

Diagnosis.   Diagnosis depends on a high index of suspicion and careful history and epidemiologic investigation. Often, symptoms subside after hospitalization, only to recur on the patient's return home. Serologic tests for precipitins and cultures of airborne fungi may be helpful; inhalational challenge testing may be necessary for some patients. If a humidifier or air conditioning unit is the source of disease, Legionnaire disease may need to be excluded from the diagnosis.

Treatment.   Therapy consists of administering steroids and helping the patient avoid exposure to the inciting agent. Proper cleaning of water sources is important. In severe cases, drastic measures to avoid environmental exposure may be necessary. The prognosis usually is good if the patient can prevent further exposure.

Allergic Bronchopulmonary Aspergillosis
See Chapter 8.

References

Behrman RE (ed): Nelson Textbook of Pediatrics. 14th ed. Philadelphia, WB Saunders, 1992, Sec. 14.65–14.68.
Bierman CW, Pierson WE, Massie FS: Nonasthmatic allergic pulmonary disease. In Chernick V, Kendig EL (eds): Disorders of the Respiratory Tract in Children. 5th ed. Philadelphia, WB Saunders, 1990, pp 601–613.

NEUROLOGIC DISORDERS AFFECTING RESPIRATORY FUNCTION

Apnea

Apnea is defined as the cessation of breathing as a result of the lack of respiratory effort (*central apnea*) or total airway obstruction (*obstructive apnea*). In many patients, apneic episodes may have both central and obstructive components (*mixed apnea*). Brief respiratory pauses usually lasting up to 10 sec, during which no respiratory effort can be detected, are common in normal infants and children, especially after a sigh. Pauses lasting longer than 15 sec, however, are considered abnormal. Normally, when a child whose airway is occluded tries to breathe, respiratory centers in the brain recruit a progressively greater amount of motor output from the respiratory center until the obstruction is overcome, but if this output fails to overcome the obstruction, an arousal impulse is triggered in the

Table 12–12. Categories of Apnea

Disease	Example	Mechanism	Signs	Treatment
Apnea of prematurity	Premature (<36 wk)	Central control, airway obstruction	Apnea, bradycardia	Theophylline, CPAP, intubation
Ondine curse	Leigh syndrome	Central control	Apnea	Mechanical ventilation
Obesity hypoventilation	Obesity, Prader Willi syndrome	Airway obstruction, central control	Obesity, somnolence, polycythemia, cor pulmonale	Theophylline, weight loss
Obstructive sleep apnea	Chronic tonsil hypertrophy, Pierre Robin syndrome, Down syndrome, cerebral palsy, myotonic dystrophy, myopathy	Airway obstruction by enlarged tonsils/adenoids, choanal stenosis/atresia, large tongue, temporomandibular joint dysfunction, micrognathia, velopharyngeal incompetence; also may be central	Daytime sleepiness, loud snoring, night insomnia and enuresis, hyperactivity, poor school performance, behavior problems, mouth breathing, inspiratory stridor	Tonsillectomy, adenoidectomy, nasal trumpets, CPAP, uvuloveloplasty
Cyanotic "breath-holding spells"	Breath holder less than 3 yr old	Prolonged expiratory apnea; hyperventilation; cerebral anoxia	Cyanosis, syncope, brief tonic–clonic movements	Reassurance that the condition is self limiting; must exclude seizure disorder
Pallid "breath-holding spells"	Breath holder	Asystole; reflex anoxic seizures	Rapid onset, with or without crying; pallor; bradycardia; opisthotonus; seizures; follows painful stimuli	Atropine?; must exclude seizure disorder; less benign than cyanotic breath holding
SIDS	Previously normal child; increased incidence with prematurity, SIDS in sibling, maternal drug abuse, cigarette smoking, males; may have preceding minor URI	Central respiratory control; Cardiac arrhythmia (prolonged QT syndrome); Central cardiac control: Prolonged expiratory apnea *Less common:* (1) Seizure (2) Parental-induced airway obstruction—suffocation (accidental or abuse) (3) RSV (4) Chemoreceptor dysfunction (5) Overheating	2–3 mo old child found cyanotic, apneic, and pulseless in bed	No treatment; prevention with home apnea monitor unproven and supine sleep position suggestive

CPAP = continuous positive airway pressure by facial mask or nasal prongs; SIDS = sudden infant death syndrome; URI = upper respiratory infection.
(Data from Southall D: Pediatrics 80:73, 1988; Mark J, Brooks J: Pediatr Clin North Am 31:907, 1984; and Gordon N: Dev Med Child Neurol 29:805, 1987.)

brain that causes the child to involuntarily move his or her head or body in order to relieve the obstruction. If any individual component of this final arousal response system fails, the apneic child will die.

The *etiology* of apnea is diverse and not well understood (Table 12–12). Premature infants commonly exhibit episodes of apnea, which may be associated with cyanosis and bradycardia (see Chapter 6). Apnea occurring in older infants warrants thorough investigation. Surgical therapy (removing adenoids, tonsils, or other obstructing tissue or bypassing the obstruction by tracheostomy) may be necessary in children who are symptomatic with obstructive apnea.

Sudden Infant Death Syndrome

Sudden infant death syndrome (SIDS) refers to the unexpected and unexplained death of an infant less than 1 yr old. In the United States, SIDS occurs in 1.6–2.3/1000 live births and is the most common cause of death between 1 and 12 mo of age. There is a peak incidence between 2 and 3 mo of age. The rates are highest in black and American Indian populations; in children of young, single impoverished mothers; in infants with near-miss SIDS; in premature infants; in infants whose mothers have abused drugs; and during the winter. SIDS is rare prior to 4 wk or after 6 mo of age.

A wide variety of mechanisms have been proposed to explain SIDS. Autonomic dysfunction, ab-

Table 12–13. Differential Diagnosis of SIDS

Fulminant infection*
Infant botulism†
Seizure disorder
Brain tumor*
Hypoglycemia†
Medium-chain acyl-coenzyme A dehydrogenase deficiency*†
Carnitine deficiency*†
Urea cycle defect†
Child abuse*
Drug intoxication†
Cardiac arrhythmia
Gastroesophageal reflux*
Midgut volvulus/shock*
Laryngospasm

 * Obvious or suspected at autopsy.
 † Requires diagnostic test.

errations in respiratory control, abnormal upper airway reflexes, cardiac arrhythmias, laryngospasm associated with gastroesophageal reflux, airway obstruction and carbon dioxide rebreathing while prone, and other mechanisms have been considered, but none is widely accepted (Table 12–12). The pathology of SIDS suggests hypoxia (acute or chronic); intrathoracic petechiae and increased pulmonary artery smooth muscle may be present.

The *risk of SIDS* is increased 3–5 times in siblings of infants who have died of SIDS. Whether this increased susceptibility is due to genetic or environmental factors is unknown. Monitoring of siblings may be warranted.

Because SIDS strikes without warning in an infant previously thought to be healthy, the impact on families is especially devastating and psychologic support is needed. Inappropriate investigation for possible child abuse should be avoided. The *differential diagnosis* is noted in Table 12–13.

Acute Life-Threatening Events ("Near-Miss SIDS")

Infants who experience acute life-threatening events, such as prolonged apnea requiring resuscitation, present the physician with challenging problems. Numerous possible etiologies (Table 12–13) warrant diagnostic evaluation, which should include an electroencephalogram; chest roentgenogram; electrocardiogram; blood gas analysis; blood chemistries, including glucose, calcium, blood urea nitrogen, and electrolytes; an evaluation for gastroesophageal reflux (barium swallow or, preferably, pH probe study); and a 12–24 hr recording of heart and respiratory activity (pneumogram).

Parents of infants ascertained to be at high risk for recurrence of such events (or siblings of SIDS victims) may be offered home monitoring with an electronic monitor. No objective guidelines exist for instituting or terminating the monitoring. The ability to predict which infant is at high risk for SIDS on the basis of a pneumogram is not established, but infants with a high percentage of periodic breathing or with apneic spells lasting longer than 15 sec may be at high risk. However, many infants with previously normal pneumograms have subsequently died of SIDS, whereas most infants with abnormal pneumograms do not die of SIDS. The parents of infants who have had acute life-threatening events should be instructed in basic cardiac life support.

Vocal Cord Paralysis

Vocal cord paralysis is an important cause of laryngeal dysfunction. Paralysis may be unilateral or bilateral and more often is due to damage of the recurrent laryngeal nerves than to a central lesion. The left recurrent laryngeal nerve passes around the arch of the aorta and thus is more susceptible to damage than the right laryngeal nerve. Trauma such as neck traction during delivery and lesions in the mediastinum are common causes of cord paralysis. Central causes include the Arnold-Chiari malformation, hydrocephalus, intracranial hemorrhage, and dysgenesis of the nucleus ambiguus.

The symptoms of vocal cord paralysis include stridor, a weak cry (in infants), hoarseness, or aphonia. Unilateral paralysis may be relatively asymptomatic. Rarely, the cords are paralyzed in the abducted position, and aspiration results. Patients with such a condition, as well as those with bilateral abductor paralysis resulting in severe airway obstruction, may require tracheostomy. The prognosis for return of vocal cord function depends on the nature of the injury and whether or not the recurrent laryngeal nerve has been disrupted.

References

AAP Task Force on Infant Positioning and SIDS: Positioning and SIDS. Pediatrics 89:1120, 1992.

Behrman RE (ed): Nelson Textbook of Pediatrics. 14th ed. Philadelphia, WB Saunders, 1992, Sec. 9.31, 14.3, 14.46, 25.1.

Holton J, Allen J, Green C, et al: Inherited metabolic diseases in sudden infant death syndrome. Am J Dis Child 66:1315, 1991.

Krongrad E: Infants at high risk for sudden infant death syndrome? Have they been identified? A commentary. Pediatrics 88:1274, 1991.

CARDIOVASCULAR DISORDERS

Pulmonary Hypertension/Cor Pulmonale

Diffuse lung disease, upper airway obstruction (such as hypertrophied tonsils or adenoids), pulmonary thromboembolism, or exposure to high altitude may produce pulmonary hypertension. Pulmonary hypertension also may result from excessive pulmonary blood flow when there is a left-to-right cardiac shunt. With prolonged hypertension, resulting from either increased flow or hypoxic vasoconstriction, permanent changes occur in the intima and media of the pulmonary artery, making the increased vascular resistance irreversible. Primary pulmonary hypertension is idiopathic, occurs in the absence of parenchymal lung or cardiac disease, is associated with autoimmune disease (SLE, scleroderma), and responds poorly to therapy.

Pulmonary hypertension resulting from lung disease leads to hypertrophy and eventually to dilation of the right ventricle, termed **cor pulmonale**. In advanced states, right heart failure may occur, with limitation of exercise capacity, hepatic congestion, fluid retention, and signs of tricuspid insufficiency. In severe disease, the ventricular septum may be displaced toward the left ventricle, reducing its volume and, thus, left ventricular function as well.

The most common causes of cor pulmonale in children are diffuse chronic lung diseases, such as CF and bronchopulmonary dysplasia. In these conditions, airway obstruction results in alveolar hypoxia, and parenchymal scarring may increase pulmonary vascular resistance.

The *diagnosis* of pulmonary hypertension should be suspected whenever there is prolonged hypoxemia or severe left-to-right shunting. In addition to the physical findings associated with pulmonary or cardiac disease, there may be an accentuated pulmonic component of the second heart sound heard in the left second interspace. Definitive diagnosis is made by cardiac catheterization, but echocardiography may confirm the presence of significant right ventricular hypertrophy, ventricular dysfunction, and tricuspid insufficiency indicative of increased pulmonary artery pressure.

Treatment is directed at the underlying condition. Relief of hypoxemia is essential and usually requires supplemental oxygen therapy. Heart failure may necessitate diuretics and restriction of salt and fluid intake. Vasodilator therapy rarely is successful. The *prognosis* is poor once chronic cor pulmonale is present; if left ventricular failure is evident, the prognosis is even worse.

Pulmonary Edema

Pathophysiology. At the alveolar–capillary interface, capillary hydrostatic forces and tissue osmotic pressures tend to push fluid into the air spaces, whereas plasma osmotic pressures and tissue mechanical forces tend to force fluid away from the air spaces. Under normal circumstances, the vectorial sum of these forces favors absorption so that the alveolar spaces remain dry. Any fluid entering the alveolus normally is removed by the pulmonary lymphatics. Pulmonary edema forms when transcapillary fluid flux exceeds lymphatic drainage. Reduced left ventricular function accompanied by pulmonary venous hypertension increases capillary hydrostatic pressure, which floods the interstitial spaces and alveoli with fluid, producing pulmonary edema. Fluid initially enters the interstitial space around the terminal bronchioles, alveoli, and arteries (*interstitial edema*), causing increased lung stiffness, premature closure of bronchioles on expiration, and dyspnea and tachypnea as a result of stimulation of lung receptors. If the process continues, fluid enters the alveolar space, reducing compliance and creating a perfused but unventilated area called a shunt. Shunting, not the presence of fluid in the alveoli, produces hypoxia.

Pulmonary hypertension as occurs in cor pulmonale rarely produces pulmonary edema, because the site of increased vascular resistance is proximal to the capillary bed. Pulmonary edema may be seen, however, when intrathoracic pressure becomes excessively negative (e.g., upper airway obstruction from hypertrophied tonsils). Pulmonary edema also may occur in patients having decreased serum oncotic pressure, in patients receiving large volumes of intravenous fluid following capillary damage (smoke inhalation, hydrocarbon aspiration), with ascent to high altitude, and in patients with a history of central nervous system injury (neurogenic).

Clinical Manifestations. Pulmonary edema typically produces dyspnea, cough (often with frothy, pink-tinged sputum), tachypnea, signs of increased respiratory effort, and diffuse rales. Chest roentgenograms show a diffuse infiltrate that classically is in a perihilar pattern but may be obscured by underlying lung disease. Signs of interstitial edema (Kerley B lines) may be seen, especially at the lung bases.

Treatment. Treatment should include positioning the patient in an upright posture and administering oxygen but otherwise is directed toward relieving the underlying problem. Morphine may relieve dyspnea and, by dilating central veins, reduce venous return to the heart. Diuretic therapy (furosemide) and rapid-acting intravenous positive inotropic agents also are helpful. In severe cases, mask continuous positive airway pressure (CPAP) or intubation with positive end-expiratory pressure (PEEP) may be required. The *prognosis* for patients with pulmonary edema depends on the nature of the underlying cause as well as on the response to therapy.

ADULT RESPIRATORY DISTRESS SYNDROME

This noncardiogenic pulmonary edema results from increases in the permeability of the alveolar–capillary interface, which allows the alveoli and interstitium to become flooded with transudate. In addition to pulmonary edema produced by classical mechanisms (see above), inflammatory mediators (vasoactive compounds, endotoxin, complement, cytokines, prostaglandins) may increase vascular permeability further and produce chemotactic factors that recruit inflammatory cells to the site of injury. Preformed and newly synthesized mediators (proteases, kinins, prostaglandins) and oxygen-free radicals cause further vascular and parenchymal damage, resulting in hypoxia and hypercapnia, which produce acute pulmonary hypertension. Therefore, ARDS becomes manifest as a composite condition of a pulmonary shunt, decreased pulmonary compliance, and pulmonary hypertension.

The *etiology* of ARDS is varied, but it often results from shock (especially septic shock), aspiration (of hydrocarbons), inhalation of toxic fumes (smoke, NO_2, SO_2, NH_3, phosgene, Cl_2), or trauma (burns, near-drowning, head injury, fat emboli from fractures). ARDS also may be associated with pneumonia, pulmonary emboli, disseminated intravascular coagulation, drug overdose, uremia, and multiple transfusions.

Patients with ARDS develop severe hypoxemia and respiratory distress. Chest roentgenograms show diffuse alveolar infiltrates, although only interstitial edema may be seen in the early stages. Often, a period of hours to even days may elapse between the original insult and the development of overt respiratory failure.

Treatment consists of mechanical ventilation accompanied by the application of PEEP, oxygen, and therapy for the underlying problem. The *mortality rate* in patients with ARDS ranges from 50% to 90%, reflecting the severity of the insult to the lungs and other organ systems that issues both from ARDS itself and from its underlying diseases.

Pulmonary Embolism

Pulmonary embolism is rare in childhood and may be associated with indwelling vascular catheters, oral contraceptives, lupus anticoagulant, trauma, abortion, or malignancy. Because the pulmonary vascular bed is very distensible, small emboli, even if multiple, usually are not detected unless they are infected, causing pulmonary infection. However, large emboli may result in acute dyspnea, pleuritic chest pain, cough, hemoptysis, and even death. Hypoxia is common, as are right-sided heart strain revealed on the electrocardiogram, an increased P2 heart sound, and occasionally a wedge-shaped pulmonary infiltrate. Ventilation–perfusion scans are useful in diagnosis by showing defects in perfusion without matching ventilation defects. For *definitive diagnosis*, however, a pulmonary angiogram is the procedure of choice.

Treatment of proven pulmonary embolism is supportive (oxygen administration) and also should be directed toward the predisposing factors. Heparin may be useful in preventing development of further emboli; thrombolytic therapy may be helpful in treating massive embolization.

References

Behrman RE (ed): Nelson Textbook of Pediatrics. 14th ed. Philadelphia, WB Saunders, 1992, Sec. 14.78–14.80.

Bernstein D, Coupey S, Schoenberg SK: Pulmonary embolism in adolescents. Am J Dis Child 140:667, 1986.

Macnaughton P, Evans T: Management of adult respiratory distress syndrome. Lancet 339:469, 1992.

Perkin RM, Anas NG: Pulmonary hypertension in pediatric patients. J Pediatr 105:511–522, 1984.

Royall J, Levin DL: Adult respiratory distress syndrome in pediatric patients. J Pediatr 112:169–180, 335–337, 1988.

ASPIRATION SYNDROMES

Aspiration of material into the lungs is common in children and may be asymptomatic or fatal.

When children with depressed levels of consciousness aspirate gastric contents from emesis, it may lead to severe pneumonia or to ARDS. The most common aspiration syndromes include foreign body aspiration, aspiration associated with gastroesophageal reflux, and near-drowning.

Foreign Body Aspiration

Aspiration of foreign bodies into the tracheobronchial tree is more common than usually is recognized. The majority of patients are less than 4 yr old, and most of the deaths also occur in this age group. Such children often put virtually anything into their mouths and frequently are out of sight of even the most diligent caretaker. Younger children most commonly aspirate food, toys, or other small objects. Older children also may aspirate objects they have held in their mouths.

Clinical Manifestations. A high percentage of children who aspirate foreign bodies will present with either a clear-cut history of choking (or witnessed aspiration) or physical or roentgenographic evidence of the foreign body. However, a small percentage of patients with foreign body aspiration will have a negative history because of unobserved or unrecognized events. Physical findings consistent with acute foreign body aspiration include unilateral absence of breath sounds, localized wheezing, stridor, and bloody sputum. Roentgenographic studies may reveal the presence of a radiopaque object or evidence of air trapping on exhalation. When aspiration is suspected, expiratory chest films should be requested, although fluoroscopy may be more helpful.

Because the right main bronchus is a more direct continuation of the trachea than is the left main bronchus, foreign bodies tend to enter the right lung preferentially. However, they also may be coughed out more readily from the right side, and, in many large reported series, nearly as many foreign bodies were found on the left as on the right. Some foreign bodies, especially nuts or seeds, may migrate from place to place in the airways and even lodge in the larynx on coughing, totally occluding the airway. Such migratory foreign bodies often are not associated with roentgenographic abnormalities and are difficult to detect.

Foreign bodies also may lodge in the esophagus and compress the trachea, producing respiratory symptoms. An esophageal foreign body should be included in the differential diagnosis of infants or young children with persistent stridor or wheezing, particularly if associated with dysphagia.

Diagnosis. The majority of foreign bodies are small and quickly coughed out, but many may remain in the lung for long periods before diagnosis, and may come to medical attention because of symptoms of fever, cough, sputum production, or chest pain. Patients with persistent wheezing unresponsive to bronchodilator therapy, persistent atelectasis, recurrent or persistent pneumonia, or persistent cough without other explanation should be suspected of harboring a foreign body. If there is good evidence (in history, physical, or roentgenographic examination) for a bronchial foreign body, the patient should undergo rigid bronchoscopy. Flexible bronchoscopy may be a very useful diagnostic technique when the presentation is not straightforward.

Prevention and Treatment. The best approach to foreign body aspiration is to educate parents and caretakers in preventing the event. Before their molar teeth have developed, infants and children should not have nuts, uncooked carrots, and other foods that may be easily broken into small pieces and aspirated. Toys should be free of small parts that also may be aspirated.

Gastroesophageal Reflux
See Chapter 11.

Near-Drowning
Near-drowning is a frequent emergency in children that may result in hypoxic organ damage and pulmonary dysfunction. In some cases, laryngospasm prevents the victim from aspirating water into the lungs, and the damage results from hypoxia alone. Usually, however, the victim aspirates water, which disturbs ventilation–perfusion relationships, causes loss of surfactant, and produces pulmonary edema.

The primary goal in *therapy* is to correct acidosis and hypoxia as rapidly as possible. In children, cardiac activity persists long after ventilation ceases, and the most urgent priority is to provide effective ventilation. Under most circumstances, water will be absorbed from the lungs quickly, and ventilation should be initiated without delay without attempting to clear water from the airways. Closed chest cardiac massage is employed, if necessary. Intubation and PEEP often are very helpful to reduce intrapulmonary shunting and improve oxygenation. Once effective ventilation is established, metabolic acidosis often corrects itself, but judicious administration of bicarbonate may be necessary in the face of profound acidosis.

Cerebral edema often results from the hypoxic insult and must be managed aggressively. Hyperventilation (to maintain P_{CO_2} in the range of 25–28 torr), fluid restriction, osmotic diuresis, and even drainage of ventricular fluid through a ventriculostomy may be necessary to prevent cerebral ischemia as a result of intracranial hypertension.

The *prognosis* for victims of near-drowning is variable and depends chiefly on the degree of initial hypoxic insult. Children who regain consciousness after they are resuscitated have an excellent prognosis. Submersion for longer than 9 min and cardiopulmonary resuscitation for longer than 25 min in the prehospital setting are associated with a high mortality and severe neurologic impairment. Exceptions to this latter observation may occur, however, in persons who have drowned in very cold water, because the cold temperature slows metabolism and limits hypoxic damage.

References

Behrman RE (ed): Nelson Textbook of Pediatrics. 14th ed. Philadelphia, WB Saunders, 1992, Sec. 6.36, 14.45, 14.59–14.63.

Quan L, Wentz KR, Gore EJ, et al: Outcome and predictors of outcome in pediatric submersion victims receiving prehospital care in King county, Washington. Pediatrics 86:586, 1990.

Steen K, Zimmerman T: Tracheobronchial aspiration of foreign bodies in children: A study of 94 cases. Laryngoscope 100:525, 1990.

HEMOSIDEROSIS

Pulmonary hemosiderosis is characterized by the accumulation of hemosiderin in the lungs as a result of bleeding into the lungs. Red blood cells are phagocytosed by alveolar macrophages and the hemoglobin is converted to hemosiderin; using special iron-staining techniques, the hemosiderin within the alveolar macrophages can be identified microscopically. Hemosiderin-laden macrophages may be found in sputum, gastric aspirate, bronchoalveolar lavage fluid, or a lung biopsy.

Etiology. Hemosiderosis may result from bleeding anywhere in the lung, airway, pharynx, nasopharynx, or mouth, but usually occurs as a result of diffuse alveolar bleeding, which may be low-grade and transient or brisk and massive.

Clinical Manifestations. The presentation is variable but often includes iron-deficiency anemia with a history of cough, tachypnea, and wheezing.

Occasionally, frank hemoptysis or hematemesis is seen. At the time of acute pulmonary bleeding, fever, leukocytosis, and an elevated sedimentation rate may occur. Some cases are associated with eosinophilia. Chest roentgenograms usually show transient infiltrates, but massive infiltrates, atelectasis, and hyperinflation may occur. In the chronic stages, an interstitial pattern suggestive of interstitial fibrosis has been seen.

Many patients are incorrectly diagnosed as having bacterial pneumonia. Iron-deficiency anemia or guaiac-positive stools in a child with pneumonia (particularly if eosinophilia is present) suggests pulmonary hemosiderosis, and sputum, gastric aspirate, and/or bronchoalveolar lavage samples should be obtained to confirm the presence of hemosiderin-laden macrophages.

The *classification* of pulmonary hemosiderosis reflects the associated findings and presumed etiology of the alveolar hemorrhage. In the majority of pediatric cases, no etiology can be identified (**"idiopathic pulmonary hemosiderosis"**). Cases of pulmonary hemosiderosis associated with glomerular basement membrane disease (**glomerulonephritis**) may be subdivided into those with circulating antigen–antibody complexes and those with antibody deposited along the basement membrane of the kidney and/or lung (Goodpasture syndrome). These antigen–antibody complexes may be associated with a number of **collagen vascular diseases** or **systemic vasculitis** (Henoch-Schönlein purpura, Wegener granulomatosis); occasionally, lung involvement with collagen vascular diseases occurs without or prior to renal involvement. Pulmonary hemosiderosis in infants also can be associated with precipitating serum antibodies to cow's milk (**Heiner syndrome**). These infants may exhibit wheezing, eosinophilia, high IgE levels, failure to thrive, and, less often, adenoidal hypertrophy with upper airway obstruction. The role of the milk sensitivity is unclear, but eliminating cow's milk from the diet often decreases the frequency and severity of the alveolar hemorrhage. Certain forms of **heart disease** associated with increased pulmonary venous and capillary pressures also may cause alveolar bleeding and pulmonary hemosiderosis.

Treatment. Management of the acute episodes of bleeding should include administering oxygen, blood transfusions, and, if necessary, mechanical ventilation accompanied by PEEP to tamponade the bleeding. Attempts should be made to identify the etiology of the bleeding; often, an open lung

Table 12–14. Differential Diagnosis of
Hemoptysis–Pulmonary Hemorrhage

Cardiovascular
Heart failure
Eisenmenger syndrome
Arteriovenous fistula (Osler-Weber-Rendu syndrome)
Pulmonary embolism

Pulmonary
Respiratory distress syndrome
Bronchogenic cyst
Sequestration
Pneumonia (bacterial, mycobacterial, fungal, parasitic)
Cystic fibrosis
Tracheobronchitis
Bronchiectasis
Abscess
Tumor (adenoma, carcinoid, hemangioma, metastasis)
Foreign body retention
Contusion–trauma

Immune
Henoch-Schönlein purpura
Heiner syndrome
Goodpasture syndrome
Wegener granulomatosis
Systemic lupus erythematosus
Allergic bronchopulmonary aspergillosis

Other
Hyperammonemia
Kernicterus
Intracranial hemorrhage (preterm infant)

biopsy is necessary (Table 12–14). Idiopathic pulmonary hemosiderosis may respond to corticosteroids. Other immunosuppressant agents, such as azathioprine and cyclophosphamide, have been used when the condition did not respond to the administration of corticosteroids over 2–3 mo. A trial period on a milk-free diet may be useful.

Prognosis. This depends on the underlying cause of the bleeding. In some children, the course of idiopathic hemosiderosis may be relentless, whereas others bleed only once. Repeated hemorrhage often results in chronic pulmonary fibrosis and respiratory insufficiency.

RESPIRATORY FAILURE

Respiratory failure occurs when the lungs are unable to deliver sufficient oxygen to the blood to meet metabolic demands. It may develop insidiously or have an abrupt onset. Usually, increased

respiratory drive leads to tachypnea, dyspnea, retractions, and the use of accessory muscles. Auscultatory findings vary with the etiology of the problem and may include diminished or absent breath sounds, wheezing or prolonged expiration, crackles and rhonchi, and grunting on exhalation. Because approximately 5 g/dL of circulating deoxygenated hemoglobin normally are required for cyanosis to be evident clinically, patients who are anemic may have seriously impaired oxygen transport without obvious cyanosis. Early in the course of the condition, tachycardia is common. Bradycardia is a late and especially ominous sign and usually is followed rapidly by hypotension and cardiac arrest. Hypoxemia may produce restlessness and irritability, which may progress to confusion, decreased levels of consciousness, seizures, and, eventually, coma. Hypercapnia results in cerebral vasodilation and often severe headache and, in later stages, profound depression of the central nervous system.

The *diagnosis* of respiratory insufficiency and failure depend on careful observation of the patient, suspicion heightened by knowledge of the history and underlying clinical circumstances, and appropriate laboratory evaluation. The single most useful laboratory study is an arterial blood gas determination. However, when clinical evidence of respiratory insufficiency or failure is present, oxygen therapy should never be withheld while awaiting a blood gas study.

Treatment of respiratory failure should be directed immediately to relieve hypoxemia and hypercapnia. In pediatric patients, it rarely is harmful to administer 100% oxygen for short periods of time, although the patient should be monitored carefully. Rarely, children having chronic respiratory insufficiency have blunted respiratory responses to hypercapnia, and function chiefly on their hypoxic drive. In such instances, the administration of high concentrations of oxygen can result in paradoxical respiratory depression.

A careful and systematic search should be made for the underlying (and potentially reversible) causes of the respiratory failure, and appropriate treatment should be instituted. In the presence of refractory hypoxia and/or significant hypercapnia ($Paco_2$ >60 mm Hg), institution of mechanical ventilation should be considered.

Patients in respiratory failure often are very unstable and must be monitored carefully. Only a few minutes separate apnea from cardiac arrest. In children, the vast majority of cardiac arrests are the direct result of hypoxemia, rather than of a primary cardiac abnormality. If respiratory failure cannot be reversed promptly by specific therapy (e.g., relief of pneumothorax or upper airway obstruction, treatment of bronchospasm), intubation and mechanical ventilation usually will be necessary.

The *prognosis* for patients with respiratory failure depends almost entirely on the nature of the underlying cause of the failure and the rapidity and efficacy of the therapy initiated. In patients with acute disease, the prognosis should be good. However, in patients with chronic disease such as CF, respiratory failure portends an ominous prognosis, al-

though most patients can survive several episodes if treated vigorously.

References

Behrman RE (ed): Nelson Textbook of Pediatrics. 14th ed. Philadelphia, WB Saunders, 1992, Sec. 14.17, 14.71.

Leatherman JW, Davies SF, Hoidal JR: Alveolar hemorrhage syndromes: Diffuse microvascular lung hemorrhage in immune and idiopathic disorders. Medicine 63:343, 1984.

Panitch H, Schidlow D: Pathogenesis and management of hemoptysis in children. Int Pediatr 4:241, 1989.

The Cardiovascular System

13

Paul C. Gillette

Today it is possible to make a correct diagnosis of the presence or absence and type of heart disease in almost every case, and in most cases this can be done noninvasively. Cardiac catheterization and angiography, however, are the gold standard when the most precise diagnosis is necessary in the most complex cases.

The origin of heart disease in children is a combination of genetic and environmental causes. Congenital heart disease may be either genetic (e.g., Down syndrome) or acquired (e.g., through maternal rubella) (Table 13–1). Acquired heart disease, such as rheumatic fever or atherosclerosis, may have genetic predispositions or may be due to systemic diseases that directly or indirectly affect the heart or vasculature (Table 13–2). Congenital heart disease is present in about 8 of every 1000 babies. It is slightly more common in premature infants and even more common in fetuses. About half of congenital heart defects are relatively insignificant but half may result in infant death or disability. Defects such as small ventricular septal defects (VSDs) or bicuspid aortic valves cause little or no disability, but the associated murmurs or clicks may cause substantial parental concern.

It may be difficult to differentiate significant from insignificant congenital cardiac defects by history and physical examination. Although the initial newborn physical exam is useful, the neonate's physiology is changing so rapidly that significant defects may be missed. Coarctation of the aorta often is missed because the pulses and leg blood pressures may be normal for the first day or so until the ductus arteriosus closes and completes the coarctation. Even lethal defects such as hypoplastic left heart syndrome may be inapparent at birth because of the palliative effects of the patent ductus arteriosus (PDA). Tests performed at the primary level in the newborn nursery, such as electrocardiography and chest roentgenography, may be nonspecific. They may be normal for the 1st wk or two of life. Many but not all serious congenital cardiac defects are associated with a lower than normal oxygen saturation. However, a normal oxygen saturation ($\geq 95\%$), as determined by pulse oximetry, is not a guarantee of a normal heart. Stenotic valve lesions often will have a normal oxygen saturation even if they are severe. Other physical signs such as tachypnea, hyperpnea, and tachycardia also are important. There are many nonpathologic heart murmurs heard at birth, so the physician must use good judgment in deciding which require further evaluation by a pediatric cardiologist. The absence of a heart murmur in a neonate is not evidence of the absence of congenital heart disease.

It is vital to diagnose serious congenital cardiac defects as early as possible. Virtually every congenital cardiac defect can be treated at least by palliation. If the defect is unrecognized, death may occur before medical or surgical palliation can be carried out. The physician caring for the infant in the newborn nursery must have a high index of suspicion regarding small signs and symptoms. It is not the pediatricians job to make the detailed anatomic or physiologic diagnosis but rather to suspect heart disease, perform initial rapid stabilization, and obtain consultation of a pediatric cardiology team. The pediatric cardiologist will use cardiac ultrasound to make the anatomic and physiologic diagnosis. Magnetic resonance imaging (MRI) and/or cardiac catheterization and angiography may be needed to clear up details prior to surgical or catheter palliation or cure.

DIAGNOSTIC EVALUATION

Congenital heart disease is the major cause of pediatric cardiovascular disease. The diagnostic evaluation of a child suspected of having congenital heart disease should proceed in an organized manner. Congenital heart disease is diagnosed accurately by careful history, physical examination, electrocardiography, chest roentgenogram, echocardiography, and cardiac catheterization.

469

Table 13–1. Congenital Malformation Syndromes Associated with Congenital Heart Disease

Syndrome	Cardiac Features
Trisomy 21 (Down syndrome)	Endocardial cushion defect
Trisomy 18	VSD, ASD, PDA
Trisomy 13	VSD, ASD, PDA
XO (Turner syndrome)	Coarctation of aorta, aortic stenosis
CHARGE association (coloboma, heart, atresia choanae, retardation, genital and ear anomalies)	TOF, endocardial cushion defect, VSD, ASD
DiGeorge syndrome	Aortic arch anomalies, conotruncal anomalies*
VATER association (vertebral, anal, tracheoesophageal, radial and renal anomalies)	VSD
Congenital rubella	PDA, peripheral pulmonic stenosis, mitral regurgitation (in infancy)
Marfan syndrome	Dilated and dissecting aorta, aortic valve regurgitation, mitral valve prolapse
Williams syndrome	Supravalvular aortic stenosis, peripheral pulmonary stenosis
Infant of diabetic mother	Hypertrophic cardiomyopathy, VSD, conotruncal anomalies
Holt-Oram syndrome	ASD, VSD
Asplenia syndrome	Complex cyanotic heart lesions, anomalous pulmonary venous return, dextrocardia, single ventricle, single AV valve
Polysplenia syndrome	Azygos continuation of inferior vena cava, pulmonary atresia, dextrocardia, single ventricle

* Conotruncal = TOF, pulmonary atresia, truncus arteriosus, transposition of great arteries.
  ASD = atrial septal defect; AV = atrioventricular; PDA = patent ductus arteriosus; TOF = tetralogy of Fallot; VSD = ventricular septal defect.

Table 13–2. Cardiac Manifestations of Systemic Diseases

Systemic Disease	Cardiac Complications
Hunter-Hurler syndrome	Valvular insufficiency, heart failure, hypertension
Fabry disease	Mitral insufficiency, coronary artery disease with myocardial infarction
Pompe disease	Short P-R interval, cardiomegaly, heart failure, arrhythmias
Friedreich ataxia	Myocardopathy, arrhythmias
Duchenne dystrophy	Myocardopathy, heart failure
Juvenile rheumatoid arthritis	Pericarditis
Systemic lupus erythematosus	Pericarditis, Libman-Sacks endocarditis; congenital A–V block
Marfan syndrome	Aortic and mitral insufficiency; dissecting aortic aneurysm
Homocystinuria	Coronary thrombosis
Kawasaki disease	Coronary artery aneurysm, thrombosis, myocardial infarction, myocarditis
Lyme disease	Arrhythmias, myocarditis
Graves disease	Tachycardia, arrhythmias, heart failure
Tuberous sclerosis	Cardiac rhabdomyoma

AV = atrioventricular.

History

In obtaining a history, it is necessary to take into account the age of the patient. For example, in the infant, congestive heart failure usually becomes manifest by feeding difficulties, easy fatigability, vomiting, lethargy, increased perspiration, and rapid respirations. Typically the baby feeds poorly. In the older child, congestive heart failure causes easy fatigability and shortness of breath and dyspnea on exertion, which is usually best described in terms of specific activities like walking on level ground, walking up steps, and bicycle riding. Orthopnea, paroxysmal nocturnal dyspnea, and edema are uncommon manifestations of heart failure in children. The family history of previous congenital cardiac defects also is important.

Physical Examination

A thoughtful, thorough, and careful cardiac examination may provide significant clues to the

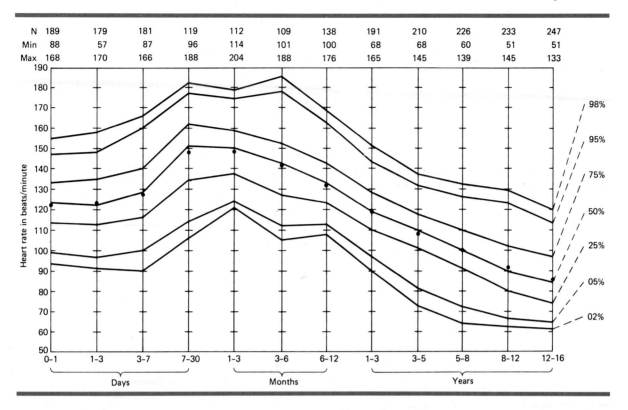

N	189	179	181	119	112	109	138	191	210	226	233	247
Min	88	57	87	96	114	101	100	68	68	60	51	51
Max	168	170	166	188	204	188	176	165	145	139	145	133

Figure 13–1. Heart rate versus age (● = mean). (From Davignon A, Rautaharju P, Boiselle E: Normal ECG standards for heart rate of infants and children. Pediatr Cardiol 1:123, 1980.)

presence of heart disease. The normal *heart rate* varies considerably according to age (Fig. 13–1). Tachycardia may be seen as a manifestation of heart failure or as a dysrhythmia. Bradycardia is seen as a normal finding in patients with high vagal tone, particularly athletes, but may be a manifestation of 2nd- or 3rd-degree atrioventricular (AV) block.

The *respiratory rate* in pediatric patients with heart disease may be increased secondary to increased lung stiffness resulting from increased lung water (decreased compliance) from a large left-to-right shunt, associated with pulmonary artery hypertension. Pulmonary venous congestion also may increase the rate. The patient's *height and weight* always should be assessed. Failure to thrive, especially when the height-to-weight ratio is increased, frequently is seen in infants with congestive heart failure and may be an important indication for surgery if medical management proves unsuccessful.

The *blood pressure* should be measured in the upper and lower extremities to identify coarctation of the aorta. If only one arm is measured, it should

be the right arm because the coarctation may involve the left subclavian artery. The appropriate size cuff for the size of the arm should be used, because a cuff that is too small (bladders that encircle less than 90% of the arm and cover less than 75% of the length) will give a blood pressure measurement that is higher than the true intravascular reading. Blood pressure may be measured by the auscultation or Doppler method. The pulse pressure, determined by subtracting the diastolic pressure from the systolic pressure, normally is less than 50 mm Hg or half the systolic pressure, whichever is less. A wide pulse pressure, as assessed by palpation, usually is seen with aorticopulmonary connections (PDA, aorticopulmonary window, truncus arteriosus) or with aortic insufficiency, fever, anemia, or complete AV block. A narrow pulse pressure is recognized in congestive heart failure, severe aortic stenosis, or pericardial tamponade.

The level of the *jugular vein venous pulsations* in the neck provides a rough assessment of the right atrial pressure. This sign is difficult to ascertain in infants and young children but may be very helpful in the school-age or older child. The veins are observed with the child sitting or lying in a relaxed manner on an examining table raised to 30 degrees. Greatly increased venous distention then can be recognized because, normally, pulsations are not visible above the clavicle in the sitting position. In complete AV block, the venous pulsations are variable and depend on the position of the tricuspid valve at the time of atrial systole; if the right atrium contracts when the tricuspid valve is closed, a large venous pulsation (cannon wave) will occur.

The presence of *rales* in the chest may be a sign of pulmonary edema resulting from increased pulmonary venous pressure; rales also may indicate infection. The absence of rales is a nonspecific sign because the patient in congestive heart failure may breath in a very shallow manner. *Hepatomegaly* is one of the cardinal signs of right-sided heart failure in the infant and child. The liver should be palpated lightly from above so as not to create a tense abdomen. *Splenomegaly* may be present in some children with long-standing congestive heart failure and may be seen in children with infective endocarditis.

Cyanosis, a bluish discoloration of the skin, nails, and mucous membranes, is apparent in infants and children with hypoxemia who have 3–5 g/dL of reduced hemoglobin. *Clubbing*, a rounding or convexity of the nails, may begin in infancy; it may become very prominent in hypoxemic adolescents and young adults. *Edema* of the lower extremities is an uncommon characteristic of heart failure in infants but may be seen in the older child or adolescent.

On inspection, *prominence of the precordial chest wall* frequently is seen in infants and children with cardiomegaly and is especially prominent when the right ventricle is involved. A *hyperdynamic precordium* suggests a volume load, usually caused by a large left-to-right shunt or semilunar or AV valve regurgitation. A *thrill*, the palpable manifestation associated with a loud murmur, is felt where the accompanying murmur is loudest.

AUSCULTATION

The art of auscultation can be improved by the practice of a careful, systematic approach. It also can be improved if the examination is carried out in a quiet room without distractions. The infant should be examined in whatever position will quiet him or her, and the stethoscope bell should be used first to avoid the startle reaction. The examiner should listen first to the entire cardiac cycle, determining the 1st sound (S_1), systole, the second sound (S_2), and diastole. The examiner then should listen carefully for each and every type of sound and murmur possible, concentrating so hard on the sound or murmur in question that nothing else is heard. This technique is called "dissection" and is done at each location over the precordium.

The 1st sound, caused by AV valve closure (Fig. 13–2), is best heard at the lower left sternal border or apex. It may be split, with the second component soft and best recognized at the lower left sternal border. The second heart sound, produced by semilunar valve closure, is best heard at the 2nd intercostal space. During inspiration, filling of the right heart is increased and the right ventricular ejection time is increased, resulting in wider splitting of the aortic and pulmonic components of the 2nd heart sound in inspiration than in expiration. Widening of the splitting is seen with right ventricular volume overload, as occurs in an atrial septal defect (ASD) as well as in pulmonic stenosis or right bundle-branch block. The pulmonary component of the 2nd heart sound is accentuated when the pulmonary artery pressure is increased, and it is decreased in intensity when low pulmonary artery diastolic pressure is present, as in pulmonary stenosis. The higher the pulmonary artery diastolic pressure, the earlier is the closure of the pulmonic valve. Therefore, when pulmonary hypertension is present, the split is narrow or may be absent. It is obviously single in the presence of pulmonic or aortic valve atresia. In aortic stenosis, left ventricular systole may be prolonged enough to delay aortic valve closure, causing a narrow split, a single S_2, or even a paradoxic split. Advanced left bundle-branch block also may cause a paradoxic split. The 4th heart sound (Fig. 13–2) is best heard with the stethoscope bell at the apex of the heart one third into diastole, but a right ventricular 3rd sound is best heard at the lower left sternal border. A 4th heart sound (Fig. 13–2) just before the 1st heart sound, best heard at the 3rd or 4th interspace, may be a sign of poor ventricular compliance.

Ejection clicks are heard early in systole and are related to dilation of the ascending aorta or pulmonary artery. Pulmonary ejection clicks are heard best at the upper left sternal border and may occur as much as 0.08 sec after the 1st sound; they also may be much closer, even simultaneous with the first sound. They are louder on expiration and may disappear on inspiration. Because S_1 normally is soft at the upper left sternal border, an apparent S_1 that is loud at the upper left sternal border, especially on expiration, is a clue that the sound is a pulmonary ejection click, not S_1. Valvular pulmonic stenosis almost always is associated with a pulmonary ejection click, and pulmonary vascular

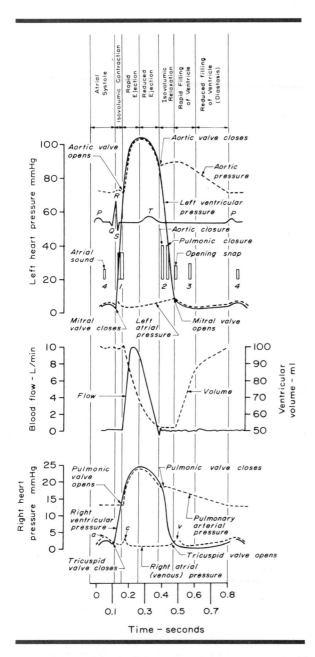

Figure 13–2. Idealized diagram of temporal events of a cardiac cycle. (From Behrman RE (ed): Nelson Textbook of Pediatrics. 14th ed. Philadelphia, WB Saunders, 1992, p 1131.)

aortic valve, valvular aortic stenosis, truncus arteriosus, and tetralogy of Fallot with pulmonary atresia.

Murmurs usually are described with regard to their intensity, timing, and pitch. The intensity of systolic murmurs is classified on a scale of 1–6. A grade 1 murmur is soft and heard with difficulty, especially when of low pitch; grade 2 is easily heard; grade 3 is louder but not associated with a thrill; grade 4 is loud and associated with a precordial thrill; grade 5 is audible with only the edge of the stethoscope on the chest; and grade 6 is very loud and audible with the stethoscope not on the chest or with the naked ear. It is important to relate the murmurs to S_1 and S_2 and to describe their length.

Systolic ejection murmurs (Fig. 13–3) typically are associated with obstruction to flow through abnormal semilunar valves or increased flow through normal semilunar valves. They begin after isovolemic contraction, about 0.08 sec after the 1st heart sound. **Regurgitant murmurs**, in contrast, typically seen with a VSD with left-to-right shunt or mitral regurgitation, vary in length and timing. With a VSD, S_1 typically is obscured, whereas in mitral regurgitation, the murmur peaks late in systole, usually with S_1 heard. Ejection murmurs tend to have a crescendo and decrescendo (diamond) shape. Regurgitant murmurs may continue at the same intensity throughout systole, may be decrescendo, may peak late, or may even be of diamond shape. A late systolic murmur, usually crescendo, beginning after a mid-systolic nonejection click, frequently is heard with mitral valve prolapse, indicating mitral regurgitation.

Diastolic murmurs (Fig. 13–3) are heard when regurgitation occurs across the semilunar valves or when stenosis of the AV valves is present. The murmur of aortic regurgitation usually is very high pitched, decrescendo beginning with the 2nd heart sound, and located along the left sternal border. Pulmonary regurgitation also begins with the 2nd heart sound but is usually of a lower pitch, unless pulmonary hypertension is present, in which case it sounds very much like aortic regurgitation. Stenotic murmurs across the AV valves usually are mid-diastolic and rumbling (very low pitch); the murmur of mitral stenosis occurs at the apex and that of tricuspid stenosis occurs along the lower left sternal border. Murmurs of relative stenosis with anatomically normal AV valves may be associated with an ASD or with high flow across either the tricuspid valve or the mitral valve; these murmurs occur in children with large left-to-right shunts at the level of either the ventricular or the great artery.

disease frequently is associated with the condition. Aortic ejection clicks, in contrast, usually are well separated from the 1st sound, do not vary in intensity with respiration, and usually are heard best at the apex (occasionally the lower left sternal border). They usually are associated with a bicuspid

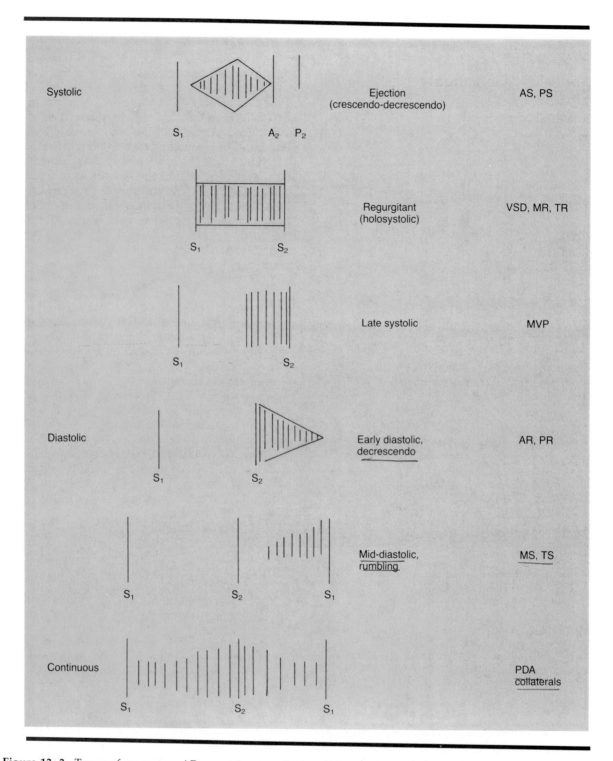

Figure 13–3. Types of murmurs. AR = aortic regurgitation; AS = aortic stenosis; MR = mitral regurgitation; MS = mitral stenosis; MVP = mitral valve prolapse; PDA = patent ductus arteriosus; PR = pulmonary regurgitation; PS = pulmonary stenosis; TS = tricuspid stenosis; VSD = ventricular septal defect.

Continuous murmurs beginning after S_1 usually peak in intensity near the end of systole and decrease in intensity a variable time into diastole. This murmur is characteristic of a persistent PDA after the newborn period. The murmur is loudest under the left clavicle and frequently is very harsh and uneven in systole. Other causes of continuous murmurs have been noted, such as cerebral AV fistula, aorticopulmonary collateral vessels, and aorticopulmonary shunts. These latter continuous murmurs tend to be of similar pitch in both systole and diastole, and they have a higher pitch than that of the PDA murmur.

A variety of normal murmurs may be heard throughout childhood. The most common is the **vibratory systolic ejection murmur** or Still murmur. This left lower sternal border ejection systolic murmur is heard most frequently in preschool-age children but also can be heard in children near the age of puberty. The murmur rarely is louder than grade 2 or 3, usually lasts about two thirds the length of systole, is heard well in the neck, and rarely is heard in the back. It is believed to originate in the root of the aorta, where everyone of all ages has a normal ejection systolic murmur. Still murmur decreases with the Valsalva maneuver. Also, a systolic murmur in the root of the pulmonary artery is present, projected onto the chest as the most common normal murmur in adolescents and adults (the normal pulmonary ejection murmur). Another type of common benign murmur is the **venous hum** heard at the right upper or, less commonly, left upper sternal border with particular radiation into the neck. This continuous, medium-pitched murmur disappears when the patient is placed in a supine position, when the jugular vein is compressed, or when the patient looks sharply to the left.

Newborns rarely have any of the aforementioned normal murmurs. For reasons not completely clear the **patent ductus arteriosus murmur**, present because the baby is premature and/or has a low P_{O_2} from lung disease, often does not sound like that of the congenital patent ductus, which becomes manifest weeks later. The newborn's PDA murmur is usually a nondescript soft systolic murmur. Another common normal murmur in newborns, often lasting 6 mo or more, is the **peripheral pulmonic stenosis murmur**; it is present because of a normal sharp angle between the main pulmonary artery and each branch. Characteristically, the murmurs are heard at the 1st or 2nd intercostal spaces, both left and right, with transmission to each axilla and to the back. Frequently, the murmurs are louder in the back than in the front.

Chest Roentgenogram

The chest roentgenogram can provide a very good estimate of the size of the heart and the size and position of the aorta and pulmonary artery (Fig. 13–4). Frequently, clues to specific cardiac anomalies also are present.

If the roentgenogram has been obtained during maximal inspiration, the cardiothoracic ratio should be less than 55% in infants under 1 yr and less than 50% in older children and adolescents. Interpretation of specific ventricular chamber enlargement is unreliable, but right atrial and left atrial enlargement frequently can be recognized.

Cardiac enlargement can be seen with any lesion that causes increased volume load to the heart or can be secondary to the presence of myocardial dysfunction. The normal large pulmonary arteries are seen in the central one third of the lung fields, with smaller vessels seen in the middle third and no pulmonary vessels seen in the lateral third of the lung fields. In the presence of a large left-to-right shunt (VSD, PDA, truncus arteriosus, or single ventricle without pulmonary stenosis), the increased pulmonary vasculature allows visualization of medium-sized vessels in the middle third and small vessels, frequently end on, in the most lateral third of the lung fields. Conversely, congenital cardiac lesions that are associated with a right-to-left shunt, where blood destined for the pulmonary circulation is diverted into the systemic circulation, result in diminished pulmonary blood flow, which can be seen as a reduction in size of pulmonary arteries in the middle third of the lung fields.

Elevated pulmonary venous pressure secondary to left-sided congestive heart failure or obstructed pulmonary venous return, as occurs in newborns with total anomalous pulmonary venous connection, results in increased lung water. In the older child, this increase in lung water results in prominence of the pulmonary veins and redistribution of pulmonary flow so that the upper lobe pulmonary arteries are fuller than the lower lobe vessels. In the infant and neonate, however, these signs are absent, and the usual pattern is a diffuse haziness resulting from increased alveolar water.

Certain other signs on the chest roentgenogram may be helpful in the diagnosis of heart disease. For example, **rib notching**, an indentation on the underside of the ribs, may be seen in older children with coarctation of the aorta as a result of large and tortuous intercostal arteries, or in children with tetralogy with pulmonary atresia when collateral vessels from the aorta to the intraparenchymal pulmonary arteries provide pulmonary blood flow.

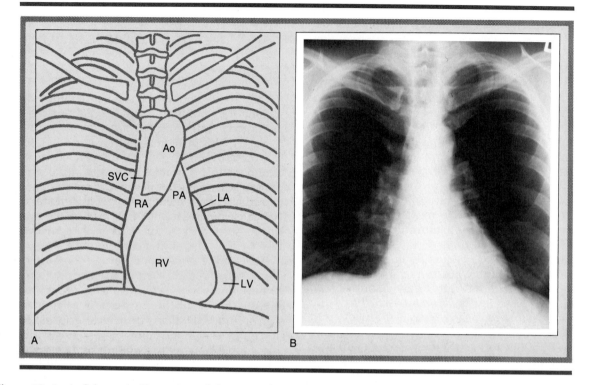

Figure 13–4. *A*, Schematic illustration of the parts of the heart whose outlines can be identified on a routine chest roentgenogram (*B*). Ao = Aorta; SVC = superior vena cava; RA = right atrium; PA = pulmonary artery; LA = left atrium; RV = right ventricle; LV = left ventricle. *B*, Routine posteroanterior roentgenogram of the normal cardiac silhouette. (From Andreoli TE, Carpenter CCJ, Plum F, et al: Cecil Essentials of Medicine. Philadelphia, WB Saunders, 1986, p 22.)

Electrocardiography

The standard 12-lead electrocardiogram (ECG) is a recording of the electrical activity from cardiac muscle cells onto each lead on the surface of the torso. The ECG is a useful screening test when used along with the chest roentgenogram and a careful physical examination. The ECG also provides insight into the metabolic state of the cardiac cell (e.g., hyperkalemia). Two children with serum potassium levels of 7.0 mEq/L may have different ECGs. One may be normal while the other may have tall peaked T waves, indicating a significant problem. The serum potassium level only reflects what is in the serum. The ECG reflects the state of the cell membrane and may be reflecting both intracellular and extracellular potassium, thus identifying the child in difficulty.

Analysis of the ECG includes the rate, rhythm, P wave, P-R interval, QRS complex, Q-T interval, and ST segment (Fig. 13–5). (Assessment of the rhythm is discussed later in the chapter.)

The **P wave** represents atrial depolarization (see Figs. 13–2 and 13–5). The first part of the P wave is due to right atrial depolarization. The best crite- rion for right atrial enlargement is an increase of the amplitude of the P wave, as is reflected best in lead II. Left atrial enlargement is best diagnosed by prolongation of the second portion of the P wave, as usually is exhibited best in the left chest leads.

The P-R interval is measured from the beginning of the P wave to the beginning of the QRS complex and represents the time it takes for electricity to travel from the high right atrium to the ventricular myocardium (Figs. 13–2 and 13–5). The greatest time is spent in the AV node. The P-R interval increases with age. The conduction time is shortened when conduction velocity is increased, as in glycogen storage disease, or when the AV node is bypassed, as in the Wolff-Parkinson-White syndrome. A prolonged P-R interval usually indicates prolonged conduction through the AV node, but disease in the atrial myocardium, bundle of His, or Purkinje system could contribute to this abnormality.

The **QRS complex** represents ventricular depolarization. Unlike the atrium, right and left ventricular activation begins virtually simultaneously in the right and left septa, halfway to two thirds

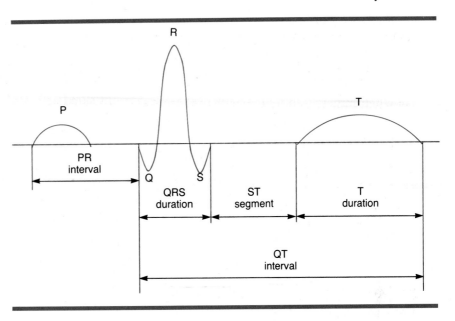

Figure 13–5. Nomenclature of electrocardiogram waves and intervals.

down, as well as in the contiguous left ventricular free wall and right ventricular endocardium. In order to interpret the ventricular ECG properly, it is necessary to understand a number of major concepts:

1. A sequence of activation is present, so that what is being depolarized (and when) must be known.
2. A greater volume of the ventricle causes greater magnitude, as does a greater mass of right or left ventricular muscle.
3. Proximity of the right ventricular wall to the chest surface accentuates that ventricle's contribution.
4. Continued changes occur in the normal ECG with time, beginning with that of the premature or full-term infant and continuing throughout childhood. The spatial magnitudes are very low in the premature infant, become higher in the full-term infant, rise sharply until age 2–3 mo, stabilize until puberty, and then decrease throughout life.
5. Normative data for each age group must be known to make diagnoses.

In the fetus and full-term newborn, the right and left ventricular masses are approximately equal, although the right ventricle may be up to one third thicker. In the premature infant compared with the full-term infant, less right ventricular dominance is exhibited. By the age of 3–6 mo, the left ventricular mass is about twice that of the right ventricle, and, when the child reaches school age, the ratio is similar to that of the adult, about 2.5:1 in favor of the left ventricle.

The **Q-T interval** is measured from the beginning of the QRS complex to the end of the T wave (see Fig. 13–5). The corrected Q-T interval (corrected for rate) should be less than 0.45 sec. It may be prolonged in children with hypocalcemia or hypokalemia (although the latter may be a Q-U interval). It also is prolonged in a group of children at risk for severe ventricular arrhythmias and sudden death (i.e., the prolonged QT syndrome); drugs such as quinidine also may prolong the Q-T interval.

Echocardiography and Doppler Ultrasonography

In the past decade, echocardiography especially with Doppler and color flow ultrasonography, has become the most important noninvasive tool for the evaluation of congenital and acquired heart disease. It is particularly useful in complex disease. The two-dimensional echocardiogram allows visualization of spatial relationships of the cardiac structures in the beating heart. Anatomic details previously requiring angiography are now easily visualized noninvasively, with little or no risk to the patient. Analysis of valve structure and function often is superior to that obtained by angiogram.

Doppler echocardiography is an adaptation of ultrasound that displays flow in cardiac chambers and vascular structures. The change in frequency imparted to sound waves caused by moving blood can be used to predict cardiac output, valve and orifice pressure gradients, and directionality of flow within structures.

Color flow Doppler encodes the flow direction and velocity in color on the two-dimensional image, allowing easy detection of small septal defects and valve regurgitation.

Cardiac Catheterization and Angiography

Catheterization is indicated for most infants who are cyanotic or in significant congestive heart failure when the etiology is not completely understood or when surgery is indicated, with the exception of some of the simpler forms of heart disease (PDA, ASD, or coarctation of the aorta), in which the physical examination, aided by noninvasive testing, makes the diagnosis obvious. Catheterization also may be appropriate when heart surgery is being considered in children with potentially progressive lesions that require careful physiologic monitoring, such as the infant with a large VSD, aortic stenosis, or various lesions that include pulmonary hypertension. Finally, certain treatments require the use of catheterization, such as balloon catheter dilation of pulmonary or aortic valve stenosis, or of peripheral pulmonary stenosis. Cathe-

terization also may be used for occlusion of PDA, ASDs, and aorticopulmonary collateral vessels, using appropriate new interventional devices.

Access to the vascular system is usually by percutaneous femoral vein catheterization, with the right-sided chambers entered sequentially. The presence of a patent foramen ovale, especially in infants, frequently allows entrance to the left side of the heart. The left side of the heart also can be entered by a transeptal technique or via retrograde arterial catheterization.

Catheterization data include evaluation of the course of the catheter compared with normal, analysis of the oxygen saturation, analysis of the pressures in cardiac structures and blood vessels, various calculations derived from the aforementioned data, and the findings on cineangiography. The normal values are shown in Figure 13–6. The oxygen saturation of the entire right side of the heart

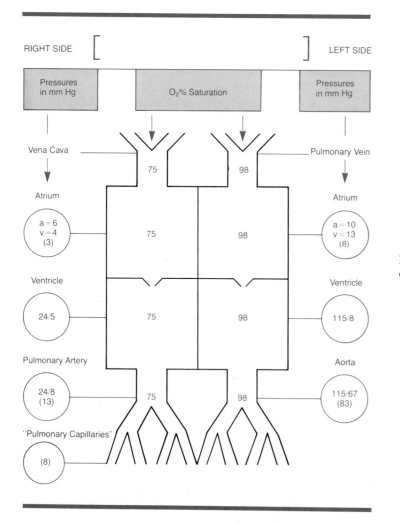

Figure 13–6. Normal data from cardiac catheterization.

reflects the mixed venous saturation and is normally 70–75%; a significant increase in oxygen saturation in a chamber or vessel on the right side indicates a *left-to-right shunt*. The left side of the heart should have a saturation of above 95%; significant decreases below the pulmonary veins suggest the presence of a *right-to-left shunt* resulting from systemic venous blood entering the left side of the heart. A decreased pulmonary venous saturation may be due to hypoventilation, pulmonary disease, or pulmonary venous congestion.

The pressures should be measured in all chambers and vessels entered. Normally, the systolic pressure in the ventricle is equal to the systolic pressure in the great arteries, and the end-diastolic pressure in the atria is equal to the end-diastolic pressure in the ventricle. If a "gradient" in pressure exists, it suggests obstruction across the valve. Analysis of the severity of the obstruction requires measurement of both the pressure gradient and the flow across that valve.

Systemic and pulmonary outputs can be measured by the Fick equation, with the cardiac output being equal to the measured oxygen consumption divided by the arteriovenous oxygen content differences between the systemic and pulmonary circulations. The pulmonary-to-systemic flow ratio can be measured by the ratio between the pulmonary and systemic arteriovenous differences, because the same oxygen consumption is in the numerator for both calculations.

Evaluation of the anatomy and physiology of the patient rarely is complete without selective angiocardiograms using a biplane system. Contrast material (approximately 1 mL/kg) is injected rapidly into the cardiac chambers or vessels.

Exercise Testing

Evaluation of the cardiovascular system normally is done at rest. However, information on cardiac reserve and the adaptation of the normal or abnormal heart to exercise can provide important data on the cardiac status that more closely approximates everyday living.

References

Behrman RE (ed): Nelson Textbook of Pediatrics. 14th ed. Philadelphia, WB Saunders, 1992, Sec. 15.1–15.10.

Braden DS, Strong WF: Cardiovascular responses to exercise in children. Am J Dis Child 144:1255, 1990.

Colan SD: Quantitative applications of Doppler cardiography in congenital heart disease. Cardiovasc Intervent Radiol 10:332, 1987.

Davignon A, Rautaharju P, Boisselle E, et al: Normal ECG standards for infants and children. Pediatr Cardiol 1:123, 1979/80.

Higgins CB, et al: Magnetic resonance imagining in patients with congenital heart disease. Circulation 70:851, 1984.

Liebman J: Diagnosis and management of heart murmurs in children. Pediatr Rev 3:321, 1982.

Rosenthal A: How to distinguish between innocent and pathologic murmurs in childhood. Pediatr Clin North Am 31:1229, 1984.

Seward JB, Tajik AJ, Edwards WD, et al: Two-Dimensional Echocardiographic Atlas. I: Congenital Heart Disease. New York, Springer-Verlag, 1987.

Sherman F, Sahn D: Pediatric Doppler echocardiography 1987: Major advances in technology. J Pediatr 110:333, 1987.

Wheller JJ, Reiss R, Allen HD: Clinical experience with fetal echocardiography. Am J Dis Child 144:49, 1990.

Wiles HB: Imaging congenital heart disease. Pediatr Clin North Am 37:115, 1990.

PRENATAL AND NEONATAL CIRCULATION

See Chapter 6.

MYOCARDIAL FUNCTION AND HEART FAILURE

Myofibril contraction is summated and translated into cardiac work or pump performance. The force generated by the muscle fiber depends on its contractile status and its basal length, which is equivalent to the preload as noted in the normal Starling curve of Figure 13–7. As the preload (fiber length, left ventricular filling pressure or volume) increases, the myocardial performance (stroke volume, wall tension) increases up to a point. The relationship is the ventricular function curve; alterations in the contractile state of the muscle lower the relative position of the curve but retain the fiber length–to–muscle work relationship. Heart rate is another important determinant of cardiac work, because the cardiac output equals stroke volume times the heart rate. Additional factors that affect cardiac performance are noted in Table 13–3.

Heart failure results when the cardiac output does not meet the metabolic needs (in terms of oxygen delivery and other factors) of the body. The term "congestive" heart failure refers to increased venous pressure in the pulmonary (left heart failure) or the systemic (right heart failure) veins. Myofibrilar failure is the result of a decline of the myofibril contractility as noted by a shift of the normal Starling curve (Fig. 13–7). The compensatory

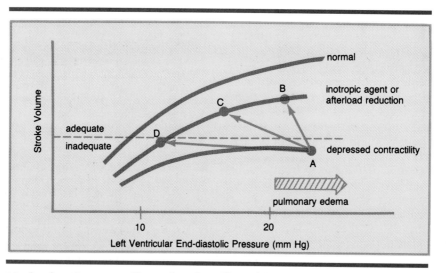

Figure 13–7. Ventricular function curve illustrating the effect of inotropic agents or arterial vasodilators. Unlike diuretics, the effect of digitalis or arterial vasodilator therapy in a patient with heart failure is to move onto another ventricular function curve intermediate between the normal and depressed curves. When the patient's ventricular function moves from A to B by the administration of one of these agents, the left ventricular end-diastolic pressure also may decrease because of improved cardiac function; further administration of diuretics or venodilators may shift the function further to the left along the same curve from B to C and eliminate the risk of pulmonary edema. A vasodilating agent that has both arteriolar and venous dilating properties (e.g., nitroprusside) would shift this function directly from A to C. If this agent shifts the function from A to D because of excessive venodilation or administration of diuretics, the cardiac output may fall too low, even though the left ventricular end-diastolic pressure would be normal (10 mm Hg) for a normal heart. Thus, left ventricular end-diastolic pressures of between 15 and 18 mm are usually optimal in the failing heart to maximize cardiac output but to avoid pulmonary edema. (From Andreoli TE, Carpenter CCJ, Plum F, et al: Cecil Essentials of Medicine. Philadelphia, WB Saunders, 1986, p 39.)

Table 13–3. Factors Affecting Cardiac Performance

Preload (left ventricular diastolic volume)	Total blood volume Venous tone (sympathetic tone) Body position Intrathoracic and intrapericardial pressure Atrial contraction Pumping action of skeletal muscle	**Contractility** (cardiac performance independent of preload or afterload)	Sympathetic nerve impulses Circulating catecholamines Digitalis, calcium, other inotropic agents Increased heart rate or postextrasystolic augmentation	} increased contractility
Afterload (impedance against which the left ventricle must eject blood)	Peripheral vascular resistance Left ventricular volume (preload, wall tension) Physical characteristics of the arterial tree (for example, elasticity of vessels or presence of outflow obstruction)		Anoxia, acidosis Pharmacologic depression Loss of myocardium Intrinsic depression	} decreased contractility
		Heart Rate	Autonomic nervous system Temperature, metabolic rate	

(From Andreoli TE, Carpenter CCJ, Plum F, et al: Cecil Essentials of Medicine. Philadelphia, WB Saunders, 1986, p 7.)

Table 13–4. Compensatory Mechanisms in Heart Failure

Mechanism	Favorable Effects	Unfavorable Effects
↑ Sympathetic activity	↑ Heart rate ↑ Contractility ↑ Venoconstriction → ↑ venous return (preload)	↑ Arteriolar constriction → ↑ afterload ↑ O_2 requirements
Cardiac hypertrophy	↑ Working muscle mass	↑ Wall tension ↓ Coronary flow ↑ O_2 requirements Abnormal systolic and diastolic properties of hypertrophic muscle

Frank-Starling mechanism	↑ Stroke volume for any given amount
	of venous return
		Pulmonary and systemic congestion:
		  ↑ LV size → ↑ wall tension and O_2
		  requirements

Renal salt and water retention	↑ Venous return	Pulmonary and systemic congestion:
		  ↑ renin–angiotension →
		  ↑ vasoconstriction (afterload)

Increased peripheral O_2 extraction	↑ O_2 delivery per unit cardiac output	

(From Andreoli TE, Carpenter CCJ, Plum F, et al: Cecil Essentials of Medicine. Philadelphia, WB Saunders, 1986, p 34.)

Table 13–5. Etiology of Heart Failure

Fetus
Severe anemia (hemolysis, fetal–maternal transfusion,
  hypoplastic anemia)
Supraventricular tachycardia
Ventricular tachycardia
Complete heart block
Congenital cardiac defects

Premature Neonate
Fluid overload
PDA
VSD
Cor pulmonale (BPD)

Full-Term Neonate
Asphyxial cardiomyopathy
Arteriovenous malformation (vein of Galen, hepatic)
Left-sided obstructive lesions (coarctation of aorta, hypo-
  plastic left heart)
Transposition of great arteries
Large mixing cardiac defects (single ventricle, truncus
  arteriosus)
Viral myocarditis

Infant–Toddler
Left-to-right cardiac shunts (VSD)
Hemangioma (arteriovenous malformation)
Anomalous left coronary artery
Metabolic cardiomyopathy
Acute hypertension (hemolytic–uremic syndrome)
Supraventricular tachycardia
Kawasaki disease

Child–Adolescent
Rheumatic fever
Acute hypertension (glomerulonephritis)
Viral myocarditis
Thyrotoxicosis
Hemochromatosis–hemosiderosis
Cancer therapy (radiation, adriamycin)
Sickle cell anemia
Endocarditis
Cor pulmonale (cystic fibrosis)
Arrhythmias
Chronic upper airway obstruction (cor pulmonale)

BPD = bronchopulmonary dysplasia.

Table 13–6. Treatment of Heart Failure

Therapy	Mechanism
General Care	
Rest	Reduces cardiac output
Oxygen	Improves oxygenation in presence of pulmonary edema
Sodium, fluid restrictions	Decreases vascular congestion; decreases preload
Diuretics	
Furosemide	Salt excretion by ascending loop of Henle; reduces preload; afterload reduced if hypertension improves; also may cause venodilation
Combination of distal tubule and loop diuretics	Greater sodium excretion
Inotropic Agents	
Digitalis	Inhibits membrane Na^+, K^+-ATPase and increases intracellular Ca^{2+}, improves cardiac contractility, increases myocardial oxygen consumption
Dopamine	Releases myocardial norepinephrine plus direct effect on beta receptor, may increase systemic blood pressure; at low infusion rates, dilates renal artery, facilitating diuresis
Dobutamine	Beta (β_1)-receptor agent; often combined with dopamine
Amrinone	Nonsympathomimetic, noncardiac glycosides with inotropic effects; also may produce vasodilation
Afterload reduction	
Hydralazine	Arteriolar vasodilator
Nitroprusside	Arterial and venous relaxation; venodilation reduces preload
Prazosin	Oral alpha-adrenergic blocking agent; arterial and venous dilator; venodilation reduces preload
Captopril/enalapril	Inhibition of angiotensin-coverting enzyme; reduces angiotensin II production

mechanisms used to improve cardiac output include augmented endogenous sympathetic activity (increases inotropy, chronotropy) and the response of the kidney to a perceived reduction of effective plasma volume, leading to salt and water retention. These compensatory mechanisms have beneficial and adverse effects (Table 13–4).

The *etiology* of heart failure is different in various stages of development (Table 13–5). Fetal causes of heart failure include arrhythmias (supraventricular tachycardia, heart block) or severe anemia secondary to hemolysis or blood loss. In the neonate, congenital heart disease, arteriovenous malformations, cardiomyopathy, and myocarditis are common causes of heart failure, whereas in the older child, myocarditis, acute hypertension (glomerulonephritis, hemolytic–uremic syndrome), and rheumatic fever are important causes of heart failure.

The *treatment* of heart failure is directed toward improving myocardial contractility, preload, and reducing afterload (Table 13–6, Fig. 13–7).

References

Behrman RE (ed): Nelson Textbook of Pediatrics. 14th ed. Philadelphia, WB Saunders, 1992, Sec. 15.73.

Friedman WF, George BL: New concepts and drugs in the treatment of congestive heart failure. Pediatr Clin North Am 31:1197, 1984.

Goldenberg I, Cohn J: New inotropic drugs for heart failure. JAMA 258:493, 1987.

Park M: Use of digoxin in infants and children with specific emphasis on dosage. J Pediatr 108:871, 1986.

Schneeweiss A: Cardiovascular drugs in children: Angiotension-converting enzyme inhibitors. Pediatr Cardiol 9: 109, 1989.

CONGENITAL HEART DISEASE

Epidemiology

Congenital heart disease affects 8:1000 births. If congenital dysrhythmias such as Wolff-Parkinson-White syndrome are included, the ratio would be 1:100. Most of these lesions occur between 18 and 50 days of gestation. At birth, VSD is the most common lesion, followed in order of decreasing frequency by transposition of the great arteries, tetralogy of Fallot, coarctation of the aorta, hypoplastic left heart syndrome, PDA, endocardial cushion defects, and heterotaxias (dextrocardia). The remaining individual lesions each represent 1–4% of congenital heart defects. Most affected neonates are full-term, appropriately grown infants of normal pregnancies.

Approximately 30% of infants with heart lesions have extracardiac malformations that also affect their morbidity and mortality (see Table 13–1). Most cases of congenital heart disease (90%) are not associated with identifiable teratogens or single-gene defects. A small number are associated with teratogens, such as congenital rubella or fetal alcohol syndrome, whereas others may be associated with gross chromosomal disorders (chromosomal deletions, trisomy), congenital anomaly syndromes (VATER, CHARGE), or maternal metabolic disorders (phenylketonuria diabetes).

The *inheritance* in most patients is multifactorial (polygenetic). The recurrence risk for congenital heart disease in the sibling of an affected infant varies from 2% to 4%. The risk is greater for the child of a parent with congenital heart disease; in this case, the risk increases to 4–5%.

Heart Disease Resulting from Abnormal Embryonic Development

The heart begins to develop in the very early embryo and circulates blood by the 3rd wk. The initial heart is a straight tube without valves. Because the heart tube grows faster than the organs around it, it loops. Abnormal looping results in abnormal cardiac position, such as dextrocardia, or other anomalies, such as congenitally corrected transposition. When a major abnormality occurs, such as looping in the wrong direction, usually, but not always, one or several smaller abnormalities occur, such as a ventricular septal defect (VSD). As the heart divides itself into four chambers and as valves develop, many other abnormalities may occur. Sometimes there is a single defect (*d*-transposition of the great arteries) and sometimes there are multiple defects (tetralogy of Fallot). Even a single defect such as transposition can be devastating after birth while having little or no effect antenatally. Conversely, some defects cause fetal death. In addition, one defect can cause another defect by altering blood flow in the fetus. Many fetuses with severe congenital cardiac defects die before birth. It is now also more clearly understood that some defects occur quite late, even in the 3rd trimester of pregnancy. Fetal cardiac diseases also may be iatrogenic. For example, maternal treatment to prevent premature labor may prematurely close the ductus arteriosus, resulting in right ventricular failure. Premature closure of the foramen ovale also can lead to the hypoplastic left heart syndrome.

ABNORMAL DEVELOPMENT OF VENOUS AND ARTERIAL SYSTEMS

The development of the venous and arterial systems in the fetus is as complex or perhaps more so than that of the cardiac chambers themselves. The single mature aorta and aortic arch develop from multiple paired aortic arches. Abnormalities in their development, such as a complete interruption of the aorta, may occur at any one of a number of sites. The fact that genetics play a great role in development is underscored by the marked difference in the incidence and site of aortic arch interruption in patients of Chinese or Japanese ancestry versus Caucasians or Filipinos. The influence of fetal hemodynamics on the development of congenital cardiovascular defects is shown by the fact that coarctation of the aorta and interruption of the aortic arch are associated with "upstream lesions" such as aortic or mitral stenosis or certain VSDs that cause less aortic blood flow.

An understanding of *fetal blood flow*, therefore, is critical to an understanding of fetal and neonatal physiology and the development of congenital cardiovascular defects. The fetus has no way to oxygenate blood or obtain nutrients on its own. It is dependent on placental blood flow. The fetus receives oxygenated, nutrient-loaded blood by way of the umbilical vein. This blood joins with the inferior cava blood and hepatic venous blood to enter the right atrium. It is preferentially but not exclusively shunted across the foramen ovale to the left atrium, the left ventricle, and out the aorta to the upper body and brain. The superior vena cava blood is preferentially but not exclusively directed to the right ventricle, the pulmonary artery, and through the ductus arteriosus to the lower half of the body and the umbilical arteries to the placenta. Only a small amount of blood perfuses the lungs during fetal life.

Fetal cardiovascular physiology explains why certain devastating defects such as transposition of the great arteries have no effect on the fetus. The same quantity of blood with a similar oxygen and nutrient concentration will reach the same organs at the same pressure no matter what chambers and vessels it passes through. An anomalous left coronary artery from the pulmonary artery will have the same pressure and a similar oxygen concentration in utero but a markedly lower pressure and lower oxygen saturation shortly after birth. In this situation, the fetal heart does not infarct but the neonatal or infant heart usually does. One congenital heart defect also can protect the neonate from the effects of another. In the infant with a large

VSD as well as an anomalous left coronary artery, the increased pressure and oxygen content in the pulmonary artery resulting from the VSD perfuses the myocardium with high-pressure oxygenated blood. If the pulmonary artery resistance drops, or if the VSD spontaneously closes or is closed surgically, the coronary artery perfusion pressure drops and an infarct results.

At birth and shortly afterward, major changes in the circulation occur. The manifestation of congenital cardiovascular defects and their timing are dependent on these changes. The umbilical venous and arterial flows are obliterated immediately at birth. The pulmonary blood flow must increase immediately and support the entire organism. It is aided in doing this by the expansion of the lungs, which greatly reduces resistance to pulmonary blood flow. Systemic vascular resistance increases as a result of loss of the low-resistance placental circuit.

Sometimes, because of lung problems such as meconium aspiration, the pulmonary vascular resistance does not decrease. The fetal circulatory pathways may persist in part. Right-to-left shunting may continue to occur at the ductus arteriosus and/or foramen ovale level, resulting in extreme cyanosis. Persistent increase in pulmonary vascular resistance may severely compromise infants with congenital cardiac defects as well. Those with anatomic defects that usually would allow a left-to-right shunt will have a large right-to-left shunt. Those with an anatomically tenuous pulmonary blood flow may have an even further diminished flow. Early aggressive management of this physiology may reverse it and/or prevent its progression.

ABNORMAL POSITIONS OF THE HEART

The location of the heart within the chest may be quite abnormal and the relationships of the chambers may be very confusing. A systematic classification (by Van Praagh) simplifies analysis. In this classification, the heart may be in the right chest (dextrocardia) or in the left chest (levocardia). The cardiac chambers are described in terms of their relationship to each other. The atrium may be *solitus,* with the right atrium to the right of the left atrium; *inversus,* with the anatomic right atrium to the left of the anatomic left atrium; or *ambiguous,* when abnormalities of systemic and pulmonary venous return make identification of the two atrial chambers impossible. The ventricles may be in their normal position (*d*) with the right ventricle to the right of the left ventricle, or they may be positioned with the anatomic right ventricle to the left of the anatomic left ventricle (*l*). The great arter-

ies may be normally related, with the pulmonary artery anterior to and to the left of the aorta; *d*-transposed, with the aorta anterior to but still to the right of the pulmonary artery; or *l*-transposed, if the aorta is anterior to and to the left of the pulmonary artery.

Classification of Congenital Cardiac Defects

Congenital cardiac defects can be classified into four groups based on their physiology (Table 13–7). Obviously this classification is an oversimplification and many variations occur. Also, the severity of each lesion is extremely variable. The timing and nature of a patient's clinical presentation are controlled by the physiology of the lesions. In each case, however, there are modifiers. An example is the size of the foramen ovale in complete *d* transposition of the great arteries. Transposition presents early with cyanosis and tachypnea, but a very small foramen ovale makes it present even earlier.

The simplest lesions are the stenoses, in which usually only one valve or artery is stenotic. In children it is usually the aortic or pulmonic valve, although the mitral and tricuspid valves, rarely, can be stenotic. Valve stenosis usually is isolated, although syndromes such as Shone syndrome of multiple left heart obstruction occur uncommonly. The right-to-left shunt lesion involves much more complex anatomy and physiology. In most cases there must also be a left-to-right shunt, which occurs as a simple defect in the septae or arterial walls. Because pulmonary vascular resistance is high at birth, neonates with congenital cardiac defects may have no shunting and thus no physical findings. The "mixing" lesions are those in which there are both right-to-left and left-to-right shunts

Table 13–7. Classification of Congenital Cardiac Defects

	Shunting		
Stenotic	*Right → Left*	*Left → Right*	Mixing
Aortic stenosis	Tetralogy	PDA	Truncus
Pulmonic stenosis	Transposition	VSD	TAPVR
Coarctation of the aorta	Tricuspid atresia	ASD	HLH

HLH = hypoplastic left heart syndrome; TAPVR = total anomalous pulmonary venous return.

without significant stenosis, resulting in an arterial saturation in the upper 80th percentile.

Hemodynamic Measurements

Representative oxygen saturations and pressures from catheterization of a child are presented in Figure 13–6. The formulas for calculating pulmonary and systemic *cardiac outputs* are

Pulmonary output
$$= \frac{O_2 \text{ consumption in (mL/min)}}{\text{pulmonary arteriovenous difference (mL/L)}}$$

and

systemic output
$$= \frac{O_2 \text{ consumption (mL/L)}}{\text{systemic arteriovenous difference (mL/L)}}$$

where pulmonary arteriovenous difference = pulmonary vein − pulmonary artery oxygen content and systemic arteriovenous difference = systemic artery − mixed venous oxygen content.

Because cardiac output increases with the size of the child, it is related to the patient's surface area in meters. For the resting child, normal cardiac output is about 4 L/min/m². In the absence of cardiac failure, the body's homeostatic mechanisms tend to keep the systemic output near normal, whatever the congenital defect. In the presence of heart failure, the systemic output usually is lowered.

The cardiac outputs and pressures in each side of the heart are critically related to each other. Thus, an elevated systolic pressure of 60 mm Hg in the pulmonary artery in the presence of a VSD is indicative of a greater degree of pulmonary hypertension when the aortic pressure is 90 mm Hg systolic than when the aortic pressure is 120 mm Hg. In the former case, pulmonary hypertension is said to be at two thirds of the systemic level, whereas in the latter, it is one half of the systemic level. When the pressure in the pulmonary artery is equal to that in the aorta, we refer to it as "systemic level" pulmonary hypertension, and when it is higher than that of the aorta it is characterized as suprasystemic pulmonary artery pressure.

A calculation of *systemic (SVR) and pulmonary vascular resistance (PVR)* also can be made. These are the resistances to flow across the resistance vessels, which are mainly small muscular arteries and arterioles. This requires knowledge of the pressures on each side of these resistance vessels. On the systemic side, ΔP is systemic artery pressure (P_{sa}) − right atrial pressure (P_{ra}). On the pulmonary side, ΔP is pulmonary artery pressure (P_{pa}) − left atrial pressure (P_{la}). The calculation is made from a modification of Poiseuille equation:

$$PVR = \frac{P_{pa} - P_{la} \text{ [pulmonary } \Delta P]}{\text{pulmonary flow}}$$

and

$$SVR = \frac{P_{sa} - P_{ra} \text{ [systemic } \Delta P]}{\text{systemic flow}}$$

If the pressure drop is measured in mm Hg and the flow in L/min/m², then the calculated resistance is in units. The normal PVR is 2–3 units, whereas the normal SVR is 15–20 units. An important concept to remember is that *blood flow goes where resistance is least.* Of course, other types of resistance are present besides vascular resistance, such as at valves, where, obviously, a narrowed valve has a greater resistance to flow than does a wide-open valve; at septal defects, where a small septal defect has a greater resistance to flow than does a large defect; and at ventricles, where a thick-walled, less compliant ventricle has a greater resistance to flow into it than does a thinner-walled, more compliant ventricle.

Acyanotic Congenital Heart Lesions

LEFT-TO-RIGHT SHUNT ACYANOTIC LESIONS

Acyanotic conditions are those in which the systemic arterial saturation is normal. Left-to-right shunt lesions have communication between the two sides of the heart through which extra blood traverses from the left to the right side. The result is an increase in pulmonary blood flow. A moderate-sized left-to-right shunt has approximately twice as much pulmonary blood flow as systemic blood flow (e.g., a 2:1 pulmonary-to-systemic [P/S] flow ratio). Assuming a normal systemic output of 4 L/min/m², the pulmonary flow is 8 L/min/m².

Hemodynamics of Common Left-to-Right Shunts

Atrial Septal Defect (Fig. 13–8). Flow from all four pulmonary veins streams through the ASD in both systole and diastole. The result is that very little increase in volume occurs in the left atrium (LA). The right atrium (RA) and the right ventricle (RV) handle twice the normal flow. The roentgenogram shows increased pulmonary artery vascularity and the ECG and echocardiogram show pure right ventricular enlargement (RVE).

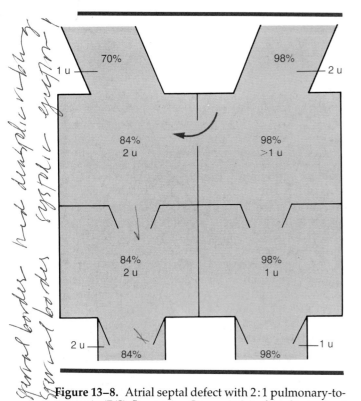

Figure 13–8. Atrial septal defect with 2:1 pulmonary-to-systemic (P/S) flow ratio. One unit (u) of cardiac output is 4 L/min/m². % is percent saturation.

No murmur is present from the low-velocity flow across the ASD, but twice the normal flow occurs across the normal tricuspid valve and normal pulmonic valve. The result is that, on the physical examination, in addition to the abnormal right ventricular impulse and widely persistently split S₂, a mid-diastolic rumbling murmur is exhibited at the lower left sternal border and a soft systolic ejection murmur is exhibited at the upper left sternal border.

Patent Ductus Arteriosus. Figure 13–9 shows normal flow through the right heart until after the blood has reached the pulmonary artery. Twice the normal flow is present in the pulmonary veins, LA, left ventricle (LV), the aorta proximal to the PDA, and pulmonary arteries distal to the PDA. The roentgenogram shows increased pulmonary artery vascularity and may also show increased pulmonary vein size. The ECG and echocardiogram show left atrial enlargement (LAE) and left ventricular hypertrophy (LVH), excluding any effects of increased pulmonary artery pressure.

If the pulmonary artery diastolic pressure is less than the aortic diastolic pressure, a continuous run-off from aorta to pulmonary artery occurs. The re-

sult is a continuous murmur. Also, twice the normal flow occurs through the normal mitral and aortic valves. The result is that, in addition to the abnormal left ventricular impulse and hyperdynamic upper left sternal edge and apex, a mid-diastolic rumble is present at that apex and a soft systolic ejection murmur is present at the upper right sternal border. If the caliber of the PDA is wide, greater transmission of systemic pressure into the pulmonary artery occurs. The wider and shorter the PDA, the higher the right ventricular pressure and the more the right ventricular hypertrophy (RVH) as well as the LVH.

Ventricular Septal Defect. Figure 13–10 shows twice as much flow as normal in the pulmonary veins, LA, and LV. The LV sends as much blood through the VSD as into the aorta so that the RV and pulmonary artery also have twice the normal flow. The roentgenogram shows increased pulmonary artery vascularity and may show increased pulmonary vein size. The ECG and echocardiogram show LAE and both LVH and RVH.

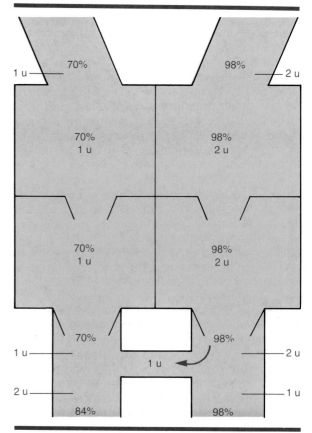

Figure 13–9. Patent ductus arteriosus with 2:1 P/S flow ratio (see Fig. 13–8).

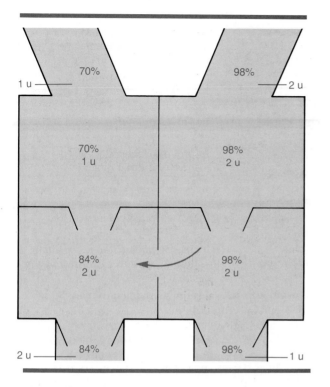

Figure 13–10. Ventricular septal defect with 2:1 P/S flow ratio (see Fig. 13–8).

A holosystolic murmur is present from left-to-right flow through the VSD. Because LV pressure rises slightly before RV pressure, the left-to-right shunt begins before mitral valve closure, resulting in S_1 being obscured by the murmur. Also, twice the flow occurs through the normal mitral and pulmonic valves, so that, in addition to the combined ventricular impulse and the hyperdynamic left sternal edge and apex, a mid-diastolic rumble is exhibited at the apex and a soft systolic ejection murmur is exhibited at the upper left sternal border.

The Natural History of Acyanotic Lesions with Left-to-Right Shunts

Atrial Septal Defect. The most common ASD (6.4:10,000 live births) is of the secundum type and makes up approximately 7% of all cases of congenital heart disease. The ratio of females to males is 2:1. The PVR is lower than normal throughout childhood and heart failure is infrequent. However, in adulthood, a significant number of individuals develop heart failure and/or atrial flutter or pulmonary vascular disease. Therefore, surgery or catheter closure, which is of extremely low risk, should be performed electively at what is deemed the appropriate psychologic age for that child. In most children, this period is after 5 yr of age. No convincing data are available to indicate the need for earlier surgery (Tables 13–8 and 13–9).

Ventricular Septal Defect. This is the most common congenital cardiac lesion, making up at least 30% of all cases of congenital heart disease. The incidence in males equals that in females. The most common position of the defect is perimembranous and subaortic, although many muscular defects may be present. VSDs in the endocardial cushion area are not rare, but supracristal defects are quite uncommon. VSD is usually a benign disease. The majority of the defects are small, most of which close spontaneously and never need catheterization. VSDs small enough to have normal pulmonary artery pressures and pulmonary to systemic flow ratios of <2:1 do not need surgery even if closure does not occur. An increase in PVR also does not occur. However, a small percentage of infants with large defects are at risk, and these infants make up a significant percentage of the infants admitted to the hospital with heart failure. Those infants who go into heart failure almost always do so by 2 mo of age.

Those with large left-to-right shunts can be divided into three groups: (1) those with half-systemic pulmonary hypertension, (2) those with two thirds–systemic pulmonary hypertension, and (3) those with systemic-level pulmonary hypertension. In the first group, medical management is almost invariably without difficulty. The left-to-right shunt also is less, rarely with more than a 2:1 P/S flow ratio, because the defect becomes smaller. Surgery is not necessary. In a few children, a mild amount of pulmonary hypertension (about 40 mm Hg) is still present with a moderate left-to-right shunt. Surgery is recommended for these children. In the second group, a small number of children are difficult to manage medically, leading to repair of the VSD within a few months after onset of the failure. However, in most, medical management is reasonably successful. In the third group, more cases occur in which medical management is unsuccessful, requiring surgery before age 6 mo.

Patent Ductus Arteriosus. The natural history of the congenital PDA is poorly defined because surgery has been available for a long time. However, three major observations should be noted. First, at the same pulmonary artery pressure, the risk of the development of pulmonary vascular disease is greater in PDA than in VSD. Second, at the same age, the risk of developing infective endocarditis is greater in PDA than in VSD because of jet

Table 13–8. Therapy of Congenital Heart Disease—Palliative Procedures

Procedure	Lesion	Comments
Blalock-Taussig Teflon tube graft or shunt (subclavian artery to ipsilateral pulmonary artery, usually right sided)	TOF, pulmonary valve atresia	Improves pulmonary blood flow; most common shunting procedure
Waterston shunt (aorta to right pulmonary artery)	TOF, pulmonary valve atresia, tricuspid atresia	Improves pulmonary blood flow
Balloon atrial septostomy (Rashkind procedure)	TGA, tricuspid atresia	Improves oxygenation with increased atrial mixing
Operative atrial septostomy (Blalock-Hanlon operation)	TGA	
Catheter balloon dilating valvotomy (balloon angioplasty)	Pulmonary valve stenosis; aortic valve stenosis	Increases valve patency
Operative valvotomy	As above for balloon plus pulmonary atresia	Increases valve patency; resultant pulmonary valve insufficiency enhances RV growth
Prostaglandin E_1 infusion	Pulmonary atresia, tricuspid atresia, TOF, coarctation of aorta, interrupted aortic arch	Maintains pulmonary blood flow via PDA
Pulmonary artery banding	Single ventricle	Decreases pulmonary blood flow, prevents heart failure
Device occlusion (embolization, umbrella); correction/closure	PDA, VSD, ASD, arteriovenous malformations	New and experimental

TGA = transposition of great arteries; TOF = tetralogy of Fallot.

Table 13–9. Therapy of Congenital Heart Disease—Corrective Procedures

Procedure	Lesion	Effect
Repair of septal defects (patching)	ASD, VSD, endocardial cushion defects	Complete repair
Valve replacement, repair	Aortic, mitral, pulmonic stenosis; Ebstein anomaly	Repair but prosthetic valve complications
Aortic graft, or subclavian flap angioplasty	Interrupted arch, coarctation of aorta	Repair but possible late recoarctation
Total correction possible	TOF; anomalous venous return; PDA	Complete repair
Mustard or Senning procedure (atrial switch by an intra-atrial baffle)	TGA	RV remains systemic ventricle
Jatene procedure (arterial switch)	TGA	Anatomic correction
Fontan procedure (right atrium–to–pulmonary artery anastomosis)	Tricuspid atresia, single ventricle, pulmonary atresia	Alleviates shunting, enhances pulmonary blood flow; atrium functions as right ventricle
Norwood procedure	Hypoplastic left heart	Two-staged procedure with variable success
Heart transplant	Hypoplastic left heart	Normal heart with risk of immune rejection
Heart–lung transplant	Eisenmenger syndrome; cor pulmonale?	Normal organs with risk of rejection

TGA = transposition of great arteries; TOF = tetralogy of Fallot.

stream–induced intimal damage. Third, the incidence of spontaneous closure of the congenital PDA is very small. Therefore, because surgery is simple and low risk, all simple congenital PDAs with a left-to-right shunt should be closed. Some PDAs may be closed by a double umbrella device; others require surgical ligation (see Tables 13–8 and 13–9). Those infants who have congestive heart failure and/or large left-to-right shunts with increased pulmonary artery pressure should be operated on at the time of diagnosis.

Endocardial Cushion Defect (A-V Canal). A broad spectrum of endocardial cushion defects has been observed, from varieties of the complete AV canal (including marked deficiency in the ventricular and atrial septa, as well as medial portions of tricuspid and mitral valves making a common AV valve) to several varieties of the partial AV canal. The simplest forms are the VSD in the endocardial cushion position and the ostium primum ASD with varying deficiencies of the anteromedial leaflet, causing mitral regurgitation. Equal numbers of males and females are affected. The more complete the defect, the more likely it is that the child has Down syndrome.

The natural history of the various partial AV canal defects depends on the size of the various atrial and ventricular defects and the amount of mitral regurgitation. The large ostium primum ASD with no mitral regurgitation has the same benign natural history as that of the simple secundum ASD. With a complete AV canal, severe heart failure and/or pulmonary vascular disease is the rule. The clinical and echocardiographic diagnosis depends on the specific anatomy. The characteristic ECG is one showing an abnormally left superior vector (formerly termed "left axis deviation"). A congenital abnormality of the anterior branch of the left bundle results in initial QRS conduction inferiorly, followed by the remainder of the conduction sequence superiorly.

In complete AV canal, left ventricular–to–right atrial communication is present in addition to the large VSD, leading to an early increase in pulmonary blood flow. If mitral regurgitation is present, early left ventricular failure may occur. The high left ventricular end-diastolic pressure causes the pulmonary venous pressure to be elevated. Therefore, three of the four major factors that slow maturation of the pulmonary resistance vessels are present. In addition, continued high pulmonary blood flow at systemic-level pulmonary artery pressure and high pulmonary venous pressure may be exhibited. Therefore, even in cases in which heart failure can be managed, the pulmonary vascular resistance eventually will increase and pulmonary vascular disease will occur. Early complete surgical repair, preferably by 3 mo of age, is strongly recommended.

OBSTRUCTIVE LESIONS

Right-Sided Lesions

The most common pure right-sided obstructive lesion is valvular pulmonic stenosis. Peripheral pulmonic stenosis that is not part of other congenital cardiac lesions (e.g., tetralogy of Fallot) occurs most commonly in association with entities such as congenital rubella, Williams syndrome, Noonan syndrome, Alagille syndrome, cutis laxa, and Ehlers-Danlos syndrome. Isolated pulmonary infundibular stenosis may exist only when a VSD is present or has been present and closed.

The majority of stenotic pulmonic valves have three leaflets with varied leaflet fusion. A less common variety is pulmonary valvular dysplasia, in which the pathology is not of fusion but of a myxomatous tissue that is disorganized, thickened, and immobile. The majority of patients with dysplastic pulmonary valves have Noonan syndrome.

The *diagnosis* of valvular pulmonic stenosis is suggested by a pulmonary ejection click that is maximal on expiration at the upper left sternal border, followed by an ejection systolic murmur and a widely split S_2. The more severe the stenosis, the longer the murmur; full-length murmurs are associated with the right ventricular pressures near systemic level. With mild stenosis the S_2 split is not much above normal and pulmonary closure may be of increased intensity. With increasing severity, the split widens and the pulmonary closure softens. In many severe cases, with suprasystemic right ventricular pressure, the murmur may extend across the aortic closure so that no 2nd sound is heard at the upper left sternal border. The ECG shows pure RVH, and the chest roentgenogram shows no significant cardiomegaly and a large dilated (poststenotic) pulmonary artery. In some severe cases, the elevated right atrial pressure may cause the flap of the foramen ovale to open, resulting in a significant right-to-left shunt. Thus, this "acyanotic lesion" would be associated with cyanosis.

Cases have been observed, especially in infancy, in which the pulmonic stenosis is so severe that marked right ventricular failure occurs, associated with venous distention, a large liver, and a large right-to-left shunt at the atrial level. This condition is termed **critical pulmonic stenosis**.

Treatment of valvular pulmonic stenosis is

straightforward. Mild pulmonic stenosis with right ventricular pressure of less than 50 mm Hg is very common, is known not to increase in severity over the years, and is associated with normal life expectancy. When the right ventricular pressure is above 60 mm Hg, the treatment is balloon valvuloplasty (see Tables 13–8 and 13–9). The success rate is very high and the risk is very low. Surgery is performed only in severe cases, such as when the balloon catheter cannot be passed through the stenotic pulmonic valve, and in most cases in which the valve is dysplastic. In the latter case, balloon valvuloplasty usually is not totally successful.

Left-Sided Lesions

Valvular Aortic Stenosis.   Left-sided lesions are very common, particularly if one includes *bicuspid aortic valve without* stenosis in this category. It is not known how common this latter lesion is (although it is known to occur in about half of patients with coarctation of the aorta). The recognition of bicuspid aortic valve (with two sinuses) is important because patients with this abnormality are very prone to infective endocarditis. The diagnosis is made readily by identifying a sharp sound well separated from S_1 and usually maximal at the apex, not varying with respiration, and less well heard at the lower left sternal border and anterior axillary line. This sound is an aortic ejection click.

Valvular Aortic Stenosis with Systolic Gradient.   This is a major lesion with tremendous variation in severity. The majority of cases do not require surgery in childhood. Although it is a potentially progressive lesion, the mild cases do not progress until adulthood. The systolic murmur usually is maximal at the upper right sternal border or sternum and often is associated with suprasternal notch and carotid systolic thrills. When the murmur is significantly less than full length and the split of S_2 is normal, indicating no significant prolongation of left ventricular systole, the condition almost certainly is mild. Such patients may have ECGs that are normal or show mild LVH. When the murmur is full length and the split of S_2 is narrow, indicating prolongation of left ventricular systole, the condition is significant. Important clues to severity include the initial QRS vector being situated to the left, LVH, and the development of ST segment and T wave abnormalities with exercise. Echo-Doppler techniques for predicting severity have become reliable, so that baseline catheterization may no longer be necessary.

If no ST or T abnormalities are present at rest and if the systolic gradient is less than 60 mm Hg,

most cardiologists agree that surgery (or balloon valvuloplasty) should not be done (see Tables 13–8 and 13–9). (The presence of ST and T abnormalities at rest, however, provides a clear indication for intervention). Most advise that children with aortic stenosis should not participate in competitive athletics. When exercise requiring sustained strength is involved (e.g., weightlifting and competitive wrestling), the end-diastolic pressure increases significantly, reducing coronary perfusion. Therefore, this type of exercise especially should be avoided. Sudden unexpected death due to valvular aortic stenosis in childhood or young adulthood is rare. Surgery, although of low risk, is palliative. A prosthetic valve is required later in life. Increasing numbers of patients are receiving balloon valvuloplasty, but long-term results are not known.

The infants who have *critical aortic stenosis*, sometimes recognized in the 1st wk of life, are very ill. They have very stenotic valves and sometimes abnormal left ventricles. All would die without surgery. Balloon valvuloplasty has been used with early success when the valve was not dysplastic (see Tables 13–8 and 13–9).

Coarctation of the Aorta.   Simple coarctation of the aorta is almost always at the level of the ductus arteriosus (or ligamentum arteriosum) and just below the origin of the left subclavian artery. (Occasionally, the origin of the left subclavian is at or below the coarctation.) Because of the position of the ductus, there is no obstruction to flow in the aorta in utero, nor while the ductus is open in the newborn period. Therefore, simple coarctation usually is not recognized in newborns.

The murmur is usually systolic, with a late peak, and can be located anywhere in the anterior chest. It usually is heard well at the apex, left axilla, and left back, but often is maximal over the left back. The ECG early in infancy may show pure RVH, although later in childhood LVH is expected.

Rarely, coarctation causes heart failure in the 1st mo of life, but often the children are asymptomatic throughout childhood. Eventually, most children have upper extremity systolic pressures in the range of 140–145 mm Hg. Because of the position of the left subclavian artery, the right arm pressure may be higher than that of the left arm. Because the pulse pressure is low below the coarctation, renal endocrine factors work to raise the pressure, both above and below the coarctation.

Treatment of simple coarctation of the aorta is indicated in Table 13–9. When heart failure is not a problem and the blood pressure is not elevated, it is wise to postpone surgery until the descending aorta is at least 50% of adult size, at about 4 yr of age. In those cases in which blood pressure is in the range of 140 mm Hg, it is probably justified to perform surgery when the child is 1 yr of age. Special problems arise when the diagnosis is missed or if surgery is not performed until later in life. First, more collateral vessels may be present, leading to increased bleeding during surgery. In addition, by adolescence, the aorta may have stiffened so that end-to-end anastomosis cannot be done. Also, a significantly higher incidence of essential hypertension and death may be present in later life.

Complicated coarctation of the aorta, a coarctation in association with another lesion (e.g., PDA arising above the coarctation or, more commonly, a VSD), commonly leads to heart failure by the 2nd wk of life. After treatment of heart failure, surgery must be performed within a few days. For those infants with a PDA, operating on both lesions successfully alleviates the problem. For the more common cases with a VSD, a decision must be made as to whether or not to place a pulmonary artery band as well as to repair the coarctation. Often, only the coarctation is operated on because it is difficult to determine the size of the VSD. If the infant remains very ill, a second operation soon may be necessary to close the VSD.

When a coarctation is corrected during infancy, the area of repair may not grow. Consequently, a situation called "restenosis" may develop. Because at the time of the original operation collateral vessels involving spinal cord arterial flow may be lost, a second operation for coarctation may include a risk of spinal cord ischemia. For this reason balloon valvuloplasty now often is recommended instead of surgery for restenosis.

Cyanotic Congenital Heart Disease

Cyanotic congenital heart disease can be divided into lesions that have decreased (Table 13–10) or

Table 13–10. Cyanotic Congenital Heart Disease with Decreased Pulmonary Blood Flow

Right Ventricular Hypertrophy
Pulmonary stenosis (severe) with ASD
Pulmonary atresia (with or without VSD)
Tetralogy of Fallot

Left Ventricular Hypertrophy
Tricuspid atresia
Pulmonary atresia and hypoplastic right ventricle

Right, Left, or Combined Ventricular Hypertrophy
Transposition of great arteries with pulmonary stenosis
Truncus arteriosus with hypoplastic pulmonary arteries

Neither Ventricle Predominant
Ebstein anomaly

Table 13–11. Cyanotic Congenital Heart Disease with Increased Pulmonary Blood Flow

Right Ventricular Hypertrophy
Hypoplastic left heart syndrome
Total anomalous venous return
Transposition of great arteries

Right, Left, or Combined Ventricular Hypertrophy
Transposition of great arteries ± VSD
Single ventricle
Tricuspid atresia with transposition
Truncus arteriosus

increased (Table 13–11) pulmonary blood flow. Because of persistent cyanosis or right-to-left shunts, these patients often have characteristic extracardiac complications (Table 13–12).

TETRALOGY OF FALLOT

The four components of this syndrome are a large nonrestrictive VSD, severe right ventricle outflow tract obstruction, overriding of the aortic root over the ventricular septum, and RVH. The RVH is secondary. Embryologically, there is one defect—hypoplasia of the conus. Because conal tissue provides the major portion of the tissue that closes the membranous ventricular septum and because the conus is hypoplastic, the result is a nonrestrictive VSD and severe infundibular pulmonic stenosis. Flow through the small conus is restricted in utero, resulting in a small annulus and small pulmonary arteries. Although the location and size of the VSD are relatively constant, the severity of the pulmonary stenosis varies considerably and accounts for the varying age at presentation and the varying clinical course. In a few infants, the pulmonary stenosis may be less severe, associated initially with a left-to-right shunt. A true tetralogy, however, has a right-to-left shunt. Occasionally, the narrowing is located almost exclusively at the infundibular level, associated with a normal pulmonary valve annulus, normal valve leaflets, and normal distal pulmonary arteries. More commonly, obstruction at the infundibular level is associated with a hypoplastic pulmonary valve annulus and a dysplastic, stenotic pulmonary valve. The main pulmonary artery and distal pulmonary arteries may be hypoplastic, and, occasionally, discrete stenoses are noted at the takeoff of the right and left pulmonary arteries or even more distally. In the most severe form, there is complete atresia of the infundibulum, the pulmonary valve, and even sometimes the main pulmonary artery. Other intracardiac anomalies are not commonly associated

Table 13–12. Extracardiac Complications of Cyanotic Congenital Heart Disease

Problem	Etiology: Therapy
Polycythemia	Persistent hypoxia: Phlebotomy
Relative anemia	Nutritional deficiency: Iron replacement
CNS abscess	Right-to-left shunting: Antibiotics, drainage
CNS thromboembolic stroke	Right-to-left shunting or polycythemia: Phlebotomy
Gum disease	Polycythemia, gingivitis, bleeding: Dental hygiene
Gout	Polycythemia, diuretic agents: Allopurinol
Arthritis, clubbing	Hypoxic arthropathy: None
Pregnancy	Poor placental perfusion, poor ability to increase cardiac output: Bed rest
Infectious disease	Associated asplenia, DiGeorge syndrome: Antibiotics Fatal RSV pneumonia with pulmonary hypertension: Ribaviran
Growth	Failure to thrive, increased oxygen consumption, decreased nutrient intake: Treat heart failure; correct defect early
Psychosocial adjustment	Limited activity, peer pressure; chronic disease, multiple hospitalizations: Counseling

CNS = central nervous system; RSV = respiratory syncytial virus.

with tetralogy, except that a right aortic arch is present in 25% of the patients.

Pathophysiology. Because of the large size of VSD, blood passing through the tricuspid and mitral valves may flow to either the aorta or the pulmonary artery; the degree of intracardiac shunting is a function of the relative outflow resistances (Fig. 13–11). The systemic resistance is composed primarily of the systemic arteriolar resistance, but the pulmonary resistance is due to the anatomic pulmonary stenosis. Because the pulmonary stenosis is severe, there is primarily or exclusively a right-to-left shunt, with blood bypassing the pulmonary artery and going to the aorta.

Although the severity of the anatomic abnormality is the primary determinant of the degree of cyanosis, changes in systemic venous oxygen saturation or pulmonary or systemic resistances also influence the degree of right-to-left shunting. For example, exercise or crying, by reducing the systemic arteriolar resistance and increasing systemic venous return, is associated with a large right-to-left shunt, more cyanosis, and a decrease in oxygen saturation. Any agent that increases systemic resistance would have the opposite effect, by decreasing systemic and increasing pulmonary blood flow and, therefore, reducing the right-to-left shunt. The child inherently learns to decrease cyanosis by assuming a squatting position. Squatting increases systemic venous return, resulting in more blood being made available to the pulmonary artery, and increases systemic resistance, driving more venous blood into the lungs.

Clinical Manifestations. The clinical findings vary depending on the degree of right ventricular outflow obstruction. Children with a less severe degree of outflow obstruction may not be cyanotic at birth and initially may have a left-to-right shunt. Usually, the right ventricular outflow tract obstruction is progressive, resulting in increasing hypoxemia and cyanosis over the first few months and years of life. Such children usually do well clinically except for dyspnea and increased cyanosis on exertion. Occasionally, children under 5 yr of age assume a squatting position.

Hypoxic ("tet") spells may occur, especially from a few months to 2 yr of life. During such spells, the child typically becomes very restless and agitated and may cry inconsolably. The child is hyperpneic, with gradually increasing cyanosis, which then often leads to a deep sleep. In severe spells, prolonged unconsciousness and even convulsions, hemiparesis, or death may occur. Treatment of these spells consists of administering oxygen, placing the child in the knee–chest position, and giving morphine sulfate. Beta-adrenergic inhibition using intravenous propranolol also is helpful, as are drugs that increase SVR without affecting the myocardium, such as intravenous methoxamine. If acidosis is present, intravenous sodium bicarbonate should be given. In severe cases, emergency surgery, either systemic-to-pulmonary artery shunt or total correction, may be necessary.

The volume work of the heart in tetralogy of Fal-

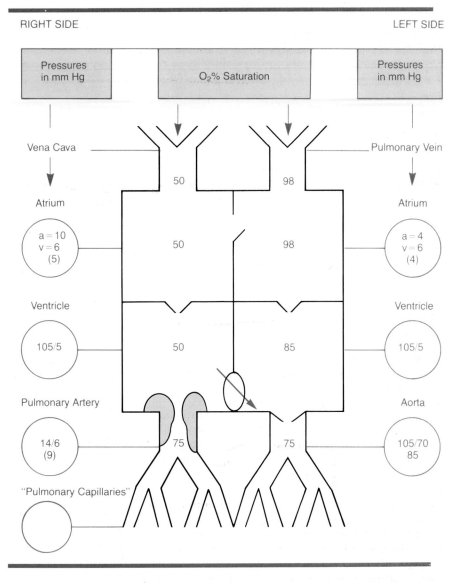

Figure 13–11. Tetralogy of Fallot.

lot is less than normal. Therefore, heart failure does not occur.

On *physical examination*, cyanosis and digital clubbing are evident. A quiet heart with a right ventricular impulse is noted. Because of the very severe pulmonic stenosis, pulmonary closure is not heard. The audible 2nd sound is that of a loud aortic closure at the lower left sternal border resulting from transmission down the descending aorta. Because no murmur occurs from a right-to-left shunt through the VSD, the only murmur heard is that of blood flowing through the pulmonic stenosis. With more severe stenosis, less blood goes through the stenotic right ventricular outflow tract and more goes through the VSD, resulting in a softer,

shorter murmur. In maximal tetralogy (pulmonary atresia), there is no systolic murmur, although there may be a loud aortic ejection click best heard at the apex. Also, a continuous murmur from either a PDA or large collateral artery off the descending aorta (best heard in the back) may be present. In the patient who has a hypoxic spell, the previously heard systolic murmur softens or disappears, returning when the spell is over.

On *chest roentgenogram*, the heart is not enlarged. Often, a concavity is found in the area usually occupied by the main pulmonary artery, and the ascending aorta is large. A right aortic arch may be present.

The *ECG* shows RVH and often RAE as well,

although in the first weeks of life the ECG may be normal. On *echocardiography*, the extent of right ventricular outflow tract obstruction and its location usually can be visualized easily, as can the VSD, the small pulmonary arteries, and the large aorta.

On *cardiac catheterization*, equal systolic pressures in the RV and LV and ascending aorta are noted (Fig. 13–11). The oxygen saturation on the right side of the heart usually is lower than normal because of systemic hypoxemia; however, the pulmonary venous and left atrial saturations are normal. Cardiac catheterization usually is not necessary in the infant, and it is not necessary to take the risk of producing hypoxic spells. Catheterization is done later when complete repair is being considered.

Angiography of the RV and LV and ascending aorta is necessary to identify specifically the anatomy of the VSD(s) and pulmonary arteries. An ascending aortogram is necessary to outline the coronary arteries, because abnormalities may be present in 5%. If the anterior descending coronary artery arises from the right rather than the left, anatomic repair may be difficult, because a large coronary artery branch may run across the right ventricular outflow tract, making patch repair of the subvalvar pulmonic stenosis difficult.

Complications. A *cerebrovascular accident* is a devastating complication of cyanotic congenital heart disease (see Table 13–11). In children less than 2 yr of age, this complication almost invariably is secondary to hypoxemia and anemia rather than to polycythemia, sludging, and in situ thrombosis, and occurs most commonly in children who are quite hypoxemic, with a relative anemia for the degree of oxygen saturation. Iron deficiency makes the red cells somewhat stiffer, and also results in less oxygen delivery. In older children, in particular, the hematocrit may rise above 65%. Even in this situation, considerable iron deficiency may be present, a diagnosis that cannot be made by examination of the red cells on the blood smear. Serum iron and iron-binding capacity must be measured. When iron therapy is given, the hemoglobin may rise but the hematocrit usually does not. Conversely, if the iron saturation is normal, the administration of iron could raise the hematocrit to dangerous levels. Although viscosity of the blood may increase significantly when the hematocrit is above 55%, there is a trade-off of improved delivery of oxygen to the tissue at the higher hematocrit. A large number of patients with congenital defects resulting in chronic cyanosis need to maintain their hematocrit level between 65 and 70% for optimal well-being. However, if questions of symptoms of polycythemia at that hematocrit have arisen or if the hematocrit goes above 70%, then partial exchange transfusion is necessary. Withdrawal of blood without continuous exchange is dangerous, the risks being the acute lowering of systemic resistance, more right-to-left shunt, and a cerebrovascular accident.

Brain abscess is a less common complication than is a cerebrovascular accident. Patients usually are more than 2 yr of age and present with headaches and localizing signs. Any central nervous system event in a cyanotic child over age 2 should be considered a brain abscess until proved otherwise because of the drastic implications. Computerized tomography scans are diagnostic. Antibiotic therapy occasionally may keep the infection localized, but surgical drainage of the abscess often is required.

Bacterial endocarditis is always a risk in children with tetralogy of Fallot prior to complete repair, particularly in patients with systemic-to-pulmonary shunts.

Treatment. The treatment of tetralogy of Fallot is surgical (see Tables 13–8 and 13–9). Although the indications for surgery have not changed very much over the years, the age for corrective surgery has been decreasing. Surgery is indicated if the affected child is significantly symptomatic, hypoxemic with an arterial oxygen saturation of less than 75%, or polycythemic with a hematocrit of more than 60%. *Palliative operations*, primarily the *Blalock-Taussig shunt* connecting the subclavian artery to the pulmonary artery, are the preferred systemic-to-pulmonary shunts, although some surgeons modify the operation by placing a conduit between the subclavian and pulmonary arteries. The Blalock-Taussig shunt is an excellent temporizing procedure but does not eliminate right-to-left shunting and has the potential of distorting the pulmonary arteries, making later repair more difficult.

Total correction of tetralogy of Fallot is performed under cardiopulmonary bypass. It usually involves a right ventriculotomy, closure of the VSD using a Dacron patch, and excision of muscle in the right ventricular outflow tract. If hypoplasia of the pulmonary annulus, main pulmonary artery, or distal pulmonary arteries is present, a patch is placed as a roof over that area. The surgical mortality is under 10%, although in institutions in which complete repair is frequently done before age 2 yr, the surgical mortality is less than 5%.

Short-term complications include a residual VSD and residual right ventricular outflow tract obstruction because of incomplete relief of the pulmonary stenosis. Pulmonary regurgitation also is expected, even with excellent surgical results. Late complications have included ventricular ectopy and even sudden death resulting from ventricular tachycardia. However, with the ready availability of electrophysiologic studies at catheterization, the identification of those infants at risk of ventricular tachycardia has made pharmacologic preventive therapy very successful. Although very long-term data are not available, the vast majority of children do quite well and remain asymptomatic at least throughout childhood and into young adulthood. Despite pulmonary regurgitation, some patients may do well for much longer periods, the unknown factor being the long-term status of the right ventricle.

d-TRANSPOSITION OF THE GREAT ARTERIES

Complete transposition of the great arteries (TGA), although less common than tetralogy of Fallot, is the most common lesion seen in the cyanotic infant in the newborn period. In this lesion, the great arteries arise off the inappropriate ventricle, the aorta from the right and the pulmonary artery from the left. The systemic venous drainage and pulmonary venous drainage are usually normal, and the right and left atria and the right and left ventricles are in their normal positions. Therefore, desaturated blood from the systemic venous return passes through the RA and RV and out to the aorta, whereas oxygenated pulmonary venous blood passes through the LA and LV and then out through the pulmonary artery (Fig. 13–12). Survival is dependent upon mixing of blood between the circulations.

Associated abnormalities of the atrial and ventricular septum, AV valves, and coronary arteries are common and may alter the physiology significantly. When a transposition is left untreated, the prognosis is poor, with 30% of affected infants dying in the 1st wk of life and 50% in the 1st mo. The clinical presentation and hemodynamics vary significantly in relation to the presence or absence of significant associated defects.

d-Transposition of the Great Arteries with an Intact Ventricular Septum

In this anomaly, the most common variant, no other intracardiac or extracardiac anomalies are present. Prior to birth, the oxygenation of the fetus is normal but, after delivery, mixing between the parallel circulations diminishes as the ductus arteri-

osus closes, and severe hypoxemia, acidosis, and death can occur rapidly.

Clinical Manifestations. Cyanosis usually is noted within the 1st day of life and progresses rapidly as the ductus arteriosus closes. The remainder of the cardiac examination may be normal, with no murmur or only a grade 2/6 ejection systolic murmur being present. The chest roentgenogram may be normal but may show mild cardiac enlargement with normal or increased pulmonary blood flow. The base of the heart is narrower than usual because of the frequent absence of a significant thymus and the more anterior–posterior relationship of the aorta and pulmonary arteries, causing an egg shape. The ECG usually is normal. The two-dimensional echocardiogram and Doppler study are diagnostic by showing the anterior great vessel branching into innominate, carotid, and subclavian arteries, and the posterior great vessel branching into the right and left pulmonary arteries.

Cardiac catheterization shows the right ventricular pressure to be at systemic levels because the RV is connected to the aorta. The left ventricular pressure may be high in the perinatal period because of elevated pulmonary vascular resistance but usually drops to a level of 30 or 40 mm Hg by the 1st or 2nd wk of life. This is the only congenital cardiac lesion in which the left ventricular pressure is less than the aortic pressure. Angiography in the RV and LV shows the great vessels arising inappropriately and rules out associated cardiac anomalies.

Treatment. The finding of cyanosis in the perinatal period in the child with *d*-TGA is a true medical emergency. As the ductus arteriosus closes, severe hypoxemia, acidosis, and death occur unless another intracardiac connection is present for mixing. The child should be started on a prostaglandin PGE_1 infusion immediately on diagnosis. By maintaining patency of the ductus arteriosus, more blood goes from the aorta into the pulmonary artery, increasing pulmonary venous and left atrial flow. Thus, more blood is available to go left to right at the atrial level. Almost any cyanotic full-term infant will be benefited by PGE_1, and very few will have adverse effects. Because apnea does occur after PGE_1, close observation and/or intubation is necessary.

The initial palliation of newborn infants who have TGA and an intact ventricular septum involves improving intracardiac mixing by tearing the fossa ovalis with a balloon catheter developed by William Rashkind (see Table 13–8). This usually is performed under fluoroscopic control but has been done in the intensive care unit using two-

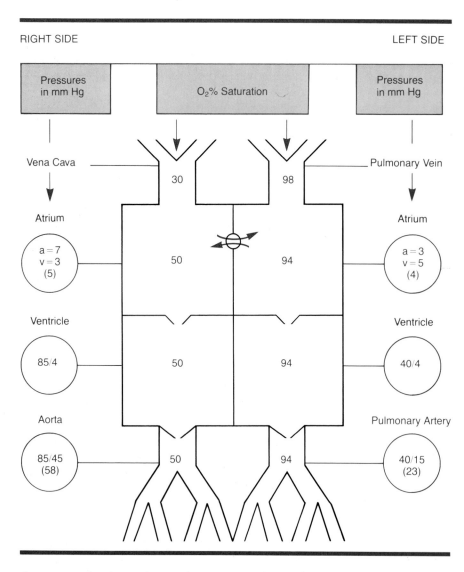

Figure 13–12. Transposition of the great arteries.

dimensional echocardiography to guide the balloon catheter into the LA. A successful *Rashkind procedure* is signaled by improvement in oxygenation and elimination of the interatrial pressure gradient.

Previously the "atrial switch" was accomplished by a *Mustard procedure*. A pantaloon-shaped baffle is inserted within the atrium to divert pulmonary venous return anteriorly through the tricuspid valve into the RV and aorta. The inferior and superior vena caval blood then can go through the mitral valve into the LV and pulmonary artery. Alternatively, the *Senning procedure* involves the same baffling but less foreign material and more autologous tissue. Both techniques switch the circulations at the atrial level so that systemic venous return passes into the pulmonary artery and pulmonary

venous return into the aorta. Long-term complications may occur, such as obstruction at either the pulmonary venous or the systemic venous portion of the baffle and a variety of interatrial arrhythmias. The most common arrhythmias are together described as the *sick sinus syndrome*. This includes sinus bradycardia or no sinus activity with atrial or A-V junctional bradycardia, together with supraventricular tachycardia or atrial flutter. The syndrome occurs in 50% of cases. This disturbing combination of tachyarrhythmias and bradyarrhythmias makes pharmacologic treatment difficult without insertion of a pacemaker.

Complications with the "atrial switch" procedure and improvements in intraoperative techniques have led to total repair of transposition by an *arterial switch technique* (see Table 13–9). The current technique for this procedure involves removing the coronary arteries along with a button of tissue from the base of the aorta and moving them posteriorly onto the pulmonary artery. The great arteries then are divided and switched so that the anterior aortic valve arises from the RV and is connected to the pulmonary arterial tree, while the posterior pulmonary valve arises from the LV and is connected to the aorta. This operation can be done only with a LV that is "prepared" to maintain a systemic pressure. This is possible in the perinatal period because, with transposition, both ventricles have been generating systemic pressure in utero. The left ventricular pressure may decrease to 30 or 40 mm Hg within a few days so that, when the child is 3 or 4 wk of age or even younger, left ventricular wall thickness may be inadequate to generate systemic pressure. Therefore, in most centers, the arterial switch is performed in the first days of life. Balloon atrial septostomy is not performed unless there is some delay before surgery can be performed. If significant valvular pulmonary stenosis is present, an arterial switch procedure usually cannot be done.

Prognosis. If the lesion is left untreated, the prognosis for TGA is poor; 30% of the infants die in the 1st wk, 50% in the 1st mo, and more than 90% in the 1st yr. This outcome has been improved markedly, first with balloon atrial septostomy and more recently by early correction. The mortality after the Senning or Mustard procedure is low, under 5%. The long-term results only now are becoming available, but it appears that survival after the Mustard operation is at least 80% at 15 yr. The short-term results for the Senning procedure appear to be equal to those for the Mustard procedure. Recent experience with the arterial switch procedure has been excellent. Many surgeons with considerable experience now can perform the operation with a mortality rate in the range of 10% and, recently, even in newborns, some centers report that the mortality rate is less than 5%. Long-term data are not yet available in this group of infants, but it would appear likely that the results will be excellent (see Tables 13–8 and 13–9).

d-Transposition of the Great Arteries with a Ventricular Septal Defect

The presence of a large VSD dramatically improves intracardiac mixing so that cyanosis is not the major problem. Infants with this abnormality develop increasing pulmonary blood flow at high pressure as the pulmonary vascular resistance

drops; they present with heart failure after a few weeks of life.

Clinical Manifestations. The clinical manifestations in the newborn who has TGA and a large VSD are dominated by signs and symptoms of heart failure. The infant usually is tachypneic and tachycardiac, with increased perspiration and poor feeding. The heart is very hyperdynamic, with prominent right and left ventricular impulses. The 2nd heart sound is single, and, frequently, a grade 3 or louder systolic murmur is present, obscuring S_1 at the 3rd or 4th left interspace, as a result of the VSD. On the chest roentgenogram, the heart is enlarged, with increased pulmonary blood flow and a haziness consistent with increased interstitial fluid from elevated pulmonary venous pressure. The base of the heart sometimes is narrow because of the more anterior–posterior relationship of the great arteries and the small thymus. The ECG shows combined ventricular hypertrophy or occasionally pure RVH. The two-dimensional echocardiogram and Doppler study are diagnostic, showing the great vessels arising off the inappropriate ventricle and a large VSD. At cardiac catheterization, left atrial pressure usually is greater than the right, but both are increased; the pressures in each ventricle are equal, and usually bidirectional shunting (right to left in systole; left to right in diastole) is found at the ventricular level. Nonetheless, left-to-right shunting at the atrial level and right-to-left shunting at the ventricular level predominate. The left and right ventricular angiograms show the great arteries arising off the inappropriate ventricles and the presence of a VSD.

Treatment. In infants with heart failure, the usual anticongestive measures, including digoxin, diuretics, increased caloric density of the formula, and afterload reduction, are useful (Table 13–6). Surgery may be necessary within the first months of life because of intractable heart failure and is indicated by 3 mo of age, because systemic-level pulmonary artery hypertension in the presence of high pulmonary blood flow invariably leads to pulmonary vascular disease. Surgeons prefer to perform the arterial switch procedure, including closure of the VSD.

PULMONARY ATRESIA WITH AN INTACT VENTRICULAR SEPTUM AND A HYPOPLASTIC RIGHT VENTRICLE

This is an uncommon condition but very important because all affected infants will expire without treatment. The pulmonary valve is atretic as a result of an obstructing diaphragm or fusion of the commissures. The RV is markedly hypoplastic. The tricuspid valve is appropriate for the size of the RV and, therefore, is small. Connections between sinusoids of the RV and the coronary arteries occasionally result in flow from the ventricle to the coronary artery in systole because of high intracavitary pressure in the RV.

Because of the atretic right ventricular outflow tract, all the systemic venous return passes through the RA into the LA where it mixes with the pulmonary venous return. The LV pumps blood to the systemic circulation and to the lungs via the ductus arteriosus. As the ductus arteriosus closes soon after birth, hypoxemia becomes progressively severe. Without intervention, death occurs rapidly.

Clinical Manifestations. Newborn infants may appear normal at birth, but as the ductus narrows, progressive cyanosis develops. On physical examination the 2nd heart sound is single. The precordium is quiet, although some children have a murmur of tricuspid insufficiency at the lower left sternal border. The chest roentgenogram shows decreased pulmonary vascular markings. The heart may be normal in size or may show dilation from RAE. The ECG shows RAE and LVH with a normal inferior vector.

The two-dimensional echocardiogram and Doppler study shows absence of the pulmonary valve, hypoplasia of the right ventricular cavity, and, frequently, significant tricuspid regurgitation. The diagnosis can be confirmed by cardiac catheterization and angiography, but these studies usually are not necessary prior to initial surgery. The oxygen saturation data show right-to-left shunting at the atrial level. The degree of hypoxemia is dependent on the pulmonary blood flow. A catheter almost invariably can be passed across the hypoplastic tricuspid valve, where the right ventricular pressure usually exceeds the left ventricular and aortic systolic pressures. Angiography of the RV shows the hypoplasia of the cavity and tricuspid valve and can illuminate right ventricular sinusoid-to-coronary artery connections.

Treatment and Prognosis. Because hypoxemia becomes worse as the ductus arteriosus closes, PGE_1 infusion, by dilating the ductus, improves the oxygen saturation and is lifesaving. A few cases have been reported of percutaneously puncturing the valve with a wire, a laser, or an electrocautery, followed by balloon dilation. In those rare instances in which the right ventricular cavity is nearly normal in size (as well as when the ventricle

is small), a pulmonary valvotomy or valvectomy is performed to allow forward flow through the ventricle, facilitating eventual growth of that ventricle. In all cases, however, an artificial connection between the aorta and pulmonary artery (e.g., a Blalock-Taussig shunt) is usually necessary, because the poor compliance of the RV forces most right atrial blood into the LA. A cardiac catheterization should be done within a few months after the first surgery, and, if the right ventricular pressure is still high, open heart surgery is performed to create unobstructed continuity between the RV and pulmonary artery. When the child is a few years of age, another catheterization is done. If the RV is large and hemodynamics are appropriate, the Blalock-Taussig connection is ligated and the foramen ovale is closed. If the right ventricular cavity remains very small, a modified Fontan procedure is needed, connecting the RA to the pulmonary artery.

The long-term prognosis for infants with pulmonary atresia with an intact ventricular septum is mixed. For those with a reasonable-sized right ventricular cavity, the prognosis is good. For those infants with severe hypoplasia, the cumulative mortality rate from the operations and waiting period probably is on the order of 20–30% in early childhood.

TRICUSPID ATRESIA

Tricuspid atresia is more common than hypoplastic RV with pulmonary atresia but is less likely to be recognized in the first days of life. The tricuspid valve is atretic (usually with hardly a dimple on the floor of the right atrium), and the right ventricular cavity is hypoplastic. Tricuspid atresia is different embryologically from pulmonary atresia. In tricuspid atresia (without TGA), a VSD always is present, which almost always is posterior, in the position of an endocardial cushion defect.

All the systemic venous return passing into the RA goes across the foramen ovale into the LA, where it mixes with pulmonary venous return and then passes into the LV. The amount of pulmonary blood flow then depends mostly on the size of the VSD, through which all pulmonary blood must flow. The LV must handle increased volume despite diminished pulmonary blood flow (Fig. 13–13). Occasionally, the VSD is large and the pulmonary blood flow almost unimpeded. In this instance, pulmonary blood flow increases as the PVR decreases after birth and may become excessive enough to cause heart failure. The VSD tends to get smaller with age so that, even in these cases,

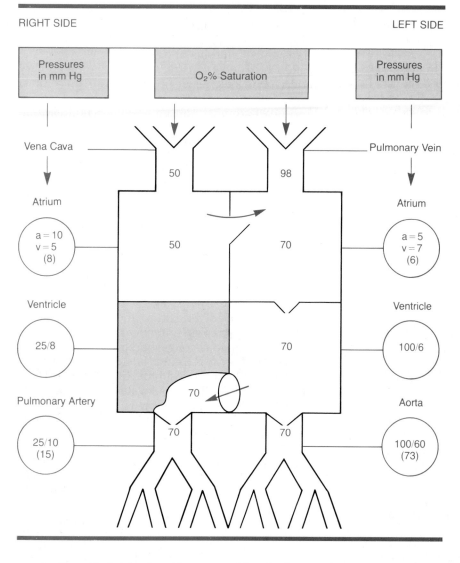

RIGHT SIDE

LEFT SIDE

| Pressures in mm Hg | O₂% Saturation | Pressures in mm Hg |

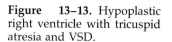

Figure   13–13. Hypoplastic right ventricle with tricuspid atresia and VSD.

eventually diminished pulmonary blood flow occurs.

Clinical Manifestations. The age of the patient and findings on presentation primarily are related to the size of the VSD and, thus, dependent on the pulmonary blood flow. In those infrequent cases in which the VSD is very small from birth, pulmonary blood flow depends on the ductus arteriosus, so that marked hypoxemia occurs when the ductus closes. In the majority of cases, however, the VSD is large enough so that the infants do well early in the 1st yr. In the infant with a small VSD, the chest roentgenogram shows a normal-sized heart with diminished pulmonary vascularity. The ECG shows considerable LVH because of the hypoplastic RV and the increased volume work of the LV.

Because the VSD is in the endocardial cushion position, abnormal conduction of the left anterior branch of the left bundle is present, resulting in an abnormally superior vector. In the newborn, this latter ECG finding is a strong clue in separating this lesion from a hypoplastic RV with pulmonary atresia.

After 2–3 yr of life, inverted T waves over the left precordium are common, suggesting a more severe LVH and fibrosis as part of left ventricular cardiomyopathy. Also, RAE is present. The echocardiogram describes the anatomy, and at catheterization (necessary only prior to consideration of Fontan types of procedures), all right atrial blood goes across the atrial opening to the LA. The catheter is easily passed into the LV and usually the aorta. Cineangiography shows the large LV, the hypoplastic RV, and the VSD. The pulmonary arteries usually are well visualized past the bifurcation into right and left branches.

Treatment and Prognosis. In the newborn period, for the child with markedly diminished pulmonary blood flow, PGE_1 infusion, by maintaining patency of the ductus arteriosus, may be lifesaving until a Blalock-Taussig shunt can be performed. Usually the administration of PGE_1 is not necessary, and for those infants who have a good VSD murmur and whose systemic arterial saturation is above 75%, administration of PGE_1 and creation of a shunt is not indicated. For those few infants with excessive pulmonary blood flow who go into heart failure in the 1st mo of life, the usual anticongestive measures are indicated (Table 13–6). Later, after the VSD gets smaller, digoxin and diuretics are discontinued.

To safely perform a *physiologic repair*, PVR must be low, the pulmonary arteries must not have been badly distorted, and the LV must be compliant. The long-term "corrective" operation is a *modified Fontan procedure* (connection of the RA to the pulmonary arteries). The surgery now usually is staged, beginning with a bidirectional systemic vein–to–pulmonary artery shunt at 1–2 yr of age. Long-term results are not yet available, but the operative risk should be less than 10%; short-term follow-up is promising. However, many patients have large congested livers for many years, and the sick sinus node syndrome also sometimes occurs.

TRUNCUS ARTERIOSUS

In this anomaly, a single arterial trunk from the base of the heart gives rise to the aorta, pulmonary arteries, and coronary arteries. A large VSD invariably is present and the single semilunar valve has a variable number of leaflets, usually between two and six. The valve may be either stenotic or regurgitant but usually is neither. The pulmonary arteries may arise as a single trunk before bifurcating (type 1) or may arise separately from the posterior wall of the aorta (type 2).

Because there is a common exit to the aorta and pulmonary artery, the saturation of blood in the systemic arteries is approximately equal to that in the pulmonary arteries. The level of arterial saturation depends on the amount of pulmonary blood flow. If the PVR is high, moderate hypoxemia may result. When the PVR is low, pulmonary blood flow may be torrential, cyanosis minimal, and heart failure severe.

Clinical Findings. Initially after birth, the PVR is high and the newborn may do well. As the PVR drops, the pulmonary blood flow increases and the signs and symptoms of heart failure develop. The runoff of blood from truncus into the pulmonary artery in diastole results in a very wide pulse pressure. The heart is hyperdynamic, with loud 1st and 2nd heart sounds, and an aortic ejection click almost always is present. A grade 2 to 3/6 systolic ejection murmur usually is noted at the upper left or right sternal border from increased flow across the semilunar valve, but if the truncal valve is stenotic, the murmur may be grade 4 and associated with a thrill. An early high-frequency diastolic murmur is present if the truncal valve is regurgitant, and a mid-diastolic rumble at the apex may be present if the pulmonary blood flow (and therefore flow across the mitral valve) is increased. In the older child who has developed increased PVR, progressive cyanosis, polycythemia, and clubbing may occur.

On chest roentgenogram, the heart usually is large, with increased pulmonary vascularity and pulmonary venous congestion; in 40% of patients, a right aortic arch is found. Because of the association with DiGeorge syndrome, the thymus shadow may be absent. When an elevated PVR and diminished pulmonary blood flow is present, the ECG shows RVH, but in the more usual cases, with very increased pulmonary blood flow, biventricular hypertrophy is expected. On echocardiogram the anatomy usually is seen well, with no demonstrable infundibulum present. At cardiac catheterization and angiography, the catheter usually can pass into the pulmonary arteries from the truncus arteriosus. Right-to-left and left-to-right shunts at the ventricular level are present, with systolic pressures equal in both ventricles.

Treatment and Prognosis. Children should be evaluated for hypocalcemia and T cell deficiencies associated with DiGeorge syndrome. Children with persistent truncus arteriosus usually present early in life, within the first few weeks. The use of vigorous anticongestive measures in an attempt to get the children to grow are worthwhile but frequently unsuccessful. A modified Rastelli procedure is performed at 3–6 mo of age. The VSD is closed so that the LV passes unimpeded into the truncal valve. The pulmonary artery is removed from the back of the aorta, usually using a button of aorta; the aortic opening is closed, and the RV is connected to the pulmonary arteries using a prosthetic conduit or aortic homograft. At selected centers, the early results have been promising, although a mortality rate of about 20% persists. Early surgery may be indicated for intractable heart failure. Successful surgery necessarily requires a later reoperation as the children "outgrow" the conduit.

TOTAL ANOMALOUS PULMONARY VENOUS CONNECTION

In this lesion there is a failure of incorporation of the common pulmonary vein into the posterior wall of the LA. During embryogenesis, the pulmonary venous return is diverted into one of the early embryonic channels returning to the right side of the heart. If the left cardinal system persists, pulmonary venous return is to the left superior vena cava, which may drain into the innominate vein or into the coronary sinus and then into the RA. If the right cardinal system persists, the pulmonary veins drain into the right superior vena cava, usually by way of a persistent ascending LV vein. Drainage directly into the RA is rare. If the umbilical–vitelline system persists, the common pulmonary veins drain inferiorly through the diaphragm, usually into the portal system of the liver. There is severe obstruction in the liver so that right atrial flow is diminished and pulmonary venous hypertension and congestion are severe. Also, severe pulmonary hypertension is present as a result of a very high PVR. When the drainage is above the diaphragm, pulmonary venous obstruction is not common and PVR usually becomes low. It is uncommon for infants with the latter condition to present before 1 mo of age. Congestive heart failure may be severe. Rarely, these children present late in a manner similar to infants who have an ASD; heart failure and cyanosis are milder than in those infants that present earlier.

Clinical Manifestations. Infants who have obstructed pulmonary veins present in the newborn period with severe cyanosis and tachypnea. Usually, no murmurs are present and the electrocardiogram shows marked RVH. On the chest roentgenogram, the heart is of normal size but interstitial fluid is increased as a result of the marked pulmonary venous congestion, often quite similar in appearance to that of respiratory distress syndrome. For children with only mild or no obstruction who present after the newborn period, cyanosis is subtle but may increase with crying or other exertion. Heart failure may be very severe with a hyperactive right ventricular impulse and a widely split 2nd heart sound that moves little with respiration. The ECG shows severe RVH; cardiac enlargement and increased pulmonary vascularity are apparent on

the chest roentgenogram. Rarely, infants in this group are asymptomatic, with the abnormality resembling a simple large ASD.

The echocardiogram is diagnostic, although the common pulmonary venous trunk may be difficult to delineate. Cardiac catheterization shows common mixing at the right atrial level, with approximately equal saturations in the RA, RV, and pulmonary artery as well as in the LA, LV, and aorta. Cineangiocardiograms usually can show the sites of drainage by injections either directly into the pulmonary artery or into the common pulmonary vein entered by way of its anomalous connection.

Treatment and Prognosis. For the newborn with obstructed pulmonary veins, emergency surgery is necessary. For those who present later in infancy or childhood, elective surgery is recommended. The usual operation is to open a wide connection between the common pulmonary vein and the back wall of the LA, after which the previously useful anomalous connection is ligated. For the infant or older child with low PVR, the prognosis is excellent, with a low surgical risk (under 2%) and a low incidence of postoperative complications. For the newborn with obstructed total veins, surgery is hazardous (10–25% mortality rate) because of difficult anatomic problems and serious cardiovascular decompensation prior to surgery. Rapid identification and diagnosis result in a lower mortality rate because the surgery is not technically difficult.

HYPOPLASTIC LEFT HEART SYNDROME

The hypoplastic left heart syndrome includes a number of closely related anomalies that are part of hypoplasia and underdevelopment of the LV. The mitral and aortic valves usually are hypoplastic, and one or both of them may be atretic. The ascending aorta usually is small, although coronary arteries are in the normal position. Discrete coarctation of the aorta may be present. After birth, the pulmonary venous return from the LA passes across the atrial septum into the RA and then to the RV and the pulmonary artery. The systemic blood flow is via the ductus arteriosus to the ascending and descending aorta. Affected fetuses do well in utero, but, after birth, the infants become ill very quickly. After birth, the pulmonary venous return comes back to the LA and must go across the atrial septum. If the atrial defect is small, as is usually the case, pulmonary venous pressure increases and the signs and symptoms of left-sided heart failure appear. The entire systemic cardiac output must pass through the ductus arteriosus, so that, when this vessel constricts, systemic cardiac output is reduced. Eventually acidosis, hypotension, and death occur.

Clinical Manifestations. The usual manifestations are a combination of heart failure resulting from excessive pulmonary blood flow and obstructed pulmonary venous return. Low cardiac output and acidosis occur after constriction of the ductus arteriosus. All peripheral pulses are weak or absent. Cyanosis usually is not prominent, but low cardiac output gives a grayish color to the cool, mottled skin. The cardiac impulse usually is hyperdynamic. Murmurs are not prominent but may be present as a result of increased flow across the tricuspid and pulmonic valves.

The ECG shows severe RVH because of the systemic right ventricular pressure, torrential pulmonary blood flow, and the hypoplastic LV. On the chest roentgenogram, the heart usually is enlarged and there are increased pulmonary vascularity and pulmonary venous congestion. The echocardiogram is diagnostic. The right side of the heart is large. A cardiac catheterization is not necessary because it merely adds undue risk for the infant.

Treatment and Prognosis. Without surgery, early death is inevitable. During the past 10 yr, a two-stage palliative approach has been done. The first stage, developed by Norwood, involves creating a large atrial opening by an atrial septectomy, dividing the pulmonary artery, and connecting the proximal segment to the ascending aorta and the distal segment to the descending aorta via a Blalock-Taussig shunt. Thus, the RV serves as the systemic ventricle, pumping blood through the pulmonary valve into the aorta with pulmonary blood flow supplied via a systemic-to-pulmonary artery shunt. As a second stage, a Fontan operation is performed when the child is about 2 yr of age.

These procedures are being done in a very limited number of institutions, with first-stage survival rates of approximately 40–75% (closer to the latter in institutions in which many operations are performed). Survival through both stages, however, is significantly lower. An alternative approach is cardiac transplantation in the newborn.

The High-Risk Newborn

A myriad of congenital heart diseases are exhibited in the neonatal period, often causing great diagnostic confusion. Despite the large varieties of possible diagnoses, approximately 70% of infants affected by these diseases have one of six lesions:

(1) hypoplastic left ventricle syndrome; (2) transposition of the great arteries with intact ventricular septum; (3) hypoplastic right ventricle with tricuspid atresia; (4) hypoplastic right ventricle with pulmonary atresia; (5) complicated coarctation of the aorta (with VSD); or (6) tetralogy of Fallot. For completeness, obstructed total anomalous veins also might be added to this list. The infants usually present with characteristic signs and symptoms that can be divided into four groups (Table 13–13). Treatment is noted in Tables 13–8 and 13–9.

Prenatal Detection and Treatment of Congenital Cardiac Defects

Congenital heart defects are being diagnosed more frequently prenatally. Cardiac ultrasound scans usually are performed first by obstetricians. An abnormal four-chamber view of the heart prompts referral to the pediatric cardiac center. Primary pediatric cardiac fetal ultrasound examinations often are performed if the mother or father had congenital heart disease or if they had a previous child with a congenital heart defect.

Fetal echocardiography is accurate in diagnosing the most severe types of congenital cardiac defects, such as valve atresia or severe stenosis. It cannot diagnose mild defects such as PDA or ASD, which are normal in the fetus. It can sometimes diagnose VSDs or coarctation of the aorta. Fetal echocardiography is still an evolving science both in a technological sense and in our understanding of fetal anatomy and physiology. It has already taught us that fetal congenital heart disease is more common than we thought, that fetal wastage is common, and that the defects progress throughout fetal life. Although the usual earliest time at which fetal echocardiography can be performed is now about 16 wk, this will decrease with improved techniques and technology.

Fetal ultrasound is useful in diagnosing arrhythmias and in following the progression and response to treatment. Both tachyarrhythmias and bradyarrhythmias occur in the fetus and may lead to fetal congestive heart failure and death. Other arrhythmias, such as premature atrial contractions, are common and probably benign. Congenital complete AV block usually is well tolerated in the fetus. The ventricles are able to compensate for the slow rate by increasing their stroke volume. If there is associated congenital heart disease, however, **fetal hydrops** (congestive heart failure) may occur. This is diagnosed by fetal scalp edema and/or ascites or other fetal edema noted by echocardiography. Congenital complete AV block without associated

Table 13–13. Categories of Cyanotic Heart Lesions in the Neonate

Group	Heart Size	Pulmonary Blood Flow	Low Cardiac Output	Respiratory Distress	Examples
I	Small	Reduced	No	None	1) Hypoplastic RV with pulmonary atresia 2) Hypoplastic RV with tricuspid atresia 3) Tetralogy of Fallot
II	Small or slight cardiomegaly	Increased	No	Moderate	Transposition of great arteries with intact ventricular septum
III	Large	Increased	Yes	Yes	1) Complicated coarctation of aorta with VSD 2) Hypoplastic LV
IV	Small	Pulmonary venous congestion	Yes	Yes	Obstructed total anomalous veins

heart defects often is associated with maternal connective tissue disorders such as lupus.

Fetal supraventricular tachycardias cause hydrops more frequently than bradycardias. Hydrops can occur within 24 hr or less. Thus, rapid effective treatment is necessary. Initial treatment may be delivery if the fetus is mature. For less mature fetuses, drug treatment through the mother is used. Different antiarrhythmics pass through the placenta to the fetus with different fetal–maternal ratios. Digitalis has the advantages of a virtual 1:1 ratio and of increasing contractility as well as slowing conduction in the AV node to attempt to stop the tachycardia. It has the disadvantage of a relatively slow onset of action and a small therapeutic–toxic ratio in the fetus and mother. If the mechanism of the tachycardia is atrial re-entry (atrial flutter), digitalis also can result in 2:1 AV block, which tends to prevent hydrops as a result of a slower ventricular rate. If digitalis fails, other drugs may be used by giving them to the mother orally. If the fetus develops hydrops, then drugs pass the placenta less well. The fetal umbilical vein may be cannulated and drugs given directly to the fetus. Amiodarone is particularly useful in this regard because it has a long half-life even when given intravenously. Very frequent follow-up using fetal ultrasound is used to control therapy.

The diagnosis of a severe congenital cardiac defect presents a major moral dilemma. Most congenital cardiac defects now can be at least well palliated after birth. The decision between fetal termination and delivery of the infant and treatment of the heart defect is a difficult and individual decision. We have begun to see fetal intervention in cases of severe aortic stenosis that are documented to be progressing to an inoperable state.

References

Behrman RE (ed): Nelson Textbook of Pediatrics. 14th ed. Philadelphia, WB Saunders, 1992, Sec. 15.11–15.61.

Jonas RA, Lang P: Open repair of cardiac defects in neonates and young infants. Clin Perinatol 15:659, 1988.

Morban BC: Incidence, etiology, and classification of congenital heart disease. Pediatr Clin North Am 25:721, 1978.

Norwood WI, Pigott JD: Recent advances in congenital cardiac surgery. Clin Perinatol 15:713, 1988.

Perry SB, Keane JF, Lock JE: Interventional catheterization in pediatric congenital and acquired heart disease. Am J Cardiol 61:109G, 1988.

Radford DJ, Thong YH: The association between immunodeficiency and congenital heart disease. Pediatr Cardiol 9:103, 1988.

Rao PS: Transcatheter therapy of cardiac defects in infants and children. Indian J Pediatr 55:137, 1988.

Van Hare GF, Soffer LL, Sivakoff MC, et al: 25 year experience with ventricular septal defect. Am Heart J 114:606, 1987.

Zeevi B, Perry SB, Keane JF, et al: Interventional cardiac procedures in neonates and infants: State of the art. Clin Perinatol 15:633, 1988.

CARDIOMYOPATHIES–MYOCARDITIS

The primary cardiomyopathies are conditions involving the myocardium. Invariably the problem for the patient is left ventricular dysfunction; however, biopsy data indicate that the right ventricle also is involved. Most of these cardiomyopathies are of the dilated type, often called congestive cardiomyopathy. Restrictive cardiomyopathies are rare, as is the slightly more common hypertrophic cardiomyopathy.

Although many cases are considered idiopathic, specific etiologies increasingly are being discov-

Table 13–14. Etiology of Myocardial Disease

Familial–Hereditary Duchenne muscular dystrophy Other muscular dystrophies (Becker, limb girdle) Myotonic dystrophy Kearns-Sayre syndrome (progressive external ophthalmoplegia) Friedreich ataxia Hemochromatosis Fabry disease Pompe disease Carnitine deficiency syndromes Endocardial fibroelastosis Mitochondrial myopathy syndromes	**Connective Tissue—Granulomatous Disease** SLE Scleroderma Churg-Strauss syndrome Rheumatoid arthritis Rheumatic fever Sarcoidosis Amyloidosis Dermatomyositis
Infections Viral (coxsackievirus, mumps, Epstein-Barr virus, varicella) Rickettsiae (psittacosis, *Coxiella*, Rocky Mountain spotted fever) Bacterial (diphtheria, *Mycoplasma, Meningococcus*, leptospirosis, Lyme disease) Parasitic (Chagas disease, toxoplasmosis, loa loa)	**Drugs–Toxins** Adriamycin Ipecac Iron overload (hemosiderosis) Irradiation **Coronary Arteries** Anomalous left coronary artery Kawasaki disease
Metabolic, Nutritional, Endocrine Beriberi (thiamine deficiency) Keshan disease (selenium deficiency) Hypothyroidism Hyperthyroidism Carcinoid Pheochromocytoma	**Other** Sickle cell anemia Hypereosinophilic syndrome Endomyocardial fibrosis Asymmetric septal hypertrophy Idiopathic

SLE = systemic lupus erythematosus.

ered. Almost all the dilated cardiomyopathies can be categorized into three types: (1) myocarditis; (2) a primary cardiomyopathy, often familial, caused by various abnormalities of mitochondrial energy metabolism; and (3) those induced by drugs, particularly Adriamycin (Table 13–14).

Myocarditis can occur at any age, including during the newborn period, and frequently is found to be related to a viral infection, such as coxsackie B virus. Myocarditis is diagnosed during the acute episode by a dilated large heart; severe heart failure, sometimes with shock; and marked ST segment abnormalities on the ECG. Before the era of intensive care units, children often died within 24 hr; if they survived when treated with digitalis and diuretics, they frequently recovered. Today, many patients survive as a result of intensive care with intubation, mechanical ventilation, positive inotropes, and various afterload-reducing drugs (see Table 13–6). Most of these children also appear to recover completely, but some develop severe chronic cardiomyopathy. Some patients who gradually develop congestive cardiomyopathy may have had asymptomatic viral myocarditis in the past, but others with this disorder have mitochondrial abnormalities and metabolic and familial disorders; fewer cases are being called idiopathic.

Another related concept is *endocardial fibroelastosis* (EFE); it is usually a secondary rather than a primary disorder. EFE occasionally is associated with a small LV and small, very abnormal aortic and mitral valves. However, EFE is also a nonspecific response to some cardiomyopathies. Primary EFE, rarely, may be seen in certain families and in infants with an anomalous left coronary artery arising from the pulmonary artery.

Patients with acute myocarditis may die. However, if they survive the difficult early period, they have an excellent chance for complete recovery. In contrast, patients with cardiomyopathy not caused by myocarditis have a poorer prognosis and are not likely to recover. Although some children may stabilize, others rapidly deteriorate. A heart transplant is the only useful therapy after unsuccessful treatment with regimens to manage congestive heart failure.

References

Behrman RE (ed): Nelson Textbook of Pediatrics. 14th ed. Philadelphia, WB Saunders, 1992, Sec. 15.68–15.72.

DeSa DJ: Isolated myocarditis in the first year. Arch Dis Child 60:484, 1985.

Kawai C, Matsumori A, Fujiwara H: Myocarditis and dilated cardiomyopathy. Annu Rev Med 38:221, 1987.

Kopecky SL, Gersh BJ: Dilated cardiomyopathy and myocarditis: Natural history, etiology, clinical manifestations, and management. Curr Probl Cardiol 12:569, 1987.

Lie J: Myocarditis and endomyocardial biopsy in unexplained heart failure: A diagnosis in search of a disease. Ann Intern Med 109:525, 1988.

ACUTE RHEUMATIC FEVER

Rheumatic fever was very common in the United States until the late 1960s and early 1970s, when a sharp decline in the incidence was reported; since the mid-1980s, multiple small outbreaks have been reported. Furthermore, acute rheumatic fever (ARF) remains very common in many developing nations. The most commonly affected group is children between 5 and 15 yr of age, but infants and adults also can be affected.

The *pathogenesis* is related to an immune reaction to untreated group A beta-hemolytic streptococcus infection. The serotype of the streptococcus and the genetically determined immune response of the host play a role in the development of ARF.

Clinical Manifestations. The wide variety of manifestations of the disease and the similarity to many other diseases may lead to difficulty in diagnosing ARF. The Jones criteria are an attempt to improve diagnosis (Table 13–15). Typically, a child presents 2–6 wk after a pharyngitis with one or more of the major or minor manifestations of ARF as described in these criteria. Arthritis may be difficult to establish. Chorea and erythema marginatum usually are easy to identify, but subcutaneous nodules are not likely to be present unless the disease is obvious and chronic. Evidence for carditis is very reliable in the hands of experienced physicians. The P-R interval widening is a weak minor criterion because it is nonspecific; if it varies with time (hourly), it is helpful. Varying QRS voltage in the chest leads provides a strong minor criterion if the voltages are measured daily. The presence of a new murmur is very strong evidence for carditis, although overdiagnosis is common because auscultation is not always specific. To diagnose carditis of ARF on the basis of heart murmur, the murmur must be (1) the murmur of mitral regurgitation, a murmur that may be as soft as grade 2, is high frequency, does not necessarily start with S_1, usually is almost full length, peaking late, and is best heard at the apex; (2) the murmur of aortic regurgitation, a high-frequency diastolic decrescendo murmur at the 3rd–5th left interspace of any intensity or length, with or without a wide pulse pressure, or (3) a mid-diastolic rumbling murmur at the apex, the Carey-Coombs murmur, believed to result from edema of the mitral valve. Finally, the erythrocyte sedimentation rate usually is elevated in ARF. Proof of streptococcal infection is critical to the diagnosis of ARF. The echocardiographic delineation of mild mitral regurgitation is not diagnostic of ARF.

Chronic rheumatic heart disease produces specific lesions: (1) mitral regurgitation, (2) mitral stenosis, (3) mitral stenosis with mitral regurgitation, (4) aortic regurgitation, or (5) aortic regurgitation with aortic stenosis. Rarely, the tricuspid valve is

Table 13–15. Major Criteria in the Jones System for Acute Rheumatic Fever[*,†]

Sign	Comments
Polyarthritis	Common: Swelling, limited motion, very tender, erythema; migratory: involves large joints but rarely small or unusual joints, such as vertebrae
Carditis	Common: Pancarditis, valves, pericardium, myocardium; tachycardia greater than explained by fever; new murmur of mitral or aortic insufficiency; Carey-Coombs mid-diastolic murmur; heart failure
Chorea (Sydenham disease)	Uncommon: Presents long after infection has resolved
Erythema marginatum	Uncommon: Pink macules on trunk and proximal extremities, evolving to serpiginous border with central clearing; evanescent, elicited by application of local heat; nonpruritic
Subcutaneous nodules	Uncommon: Associated with repeated episodes and severe carditis; present over extensor surface of elbows, knees, knuckles, and ankles or scalp and spine; firm, nontender

[*] Minor criteria include fever (101–102°F [38.2–38.9°C]), arthralgias, previous rheumatic fever, leukocytosis, elevated erythrocyte sedimentation rate/C-reactive protein, prolonged P-R interval.

[†] One major plus two minor, or two major criteria with evidence of recent group A streptococcal disease (scarlet fever, positive throat culture, or elevated antistreptolysin O or other antistreptococcal antibodies), strongly suggests the diagnosis of acute rheumatic fever.

involved. The pulmonary valve is not known to be involved, and pure or dominant aortic stenosis does not occur.

In pure mitral regurgitation, the mid-diastolic low-frequency murmur does not extend into late diastole. When pure mitral stenosis (and sinus rhythm) is present, the diastolic low-frequency murmur extends into late diastole, often with pre-systolic accentuation. If mitral regurgitation with stenosis is present, a long diastolic murmur extending into late diastole also is present. Aortic regurgitation may distort the anterior leaflet of the mitral valve as the blood leaks back into the LV, resulting in the low-frequency mid-diastolic murmur called the Austin Flint murmur.

Treatment. The management of ARF consists almost entirely of nonspecific measures—bed rest, penicillin to eradicate the beta-hemolytic streptococcus, and aspirin for the arthritic pain. Steroids have not proved effective in minimizing valve damage, and they should not be used except for patients with severe life-threatening carditis.

Once the diagnosis is made, whether valvulitis is present or not, permanent penicillin prophylaxis is essential. Intramuscular penicillin G benzathine (Bicillin) given every 28 days is more reliable than low-dose oral penicillin given twice a day. Patients on a continuous Bicillin regimen for 10 yr usually improve; only 30% of patients with mitral regurgitation on initial evaluation still have a murmur, although fewer patients with aortic regurgitation lose their murmur. Few treated patients develop mitral stenosis, but poor compliance is associated with the development of mitral stenosis. The development of a stenotic valvular lesion probably is usually due to repeated episodes of ARF. Prevention of such attacks with penicillin should eliminate this late sequela.

Treatment of valve disease includes balloon valvotomy, valve replacement, and vigilant antimicrobial prophylaxis to prevent bacterial endocarditis.

References

Behrman RE (ed): Nelson Textbook of Pediatrics. 14th ed. Philadelphia, WB Saunders, 1992, Sec. 11.75, 15.67.

Gillum RF: Trends in acute rheumatic fever and chronic rheumatic heart disease: A national perspective. Am Heart J 111:430, 1986.

Markowitz M: Rheumatic fever in the eighties. Pediatr Clin North Am 33:1141, 1986.

Tadzynski LA, Ryan ME: Diagnosis of rheumatic fever. A guide to the criteria and manifestations. Postgrad Med 79:295, 1986.

Veasy L, Wiedmeier S, Orsmond G, et al: Resurgence of acute rheumatic fever in the intermountain area of the United States. N Engl J Med 316:421, 1987.

PERICARDITIS

Pericardial diseases and inflammatory responses of the pericardium may be caused by common and uncommon disorders. Inflammatory processes, such as viral or bacterial infections and immune-mediated disease (postinfectious immune complexes, connective tissue diseases, the presence of autoantibody), are the most common pathogenic mechanisms in pediatric patients. Other causes include uremia, hypothyroidism, trauma, postpericardiotomy, and malignancy.

The *clinical manifestations* of pericarditis as it progresses from a simple inflammatory response of the pericardium with no cardiovascular compromise to cardiac tamponade and constrictive pericarditis are noted in Table 13–16. Laboratory diagnosis is obtained by evaluation of the ECG and chest roentgenogram but is confirmed by echocardiography

Table 13–16. Manifestations of Pericarditis

Symptoms
Chest pain (worsened if lying down or with inspiration)
Dyspnea
Malaise
Patient assumes sitting position

Signs
Nonconstrictive
  Fever
  Tachycardia
  Friction rub (accentuated by inspiration, body position)
  Enlarged heart by percussion
  Distant heart sounds

Tamponade: as above plus
  Distended neck veins
  Hepatomegaly
  Pulsus paradoxus (greater than 10 mm Hg with inspiration)
  Narrow pulse pressure
  Weak pulse, poor peripheral perfusion

Constrictive Pericarditis
  Distended neck veins
  Kussmaul sign (inspiratory increase of jugular venous pressure)
  Distant heart sounds
  Pericardial knock
  Hepatomegaly
  Ascites
  Edema
  Tachycardia

Table 13–17. Laboratory Evidence of Pericarditis

ECG	Elevated ST segments, T wave inversion (late), tachycardia, reduced QRS voltage, electrical alternans (variable QRS amplitudes)
Chest roentgenogram	Cardiomegaly ("water bottle heart")
Echocardiogram	Pericardial fluid
Pericardiocentesis	Gram and acid-fast stains, culture (virus, bacteria, mycobacteria, fungus). Cytology, cell count, glucose, protein, pH
Blood tests	ESR, viral titers, ANA, ASO titers, EBV titers

ANA = antinuclear antibodies; ASO = antistreptolysin O; EBV = Epstein-Barr virus; ESR = erythrocyte sedimentation rate.

and eventually by examination of the pericardial fluid obtained by pericardiocentesis (Table 13–17). *Treatment* is directed at the underlying disease process, alleviation of pericardial fluid accumulation by pericardiocentesis or pericardial drainage, or surgical stripping of the pericardium in patients with constrictive pericarditis.

References

Behrman RE (ed): Nelson Textbook of Pediatrics. 14th ed. Philadelphia, WB Saunders, 1992, Sec. 15.75.

Permanyer-Miralda G, Sagrist A, Sauleda J, Soler J: Primary acute pericardial disease: A prospective series of 231 consecutive patients. Am J Cardiol 56:623, 1985.

Sinzobahamvya N, Ikeogu MO: Purulent pericarditis. Arch Dis Child 62:696, 1987.

INFECTIVE ENDOCARDITIS
(See Chapter 10)

Bacterial endocarditis is infrequent in pediatric patients and occurs on native valves, valves damaged by rheumatic fever, congenitally abnormal valves, acquired valvular lesions (mitral valve prolapse), and prosthetic replacement valves and as a consequence of jet streams of turbulent blood (PDA, VSD, systemic-to-pulmonary shunts). A listing of predisposing factors for the preceding bacteremia, laboratory tests, and *clinical manifestations* of bacterial endocarditis is presented in Table 13–18. Because of the endovascular nature of endocarditis, bacteremia is usually of a continuous nature, may be low grade (few bacteria per milliliter of blood), and is not necessarily altered during episodes of fever or chills. Therefore, the volume of the blood culture probably is more important than the frequency of obtaining cultures. The pathogens responsible for endocarditis depend on the status of the heart valve and the presence or absence of a predisposing procedure. Because some bacterial agents have unusual nutritional requirements and others may need longer than the usual incubation period to demonstrate growth in vitro, the blood samples should be labeled so that, when endocarditis is suspected, the sample can be observed for a longer time. Despite adequate blood culture techniques, 10–15% of cases of endocarditis are culture negative.

Treatment of culture-negative patients requires knowledge of the epidemiology and historic risk factors for that patient. Treatment of culture-positive patients is directed against the particular bacteria (*S. aureus*, *S. viridens*, enterococcus, HACEK

Table 13–18. Manifestations of Infective Endocarditis

History
Prior congenital or rheumatic heart disease
Preceding dental, urinary, or intestinal procedure
Intravenous drug abuse
Central venous catheter
Prosthetic heart valve

Symptoms
Fever
Chills
Chest pain
Arthralgia/myalgia
Dyspnea
Malaise

Signs
Fever
Tachycardia
Embolic phenomena (Roth spots, petechiae, Osler nodes, CNS lesion)
Janeway lesions
New or changing murmur
Splenomegaly
Arthritis
Heart failure
Arrhythmias

Laboratory Tests
Positive blood culture
Elevated ESR, CRP
Leukocytosis
Immune complexes
Rheumatoid factor
Hematuria
Echocardiographic evidence of valve vegetations

CNS = central nervous system; CRP = C-reactive protein; ESR = erythrocyte sedimentation rate.

group bacteria, etc.) using bactericidal antibiotics. Therapy is continued for 4–8 wk (see Chapter 10). Surgery for endocarditis is indicated if medical treatment is unsuccessful or for an unusual pathogen, myocardial abscess formation, refractory heart failure, serious embolic complications, or refractory prosthetic valve disease.

Prevention of endocarditis is necessary for all patients with structural congenital heart disease, rheumatic valve lesions, prosthetic heart valves, mitral valve prolapse with a regurgitant valve, idiopathic hypertrophic subaortic stenosis, transvenous pacemaker leads, or surgical systemic-to-pulmonary shunts, and for patients with previous endocarditis. Antimicrobial prophylaxis is not indicated for an isolated secundum ASD, a repaired secundum ASD 6 mo after patch placement, or a divided and ligated PDA 6 mo after repair. Antibiotic regimens to prevent endocarditis during dental or respiratory procedures include oral amoxicillin or parenteral ampicillin plus gentamicin. The latter recommendation is for high-risk patients, such as those with prosthetic heart valves, systemic-to-pulmonary shunts, or previous endocarditis. Preventive treatment for gastrointestinal or genitourinary manipulation includes parenteral ampicillin and gentamicin or oral amoxicillin. Vancomycin can be added to gentamicin in penicillin-allergic patients (see Appendix I for dosages).

References

Behrman RE (ed): Nelson Textbook of Pediatrics. 14th ed. Philadelphia, WB Saunders, 1992, Sec. 15.66.

Kavey RE, Frank DM, Byrum CJ, et al: Two-dimensional echocardiographic assessment of infective endocarditis in children. Am J Dis Child 137:851, 1983.

Sanyal SK, Saleh MA, Abu-Melha A: Infective endocarditis during infancy and childhood: Current status. Indian J Pediatr 55:51, 1988.

Van Hare G, Ben-Shachar G, Liebman J, et al: Infective endocarditis in infants and children during the past 10 years: A decade of change. Am Heart J 107:1235, 1984.

Weinstein M, Stratton C, Ackley A, Hawley H, et al: Multicenter collaborative evaluation of a standardized serum bactericidal test as a prognostic indicator in infective endocarditis. Am J Med 78:262, 1985.

DYSRHYTHMIAS

Cardiac dysrhythmias are a frequent occurrence in children. A dysrhythmia is an abnormal rhythm; the term *arrhythmia* often is used as a synonym.

Table 13–19. Etiology of Arrhythmias

Drugs
Intoxication (cocaine, tricyclic antidepressants, others)
Antiarrhythmic agents (proarrhythmic agents, e.g., quinidine)
Sympathomimetic agents (caffeine, theophylline, ephedrine, others)
Digoxin

Infections/Postinfections
Endocarditis
Lyme disease
Diphtheria
Myocarditis
Guillain-Barré syndrome
Rheumatic fever

Metabolic–Endocrine
Cardiomyopathy
Electrolyte disturbances ($\downarrow \uparrow K^+$, $\downarrow \uparrow Ca^{2+}$, $\downarrow Mg^{2+}$)
Uremia
Thyrotoxicosis
Pheochromocytoma
Porphyria

Structural Lesions
Mitral valve prolapse
Ventricular tumor
Ventriculotomy
Pre-excitation/aberrant conduction system
Congenital heart defects
Arrhythmogenic right ventricle

Other
Adrenergic induced
Prolonged QT interval
Maternal SLE
Idiopathic
Central venous catheter

SLE = systemic lupus erythematosus.

The diverse etiologies are presented in Table 13–19 and the common types and their treatment in Table 13–20. Many pediatric dysrhythmias do not present a risk to the patient and are normal variants.

Some cardiac abnormalities are subtle, such as the prolonged Q-T interval, arrhythmogenic right ventricular dysplasia, and mild cardiomyopathy or myocarditis. Ventricular dysrhythmias that require treatment usually are treated with antiarrhythmic drugs (Table 13–21). A specific treatable etiology rarely is found. Infants and young children (≤4 yr) are the exception, often having small tumors that can be treated with surgery.

Sinus Arrhythmia and Wandering Atrial Pacemaker

These are phasic variations with respiration that are heard in virtually all normal children. They are

Table 13–20. Arrhythmias in Children

Type	ECG Characteristics	Treatment
Complete heart block	Atria and ventricles have independent pacemakers; atrioventricular dissociation; escape-pacemaker is at atrioventricular junction if congenital	Awake rate <55 in neonate or <40 in adolescent or hemodynamic instability requires permanent pacemaker
First-degree heart block	Prolonged P-R interval for age	Observe, obtain digoxin level if on therapy
Mobitz type I (Wenckebach) second-degree block	Progressive lengthening of P-R interval until P wave is not followed by conducted QRS complex	Observe, correct underlying electrolyte or other abnormalities
Mobitz type II second-degree heart block	Sudden nonconduction of P wave with loss of QRS complex without progressive P-R interval lengthening	Consider pacemaker
Sinus tachycardia	Rate less than 240	Treat fever, remove sympathomimetic drugs
Supraventricular tachycardia	Rate usually greater than 200 (180–320); abnormal atrial rate for age; ventricular rate may be slower due to AV block; P waves usually present and are related to QRS complex; normal QRS complexes unless aberrant conduction is present	Increase vagal tone (ice water to face, Valsalva maneuver); digoxin; adenosine; electrical cardioversion if acutely ill; catheter ablation
Atrial flutter	Atrial rate usually 300, with varying degrees of block; sawtooth flutter waves	Digoxin, cardioversion
Premature ventricular contraction (PVC)	Premature, wide, unusually shaped QRS complex, with large inverted T wave	None if normal heart and PVCs disappear on exercise; Lidocaine, procainamide, quinidine
Ventricular tachycardia	Three or more premature ventricular beats; AV dissociation; fusion beats, blocked retrograde AV conduction; sustained if longer than 30 sec; rate 120–240	Lidocaine, cardioversion, procainamide, propranolol, bretylium, phenytoin
Ventricular fibrillation	No distinct QRS complex or T waves; irregular undulations with varied amplitude and contour; no conducted pulse	Nonsynchronized cardioversion

Table 13–21. Classification of Drugs for Antiarrhythmia

Class	Action	Examples
I	Depresses phase O depolarization; sodium channel blockers	
Ia	Prolong QRS complex and Q-T interval	Quinidine, procainamide
Ib	Significant effect on abnormal conduction	Lidocaine, mexiletine, phenytoin
Ic	Prolong QRS complex and P-R interval	Flecainide, propafenone
II	Beta-blockade, sinus rate slowing, prolonged P-R interval	Propranolol, atenolol, acebutolol
III	Prolonged action potential; prolonged P-R, Q-T intervals, QRS complex; sodium and calcium channel blocker	Bretylium, amiodarone, sotolol
IV	Calcium channel blockade; reduced sinus and AV node pacemaker activity and conduction; prolonged P-R interval	Verapamil

accentuated in athletic children and diminished during most illnesses. Sinus arrhythmia is differentiated from wandering atrial pacemaker by the continuous normal morphology of the P wave preceding each QRS complex in the former compared to the continuously changing P wave morphology in the latter (Figure 13–5). These two arrhythmias are thought to be controlled by an interaction of the vagal and sympathetic divisions of the autonomic nervous system.

Premature Beats

Premature atrial contractions (PACs) are common in fetuses, neonates, and infants and less so in children. They often are of little concern. If they are extremely frequent or early in the cardiac cycle, they may predispose the neonate to atrial flutter. PACs often decrease in frequency very rapidly after birth; thus a short period of observation plus parental counseling about the presentation and significance of atrial flutter a neonate may be all that is necessary. If a PAC occurs after each sinus beat, and if it fails to conduct to the ventricle (a blocked PAC), a relative bradycardia will develop. Thus the ST segment and T wave should be searched for blocked PACs in bradycardic neonates. If the PACs do not stop or decrease, treatment with digoxin may suppress them. In any case, it will not worsen the bradycardia.

Premature ventricular contractions (PVCs) are more common in adolescents and are found infrequently in neonates or infants. Benign PVCs are single (i.e., not 2 or 3 consecutively), uniform, disappear with exercise, and occur in patients with normal hearts. Any deviations require extensive evaluation. Bigeminal patterns and frequent PVCs are not considered deviations from benignness, nor is the R-on-T phenomenon. Benign PVCs of childhood do not cause serious dysrhythmias but are present at 5 yr follow-up in 50% of patients. Multiform PVCs, triplets or longer runs, and any type of cardiac abnormality are associated with more sustained dysrhythmias and symptoms, syncope, and death.

Supraventricular Tachycardia

Supraventricular tachycardia (SVT) is the most frequent sustained dysrhythmia in pediatrics. Although it is not immediately life threatening, it can lead to serious symptoms if it persists. It most commonly occurs in neonates and infants but also is common in fetuses and older children. The mechanism is usually re-entry, although enhanced automaticity accounts for 5–10% of cases. Re-entry most often involves an accessory connection (bundle of Kent) but may occur in the AV node, sinus node, or atrial muscle (atrial flutter).

Pediatric SVT is characterized by a rate of greater than 210 bpm, a normal narrow QRS complex, and extreme regularity. If the QRS complex is even slightly wide or abnormal in morphology, the diagnosis is likely ventricular tachycardia. There is usually a 1:1 relationship between the atrium and ventricle, but the atrium can be either faster (atrial flutter) or slower (junctional automaticity).

The initial treatment of pediatric SVT involves enhancing vagal tone by the diving reflex (Table 13–20). This involves applying a cold stimulus to the face. If this fails to convert, intravenous adenosine usually is effective at a dose of 50–250 micrograms/kg. In patients in whom the AV node or sinus node is not part of the re-entry circuit, adenosine may only temporarily (5–10 sec) slow the rate by creating AV block. Atrial overdrive pacing (intra-atrial or transesophageal) often is effective in atrial re-entry tachycardia. It also can be used to create temporary AV block and stabilize the blood pressure. Direct-current synchronized cardioversion at 0.25–1 W·S/kg is the gold standard for converting resistant re-entrant tachycardias.

Once SVT is converted in a child, there is an approximately 90% chance it will recur; therefore, prophylactic pharmacologic therapy is warranted for 6–12 mo. In patients with manifest Wolff-Parkinson-White (WPW) syndrome, digitalis often is not used for fear of precipitating a worse dysrhythmia; otherwise, it is the drug of choice. Propranolol and verapamil also may be used orally in older children.

In cases of SVT that are resistant to medical therapy or have life-threatening components (WPW), or when the patient does not want to take medication, the dysrhythmogenic substrate frequently (90%) can be destroyed by catheter ablation.

Bradydysrhythmias

These dysrhythmias may be classified as congenital, surgically acquired, or, rarely, caused by infection (Table 3–19). The surgically acquired type are by far the most common. Despite improving knowledge of the location of the heart's electrical system in various heart defects and improving surgical results, both acute and chronic abnormalities of the conduction system and the sinus node occur. Modern pacemakers and leads have improved treatment of these problems greatly.

Congenital complete AV block often is due to maternal antibodies to connective tissues that cross the placenta. Association with morphologic cardiac defects is the other common etiology.

References

Behrman RE (ed): Nelson Textbook of Pediatrics. 14th ed. Philadelphia, WB Saunders, 1992, Sec. 15.62–15.65.

Campbell R, Jammon J, Echt D, Graham T: Surgical treatment of pediatric cardiac arrhythmias. J Pediatr 110:501, 1987.

Dick M, Scott WA, Serwer GS, et al: Acute termination of supraventricular tachyarrhythmias in children by transesophageal atrial pacing. Am J Cardiol 61:925, 1988.

Garson A: Arrhythmias in pediatric patients. Med Clin North Am 68:1171, 1984.

Ruckman R: Cardiac causes of syncope. Pediatr Rev 9:101, 1987.

Zales VR, Dunnigan A, Benson DW, Jr: Clinical and electrophysiologic features of fetal and neonatal paroxysmal atrial tachycardia resulting in congestive heart failure. Am J Cardiol 62:22, 1988.

SUDDEN DEATH

Sudden death is a rare but important problem in pediatrics. Most pediatric sudden deaths occur in patients with known heart disease. Unoperated congenital heart disease used to be a prime cause of pediatric sudden death. Because most congenital heart defects now are repaired or palliated early in life, postoperative dysrhythmias are assuming increasing importance. A combination of earlier, more precise repairs with improved myocardial protection, and postoperative screening for dysrhythmias together with pacemaker and medical treatment, has improved the outlook for postoperative patients.

Infrequently, a child without known heart disease dies suddenly from anomalous coronary arteries, arrhythmias, or cardiomyopathy. This often occurs in relation to athletics. More than one half of these deaths probably could be prevented by including a screening ECG with a proper preparticipation history and physical exam, although this would be expensive. Attention to the symptoms of exercise-related syncope could prevent many others.

CHEST PAIN IN CHILDHOOD AND ADOLESCENCE

Chest pain among pediatric patients usually does not represent serious cardiovascular disease as it does in adult patients. Many patients are preadolescents or adolescents who have pain at rest of

Table 13–22. Differential Diagnosis of Pediatric Chest Pain

Musculoskeletal (Common)
Trauma
Exercise, overuse injury (bursitis)
Costochondritis (Tietze syndrome)
Herpes zoster (cutaneous)
Pleurodynia

Pulmonary (Common)
Pneumonia
Asthma
Pneumothorax
Infarction (sickle cell anemia)
Embolism
Hyperventilation
Tumor
Pleuritic catch

Gastrointestinal
Esophagitis (gastroesophageal reflux)
Cholecystitis
Subdiaphragmatic abscess
Peptic ulcer disease

Cardiac (Rare)
Pericarditis
Endocarditis
Mitral valve prolapse
Arrhythmias
Marfan syndrome (dissecting aortic aneurysm)
Anomalous coronary artery
Kawasaki disease

Idiopathic
Anxiety

noncardiac origin (Table 13–22). A careful history (including family history), physical examination, and screening laboratory tests are indicated to reassure the patient and family. These tests should be based on the history and physical findings and be directed to musculoskeletal, pulmonary, gastrointestinal, or cardiac signs and symptoms. Chest pain suggestive of cardiac pain that is associated with syncope, exertional dyspnea, or an irregular pulse requires more detailed evaluation, such as 24-hr continuous ECG monitoring (Holter monitor).

Chest pain is a very frequent symptom in children, as it is in adults. The most frequent cause of cardiac chest pain may be pericarditis. It usually is associated with a febrile illness, and the young age of a patient may result in the chest pain being expressed nonspecifically. Exercise-induced chest pain may indicate exercise induced asthma but rarely may indicate cardiac disease, including coronary artery anomalies. The chest wall is a common cause of chest pain in children. Costochondritis may be diagnosed by finding tenderness of one or more costochondral joints. Esophagogastritis is another frequent cause of chest pain in children. The "pleuritic catch" may be the most frequent benign cause of chest pain in children; it is brief but may recur for years. The popularization of this important symptom in the adults media in an attempt to help recognize coronary artery disease also may confuse children and their parents. Children with chest pain may be mimicking their parents or grandparents.

Cardiac Pain in Infancy

This condition may be due to an **anomalous origin of the left coronary artery** from the pulmonary artery.

The *clinical manifestations* include marked irritability, pallor, diaphoresis, apnea, or shock during or following nursing. These paroxysmal episodes of discomfort are similar to attacks of angina pectoris in adults. Heart failure may develop from poor myocardial performance. There usually is no murmur unless mitral regurgitation is present as a result of papillary muscle ischemia. If there are large collateral vessels (a left-to-right shunt through the coronary artery to the pulmonary arteries), a continuous murmur may be present, but these children usually are not ill. Thus, the diagnosis often is made after infancy.

Laboratory evidence reveals ECG signs of myocardial ischemia or infarction. Cardiomegaly is present on chest roentgenogram, and the echocardiogram and angiography reveal the anomalous coronary artery. The differential diagnosis includes SVT, myocarditis, and cardiomyopathy.

Treatment of the acute condition includes oxygen, intravenous inotropic agents, and morphine. Surgical ligation of the artery at its origin from the pulmonary artery may be successful if there are a large left-to-right shunt during systole and diastole, absence of ischemic ECG changes, and large collateral vessels. Other operative procedures include transplantation of a cuff of the pulmonary artery with the coronary ostium to the subclavian artery or aorta. The *prognosis* is poor because of myocardial ischemia and severe heart failure.

References

Brenner JI, Ringel RE, Berman MA: Cardiologic perspectives of chest pain in childhood: A referral problem? To whom? Pediatr Clin North Am 31:1241, 1984.

Selbst S: Chest pain in children. Pediatrics 75:1068, 1985.

SYNCOPE

Syncope is an increasingly important symptom in cardiologic and neurologic evaluation. It has been estimated that two thirds of children will have syncope. Most importantly, it can be a precursor to sudden death. In this instance, there usually is associated diagnosable heart disease. The second type of important syncope is *vasodepressor syncope*, which, although it does not lead to death, is very frequent. There are many other causes of syncope (dehydration, viral illness), and the presence of heart disease and exercise induction of the syncope are helpful to distinguish the rare patient who needs treatment from the majority with benign transient syncope.

When the heart ceases effective function, the patient may develop either syncope or seizures. Thus, some pediatric patients with seizures also should be evaluated for syncope. Several cardiological diseases, including the *long QT syndrome* and *hypertrophic cardiomyopathy*, frequently cause syncope. The evaluation of syncope should include a detailed history, including family history. Physical examination may reveal signs of heart disease. ECG and echocardiography are useful in diagnosing electrical and structural heart disease.

In the patient having recurrent syncope with a normal heart, testing of the response of the autonomic nervous system to assuming the upright posture is useful. If a cardiac cause of syncope is found, it should be treated directly. If vasodepressor syncope is diagnosed by autonomic testing, it may be treated by salt and fludrocortisone or beta-blockers. Treatment of vasodepressor syncope usually is temporary. The rare form of autonomic syncope, *cardioinhibitory syncope*, may require a combination of pacemaker and medical treatment.

Hematology

14

J. Paul Scott

Hematologic disorders are caused by quantitative or qualitative abnormalities of the formed elements of the blood, of the circulating proteins, or of the vascular wall. Diseases of the blood are either congenital or acquired. Hereditary abnormalities in molecular structure may lead to decreased stem cell production (Fanconi anemia), abnormal cell membrane function (hereditary spherocytosis, Glanzmann thrombasthenia), deficiency of an essential enzyme (glucose-6-phosphate dehydrogenase [G6PD] deficiency, chronic granulomatous disease), or dysfunction of a cytosolic (sickle cell anemia) or plasma (hemophilia) protein. Secondary causes of hematologic disease include infiltration of normal structures (leukemia, neuroblastoma), nutritional deficiency (iron, vitamins K, E, B_{12}, and folate), autoimmune disease (immune thrombocytopenic purpura), exogenous drugs (antimetabolites, penicillin, anti-inflammatory agents), and altered vascular matrix (thrombosis with vasculitis).

Hematologic disorders have characteristic clinical presentations related to the specific affected blood component or factor (Table 14-1). These manifestations are not diagnostic of the cause of the disorder, but certain characteristic signs and symptoms point to a likely diagnosis, such as spoonshaped nails or pica with iron deficiency, mental and neurologic manifestations with anemia in vitamin B_{12} deficiency, vaso-occlusive crises in sickle cell anemia, and progressive pancytopenia in association with congenital abnormalities in Fanconi's anemia.

DEVELOPMENTAL HEMATOPOIESIS

Hematopoiesis begins by the 3rd wk of gestation with erythropoiesis in the yolk sac. By 2 mo gestation, the primary site of hematopoiesis has migrated to the liver. Red cells, platelets, and leukocytes are synthesized at that site. During the 3rd trimester, the process of hematopoiesis shifts from the liver to the bone marrow. Therefore, an extremely premature infant may have significant extramedullary hematopoiesis with limited bone marrow hematopoiesis. During infancy, virtually all marrow cavities are actively hematopoietic, and the proportion of hematopoietic to stromal elements is very high. As the child grows, hematopoiesis moves to the central bones of the body (vertebrae, sternum, ribs, pelvis), and the marrow of the extremities and the skull is replaced with fat. This replacement of marrow with fat is a gradual and partially reversible process. Hemolysis or marrow damage may result in marrow repopulation of cavities where hematopoiesis had previously ceased or cause a delay in the shift of hematopoiesis. Children with thalassemia and other chronic hemolytic diseases may have large head circumferences and prominent skull bones as a result of erythropoiesis within the medullary cavities of the skull. Furthermore, hepatosplenomegaly in patients with chronic hemolysis may represent extramedullary hematopoiesis. Because of the extensive utilization of all bone marrow cavities, very young children do not have the marrow reserves of older children and adults. In hematologic disorders, bone marrow examination provides valuable information about the processes that result in underproduction of circulating cells. In addition, bone marrow infiltration by neoplastic elements or storage cells often occurs in concert with similar infiltration in the liver, spleen, and lymph nodes.

The hematopoietic cells consist of: a small compartment of pluripotential progenitor stem cells that morphologically resemble small lymphocytes and are capable of forming all myeloid elements; a large compartment of committed, proliferating cells of myeloid, erythroid, and megakaryocytic lineage; and a large compartment of postmitotic maturing cells (Fig. 14–1). The bone marrow is the major storage organ for mature neutrophils and contains about 7 times the intravascular pool of neutrophils; it contains 2.5–5 times as many cells of myeloid lineage as that of erythroid lineage. In addition, smaller numbers of megakaryocytes and plasma cells, histiocytes, lymphocytes, and stromal cells are stored in the marrow.

Table 14–1. Presentation of Hematologic Disorders

Condition	Symptoms and Signs	Common Examples
Anemia	Pallor, fatigue, heart failure, jaundice	Iron deficiency, hemolytic anemia
Polycythemia	Irritability, cyanosis, seizures, jaundice, stroke, headache	Cyanotic heart disease, infant of diabetic mother
Neutropenia	Fever, pharyngitis, oral ulceration, cellulitis, lymphadenopathy, bacteremia	Congenital or drug-induced agranulocytosis, leukemia
Thrombocytopenia	Petechiae, ecchymosis, gastrointestinal hemorrhage epistaxis	ITP, leukemia
Coagulopathy	Bruising, hemarthrosis, mucosal bleeding	von Willebrand disease, hemophilia
Thrombosis	Pulmonary embolism, deep venous thrombosis	Lupus anticoagulant; protein C, protein S, or antithrombin III deficiency

ITP = idiopathic thrombocytopenic purpura.

Erythropoiesis (red cell production) is controlled by erythropoietin, a hormone made by the juxtaglomerular apparatus of the kidney in response to local tissue hypoxia (Fig. 14–1). Control of erythropoiesis by erythropoietin begins at the time of hepatic hematopoiesis in early gestation. The normally high hemoglobin level of the fetus is due to fetal erythropoietin production in the liver in response to low PO_2 in utero. Erythropoietin is a glycoprotein that stimulates the primitive pluripotent stem cell to differentiate along the erythroid line, leading to production of what is recognized in vitro as the erythroid colony-forming unit (CFU-E). The earliest recognizable erythroid cell in vivo is the erythroblast, which forms eight or more daughter cells. During maturation, the immature red cell nucleus becomes gradually pyknotic as the cell matures and eventually is extruded before the cell is released from the marrow as a reticulocyte. The reticulocyte maintains residual mitochondrial and protein synthetic capacity. These highly specialized red cell precursors are engaged primarily in the production of globin chains, glycolytic enzymes, and heme. Iron is taken up via transferrin receptors and incorporated into the heme ring, which then combines with globin chains synthesized within the immature red blood cell. Once the messenger RNA and mitochondria are gone from the red cell, it is no longer capable of heme or protein synthesis but continues to function for its normal life span of about 120 days in older children and adults.

During embryonic and fetal life, the globin genes are sequentially activated and inactivated. The control mechanism of globin chain switching remains incompletely understood. Embryonic hemoglobins are produced during yolk sac erythropoiesis and then are replaced by fetal hemoglobin (hemoglobin F, $\alpha_2\gamma_2$) during the hepatic phase. During the 3rd trimester, gamma chain production gradually diminishes and is replaced by beta chains, resulting in hemoglobin A ($\alpha_2\beta_2$). Some fetal factors (e.g., being an infant of diabetic mother) delay onset of beta chain production, but premature birth does not affect its timing. Just after birth, with the expansion of the lungs and establishment of normal neonatal cardiorespiratory function, the oxygen saturation rapidly rises from 65% in utero to nearly 100%. Erythropoietin production ceases and shuts down erythropoiesis. In normal circumstances, there is a gradual decline in hemoglobin levels, with a nadir at 6–8 wk of life. This nadir is accentuated in premature infants. As the hemoglobin approaches its nadir, erythropoietin is produced and there is a subsequent resumption of erythropoiesis, with a rise in the reticulocyte court and a gradual rise in the hemoglobin level accompanied by the synthesis of increasing amounts of hemoglobin A. By 6 mo of age in healthy infants, only trace gamma chain synthesis occurs.

Fetal red cells have a relatively short survival time compared with that of red cells of children and adults (60 days vs. 120 days). Fetal red cells have less deformable membranes and possess enzymatic differences from the cells of older children. Senescent cells are destroyed in the liver and spleen, where they are recognized as abnormal by changes in their membrane sialic acid content and the metabolic depletion that occurs as they age.

Production of neutrophil precursors is controlled by two different colony-stimulating factors (Fig. 14–1). The most immature neutrophil precursors are controlled by granulocyte–monocyte colony-stimulating factor (GM-CSF), which is produced by monocytes and lymphocytes. GM-CSF increases the entry of primitive precursor cells into the myeloid line of differentiation. Granulocyte colony-stimulating factor (G-CSF) augments the produc-

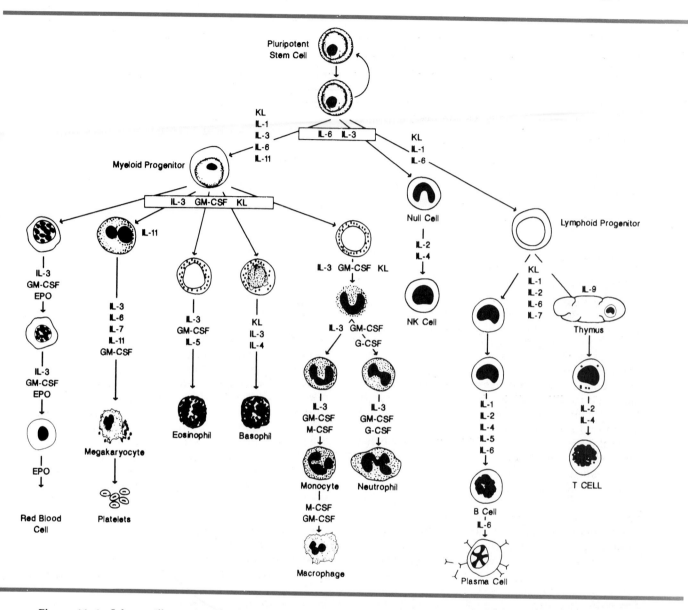

Figure 14–1. Schema illustrating the current understanding of hematopoietic growth and differentiation and the hemopoietins that control each step. EPO = erythropoietin; G-CSF = granulocyte colony-stimulating factor; GM-CSF = granulocyte–macrophage colony-stimulating factor; IL = interleukin; KL = kit ligand (also called stem cell growth factor or mast cell growth factor); M-CSF = macrophage colony-stimulating factor; NK = natural killer. (From Furman WL, Crist WM: Biology and clinical applications of hemopoietins in pediatric practice. Pediatrics 90:716, 1992.)

tion of more mature granulocyte precursors. Both, working in concert, can augment production of neutrophils and shorten the usual baseline 10–14 day production time from stem cell to mature neutrophil. The rapid increase in neutrophil count that occurs with infection is due to release of stored neutrophils from the bone marrow; this is also under the control of GM-CSF. The mitotic pool within the marrow consists of myeloblasts, promyelocytes, and myelocytes. Primary granules are found in immature myeloid cells; secondary granules develop in more mature daughter cells. Metamyelocytes, band forms, and mature polymorphonuclear leukocytes are postmitotic cells, but only bands and mature neutrophils are fully functional with regard to phagocytosis, chemotaxis, and bacterial killing. Eosinophil production is under the control of a related glycoprotein hormone, interleukin-3 (IL-3).

Neutrophils migrate from the bone marrow, circulate for 6–7 hr, and then enter the tissues, where they become end-stage cells that do not recirculate. The ability to adhere to endothelium is controlled by the interaction of adhesive molecules/receptors on the endothelial and leukocyte membrane modulated by cytokines. Neutrophils respond to chemotactic stimuli, especially C5a, then migrate toward inflammatory stimuli, where they ingest and kill invading micro-organisms. Monocytes migrate into tissues, where they become macrophages and may live from months to years. Eosinophils, which play a role in host defense against parasites, also are capable of living in tissues for prolonged periods and, like monocytes, are less streamlined but more durable than neutrophils, which form the first line of defense against infection.

Megakaryocytes are giant, multinucleated cells that derive from the primitive stem cell and are polyploid (16–32 times the normal DNA content) because of nuclear but not cytoplasmic cell division. Platelets form by invagination of the megakaryocytic cell membrane and bud off from the periphery. Platelets possess specific membrane receptors to which plasma adhesive proteins bind. Platelets also have specific granules that readily release their contents following stimulation and trigger the process of platelet aggregation. Platelets circulate for 7–10 days and, like red cells, have no nucleus.

Lymphocytes are particularly abundant in the bone marrow of young children, although they are a significant component of normal bone marrow of all ages. These are primarily B lymphocytes arising in the spleen and lymph nodes, but T lymphocytes also are present (see Chapter 8).

The stroma of the bone marrow is of major importance for the marrow's normal function. Less is known about details of its function than about the function of the other hematopoietic components because of difficulties in growing these cells in culture.

An essential element to the understanding of the hematology of pediatric patients is a detailed knowledge of normal hematologic values during infancy and childhood. These values vary according to age and also according to sex after puberty (Table 14–2).

The *coagulation factors* and *anticoagulant proteins* are synthesized primarily in the liver. Levels of most of these factors increase throughout gestation, although levels of factor VIII, von Willebrand factor, and fibrinogen reach adult normal values by the 2nd trimester.

ANEMIA

Anemia may be defined either quantitatively or functionally (physiologically). The presence of anemia usually is determined by comparison of the patient's hemoglobin with age- and sex-specific normal values. The data presented in Table 14-2 provide the normal ranges, and hemoglobin values below those ranges would represent a perfectly acceptable definition of anemia in most circumstances. However, under certain pathologic states, anemia may be present when the hemoglobin level is within the "normal range," such as in cyanotic cardiac or pulmonary disease or when a hemoglobin with an abnormally high affinity for oxygen is present. In these circumstances the physiologic definition is more appropriate. It is important to recognize that anemia is not a disease per se, but rather a manifestation of some other primary pro-

Table 14–2. Hematologic Values during Infancy and Childhood

	Hemoglobin (g/dL)		Hematocrit (%)		Reticulocytes (%)	Leukocytes (mm³)		Neutrophils (%)		Differential Counts Lymphocytes (%)	Eosinophils (%)	Monocytes (%)	Nucleated Red Cells/ 100 WBC
Age	*Mean*	*Range*	*Mean*	*Range*	*Mean*	*Mean*	*Range*	Mean	Range	Mean	Mean	Mean	*100 WBC*
Cord blood	16.8	13.7–20.1	55	45–65	5.0	18,000	(9–30,000)	61	(40–80)	31	2	6	7.0
2 wk	16.5	13.0–20.0	50	42–66	1.0	12,000	(5–21,000)	40		48	3	9	(3–10)
3 mo	12.0	9.5–14.5	36	31–41	1.0	12,000	(6–18,000)	30		63	2	5	0
6 mo–6 yr	12.0	10.5–14.0	37	33–42	1.0	10,000	(6–15,000)	45		48	2	5	0
7–12 yr	13.0	11.0–16.0	38	34–40	1.0	8000	(4500–13,500)	55		38	2	5	0
Adult													
Female	14	12.0–16.0	42	37–47	1.6	7500	(5–10,000)	55	(35–70)	35	3	7	0
Male	16	14.0–18.0	47	42–52									

* Relatively wide range.
WBC = white blood cells.
(From Behrman RE (ed): Nelson Textbook of Pediatrics. 14th ed. Philadelphia, WB Saunders, 1992, p 1232.)

cess. Anemia is a common complication that may accentuate other organ dysfunction. The easiest quantitative definition of anemia is any value for the hemoglobin or hematocrit 2 standard deviations (95% confidence limits) below the mean for age and sex. This value is less easily determined in young children than in adults because the normal range varies considerably with age. The normal hemoglobin concentration is higher at high altitudes (lower inspired oxygen content) than at sea level and in males after puberty because high levels of androgen result in greater red cell synthesis.

Pathophysiology. The physiologic consequences of anemia can be determined from the history and physical examination. Anemia that is acute in onset often is poorly compensated in terms of cardiovascular function. An elevated pulse, hemic flow murmur, poor exercise tolerance, headache, excessive sleeping (especially in infants), poor feeding, and syncope may occur. These findings all are suggestive of acute onset of anemia. Chronic anemia often is exceptionally well tolerated in children because of their cardiovascular reserve. Anemia that would induce angina in an adult may be asymptomatic in a young child. The extent of cardiovascular or functional impairment, more so than the absolute level of hemoglobin, should dictate the urgency of diagnostic and therapeutic intervention, especially the use of transfusion to correct a low hemoglobin level.

Etiology. Common etiologies and mechanisms leading to anemia and an approach to their organization are presented in Figure 14–2 and Table 14–3. The causes for anemia can often be suspected from a careful history and physical examination. Often the focus of the history is dictated by the patient's age (Table 14–4). In a newborn, a history of jaundice, pallor, previously affected siblings, drug ingestion by the mother, or excessive blood loss at the time of birth provides important clues to the diagnosis. In a young infant, a careful *dietary history* is crucial. A history of jaundice, blood loss, drug injection, or acute or chronic illnesses also will indicate probable causes of anemia. In later childhood and in teenagers, the presence of constitutional symptoms, unusual diets, drug ingestion, or blood loss, especially from menstrual bleeding, often will point to a diagnosis. Congenital red cell disorders (e.g., enzyme deficiencies and membrane problems) often present in the first 6 mo of life and frequently are associated with neonatal jaundice, although they often go undiagnosed. A careful drug history is essential for detecting problems that may be drug-induced (hemolysis in G6PD defi-

Table 14–3. Mechanisms of Childhood Anemia

Reduced Capacity to Produce RBCs
Bone marrow failure
  Aplastic anemia (congenital, acquired)
  Marrow infiltration (leukemia, neuroblastoma)
  Parvovirus infection
  Drugs (antimetabolites, penicillin, anti-inflammatory
    agents)
  Fanconi anemia
  Chronic disease
Deficiency syndromes
  Iron
  Folate
  Vitamin B_{12}
  Vitamin E
  Vitamin B_6

Hemolysis
Intrinsic membrane defects
Hemoglobinopathy
RBC enzyme defects
Microangiopathic (DIC, HUS)
Isoimmune (Rh, ABO in neonate)
Autoimmune
Drug-induced
Intravascular (transfusion reaction)

Blood Loss
Gastrointestinal
Menstrual
Trauma

DIC = disseminated intravascular coagulation; HUS = hemolytic–uremic syndrome; RBC = red blood cell.

ciency, bone marrow suppression, antibody-mediated hemolysis). Pure dietary iron deficiency is rare except in infancy, wherein cow's milk protein intolerance causes gastrointestinal blood loss and complicates an inadequate iron intake. A careful history justifies providing replacement therapy without performing an extensive search for blood loss (Table 14–4).

Clinical Manifestations. The *physical examination* also suggests the presence of anemia and the potential causes of the anemia (Table 14–5). Presence of jaundice suggests hemolysis. Petechiae and purpura indicate a bleeding tendency. Hepatosplenomegaly and adenopathy suggest infiltrative disorders. Growth failure or poor weight gain suggest an anemia of chronic disease or organ failure. An essential element of the physical examination in a patient with anemia is the investigation of the stool for the presence of occult blood.

The initial *laboratory evaluation* of anemia includes a hemoglobin or hematocrit test to indicate the severity of the anemia. Once the diagnosis of anemia has been substantiated, the work-up should in-

ANEMIA

HEMOGLOBIN AND INDICES
RETICULOCYTE COUNT AND MORPHOLOGY

Inadequate response (RPI <2)   Adequate Response
                                                                (RPI >3)

HYPOCHROMIC, MICROCYTIC	NORMOCHROMIC, NORMOCYTIC	MACROCYTIC	R/O BLOOD LOSS
Iron deficiency	*Anemia of chronic*	*Vitamin B$_{12}$ deficiency*	HEMOLYSIS
−Chronic blood loss	*inflammatory disease*	−Pernicious anemia	
−Poor dietary intake	−Infection	−Ileal resection	*Hemoglobinopathy*
−Cow's milk protein	−Collagen vascular	−Strict vegetarian	−Hemoglobin SS, S-C,
intolerance	disease	−Abnormal intestinal transport	S-thal
		−Congenital intrinsic factor	
Thalassemia	*Malignancy/marrow*	deficiency	*Enzymopathy*
−β minor, major	*infiltration*	−Congenital transcobalamin	−Pyruvate kinase deficiency
−α minor		deficiency	−G6PD deficiency
	Recent blood loss		
Chronic inflammatory		*Folate deficiency*	*Membranopathy*
disease	*Uremia*	−Poor diet	−Hereditary spherocytosis
		−Malabsorption	−Elliptocytosis
Copper deficiency	*Transient*	−Antimetabolite	−Ovalocytosis
Sideroblastic anemia	*erythroblastopenia of*	−Phenytoin	−Acquired hemolytic
Aluminum, ? lead	*childhood (TEC)*	−Trimethoprim−sulfamethoxazole	disease
intoxication		−Chronic hemolysis	−DIC, HUS
	Marrow aplasia/hypoplasia		−Autoimmune hemolytic
		Hypothyroidism	anemia (AIHA)
	Hemophagocytic		−Burns
	syndromes	*Oroticaciduria*	−Abetalipoproteinemia
		Lesch-Nyhan syndrome	
		Chronic liver disease	
		Marrow failure	
		−Preleukemia	
		−Fanconi anemia	
		−Aplastic anemia	
		−Myelodysplasia	
		Drugs	
		−Azidothymidine	

Figure 14–2. Use of the complete blood count, reticulocyte count, and blood smear to diagnose anemia. DIC = disseminated intravascular coagulation; HUS = hemolytic–uremic syndrome; RPI = reticulocyte production index (see text).

clude a complete blood count with differential, platelet count, indices, and reticulocyte count. The blood smear should be studied for morphologic abnormalities (Fig. 14–3). Using data obtained from the indices and reticulocyte count, one can organize the work-up for anemia on the basis of whether there is adequate or inadequate red cell production (Table 14–3) and whether the cells are microcytic, normocytic, or macrocytic (Fig. 14–2). Examination of the peripheral blood smear is critical in assessing the red cell morphology, the white cell number and the presence or absence of abnormal leukocytes, and the platelet number and size. These data indicate whether the anemia is due to

Table 14–4. Historical Clues in Evaluation of Anemia

Variable	Comments
Age	Iron deficiency rare in the absence of blood loss prior to 6 mo in term or prior to doubling birth weight in preterm infants
	Neonatal anemia with reticulocytosis suggests hemolysis or blood loss; with reticulocytopenia, it suggests bone marrow failure
	Sickle cell anemia and beta-thalassemia appear as fetal hemoglobin disappears (4–8 mo of age)
Family history and genetic considerations	X-linked: G6PD deficiency
	Autosomal dominant: spherocytosis
	Autosomal recessive: sickle cell, Fanconi anemia
	Family member with early age of cholecystectomy (bilirubin stones) or splenectomy
	Ethnicity (thalassemia with Mediterranean origin), (G6PD deficiency in blacks, Greeks, and sephardic Jews)
	Race (beta-thalassemia in white, alpha-thalassemia in blacks and Orientals, and SC and SS in blacks)
Nutrition	Cow's milk diet and iron deficiency
	Strict vegetarian and vitamin B_{12} deficiency
	Goat's milk and folate deficiency
	Pica, plumbism, and iron deficiency
	Cholestasis, malabsorption, and vitamin E
Drugs	G6PD-susceptible agents
	Immune-mediated hemolysis (e.g., penicillin)
	Bone marrow suppression
	Phenytoin increasing folate requirements
Diarrhea	Malabsorption of vitamins B_{12} and E and iron
	Inflammatory bowel disease and anemia of chronic disease or blood loss
	Milk protein allergy–induced blood loss
	Intestinal resection and vitamin B_{12} deficiency
Infection	*Giardia* and iron malabsorption
	Intestinal bacterial overgrowth (blind loop) and vitamin B_{12} deficiency
	Fish tapeworm and vitamin B_{12} deficiency
	Epstein-Barr virus, cytomegalovirus, and bone marrow suppression
	Mycoplasma and hemolysis
	Parvovirus and bone marrow suppression
	Chronic infection
	Endocarditis
	Malaria and hemolysis
	Hepatitis and aplastic anemia

a process limited to the erythroid line or to one that is affecting other marrow elements.

The reticulocyte production index (RPI), which corrects the reticulocyte count for the degree of anemia, indicates whether the bone marrow is responding appropriately to the anemia. Reticulocytes routinely are counted per 1000 red cells; hence a reduction in the denominator, which occurs in anemia, will falsely increase the reticulocyte count. The formula for calculating the RPI is:

$$RPI = Retic\ ct \times \frac{Hgb_{observed}}{Hgb_{normal}} \times 0.5$$

An RPI greater than 3 suggests increased produc-

tion and implies either hemolysis or blood loss, whereas an index less than 2 suggests decreased production or ineffective production for the degree of anemia. Reticulocytopenia signifies either that the anemia is so acute in onset that the marrow has not had adequate time to respond, that reticulocytes are being destroyed (antibody mediated), or that intrinsic bone marrow disease is present.

Hypochromic, Microcytic Anemia with Inadequate Red Cell Production

This type of anemia is caused by an inadequate production of hemoglobin (Table 14–6).

Table 14–5. Physical Findings in the Evaluation of Anemia

System	Observation	Significance
Skin	Hyperpigmentation	Fanconi, dyskeratosis congenita
	Café-au-lait spots	Fanconi anemia
	Vitiligo	Vitamin B_{12} deficiency
	Partial oculocutaneous albinism	Chédiak-Higashi syndrome
	Jaundice	Hemolysis
	Petechiae, purpura	Bone marrow infiltration, autoimmune hemolysis with autoimmune thrombocytopenia, hemolytic uremic syndrome
	Erythematous rash	Parvovirus, Epstein-Barr virus
	Butterfly rash	SLE autoantibodies
Head	Frontal bossing	Thalassemia major, severe iron deficiency, chronic subdural hematoma
	Microcephaly	Fanconi anemia
Eyes	Microphthalmia	Fanconi anemia
	Retinopathy	SS, SC disease
	Optic atrophy	Osteopetrosis
	Blocked lacrimal gland	Dyskeratosis congenita
	Kayser-Fleischer ring	Wilson disease
	Blue sclera	Iron deficiency
Ears	Deafness	Osteopetrosis
Mouth	Glossitis	B_{12} deficiency, iron deficiency
	Angular stomatitis	Iron deficiency
	Cleft lip	Diamond-Blackfan syndrome
	Pigmentation	Peutz-Jeghers syndrome (intestinal blood loss)
	Telangiectasia	Osler-Weber-Rendu syndrome (blood loss)
	Leukoplakia	Dyskeratosis congenita
Chest	Shield chest or widespread nipples	Diamond-Blackfan syndrome
	Murmur	Endocarditis: prosthetic valve hemolysis
Abdomen	Hepatomegaly	Hemolysis, infiltrative tumor, chronic disease, hemangioma, cholecystitis
	Splenomegaly	Hemolysis, sickle cell disease, (early) thalassemia, malaria, lymphoma, Epstein-Barr virus, portal hypertension
	Nephromegaly	Fanconi anemia
	Absent kidney	Fanconi anemia
Extremities	Absent thumbs	Fanconi anemia
	Triphalangeal thumb	Diamond-Blackfan syndrome
	Spoon nails	Iron deficiency
	Beau line (nails)	Heavy metal intoxication, severe illness
	Mees line (nails)	Heavy metals, severe illness, sickle cell anemia
	Dystrophic nails	Dyskeratosis congenita
Rectal	Hemorrhoids	Portal hypertension
	Heme positive stool	Intestinal hemorrhage
Nerves	Irritable, apathy	Iron deficiency
	Peripheral neuropathy	Deficiency of vitamins B_1, B_{12}, and E, lead poisoning
	Dementia	Deficiency of vitamins B_{12} and E
	Ataxia, posterior column signs	Vitamin B_{12} deficiency
	Stroke	Sickle cell anemia, paroxysmal nocturnal hemoglobinuria

SLE = systemic lupus erythematosus.

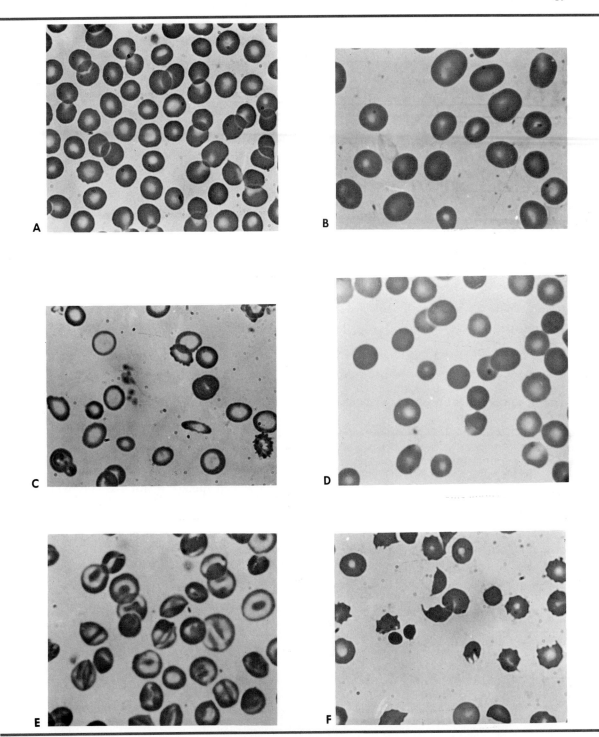

Figure 14–3. Morphologic abnormalities of the red cell. *A*, Normal. *B*, Macrocytes (folic acid deficiency). *C*, Hypochromic microcytes (iron deficiency). *D*, Spherocytes (hereditary spherocytosis). *E*, Target cells (Hgb CC disease). *F*, Schistocytes (hemolytic–uremic syndrome). (From Behrman RE, (ed): Nelson Textbook of Pediatrics, 14th ed. Philadelphia, WB Saunders, 1992, p 1237.)

Table 14–6. Differentiating Features of Microcytic Anemias*

Tests	Iron-Deficiency Anemia	Thalassemia	Sideroblastic Anemia†	Anemia of Chronic Disease‡
Serum iron	Low	Normal	High or normal	Low
Serum iron-binding capacity	High	Normal	Normal or high	Low or normal
Serum ferritin	Low	Normal or high	High	Normal or high
Marrow iron stores	Low or absent	Normal or high	High	Normal or high
Marrow sideroblasts	Decreased or absent	Normal or increased	Increased	Decreased
Free erythrocyte protoporphyrin	High	Normal	High	High
Hemoglobin A_2 or F	Normal	High β-thal; normal α-thal	Normal	Normal
Red cell distribution width (RDW)§	High	Normal	—	Normal

* See Table 14–7 for definition of microcytosis.
† Thrombocytopenia and neutropenia develop as the disease progresses.
‡ Usually normochronic; 25% are microcytic.
§ RDW quantitates the degree of anisocytosis (different sizes) of red blood cells.

IRON-DEFICIENCY ANEMIA

Dietary iron-deficiency anemia is most common in bottle-fed infants who are receiving large volumes of cow's milk. They ingest little in the way of dietary substances high in iron, such as meat and green vegetables (see Chapter 2). Iron deficiency is the single most common cause of anemia in the world. Breast-fed infants develop iron deficiency less commonly than bottle-fed infants because, although there is less iron in breast milk, this iron is more effectively absorbed. The sequence of events in the development of iron-deficiency anemia is noted in Table 14–7. In addition to the manifestations of anemia, central nervous system (CNS) abnormalities (apathy, irritability, poor concentra-tion) have been linked to iron deficiency, presumably resulting from alterations of iron-containing enzymes (monoamine oxidase) and cytochromes. Poor muscle endurance, gastrointestinal dysfunction, and impaired white blood cell and T cell function also have been noted in association with iron deficiency. Increasing evidence has been found that mild iron deficiency in infancy may be associated with later cognitive deficits.

A detailed dietary history usually will disclose the child's poor diet. If the dietary history suggests iron deficiency, a therapeutic trial of iron is appropriate with or without laboratory confirmation. In an otherwise healthy child, a therapeutic trial is the best diagnostic study for iron deficiency so long as

Table 14–7. Stages in Development of Iron-Deficiency Anemia

Hemoglobin (g/dL)	Peripheral Smear*	Serum Iron (μg/dL)	Bone Marrow	Serum Ferritin (ng/mL)
13+ (normal)	nc/nc	50–150	Fe^{2+}	40–340 (male) 14–150 (female)
10–12	nc/nc	↓	Fe^{2+} absent, erythroid hyperplasia	<12
8–10	hypo/nc	↓	Fe^{2+} absent, erythroid hyperplasia	<12
<8	hypo/micro†	↓	Fe^{2+} absent, erythroid hyperplasia	<12

* nc/nc = normochromic, normocytic; hypo/nc = hypochromic, normocytic; hypo/micro = hypochromic, microcytic.
† Microcytosis, determined by a mean corpuscular volume (in fL) less than 2 standard deviations (SD) below the mean, must be adjusted for age (e.g., −2 SD at 3–6 mo = 74, at 0.5–2 yr = 70, at 2–6 yr = 75, at 6–12 yr = 77, and at 12–18 yr = 78).
(From Andreoli TE, Carpenter CCJ, Plum F, et al: Cecil Essentials of Medicine. Philadelphia, WB Saunders, 1993, p 360.)

the child is re-examined and a response documented. The response to oral iron includes rapid subjective improvement, especially in neurologic function (24–48 hr), reticulocytosis (48–72 hr), increase in hemoglobin (4–30 days), and repletion of iron stores (1–3 mo). A usual therapeutic dose of 3–6 mg/day of elemental iron will induce an increase in hemoglobin of 0.25–0.4 g/dL/day (1%/day rise in hematocrit). In the absence of a rise in hemoglobin within 2 wk after the institution of iron treatment, the clinician should carefully re-evaluate the patient for ongoing blood loss, development of infection, poor compliance, or other causes of microcytic anemia (Fig. 14–2, Table 14–6).

THALASSEMIA MINOR

The thalassemia minor syndromes are characterized by a mild hypochromic, microcytic anemia with a low RPI (Table 14–8, Fig. 14–2) *Alpha-thalassemia* occurs in 1.5% of African–Americans and is a common cause of microcytosis either without anemia or with a mild hypochromic, microcytic anemia. Alpha-thalassemia is common in Southeastern Asians, and an Oriental variant is associated with a risk of homozygous alpha-thalassemia, Bart hemoglobin in the newborn ($\gamma4$ tetramers), and hemoglobin H ($\beta4$ tetramers) in older children. The blood smear is normal in alpha-thalassemia ex-

Table 14–8. Comparison of the Thalassemia Syndromes

Genetic Abnormality	Percent Hemoglobin			Other	Clinical Syndrome
	Hb A	*Hb A$_2$*	*Hb F*		
Normal $\alpha\beta$	90–98	2–3	2–3		None
Beta-Thalassemias					
Thalassemia major					
β-thal^0 β-thal^0	0	2–5	95	—	Severe anemia, abnormal growth, iron overload, needs transfusion, Cooley anemia.
β-thal$^+$ β-thal$^+$	Very low	2–5	20–80	—	Severe hypo/micro anemia with Hb 7–9 g/dL, hepatosplenomegaly, bone changes, iron overload, less need for transfusion
Thalassemia intermedia (varied genetic globin abnormalities)	overlaps with thalassemia major				
Thalassemia minor					
β β-thal^0 or β β-thal$^+$	90–95	5–7	2–10	RBC	Hypo/micro blood smear, mild to no anemia
Alpha-Thalassemias					
Homozygous α-thalassemia $- -/- -$	—	—	—	Hb H ($\beta4$) Hb Bart ($\gamma4$)	Hydrops fetalis, stillborn
Hemoglobin H disease $- -/- \alpha$	60–70	2–5	2–5	Hb H 30–40	Hypo/micro anemia, Hb 7–10 g/dL, Heinz bodies
Alpha-thalassemia trait $- \alpha/- \alpha$ $\alpha \alpha/- -$	90–98	2–3	2–3		Hypo/micro smear, no anemia
Silent carrier $- \alpha/\alpha \alpha$	90–98	2–3	2–3		Normal
Hemoglobin Lepore ($\delta\beta$ fusion)					
Heterozygote	70–80	1–2	5–20	Hb Lepore 5–15	Mild hypo/micro anemia
Homozygote	0	0	70–90	Hb Lepore 10–30	Severe thalassemia major

(From Andreoli TE, Carpenter CCJ, Plum F, et al: Cecil Essentials of Medicine. Philadelphia, WB Saunders, 1993, p. 373.)

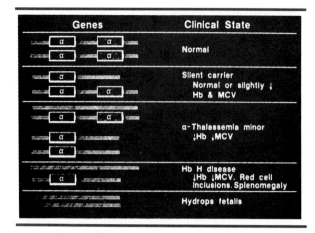

Genes	Clinical State
α α / α α	Normal
α α / α	Silent carrier Normal or slightly ↓ Hb & MCV
α α /	α-Thalassemia minor ↓Hb ↓MCV
	α
	α
α /	Hb H disease ↓Hb ↓MCV. Red cell inclusions. Splenomegaly
	Hydrops fetalis

Figure 14–4. Schematic illustration of alpha-globin gene deletions and their clinical consequences. HB = hemoglobin; MCV = mean corpuscular volume. (From Beutler E: The common anemias. JAMA 259:2433, 1988. Copyright 1988, American Medial Association.)

cept for microcytosis. No basophilic stippling is present. Hemoglobin electrophoresis usually is normal in alpha-thalassemia minor, although Bart hemoglobin may be present in the neonatal period. Homozygous alpha-thalassemia results in fatal hydrops fetalis (Fig. 14–4).

Beta-thalassemia minor is prevalent throughout the Mediterranean region, the Middle East, India, and southeast Asia. There is basophilic stippling of the red cells in addition to hypochromic, microcytic anemia. The stippling is caused by precipitation of alpha-chain tetramers. The diagnosis is based on an elevation of hemoglobin A_2 and F.

LEAD POISONING

This may be associated with a hypochromic, microcytic anemia, although most patients have concomitant iron deficiency. The history of a child with pica who lives in a disadvantaged urban area should raise suspicion of leading poisoning. Basophilic stippling on the blood smear is common. Detection by routine screening, removal from exposure, chelation therapy, and correction of iron deficiency are of utmost importance to the potential development of these children (see Chapter 3).

Normocytic Anemia with Inadequate Red Cell Production

Normocytic anemias include a wide variety of red cell disorders in which the marrow fails to synthesize adequate numbers of red blood cells as a result of a systemic illness. The bone marrow function is impaired by fibrosis, tumor, storage cells, transient or prolonged marrow failure (transient erythroblastopenia of childhood, aplastic anemia), or failure to synthesize erythropoietin (renal failure). Normocytic anemias also occur in the presence of acute blood loss before the marrow has had time to respond. The site of blood loss usually is quite clear cut, and commonly in the gastrointestinal tract (see Chapter 11).

Anemia is a common component of *chronic inflammatory disease,* in which cytokines trigger a reticuloendothelial blockade within the marrow. Iron is taken up by the reticuloendothelial cells but is not available for erythroid synthesis. Typically, the anemia may be normocytic or, less often, microcytic. At times this poses a clinical challenge when children with inflammatory disorders that may be associated with blood loss (e.g., inflammatory bowel disease) present with a microcytic anemia. In these circumstances the only specific diagnosis test that can clearly differentiate the two entities is a bone marrow aspiration with staining of the sample for iron (Table 14–6). Serum ferritin levels also may be helpful. A trial of iron therapy is not indicated without a specific diagnosis in children who appear to be systemically ill.

Bone marrow *infiltration by malignant cells* commonly results in a normochromic, normocytic anemia. The mechanism by which neoplastic cells interfere with red cell and other marrow cell synthesis is unclear. The reticulocyte count is low. There may be release of immature myeloid elements into the peripheral blood as a result of the presence of the offending tumor cells. An examination of the peripheral blood may disclose lymphoblasts; when solid tumors metastasize to the marrow, these cells seldom are seen in the peripheral blood. Teardrop cells may be seen in the peripheral blood. Performance of a bone marrow examination frequently is necessary in the face of normochromic, normocytic anemia.

Congenital pure red cell aplasia (Diamond-Blackfan syndrome) usually presents in the first few months of life or even at birth (see Table 14–9). This is a lifelong disorder. Most patients respond to corticosteroid treatment but must receive therapy indefinitely. At the time of presentation the patient may have mild macrocytosis or may be normocytic. Those who do not respond to steroid treatment are transfusion dependent and are at risk of the multiple complications of chronic transfusion therapy, including blood-borne virus-associated illnesses and iron overload.

Table 14–9. Differentiation of Red Cell Aplasias and Aplastic Anemias

Disorder	Age of Onset	Characteristics	Treatment
Congenital			
Diamond-Blackfan syndrome (congenital hypoplastic anemia)	Newborn–1 mo; 90% <1 yr age	Pure red cell aplasia, autosomal recessive trait, elevated fetal hemoglobin, fetal i antigen present, macrocytic, thrombosis, short stature, web neck, cleft lip, triphalangeal thumb; late-onset leukemia	Prednisone, transfusion
Acquired			
Transient erythroblastopenia	6 mo–5 yr age; 85% >1 yr age	Pure red cell defect; no anomalies, fetal hemoglobin, or i antigen; spontaneous recovery, normal MCV	Expectant transfusion for symptomatic anemia
Idiopathic aplastic anemia (s/p hepatitis, drugs, unknown)	All ages	All cell lines involved; chloramphenicol, phenylbutazone, radiation	Bone marrow transplant, antithymocyte globulin, cyclosporine, androgens
Familial			
Fanconi syndrome	Before 10 yr age; mean is 8 yr	All cell lines; microcephaly, absent thumbs, café-au-lait spots, cutaneous hyperpigmentation, short stature; chromosomal breaks, high MCV and hemoglobin F; horseshoe or absent kidney; leukemic transformation; autosomal recessive trait	Androgens, corticosteroids, bone marrow transplant
Paroxysmal nocturnal hemoglobinuria	After 5 yr	Initial hemolysis followed by aplastic anemia; increased complement-mediated hemolysis; thrombosis; iron deficiency	Iron, bone marrow transplant, androgens, steroids
Dyskeratosis congenita	Mean 10 yr for skin; mean 17 yr for anemia	Pancytopenia; hyperpigmentation, dystrophic nails, leukoplakia; X-linked recessive; lacrimal duct stenosis; high MCV and fetal hemoglobin	Androgens, splenectomy, bone marrow transplant
Familial hemophagocytic lymphohistiocytosis	Before 2 yr	Pancytopenia; fever, hepatosplenomegaly, hypertriglyceridemia, CSF pleocytosis	Transfusion; often lethal. VP-16 bone marrow transplantation
Infectious			
Parvovirus	Any age	Any chronic hemolytic anemia, typically sickle cell; new-onset reticulocytopenia	Transfusion
Epstein-Bar virus (EBV)	Any age; usually <5 yr	X-linked immunodeficiency syndrome, pancytopenia	Transfusion, bone marrow transplantation
Viral-associated hemophagocytic syndrome (CMV, HHV–6, EBV)	Any age	Pancytopenia; hemophagocytosis present in marrow	Transfusion, antiviral therapy (see Chapter 10), intravenous immunoglobulin

CMV = cytomegalovirus; CSF = cerebral spinal fluid; HHV–6 = human herpesvirus-6; MCV = mean corpuscular volume.

In contrast to the congenital hypoplastic anemias, *transient erythroblastopenia of childhood* (TEC) usually appears after 6 mo of age (Table 14–9). This is a normocytic anemia caused by bone marrow suppression. Viral infections are thought to be the major cause of TEC, but no specific etiology has been identified. The onset is gradual; however, the anemia may become severe. Recovery usually is spontaneous; transfusion of packed red cells may be necessary pending recovery. Differentiation from Diamond-Blackfan syndrome, in which erythroid precursors also are absent or diminished in the bone marrow, is noted in Table 14–9.

Aplastic crises, which may complicate any chronic hemolytic anemia, are periods of reticulocytopenia during which the usual high rate of red cell destruction leads to an acute exacerbation of the anemia, potentially precipitating cardiovascular decompensation. Human parvovirus B-19 (the cause of fifth disease [erythema infectiosum]) infecting erythroid precursors accounts for many of these episodes. Transient erythroid aplasia is without consequence in individuals with normal red cell survival. Recovery from parvovirus infection in hemolytic disease is spontaneous, but patients may need transfusion if the anemia is severe.

Macrocytic Anemia

Vitamin B_{12} and folic acid deficiencies lead to macrocytic anemia and are discussed in Chapter 2 (see also Figs. 14–2 and 14–3).

Hemolytic Anemias

Hemolytic diseases are mediated either by intrinsic disorders of the red cell or by disorders extrinsic to the red cell itself.

HEMOLYTIC ANEMIA CAUSED BY INTRINSIC RED CELL DISORDERS

Membrane Disorders

Hereditary spherocytosis and hereditary elliptocytosis are the most common red cell membrane disorders. These frequently are associated with neonatal jaundice, although the disorder often goes undiagnosed in the neonate. *Hereditary spherocytosis* varies greatly in clinical severity, ranging from a severe hemolytic anemia with growth failure, splenomegaly, and chronic transfusion requirements in infancy necessitating early splenectomy to an asymptomatic, well-compensated, mild hemolytic anemia that may be discovered incidentally. The biochemical bases of the defects probably are similar and appear to have in common a defect in the protein lattice (spectrin, ankyrin, protein 4.2) that underlies the red cell lipid bilayer and provides stability of the membrane shape. The amount or the function of the spectrin may be abnormal; the greater the abnormality the more severe the symptoms. When the red cell loses membrane, the shape changes from a biconcave disc to a spherocyte; the spherocyte shape has the lowest ratio of surface area to volume. The red cell therefore is less deformable when passing through narrow passages in the spleen. The transmission of this disorder usually is autosomal dominant but occasionally is recessive. There is a high, spontaneous mutation rate. The diagnosis should be suspected in patients with even a few spherocytes exhibited on the blood smear because the spherocytes are removed preferentially by the spleen. An incubated osmotic fragility test confirms the diagnosis, but it is important to note that the osmotic fragility test frequently is abnormal in any hemolytic disease in which spherocytes are present, especially in antibody-mediated hemolysis.

Splenectomy corrects the anemia and normalizes the red cell survival, but the morphologic abnormalities persist. Splenectomy should be considered for any child with symptoms referable to anemia or growth failure, but should be deferred until age 5, if at all possible, to minimize the risk of overwhelming postsplenectomy sepsis and maximize the antibody response to the polyvalent pneumococcal vaccine. Vaccinations against *Haemophilus influenzae* type B should be given according to current recommendations at 2, 4, and 6 mo of age. Gallstones (bilirubinate), resulting from chronic hemolysis, may be asymptomatic or may be the cause of vague abdominal pain.

Hereditary elliptocytosis is a disorder of spectrin dimer interactions that occurs primarily in individuals of African descent. The most common variant is a clinically insignificant, morphologic abnormality without shortened red cell survival. The less common variant is associated with spherocytes, ovalocytes, and elliptocytes and with a moderate, usually compensated, hemolysis. Both variants are transmitted as autosomal dominant traits. Far more significant hemolysis occurs in a very small percentage of patients with elliptocytes, spherocytes, fragmented red cells, and striking microcytosis. This disorder is termed *hereditary pyropoikilocytosis* and is due to a structural abnormality of spectrin. The term "pyropoikilocytosis" refers to the unusual instability of the erythrocytes when exposed to heat (45°C).

Red Cell Enzyme Deficiencies

There are numerous red cell enzyme deficiencies but only a few are clinically important disorders. The most common is **glucose-6-phosphate dehydrogenase deficiency,** an abnormality in the hexose monophosphate shunt pathway of glycolysis that results in the depletion of NADPH and the inability to regenerate reduced glutathione. Reduced glutathione plays a critical role in the reduction of oxidants generated within a red cell; therefore, children with G6PD deficiency develop episodic hemolysis when exposed to oxidant stress. The severity of the hemolysis depends on the enzyme variant. In many G6PD variants, the enzymes become unstable with aging. Young red cells have normal G6PD activity that is lost as the cell ages and cannot be replaced because the cell is anucleated. Older cells are most susceptible to oxidant-induced hemolysis. In other variants, the enzyme is kinetically abnormal. The most common variants of G6PD have been found in areas where malaria is endemic. G6PD deficiency protects against parasitism of the erythrocyte. The most common variant with normal activity is termed type B and defined by its electrophoretic mobility. The approximate gene frequencies in African–Americans are 70% type B, 20% type A+, and 10% type A−. Only the A− variant is unstable. The A− variant is termed the "African" variant, and 10% of black males are affected. A group of variants found in Sardinians, Sicilians, Greeks, sephardic and Oriental Jews, and Arabs is termed the "Mediterranean" variant and is associated with chronic hemolysis and potentially life-threatening hemolytic disease. The gene for G6PD is carried on the X chromosome. Clinical hemolysis is most common in males, who will possess a single abnormal X chromosome. Heterozygous females who have randomly inactivated a higher percentage of the normal gene may become symptomatic, as may homozygous females with the A− variant, which occurs in 1% of females of African descent.

When a patient with G6PD is exposed to significant oxidant stress, hemoglobin is oxidized and the sulfhemoglobin is denatured and forms Heinz bodies visible on specially stained preparations. The morphology of acute hemolysis is striking. Red cells appear to have "bites" (cookie cells) taken out of them. These are areas of absent hemoglobin caused by phagocytosis of Heinz bodies by splenic macrophages; as a result, the red cells appear blistered. Jaundice, dark urine resulting from both bilirubin pigments and hemoglobinuria when hemolysis is intravascular, and decreased haptoglobin are common during hemolytic episodes. Because 5% of African–Americans lack haptoglobin, absent haptoglobin is meaningful only in the context of the other abnormalities. Early on, the hemolysis usually exceeds the ability of the bone marrow to compensate, so the reticulocyte count may be low for 3–4 days.

The *diagnosis* of G6PD deficiency is based on decreased NADPH formation. However, G6PD levels may be normal in the setting of acute, severe hemolysis because the most deficient cells have been destroyed. Repeating the test at a later time when the patient is in a steady state condition, testing the mothers of boys with suspected G6PD deficiency, and/or performing electrophoresis to identify the precise variant present will facilitate early diagnosis.

The *treatment* of G6PD deficiency is supportive, including transfusion when significant cardiovascular compromise is present, and protecting the kidneys against damage from precipitated free hemoglobin by maintaining hydration and urine alkalization. *Prevention* of hemolysis is achieved by avoiding known oxidants, particularly long-acting sulfonamides, nitrofurantoin, primaquine, and dimercaprol; fava beans (favism) have triggered hemolysis, particularly in patients with the Mediterranean variant. Infection also is a major precipitant of hemolysis in young children. Patients with the most severe degrees of G6PD deficiency not only have chronic hemolysis, but their neutrophils demonstrate defective oxidative killing because of depletion of NADPH, which serves as an electron donor to the membrane-bound oxidase that produces bactericidal oxygen species (see Chapter 8).

Pyruvate kinase (PK) deficiency is much less common than G6PD deficiency and also represents a clinical spectrum of disorders caused by the functional deficiency of PK. Some individuals have a true deficiency state and others have abnormal enzyme kinetics. This enzyme in the Embden-Meyerhof pathway of glycolysis is important for the production of two moles ATP/mole of glucose metabolized. The metabolic consequence of PK deficiency is ATP depletion, thus impairing red cell survival. PK is an autosomal disorder, and most children who are affected (and are not products of inbreeding) are double heterozygotes for two abnormal enzymes. Hemolysis is not aggravated by oxidant stress because these patients tend to have a profound reticulocytosis. Aplastic crises potentially are life-threatening. The spleen is the site for red cell removal in PK deficiency. Most patients have amelioration of the anemia and a reduction of transfusion requirements after splenectomy.

Major Hemoglobinopathies

Because alpha chains are needed for fetal erythropoiesis and production of hemoglobin F ($\alpha_2 \gamma_2$), alpha chain hemoglobinopathies present in utero. There are a total of four alpha genes present on the two number 16 chromosomes (see Fig. 14–4 and Table 14–8). Single-gene deletions produce no disorder (the silent carrier state) but can be detected by measuring the rates of alpha and beta synthesis or by using molecular biologic techniques. Deletion of two genes produces alpha-thalassemia minor with mild or no anemia and microcytosis. In the black population, the gene deletions occur on different chromosomes (trans) and the disorder is benign, with virtually no individuals of African descent having more than two genes deleted. In the Oriental population, deletions may occur on the same chromosome (cis) and, therefore, infants may inherit two number 16 chromosomes lacking three or even four genes. Deletion of all four genes results in hydrops fetalis, severe intrauterine anemia, and death. Deletion of three genes produces a mild to moderate hemolytic anemia with $\gamma 4$ tetramers (Bart hemoglobin) in the fetus and $\beta 4$ tetramers (hemoglobin H) in older children and adults (Table 14–8).

A greater number of disorders occur in beta chain hemoglobinopathies because these abnormalities are not symptomatic in utero. In contrast, severe gamma chain abnormalities would be expected to be lethal. The major group of beta-hemoglobinopathies include those that alter hemoglobin function, including hemoglobins S, C, E, D, and G, and those that alter beta chain production—the beta-thalassemias. Because each red cell has two copies of chromosome 11 and the beta-globin genes are both expressed, most of the disorders of beta chains are not clinically severe unless both beta chains are abnormal. Disorders of the beta chain usually manifest between 6 and 12 mo of age unless they have been detected prenatally or by cord blood screening.

Beta-Thalassemia Major (Cooley Anemia).

This hemoglobinopathy is caused by mutations that alter beta chain synthesis (Table 14–8); excess gamma and beta chains do not damage the red cells, whereas excess alpha chains are toxic. Alpha chains precipitate within the cells, resulting in cell destruction either in the bone marrow or in the spleen once the cell is released. The clinical severity of the illness varies to some extent on the basis of the molecular defect; however, the majority of the patients are transfusion dependent from infancy. An uncommon mutation that results in deletion of both beta and delta chains results in **hereditary persistence of fetal hemoglobin** (HPFH), in which gamma chain synthesis represents about 30% of non–alpha chain synthesis in adult life. HPFH usually is asymptomatic.

Clinical manifestations of beta-thalassemia major result from the combination of chronic hemolytic disease, decreased production of normal hemoglobin, and ineffective erythropoiesis in the marrow. The anemia is severe and results in growth failure and heart failure. Ineffective erythropoiesis causes increased expenditure of energy and expansion of the bone marrow cavities of all bones, resulting in osteopenia, pathologic fractures, extramedullary erythropoiesis, and an increase in the rate of iron absorption. Patients usually are transfusion dependent from the end of the 1st yr of life. Adolescents develop complications from iron overload (hemochromatosis), including diabetes mellitus, cirrhosis, heart failure, bronzing of the skin, and multiple endocrine abnormalities (thyroid, gonad). The amount of iron the patient acquires from transfusion may be estimated by the formula that each milliliter of packed red blood cells contains approximately 1 mg of iron.

Treatment of beta-thalassemia major is based on hyper-transfusion program that corrects the anemia and suppresses the patient's own inadequate erythropoiesis, thus limiting the stimulus for increased iron absorption. This suppression permits the bones to heal, decreases the metabolic expenditures, increases growth, and limits dietary iron absorption. Splenectomy may reduce the transfusion volume but adds to the risk of serious infection. Chelation therapy, started by 10 yr of age, with deferoxamine removes excess iron and prolongs life when appropriately administered. With such therapy, life expectancy approaches 40 yr. Bone marrow transplantation in childhood prior to organ dysfunction induced by iron overload has had a high success rate in beta-thalassemia major.

Sickle Cell Disease. The common sickle cell syndromes include hemoglobin SS disease, hemoglobin S–hemoglobin C disease, hemoglobin S–beta-thalassemia, and rare variants (Table 14–10). It is important to identify the specific hemoglobin phe-

Table 14–10. Comparison of Sickle Cell Syndromes

Genotype	Clinical Condition	Percent Hemoglobin					Other Findings
		Hb A	Hb S	Hb A$_2$	Hb F	Hb C	
SA	Sickle cell trait	55–60	40–45	2–3	—	—	Usually asymptomatic
SS	Sickle cell anemia	0	85–95	2–3	5–15	—	Clinically severe anemia; Hb F heterogeneous in distribution
S-β^0 thal	Sickle cell–beta thalassemia	0	70–80	3–5	10–20	—	Moderately severe anemia; splenomegaly in 50%; smear: hypo, micro anemia
S-β$^+$ thal	Sickle cell–beta thalassemia	10–20	60–75	3–5	10–20		Hb F distributed heterogeneously
SC	Hb SC disease	0	45–50	—	—	45–50	Moderately severe anemia; splenomegaly; target cells
S-HPFH	Sickle—hereditary persistence of Hb F	0	70–80	1–2	20–30	—	Asymptomatic; Hb F is uniformly distributed

(From Andreoli TE, Carpenter CCJ, Plum F, et al: Cecil Essentials of Medicine. Philadelphia, WB Saunders, 1993, p 371.)

notype because the clinical complications differ in frequency, type, and severity.

Sickle cell disease manifests as a chronic hemolytic anemia on which is superimposed sudden, occasionally severe, and life-threatening complications caused by the acute intravascular sickling of the red cells, with resultant pain or organ dysfunction.

Pathophysiology. As a result of a single amino acid substitution (valine for glutamic acid at the β6 position), hemoglobin S cells change from a normal biconcave disc when oxygenated to a sickled form, with resultant decreased deformability in deoxygenated conditions. Sickle hemoglobin crystallizes and forms a gel in the deoxy state. When reoxygenated, the sickle hemoglobin is normally soluble. The so-called reversible sickle cell is capable of entering the microcirculation. However, as the oxygen saturation falls, sickling may occur with resultant occlusion of the microvasculature. The surrounding tissue undergoes infarction, inducing pain and/or dysfunction. This sickling phenomenon is accentuated by hypoxia, acidosis, increased or decreased temperature, and dehydration (increased concentration of erythrocyte hemoglobin S). The clinical manifestations may be due to infection, anemia, and/or vaso-occlusion (Table 14–11).

Clinical Manifestations. The child with sickle cell anemia is vulnerable to life-threatening infection as early as 4 mo of age because of splenic dysfunction, which results from sickling of the red cells within the spleen with resultant inability of the spleen to filter micro-organisms from the bloodstream. Splenic dysfunction is followed eventually by splenic infarction, usually by 2–4 yr of age. In the absence of normal splenic function, the patient is susceptible to overwhelming infection by encapsulated organisms, especially *Streptococcus pneumoniae* and other pathogens (Table 14–11). The hallmark of infection is fever. The patient with a sickle cell syndrome who has a temperature greater than 38.5°C (101.5° F) must be evaluated immediately (see Chapter 10). Current precautions to prevent infections include prophylactic *amoxicillin (or penicillin)* begun at diagnosis and vaccinations against *pneumococcus, H. influenzae* type b, hepatitis B virus, and influenza virus.

The anemia of SS disease is usually a chronic, well-compensated, severe anemia that is not routinely transfusion dependent. The severity depends in part on the patient's phenotype (Table 14–10). Decisions about transfusion should be made on the basis of the patient's clinical condition, the hemoglobin level, and the reticulocyte count. Patients have multiple manifestations of chronic anemia, including jaundice, pallor, variable splenomegaly in infancy, a cardiac flow murmur, and delayed sexual maturation and growth (Table 14–11).

In three different clinical situations, an acute, potentially life-threatening decline in hemoglobin may be superimposed on the chronic compensated anemia. *Splenic sequestration crisis* is a life-threatening hyperacute fall in hemoglobin secondary to splenic pooling of the patient's red cells and sickling within the spleen. The spleen is moderately to markedly enlarged and the reticulocyte count is

Table 14–11. Clinical Manifestations of Sickle Cell Anemia*

Manifestation	Comments
Anemia	Chronic, onset 3–4 mo of age; may require folate therapy for chronic hemolysis. Hematocrit usually 18–26%
Aplastic crisis	Parvovirus infection, reticulocytopenia; acute and reversible
Sequestration crisis	Massive splenomegaly, shock; treat with transfusion
Hemolytic crisis	May be associated with G6PD deficiency
Dactylitis	Hand–foot swelling in early infancy
Painful crisis	Microvascular painful vaso-occlusive infarcts of muscle, bone, bone marrow, lung, intestines
Cerebral vascular accidents	Large- and small-vessel sickling and thrombosis (stroke); requires chronic transfusion
Acute chest syndrome	Infection and/or infarction, severe hypoxemia, infiltrate, dyspnea, rales
Chronic lung disease	Pulmonary fibrosis, restrictive lung disease, cor pulmonale
Priapism	Causes eventual impotence; treat with transfusion, oxygen, or corpora cavernosa–to–spongiosa shunt
Ocular	Retinopathy
Gall bladder disease	Bilirubin stones; cholecystitis
Renal	Hematuria, papillary necrosis, renal-concentrating deficit; nephropathy
Cardiomyopathy	Heart failure (fibrosis)
Leg ulceration	Seen in older patients
Infections	Functional asplenia, defects in properdin system; pneumococcal bacteremia, meningitis, and arthritis; deafness from meningitis in 35%; *H. influenzae* sepsis, *Salmonella*, and *Staphylococcus aureus* osteomyelitis; severe *Mycoplasma* pneumonia; transfusion-acquired HIV, hepatitis A, B, C, D, and E, EBV, CMV
Growth failure, delayed puberty	May respond to nutritional supplements
Psychologic problems	Narcotic addiction, dependence unusual; chronic illness

* Clinical manifestations with sickle cell trait are unusual but include renal papillary necrosis (hematuria), sudden death on exertion, intraocular hyphema extension, and sickling in unpressurized airplanes.

CMV = cytomegalovirus; EBV = Epstein-Barr virus; HIV = human immunodeficiency virus.

elevated. In an *aplastic crisis*, parvovirus B19 infects red cell precursors in the bone marrow and induces transient red cell aplasia with reticulocytopenia. In the *"hyperhemolytic crisis,"* patients may have an acute fall in hemoglobin associated with medications or infection. There is an increase in bilirubin, reticulocytosis, and accentuated jaundice. These patients usually have G6PD deficiency. For sequestration, aplastic, and hemolytic crises, simple transfusion therapy is indicated when the anemia is symptomatic.

Vaso-occlusive crises may occur in any organ of the body, where they are manifested by pain and/or significant dysfunction (Table 14–11). The acute chest syndrome is a vaso-occlusive crisis within the lungs, often in association with infection/infarction. The patient may present with pain but within

a few hours develops cough, increasing respiratory and heart rates, hypoxia, and progressive respiratory distress. Physical examination of the chest reveals area(s) of decreased breath sounds, rales, and dullness to percussion. Treatment includes early recognition and prevention of arterial hypoxemia. Oxygen, fluids, judicial use of analgesic medications, antibiotics, and blood transfusion (occasionally exchange transfusion) usually are indicated in therapy of acute chest syndrome. Patients also may develop large cerebral vessel vaso-occlusive crises within the CNS (stroke); they present with the sudden onset of an altered state of consciousness, seizures, or focal paralysis. Priapism occurs most typically in boys between 6 and 20 yr of age. The child develops sudden, painful onset of a tumescent penis that will not relax. Therapeutic steps for stroke, priapism, and other potentially life-threatening complications include administration of oxygen, fluids, transfusion to achieve a hemoglobin S less than 30% (often by exchange transfusion), and analgesia when appropriate. Fluid management requires recognition that renal medullary infarction results in loss of the ability to concentrate urine. Vaso-occlusive crises may result in avascular necrosis of the femoral head and chronic hip disease.

Pain crisis is the most common type of vaso-occlusive crisis. The pain usually localizes to the long bones of the arms or legs, but may occur in smaller bones of the hands or feet in infancy. These painful crises usually last 2–7 days. The treatment of a pain crisis includes fluids, analgesia usually with narcotics or nonsteroidal anti-inflammatory agents, oxygen if the patient is hypoxic, and monitoring of arterial oxygen saturations. The clinician must maintain a sympathetic attitude toward the patient in pain crisis because pain is impossible to quantitate and the risk of developing drug dependency is highly overrated.

Diagnosis. This is made by the presence of a positive sickle cell solubility test (Sickledex) demonstrating that the patient's red cells sickle (change shape at low oxygen tension) and by a precise characterization of the hemoglobin abnormality using hemoglobin electrophoresis. Every member of an at-risk population should have a precise hemoglobin phenotype (electrophoresis) performed at birth or during early infancy.

Methemoglobinemia. Methemoglobinemia, in which ferrous iron has been oxidized to the ferric state, may be either congenital or acquired. Congenital methemoglobinemia may be due to abnormalities in either the alpha or beta chain. Homozygosity is lethal, whereas heterozygotes usually have a level of 20–30% methemoglobin and are cyanotic in the face of normal Pao_2. Homozygous deficiency of NADH reductase (diaphorase) is common in Navajo Indians and results in chronic methemoglobinemia. Infants under the age of 3 mo, whose antioxidant mechanisms are poorly developed, are especially vulnerable.

Acquired methemoglobinemia is seen with ingestion of certain oxidants. Nitrates and nitrites, derived from fertilizer and disinfectants in well water and foods or from enteric bacteria during diarrhea, are major causes of acquired methemoglobinemia. If sufficiently severe, this condition may be life threatening. Methemoglobinemia should be suspected in a deeply chocolate-colored cyanotic infant without cardiopulmonary disease in whom metabolic acidosis, a high Pao_2, and un-saturated hemoglobin are present. The methemoglobin levels should be measured; treatment with methylene blue or ascorbate usually rapidly reduces Fe^{3+} to Fe^{2+}, correcting this condition.

HEMOLYTIC ANEMIA CAUSED BY DISORDERS EXTRINSIC TO THE RED CELL

Immune-mediated hemolysis may be extravascular, because red cells coated with antibodies or complement are phagocytosed by the reticuloendothelial system, or intravascular, mediated by complement fixation to antibody-coated cells.

Isoimmune hemolysis is caused by active maternal immunization against fetal antigens that the mother's erythrocytes do not express (see Chapter 6). Examples include antibody to the A, B, and Rh D antigens, other Rh antigens, and the Kell, Duffy, and other blood groups. Anti-A and anti-B hemolysis usually is due to the placental transfer of naturally occurring maternal antibodies from mothers who lack A or B antigen (usually blood type O). Positive results of the direct antiglobulin (Coombs) test on the baby's red cells (Figure 14–5) and the indirect antiglobulin test on the mother's serum,

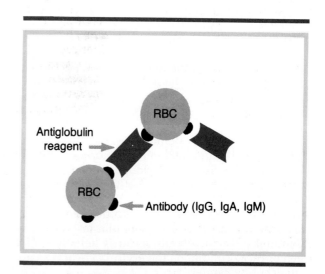

Figure 14–5. Coombs or antiglobulin test. In the Coombs test, an antibody directed against human immunoglobulin (Ig) is used to detect the presence of antibody on the surface of the red cells by agglutination. Complement coating on the red cells (C_3) similarly can be detected by an anticomplement Coombs reagent. Broad-spectrum Coombs reagents can be prepared that detect either immunoglobulin or complement, or both; these are used for screening. (From Andreoli TE, Carpenter CCJ, Plum F, et al: Cecil Essentials of Medicine. Philadelphia, WB Saunders, 1993, p. 367.)

and the presence of spherocytes and immature erythroid precursors (erythroblastosis) on the infant's blood smear confirm this diagnosis. Isoimmune hemolytic disease may be highly variable in its clinical severity. No clinical manifestations may be present, or the infant may present with jaundice, severe anemia, and hydrops fetalis.

Autoimmune hemolytic anemia (AIHA) is usually an acute, self-limited process that develops after an infection (*Mycoplasma,* Epstein-Barr, or other viral infections). Over 80% of patients spontaneously recover. AIHA also may be the presenting symptom of a chronic autoimmune disease (e.g., systemic lupus erythematosus [SLE], lymphoproliferative disorders, or immune deficiency). Transfusion is challenging because cross-matching is difficult as the autoantibodies react with virtually all red cells. The peripheral blood smear usually demonstrates spherocytes and occasionally nucleated red cells. The reticulocyte count is variable, because some patients have relatively low reticulocyte counts as a result of autoantibody that cross-reacts with red cell precursors. Management of this potentially life-threatening condition includes administration of corticosteroids and perhaps intravenous immunoglobulin (IVIG). The corticosteroids reduce the clearance of the sensitized red cells in the spleen.

Drugs also may induce a Coombs-positive hemolytic anemia. Withdrawal of the drug usually results in resolution of the hemolytic process. Drugs may form a hapten on the red cell membrane (penicillin). Alternatively, drugs may form immune complexes (quinidine) that attach to the red cell membrane. Antibodies then activate complement-induced intravascular hemolysis. The third type of drug-induced immune hemolysis occurs during treatment with alpha-methyldopa and a few other drugs and is due to alteration of the red cell membrane after prolonged exposure to the drug. Antibodies are produced that bind to the neoantigen; this produces a positive antiglobulin test far more commonly than it actually induces hemolysis. In each of these conditions the erythrocyte acts as an "innocent bystander."

A second form of acquired hemolytic disease is not immune in nature and is caused by mechanical damage to the membrane of the red cells during circulation. In **microangiopathic hemolytic anemia** (MAHA), the red cells are trapped by fibrin strands in the circulation and physically broken by shear stress as they pass through these strands. Hemolytic–uremic syndrome, disseminated intravascular coagulation (DIC), thrombotic thrombocytopenic purpura, malignant hypertension, toxemia,

and renal graft rejection all produce MAHA. Platelets usually are large, indicating that they are young. These platelets have a decreased survival even if the numbers are normal. Consumption of clotting factors is more prominent in DIC than in the other forms of MAHA. The smear shows red cell fragments (schistocytes), microspherocytes, teardrop forms, and polychromasia. The red cells also may be damaged by exposure to nonendothelialized surfaces (e.g., as in artificial heart valves [the "Waring blender" syndrome]) or as a result of high flow and shear rates in arteriovenous malformations (Kasabach-Merritt syndrome).

Alterations in the plasma lipids, especially cholesterol, may result in damage to the red cell membrane and shorten red cell survival. Lipids in the plasma are in equilibrium with those in red cell membrane; high cholesterol levels increase the membrane cholesterol and the total membrane surface without affecting the volume of the cell. This condition produces spur cells. These are seen in abetalipoproteinemia and liver diseases. Hemolysis occurs in the spleen, where poor red cell deformability results in erythrocyte destruction. *Circulating toxins* such as snake venoms and heavy metals that bind sulfhydryl groups (copper, arsenic) may damage the red cell membrane and induce hemolysis. Irregularly spiculated red cells (burr cells) are seen in renal failure. *Vitamin E deficiency* also can cause an acquired hemolytic anemia as a result of abnormal sensitivity of membrane lipids to oxidant stress. Vitamin E deficiency may occur in premature infants who are not being supplemented with vitamin E or who have insufficient nutrition, in severe malabsorption syndromes (including cystic fibrosis), and in transfusional iron overload, which can result in severe oxidant exposure.

PANCYTOPENIA

Pancytopenia is a decrease in the number of all the formed elements of the blood—erythrocytes, leukocytes, and platelets. Patients present with petechiae, purpura, pallor, dyspnea, or fever. Individual formed elements, or a combination of elements, may be decreased in numbers because of failure of production (implying intrinsic bone marrow disease), sequestration (as in hypersplenism), or increased peripheral destruction. *Features that suggest bone marrow failure* and mandate an examination of bone marrow include a low (less than 2%) RPI, teardrop forms of red cells (implies marrow replacement, not just failure), the presence of abnormal forms of leukocytes or myeloid elements less mature than band forms, small platelets, and an elevated mean corpuscular volume in the face of a low reticulocyte count. Pancytopenia resulting from bone marrow failure is usually a gradual process. Patients may present with one or two involved cell lines but later progress to involvement of all three cell lines. *Features suggesting increased destruction* include reticulocytosis, jaundice, immature erythroid or myeloid elements on the blood smear, large platelets, and increased serum bilirubin and lactic dehydrogenase.

Aplastic Anemia

In this disorder, pancytopenia evolves as the hematopoietic elements of the bone marrow disappear and the marrow is replaced by fat. A biopsy is crucial to determine the extent of depletion of the hemopoietic elements. Aplastic anemia may be idiopathic. Alternatively, this disorder may be induced by drugs such as chloramphenicol or by toxins such as benzene. Aplastic anemia also may follow infections, particularly hepatitis and infectious mononucleosis (Table 14–9). **Fanconi anemia,** a constitutional aplastic anemia, usually presents in the latter half of the first decade of life and may evolve over a period of years. The repair mechanism for DNA damage is abnormal in all cells in Fanconi anemia, a finding that facilitates the diagnosis but also may contribute to the development of malignancies (terminal acute leukemia develops in 10% of cases). These patients have a number of characteristic clinical findings (Table 14–9).

For children with severe aplastic anemia, as defined by an RPI less than 1%, absolute neutrophil count less than 500/mm³, platelet count less than 20,000/mm³, and bone marrow cellularity on biopsy less than 10%, the *treatment* of choice is bone marrow transplantation from a human leukocyte antigen (HLA)–identical, mixed lymphocyte–compatible sibling. With supportive care alone, survival is only about 20% in severe aplastic anemia, although the duration of survival may be years when vigorous blood product and antibiotic support are provided. When bone marrow transplantation takes place prior to sensitization of the recipient to blood products by repeated transfusion, survival rate is in excess of 80%. Positive results may be attained by bone marrow transplantation from HLA-compatible, nonrelated donors. Graft-versus-host disease is a complication of bone marrow transplantation (see Chapter 8). The treatment of aplastic anemia without transplantation is unsatisfactory (Table 14–9). Most patients with Fanconi anemia and about 20% of children with aplastic

anemia appear to respond to androgenic therapy, which unfortunately induces masculinization and may cause liver injury and liver tumors. Androgenic therapy increases red cell synthesis and may diminish transfusion requirements. The effect on granulocytes, and especially the platelet count, is less impressive.

Immune suppression of hematopoiesis is postulated to be an important mechanism in patients with postinfectious and idiopathic aplastic anemia. Therapies with antithymocyte globulin, corticosteroids, cyclosporine, and various immunosuppressive drugs in combination with hematopoietic growth factors (Fig. 14–1) have been successful in occasional patients. None of these drugs is curative, and they are associated with toxicity and relapse.

Marrow Replacement

This condition may occur as a result of leukemia, solid tumors (especially neuroblastoma), osteopetrosis in infants, and myelofibrosis, which is rare in childhood. The mechanism(s) by which malignant cells impair marrow synthesis of normal hemopoietic elements are unclear. Bone marrow aspirate and biopsy are needed for precise diagnosis that then determines appropriate therapy.

Pancytopenia Resulting from Destruction of Cells

This condition may be caused by intramedullary destruction of hemopoietic elements, as occurs in myeloproliferative disorders, folic acid, and vitamin B₁₂ deficiency, or as a result of peripheral destruction of mature cells. The usual site of peripheral destruction of blood cells is the spleen, although the liver and other parts of the reticuloendothelial system may participate. *Hypersplenism* may be due to anatomic causes such as portal hypertension or splenic hypertrophy from thalassemia, infections (including malaria), storage diseases such as Gaucher disease, lymphomas, and histiocytosis. Splenectomy is indicated only when the pancytopenia is of clinical significance, causing the patients to have increased susceptibility to bleeding or infection or producing a high transfusion requirement.

References

Behrman RE (ed): Nelson Textbook of Pediatrics. 14th ed. Philadelphia, WB Saunders, 1992, Sec. 16.1–16.32.
Berkowitz FE: Hemolysis and infection: Categories and

mechanisms of their interrelationship. Rev Infect Dis 13: 1151, 1991.

Beutler E: Glucose-6-phosphate dehydrogenase: New perspectives. Blood 73:1397, 1990.

Colon-Otero G, Menke D, Hook CC: A practical approach to the differential diagnosis and evaluation of the adult patient with macrocytic anemia. Med Clin North Am 76: 581, 1992.

Eber SW, Armbrust R, Schroter W: Variable clinical severity of hereditary spherocytosis: Relation to erythrocytic spectrin concentration, osmotic fragility, and autohemolysis. J Pediatr 117:409, 1990.

Ehlers KH, Giardina PJ, Lesser ML, et al: Prolonged survival in patients with beta-thalassemia major treated with deferoxamine. J Pediatr 118:540, 1991.

Furman WL, Crist WM: Biology and clinical applications of hemopoietins in pediatric practice. Pediatrics 90:716, 1992.

Frickhofen, N, Kaltwasser JP, Schrezenmeier H, et al: Treatment of aplastic anemia with antilymphocyte globulin and methylprednisolone with or without cyclosporine. N Engl J Med 324:1297, 1991.

Leikin SL, Gallagher D, Kinney TR, et al: Mortality in children and adolescents with sickle cell disease. Pediatrics 84:500, 1989.

Massey AC: Microcytic anemia: Differential diagnosis and management of iron deficiency anemia. Med Clin North Am 76:549, 1992.

Pearson H: Sickle cell diseases: Diagnosis and management in infancy and childhood. Pediatr Rev 9:121, 1987.

Platt OS, Thorington BD, Brambilla DJ, et al: Pain in sickle cell disease: Rates and risk factors. N Engl J Med 325: 11, 1991.

Raunikar RA, Sabio H: Anemia in the adolescent athlete. Am J Dis Child 146:1201, 1992.

Rodgers GP: Recent approaches to the treatment of sickle cell anemia. JAMA 265:2097, 1991.

Sears DA: Anemia of chronic disease. Med Clin North Am 76:567, 1992.

Steingart R: Management of patients with sickle cell disease. Med Clin North Am 76:669, 1992.

Stevens D: Epidemiology of hypochromic anaemia in young children. Arch Dis Child 66:886, 1991.

Stewart FM: Hypoplastic, aplastic anemia: Role of bone marrow transplantation. Med Clin North Am 76:683, 1992.

Tabbara IA: Hemolytic anemias: Diagnosis and management. Med Clin North Am 76:649, 1992.

Webb DKH, Mann IM, Chessells JM: Acquired aplastic anaemia: Still a serious disease. Arch Dis Child 66:858, 1991.

DISORDERS OF LEUKOCYTES

The major function of phagocytic cells is to ingest and kill pathogens (see Chapters 8 and 10). The major manifestation of neutropenia or neutrophil dysfunction is increased susceptibility to infection with bacterial and/or fungi.

Neutropenia

The normal neutrophil count varies with age (see Table 14–2). Neutropenia is defined as an absolute neutrophil count less than 1500/mm³ for white children over 1 yr of age. Black children normally have somewhat lower total white blood cell (WBC) and neutrophil counts.

The impact of neutropenia depends on its severity. The susceptibility to infection is unaffected until the absolute neutrophil count (ANC) is less than 1000/mm³. Patients do quite well as long as the ANC is greater than 500/mm³. At these levels of circulating neutrophils, localized infections are more common than generalized bacteremia. With an ANC less than 200/mm³, serious bacterial infections are quite common. Episodes of bacteremia also are associated with the presence of indwelling catheters, mucosal injury secondary to cytotoxic agents, and immunosuppressive agents. The presence of an underlying malignancy or immunodeficiency disorder also increases the risk for serious bacterial or fungal infection. In the absence of an adequate neutrophil count, there is a subsequent delay in migration of neutrophils to areas of damage in the skin and mucous membrane. The major types of infection associated with neutropenia include cellulitis, pharyngitis, gingivitis, lymphadenitis, abscesses (cutaneous or perianal), enteritis (typhlitis), and pneumonia. These sites usually all are colonized heavily with normal bacterial flora that become invasive in the presence of neutropenia. Meticulous attention to oral and skin hygiene and prevention of colonization with fungi are helpful in minimizing such infections.

Neutropenia may be congenital or acquired. Neutropenia may be classified mechanistically (Table 14–12) and commonly may be associated with specific diseases, especially infections (Table 14–13), or drugs (Table 14–14).

Congenital Neutropenia. Most congenital neutropenias are caused by an inadequate production of cells. The most severe clinical disorders are *reticular dysgenesis* (severe combined immunodeficiency with agranulocytosis) and *infantile genetic agranulocytosis* (IGA, or Kostmann syndrome). Both are inherited as autosomal recessive disorders and frequently are fatal in infancy. IGA is marked by monocytosis in up to 50% of the circulating leukocytes. Growth of myeloid cultures in vitro is normal, suggesting a defect in control mechanisms; G-CSF levels are undetectable while exogenous G-CSF produces a rise in the neutrophil count. Transfusion of granulocytes and administration of G-CSF during severe infections may be lifesaving. Rare

Table 14–12. Mechanisms of Neutropenia

Abnormal Bone Marrow
Marrow injury
  Drugs: idiosyncratic, cytotoxic (myelosuppressive)
  Radiation
  Chemicals: DDT, benzene
  Hereditary
  Immune-mediated: T and B cell and immunoglobulin
  Infection: HIV, hepatitis
  Infiltrative processes: tumor, storage disease

Maturation defects
  Folic acid deficiency
  Vitamin B_{12}
  Glycogen storage disease type Ib
  Shwachman syndrome
  Organic acidemias
  Clonal disorders: congenital
  Cyclic neutropenia

Peripheral Circulation
Pseudoneutropenia: shift to bone marrow
  Hereditary
  Severe infection

Intravascular
  Destruction: neonatal isoimmune, autoimmune, hypersplenism
  Leukoagglutination: lung, after cardiac bypass surgery

Extravascular Mechanisms
Increased utilization: Severe infection, anaphylaxis

Destruction: antibody-mediated, hypersplenism

DDT = chlorophenothane; HIV = human immunodeficiency virus.
(Adapted from Bagby G: In Andreoli TE, Carpenter CCJ, Plum F, et al (eds): Cecil Essentials of Medicine. 18th ed. Philadelphia, WB Saunders, 1988.)

Table 14–13. Infections Associated with Neutropenia

Bacterial
Typhoid—paratyphoid
Brucellosis
Neonatal sepsis
Meningococcemia
Overwhelming sepsis
Congenital syphilis
Tuberculosis

Viral
Measles
Hepatitis A and B
HIV
Rubella
CMV
Influenza A and B
Epstein-Barr virus

Rickettsial
Rocky Mountain spotted fever
Typhus
Rickettsialpox

CMV = cytomegalovirus; HIV = human immunodeficiency virus.

cant abnormality is neutropenia because of the short half-life of neutrophils (6–7 hr) in comparison to platelets (10 days) and red cells (120 days). The usual neutropenic cycle is 21 days, with agranulocytosis lasting 4–6 days accompanied by monocytosis and often by eosinophilia. Clinical manifestations include stomatitis or oral ulcers, pharyngitis, lymphadenopathy, fever, and cellulitis at the time of neutropenia. Severe debilitating bone pain is common in these patients when the neutrophil count is low. Cyclic neutropenia re-

Table 14–14. Drugs Associated with Neutropenia

Cytotoxic
Myelosuppressive agents
Chemotherapy
Immunosuppressive agents

Idiosyncratic
Chloramphenicol
Sulfonamides
Propylthiouracil
Penicillins
Trimethoprim–sulfamethoxazole
Carbamazepine
Phenytoin
Cimetidine
Methyldopa
Indomethacin
Chlorpromazine
Penicillamine
Gold salts

patients who have survived into adolescence have developed acute myeloid leukemia. Bone marrow transplantation may be curative.

Other congenital neutropenias caused by deficient production of neutrophils vary in severity and are poorly characterized. *Benign congenital neutropenia* is a functional diagnosis for patients with significant neutropenia who do not develop major infectious complications. Many patients whose ANCs range from 100 to 500/mm³ have an increased frequency of infections, particularly respiratory infections, but the major problem is the slow resolution of the infections that develop. These disorders may be sporadic or familial and, in some instances, they are transmitted as an autosomal dominant disorder.

Cyclic neutropenia may be transmitted as an autosomal dominant, recessive, or sporadic disorder. This is a stem cell disorder in which all marrow elements cycle. However, the only clinically signifi-

sponds to G-CSF with a reduced number of days of neutropenia and an overall increase of neutrophils.

Pancreatic insufficiency accompanying bone marrow dysfunction (Shwachman-Diamond syndrome) is also a panmyeloid disorder in which neutropenia is the most prominent manifestation. In this autosomal recessive condition, patients may have all the common complications of neutropenia. A major complication is gingivitis, which may be severe and lead to serious oral infections and alveolar bone destruction. Patients may become edentulous at an early age. Metaphyseal dysostosis and dwarfism also may occur. Patients may respond to G-CSF.

Acquired Neutropenias. These conditions may be caused by either marrow hypoplasia or peripheral neutrophil destruction. *Isoimmune neutropenia* occurs in up to 3% of neonates and is due to transplacental transfer of maternal antibodies to fetal neutrophil antigens. In isoimmune neonatal neutropenia, the mother is sensitized to specific neutrophil antigens (NA1, NA2, NB1, and NC1) on fetal leukocytes inherited from the father and not present on maternal cells. Isoimmune neonatal neutropenia, like isoimmune anemia and thrombocytopenia (see Chapter 6), is a transient process. Early treatment of infection (cutaneous is most common; sepsis is rarer) while the infant is neutropenic is the major goal of therapy. Administration IVIG may decrease the duration of neutropenia.

Autoimmune neutropenia usually develops early in childhood (5–24 mo of age) and often persists for prolonged periods. Neutrophil autoantibodies may be immunoglobulin (Ig) M, IgG, IgA, or a combination of these. Usually there is resolution in 6 mo to 4 yr. Clinical symptoms may dictate treatment. IVIG or corticosteroids have been used in some circumstances. Other patients have responded to G-CSF. Most patients do not progress to more generalized autoimmune disorders; however, rarely, autoimmune neutropenia may be an early manifestation of SLE or rheumatoid arthritis. The marrow in autoimmune neutropenia and SLE shows myeloid hyperplasia, except that if antibody is directed against myeloid precursors, it reveals hypoplasia. The differential diagnosis of autoimmune neutropenia includes SLE, rheumatoid arthritis (Felty syndrome), bone marrow transplantation, or drug induced neutropenia.

Neutropenia is common in *stressed neonates*. Virtually any major illness, including asphyxia, may precipitate transient neonatal neutropenia. Infected neonates are prone to develop significant neutropenia at least in part on the basis of depletion of bone marrow stores. These bone marrow stores, which constitute 7 times the circulating pool of neutrophils in adults, are far less extensive in neonates. Therefore, their marrow reserve is readily depleted by infectious processes.

Diagnosis. Neutropenia is confirmed by a complete blood count and differential. The evaluation of the neutropenic child depends on associated clinical abnormalities, such as signs of infection, family and medication history, age of the patient, cyclic or persistent nature of the condition, signs of bone marrow infiltration (malignancy, storage disease), and evidence of involvement of other cell lines. An algorithm for the work-up of the child with neutropenia is presented in Figure 14–6.

Treatment. Therapy of neutropenia is dependent on the underlying cause. Patients with severe bacterial infections require broad-spectrum antibiotics; the resolution of neutropenia during an infection is a good prognostic sign. Unfortunately, granulocyte transfusions have been relatively unsuccessful in improving survival in instances of overwhelming infections in neutropenic patients. Chronic mild neutropenia not associated with immunosuppression can be managed expectantly with prompt antimicrobial treatment of soft tissue infections (*Staphylococcus aureus*, *Streptococcus*). Specific therapies of neutropenia may include steroids (to decrease antibody production or splenic destruction), lithium (to increase bone marrow release), splenectomy, intravenous immunoglobulin (to decrease autoantibody production or decrease clearance of sensitized neutrophils), or G-CSF (to increase production). The treatment of clinically significant congenital neutropenia has been improved by the development of recombinant G-CSF and GM-CSF.

Leukocytosis or Neutrophilia

This condition most often is associated with infection ($>15,000$ WBC/mm^3). When acute infection occurs, particularly bacterial infection, neutrophils are released from bone marrow stores to induce a rapid increase in the circulating WBC count. Chronic infection, such as tuberculosis, osteomyelitis, and abscesses, also may cause neutrophilia. A shift in the distribution of the cells, with a greater number circulating than adhering to blood vessel walls, is a common mechanism for neutrophilia associated with drugs, including corticosteroids and epinephrine. Certain disorders of neutrophil function, especially the lack of the complement receptor

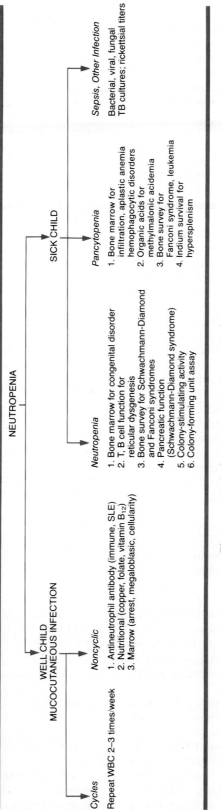

Figure 14–6. Laboratory evaluation of neutropenia.

CR3 (*Mo-1 deficiency*) are associated with a marked leukocytosis. Leukocytosis also may be a normal variant in some families in which several members have an increase in total neutrophil counts without apparent underlying pathology. Chronic myelogenous leukemia also is characterized by neutrophilia. However, immature forms of granulocytes usually are present.

Defects in Neutrophil Function

These relatively rare inherited disorders tend to be associated with a marked susceptibility to bacterial infection (see Chapter 8). Some acquired functional disorders also occur and may be quite severe. Leukocyte adhesion deficiency is due to defective neutrophil chemotaxis, ingestion of particles opsonized with complement, and adherence to surfaces. It is a consequence of lack of CR3, the receptor for C3Bi. This disorder presents in early infancy with failure of separation of the umbilical cord, often until as late as 2 mo after birth, with attendant omphalitis and sepsis. The neutrophil count usually is greater than 20,000 per mm³ because of failure of the neutrophils to adhere normally to vascular endothelium and to migrate out of blood to the tissues. Affected children develop cutaneous, respiratory, and mucosal infections and usually have severe gingivitis. Sepsis usually leads to death in early childhood. This disorder is transmitted as an autosomal recessive trait that has an unknown frequency. Bone marrow transplantation may improve the outcome.

Defective bacterial killing, because the phagocytes are unable to generate reactive oxygen species such as hydrogen peroxide, hydroxyl radical, and superoxide anion, is the major feature of *chronic granulomatous disease* (see Chapter 8). Nonoxidative killing is abnormal in *secondary granule deficiency*, a rare disorder in which bacterial killing also is delayed. An acquired form of secondary granule deficiency occurs in patients with severe burn injuries; it occurs about 2 wk after the original trauma. This poor killing ability may contribute to the increased susceptibility to bacterial infection of burn patients (see Chapter 3). The acquired defect is reversible.

Another abnormality of secondary granules is *Chédiak-Higashi syndrome*, an autosomal recessive disorder that results in fusion of the primary and secondary granules of the neutrophil. Giant granules are present in many cells, including lymphocytes, platelets, and melanocytes. Patients usually have partial oculocutaneous albinism. Although most patients have frequent fevers in infancy and early childhood, documented bacterial infection is not common. Infection with the Epstein-Barr virus (EBV) produces a loss of natural killer cells and results in a *lymphoproliferative syndrome* characterized by hepatomegaly, adenopathy, and pancytopenia. This may lead to an "accelerated phase," which usually is rapidly fatal. Children who avoid EBV infection may live into adulthood without major clinical problems, except for gingivitis.

A variety of conditions also are associated with chemotactic defects in neutrophils. *Job's syndrome* usually is acquired and may be seen in childhood. The major manifestations are eczema, hyperimmunoglobulin E, an extrinsic chemotactic defect, a T cell defect with reduced interferon production, and recurrent "cold" boils (*S. aureus*) that do not become markedly red or drain. In some patients, identifying offending allergens or removing them has resulted in resolution of the chemotactic defect as well as the eczema and boils. The *"lazy leukocyte syndrome"* is caused by a chemotactic defect resulting from failure of neutrophil egress from the bone marrow and consequent neutropenia. Several systemic disorders, including uremia, SLE, Hodgkin disease, liver disease, and poorly controlled diabetes mellitus, also have associated chemotactic defects.

References

Behrman RE (ed): Nelson Textbook of Pediatrics. 14th ed. Philadelphia, WB Saunders, 1992, Sec. 16.34–16.62.

Conway L, Clay M, Kline W, et al: Natural history of primary autoimmune neutropenia in infancy. J Pediatr 79: 728, 1987.

Dunkel I, Bussel J: New developments in the treatment of neutropenia. AJDC 147:994, 1993.

Glasser L, Duncan BR, Corrigan JJ: Measurement of serum granulocyte colony-stimulating factor in a patient with congenital agranulocytosis (Kostmann's syndrome). Am J Dis Child 145:925, 1991.

Jonsson OG, Buchanan GR: Chronic neutropenia during childhood. A 13 year experience in a single institution. Am J Dis Child 145:232, 1991.

Metcalf D: Control of granulocytes and macrophages: Molecular, cellular, and clinical aspects. Science 254:529, 1991.

Yang KD, Hill HR: Neutrophil function disorders: Pathophysiology, prevention, and therapy. J Pediatr 119:343, 1991.

HEMOSTATIC DISORDERS

Normal Hemostasis

Hemostasis is the dynamic process by which coagulation occurs on areas of vascular injury and is limited to areas of injury so that the clot does not extend beyond the initial site of vascular damage. This process involves the carefully modulated interaction of platelets, vascular wall, and procoagulant and anticoagulant proteins. Following injury to the vascular endothelium, subendothelial collagen induces a conformational change in von Willebrand factor, an adhesive protein to which platelets bind via their glycoprotein Ib receptor. Following adhesion, platelets undergo activation and release a number of intracellular contents, including ADP, that subsequently induce aggregation of additional platelets. Simultaneously, subendothelial collagen

and other matrix proteins in the tissue activate the coagulation cascade, leading to the formation of the enzyme thrombin (Fig. 14–7). Thrombin has multiple effects on the coagulation mechanism, including further aggregation of platelets, a positive feedback activation of factors V and VIII, the conversion of fibrinogen to fibrin, the activation of factor XIII, and the eventual limitation of the thrombus by activating plasminogen to plasmin (Fig. 14–8). The platelet plug forms and bleeding ceases usually within 3–7 min. The generation of thrombin results in formation of a permanent clot by the activation of factor XIII, which crosslinks fibrin and results in

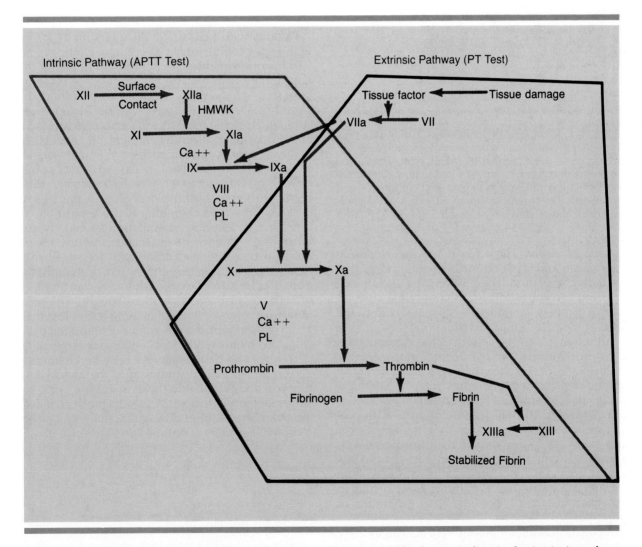

Figure 14–7. Simplified pathways of blood coagulation. The area inside the green line is the intrinsic pathway, measured by the activated partial thromboplastin time (APTT). The area inside the black line is the extrinsic pathway, measured by the prothrombin time (PT). The area encompassed by both lines is the common pathway. (From Andreoli, TE, Carpenter CCJ, Plum F, et al: Cecil Essentials of Medicine. Philadelphia, WB Saunders, 1993, p 409.)

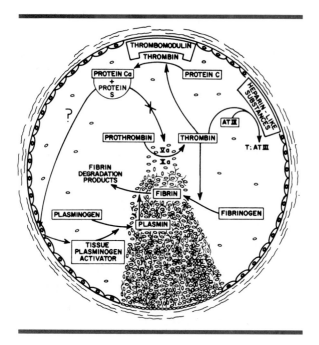

Figure 14–8. Formation of the hemostatic plug at the site of vascular injury. Three major physiologic anticoagulant mechanisms—antithrombin III (AT III), protein C, and the fibrinolytic system—are activated to limit clot formation to the site of damage and to prevent generalized thrombosis. T = thrombin. (From Schafer A: The hypercoagulable states. Ann Intern Med 102:814, 1985, p. 815.)

a stable thrombus. These two processes are closely interwoven and occur on the biologic surfaces that mediate coagulation: the platelet, the endothelial cell, and the subendothelium. As a final element to this process, contractile elements within the platelet mediate clot retraction.

Although it is convenient to think of coagulation as having "intrinsic" and "extrinsic" pathways, the reality is that these pathways are closely interactive and do not react independently (Fig. 14–7). Negatively charged surfaces (glass, collagen, or kaolin) activate factor XII, which then interacts with prekallikrein and high-molecular-weight kininogen to activate factor XI and initiate the intrinsic system. Tissue factor, in combination with calcium and factor VII, activates the extrinsic pathway. In vivo, the extrinsic pathway, however, most likely results in activation of factor IX and eventual generation of thrombin.

As the procoagulant proteins are activated, there are a series of inhibitory factors that serve to regulate the activation of coagulation tightly (Fig. 14–8). Antithrombin III inactivates thrombin and factors Xa, IXa, and XIa. The protein C and protein S sys-

tem serves to inactivate activated factors V and VIII, which are cofactors localized in the "tenase" and "prothrombinase" complexes. The tissue factor pathway inhibitor (TFPI), an anticoagulant protein, serves to limit the activation of the coagulation cascade by factors VIIa and Xa. *Fibrinolysis* is initiated by the action of tissue plasminogen activator (urokinase) on plasminogen, producing plasmin, the active enzyme that degrades fibrin into split products (Fig. 14–8). It is fibrinolysis that eventually dissolves the clot and allows normal flow to resume.

Approach to the Patient with a Hemostatic Disorder

Patients with hemostatic disorders may present with either complaints of bleeding or clotting. Certain historic variables are paramount in taking the appropriate history. The age at onset of bleeding (acquired, congenital), the sites of bleeding, the amount of trauma required, aspirin (drug) exposure, and the characteristics of symptoms (mucocutaneous or deep bleeding) are critical. A detailed family history is quite important. When investigating thrombotic disorders, a personal and family history of early-onset stroke, heart attack, cutaneous thrombosis, and blood clots in the legs or lungs suggests a hereditary predisposition to thromboses. Physical examination should characterize the presence of cutaneous, synovial, and mucosal bleeding, in addition to deeper sites of hemorrhage. Evidence of malignancy (lymphadenopathy, hepatosplenomegaly) or chronic hepatic or renal disease also should be sought. The term **petechiae** refers to a nonblanching lesion less than 2 mm in size, **purpura** are groups of adjoining petechiae, **ecchymoses** are isolated lesions larger than petechiae, and **hematomas** are raised ecchymoses. Screening laboratory studies after the history and physical should include those in Table 14–15. No single laboratory test study can diagnose all bleeding disorders. A brief differential diagnosis of hemostatic disorders is outlined in Figure 14–9.

Disorders of Platelets

THROMBOCYTOPENIA
(Table 14–16), Fig. 14–9)

Platelet counts below 150,000/mm³ constitute thrombocytopenia. Mucocutaneous bleeding is the hallmark of platelet disorders, including thrombocytopenia. The risk of bleeding, however, corre-

Table 14–15. Screening Tests for Bleeding Disorders

Test	Mechanism Tested	Normal	Disorder
Prothrombin time (PT)	Extrinsic and common pathway	<12 sec beyond neonate; 12–18 sec in term neonate	Defect in vitamin K–dependent factors; hemorrhagic disease of newborn, malabsorption, liver disease, DIC, oral anticoagulants, ingestion of rat poison
Activated partial thromboplastin time (APTT; PTT)	Intrinsic and common pathway	25–40 sec beyond neonate; 70 sec in term neonate	Hemophilia; von Willebrand disease, heparin; DIC; deficient factor XII, IX, and XI, lupus anticoagulant
Thrombin time (TT)	Fibrinogen to fibrin conversion	10–15 sec beyond neonate; 12–17 sec in term neonate	Fibrin split products, DIC, hypofibrinogenemia, heparin
Bleeding time (BT)	Hemostasis, capillary and platelet function	3–7 min beyond neonate	Platelet dysfunction, thrombocytopenia, von Willebrand disease, aspirin
Platelet count	Platelet number	150,000–450,000/mm³	Thrombocytopenia differential diagnosis (see Table 14–16)
Blood smear	Platelet number and size; RBC morphology	—	Large platelets suggest peripheral destruction; fragmented, bizarre RBC morphology suggests microangiopathic process (e.g., hemolytic–uremic syndrome, hemangioma, DIC)

RBC = red blood cells.

lates imperfectly with the platelet count. In general, children with platelets counts greater than 80,000/mm³ are able to withstand all but the most extreme hemostatic challenges, such as surgery or major trauma. In contrast, those with platelet counts less than 20,000/mm³ are at risk for spontaneous bleeding. These generalizations are modified by factors such as the age of the platelets (young, large platelets usually function better than old ones), and the presence of inhibitors of platelet function, such as antibodies, drugs (especially aspirin), fibrin degradation products, and toxins in hepatic or renal disease. The etiology of thrombocytopenia may be organized into disorders of decreased platelet production, increased destruction, and sequestration.

Thrombocytopenia Resulting from Decreased Platelet Production. As a primary disorder, this is rare in childhood, other than as part of an aplastic syndrome. Congenital hypoplastic thrombocytopenia is part of several constitutional disorders. *Thrombocytopenia with absent radii syndrome* is characterized by severe thrombocytopenia in association with orthopedic abnormalities, especially of the upper extremity. The thrombocytopenia usually improves over time. The *Wiskott-Aldrich syndrome* is an X-linked disorder characterized by hypogammaglobinemia, eczema, and thrombocytopenia (see Chapter 8). The platelets on peripheral blood smear are small. Bone marrow transplantation results in a complete cure of the immunodeficiency and thrombocytopenia and resolution of the eczema.

Acquired thrombocytopenia due to decreased production is rarely an isolated finding. It is more often seen in the context of *pancytopenia due to bone marrow failure.* Certain chemotherapeutic agents may affect megakaryocytes selectively more than other marrow elements. *Cyanotic congenital heart disease with polycythemia* often is associated with thrombocytopenia, but this is rarely severe or associated with significant clinical bleeding. Both congenital (TORCH) and acquired *viral infections* (human immunodeficiency virus, [HIV], EBV, measles) and some *drugs* (anticonvulsants, antibiotics, cytotoxic agents heparin, quinidine) may induce thrombocytopenia. Postnatal infections (other than HIV) and drug reactions usually cause transient thrombocytopenia, whereas congenital infections may pro-

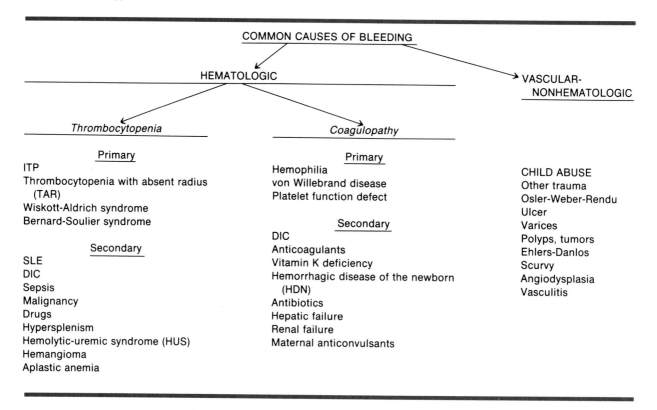

Figure 14–9. Diagnostic considerations for the bleeding patient.

duce prolonged suppression of bone marrow function.

Thrombocytopenia Resulting from Peripheral Destruction.   In a well-appearing child, immune-mediated mechanisms are the most common cause of thrombocytopenia. Thrombocytopenia results from increased rates of antibody-dependent platelet destruction. *Neonatal alloimmune thrombocytopenic purpura* (NATP) occurs as a result of sensitization of the mother to antigens present on fetal platelets during gestation. Antibodies cross the placenta and attack the fetal platelet (see Chapter 6). *Mothers with idiopathic thrombocytopenic purpura* (ITP) or with a previous history of ITP may have passive transfer of antiplatelet antibodies that react with fetal platelets, with resultant neonatal thrombocytopenia (see Chapter 6). The maternal platelet count is sometimes a useful indicator of the probability the infant will be affected. If the mother had a splenectomy, the maternal platelet count may be normalized and is a poor predictor of the likelihood of severe neonatal thrombocytopenia because maternal antibody will trigger destruction of the fetal platelets in the fetal spleen. In NATP, the infant is at risk in utero and during the immediate delivery process. In ITP, the greatest risk appears to be during passage through the birth canal, during which molding of the head may induce intracranial hemorrhage. Fetal scalp sampling or percutaneous umbilical blood sampling may be performed to measure the fetal platelet count. Administration of IVIG prior to delivery has been shown to be effective in raising fetal platelets counts and may alleviate thrombocytopenia in the infant in both NATP and ITP. Delivery by cesarean section is recommended to prevent CNS bleeding (see Chapter 6). Those neonates with severe thrombocytopenia (platelet counts <20,000) may be treated with IVIG and/or corticosteroids until the period of thrombocytopenia remits. If necessary, infants with NATP may receive maternal platelets.

Autoimmune thrombocytopenic purpura of childhood (childhood ITP) is a common disorder in children that usually follows an acute viral infection and is caused by an antibody (IgG or IgM) that binds to the platelet membrane and results in splenic destruction of antibody-coated platelets. Rarely, ITP may be the presenting symptom of an autoimmune disease such as SLE. Approximately 80% of children have a spontaneous resolution of ITP within 6 mo following diagnosis. Young children typically

Table 14–16. Causes of Thrombocytopenia

Neonate
Maternal ITP,* SLE, drugs, pre-eclampsia
Isoimmune*
Congenital megakaryocytic hypoplasia (thrombocyto-
   penia absent radius)
Giant hemangioma
Sepsis*
DIC
TORCH infections

Infant
Wiskott-Aldrich syndrome
Viral infections* ± hemophagocytic syndrome
Drugs
Neuroblastoma
Leukemia*
Hemolytic–uremic syndrome
Sepsis
ITP*

Childhood
ITP*
Drugs*
Aplastic anemia
Leukemia*
Hypersplenism (thalassemia, Gaucher, portal hyper-
   tension)
Sepsis
SLE
Virus-induced hemophagocytic syndrome
ITP with autoimmune hemolytic anemia (Evans syn-
   drome)
AIDS

* Common
AIDS = acquired immunodeficiency syndrome; ITP = idiopathic thrombocytopenic purpura.

present 1–4 wk after viral illness with abrupt onset of petechiae, purpura, and epistaxis. The thrombocytopenia usually is severe. Significant adenopathy or hepatosplenomegaly is unusual, and the red cell and white cell counts are normal. Diagnosis of ITP usually does not require a bone marrow examination. However, if there are atypical findings, marrow examination is indicated to rule out leukemia or aplastic anemia. In ITP, the bone marrow reveals increased megakaryocytes and normal erythroid and myeloid elements.

For clinical bleeding or severe thrombocytopenia (platelet counts <20,000), there are several options for treatment. Corticosteroids, (prednisone 2 mg/kg/day for 2 wk) or IVIG 1 g/kg/day for 1–2 days decreases the duration of severe thrombocytopenia but does not affect the long-term outcome of the ITP. Both work by decreasing the rate of clearance of sensitized platelets rather than decreasing production of antibody. IV anti-D (Rhogam) is effec-

tive in roughly 80% of patients with ITP who are Rh positive and also impairs splenic clearance of sensitized platelets. It is estimated that serious bleeding, especially intracranial bleeding, occurs in less than 1% of patients with acute ITP. Therapy seldom is indicated for platelet counts greater than 30,000/mm^3. Splenectomy is indicated in acute ITP only for life-threatening bleeding.

Chronic ITP is diagnosed following 6–12 mo of persistent thrombocytopenia. Repeated treatments with IVIG or IV anti-D have been effective in delaying splenectomy. Splenectomy is effective in inducing a remission in 70–80% of childhood ITP. The risks of splenectomy (surgery, sepsis from encapsulated bacteria [e.g., *pneumococcus*]) must be weighed against the risk of severe bleeding.

Microangiopathic hemolytic anemia (MAHA) generally is associated with thrombocytopenia, anemia secondary to intravascular red cell destruction, and depletion of clotting factors. Children with MAHA usually are quite ill (see Anemia). In *DIC*, the deposition of fibrin strands within the vasculature and activation of both thrombin and plasmin result in a wide-ranging hemostatic disorder with activation and clearance of platelets. In *thrombotic thrombocytopenic purpura*, platelet consumption precipitated or aggravated by a plasma factor or lack of an inhibitory factor appears to be the primary process, with a modest deposition of fibrin and red cell destruction. *Hemolytic–uremic syndrome* occurs as a result of exposure to a toxin that induces endothelial injury, fibrin deposition, and platelet activation and clearance (see Chapter 16).

DISORDERS OF PLATELET FUNCTION

These disorders present with mucocutaneous bleeding and a prolonged bleeding time and may be primary or secondary. The former are rare. Secondary disorders caused by toxins and drugs (uremia, salicylates, nonsteroidal anti-inflammatory agents, and infections) may cause a broad spectrum of platelet dysfunction.

Disorders of Clotting Factors

Hereditary deficiencies of procoagulant proteins result in bleeding. Only deficiencies of prekallikrein and Hageman factor are not associated with a predisposition toward bleeding. The genes for factors VIII and IX are on the X chromosome, whereas virtually all the other clotting factors are coded on autosomal chromosomes and therefore inherited autosomally. Factor VIII and factor IX deficiencies are the most common severe inherited bleeding disorders. Of the mild congenital coagulopathies, von Willebrand disease is most common.

HEMOPHILIA

Hemophilia A (factor VIII deficiency) occurs in 1:5000 males. *Hemophilia B* (factor IX deficiency) occurs approximately one fifth as often. Clinically, the two disorders are indistinguishable other than in their therapy. Because of a lack of factor VIII or IX, there is a delay in generation of thrombin, which is crucial to forming a normal, functional fibrin clot and solidifying the platelet plug that has formed in areas of vascular injury. The severity of the disorder is determined by the degree of clotting factor deficiency. Patients with less than 1% (severe hemophilia) factor VIII or factor IX may have spontaneous bleeding or bleeding with very minor trauma. Patients with 1–5% (moderate hemophilia) factor VIII or factor IX usually require moderate trauma to induce bleeding episodes. In mild hemophilia (>5% factor VIII or IX), significant trauma is necessary to induce bleeding; spontaneous bleeding does not occur. Mild hemophilia may go undiagnosed for many years, whereas severe hemophilia manifests in infancy. In severe hemophilia spontaneous bleeding occurs, usually in the muscles or joints (hemarthroses). Prevention of long-term crippling orthopedic abnormalities is a major goal of care. Early institution of factor replacement therapy has prevented the vast majority of crippling orthopedic abnormalities.

Diagnosis. The diagnosis of hemophilia is based on a prolonged activated partial thromboplastin time (APTT). In the APTT, a surface-active agent activates the intrinsic system of coagulation, of which factors VIII and IX are critical components. With factor VIII or IX deficiency, the APTT is quite prolonged. Once an abnormal APTT is obtained, specific factor assays are needed to make a precise diagnosis, which is critical to decide on the appropriate factor replacement therapy (Table 14–17). Both prenatal diagnosis and carrier diagnosis now are possible using either coagulation-based methods or molecular biologic techniques.

Treatment. Early appropriate replacement treatment is the aim of optimal hemophilia care. Acute bleeding episodes are best treated in the home once the patient has attained the appropriate age and the parents have learned home treatment. Bleeding associated with surgery, trauma, or dental extraction often can be anticipated and excessive bleeding prevented with appropriate replacement therapy. For life-threatening bleeding, levels of 80–100% of normal factor VIII or IX are necessary. For mild to moderate bleeding episodes (e.g., hemarthroses), a 40% level for factor VIII or a 30–40% level for factor IX is appropriate. The dose can be calculated by knowing that 1 unit/kg body weight of factor VIII will raise the plasma level 2%, whereas 1 unit/kg of factor IX will raise the plasma level 1%. Therefore, dose = desired level (%) × weight (kg) × 0.5 (for factor VIII) or × 1.0 (for factor IX). Aminocaproic acid or tranexamic acid are inhibitors of fibrinolysis that may be useful for oral bleeding. Desmopressin acetate (DDAVP) is a synthetic vasopressin analogue with minimal vasopressor effect. DDAVP triples or quadruples the initial factor VIII level of a patient with hemophilia A, but has no effect on factor IX levels. When adequate hemostatic levels can be attained, DDAVP is the treatment of choice for individuals with mild and moderate hemophilia A.

Patients treated with older factor VIII or IX concentrates were at high risk for hepatitis B, C, and D and HIV. Newer concentrates are safe from virally transmitted illnesses. Also, recombinant factor VIII should be completely safe from all viral agents. Older patients who were exposed to factor concentrates or, less often, cryoprecipitate prior to HIV testing have a high prevalence of HIV infection. Acquired immunodeficiency syndrome is the most common cause of death in older patients with hemophilia. Many older patients also have chronic non-A, non-B hepatitis (hepatitis C).

Inhibitors are IgG antibodies directed against transfused factor VIII or IX in congenitally deficient patients. Inhibitors arise in 15% of severe factor VIII and much less commonly in factor IX hemophiliacs. They may be high or low titer and demonstrate an anamnestic response to treatment. The treatment of bleeding patients with an inhibitor is difficult. For low-titer inhibitors, options include continuous factor VIII infusions or administration of porcine factor VIII. For high-titer inhibitors, it usually is necessary to administer a product that bypasses the inhibitor, such as activated prothrombin complex concentrates or recombinant factor VIIa. The use of frequent high doses of prothrombin complex concentrates, and especially the activated products, paradoxically increases the risks of thrombosis, which has resulted in fatal complications like myocardial infarction. Induction of immune tolerance with continuous antigen exposure plus immunosuppression may be beneficial.

Table 14–17. Comparison of Hemophilia A, Hemophilia B, and von Willebrand Disease

	Hemophilia A	Hemophilia B	von Willebrand disease
Inheritance	X-linked	X-linked	Autosomal dominant
Factor deficiency	Factor VIII	Factor IX	von Willebrand factor and VIIIC
Bleeding site(s)	Muscle, joint, surgical	Muscle, joint, surgical	Mucous membranes, skin, surgical, menstrual
Prothrombin time (PT)	Normal	Normal	Normal
Partial thromboplastin time (APTT)	Prolonged	Prolonged	Prolonged or normal
Bleeding time	Normal	Normal	Prolonged or normal
Factor VIII coagulant activity (VIIIC)	Low	Normal	Low or normal
von Willebrand factor antigen (vWF:Ag)	Normal	Normal	Low
von Willebrand factor activity (vWF:Act)	Normal	Normal	Low
Factor IX	Normal	Low	Normal
Ristocetin-induced platelet agglutination	Normal	Normal	Normal or low
Platelet aggregation	Normal	Normal	Normal

von Willebrand Disease

This common disorder is caused by a deficiency of von Willebrand factor (vWF), an adhesive protein that serves two functions: to bridge between subendothelial collagen and platelets, and, circulating in conjunction with factor VIII, to protect factor VIII from rapid clearance from circulation. von Willebrand disease usually is inherited as an autosomal dominant trait and rarely as an autosomal recessive trait. vWF is either quantitatively deficient (partial or absolute) or quantitatively abnormal (dysproteinemia).

The *clinical manifestations* of von Willebrand disease include mucocutaneous bleeding, epistaxis, gingival bleeding, cutaneous bruising, and menorrhagia. In severe von Willebrand disease, factor VIII deficiency may be profound and the patient also may have manifestations similar to hemophilia A (e.g., hemarthrosis).

Approximately 80% of patients with von Willebrand disease have classic (type I) disease (i.e., a mild to moderate deficiency of vWF). There are several other clinically important subtypes each of which requires somewhat different therapy. vWF testing requires measurement of the amount of protein, usually done immunologically as the von Willebrand factor antigen (vWF:ag). von Willebrand factor activity (vWF:Act) is measured functionally in the ristocetin cofactor assay (vWFR:Co)

that utilizes the antibiotic ristocetin to induce vWF to bind to platelets. In Table 14–17, the findings in classic von Willebrand disease are compared with those in hemophilia A and B.

The *treatment* of von Willebrand disease depends on the severity of the bleeding. DDAVP is the treatment of choice for the majority of bleeding episodes in patients with type I disease and some patients with type II disease. When high levels of vWF are needed and the patient cannot be satisfactorily treated with DDAVP, treatment with a virally attenuated vWF-containing concentrate (e.g., Humate P) may be appropriate, and the dosage can be calculated as for factor VIII in hemophilia. Cryoprecipitate also may be used; however, cryoprecipitate cannot be virally attenuated. Hepatitis B vaccine should be given prior to exposure to plasma-derived products. As in all bleeding disorders, aspirin should be avoided for patients with von Willebrand disease.

VITAMIN K DEFICIENCY

See Chapters 2 and 6.

DISSEMINATED INTRAVASCULAR COAGULATION

DIC refers to a disorder in which a severely ill patient sustains widespread activation of the coag-

Table 14–18. Conditions Associated with Disseminated Intravascular Coagulation

Acute	Chronic
Sepsis	Polycythemia
Congenital infection	Hemangioma
Asphyxia–hypoxia	Arteriovenous
Trauma	malformation
Shock	Retained dead fetus
Burns	Malignancy
Heat stroke	Pre-eclampsia
Snake bites	Malignant hypertension
Transfusion reactions	Cirrhosis
Promyelocytic leukemia	Renal vein thrombosis
Respiratory distress syndrome	
Adult respiratory distress syndrome	
Hepatitis/hepatic failure	

ulation mechanism usually associated with shock. Bleeding or clotting manifestations may be present. Normal hemostasis is a balance between hemorrhage and thrombosis. In DIC, this balance is altered by the severe illness so that the patient has activation of both coagulation (thrombin) and fibrinolysis (plasmin). Coagulation factors, especially platelets, fibrinogen, and factors II, V, and VIII, are consumed, as are the anticoagulant proteins, especially antithrombin III, protein C, and plasminogen. Endothelial injury, tissue release of thromboplastic procoagulant factors, or, rarely, exogenous factors (e.g., snake venoms) directly activate the coagulation mechanism (Table 14–18).

The *diagnosis* of DIC is a clinical one sustained by laboratory findings (Table 14–19). In some patients, the DIC may evolve more slowly and there may be a degree of compensation. In an acutely ill patient, the sudden occurrence of bleeding from a venipuncture or incision site, gastrointestinal or pulmonary hemorrhage, petechiae, ecchymosis, and/or evidence of peripheral gangrene or thrombosis suggests the diagnosis of DIC.

The *treatment* of DIC is problematic. The disorder inducing the DIC should be treated effectively and hypoxia, acidosis, and poor perfusion should be

Table 14–19. Laboratory Evidence of DIC

Prolonged prothrombin, partial thromboplastin, and thrombin times
Thrombocytopenia
Low fibrinogen, factors V and VIII
Elevated fibrin degradation (split) products and D-dimers
Microangiopathic RBC morphology

RBC = red blood cell.

corrected. Depleted blood clotting factors, platelets, and anticoagulant proteins then should be replaced. Heparin may be useful in the presence of significant arterial or venous thrombotic disease unless sites of life-threatening bleeding coexist. In addition, heparin may be useful for the treatment of DIC induced by meningococcemia, purpura fulminans, or acute promyelocytic leukemia.

THROMBOSIS

Deficiencies of the anticoagulant proteins, especially protein C, protein S, and antithrombin III (AT-III), are the most common causes of an inherited predisposition to thrombosis. Their functions are outlined in Figure 14–8. Deficiency syndromes may present in neonates, especially homozygous protein C deficiency, which presents with purpura fulminans or arterial thrombosis in the major vessels and requires plasma replacement therapy. Patients with heterozygous deficiencies of anticoagulant proteins usually present in adolescence or early adulthood. Protein C deficiency that presents in adulthood usually is inherited as an autosomal

Table 14–20. Hypercoagulable States

Primary Disorders
Antithrombin III deficiency
Protein C deficiency
Protein S deficiency
Dysfibrinogenemia
Plasminogen deficiencies

Secondary Disorders
Coagulopathies
  Nephrotic syndrome
  Oral contraceptives (estrogen)
  Malignancy
  Therapy with activated prothrombin complex concentrates
  Pregnancy
  Lupus anticoagulant (antiphospholipid antibody)

Platelet Disorders
  Diabetes mellitus
  Myeloproliferative disorders
  Thrombocytosis
  Paroxysmal nocturnal hemoglobinuria

Flow and Vessel Disorders
  Polycythemia–hyperviscosity
  Homocystinuria
  Marfan syndrome
  Vasculitis
  Vessel grafts
  Vascular stasis

(Adapted from Schafer A: The hypercoagulable states. Ann Intern Med 102:814, 1985.)

Table 14–21. Evaluation of Transfusion Reactions

Type of Reaction	Clinical Signs	Management of Problems
Major hemolytic (1:100,000) (incompatibility)	Acute shock, back pain, flushing, early fever, intravascular hemolysis, hemoglobinemia, hemoglobinuria; may be delayed 5–10 days if anamnestic response is present	1. Stop transfusion; return blood to bank with fresh sample of patient's blood 2. Hydrate IV; support BP, maintain high urine flow, alkalinize urine 3. Check for hemoglobinemia, hemoglobinuria, hyperkalemia 4. Jaundice, anemia if delayed
Febrile (1:100)	Fever at end of transfusion, urticaria (usually due to sensitization to WBC HLA antigens), chills	Pretreat with hydrocortisone, antipyretics, Benadryl or all three; use buffy coat–poor RBC, washed RBC, filtered or frozen RBC
Allergic	Fever, urticaria, anaphylactoid reaction (often due to sensitivity to donor plasma proteins)	Benadryl, hydrocortisone; use washed RBC or frozen RBC

BP = blood pressure; RBC = red blood cells.
(Adapted from Andreoli TE, Carpenter CCJ, Plum F, et al: Cecil Essentials of Medicine. Philadelphia, WB Saunders, 1993, p 377.)

dominant trait, whereas the homozygous form usually is autosomal recessive. Protein S and AT-III deficiencies are inherited as autosomal dominant traits. Acquired antiphospholipid antibodies (anticardiolipin, lupus anticoagulant) also produce thrombosis.

Clinical manifestations of thromboembolic disease in pediatrics occur most frequently in neonates or in adolescents. Indwelling catheters, vasculitis, sepsis, immobilization, nephrotic syndrome, coagulopathy, trauma, infection, surgery, inflammatory bowel disease, oral contraceptive agents, pregnancy, and abortion all predispose to thrombosis (Table 14–20). The diagnosis of venous thrombosis can be made noninvasively by Doppler flow compression studies or plethysmography; however, the gold standard remains the venogram. The manifestations of pulmonary emboli may be highly variable, including sudden chest pain, diminished breath sounds, increased pulmonic 2nd heart sound, cyanosis, tachypnea, and hypoxemia or minimal or no findings. An abnormal opacity on chest roentgenogram (the roentgenogram also may be normal) and an abnormal ventilation–perfusion scan are frequent findings.

Treatment of thrombotic disorders depends on the underlying condition and usually includes heparin and then longer term anticoagulation with coumarin. Major vessel thrombosis or life-threatening thrombosis may require treatment with fibrinolytic agents (e.g., streptokinase, urokinase, or tissue plasminogen activator). Inherited deficiency syndromes may present as emergencies and require plasma, AT-III concentrates, and protein C concentrates. Protein C, protein S, and AT-III deficient patients are usually chronically anticoagulated with coumarin.

Blood Component Therapy

Transfusion of red blood cells, granulocytes, platelets, and coagulation factors can be lifesaving or life maintaining. Whole blood is indicated only when acute hypovolemia and reduced oxygen-carrying capacity are present. Otherwise, packed red blood cells are indicated to treat anemia to increase oxygen carrying capacity. Blood cell transfusions should not be used to treat asymptomatic nutritional deficiencies that can be corrected by administering the appropriate deficient nutrient (e.g., iron, folic acid). Blood component therapy requires proper anticoagulation of the blood, screening for a variety of infectious agents, and blood group compatibility testing prior to administration. Typical transfusion reactions are listed in Table 14–21. Long-term complications of transfusions include iron overload, alloimmunization to red and white blood cells or platelets and plasma proteins (1:100), graft-versus-host disease, and infectious diseases (hepatitis [1:250], HIV [<1:250,000] malaria, syphilis, babesiosis, brucellosis, Chagas disease). Transfusional therapy also may result in circulatory overload, especially in the presence of chronic cardiopulmonary deficiency.

References

Behrman RE (ed): Nelson Textbook of Pediatrics. 14th ed. Philadelphia, WB Saunders, 1992, Sec. 16.65–16.89.

Bussel JB: Autoimmune thrombocytopenic purpura. Hematol Oncol Clin North Am 4:179, 1990.

Dubansky AS, Boyett JM, Falletta J, et al: Isolated thrombocytopenia in children with acute lymphoblastic leukemia: A rare event in a pediatric oncology group study. Pediatrics 84:1068, 1989.

Eden OB, Lilleyman JS: Guidelines for management of idiopathic thrombocytopenic purpura. Arch Dis Child 67:1056, 1992.

Goldhaber SZ, Morpurgo M: Diagnosis, treatment, and prevention of pulmonary embolism: Report of the WHO/International Society and Federation of Cardiology Task Force. JAMA 268:1727, 1992.

Halperin D, Doyle JJ: Is bone marrow examination justified in idiopathic thrombocytopenic purpura? Am J Dis Child 142:508, 1988.

Jones PK, Ratnoff OD: The changing prognosis of classic hemophilia (factor VIII "deficiency"). Ann Intern Med 114:641, 1991.

Katsanis E, Luke K-H, Hsu E, et al: Prevalence and significance of mild bleeding disorders in children with recurrent epistaxis. J Pediatr 113:73, 1988.

Lockshin MD: Antiphospholipid antibody syndrome. JAMA 268:1451, 1992.

Mannucci PM: Desmopressin: A non-transfusional form of treatment for congenital and acquired bleeding disorders. Blood 72:1449, 1988.

Schwartz RS, Abildgaard CF, Aledort LM, et al: Human recombinant DNA-derived antihemophilic factor (factor VIII) in the treatment of hemophilia A. N Engl J Med 323:1800, 1990.

Werner EJ, Abshire TC, Giroux DS, et al: Relative value of diagnostic studies for von Willebrand disease. J Pediatr 121:34, 1992.

Oncology

15

Herbert T. Abelson

Childhood cancers represent a group of approximately a dozen common malignancies, each with a distinct epidemiology, pathology, and mortality rate. Malignancy is the most common disease causing death among children between 1 and 16 yr of age; of the approximately 1 million new cases of cancer in the United States each year (exclusive of carcinoma in situ and nonmelanoma skin cancer), 6000–7000 (less than 1%) occur in children. A coordinated multidisciplinary team effort is needed for detecting and managing childhood malignancies. This often is provided in specialized pediatric cancer centers by staff that include oncologists, surgeons, radiotherapists, chemotherapists, psychologists, social workers, epidemiologists, and oncology nurses.

GENERAL CONSIDERATIONS

Epidemiology

The types of childhood cancers tend to differ more than those that occur in adults. Adults characteristically develop cancer of solid organs, such as the lung, the colon, the breast, and the genitourinary system. However, leukemia and brain tumors are the predominant malignancies among children (Table 15–1). The annual incidence of all cancers among white children is approximately 12:100,000, whereas the incidence is 9:100,000 among black children. The incidence of cancer is slightly increased among boys compared with girls, with an overall sex ratio of 1.2:1. However, for lymphoma the incidence is higher in boys by 2:1. Leukemia and various embryonal tumors, such as neuroblastoma, Wilms tumor, retinoblastoma, and hepatic tumors, are more common in infancy and early childhood; Hodgkin disease, gonadal malignancy, and bone tumors are seen more commonly during adolescence. It is rare for a newborn infant to have a malignancy; neuroblastoma, congenital leukemia, mesoblastic nephroma, teratoma (sacrococcygeal, mediastinal, gonadal), and the potentially large but nonmalignant lymphangioma or hemangioma (cutaneous, hepatic) are the predominant neonatal neoplasms. Metastasis of malignant disease from the mother to the fetus is very rare and, when present, occurs most often from maternal malignant melanoma.

Most of the common childhood cancers occur sporadically and only rarely are associated with increased host susceptibility resulting from predisposing environmental (Table 15–2) or familial factors (Table 15–3). Nonetheless, environmental risks, single gene or gross chromosomal defects, neurocutaneous or immunodeficiency syndromes, and familial or hereditary conditions associated with malignancy are important disorders to identify among pediatric patients because careful screening, examination, and counseling can detect early signs of cancer and improve the chance for successful treatment.

Etiology

Cancer begins with the onset of unregulated, often rapid growth and proliferation of usually a single somatic cell. One theory of carcinogenesis,

Table 15–1. Common Childhood Malignancies

	Percentage of Total Malignancies	
	White Children	*Black Children*
Leukemia	34	25
CNS tumors*	19	24
Lymphoma	11	14
Neuroblastoma	8	7
Sarcoma†	7	4
Wilms tumor	6	8
Bone tumors‡	4	5
Retinoblastoma	3	3
Other tumors§	8	10

* Cerebellar astrocytoma, glioblastoma, medulloblastoma, brain stem glioma.

† Rhabdomyosarcoma (embryonal, botryoid, alveolar), fibrosarcoma.

‡ Osteosarcoma, Ewing sarcoma.

§ Hepatic, ovarian, testicular, endocrine, melanoma, teratoma.

Table 15–2. Environmental Causes of Cancer

Etiology	Cancer
Physical Agents	
Ionizing radiation	Leukemia, thyroid, breast
Ultraviolet irradiation	Melanoma, basal and squamous cell in xeroderma pigmentosum
Chemical Agents	
Cigarette, tobacco	Lung, oropharynx, larynx
Diethylstilbestrol	Vaginal carcinoma
Asbestos	Mesothelioma
Androgens	Hepatoma
Alkylating agents	Leukemia
Immunosuppressant drugs	Lymphoma
Aflatoxin	Hepatic carcinoma
Vinyl chloride	Hepatic angiosarcoma
Phenytoin	Lymphoma
Cyclophosphamide	Bladder cancer
Alcohol (fetal alcohol syndrome)	Neuroblastoma
Benzene	Leukemia
Microbiologic Agents	
Hepatitis B, C viruses	Hepatic carcinoma
Human immunodeficiency virus	Kaposi sarcoma, lymphoma
Schistosoma haematobium	Bladder carcinoma
Epstein-Barr virus	African Burkitt lymphoma, X-linked immunodeficiency–associated lymphoma, nasopharyngeal carcinoma
Papillomavirus	Cervical cancer
Human T lymphotropic virus I	T cell lymphoma
SV40 virus	Possible ependymoma, choroid plexus tumor

the clonal initiation of malignancy, proposes that the genetic regulation of growth of a single precursor cell becomes abnormal and results in autonomous, uncontrolled proliferation of the transformed cell line. Alternatively, a "two-hit" theory (Knudson hypothesis) has been postulated for initiating the malignant process in many cancers. For example, in familial retinoblastoma, a mutation of one gene in the germ cell line occurs. A subsequent second "hit" in the somatic cell line results in the mutation of the other retinoblastoma gene on the second chromosome. This double-gene mutation produces neoplastic transformation of retinal cells. The second "hit" may be a carcinogen or spontaneous DNA recombination events in the somatic cell during mitosis. There is probably a sequence of multiple steps needed in the initiation and progression of malignant cell transformation. Unidentified carcinogenic factors, in the presence of unknown genetic susceptibility and a cellular environment favorable to carcinogenesis, may initiate tumor growth in the presence or absence of identifiable extrinsic (Table 15–2) or familial (Table 15–3) factors.

Human cellular genes that may regulate normal cell growth and that are homologous to the genetic material of transforming RNA tumor viruses are called *proto-oncogenes*. Mutagenesis may be initiated by incorporation of the retroviral genome into host DNA (insertional mutagenesis), but more likely tumorigenesis results from unregulated activation of the related endogenous *oncogene* (activated proto-oncogene) present in the host genome. A somatic mutation near a proto-oncogene may cause its uncontrolled expression and amplification as an activated oncogene, which results in neoplastic growth. Alternately, a mutation involving the expression of antioncogenes or tumor suppressor genes may result in loss of inhibition of an oncogene. Chromosome translocation provides another mechanism for tumorigenesis because it may move one gene from its normal position to an abnormal unregulated site, resulting in uncontrolled cell growth. For example, in Burkitt lymphoma, a break point at the site of the c-myc oncogene occurs, with a translocation between chromosome 8 and the immunoglobulin genes on either chromosome 2, 14, or 22. The c-myc oncogene is now next to the immunoglobulin gene. The end result is B cell–malignant transformation. Familial retinoblastoma is associated with an inherited mutation or deletion of a tumor suppressor gene on one of the pairs of chromosome 13. Subsequently, somatic inactivation of the allele (RB gene) on the other chromosome pair results in carcinogenesis.

During carcinogenesis, the oncogene controls the synthesis of various protein products that contribute to the malignant alteration of the cell. Oncogene products may be proteins that are similar to various growth factors, growth factor receptors, or enzymes that activate these receptors. The end result may be a perpetual signal to the cell to transform and proliferate in the absence of the true growth factor.

Other virus-induced tumors have been associ-

Table 15–3. Familial or Genetic Susceptibility to Malignancy

Disorder	Tumor/Cancer	Comment
Chromosomal Syndromes		
Chromosome 11p − (deletion) with sporadic aniridia	Wilms tumor	Associated with genitourinary anomalies, mental retardation
Chromosome 13q − (deletion)	Retinoblastoma	Associated with mental retardation, skeletal malformations: autosomal dominant (bilateral) or sporadic new mutation
Trisomy 21	Lymphocytic or nonlymphocytic leukemia	Risk is 15 times normal
Klinefelter syndrome (47, XXY)	Breast cancer	
Gonadal dysgenesis XO/XY	Gonadoblastoma	Gonads must be removed; 25% chance of gonadal malignancy
DNA Fragility		
Xeroderma pigmentosum	Basal, squamous cell skin cancers	Autosomal recessive; failure to repair solar-damaged DNA
Fanconi anemia	Leukemia	Autosomal recessive; 10% risk for AML; chromosome fragility, positive diepoxybutane test
Bloom syndrome	Leukemia, lymphoma	Autosomal recessive; chromosome fragility; high risk for malignancy
Ataxia–telangiectasia	Lymphoma, leukemia	Autosomal recessive; sensitive to X-radiation, radiomimetic drugs; chromosome fragility
Dysplastic nevus syndrome	Melanoma	Autosomal dominant
Immunodeficiency Syndromes		
Wiskott-Aldrich syndrome	Lymphoma	Immunodefiency; X-linked recessive
X-linked immunodeficiency (Duncan syndrome)	Lymphoma	Epstein-Barr virus is inciting agent
Severe combined immunodeficiency	Leukemia, lymphoma	Immunodeficiency; x-linked recessive
Others		
Neurofibromatosis	Neurofibroma, optic glioma, acoustic neuroma, astrocytoma, meningioma, pheochromocytoma	Autosomal dominant
Tuberous sclerosis	Fibroangiomatous nevi, myocardial rhabdomyoma	Autosomal dominant
Retinoblastoma	Sarcoma	Increased risk of secondary malignancy 10–20 years later
Familial adenomatous polyposis coli	Adenocarcinoma of colon	Autosomal dominant
Gardner syndrome	Adenocarcinoma of colon; skull and soft tissue tumors	Autosomal dominant
Peutz-Jeghers syndrome	Gastrointestinal carcinoma	Autosomal dominant
Hemihypertrophy ± Beckwith syndrome	Wilms tumor, hepatoblastoma, adrenal carcinoma	25% develop tumor, most in first 5 yr of life
Tyrosinemia galactosemia	Hepatic carcinoma	Nodular cirrhosis; autosomal recessive
Multiple endocrine neoplasia (MEN) syndrome I (Wermer syndrome)	Parathyroid adenoma, pancreatic islet tumor, pituitary adenoma carcinoid	Autosomal dominant; Zollinger-Ellison syndrome
Multiple endocrine neoplasia syndrome II (Sipple syndrome)	Medullary carcinoma of the thyroid, hyperparathyroidism, pheochromocytoma	Autosomal dominant; monitor calcitonin and calcium levels
Multiple endocrine neoplasia III (multiple mucosal neuroma syndrome)	Mucosal neuroma, pheochromocytoma, medullary thyroid carcinoma; Marfan habitus; neuropathy	Autosomal dominant
von Hippel-Lindau disease	Hemangioblastoma of the cerebellum and retina, pheochromocytoma	Autosomal dominant; mutation of tumor suppressor gene
Cancer family syndrome	Colonic, uterine carcinoma	Autosomal dominant
Li-Fraumeni syndrome	Bone, soft tissue sarcoma, breast	Possible mutation of p53 tumor suppressor gene

ated with DNA viruses, such as Epstein-Barr virus, papillomavirus, and hepatitis B virus. The mechanism of action of these viruses may include insertional mutagenesis, point mutation, and oncogene activation. Viral DNA has been recovered in the transformed cells from tumors produced by Epstein-Barr virus (Burkitt lymphoma, nasopharyngeal carcinoma), papillomavirus (cancer of the cervix), and hepatitis B virus (hepatocellular carcinoma).

Clinical Manifestations and Diagnosis

Malignancy may produce nonspecific systemic effects, such as anorexia, weight loss, malnutrition, or fever. Specific manifestations of various malignancies include hematologic, systemic, intracranial, or ocular signs and symptoms (Table 15–4). These manifestations may be a direct effect of local tumor extension (pain, obstruction, pressure) or the results of metastasis. Alternately, tumor products may produce neuroendocrine effects such as

Table 15–4. Common Manifestations of Childhood Malignancy

Sign/Symptom	Significance	Example
Hematologic		
Pallor, anemia	Bone marrow infiltration	Leukemia, neuroblastoma
Petechiae, thrombocytopenia	Bone marrow infiltration	Leukemia, neuroblastoma
Fever, pharyngitis, neutropenia	Bone marrow infiltration	Leukemia, neuroblastoma
Systemic		
Bone pain, limp, arthralgia	Primary bone tumor, metastasis to bone	Osteosarcoma, Ewing sarcoma, leukemia, neuroblastoma
Fever of unknown origin, weight loss, night sweats	Lymphoreticular malignancy	Hodgkin disease, non-Hodgkin lymphoma
Painless lymphadenopathy	Lymphoreticular malignancy	Leukemia, Hodgkin disease, non-Hodgkin lymphoma, Burkitt lymphoma
Cutaneous lesion	Primary or metastatic disease	Neuroblastoma, leukemia, histiocytosis X, melanoma
Abdominal mass	Adrenal–renal tumor	Neuroblastoma, Wilms tumor
Hypertension	Sympathetic nervous system tumor	Neuroblastoma, pheochromocytoma, Wilms tumor
Diarrhea	Vasoactive intestinal polypeptide (VIP)	Neuroblastoma, ganglioneuroma
Soft tissue mass	Local or metastatic tumor	Ewing sarcoma, osteosarcoma, neuroblastoma, rhabdomyosarcoma, eosinophilic granuloma Askin tumor
Emesis, visual disturbances, ataxia, headache, papilledema	Increased intracranial pressure	Primary brain tumor; metastasis
Ophthalmologic Signs		
Leukokoria	White pupil	Retinoblastoma
Periorbital ecchymosis	Metastasis	Neuroblastoma
Miosis, ptosis, heterochromia	Horner syndrome: compression of cervical sympathetic nerves	Neuroblastoma
Opsoclonus/ataxia	Neurotransmitters? Autoimmunity?	Neuroblastoma
Exophthalmos, proptosis	Orbital tumor	Rhabdomyosarcoma
Thoracic Mass		
Anterior mediastinal	Cough, stridor, pneumonia, tracheal–bronchial compression	Thymoma, teratoma, T cell lymphoma, thyroid
Posterior mediastinal	Vertebral or nerve root compression; dysphagia	Neuroblastoma, neuroenteric cyst

Table 15–5. Cancer Chemotherapy

Drug*	Action	Metabolism	Excretion	Indication	Toxicity
Antimetabolites					
Methotrexate	Folic acid antagonist; inhibits dihydrofolate reductase	Hepatic	Renal, 50–90% excreted unchanged; biliary	ALL, lymphoma, medulloblastoma, osteosarcoma	Myelosuppression (nadir 7–10 days), mucositis, stomatitis, dermatitis, hepatitis; renal and CNS with high-dose administration; prevent with leucovorin, monitor levels
6-Mercaptopurine	Purine analogue	Hepatic; allopurinol inhibits metabolism	Renal	ALL	Myelosuppression; hepatic necrosis; mucositis; allopurinal increases toxicity
Cytosine arabinoside (Ara-C)	Pyrimidine analogue; inhibits DNA polymerase	Hepatic	Renal	ALL, lymphoma	Myelosuppression, conjunctivitis, mucositis, CNS dysfunction
Alkylating Agents					
Cyclophosphamide (Cytoxan)	Alkylates guanine; inhibits DNA synthesis	Hepatic	Renal	ALL, lymphoma, sarcoma	Myelosuppression; hemorrhagic cystitis; pulmonary fibrosis, inappropriate ADH secretion, bladder cancer, anaphylaxis
Ifosfamide	Similar to Cytoxan	Hepatic	Renal	Lymphoma, Wilms tumor, sarcoma, germ cell and testicular tumors	Similar to Cytoxan; CNS dysfunction, cardiac toxicity
Antibiotics					
Doxorubicin (Adriamycin) and Daunorubicin (Cerubidine)	Binds to DNA, intercalation	Hepatic	Biliary, renal	ALL, AML, osteosarcoma, Ewing sarcoma, lymphoma, neuroblastoma	Cardiomyopathy, red urine, tissue necrosis on extravasation, myelosuppression, conjunctivitis, radiation dermatitis, arrhythmia
Dactinomycin (Actinomycin-D)	Binds to DNA, inhibits transcription	—	Renal, stool, 30% excreted unchanged drug	Wilms tumor, rhabdomyosarcoma, Ewing sarcoma	Tissue necrosis on extravasation, myelosuppression, radiosensitizer
Bleomycin	Binds to DNA, cuts DNA	Hepatic	Renal	Hodgkin disease, lymphoma, germ cell tumors	Pneumonitis, stomatitis, Raynaud phenomenon, pulmonary fibrosis, dermatitis
Vinca Alkaloids					
Vincristine (Oncovin)	Inhibits microtubule formation	Hepatic	Biliary	ALL, lymphoma, Wilms tumor, Hodgkin disease, Ewing sarcoma, neuroblastoma, rhabdomyosarcoma	Local cellulitis, peripheral neuropathy, constipation, ileus, jaw pain, inappropriate ADH secretion, seizures, ptosis, minimal myelosuppression
Vinblastine (Velban)	Inhibits microtubule formation	Hepatic	Biliary	Hodgkin disease; Langerhans cell histiocytosis	Local cellulitis, leukopenia
Enzymes					
L-Asparaginase	Depletion of L-asparagine	—	Reticuloendo-thelial system	ALL	Allergic reaction; Pancreatitis, hyperglycemia, platelet dysfunction and coagulopathy, encephalopathy
Hormones					
Prednisone	Unknown; lymphocyte modification?	Hepatic	Renal	ALL; Hodgkin disease, lymphoma	Cushing syndrome, cataracts, diabetes, hypertension, myopathy, osteoporosis, infection, peptic ulceration, psychosis

Continued

Table 15–5. *Continued*

Drug*	Action	Metabolism	Excretion	Indication	Toxicity
Miscellaneous					
BCNU (carmustine, nitrosourea)	Carbamylation of DNA; inhibits DNA synthesis	Hepatic; phenobarbitol increases metabolism, decreases activity	Renal	CNS tumors, lymphoma, Hodgkin disease	Delayed myelosuppression (4–6 wk); pulmonary fibrosis, carcinogenic, stomatitis
Cis-platinum	Inhibits DNA synthesis	—	Renal	Gonadal tumors; osteosarcoma, neuroblastoma, CNS tumors, germ cell tumors	Nephrotoxic; myelosuppression, ototoxicity, tetany, neurotoxicity, hemolytic–uremic syndrome; aminoglycosides may increase nephrotoxicity, anaphylaxis
Etoposide (VP–16)	Topoisomerase inhibitor	—	Renal	ALL, lymphoma, germ cell tumor	Myelosuppression, secondary leukemia
Etretinate (vitamin A analogue) and Tretinoin	Enhances normal differentiation	Liver	Liver	Some leukemias; neuroblastoma	Dry mouth, hair loss, pseudo tumor cerebri, premature epiphyseal closure

* Many drugs produce nausea and vomiting during administration, and many cause alopecia with repeated doses.
ADH = antidiuretic hormone; ALL = acute lymphocytic leukemia; AML = acute myelogenous leukemia; CNS = central nervous system.
(Data from Med Lett 35:43, 1993; W. Archie Bleyer: Cancer chemotherapy in infants and children In Altman AJ (ed): Pediatric oncology. Pediatr Clin Norh Am 32:557, 1985.)

hypertension (neuroblastoma, pheochromocytoma), diarrhea (vasoactive intestinal polypeptide, pancreatic tumor), hypoglycemia (islet cell adenoma), or Cushing syndrome (adrenal, lung, pituitary tumors). Signs and symptoms of malignancy may be confused with less severe diseases so that, for example, nasal infections may be confused with nasopharyngeal cancer, lymphadenopathy with lymphoma, anemia or idiopathic thrombocytopenic purpura with leukemia, and diarrhea with neuroblastoma. Leg pain and limp associated with trauma in the athletic adolescent are common manifestations of osteosarcoma and Ewing sarcoma.

Persistent localized pain, unexplained fever, persistent lymph node swelling, signs of increased intracranial pressure, and soft tissue mass warrant evaluation for suspected malignancy. For most childhood cancers, a tissue biopsy is needed to confirm the diagnosis. This biopsy may include a bone marrow examination for leukemia, malignant histiocytosis, metastatic neuroblastoma, and lymphoma. Tissue obtained at the time of operative resection or during a more limited incisional biopsy of a solid tumor must be classified by histologic type and by the extent to which the tumor mass has invaded adjacent tissue. After identifying the tumor type, staging the tumor and determining metastatic foci are both critical diagnostic principles that will guide the therapeutic approach.

Principles of Cancer Treatment

The choice of cancer therapy is based on the type, stage, and extent of spread of the malignancy. The goal may be curative, palliative, or supportive, but it always involves specific anticancer modalities plus supportive care. Anticancer modalities include surgical excision, radiation therapy, chemotherapy (Table 15–5), or a combination of these three modalities.

Adjuvant chemotherapy is an appropriate therapeutic strategy for many solid tumors and for micrometastatic disease. Immunotherapy (interleukins, lymphokine-activated killer cells, radiolabeled antibodies) has not yet achieved wide clinical applicability. Bone marrow transplantation (permitting high dose anticancer therapy) has become the treatment of choice for children with acute myelogenous leukemia in first remission, juvenile chronic myelogenous leukemia, and adult-type chronic myelogenous leukemia in chronic phase. Supportive care includes treatment of malignancy- and therapy-induced emergencies (Table 15–6) and infectious complications (Table 15–7), as well as appropriate pain and symptom control.

Tumor growth is governed by the typical cell cycle of normal tissues: phases M, G1, S, and G2. M is cell division; G1 is normal cell metabolism with protein and RNA synthesis; G0 is a spinoff of the G1 phase and refers to irreversible differentiation. DNA synthesis and chromosome replication occur in the S phase, whereas G2 is the preparative phase for the next cell division in M phase. At any given time, cancer cells in a particular malignancy are usually in different cell phases. Most drugs will affect a particular cell phase, usually the S phase. Some drugs affect the cell cycle of tumor cells to a greater extent than the cycle of normal cells. Resistance to the effects of cancer chemotherapy may be due to the malignant cells' being out of phase (not

Table 15–6. Oncologic Emergencies

Condition	Manifestations	Etiology	Malignancy	Treatment
Metabolic				
Hyperuricemia	Uric acid nephropathy, gout	Tumor lysis syndrome	Lymphoma, leukemia	Allopurinol; alkalinize urine; hydration and diuresis
Hyperkalemia	Arrhythmias, cardiac arrest	Tumor lysis syndrome	Lymphoma, leukemia	Kayexalate; sodium bicarbonate, glucose and insulin; check for pseudohyperkalemia from leukemic cell lysis in test tube
Hyperphosphatemia	Hypocalcemic tetany; metastatic calcification, photophobia, pruritus	Tumor lysis syndrome	Lymphoma, leukemia	Hydration, forced diuresis; stop alkalinization; oral aluminum hydroxide to bind phosphate
Hyponatremia	Seizure, lethargy; asymptomatic	Syndrome of inappropriate ADH secretion (SIADH); fluid, sodium losses in vomiting, diarrhea, diuresis	Leukemia; CNS tumor	Restrict free water for SIADH; replace sodium if depleted
Hypercalcemia	Anorexia, nausea, polyuria, pancreatitis, gastric ulcers; prolonged PR, shortened QT interval	Bone resorption; ectopic parathormone, vitamin D, or prostaglandins	Hodgkin disease; metastasis to bone	Hydration and furosemide diuresis; corticosteroids; mithramycin; calcitonin; diphosphonates
Hematologic				
Anemia	Pallor, weakness, heart failure	Bone marrow suppression or infiltration; blood loss	Any with chemotherapy	Packed red blood cell transfusion
Thrombocytopenia	Petechiae, hemorrhage	Bone marrow suppression or infiltration	Any with chemotherapy	Platelet transfusion
Disseminated intravascular coagulation	Shock, hemorrhage	Sepsis, hypotension tumor factors	Promyelocytic leukemia; others	Fresh frozen plasma; platelets, correct infection, etc
Neutropenia	Infection	Bone marrow suppression or infiltration	Any with chemotherapy	If febrile, give broad-spectrum antibiotics and G-CSF if appropriate
Hyperleukocytosis ($>50,000/mm^3$)	Hemorrhage, thrombosis; pulmonary infiltrates, hypoxia; tumor lysis syndrome	Leukostasis; vascular occlusion	Leukemia	Leukapheresis; chemotherapy
Graft-versus-host disease	Dermatitis, diarrhea, hepatitis	Immunosuppression and nonirradiated blood products; bone marrow transplantation	Any with immunosuppression	Corticosteroids; cyclosporine; antithymocyte globulin
Space-Occupying Lesions				
Spinal cord compression	Back pain ± radicular. *Cord above T10:* Symmetric weakness, increased deep tendon reflex (DTR); sensory level present; toes up *Conus medullaris* (T10–L2): Symmetric weakness, increased knee reflexes, decreased ankle reflexes; saddle sensory loss; toes up or down *Cauda equina* (below L2): Asymmetric weakness, loss of DTR and sensory deficit; toes down	Metastasis to vertebra and extramedullary space	Neuroblastoma; medulloblastoma	Magnetic resonance imaging (MRI) or myelography for diagnosis; corticosteroids; radiotherapy; laminectomy; chemotherapy
Increased intracranial pressure	Confusion, coma, emesis, headache, hypertension, bradycardia, seizures, papilledema, hydrocephalus; III and VI nerve palsies	Primary or metastatic brain tumor	Neuroblastoma, astrocytoma; glioma	Computerized tomography or MRI for diagnosis; corticosteroids; phenytoin; ventricular–peritoneal shunt; radiotherapy; chemotherapy
Superior vena cava syndrome	Distended neck veins, plethora, edema of head and neck, cyanosis; proptosis; Horner syndrome	Superior mediastinal mass	Lymphoma	Chemotherapy; radiotherapy

ADH = antidiuretic hormone; G-CSF = granulocyte colony stimulation factor.

Table 15–7. Infectious Complications of Malignancy

Predisposing Factor	Etiology	Site of Infection	Infectious Agents
Neutropenia	Chemotherapy, bone marrow infiltration	Sepsis, shock, pneumonia, soft tissue, proctitis, mucositis	*Staphylococcus aureus, Staphylococcus epidermidis; Escherichia coli, Pseudomonas aeruginosa, Candida, Aspergillus;* anaerobic oral and rectal bacteria
Immunosuppression, lymphopenia, lymphocyte–monocyte dysfunction	Chemotherapy, prednisone	Pneumonia, meningitis, disseminated viral infection	*Pneumocystis carinii, Cryptococcus neoformans, Mycobacterium; Nocardia, Listeria monocytogenes, Candida, Aspergillus, Strongyloides; Toxoplasma, varicella-zoster,* cytomegalovirus, herpes simplex
Splenectomy	Staging of Hodgkin disease	Sepsis, shock, meningitis	Pneumococcus, *Haemophilus influenzae*
Indwelling central venous catheter	Nutrition, administration of chemotherapy	Line sepsis, tract or tunnel infection, exit site infection	*S. aureus, S. epidermidis, Candida albicans; P. aeruginosa; Aspergillus; Corynebacterium* JK, *Streptococcus faecalis, Mycobacterium fortuitum, Propionibacterium acnes*

(Data from Englehard D, Marks MI, Good RA: Infections in bone marrow transplant recipients. J Pediatr 108:335, 1986; Bodey GP: Infection in cancer patients–a continuing association. Am J Med 81 (suppl 1A): 11, 1986; Whimbey E, Kiehn TE, Brannon P, et al: Bacteremia and fungemia in patients with neoplastic disease. Am J Med 82:723, 1987; Pizzo PA: After empiric therapy: What to do until the granulocyte comes back. Rev Infect Dis 9:214, 1987; Johnson PR, Decker MD, Edwards KM, et al: Frequency of broviac catheter infections in pediatric oncology patients. J Infect Dis 154:570, 1986.)

synchronized) at the time of exposure to the particular chemotherapeutic agent; resistance to therapy also may be due to the presence of tumor cells in a sanctuary site, such as the brain or testis, which the drugs cannot enter. In addition, tumor cells may develop resistance to drugs by producing enzymes that inactivate the drugs or by creating transport barriers that prevent the penetration of the drug into the cell, or, in the case of P-glycoprotein expression (product of multidrug resistant gene MDR-1) a membrane pump decreases intracellular drug concentration by pumping drug out of the cell.

Resistance to treatment may be overcome by debulking the tumor mass and by bypassing sanctuary barriers (e.g., intrathecal administration of chemotherapeutic agents). Drug resistance also can be reduced by early treatment with multiple agents. The Goldie-Coldman model proposes use of as many drugs as available for the particular cancer at the highest possible doses to prevent cancer cell resistance. Combinations of various drugs acting at different intracellular targets, with treatment lasting for several years, may provide greater success without the emergence of resistant tumor cells.

Complications

Chemotherapeutic agents produce distinct manifestations of toxicity particularly associated with a specific drug (see Table 15–5) but also may produce complications typical of most antineoplastic agents, such as alopecia, bone marrow suppression, and immunosuppression. The latter two significant problems are responsible for the infectious complications of cancer therapy (Table 15–7). Late sequelae also occur in survivors of childhood cancer (Table 15–8). Some complications may be avoided by monitoring the blood level of drugs, by using leucovorin following methotrexate therapy, by using zoster immune globulin as a prophylactic agent when the patient is exposed to varicella, or by using trimethoprim–sulfamethoxazole as a prophylactic agent against *Pneumocystis carinii*. Over 50% of childhood malignancies may be cured with a minimum of long-term consequences.

LEUKEMIA

Each year, 2000–2500 new cases of childhood leukemia develop in the United States; about 40 children per million are affected under the age of 15 yr. Three quarters of these children will have acute lymphoblastic leukemia (ALL); 15–20%, acute myelogenous leukemia (AML); and the remainder, other forms of acute nonlymphocytic leukemia (ANLL) (Table 15–9).

Etiology and Epidemiology. The acute leukemias are heterogeneous diseases representing the malig-

Table 15–8. Long-Term Sequelae of Cancer Therapy

Problem	Etiology
Infertility	Alkylating agents; radiation
Second cancers	Genetic predisposition; radiation, alkylating agents
Sepsis	Splenectomy
Hepatotoxicity	Methotrexate, 6-mercaptopurine, radiation
Hepatic veno-occlusive disease	High-dose, intensive chemotherapy (busulfan, cyclophosphamide) ± bone marrow transplant
Scoliosis	Radiation
Pulmonary (pneumonia, fibrosis)	Radiation, bleomycin, busulfan
Myocardiopathy pericarditis	Adriamycin, daunomycin, radiation
Leukoencephalopathy	Cranial irradiation ± methotrexate
Cognition/intelligence	Cranial irradiation ± methotrexate
Pituitary dysfunction (isolated growth hormone deficiency, panhypopituitary)	Cranial irradiation
Psychosocial	Stress, anxiety, death of peers; conditioned responses to chemotherapy

nant transformation and clonal expansion of hematopoietic cells that are blocked at a particular stage of differentiation and unable to progress to more mature forms. Although much is known about the taxonomy of leukemia, the etiology remains elu-

Table 15–9. Acute Nonlymphocytic Leukemia Subtypes

	FAB Classification
Myeloblastic without maturation	M1
Myeloblastic with some maturation	M2
Hypergranular promyelocytic	M3
Myelomonocytic	M4
Monocytic	M5
Erythroleukemia	M6
Megakaryocytic	M7

sive. Epstein-Barr virus is associated with African Burkitt lymphoma, whereas a retrovirus, human T lymphotropic virus I, is associated with some cases of T cell leukemia in adults. Nonetheless, no specific agent(s) has been found for ALL or ANLL of childhood.

Certain groups of patients, however, are recognized as being at increased risk for developing leukemia. Those in the increased risk group include the identical twin of a leukemic patient under the age of 4 yr; children with trisomy 21, Fanconi anemia, Bloom syndrome, and ataxia–telangiectasia (see Table 15–3); and children exposed to radiation and some chemotherapeutic agents (see Table 15–2).

Clinical Manifestations. Leukemia can be quite varied in its presentation and may mimic other diseases. Most signs and symptoms are due to infiltration of leukemic cells, resulting in either bone marrow failure (anemia, neutropenia, thrombocytopenia) or specific tissue infiltration (lymph nodes, liver, spleen, brain, bone, skin, gingiva, testis) (see Table 15–4). Common presenting symptoms include fever, pallor (anemia), overt signs of bleeding such as petechiae or ecchymoses, lethargy, malaise, anorexia, and extremity or joint pain. In support of findings suggested by the history, physical examination frequently reveals lymphadenopathy and hepatosplenomegaly. At the time of diagnosis extramedullary involvement may be present—for example, central nervous system (CNS) involvement, which may result in diffuse or focal neurologic signs and symptoms, including headache, vomiting, papilledema, and VIth nerve palsy. In patients with AML, a soft tissue tumor may be found in the spinal cord or in other extramedullary sites. The presence of myeloperoxidase in these tumors may impart a greenish hue, and they are known as chloromas. The testicle is another common extramedullary site for ALL; it presents as a painless enlargement of one or both testes. The CNS and testes are referred to as "sanctuaries" because they are relatively impermeable to treatment with chemotherapeutic agents.

Diagnosis. Initial laboratory data provide a broad spectrum of abnormal findings in leukemia. Anemia, abnormal white blood cell and differential counts, and thrombocytopenia are the rule. A reactive eosinophilia may be present. As many as 10% of children with ALL may have normal routine blood counts at the time of diagnosis. Subtle changes may be present in the peripheral smear, however, that identify the underlying abnormality. There may be teardrop-shaped red blood cells, nucleated red blood cells, and immature myeloid forms, a constellation referred to as "leuko-erythroblastic" that strongly suggests leukemia, metastatic disease, myelofibrosis, or infection involving the bone marrow. The differential diagnosis of leukemia includes aplastic anemia, idiopathic thrombocytopenic purpura, other malignancies, collagen vascular or rheumatologic diseases, virus-induced or familial hemophagocytic syndromes, and Epstein-Barr virus infection.

When the total white blood cell count is less than 5000/mm^3, blast cells may not be seen in the peripheral blood, a fact that may delay diagnosis. When the white blood cell count is greater than 5000/mm^3, some leukemic blasts almost always are seen in the peripheral blood. It is critical to look at the bone marrow in every case, because the morphology of blasts in the peripheral blood may not reflect their bone marrow morphology, which is diagnostic. Electrolyte and other biochemical abnormalities, especially hyperuricemia, may be present at diagnosis or after the initiation of therapy (see Table 15–6). It is particularly important to treat existing hyperuricemia with allopurinol and to ensure adequate renal function prior to the onset of antileukemic therapy.

It is possible to recognize stages of human lymphocyte and granulocyte differentiation utilizing specific monoclonal antibodies to define cell surface antigens. When this application is combined with cytochemical histology, with molecular probes, and with morphology (traditional cell surface markers, such as surface membrane immunoglobulin [SmIg], cytoplasmic immunoglobin [CIg] on B lymphocytes, or sheep erythrocyte receptors on T lymphocytes), the diagnostic classification, treatment, and prognosis become more specific. Precisely diagnosing the type of leukemia is extremely important because it enables the physician to devise a specific therapy tailored to the particular phenotype (Table 15–10).

Structural abnormalities such as translocations (e.g., t(8;14)(q24;q23) associated with B-cell [SmIg$^+$] disease), and increased chromosome number or ploidy (e.g., hyperdiploidy in excess of 50 chromosomes), occur most often in CALLA$^+$ early B-cells.

Prognosis. Factors have been identified that have a bearing on the intensity of treatment and on the outcome of the disease (Table 15–11). "Standard risk" children have the most favorable prognosis and require less intensive therapy. Overall, the initial white blood cell count and age of the child are the most significant variables. Fab status L2, the presence of massive organomegaly, T cell leukemia, and CNS disease also may be important factors.

Treatment. The principles of treatment for ALL are outlined in Table 15–12. The combination of weekly intravenous vincristine and daily oral prednisone has nonoverlapping toxicities, is not myelosuppressive, and can induce complete remission in more than 90% of patients with ALL within 3–4 wk. Virtually all new patients with ALL have a third agent added for induction therapy (e.g., L-asparaginase). Complete remission is defined as disappearance of clinical signs and symptoms of disease, normalization of blood counts, and restoration of the bone marrow to normal cellularity, registering 5% or fewer blasts (M1). At this time about 10^9–10^{10} leukemic cells remain, which represents a 99–99.9% decrease in tumor cells.

After complete remission has been achieved, CNS prophylaxis is begun. This is a crucial part of the treatment because, without routine CNS prophylaxis, approximately 60% of patients with ALL will develop CNS leukemia while still in bone marrow remission. CNS leukemia is difficult to treat once it becomes symptomatic, because it predisposes the patient to bone marrow relapse. Prophylaxis is accomplished with intrathecal drugs alone for most patients and with chemotherapy plus cranial radiation for patients at high risk.

Maintenance therapy or treatment during remission is required to completely eliminate the 10^9–10^{10} leukemic cells remaining after the initial induction of remission. All leukemia cells must be eliminated to prevent relapse. Combinations of active agents are used during maintenance therapy to prevent the development of drug resistance and to exploit the effects of drugs having different mechanisms of action.

Fifty to 60% of patients with ALL who are treated with standard therapy achieve long-term disease-free survival. For children between 2 and 9 yr of age who have low white blood cell counts, the rate of survival is 85% with mild to moderately intense therapy; those with a larger tumor burden, evidenced by high white blood cell counts and extramedullary disease, have a 60–80% survival rate with more aggressive therapy. Five-year survival without relapse usually is considered a cure.

Relapses occur most commonly in bone marrow but also may present in the CNS, testis, or other extramedullary sites. If relapse occurs while the patient is still receiving modern first-line maintenance chemotherapy, the prognosis is worse than for relapse following discontinuation of therapy. Al-

Table 15–10. Classification of Acute Lymphocytic Leukemia

Cell of Origin	Ia*	CALLA†	CIg‡	SmIg§	LEU-9‖	Incidence (%)	Clinical Characteristics	Prognosis
T cell	−	−/+	−	−	+	15	Mediastinal mass, high WBC count, predominantly males	Variable
B cell	+	+/−	+/−	+	−	1	Burkitt-like	Poor
Pre-B cell	+	+	−/+	−	−	20 ⎫		
Early Pre-B cell	+	+	−	−	−	60–65 ⎬ Protean		Good
Null cell	+	−	−	−	−	5–10 ⎭		

* Immune-associated antigen.
† Common ALL antigen.
‡ Cytoplasmic immunoglobulin.
§ Surface immunoglobulin.
‖ Monoclonal antibody against T cells.
WBC = white blood cell.

Table 15–11. Prognostic Factors in Acute Lymphoblastic Leukemia of Childhood

Factor	Favorable (Standard Risk)	Unfavorable (High Risk)
Demographic		
Age	2–9 yr	<2, >10 yr
Race	White	Black
Sex	Female	Male
Leukemic Burden		
Initial WBC count	$<10 \times 10^9$/L	$>50 \times 10^9$/L
Adenopathy	Absent	Present
Hepatosplenomegaly	Absent to mild (<3 cm)	Marked (>3 cm)
CNS disease at diagnosis	Absent	Present
Hemoglobin	<7 g/dL	>10 g/dL
Platelet count	$>100 \times 10^9$/L	$<100 \times 10^9$/L
Mediastinal mass	Absent	Present
LDH	Not high	High
Morphology, Histochemistry, Cytogenetics, and Biochemistry		
Lymphoblasts*	L1*	L2* or L3*
Periodic acid–Schiff stain	Positive	Negative
Cytogenetics†	Modal number: 50	t(1;19) *or* t(8;14), 22q−, 9q+
Mitotic and labeling index	Low	High
Immunologic Factors		
Immunoglobulins	Normal IgG, IgA, IgM	Decreased IgG, IgA, IgM
Surface markers	Non-T–non-B cell ALL, CALLA+	T or B cell ALL *or* Pre-B
Glucocorticoid receptors	High number	Lower number
Response to induction therapy	M2 marrow (5% blasts) on day 14	M3 marrow (25% blasts) on day 14

* FAB classifiction: L1 typical (85%) = small cells, little cytoplasm; L2 undifferentiated (15%) = large cells, large cytoplasm; L3 Burkitt type (1%) = cytoplasmic vacuoles.
† Cytogenetics refers to chromosome changes; t is transposition (see Chapter 4).
LDH = lactic dehydrogenase; WBC = white blood cell.
(Modified from Miller DR: Acute lymphoblastic leukemia. Pediatr Clin North Am 27:269, 1980.)

Table 15–12. Treatment of Childhood ALL

Induction (4 wk)
(1) Hydration
(2) Treat hyperuricemia and prevent renal complications by using allopurinol
(3) Weekly IV vincristine and daily oral prednisone
(4) Most centers add a third agent, such as L-asparaginase or daunorubicin
(5) Irradiation for mediastinal mass, spinal tumor, other mass-like lesions

CNS Prophylaxis
(1) Intrathecal methotrexate
or
(2) Intrathecal methotrexate and Ara-C
or
(3) Intrathecal chemotherapy plus cranial irradiation for high-risk patients

Consolidation Treatment for High-Risk Groups (2–4 wk)
Removes residual or resistant leukemic cells

Maintenance Therapy (2–5 yr) or Treatment in Remission
Combinations of drugs with differential modes of activity, such as vincristine, prednisone, methotrexate, and 6-mercaptopurine

Bone Marrow Relapse
Autologous, purged bone marrow transplant
Allogeneic bone marrow transplant
Multiple drug reinduction, intensive chemotherapy, CNS irradiation

Local Tissue Relapse
CNS: irradiation, intrathecal or intraventricular methotrexate plus reinduction chemotherapy
Testis: irradiation plus reinduction chemotherapy

though additional remissions are relatively easy to induce, their duration often is short despite intensive therapy. Bone marrow transplantation has been used in second or subsequent remission for children having matched sibling or unrelated donors with 20–40% long-term disease-free survival.

The treatment of AML and ANLL entails a very different philosophy from that for ALL. During induction, intensive multiagent chemotherapy (e.g., an anthracycline, 6-mercaptopurine, and cytosine arabinoside) leads to transient bone marrow aplasia. Following induction, limited further intensive chemotherapy has been used with allogeneic bone marrow transplantation offered as an alternative if a matched sibling or unrelated donor is available.

Complications. Therapy for either ALL or ANLL may cause (1) bone marrow hypoplasia, resulting in thrombocytopenia and bleeding requiring platelet transfusions; (2) anemia, necessitating blood transfusion; and (3) granulocytopenia, which rarely requires transfusion of white blood cells. Infection also may occur (Tables 15–5 and 15–7). Metabolic derangements must be anticipated and prevented, if possible, or treated appropriately when present (see Table 15–6). Long-term sequelae are uncommon (see Table 15–8).

LYMPHOMAS

Malignant lymphomas are the third most common tumor in childhood and are broadly categorized into Hodgkin disease (5.7 cases/million) and non-Hodgkin lymphoma (NHL; 7.4 cases/million).

Non-Hodgkin Lymphoma

Epidemiology. NHL occurs at least three times as frequently in boys as in girls and has a peak incidence between the ages of 7 and 11 yr. NHL in children differs from adult NHL in a number of important features. Most cases of NHL in childhood are diffuse, highly malignant, and very aggressive and show little differentiation beyond primitive cells; highly differentiated, nodular lymphomas that occur in adults are rare in children. Distant noncontiguous metastases are common in childhood NHL, making adult staging systems that depend primarily on nodal involvement of little relevance and mandating that systemic therapy be given to all patients. NHL in childhood resembles acute lymphoblastic leukemia more than it resembles adult-onset NHL or Hodgkin disease. Almost half the cases of NHL in childhood are of T cell origin, compared with approximately 5% of those in adults.

NHLs have been described in association with congenital or acquired immunodeficiency states, chronic immune stimulation, autoimmune disease, and Epstein-Barr virus–induced lymphoproliferation (see Tables 15–2 and 15–3). Acquired immunodeficiency syndrome may be associated with B cell NHL.

Clinical Manifestations. The abdomen is the most common site of the initial manifestation of B cell NHL, whereas the anterior mediastinum is the primary site for T cell lymphomas. In the former site, usually an abdominal mass or evidence of gastrointestinal obstruction or intussusception is present, whereas mediastinal tumors may produce airway or superior vena cava compression and pleural effusion. Painless lymphadenopathy of the cervi-

Table 15–13. Distribution of Childhood NHL by Histopathologic Type

Histologic Type	Marker	Incidence (%)
Lymphoblastic	T cell	30–50
Histiocytic (large cell)	B cell, non-T–non-B cell	14–20
Undifferentiated (small cell)		
Burkitt	B cell	12–20
Pleomorphic	B cell	15–20
Other		1–12

cal, supraclavicular, and axillary nodes often is noted in association with an anterior mediastinal tumor. The diagnosis is established by tissue biopsy. The differential diagnosis of lymphadenopathy is extensive and includes infectious, autoimmune, and malignant diseases. Fever and weight loss may be present, and immunosuppressed patients may demonstrate signs and symptoms of primary CNS lymphoma.

No generally agreed on staging classification for childhood NHL is available. It is essential to ascertain whether a patient has local disease (nodal or extranodal) in one site, which has an excellent prognosis, or disseminated disease, which has a less favorable prognosis. Childhood NHL has a high frequency of dissemination to extranodal sites such as the CNS, bone marrow, or other noncontiguous areas. The progression of disease in childhood NHL does not follow an orderly anatomic sequence of spread as seen with Hodgkin disease. Evaluation prior to therapy should include complete blood count (CBC), bone marrow aspiration and biopsy, chest roentgenograms, lumbar puncture with cerebrospinal fluid cytology, radionuclide bone scan, evaluation of renal and hepatic function, and appropriate CT and ultrasound studies. Staging laparotomy with splenectomy and liver biopsy is not indicated in childhood NHL. Tumor cells should be obtained for histologic type and for surface and cytoplasmic marker evaluation, because this classification may be relevant to therapy and prognosis (Table 15–13).

Treatment. Systemic disease, occult or overt, is present in about 80% of children with NHL. The dramatic improvement in survival for these patients stems in large part from the use of aggressive multidrug combination chemotherapy with agents known to be effective in childhood ALL. Induction produces remission in 90% of affected children, and maintenance chemotherapy reduces the incidence of relapse. With radiotherapy alone, 30% of patients develop leukemic transformation and bone marrow relapse. CNS prophylaxis is essential. Local radiation therapy and surgery to debulk large tumors may be integrated into the treatment plan. Patients with localized disease have a significantly better survival rate than that of patients with nonlocalized tumors. Patients with a large tumor burden, often identified by hyperuricemia or by a serum lactic dehydrogenase greater than 1000 IU, are at risk for the tumor lysis syndrome (see Table 15–6). When all patients are considered, 50–75% of patients are long-term survivors.

Hodgkin Disease

Hodgkin disease in children is similar to that in adults. It has a bimodal incidence at age 15–30 yr and after the age of 50, and is rare before 10 yr of age. There is a 3:1 male predominance in early childhood Hodgkin disease; the sex ratio diminishes after puberty to the 1.4:1 ratio seen in adult Hodgkin disease. Hodgkin disease in childhood has a very good prognosis. The cause of Hodgkin disease is unknown, but indirect evidence has been uncovered suggesting an infectious agent. Hodgkin disease occurs in clusters and within families.

Clinical Manifestations. Painless, firm lymphadenopathy, often confined to 1–2 lymph node areas, usually the supraclavicular and cervical nodes, is the most common clinical presentation. Mediastinal lymphadenopathy is another frequent initial presentation. Fever, night sweats, occasionally pruritis, and weight loss are noted in 30% of children. Anemia and thrombocytopenia are unusual, but leukocytosis with eosinophilia may occur. Elevation of the erythrocyte sedimentation rate (ESR) and serum copper level are nonspecific but may correlate with disease activity. Cellular immunity as determined by cutaneous antigen testing reveals anergy and predisposes the patient to protozoal (*Toxoplasma, P. carinii*), fungal (cryptococcal), or viral (disseminated varicella-zoster) infections. Autoimmune hemolytic anemia or thrombocytopenia and the nephrotic syndrome are rare manifestations of Hodgkin disease.

Diagnosis and Staging. The hallmark of diagnosis is the identification of Reed-Sternberg cells in tumor tissue. Histopathologic subtypes in childhood Hodgkin disease are similar to those in adults, with 10–20% lymphocyte predominance, 40–60% nodular sclerosis, 20–40% mixed cellularity, and 1–10% lymphocyte depletion. As in adults, lymphocyte predominance is most favorable and lymphocyte depletion least favorable.

Table 15–14. Ann Arbor Staging Classification for Hodgkin Disease*

Stage I
Involvement of a single lymph node region (I), or a single extralymphatic organ or site (I$_E$)

Stage II
Involvement of two or more lymph node regions on the same side of the diaphragm (II), or localized involvement of an extralymphatic organ or site and of one or more lymph node regions on the same side of the diaphragm (II$_E$)

Stage III
Involvement of lymph node regions on both sides of the diaphragm (III), which may be accompanied by localized involvement of an extralymphatic organ or site (III$_E$), by involvement of the spleen (III$_S$), or both (III$_{SE}$)

Stage IV
Diffuse or disseminated involvement of one or more extralymphatic organs or tissues, with or without associated lymph node enlargement

* Each stage is divided into "A" and "B" categories, where A indicates no systemic symptoms and B indicates the presence of one or more of the following: (1) unexplained weight loss greater than 10% of body weight in preceding 6 mo, (2) fever higher than 38°C, and (3) night sweats.
E = extralymphatic; S = splenic involvement.

Unlike the case with NHL, it is of critical importance to accurately stage patients with Hodgkin disease, because both the type of therapy and the prognosis are directly related to the stage of disease (Table 15–14). Staging is accomplished by clinical (e.g., fever, night sweats) and surgical evaluation. Clinical staging includes the history, physical examination, and initial chest roentgenogram for evaluation of mediastinal, hilar, or pulmonary parenchymal involvement. Evaluation includes determining CBC, ESR, and serum copper level; tests of hepatic and renal function; lymphangiography or computerized tomography (CT) evaluation of the retroperitoneal nodes; appropriate radionuclide scans; and bone marrow biopsy (rather than an aspiration). The disease may arise in a unifocal node and then spread through contiguous lymph node chains by the lymphatic channels. Right-sided cervical nodal involvement is associated with mediastinal disease, and bilateral or left-sided cervical nodes are associated with splenic disease.

Surgical staging is not indicated unless therapy will be influenced by the findings. If the patient clearly has disseminated disease (stage IIIB or IV) or disease demonstrated on bone marrow biopsy, surgical staging is unnecessary. With surgical staging, as many as 30% of stage I and II patients are reclassified to higher stages, thus necessitating different therapy (Table 15–15). The most common site of abdominal involvement is the spleen and splenic hilar nodes.

The major *differential diagnoses* for Hodgkin disease and NHL are lymphadenitis, infectious mononucleosis, tuberculosis, atypical mycobacteria, cat-scratch disease, acquired immunodeficiency disease, and toxoplasmosis.

Treatment. Table 15–15 shows the indicated therapy for various stages of Hodgkin disease. With appropriate therapy, 80–90% of patients survive 5 yr. Irradiation has been the cornerstone of treatment for Hodgkin disease in adults; however, smaller fields and lower doses often are used in prepubertal teenagers. Radiation fields used in the treatment of the disease are illustrated in Figure 15–1. Localized disease is treated successfully by irradiation alone, but patients with systemic symptoms or disseminated disease require chemotherapy. Although some institutions avoid using staging laparotomy for children and offer systemic chemotherapy to most patients, the combination of irradiation and chemotherapy for all patients may be unacceptably toxic. MOPP (nitrogen mustard, vincristine, prednisone, procarbazine) has been the

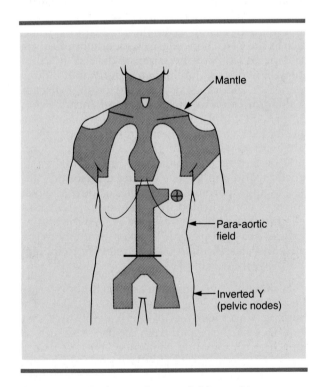

Figure 15–1. Radiation therapy fields used in treatment of Hodgkin disease.

Table 15–15. Recommended Therapy for Patients with Hodgkin Disease

	Patient Features	Recommended Therapy
Stages IA, IB, IIA	Attained full growth; no unfavorable signs	Full-dose radiotherapy*
	Still growing or large mediastinal mass or chest wall or pericardial invasion	Low-dose radiotherapy plus 6 courses of MOPP Other chemotherapy (experimental)
Stages IIB, IIIA	Attained full growth; no unfavorable signs	Full-dose radiotherapy; definitive hepatic radiotherapy for patients with splenic involvement treated with radiation alone
	Still growing or large mediastinal mass†	Low-dose radiotherapy plus 6 courses of MOPP; other chemotherapy (experimental)
Stages IIIA$_2$, IIIB, IVA, IVB		6 courses MOPP ± full dose IF radiotherapy; or 12 courses alternating MOPP/ABVD; or 6 courses MOPP + low-dose TNLI; or other chemotherapy (experimental)

* Full-dose radiotherapy = 3500–4400 cGy; low-dose = ≤2500 cGy.
† Some would treat these patients as though they had advanced (stage IIIA$_2$–IV) disease.
ABVD = Adriamycin, bleomycin, vinblastine, and dacarbazine; MOPP = nitrogen mustard, vincristine, prednisone, and procarbazine; TNLI = Total nodal-lymphoid irradiation.
(From Leventhal BG, Donaldson SS: Hodgkin's disease. In Pizzo PA, Poplack DG (eds): Principles and Practice of Pediatric Oncology. Philadelphia, JB Lippincott, 1989, p 471.)

most commonly used combination of agents, but other 4-drug combinations may be as effective and may have fewer adverse effects. To avoid emergence of resistant cells and decrease side effects, studies are underway utilizing alternating cycles of MOPP and ABVD (Adriamycin, bleomycin, vinblastine, and dacarbazine [DTIC]) or variants.

Complications. Complications include recurrent disease; chronic immune deficiency; pneumococcal and *Haemophilus influenzae* sepsis; growth retardation and restrictive lung disease secondary to irradiation; thyroid, testicular, and ovarian dysfunction; amenorrhea; and development of secondary tumors (see Table 15–3). Although Hodgkin disease is one of the most curable malignant tumors in childhood, concern now must be directed increasingly toward minimizing the serious side effects of successful antitumor treatment.

Splenectomy in young children leaves them susceptible to bacterial sepsis, and for this reason physicians are reluctant to remove spleens routinely in young patients. If splenectomy is anticipated, immunizing all patients with polyvalent pneumococcal vaccine, meningococcal vaccine, and *H. influenzae* vaccine routinely should precede the operation.

PRIMARY CENTRAL NERVOUS SYSTEM TUMORS

CNS tumors are the most common solid tumors in children and are second to leukemia in overall incidence of malignant diseases. There are about 1200 new cases per year, or approximately 24 cases per million children under the age of 15. Brain tumors in children differ from those in adults in that, rather than being supratentorial tumors as in adults, they are predominantly infratentorial tumors (posterior fossae) involving the cerebellum, mid-brain, and brain stem (Table 15–16). Childhood brain tumors are differentiated further from those in adults in that they are usually low-grade astrocytomas or embryonic neoplasms (medulloblastomas, ependymomas, or germ cell tumors), whereas most CNS tumors in adults are malignant astrocytomas and metastatic carcinomas.

Clinical Manifestations. Common presenting signs and symptoms of CNS tumors in childhood often are dismissed initially as intercurrent viral or nonspecific illnesses. Signs of increased intracranial pressure and focal neurologic deficits eventually suggest intracranial pathology (Table 15–17). Headache is not localizing but is suggestive of increased intracranial pressure if it is present at night or on awakening, worsens with cough or straining, and is intermittent but recurs with increasing frequency and intensity. Vomiting without nausea, another nonspecific sign of increased intracranial pressure, usually is intermittent and occurs on arising in the morning. Strabismus with diplopia is the result of VIth nerve palsy caused by increased intracranial pressure. Double vision resulting from a VIth nerve deficit is not a localizing finding. Papilledema or choked optic discs may be a late but

Table 15–16. Location, Incidence, and Prognosis of CNS Tumors in Children

Location	Incidence (%)	5-Yr Survival (%)
Infratentorial	55–60	
(Posterior fossa)		
Astrocytoma (cerebellum)		90
Medulloblastoma		44–55
Glioma (brain stem)		0–5 (high grade)
		30 (low grade)
Ependymoma		50–60
Supratentorial	40–45	
(Cerebral hemispheres)	25–30	
Astrocytoma		10–50
Glioblastoma multiforme		0–5
Ependymoma		50–60
Choroid plexus papilloma		60–80
Midline	15	
Craniopharyngioma		70–90
Pineal (germinoma)		65–75
Optic nerve glioma		50–90

specific sign of increased intracranial pressure. Obstructive hydrocephalus may produce a large cranium if it occurs before the sutures have fused. Focal signs may be present, with or without signs of increased intracranial pressure. Nystagmus usually is due to cerebellovestibular pathway irritative or destructive lesions, but nystagmus also may be seen with a marked visual deficit (peripheral or cortical blindness). Cranial nerve deficits other than VIth nerve deficits localize the lesion to the brain stem. Head tilt, as a compensation for loss of binocular vision, is noted with extraocular muscle weakness.

Personality changes, poor school performance, and change in hand preference should suggest a cortical lesion, whereas ataxia suggests a cerebellar or brain stem lesion. Babinski sign, hyperreflexia, spasticity, and loss of dexterity are suggestive of brain stem or cortical tumors, whereas seizures are noted with cortical lesions. Endocrine abnormalities are noted with pituitary, hypothalamic, or pineal tumors.

Diagnosis. History, physical examination, and neurologic examination, including that of visual fields and fundi, are fundamental for evaluation, but CT scan and magnetic resonance imaging (MRI) of the head have revolutionized the field of neurodiagnosis. They are the procedures of choice for diagnosing and localizing tumors as well as other intracranial masses.

MRI may be of additional diagnostic benefit, particularly in posterior fossa and spinal tumors, in which CT scans are least effective because the surrounding bone often limits resolution. Examination of cerebrospinal fluid by cytocentrifuge histology is essential to determine the presence of metastasis in medulloblastoma and pinealoma.

Differential diagnosis should include arteriovenous malformation, aneurysm, brain abscess, echinococcal or cysticercosal or other parasite infestation, herpes simplex encephalitis, granulomatous disease (tuberculosis, cryptococcal, sarcoid), intracranial hemorrhage, pseudotumor cerebri, primary cerebral lymphoma, vasculitis, and, rarely, metastatic tumors.

Treatment. Once diagnosis is established, corticosteroids often are administered to reduce tumor edema. With improvements in neurodiagnosis, lessened surgical morbidity, and better chemotherapy programs, an aggressive approach to treatment of pediatric brain tumors has improved outcome (Tables 15–16 and 15–17). Utilizing improved neurosurgical techniques, surgical objectives include biopsy, debulking or complete excision if possible, and treatment of hydrocephalus. Radiation therapy has been the mainstay of treatment of malignant CNS tumors. Medulloblastomas, ependymomas, germ cell tumors, and some low-grade astrocytomas are responsive to radiation in doses of 4500–6500 cGy. About 50% of patients with medulloblastoma will be cured by a combination of surgery and radiation therapy to the posterior fossa, whole brain, and spinal axis. Trials of single and multiagent chemotherapy for brain tumors are under way; however, the definitive role of chemotherapy in treatment of brain tumors has not been clarified. Objective tumor responses for a number of chemotherapeutic programs have been observed in several tumors.

Prognosis. The 5-yr survival rate associated with all childhood CNS tumors is approximately 50%, resulting in large measure from the high curability of cerebellar astrocytomas and some medulloblastomas (see Table 15–16). The best prognosis is noted following simple surgical total excision of a cystic cerebellar astrocytoma.

WILMS TUMOR

Wilms tumor is the most common intrarenal malignant tumor of childhood, with a yearly incidence of 7.8 new cases per million children.

Table 15–17. Manifestations and Treatment of Primary CNS Tumors

Tumor/Site	Manifestations	Treatment	Comments
Cerebellar astrocytoma	Onset between 5 and 8 yr of age; ↑ ICP, ataxia, nystagmus, head tilt, intention tremor	Surgical excision plus adjuvant radiotherapy if a solid tumor; corticosteroids to ↓ tumor edema	Symptoms present for 2–7 mo; cystic tumors have favorable outcome
Medulloblastoma Cerebellar vermis and floor of 4th ventricle	Onset between 3 and 5 yr of age; ↑ ICP, obstructive hydrocephalus, ataxia, cerebrospinal fluid metastasis, and spinal cord compression	Surgical excision and radiotherapy plus adjuvant chemotherapy*; corticosteroids to ↓ tumor edema	Acute onset of symptoms; tumor is radiosensitive; cerebrospinal fluid checked for metastatic cells
Ependymoma Floor of 4th ventricle	↑ ICP, obstructive hydrocephalus; rarely seeds spinal fluid	Surgical excision, radiotherapy, chemotherapy*; corticosteroids to ↓ tumor edema	Onset intermediate between astrocytoma and medulloblastoma
Brain stem glioma	Onset between 5 and 7 yr of age; triad of multiple cranial nerve deficit (VII, IX, X, V, VI) pyramidal tract, and cerebellar signs; skip lesions common; ↑ ICP is late	Excision impossible; radiotherapy is palliative; corticosteroids to ↓ tumor edema; experimental chemotherapy*	Small size but critical location makes this tumor highly lethal
Pinealoma	Paralysis of upward gaze (Parinaud syndrome); lid retraction (Collier sign); hearing loss; precocious puberty; ↑ ICP; may seed spinal fluid	Radiotherapy, chemotherapy; shunting of CSF	Germ cell line; germinoma, dermoid, teratoma, mixed lesions may calcify or secrete hCG or alpha-fetoprotein
Diencephalic glioma Hypothalamus	Onset between 2 and 5 mo of age; alert, euphoric but emaciated appearance; emesis, optic atrophy, nystagmus	Radiotherapy	Patient may become obese after treatment
Astrocytoma/glioma Cerebral cortex	Onset between 5 and 10 yr of age; personality changes; headache, motor weakness, seizures, ↑ ICP later	Location determines surgical or radiotherapy; anticonvulsant and corticosteroids; chemotherapy*	*Differential diagnosis:* Abscess, hydatid or porencephalic cyst; herpes simplex encephalitis, granuloma (TB, cryptococcus); arteriovenous malformation; hematoma; lymphoma
Optic glioma	Onset before 2 yr of age; poor visual acuity, exophthalmos, nystagmus; ↑ ICP; optic atrophy, strabismus	Surgical resection or radiotherapy; chemotherapy*	Neurofibromatosis in 25% of patients
Craniopharyngioma Pituitary fossa	Onset between 7 and 12 yr of age; ↑ ICP, bitemporal hemianopia, sexual and growth retardation; growth hormone and gonadotropic deficiency	Begin cortisol replacement prior to surgery; total excision, adjuvant radiotherapy if extensive	Calcification above sella turcica; diabetes insipidus common postoperatively

CSF = cerebral spinal fluid; hCG = human chorionic gonadotropin; ↑ ICP = increased intracranial pressure: headache, vomiting (papilledema, IIIrd and VIth nerve palsies, wide sutures); TB = tuberculosis.

* Chemotherapy may delay need for radiotherapy thus avoiding treatment related neurotoxicity. Chemotherapy includes alternating cycles of cyclophosphamide plus vincristine with cisplatin plus etoposide.

Epidemiology. The mean age at diagnosis is 3–3½ yr, and no sex predilection is apparent. A hereditary form of Wilms tumor may be associated with a bilateral presentation and with some unilateral tumors. A number of congenital anomalies frequently are identified in children with Wilms tumor, including sporadic aniridia (1:100 in patients with Wilms tumor versus 1:50,000 in the general population), hemihypertrophy (2:100 in patients with Wilms tumor versus 3:100,000 in the general population), and genitourinary anomalies (5:100 in patients with Wilms tumor), including hypospadias, cryptorchidism, horseshoe or fused kidneys, ureteral duplication, and polycystic kidneys. Wilms tumor with aniridia often is associated with a deletion of part of chromosome 11 [del (11p13)].

Clinical Manifestations. Over 80% of children with Wilms tumor present with an abdominal mass, which usually is discovered incidentally by the parents while bathing or dressing the child or during a routine well child examination. Associated symptoms and laboratory abnormalities may include abdominal pain, fever, hypertension, and microscopic or gross hematuria. Polycythemia is a rare paraneoplastic complication.

Other manifestations include signs of complete or partial aniridia, hemihypertrophy, and a history of any genitourinary abnormalities. A CBC, urinalysis, liver and renal function studies, and a search for sites of metastases (lung, liver, nodes, kidney, bone, brain) should be performed. Ultrasound studies of the abdomen, plain abdominal roentgenograms, and intravenous pyelograms (IVPs) often reveal a mass that distorts the calyces, displaces the kidney, and does not cross the midline. CT is helpful for identifying metastasis or local spread (to the inferior vena cava and retroperitoneum) and for evaluating the contralateral kidney.

Diagnosis. A sample of tumor tissue is required for definitive diagnosis. The differential diagnosis of Wilms tumor includes benign lesions, such as hydronephrosis, polycystic disease of the kidney, and splenomegaly, as well as malignant tumors, such as renal cell carcinoma, neuroblastoma, lymphoma, retroperitoneal rhabdomyosarcoma, and ovarian tumors. Prognostic factors include tumor stage (Table 15–18) and tumor histology (classic nephroblastoma, with a favorable histology and 88% survival, versus anaplastic or sarcomatous variant, with an unfavorable histology and 12% survival). The 4-yr relapse-free survival of patients with tumors of favorable histology is directly related to stage and, with treatment, can be expected

Table 15–18. National Wilms Tumor Study Staging System*

Stage I
Tumor limited to the kidney and completely excised
The surface of the renal capsule is intact; the tumor is not ruptured before or during removal
No residual tumor is apparent beyond the margins of excision

Stage II
Tumor extends beyond the kidney but is completely excised
Regional extension of the tumor is present (i.e., penetration through the outer surface of the renal capsule into the perirenal soft tissues); vessels outside the kidney substance are infiltrated or contain tumor thrombus; the tumor may have been biopsied or local spillage of tumor confined to the flank has occurred; no residual tumor is apparent at or beyond the margins of excision

Stage III
Residual nonhematogenous tumor confined to the abdomen
Any of the following may occur:
  a. Lymph nodes on biopsy are found to be involved in the hilus, the periaortic chains, or beyond
  b. Diffuse peritoneal contamination by the tumor has occurred, such as by spillage of tumor beyond the flank before or during surgery, or by tumor growth that has penetrated through the peritoneal surface
  c. Implants are found on the peritoneal surfaces
  d. The tumor extends beyond the surgical margins either microscopically or grossly
  e. The tumor is not completely resectable because of local infiltration into vital structures

Stage IV
Hematogenous metastases; deposits beyond Stage III (e.g., lung, liver, bone, and brain)

Stage V
Bilateral renal involvement at diagnosis
An attempt should be made to stage each side according to the above criteria on the basis of extent of disease prior to biopsy

* The clinical stage is decided by the surgeon in the operating room and is confirmed by the pathologist, who also evaluates the histology. It is done on the basis of gross and microscopic tumor distribution and is the same for tumors with favorable and with unfavorable histologic features. The patient is characterized, however, by a statement of both criteria (e.g., Stage II, favorable histology, or Stage II, unfavorable histology).

to be 97%, 92%, 87%, and 73% for stages I, II, III, and IV, respectively.

Treatment. Surgery continues to be the cornerstone of therapy. Gentle technique is required to prevent rupture of the tumor during removal. A large transabdominal incision facilitates the search for metastatic disease, examination of the opposite kidney, approach to the inferior vena cava if necessary, and removal of the tumor en bloc when feasible. Radiation is begun postoperatively, with the therapeutic plan being dependent on the stage of the disease and age of the patient. In patients with stage III or IV disease, the tumor bed or full abdomen, if necessary, is irradiated with total doses of approximately 1000 cGy. Care must be taken to minimize radiation effects to the liver, because radiation hepatotoxicity is potentiated by subsequent chemotherapy. Chemotherapy utilizing vincristine, dactinomycin, and Adriamycin has significantly improved the relapse-free survival rate. The first two drugs are used in all stages and Adriamycin is used in stages III and IV.

Bilateral Wilms tumor is present in about 5% of children on initial presentation, whereas recurrent disease affects the opposite kidney in 4–5% of patients. Treatment must be individualized but may require excisional biopsy or heminephrectomy on one side and radical nephrectomy on the more involved side, with the objective to preserve as much normal kidney as possible. Preoperative chemotherapy with dactinomycin and vincristine often aids the surgeon in determining the appropriate procedure. If pulmonary metastases are present, lung irradiation is added to the therapy of the primary tumor.

NEUROBLASTOMA

Neuroblastoma is the most enigmatic of childhood tumors. It arises from the primitive neural crest cells that form the adrenal medulla and the sympathetic nervous system of the cervical sympathetic chain, the thoracic chain, and the abdominal organ of Zuckerkandl. Despite the fact that it is responsive to a variety of aggressive chemotherapy treatment protocols, the outlook for children with this tumor has not changed materially in the last three decades.

Epidemiology. Neuroblastoma is the most common malignant tumor in infancy (median age of onset is 20 mo of life) and, in childhood, ranks fourth in frequency to leukemia, lymphoma and CNS tumors. Although neuroblastoma represents less than 8% of childhood cancer, it is responsible for 15% of cancer deaths in children. The incidence of neuroblastoma is estimated to be 1:100,000 infants, and it may be associated with fetal hydantoin syndrome, von Recklinghausen disease, and Hirschsprung disease.

Clinical Manifestations. The most common presentation is an abdominal mass that is hard, smooth, nontender, and most often palpated in the flank. In the abdomen, 45% of tumors arise in the adrenal gland and 25% in retroperitoneal sympathetic ganglia. Other sites include the pelvis (4%), the posterior mediastinum (20%), and the neck (4%). Calcification within the tumor often is observed on plain films of the abdomen, and IVP shows displacement of a kidney with minimal distortion of the calyceal system if the tumor arises in the adrenal gland. The presentation must be differentiated from that of Wilms tumor, which also presents as an abdominal flank mass. In contrast to neuroblastoma, Wilms tumors are often lobulated rather than smooth, and they are seen to displace and distort the urinary collecting system on IVP. Neuroblastoma may become manifest at birth as a flank mass or malignant ascites with nonimmune hydrops fetalis.

Neuroblastoma may spread to the liver, producing hepatomegaly, and may metastasize to bone and bone marrow, producing limp and bone pain. Primary involvement of the cervical sympathetic chain produces ipsilateral Horner syndrome with heterochromia of the iris; posterior mediastinal tumors produce pain, spinal cord compression, and airway obstruction. Esthesioneuroblastoma of the olfactory bulb produces epistaxis and nasal obstruction. Metastasis may produce blanching skin nodules, periorbital ecchymosis, and proptosis. Vasoactive intestinal polypeptide secretion may produce watery diarrhea. Rapid multidirectional eye movements (opsoclonus), myoclonus, and cerebellar ataxia also are noted occasionally.

Diagnosis. In addition to the history and the physical examination with blood pressure, evaluation should include a CBC, renal and hepatic function tests, chest roentgenogram, abdominal plain film, radionuclide scan of bone and liver, ultrasonogram and CT scan, and a careful search for products of catecholamine metabolism. Most neuroblastomas secrete one or more catecholamines or their metabolic by-products (vanillylmandelic acid [VMA] and homovanillic acid [HVA]). Bone marrow examination may demonstrate neuroblastoma cells forming typical rosettes.

Prognosis. Age at presentation, stage of disease, primary site, site of metastases, amplification of the N-myc oncogene (poor prognosis) or TRK (good prognosis), ferritin concentration, degree of cell differentiation, lymphocyte infiltration of the tumor, and the presence of peripheral lymphocytosis all affect survival. In general, children under 1

Table 15–19. Neuroblastoma Staging System Proposed by the International Staging System Working Party

	Staging Criteria	Incidence (%)	Survival at 5 Yr
Stage I	Localized tumor confined to the area of origin, complete gross excision, with or without microscopic residual disease; identifiable ipsilateral and contralateral lymph nodes negative microscopically	5	90% or greater
Stage IIa	Unilateral tumor with incomplete, gross excision; identifiable ipsilateral and contralateral lymph nodes negative microscopically		
Stage IIb	Unilateral tumor with complete or incomplete gross excision; with positive ipsilateral regional lymph nodes; identifiable contralateral lymph nodes negative microscopically	10	70–80%
Stage III	Tumor infiltrating across the midline with or without regional lymph node involvement; or, midline tumor with bilateral regional lymph node involvement	25	40–70% (depending on completeness of surgical resection)
Stage IV	Dissemination of the tumor to distant lymph nodes, bone, bone marrow, liver, and/or other organs (except as defined in stage IVS)	60	More than 60% if age at diagnosis is younger than 1 yr; 20% if age at diagnosis is older than 1 yr and under 2 yr; 10% if age at diagnosis is over 2 yr
Stage IVS	Localized primary tumor as defined for stage I or II with dissemination limited to liver, skin, and/or bone marrow	5	More than 80

(From Philip T: Overview of current treatment of neuroblastoma. Am J Pediatr Hematol Oncol 14:97, 1992.

yr of age have a good prognosis, whereas children over 2 yr of age have a much poorer prognosis (Table 15–19). Older patients generally have more extensive disease. Children with tumors arising in the neck and posterior mediastinum have a better prognosis than those with abdominal primaries. Metastatic lesions in bone or positive ipsilateral lymph nodes carry a poor prognosis.

Treatment. Total surgical excision offers the best hope of cure, but the presence of metastatic disease in over 70% of patients at diagnosis limits the effectiveness of this modality alone. The role of radiation therapy is not precisely defined, although it clearly plays a role in the palliative treatment of patients with advanced disease. A wide range of chemotherapeutic agents have been used for patients with extensive local or disseminated disease at diagnosis. Although chemotherapy has significantly increased the tumor response rate, the cure rate for children has remained essentially unchanged. The most active agents include vincristine, cyclophosphamide, Adriamycin, cis-platinum, and VM-26. Experimental protocols with radiolabeled monoclonal antibodies to the neuro-

blastoma cell line or with total body irradiation and high-dose chemotherapy followed by purged autologous bone marrow transplantation are newer approaches to therapy.

There are a number of curious issues relating to neuroblastoma. Occasionally, one cannot find evidence of a primary tumor but only evidence of metastases to the orbit. Furthermore, a small percentage of neuroblastomas, especially in very young children, appear to regress spontaneously without any treatment; this regression has been documented more frequently in neuroblastoma than in any other malignancy. In addition, as many as 1:200 neonates demonstrate neuroblastoma in situ at autopsy. Also, numerous reports have been made of tumors initially considered to be malignant neuroblastomas that, after treatment, were found to be clearly benign ganglioneuromas. The stage IV-S designation also is unique in that it refers to a small primary tumor with disseminated disease but without bone involvement. Symptomatic therapy only is needed (usually to control hepatomegaly), and outcome may be compromised by aggressive chemotherapy. Recently, screening all infants at 6 mo of age for urine spot tests of VMA or HVA has been initiated in an attempt to identify patients before widespread dissemination of the tumor has occurred.

SOFT TISSUE SARCOMAS

Rhabdomyosarcoma

Rhabdomyosarcoma is the most common soft tissue sarcoma in children and has an incidence of about 4.5 cases/million (1.3/million black children), with a peak occurrence in children 2–6 yr of age and a second peak in adolescence. The tumor arises primarily in skeletal muscle but may occur in any tissue derived from mesenchyme. The early peak is associated with tumors in the prostate, vagina, bladder, and head and neck, whereas the later peak is associated with tumors in the extremities, trunk, and male genitourinary tract. Tumors of the head and neck (35–40%) occur in the orbit, sinuses, nasopharynx, and soft tissues.

Clinical Manifestations. The clinical presentation of rhabdomyosarcoma varies depending on the site of origin and the subsequent mass effect. For example, in the *orbit,* swelling, proptosis, and limitation of extraocular motion may be exhibited; in *other head and neck sites,* nasal mass, chronic otitis media, hemorrhage, ear discharge, obstruction, dysphagia, hearing abnormalities, and cranial nerve involvement may be noted; in the *retroperitoneum,* symptoms associated with a mass are seen; in the *genitourinary tract,* urethral, vaginal (polypoid) masses, peritesticular swelling, hematuria, and urinary frequency or retention may be exhibited; and in the *extremities and trunk,* painful or asymptomatic masses may be the main features. Evaluation must be directed toward the particular site of involvement, but additionally should include CBC, liver and renal function tests, urinalysis, radionuclide bone scan, bone marrow biopsy, lumbar puncture with spinal fluid cytology for craniospinal sites, and other tests for identifying occult and metastatic disease.

Diagnosis. Tissue biopsy is needed for definitive diagnosis. The staging system has prognostic significance. Histopathology also is important, because patients with alveolar histology have a consistently higher mortality rate than patients with embryonal histology, irrespective of the primary site of involvement. Embryonal histopathology predominates, especially in younger patients.

Treatment. Treatment must be tailored to the site of involvement but includes integration of surgery, radiation therapy, and chemotherapy. If it is possible to remove the tumor completely with a wide margin of resection, the chance for local control is good. Radiation therapy combined with chemotherapy can provide local control of gross residual or microscopic disease in 90% of patients. Administering the combination of cyclophosphamide, vincristine, dactinomycin, and Adriamycin has dramatically improved survival over that achievable by radiation therapy and surgery alone. Although primary site and histology are strong prognostic indicators, the most important determinant of outcome is the extent of disease at diagnosis. Preliminary data suggest that patients with group I (localized tumor, completely resected, and no lymph node involvement) and II (regional disease, completely or grossly resected) tumors can be treated effectively with vincristine and dactinomycin and have a 2-yr relapse-free survival of 83–87% for group I tumors and 70–81% for group II tumors. Chemotherapy for groups III (incomplete resection or biopsy with residual disease) and IV (distant metastatic disease at onset) is not yet satisfactory despite the addition of Adriamycin to vincristine, cyclophosphamide, and dactinomycin. The 2-yr survival rate for patients with group III tumors treated with all four drugs is 71–79%, and, for patients with group IV tumors, it is 37–40%.

Less common soft tissue sarcomas of infancy and childhood are fibrosarcoma (11% of soft tissue sarcomas), neurofibrosarcoma (3%), synovial sarcoma (5%), liposarcoma (4%), malignant fibrous histiocytoma (4%), hemangiopericytoma (3%), and leiomyosarcoma (<2%).

MALIGNANT BONE TUMORS

The two most important malignant bone tumors in children are osteosarcoma and Ewing sarcoma. Less commonly encountered are chondrosarcoma, fibrosarcoma, reticulosarcoma, reticulum cell sarcoma, non-Hodgkin lymphoma of bone, hemangiosarcoma, and malignant giant cell tumor.

Osteosarcoma

Osteosarcoma is a rare tumor; in children less than 15 yr old, only about 300 new cases occur each year in the United States. Males are affected 1½ times more often then females.

Epidemiology and Etiology. The disease most commonly affects adolescents, with the peak incidence occurring during the period of maximum growth velocity. The primary tumor most often is located at the epiphysis or metaphysis of anatomic sites that are associated with maximum growth velocity—the distal femur, the proximal tibia, and the proximal humerus—but any bone may be involved.

The cause of osteosarcoma is unknown, but the correlation of the location of most tumors with the period of maximum bone growth suggests some relation to increased osteoblastic activity. Genetic factors may have a role in osteosarcoma; 16 sets of siblings with the disease have been identified. Among patients with hereditary retinoblastoma, the incidence of osteosarcoma is increased 500 times, and deletions on the long arm of chromosome 13, which can occur in patients with retinoblastoma, recently have been found in some osteosarcoma tumors, implicating the RB allele as in retinoblastoma. Osteosarcoma also may occur following radiotherapy.

Clinical Manifestations. Osteosarcomas arise in either the medullary cavity or the periosteum. The tumor occurs most frequently in the femur (43% of cases), followed by the tibia (19%) and the humerus (10%). The tumor usually comes to attention as a painful swelling or pain near the knee without other symptoms. Often a history of trauma is noted, but this is only an incidental finding. Gait disturbances and pathologic fractures also may be present. Evaluation should be based on plain films of the affected area, chest roentgenogram, radionuclide bone scan, and MRI scan of the involved bone. These tests may demonstrate sclerosis, periosteal new bone formation, and soft tissue extension of tumor. Because of the frequent presence of pulmonary metastasis (10–15%), CT of the chest is essential to detect small lesions; these lesions often appear as calcified nodules. Micrometastatic disease is present at diagnosis in 80–90% of patients but is undetectable with any of our present tests. Serum alkaline phosphatase levels may be elevated and may be used as a marker of the response to treatment. ESR is normal. Arteriography may be useful when limb-sparing procedures are contemplated. Biopsy is essential for accurate diagnosis. Osteosarcoma must be differentiated from Ewing sarcoma, benign and malignant bone tumors, and chronic osteomyelitis.

Treatment. Prior to the onset of effective adjuvant chemotherapy, only about 20% of patients with osteosarcoma survived. Aggressive combination adjuvant chemotherapy preceding and following surgical resection dramatically improves the survival of patients with osteosarcoma, with more than 50–60% of patients now identified as long-term, relapse-free survivors. Chemotherapy includes the use of high-dose methotrexate, Adriamycin, cis-platinum, and possibly ifosfamide. The tumor is not radiosensitive at conventional doses. In addition, about one third of patients can be successfully treated if they have a limited relapse in the lung by utilizing a combination of surgery, to remove each pulmonary metastatic lesion, and additional chemotherapy. Poor prognostic findings include age less than 10 yr, large tumor (>15 cm), osteoblastic cell type, involvement of the axial skeleton or humerus, elevated serum lactic dehydrogenase, presence of symptoms for less than 2 mo, and metastasis.

The improvement in survival for these patients has generated many attempts to lessen the morbidity of surgery by attempting to resect tumors and implant protheses of various sorts rather than simply amputating or disarticulating an extremity. These limb-sparing procedures include the use of bone grafting and an internal prosthesis in selected patients. Postoperative rehabilitation therapy is critical after amputation.

Ewing Sarcoma

Ewing sarcoma is a highly malignant, nonosseous, small round cell tumor (as in neuroblastoma, primitive neuroectodermal tumor [PNET], lymphoma, and rhabdomyosarcoma) that frequently has metastasized at the time of diagnosis. The clonal nature of the malignant cells is revealed by the consistent t(11;22) chromosomal abnormality. The incidence of Ewing sarcoma in white children is about 1.9/million, but the disease is almost unknown in blacks. It occurs in younger children as well as in adolescents. The tumor most often involves the diaphyseal portion of long bones. The femur and pelvis are the most common sites, but lesions of the tibia, fibula, ribs, humerus, scapula, and clavicle also are encountered.

The *clinical manifestations* of the disease are similar to those of osteosarcoma; however, systemic symptoms, such as weight loss, fatigue, and fever, are found more commonly in Ewing sarcoma. The diagnostic evaluation is similar to that for osteosarcoma. ESR is elevated. Plain roentgenograms of the bone reveal calcified periosteal elevation (onionskin), osteolytic lesions, and sclerosis. Osteomyelitis and eosinophilic granuloma are part of the differential diagnosis. Metastasis to the bone by neuroblastoma or rhabdomyosarcoma should be considered in younger children with a solitary bone lesion.

Because the majority of patients with Ewing sarcoma have micrometastatic disease at the time of diagnosis, chemotherapy is a critical component of the *treatment*. Chemotherapy includes vincristine, cyclophosphamide, dactinomycin, and doxorubicin, with agents like ifosfamide under evaluation. Local control of the tumor initially is obtained with a combination of surgery, chemotherapy, and radiation therapy to the involved bone. If tumors affect expendable bones (e.g., fibula, rib, or clavicle), complete surgical excision may be warranted. If the initial combination treatment and the complete surgical excision are unsuccessful, radiation therapy to the involved bone, and aggressive multiagent chemotherapy result in an 80–90% likelihood of local control. The presence or absence of demonstrable metastatic disease at the time of diagnosis is the most important prognostic variable. Other, less favorable features include soft tissue extension, a low lymphocyte count, and elevated serum lactic dehydrogenase. Patients with primary tumors of the pelvis do less well than those having tumors at other sites. Without metastatic disease, 40–70% will have long-term survival.

LANGERHANS CELL HISTIOCYTOSIS

Langerhans cell histiocytosis (LCH) includes a group of diseases in which progression is due to proliferation and tissue infiltration of differentiated Langerhans cell histiocytes, which may mimic malignant neoplasms. The disorders probably are not malignancies and are of unknown etiology. Abnormalities of immune regulation, such as reduced suppressor and increased helper lymphocyte counts, have been reported with LCH. The pathology reveals granuloma formation composed of histiocytes with characteristic large cell size, grooved nuclei, absence of an obvious malignant cytology, and the presence of characteristic multilaminar Birbeck granules in electron micrographs.

Three classic disease types occur. *Letterer-Siwe disease* often is noted in young children who exhibit multisystemic involvement, including skin (seborrhea, rash), lung (interstitial pneumonia), hepatosplenomegaly, bone marrow infiltration (pancytopenia), and bone (osteolytic, punched-out lesions). *Hand-Schüller-Christian disease* is less serious, noted in older children, and exhibited as granulomatous lesions in bone, tooth loss (mandible), exophthalmos (orbital), diabetes insipidus, and growth hormone deficiency (both factors, hypothalamus). The solitary *eosinophilic granuloma* has the most favorable prognosis, and patients have dull pain, a mass

in the skull, or a localized lytic lesion of the mandible, mastoid, and proximal long bones. Vertebral involvement and collapse may cause spinal cord compression. Involvement of skin and multiple visceral organs with organ system dysfunction (e.g., jaundice, anemia, or hypoxia) has the poorest prognosis.

The differential diagnosis includes primary or metastatic bone tumors; leukemia; viral or familial hemophagocytic lymphohistiocytosis; storage diseases, such as Gaucher or Niemann-Pick disease; chronic or recurrent multifocal osteomyelitis; and granulomatous infections of mycobacterial or fungal origin.

Severe systemic disease with multiorgan involvement should be treated with chemotherapy. Localized granuloma, if of large size, may be treated with excision and bone grafting; rarely, low-dose radiotherapy also is used. Long-term survival is possible, but bone lesions may recur. Long-term sequelae of the disease or its treatment, such as diabetes insipidus, growth failure, pulmonary fibrosis, and cirrhosis, require ongoing management.

References

Altman AJ (ed): Pediatric oncology. Pediatr Clin North Am 32:541, 1985.

Anonymous: Ewing's sarcoma and its congeners: an interim appraisal. Lancet 339:99, 1992.

Behrman RE (ed): Nelson Textbook of Pediatrics. 14th ed. Philadelphia, WB Saunders, 1992, Sec. 17.1–17.30.

Bergsagel DJ, Finegold MJ, Butel JS, et al: DNA sequences similar to those of simian virus 40 in ependymomas and choroid plexus tumors of childhood. N Engl J Med 25: 988, 1992.

Canellos GP, Anderson JR, Propert KJ, et al: Chemotherapy of advanced Hodgkin's disease with MOPP, ABVD, or MOPP alternating with ABVD. N Engl J Med 327:1478, 1992.

Crist WM, Kun LE: Common solid tumors of childhood. N Engl J Med 324:461, 1991.

Duffner PK, Horowitz ME, Krischer JP, et al: Postoperative chemotherapy and delayed radiation in children less than three years of age with malignant brain tumors. N Engl J Med 328:1725, 1993.

Fernandes ET: Wilms' tumor in children. Int J Pediatr 7: 303, 1992.

Fernbach DJ, Vietti TJ (eds): Clinical Pediatric Oncology. 4th ed. Philadelphia, Mosby-Year Book, 1991.

Link M, Gourin A, Miser A, et al: The effect of adjuvant chemotherapy on relapse-free survival in patients with osteosarcoma of the extremity. N Engl J Med 314:1600, 1986.

Nakagawara A, Arima-Nakagawara M, Scavarda NJ, et al: Association between high levels of expression of the TRK gene and favorable outcome in human neuroblastoma. N Engl J Med 328:847, 1993.

Robertson CM, Stiller CA, Kingston JE: Causes of death in children diagnosed with non-Hodgkin's lymphoma between 1974–1985. Arch Dis Child 67:1378, 1992.

Saha V, Love S, Eden T, et al: Determinants of symptom interval in childhood cancer. Arch Dis Child 68:771, 1993.

Writing Group of the Histiocyte Society. Histiocytosis syndrome in children. Lancet 1:208, 1987.

Yellin A, Mandel M, Rechavi G et al: Superior vena cava syndrome associated with lymphoma. AJDC 146:1060, 1992.

Nephrology: Fluids and Electrolytes

16

John E. Lewy

Renal dysfunction is common in children. *Primary* dysfunction may be due to diseases originating in the kidney (pyelonephritis, Wilms tumor, dysplasia, minimal change nephrotic syndrome); *secondary* dysfunction may be due to systemic illnesses that alter renal function, such as systemic lupus erythematosus (SLE), dehydration (acute tubular necrosis), heart failure (prerenal azotemia), hemolysis (hemoglobinuria), or nephrolithiasis (hyperparathyroidism). Renal involvement may be one manifestation of a systemic disorder (galactosemia, hemolytic–uremic syndrome), or the kidney may be the target organ for immune-mediated injury (poststreptococcal glomerulonephritis), but a limited number of manifestations of either primary or secondary renal disease exist (Table 16–1). Abnormalities of the many functions of the kidney appear predominantly as alterations in urine appearance or volume, and/or disturbances of fluid and electrolyte or acid–base balance. Renal malformations and tumors (see Chapter 15) may be noted as flank or abdominal masses.

Because fetal urine production contributes to amniotic fluid volume, renal anomalies often are associated with reduced amniotic fluid volume, or oligohydramnios. Renal and ureter anomalies are present in 3–4% of infants.

RENAL PHYSIOLOGY

The major functions of the kidney are to maintain body fluid and electrolyte homeostasis and to remove waste products of metabolism. This organ system has metabolic (gluconeogenesis) and endocrine functions (vitamin D activation) that also are important.

Renal blood flow constitutes approximately 20% of cardiac output. The majority of this 20% (approximately 90%) is distributed to the renal cortex. The internal redistribution of blood flow within the kidney as well as the overall renal blood flow itself is affected by the intrarenal production of *prostaglandins*. The autoregulation of regional blood flow,

particularly during sodium depletion and reduced cardiac output, may be critically influenced by *angiotensin II*, a potent renal vasoconstrictor. *Atrial natriuretic peptides* have an important role as vasodilators and natriuretic agents. Autoregulation of renal blood flow is influenced by a feedback mechanism that coordinates alterations in distal tubular flow or sodium concentrations with the release of angiotensin II within the kidney and by changes in arterial smooth muscle tone in response to changes in vascular wall tension.

The major homeostatic functions of the kidney are carried out by the processes of glomerular ultrafiltration, tubular reabsorption, and secretion. *Glomerular ultrafiltration* is the net result of opposing pressures acting within the glomeruli, those pressures moving fluid across the glomerular capillary wall and those opposing this filtration.

Glomerular capillary hydrostatic pressure results from the systemic arterial pressure, which is modified by the afferent and efferent arteriolar tone. Because only minimal amounts of protein are filtered by the glomerulus, the oncotic pressure of the urinary space at the beginning of the proximal tubule generally is zero, and thus the pressure favoring filtration is essentially that of the capillary hydrostatic pressure. The hydrostatic pressure within the lumen of the urinary space of the early proximal tubule plus the mean glomerular capillary oncotic pressure oppose filtration. The hydrostatic pressure remains constant, but the oncotic pressure of the glomerular capillary progressively rises from the afferent to the efferent end as a result of the removal of fluid during filtration. Thus the pressures favoring filtration are maximal at the afferent end of the glomerulus and minimal at the efferent end. Alterations in systemic blood flow or in the internal regulation of glomerular pressures also will alter the glomerular filtration rate. Obstruction of the renal tubules, ureter, or bladder may raise intratubular pressure and retard filtration. Changes in glomerular capillary protein concentration or in the permeability of the capillary wall also affect the glomerular filtration rate.

Table 16–1. Common Manifestations of Renal Disease

Neonate

Flank mass	Dysplasia, polycystic disease, hydronephrosis, tumor
Hematuria	Asphyxia, malformation, trauma
Anuria/oliguria	Agenesis, obstruction, asphyxia

Child and Adolescent

Cola-red–colored urine	Hemoglobinuria (hemolysis); myoglobinuria (rhabdomyolysis); pigmenturia (porphyria, urate, beets, drugs); hematuria (glomerulonephritis, Henoch-Schönlein purpura)
Gross hematuria	Glomerulonephritis, benign hematuria, trauma, cystitis, tumor
Edema	Nephrotic syndrome, nephritis, acute/chronic renal failure, cardiac or liver disease
Hypertension	Acute glomerulonephritis, acute/chronic renal failure, dysplasia, coarctation of the aorta, renal artery stenosis
Polyuria	Diabetes mellitus, central and nephrogenic diabetes insipidus, hypokalemia, hypercalcemia, psychogenic polydipsia, sickle cell anemia, polyuric renal failure, diuretic abuse
Oliguria	Dehydration, acute tubular necrosis, interstitial nephritis, acute glomerulonephritis
Urgency	Urinary tract infection, vaginitis, foreign body

Glomerular filtration begins during the 3rd mo of gestation. Glomerulogenesis is completed at about 34 wk of gestation, and subsequently the glomerular filtration rate increases more rapidly than body size.

Glomerular filtration rate (GFR) is measured most accurately by the infusion of a substance that is freely filtered by the glomerulus but is neither reabsorbed nor secreted, as is inulin. Clinically, creatinine is used to approximate GFR because it is excreted primarily through glomerular filtration and has little tubular reabsorption or secretion except in renal insufficiency. The glomerular filtration rate is calculated as:

$$GFR = \frac{UV}{P} \times \frac{1.73}{SA}$$

in which U = urine creatinine (mg/dL), V = volume collected over time (mL/min), P = serum creatinine (mg/dL), and SA = body surface area. This equation must be corrected for body surface area to achieve the standard nomenclature of mL/min/1.73 m². Creatinine clearance is therefore approximately 40 mL/min/1.73 m² in the full-term newborn. GFR increases during the first 2 yr of life more rapidly than body size and achieves adult values/1.73 m² at this time (110–125 mL/min/1.73 m²). Subsequently GFR and body size increase proportionately and thus GFR/1.73 m² remains stable throughout the remainder of childhood to adulthood (95–105 mL/min/1.73 m²).

Plasma creatinine concentration alone is not an adequate measure of renal function. The "normal" levels of creatinine in most laboratories vary from 0.3 to 1.5 mg/dL, a range that encompasses individuals of all ages and sizes. The plasma creatinine concentration in a newborn equals the maternal value at delivery because of equilibration across the placenta. The neonate's own plasma creatinine is achieved by 2 wk of age in full-term infants.

Plasma creatinine depends on body mass as well as on renal function; hence, normal creatinine concentration is a gradually increasing absolute value throughout childhood. In order to determine the relationship between plasma creatinine and GFR in any given child, one classically must measure creatinine clearance or another indicator of GFR. Because urine collections are somewhat difficult to obtain in the young child, another method is used to estimate glomerular filtration rate: it has been demonstrated that plasma creatinine (P_{CR}), length in centimeters (L), and a constant of proportionality (k) reflect the relationship between urinary creatinine excretion and units of body size. The formula is:

$$GFR \text{ (mL/min/1.73 m}^2\text{)} = k \times L \text{ (cm)} / P_{CR} \text{ (mg/dL)}$$

The value for k is 0.33 in preterm infants, 0.45 in full-term infants, 0.55 in children and adolescent girls, and 0.7 in adolescent boys. This formula is useful only in infants and children whose body habitus is reasonably normal and renal function is stable. Once one has measured or estimated basal GFR and basal plasma creatinine, subsequent plasma creatinine levels can be used to follow changes in renal function over a short period of time.

FUNCTIONAL MORPHOLOGY

The *proximal tubule* is characterized by iso-osmotic reabsorption of the glomerular ultrafiltrate

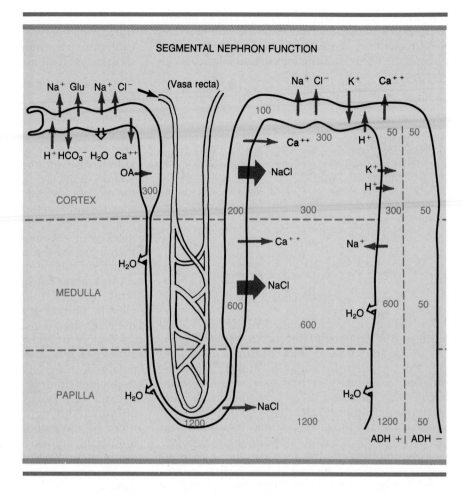

SEGMENTAL NEPHRON FUNCTION

Figure 16–1. Major transport functions of each nephron segment, including representative osmolalities (color) in vasa recta, interstitium, and tubule at different levels within the kidney. Glu, glucose; OA, organic acid. (From Andreoli TE, Carpenter CCJ, Plum F, et al: Cecil Essentials of Medicine. Philadelphia, WB Saunders, 1986, p 185.)

(Fig. 16–1). Normally approximately two thirds of the glomerular ultrafiltrate is reabsorbed from the proximal tubule; a number of solutes, such as glucose and amino acids, are reabsorbed completely, and potassium is reabsorbed nearly completely. Most phosphate also is reabsorbed from the proximal tubule, and calcium is absorbed in parallel with sodium reabsorption. The straight portion of the proximal tubule is responsible for secreting organic acids, including drugs such as penicillin.

The *loop of Henle* serves a major role in that 25% of filtered sodium chloride is absorbed in this segment (Fig. 16–1). Differential permeabilities convert the isotonic fluid entering the loop of Henle from the proximal tubule into a hypotonic fluid delivered to the distal tubule. Preferential sodium chloride absorption (probably associated with active chloride transport) is the principal mechanism by which the countercurrent multiplier is activated and by which the medullary interstitial hypertonicity, required for urinary concentration, is accomplished. This principally occurs in the thick ascend-

ing limb. Salt and water movement across the thin limbs is driven primarily by osmotic gradients.

The *distal tubule* is made up of the *distal convoluted tubule,* which is water impermeable and continues to carry out the dilution of luminal fluid by way of active sodium chloride absorption, and the *collecting ducts,* which are the primary sites of *antidiuretic hormone* (ADH) activity. These distal segments are the site of potassium secretion, which is virtually all the potassium excreted within the nephron system. Hydrogen ion secretion, which is responsible for the final acidification of the urine, also occurs at the distal convolution. The processes of sodium reabsorption and potassium and hydrogen ion secretion all are stimulated by aldosterone.

The maximum *urinary concentrating capacity* is less in the newborn (600–800 mOsm/L in the full-term newborn and approximately 400 mOsm/L in the preterm infant) than in children older than 1 yr of age (greater than 1200 mOsm/L). The neonate's ability to dilute the urine is fully developed, but the capacity to excrete a water load is quantitatively less. The newborn exhibits numerous other quantitative limitations, which include the rate of excretion of sodium, potassium, hydrogen ion, and phosphate, but renal functions are qualitatively operative.

References

Behrman RE (ed): Nelson's Textbook of Pediatrics. 14th ed. Philadelphia, WB Saunders, 1992, Sec. 6.8, 18.1–18.2.
Jones DP, Chesney RW: Development of tubular function. Clin Perinatol 19:33, 1992.
Robillard JE, Segar JL, Smith FG, et al: Regulation of sodium metabolism and extracellular fluid volume during development. Clin Perinatol 19:15, 1992.

CONGENITAL AND DEVELOPMENTAL ABNORMALITIES OF THE URINARY TRACT

Bilateral renal agenesis, which occurs in 1:4000 births, is due to failure of development of or degeneration of the ureteric bud. Features associated with this condition are **Potter syndrome** (flat facies, clubfoot, pulmonary hypoplasia) resulting from oligohydramnios and fetal compression by the uterus (see Chapter 19). Infants with bilateral renal agenesis usually die of respiratory insufficiency in the 1st wk of life as a result of pulmonary hypoplasia, pneumothoraces, and pulmonary hypertension. *Unilateral renal agenesis* (1:1000 births) is associated with compensatory hypertrophy in the contralateral kidney and normal or minimally reduced renal function. Although this condition is compatible with normal renal function and normal life expectancy, an associated incidence of other abnormalities exists with unilateral renal agenesis, including abnormalities of the genital tract, skeletal system, and cardiovascular system. Unilateral renal agenesis also has been described as a component of the VATER association, Turner syndrome, and Poland syndrome.

Renal hypoplasia refers to kidneys that are present but small in size, which, because of their reduced renal mass, over time predispose a child to progressive renal insufficiency. Hypoplastic kidneys frequently are scarred and difficult to distinguish from those that are chronically infected. Renal hypoplasia also may be associated with poor growth, which is most common in the second decade of life.

Renal dysplasia usually is unilateral and may be associated with hypoplasia. It is a developmental abnormality with abnormal organization and ductal differentiation. A majority of children with this disorder have obstructive anomalies of the urinary tract. It has been suggested that obstruction early in gestation is the primary factor that leads to the dysplastic changes.

Cystic Dysplasias of the Kidney

Polycystic kidney disease is an inherited disease affecting both kidneys. The two major forms include an autosomal recessive type, "infantile" polycystic kidney disease, and an autosomal dominant type, "adult" polycystic disease. The two conditions differ morphologically and clinically, although both may occur in infancy or in older children. The *autosomal recessive,* or infantile, type is characterized by marked enlargement of both kidneys with innumerable cysts throughout the cortex and medulla, which are dilated collecting ducts. Interstitial fibrosis and tubular atrophy may not be present at birth but progress with time, frequently to renal failure. Hepatic fibrosis is present and may lead to portal hypertension. Bile duct ectasia and biliary dysgenesis also occur. The kidneys of the newborn with the autosomal recessive form are spongy and markedly enlarged and maintain the usual renal configuration; older children have less severe cyst formation but still show progressive renal fibrosis and tubular atrophy. Although this form can be diagnosed in utero by ultrasonography, many of the live-born infants die in the neonatal period, often from respiratory distress resulting from pulmonary hypoplasia. Eighty percent of infants have clinical manifestations, such as flank mass, hepatomegaly, pneumothorax, proteinuria, or hematuria. Intravenous pyelography (IVP) reveals opacification of dilated collecting ducts, which appear as radial streaks. Treatment of this condition is supportive, including the management of hypertension and renal failure. The prognosis is poor, in terms of both renal insufficiency and hepatic fibrosis. Renal transplantation and portosystemic shunts may be beneficial.

The *autosomal dominant,* or adult, type of polycystic kidney disease characteristically appears in the fourth or fifth decade of life, but also occurs in infancy or childhood. Infants have a clinical picture similar to that of autosomal recessive polycystic kidney disease, but older children may show a pattern similar to that of adults. *Renal biopsy* shows a predominantly glomerular pattern of cyst formation. Family history is positive. Hepatic cysts are present in this disease but they usually are not of clinical significance, whereas cerebral aneurysms are common; splenic and pancreatic cysts also occur.

References

Behrman RE (ed): Nelson's Textbook of Pediatrics. 14th ed. Philadelphia, WB Saunders, 1992, Sec. 18.17, 18.34.

Chevalier RL, Garland TA, Buschi HA: The neonate with autosomal dominant polycystic kidney disease. Int J Pediatr Nephrol 2:73, 1981.

Kissane JM: Renal cysts in pediatric patients. A classification and overview. Pediatr Nephrol 4:69, 1990.

Vesicoureteral Reflux

Vesicoureteral reflux, the abnormal backflow of urine from the bladder to the ureter or kidney, usually results from a congenital incompetence of the vesicoureteral junction or, less often, from incompetence of the junction secondary to obstruction or infection. Reflux may be familial.

Pathophysiology. Reflux is potentially harmful because of the exposure of the kidney to *increased hydrodynamic pressure* during voiding. In addition, the incomplete emptying of the ureter and bladder on voiding predisposes the patient to *urinary tract infection* because, in the presence of lower urinary tract infection, reflux allows bacteria to gain access easily to the pelvocalyceal system. *Reflux nephropathy* refers to the development and/or progression of *renal scarring*, often secondary to prolonged reflux, particularly if associated with infection or obstruction (bladder neck obstruction or posterior urethral valves). A significant number of children have end-stage renal disease as a result of reflux nephropathy, which also may be an important precursor to hypertension.

The normal vesicoureteral junction prevents reflux because of the oblique entry of the ureter into the bladder, the length of the ureteral tunnel traversing the bladder wall, and the 4–5:1 ratio of the length of this tunnel to the ureteral diameter. Primary reflux results from a short intramural tunnel ratio, as low as 1.5:1, and is characteristically associated with a lateral position of the ureteral orifice and an underdeveloped trigone. The shortened intramural tunnel decreases the efficiency of the valvular mechanism, allowing reflux to occur. Less often, duplications of the ureters that also exhibit ureterocele may obstruct the upper collecting system. Reflux may be associated with ureteral diverticulum. Abnormalities of the neurogenic bladder associated with myelomeningocele are complicated by reflux in approximately one third to one half of affected children. Reflux also may be secondary to increased intravascular pressure when the bladder outlet is obstructed, to inflammation of the bladder (cystitis), or to surgical procedures performed on the bladder.

Clinical Manifestations. Reflux is characteristically discovered during radiologic evaluation following a urinary tract infection. Severe reflux may begin in utero and be associated with neonatal renal insufficiency resulting from renal parenchymal loss. A high incidence of reflux also occurs in neonates with urinary tract infection. Reflux may resolve with time. Females up to 1 yr of age have a 57% incidence, whereas reflux is noted in 36% of girls between 2 and 16 yr of age. Males 2–12 mo and 2–16 yr of age have a 30% and an 18% frequency of reflux, respectively. The finding of reflux has been associated with the finding of renal scars, on Tc-dimercaptosuccinic acid (DMSA) renal scan, in children with urinary tract infection. A 15% incidence of scars exists in patients with grade 1 reflux, 18% in grade 2, 27% in grade 3, and 64% in grade 4 or 5 (Fig. 16–2). Long-term follow-up (7–15 yr) demonstrated that the reflux ceased in 89% of patients with grade 1, in 86% with grade 2, in 83% with grade 3, but in only 41% of those with grade 4 (or 5) reflux. The *voiding cystourethrogram* should be performed approximately 3–4 wk after an acute

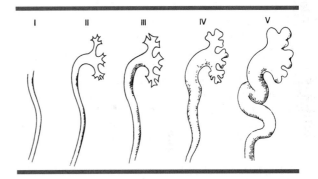

Figure 16–2. International Classification of Vesicoureteral Reflux: Grade I, ureter only. Grade II, ureter, pelvis, and calyces. No dilation, normal calyceal fornices. Grade III, mild to moderate dilation and/or tortuosity of the ureter, and mild to moderate dilation of the renal pelvis; slight or no blunting of the fornices. Grade IV, moderate dilation or tortuosity of the ureter and moderate dilation of the renal pelvis and calyces. Complete obliteration of sharp angle of fornices but maintenance of the papillary impressions in the majority of calyces. Grade V, gross dilation and tortuosity of the ureter. Gross dilation of the renal pelvis and calyces. The papillary impressions are no longer visible in most of the calyces. Some authors consider grade IV or V with intrarenal reflux into the collecting ducts a high risk for scarring. (From Duckett JW, Bellinger MF: Cystographic grading of primary reflux as an indicator of treatment. In Johnston JH [ed]: Management of Vesicoureteral Reflux. International Perspectives in Urology. Vol 10. Baltimore, Williams & Wilkins, 1984; with permission.)

urinary tract infection, because the passage of that amount of time allows resolution of the mucosal changes (edema) present during the active infection that may lead to *transient* reflux.

Treatment. The finding of reflux indicates the need for long-term prophylactic antibiotic therapy that includes trimethoprim–sulfamethoxazole, sulfisoxazole, or nitrofurantoin. The urine should be cultured frequently (at monthly intervals) at the onset of therapy. When a cumulative number of three monthly cultures are negative, cultures can be repeated at 3-mo intervals. As noted above in grade 1 through grade 3 reflux, if IVP or nephrosonography is normal, reflux generally disappears with time. More severe reflux, which is associated with significant ureteral dilation or upper tract changes on IVP or renal ultrasound or scan, frequently requires surgical intervention. In general, reflux of any grade found on voiding cystourethrography associated with a normal nephroson organ or scan can be treated medically with long-term prophylactic antibiotics and serial urine cultures. However, if the IVP or renal scan reveals renal scarring and dilation or clubbing of the pelvocalyceal system, surgical intervention most likely is indicated at the outset. Surgical intervention also is employed commonly if reinfection occurs while the patient is on antibiotics. Surgical intervention clearly is needed if the reflux is associated with a ureterocele or other urinary tract obstruction. The presence of grade 4 to grade 5 reflux and the failure of medical management to resolve reflux over several years remain controversial indications for medical or surgical treatment.

Complications of reflux nephropathy include hypertension and end-stage renal disease. The latter is predicted by proteinuria (>1 g/day) and is due to the development of focal and segmental *glomerulosclerosis* and interstitial scarring.

Urinary Tract Obstruction

Obstruction of the urinary tract may occur at any anatomic level of the genitourinary system (Table 16–2). Severe obstruction early in gestation is thought to result in **renal dysplasia**. Ureteral obstruction later in fetal life or after birth results in dilation of the ureter and collecting system, often with alterations in renal parenchyma that may range from dilation to scarring and glomerular atrophy. The obstructed urinary tract is susceptible to infections, which may further complicate the problem.

Table 16–2. Site and Etiology of Urinary Tract Obstruction

Site	Etiology
Infundibula	Congenital
	Calculi
	Infection
	Trauma
	Tumor
Pelvis	Congenital stenosis
	Infection
	Calculi
	Tumor
Ureteropelvic junction	Congenital stenosis*
	Calculi
	Tumor
	Trauma
Ureter	Obstructive megaureter*
	Ectopic ureter
	Ureterocele
	Valves
	Calculi*
	Primary renal tumor (Wilms tumor)
	Retroperitoneal tumor (lymphoma)
	Inflammatory bowel disease
	Retroperitoneal fibrosis
	Chronic granulomatous disease
Bladder	Neurogenic dysfunction*
	Tumor (rhabdomyosarcoma)
	Diverticula
	Ectopic ureter
Urethra	Posterior valves*
	Diverticula
	Strictures
	Atresia
	Ectopic ureter
	Foreign body
	Phimosis*

* Relatively common.

Clinical Manifestations. Obstructions may be silent but usually are discovered as a urinary tract infection or flank masses. In a newborn, bilateral abdominal masses frequently are hydronephrotic kidneys.

Diagnosis. *Intravenous urography* and *voiding cystourethrography* have been the standard tests for diagnosis of urinary tract obstruction, but a marked reduction in renal function often is associated with poor or nonvisualization of the kidney on the IVP. *Renal ultrasound* facilitates the identification of renal agenesis, renal hypoplasia, or cystic changes in the presence of obstruction, scarring, and dilation. The dilated upper urinary tract may or may not be obstructed. The radioisotope (hippuran) renogram, particularly used in conjunction with a diuretic, frequently can allow differentiation of patients with a dilated urinary tract, which empties rapidly, from those with obstruction. Technetium-99m–labeled DMSA (dimercaptosuccinic acid) scans are the most useful test to evaluate for the presence of renal scars.

Obstruction of the urinary tract may be at multiple anatomic levels (Table 16–2). An obstruction of the ureteropelvic junction is the most common lesion in childhood. Such an obstruction may present as a palpable renal mass, urinary tract infection, hematuria (with or without trauma), or flank pain or may be discovered on routine fetal ultrasonography. Twenty percent of ureteropelvic junction obstructions are bilateral.

Treatment.   An obstructed ureteropelvic junction requires surgery. The success rate of pyeloplasties in relieving obstruction is high, although the dilated calyces may persist.

Obstructions of the ureter also may occur at midureter or at the lower ureter in association with a ureterocele or with an ectopic ureteral orifice, which, in turn, frequently is associated with reflux. Ectopic ureters may drain a single collecting system or drain the upper portion of a duplicated collecting system. Ectopic ureters frequently are obstructed and require prompt surgical intervention.

Prune Belly Syndrome (Eagle-Barrett Syndrome)

The absence or severe reduction in abdominal musculature associated with undescended testes and urinary tract abnormalities occurs in approximately 1:40,000 births. The characteristic dilatation of the prostatic urethra without posterior urethral valves suggests severe, but possibly transient, urethral obstruction in fetal life. The reduced abdominal musculature may be due to transient tense fetal ascites. Oligohydramnios and pulmonary hypoplasia may be present.

Urinary abnormalities include marked dilation of the ureters and calyceal system, a large bladder, and often a patent urachus. The kidneys may be dysplastic and the testes usually are undescended in the abdomen. Anomalies of the bowel, heart, and musculoskeletal system may occur. The condition is rare in females. There usually is no demonstrable obstruction of the urinary tract at birth. Initial *treatment* consists of stabilization of the cardiopulmonary status and prevention of urinary tract infection. Renal ultrasound, measurement of renal function, renal scan, and voiding cystourethrogram facilitate full assessment of the abnormalities. Therapy then is individualized in order to maintain renal function and prevent infection.

Posterior Urethral Valves

This is the most common cause of **bladder outlet obstruction** in males, present in 1:50,000 boys. The valves are sail-shaped membranes that arise from the verumontanum and attach to the contralateral wall of the urethra. In the presence of persistent valves, the prostatic urethra becomes dilated, vesicoureteral reflux may be present, and a small bladder with hypertrophied walls develops. Renal dilation varies in degree from mild hydronephrosis to severe hydronephrosis with dysplasia. Severe obstruction may be associated with oligohydramnios and subsequent lethal pulmonary hypoplasia. The male infant may present in the newborn period with a urinary tract infection, bilateral flank masses (hydronephrosis), a poor voiding stream, or little urinary output. Rupture of the renal pelvis will produce **urinary ascites**, the most common cause of ascites in the newborn period. A child may come to medical attention later in infancy with a poor urinary stream, failure to thrive secondary to renal failure, urinary tract infection, or renal tubular acidosis. Infants with pulmonary hypoplasia usually die within 2 days of life.

The *diagnosis* and extent of renal damage are established by ultrasonography and by voiding cystourethrography. Many infants are diagnosed prior to birth by fetal ultrasonography. Once the infant is medically stabilized, *treatment* consists of either preliminary decompression and/or valve ablation, depending on the individual circumstances. Valve ablation is successful in most infants, and the serum creatinine returns to normal by 1 yr of age. Children having persistent elevated creatinine levels also may have associated renal dysplasia. Immediately after relief of the obstruction, a marked diuresis resulting from a defect in urine concentration often may be present.

References

Behrman RE (ed): Nelson Textbook of Pediatrics. 14th ed. Philadelphia, WB Saunders, 1992, Sec. 18.39–18.42.

Jakobsson B, Söderlundhs S, Bert U: Diagnostic significance of ^{99m}Tc-dimercaptosuccinic acid (DMSA) scintigraphy in urinary tract infections. Arch Dis Child 67:1138, 1992.

Swartz GW, Brion LT, Spitzer A: The use of plasma creatinine concentration for estimating glomerular filtration rate in infants, children and adolescents. Pediatr Clin North Am 34:571, 1987.

DISTURBANCES OF ELECTROLYTES, ACID–BASE BALANCE, AND FLUIDS

Because sodium is the principal extracellular cation, regulation of extracellular fluid parallels regulation of sodium balance. Sodium conservation is regulated by receptors in the juxtaglomerular apparatus that sense hypovolemia or decreased effective renal blood flow and respond by releasing renin. Renin acts on angiotensinogen to produce angiotensin I. Angiotensin-converting enzyme then converts angiotensin I to angiotensin II, which stimulates the release of aldosterone. Aldosterone increases distal tubule sodium reabsorption. In conditions of severe sodium restriction, decreased intravascular volume (hemorrhage, sepsis), or decreased effective renal blood flow (heart failure), the urinary excretion of sodium approaches zero. In addition, baroreceptors in the atria, aortic arch, carotid bifurcations, and pulmonary vessels also sense volume depletion and signal the brain via cranial nerves IX and X. This signaling results in increased central nervous system (CNS) efferent sympathetic discharge, which regulates renal blood flow, vascular resistance, angiotensin II, and, thus, aldosterone release; the net result is sodium conservation.

The ADH system also senses volume changes. In conditions of hypovolemia, ADH, which will increase renal reabsorption of water, is released. Usually, this system functions to conserve osmolality, because ADH secretion is stimulated during normovolemic states characterized by high serum osmolality.

Parenteral Fluid Therapy

Illnesses that result in imbalances in fluids and electrolytes are a greater risk for children than for adults. The younger the child, the greater the vulnerability to such disturbances because of the larger daily turnover of water relative to the total body water, the large extracellular fluid space, and the developmental limitations of renal function. The untoward effects of vomiting (reduced intake) and diarrhea (increased losses) appear much more rapidly in the infant than in the adult.

Fluid and electrolyte requirements and their provision are conveniently considered in terms of *maintenance, deficit,* and *supplemental* therapy. Therapeutic plans based on calculations of these needs must be modified constantly based on a continuing clinical reassessment of the child's physical and mental status and the serial monitoring of serum electrolytes, acid–base balance, blood urea nitrogen, and serum creatinine.

MAINTENANCE THERAPY

Ongoing obligatory normal and abnormal losses of fluids and electrolytes from urine, sweat, feces, and lung must be replaced so that deficits will not occur. Disease states may modify the amount and type of such losses. Protein and calories also must be replaced when oral intake is restricted for a protracted time (see Chapter 2). Losses should be replaced orally, when possible, or by intravenous administration.

Maintenance requirements of fluid and electrolytes are directly related to metabolic rate. An increased metabolic rate increases catabolism of metabolic fuels. This leads to increases in the rate of production of water of oxidation from carbohydrate, fat, and protein; in urinary excretion of solute and water; and in heat production, which increases water loss in sweat and respiratory gases. The turnover rates of electrolytes also are related closely to water loss and metabolic rate. Thus, maintenance requirements for fluid and electrolytes can be calculated from a child's caloric expenditures.

Calculation of Normal Maintenance Requirements

A child's metabolic rate or caloric expenditure will depend on age, body weight, degree of activity, temperature, and any pathologic state. Adjustments above basal caloric expenditures for activity are made by observing the patient. Although no increase above the basal level is needed for adjustments in calculations for patients in coma, usual bed activity increases basal caloric expenditure by 25–30%. Fever increases basal caloric expenditure by about 12%/1° C rise in temperature, and salicylism and hyperthyroidism increase it by 25–75%. Conversely, hypothermia results in similar decreases in caloric expenditure per incremental fall in temperature, and hypothyroidism results in a 10–25% decrease in basal metabolism.

Table 16–3 provides a simplified means of calculating expenditure for the average hospitalized child (non-neonate) engaged in the usual bed activity. Additional adjustments should be made for further activity, temperature, and disease states. The usual fluid and electrolyte losses that occur for each

Table 16–3. Calculation of Caloric Expenditure from Body Weight

Body Weight (kg)	Caloric Expenditure*
Up to 10	100 kcal/kg
11–20	1000 kcal + 50 kcal/kg for each kg above 10 kg
Above 20	1500 kcal + 20 kcal/kg for each kg above 30 kg

* 1 kcal (kilocalorie) = 1000 calories.
(Modified from Holliday and Segar: In Nelson Textbook of Pediatrics. 14th ed. Philadelphia, WB Saunders, 1992, p 196.)

100 kcal metabolized then also can be estimated. Using this approach for replacing losses resulting from ongoing metabolism, 100 mL of fluid should be provided for every 100 kcal expended, and the solution should contain 35 mEq of sodium and 20 mEq of potassium per liter, and 5% dextrose. This approach to providing maintenance requirements assumes there is no kidney damage or disease state that would limit renal capacity to adjust urine flow rates and electrolyte excretion over wide ranges.

Modification of Maintenance Therapy as a Result of Disease

Maintenance requirements are decreased (30–45 mL/100 kcal of exogenous water to replace insensible water losses is required) in conditions of anuria or extreme oliguria or when excessive or inappropriate release of ADH occurs, such as during meningitis; and for children who are in congestive heart failure. Requirements for fluid and electrolytes are increased as a result of abnormal losses from gastrointestinal drainage, heat stress, adrenal insufficiency, diabetes mellitus, hyperventilation, loss of renal concentrating and diluting ability, hypothalamic diabetes insipidus, and burns. The amount and nature of the losses depend on the underlying disorder and the site of the loss.

DEFICIT THERAPY

Deficits in body water and electrolytes occur from decreased intake and continuing normal losses, from increased losses with or without the usual intake, or from a combination of these events. Because deficits reflect ongoing physiologic readjustments as well as direct losses, the amount of the deficits often is similar for a variety of precipitating conditions; therefore, they usually can be treated in a similar manner. Fluid and electrolyte treatment is related to a greater extent to the sever-

ity and type of deficit than to the underlying cause. The etiology also must be addressed specifically.

Severity (Table 16–4)

A loss of body weight greater than 1%/day reflects a loss of body water. The more rapidly a deficit develops, the less well it will be tolerated. Severe dehydration is frequently associated with shock, but even moderate deficits may cause circulatory instability if they develop over the course of a day.

Pathophysiologic Types of Dehydration

Deficits from dehydration are classified as isonatremic (130–150 mEq serum Na^+/L), hyponatremic (<130 mEq Na^+/L), or hypernatremic (>150 mEq Na^+/L). Because plasma osmolality usually mirrors sodium concentration, these forms usually are isotonic, hypotonic, and hypertonic, respectively. This may not be the case when another serum solute such as glucose is elevated, as occurs in diabetic ketoacidosis, which may result in hyponatremia and hypertonicity.

In isonatremic dehydration, approximately proportional fluid and electrolyte losses occur from the extracellular compartment, and because no resulting osmotic gradient across the cell walls takes place, intracellular fluid volume is not significantly changed. In hypernatremic dehydration, more water than sodium is lost from the extracellular space, or excess sodium is provided, increasing the osmolality of this fluid and causing water to move out of cells, a movement that adds to the extracellular volume so that its depletion is less than expected. In hypotonic dehydration, relatively more sodium than water is lost from the extracellular space, or excess water is provided. This leads to movement of water into cells, which further depletes the extracellular fluid, aggravating circulatory insufficiency.

Clinical Assessment of Deficit

The history is the first critical step in this evaluation. Table 16–5 indicates some of the important information that should be sought. For example, a history of fever and high-solute feedings in the presence of watery diarrhea favors hypernatremic dehydration. Physical examination may be complementary to the history and may be particularly helpful in characterizing the severity of dehydration (Table 16–6). Laboratory data may reflect hemoconcentration, although this may be masked by pre-existing anemia or malnutrition. Blood urea ni-

Table 16–4. Assessment of Degree of Dehydration

	Mild	**Moderate**	**Severe**
Infant	5%	10%	15%
Adolescent	3%	6%	9%
Signs and Symptoms			
General appearance and condition			
Infants/young children	Thirsty; alert; restless	Thirsty; restless or lethargic but irritable or drowsy	Drowsy; limp, cold, sweaty, cyanotic extremities; may be comatose
Older children	Thirsty; alert; restless	Thirsty; alert (usually)	Usually conscious (but at reduced level), apprehensive; cold, sweaty, cyanotic extremities; wrinkled skin on fingers/toes; muscle cramps
Tachycardia	Absent	Present	Present
Palpable pulses	Present	Present (weak)	Decreased
Blood pressure	Normal	Orthostatic hypotension	Hypotension
Cutaneous perfusion	Normal	Normal	Reduced/mottled
Skin turgor	Normal	Slight reduction	Reduced
Fontanel	Normal	Slightly depressed	Sunken
Mucous membrane	Moist	Dry	Very dry
Tears	Present	Present/absent	Absent
Respirations	Normal	Deep, may be rapid	Deep and rapid
Urine output	Normal	Oliguria	Anuria/severe oliguria

(Modified from World Health Organization Guide.)

trogen may be increased as a result of decreased blood flow and enhanced recycling of urea if the circulation is compromised, and creatinine levels usually are increased as a result of a decrease in glomerular filtration. Urine usually is concentrated and may transiently contain abnormal amounts of protein, casts, and cells. Serum electrolytes and acid–base data will reflect specific deficits and their etiologies.

Table 16–5. Historic Data for Evaluating Deficits

Weight change (preillness vs. dehydrated weight)
Intake—quantity and composition of fluids and solids (including drugs) taken during illness
Output—quantity and pattern of output or urine, emesis, diarrhea, sweating, and drainage during illness
General medical status—respiratory function, cardiovascular status, renal function, central nervous system disease, and metabolic state (temperature) are especially relevant

(Modified from Behrman RE [ed]: Nelson Textbook of Pediatrics. 14th ed. Philadelphia, WB Saunders, 1992, p 199.)

SUPPLEMENTAL THERAPY

In certain disorders, specific fluids and electrolytes may be needed in addition to those required to replace deficits and maintain homeostasis. For example, in pyloric stenosis, sodium and potassium should be replaced as chloride salts because of gastric losses of hydrochloric acid, and burns may require special replacement of the plasma lost by surface oozing or ultrafiltrate sequestrations around the burn site as well as renal nitrogen losses.

PRINCIPLES OF THERAPY

Shock always must be treated as a medical emergency, with intravenous or, rarely, with intraosseous infusions (see Chapter 3). *Oral rehydration* may be appropriate in patients with mild to moderate dehydration (Table 16–7); this decision requires judgment about the etiology of the illness, the child's condition, and the capacity of the care givers to provide adequate supervision of care.

Table 16–6. Typical Patterns of Physical Signs in Moderate–Severe Dehydration

Sign	Isonatremic	Hyponatremic	Hypernatremic
Skin			
Color	Gray	Gray	Gray
Temperature	Cold	Cold	Cold
Turgor	Poor	Very poor	Fair
Feel	Dry	Clammy	Thick, doughy
Mucous membrane	Dry	Dry	Parched
Eyeball	Sunken and soft	Sunken and soft	Sunken
Fontanel	Sunken	Sunken	Sunken
State of consciousness	Lethargic	Very lethargic	Hyperirritable
Pulse	Rapid	Rapid	Moderately rapid
Blood pressure	Low	Very low	Moderately low

(Modified from Behrman RE [ed]: Nelson Textbook of Pediatrics. 14th ed. Philadelphia, WB Saunders, 1992, p 200.)

Intravenous therapy should be provided for children when there is shock, severe dehydration, uncontrollable vomiting, diarrhea exceeding 10 mL/kg/hr, extreme fatigue, stupor, coma, severe gastric distention, or other serious complications. The goal of *initial therapy* is to treat or prevent shock by rapidly expanding the vascular volume by administering 10–30 mL/kg of an electrolyte solution, such as isotonic saline (0.9%; Na^+ and Cl^- both 155 mEq/L) or Ringer lactate. This solution is given immediately, even before knowing electrolyte values, because it is equally appropriate for iso-, hypo-, or hypernatremic dehydration and usually will return the serum sodium toward normal. It is given as rapidly as possible for shock or over 1–3 hr for less severely ill patients. Ordinarily 20 mL/kg will re-store circulatory stability; if signs of shock persist, a second infusion of fluid (10–30 mL/kg) may be needed.

When the circulation is stabilized, *subsequent treatment* is directed at correcting the remaining water and sodium deficits and replacing ongoing abnormal and obligatory losses. Treatment usually is based on knowing serum electrolytes. Unless hypokalemia is demonstrated or a condition known to be associated with severe potassium losses is present (pyloric stenosis, prolonged diarrhea, diabetic acidosis), potassium losses are not replaced until urinary output is established.

Isonatremic Dehydration

In this condition, sodium is lost from the extracellular space to the external environment and to the intracellular space, where it moves to compensate for intracellular potassium losses. To avoid subsequent overexpansion of the extracellular space after replacement of potassium as a result of sodium shift from the cells, one half of the deficit is replaced in the first 12-hr period, one quarter in the second, and one quarter in the third 12-hr period. In addition, the child should receive replacements for both ongoing normal losses (maintenance water, sodium, and potassium) and continuing abnormal losses during this 24-hr period.

Subsequently, there should be 100% replacement of losses. Careful monitoring of weight is the best guide to successful fluid replacement. Serum electrolytes also should be monitored. Potassium losses should be replaced slowly (over 36–48 hr) to avoid hyperkalemia. Potassium concentration in intravenous fluids should usually not exceed 40 mEq/L at a rate not greater than 3 mEq/kg/24 hr.

Table 16–7. Oral Rehydration*

Status†	Mild Dehydration	Moderate Dehydration
Initial	50 mL/kg (over 4 hr)	100 mL/kg (over 6 hr)
Subsequent‡	100 mL/kg/24 hr	100 mL/kg/24 hr

* Amounts and rates should be increased or decreased based on evaluation of patient. Breast feeding or plain water should be offered as needed.

† World Health Organiztion oral rehydration solution (ORS) is composed of 2 g glucose (CHO)/100 mL, 90 mEq Na^+/100 mL, 20 mEq K^+/100 mL, and 30 mEq HCO_3^-/100 mL. In the United States, commercially available oral rehydration solutions for the first 12 hr contain 2.0–2.5 g CHO/100 mL, 75 mEq Na^+/100 mL, 20 mEq K^+/100 mL, and 30 mEq HCO_3^-/100 mL. Solutions for subsequent use contain 2.0–2.5 g CHO/100 mL, 45–50 mEq Na^+/100 mL, 20 mEq K^+/100 mL, and 30 mEq HCO_3^-/100 mL.

‡ Continue until diarrhea stops. Volume of ORS ingested should equal volume of stool losses. If losses cannot be measured, administer 10–15 mL ORS/kg/hr. Weigh child for best estimate of loss and repair.

Disturbances of Sodium

HYPONATREMIA (Na$^+$ <130 mEq/L)

Etiology and Pathophysiology.   Reduced serum sodium content usually is associated with one of three mechanisms (Fig. 16–3). Because sodium is the main extracellular fluid cation, hyponatremia usually is associated with hypo-osmolality. Occasionally, *pseudohyponatremia* is noted with isotonicity when plasma protein or triglyceride levels are elevated, or with hyperosmolality when hypertonic infusions (mannitol, diatrizoate sodium) are given or during hyperglycemia. For every 100-mg/dL increment of glucose, sodium will decline by 1.6

mEq/L. *Hyperosmolar hyponatremia* is due to osmotic fluid shifts from the intracellular space to the extracellular space, whereas *isosmolar hyponatremia* is due to an artifact of the laboratory analysis of sodium that measures the sodium content in serum drawn off after centrifugation, which contains both the plasma water and that component represented by excess lipid (hyperlipidemia) or protein (macroglobulinemia). Because sodium is present only in plasma (or serum) water and not in the lipid phase, measurements based on total volume (flame ionization) but not on plasma water will yield pseudohyponatremia.

One frequent etiology of true hyponatremia is the **syndrome of inappropriate ADH** secretion

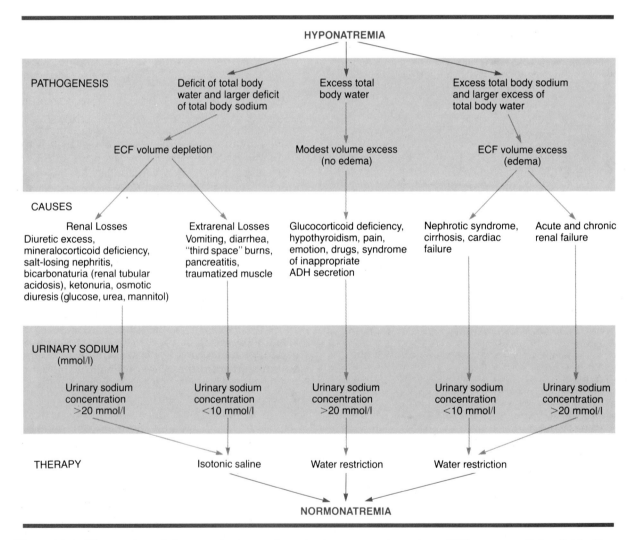

Figure 16–3. Diagnostic and therapeutic approach to the hyponatremic patient. ECF = extracellular fluid. (From Schrier RW, Berl T: Disorders of water metabolism. In Schrier RW [ed]: Renal and Electrolyte Disorders. 2nd ed. Boston, Little, Brown & Co., 1980.)

(SIADH), which may be due to a variety of disorders, including unregulated tumor production of ADH-like peptides, pulmonary disorders (pneumonia, positive end-expiratory pressure ventilation, asthma, cystic fibrosis, pneumothorax), inappropriate hypothalamic–pituitary release of ADH related to a perceived volume deficit, drugs (vincristine, opiates, carbamazepine, cyclophosphamide), and direct irritation of the CNS (meningitis, encephalitis, hemorrhage, hypoxia, trauma).

Hyposmolal hyponatremia accompanied by increased extracellular volume also is common in various edematous states, such as cardiac failure or cirrhosis. In these states, water retention may be due to a combination of reduced effective plasma volume, which is sensed by the aortic and carotid baroreceptors, and increased activity of the juxtaglomerular apparatus, which signals both ADH and renin secretion. The net result is both water and sodium retention and, thus, the formation of edema. Water retention in excess of sodium produces hyponatremia. This often is intensified when natriuretic (diuretic) agents are prescribed and the fluid intake is hyponatremic.

Hyponatremia occurs in infants as a result of excessive dilution of formula caused by errors in formula preparation and by intentional formula dilution for the treatment of diarrhea or for reasons of financial difficulty. Hyponatremic dehydration may result during diarrhea when fluid replacement is more hypotonic than the diarrheal losses.

Clinical Manifestations.   The symptoms of hyponatremia may include lethargy, apathy, disorientation, muscle cramps, anorexia, and agitation. The signs may include reduced mental status, decreased deep tendon reflexes, hypothermia, seizures, and pseudobulbar palsies. No clinical manifestations may be apparent. Symptoms rarely occur unless the serum sodium level falls below 120 mEq/L.

Treatment.   The treatment to be used depends on the mechanism of hyponatremia and presence or absence of serious clinical manifestations (Fig. 16–3). Acute-onset hyponatremia is more likely to be symptomatic than chronic stable hyponatremia. Initial therapy should be calculated to raise the serum Na$^+$ to 120 mEq/L rapidly, which usually will stop the seizures. Subsequent correction to 130 mEq Na$^+$/L can be carried out over the next 24–36 hr. Rapid correction to levels greater than 130 mEq/L may rarely be associated with severe adverse effects, such as central pontine myelinolysis. Most patients with *acute SIADH* respond to fluid restric-

tion, although sodium chloride infusion may be needed if hyponatremia is symptomatic.

Hyponatremic dehydration requires both sodium and fluid replacement in addition to the provision of supplements for ongoing losses and maintenance. Therapy is similar to that for isonatremic dehydration except that, when calculating the sodium to be infused, the extra loss of this ion should be taken into account. This replacement usually should be spread over 36 hr. The sodium deficit in hyponatremic dehydration can be estimated by using the following equation:

$$(\text{Desired Na}^+ - \text{current Na}^+) \times 0.6$$
$$\times \text{ wt (kg)} = \text{mEq required}$$

Symptomatic hyponatremia may be treated with hypertonic (3%) saline (or normal saline) to raise the serum to 120 mEq/L.

In situations of symptomatic hyponatremia without edema but with excess total body water, water diuresis may be helpful (diuretics). The volume of diuresis needed to correct hyponatremia may be calculated by using the following equation:

$$\text{Total body water (TBW)} = 0.6 \times \text{wt (kg)}$$

$$\text{Excess water} = \text{TBW} - \frac{\text{current Na}^+}{\text{desired Na}^+} \times \text{TBW}$$

With this regimen, urine electrolytes also must be replaced with 3% or normal saline and sufficient KCl to avoid additional electrolyte depletion.

HYPERNATREMIA (Na$^+$ >150 mEq/L)

Etiology and Pathophysiology.   The serum sodium level is regulated by both ADH secretion and thirst. High serum sodium may be due to water loss in excess of sodium loss (increased insensible water losses), insufficient ADH production (central diabetes insipidus) or reduced renal response to ADH (nephrogenic diabetes insipidus), poor response to thirst (hypodipsia), salt poisoning, or, less likely, excessive sodium retention (Fig. 16–4).

Central diabetes insipidus (absent ADH release) may be acquired (CNS trauma, tumor, autoimmunity, infection, hypoxia, histiocytosis) or hereditary and associated with craniofacial anomalies. *Nephrogenic diabetes insipidus* (absent or reduced renal response to ADH) may be due to renal pathology (interstitial nephritis, acute tubular necrosis), electrolyte disorders (hypercalcemia, hypokalemia), or drugs (lithium, demeclocycline) or may be hereditary. The hereditary illness appears in infants and is associated with polyuria, polydipsia,

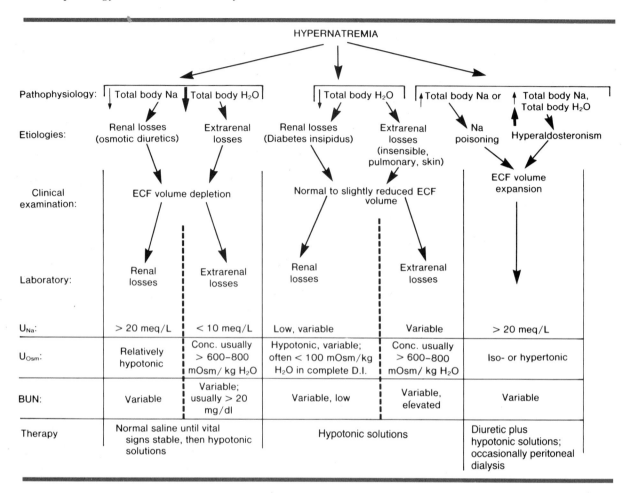

	HYPERNATREMIA				
Pathophysiology:	↓ Total body Na ↓ Total body H₂O		↓ Total body H₂O	↑ Total body Na or	↑ Total body Na, Total body H₂O
Etiologies:	Renal losses (osmotic diuretics)	Extrarenal losses	Renal losses (Diabetes insipidus)	Extrarenal losses (insensible, pulmonary, skin)	Na poisoning Hyperaldosteronism
Clinical examination:	ECF volume depletion		Normal to slightly reduced ECF volume		ECF volume expansion
Laboratory:	Renal losses	Extrarenal losses	Renal losses	Extrarenal losses	
U_{Na}:	> 20 meq/L	< 10 meq/L	Low, variable	Variable	> 20 meq/L
U_{Osm}:	Relatively hypotonic	Conc. usually > 600–800 mOsm/ kg H₂O	Hypotonic, variable; often < 100 mOsm/kg H₂O in complete D.I.	Conc. usually > 600–800 mOsm/ kg H₂O	Iso- or hypertonic
BUN:	Variable	Variable; usually > 20 mg/dl	Variable, low	Variable, elevated	Variable
Therapy	Normal saline until vital signs stable, then hypotonic solutions		Hypotonic solutions		Diuretic plus hypotonic solutions; occasionally peritoneal dialysis

Figure 16–4. Approach to hypernatremia. BUN = blood urea nitrogen; ECF = extracellular fluid; U_{Na} = urinary sodium; U_{Osm} = urinary osmolality; ↓ Less reduction; ↓ more severe reduction. (From Norman M: In Fleisher G, Ludwig S [eds]: Textbook of Pediatric Emergency Medicine. Baltimore, Williams & Wilkins, Inc., 1983, p 423.)

dehydration, fever, and growth and developmental retardation; males have a complete deficit, whereas females have a partial disorder.

Hypernatremic dehydration may occur in infants with a poor thirst mechanism or in breast-fed neonates of mothers whose milk supply is inadequate, if these children have limited supplemental fluid intake. Failure to thrive, dehydration, hyperglycemia, and prerenal azotemia are common associated findings. Infants with diarrhea and fever or those exposed to excessive environmental heat lose water in excess of sodium, placing them at risk for hypernatremia, if fluid replacement is hypertonic to losses.

Clinical Manifestations. The signs and symptoms relate to the primary disorder, dehydration. In hypernatremic dehydration, intravascular vol-

ume is conserved as a result of the hyperosmotic state, which results in a shift of water from the intracellular to the extracellular space. Therefore, the signs of dehydration are not as apparent as they are for an equivalent degree of isotonic dehydration. Based on skin turgor, tachycardia, and blood pressure, the severity of dehydration may be underestimated. Weight change remains the most reliable indicator of the degree of dehydration. Patients with salt poisoning may present in shock with seizures.

Treatment. *Hypernatremic dehydration* requires replacement of water in excess of sodium, which must be done carefully, because rapidly lowering serum sodium will lower serum osmolality faster than intracellular osmolality is lowered, resulting in fluid crossing the cell membrane into the cell to re-establish osmotic equilibrium. This produces cellular swelling, which, in the brain, may result in cerebral edema. Hemorrhage and thrombosis also may occur when the correction is too rapid, further contributing to the risk of seizures, coma, and death. Therefore, the serum sodium level should be lowered slowly toward normal at a rate of not more than 10 mEq/L/24 hr. The water deficit in hypernatremic dehydration can be estimated by using the following equation:

$$\text{Normal TBW} = 0.6 \times \text{normal weight (kg)}$$

$$\frac{\text{Normal Na}^+}{\text{Current Na}^+} \times \text{TBW} = \text{current TBW}$$

$$\text{Deficit} = \text{normal TBW} - \text{current TBW}$$

The total fluid deficit should be corrected over 36–48 hr.

Central *diabetes insipidus* requires ADH replacement. Nephrogenic diabetes insipidus will not respond to ADH and is treated with a low-salt and high-water diet. Chlorothiazides may reduce urine output in children with nephrogenic diabetes insipidus by reducing intravascular volume, which may enhance proximal tubular salt and water reabsorption.

Disturbances of Potassium

HYPOKALEMIA (K$^+$ <3.0 mEq/L)

Etiology and Pathophysiology. Reduced serum potassium concentration may be due to redistribution between the large intracellular potassium compartment and the smaller extracellular potassium space. Shifts of transcellular potassium from serum to cells are noted with acute alkalosis, insulin therapy, sympathomimetic agents, vitamin B$_{12}$ therapy, and familial hypokalemic periodic paralysis.

Net renal loss of potassium is associated with the use of most diuretics, gentamicin, amphotericin B, cisplatinum, excessive mineralocorticoid administration, renal disease such as renal tubular acidosis, hypomagnesemia, and **Bartter syndrome**. The latter is characterized by hypokalemic, hypochloremic metabolic alkalosis, hyperaldosteronism, hyperreninemia, increased urine chloride excretion, growth failure, normal blood pressure, hyperplasia of the juxtaglomerular apparatus, and increased urine prostaglandin E$_2$ excretion. It may be caused by a defect in chloride reabsorption in the ascending loop of Henle. Bartter syndrome is exhibited in infancy as failure to thrive, salt craving, polyuria, muscle weakness, tetany, and constipa-

tion. *Gastrointestinal losses,* such as vomiting (which also results in renal potassium wasting secondary to alkalosis) and diarrhea in previously healthy children, frequently result in hypokalemia.

Clinical Manifestations. The manifestations of hypokalemia include ileus, muscle weakness, nephrogenic diabetes insipidus, areflexic paralysis, and, especially with the use of digitalis, arrhythmias. The electrocardiogram in hypokalemia reveals ST segment depression, T wave reduction, and an elevated U wave. An approach to the evaluation of patients with hypokalemia is presented in Figure 16–5.

Treatment. The type of treatment selected depends on the underlying etiology. Renal and gastrointestinal loss usually can be replaced by providing additional KCl administered orally or intravenously. Bartter syndrome is treated with prostaglandin synthetase inhibitors (indomethacin, ibuprofen) together with KCl and a potassium-sparing diuretic. Total potassium losses should be replaced slowly to avoid hyperkalemia, because potassium must pass through the extracellular space in order to replete the larger intracellular deficits.

HYPERKALEMIA (K$^+$ >5.5 mEq/L)

Increased serum potassium may be due to transcellular shifts, increased potassium loss from cells, or decreased excretion (Table 16–8). The *clinical manifestations* of hyperkalemia include paresthesias, weakness, flaccid paralysis, and cardiac arrhythmias. The earliest electrocardiographic sign of hyperkalemia is peaked or tented T waves (K$^+$ 5.5–7.0 mEq/L). Higher levels (7.0–8.0 mEq/L) are associated with a prolonged P-R interval, ST depression, and the initial widening of the QRS complex. The P wave may flatten as the potassium level increases. When the potassium level exceeds 8.0 mEq/L, the P wave may disappear and the QRS complex widens and merges with the T wave, producing a sine wave pattern. Without treatment, asystole or ventricular fibrillation may occur. Hyponatremia, hypocalcemia, and acidosis intensify hyperkalemic cardiac effects.

The *treatment* of hyperkalemia includes providing measures to directly antagonize the membrane effects (calcium), redistribute potassium to the intracellular space (sodium bicarbonate, albuterol, glucose, with or without insulin), or remove potassium from the body. The administration of calcium gluconate, sodium bicarbonate, albuterol, and glucose is a temporary measure that must be followed

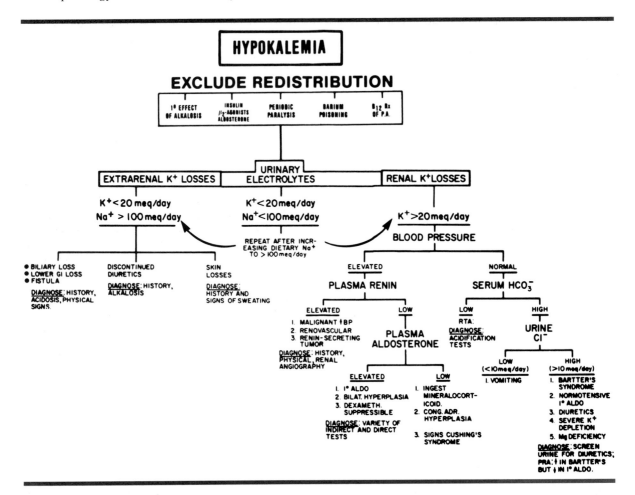

Figure 16–5. Diagnostic approach to hypokalemia. ALDO = aldosteronism; BP = blood pressure; CONG. ADR. = congenital adrenal; GI = gastrointestinal; PA = pernicious anemia; PRA = plasma renin–angiotensin; RTA = renal tubular acidosis; 1° = primary. (From Narins RG, Jones ER, Stom MC, et al: Diagnostic strategies in disorders of fluid, electrolyte, and acid-base homeostasis. Am J Med 72:496, 1982.)

by procedures to remove potassium from the body. This can be accomplished by providing peritoneal dialysis, hemodialysis, or forced diuresis, or by administering a cation exchange resin (Kayexalate) that exchanges sodium for potassium and binds potassium, which then is eliminated in the stool.

Disturbances of Acid–Base Balance

Maintaining acid–base balance depends acutely on respiratory compensation (Table 16–9) and the tissue buffering capacity of hemoglobin, albumin, bicarbonate, and bone. More chronic mechanisms involve increased renal excretion or reabsorption of bicarbonate by adding or subtracting bicarbonate molecules to or from the buffering system. Pure acid–base disturbances are due to alterations of only one of these functions, resulting in primary metabolic acidosis or alkalosis or primary respiratory acidosis or alkalosis. Compensating mechanisms rarely completely correct a pure disorder, but they can provide significant improvement of pH. Mixed disturbances involve two or more primary disorders, such as occurs in a patient who has mixed respiratory–metabolic acidosis following a cardiopulmonary arrest.

METABOLIC ALKALOSIS

A net gain of base or a net loss of acid produces metabolic alkalosis (Table 16–10). In time, renal compensation occurs unless these renal mecha-

Table 16–8. Etiology of Hyperkalemia

Transcellular Shift
Acute acidosis, hyperkalemic familial periodic paralysis

Increased Endogenous Cell Release
Hemolysis, rhabdomyolysis, lysis of massive leukocytosis (leukemia)

Decreased Excretion
Renal failure
Reduced renin–aldosterone production (Addison disease, adrenal genital syndrome, hypoaldosteronism, hyporeninemia)
Reduced tubular excretion (sickle cell anemia, SLE, obstructive uropathy, postrenal transplant)
Inhibition of tubular secretion by drugs (digitalis, spironolactone, amiloride, angiotension-converting–enzyme inhibitors

nisms encounter interference from factors that maintain the alkalosis. For example, loss of hydrochloric acid from gastric emesis in patients with pyloric stenosis increases serum pH and bicarbonate levels. Increased renal bicarbonate excretion should correct the disorder. However, in the presence of volume contraction, reduced effective renal blood flow, and reduced GFR, a hyperaldosterone state will develop and decreased bicarbonate filtration and increased bicarbonate reabsorption will take place. Furthermore, the accompanying hypokalemia, when severe, results in increased hydrogen ion excretion in the distal tubule, with the net effect of additional bicarbonate reabsorption and **paradoxic aciduria.** The final result is an inability to excrete the excessive amount of serum bicarbonate with persistent metabolic alkalosis.

The *clinical manifestations* of metabolic alkalosis include mental confusion, tetany, poor cardiac output, enhanced digitalis toxicity, hypoventilation, and a shift of the hemoglobin oxygen curve to the left. The *treatment* of a metabolic alkalosis depends on the cause. Most cases caused by diuretics, vomiting, bicarbonate therapy, or nasogastric tube losses are "chloride responsive" and can be treated primarily with normal saline, and, if needed, KCl. Chloride repletion results in enhanced renal bicarbonate excretion. Rarely, ammonium chloride is needed in acutely symptomatic patients. "Chloride-unresponsive" patients may be hypertensive (primary hyperaldosteronism, Cushing syndrome) or normotensive (Bartter syndrome, magnesium deficiency, severe hypokalemia) and require specific therapy for these disease states.

Table 16–9. Characteristics of Primary Acid–Base Disturbances

Disorder	Etiology	Example	Compensation Mechanisms	Prediction of Pure Compensation
Metabolic				
Acidosis	$\downarrow HCO_3^-$	Hypoxia, drug ingestion	$\downarrow P_{CO_2}$ (acute) $\uparrow$ renal bicarbonate reabsorption (late)	1 mEq fall of HCO_3^- = 1–1.3 mm Hg fall of P_{CO_2}
Alkalosis	$\uparrow HCO_3^-$ $\downarrow HCl$	$\uparrow$ Bicarbonate/citrate pyloric stenosis	$\uparrow P_{CO_2}$ (acute), renal bicarbonate excretion (late)	P_{CO_2} increases 6 mm Hg for 10-mEq increase of HCO_3^-
Respiratory				
Acidosis				
Acute (hr)	$\uparrow P_{CO_2}$	Hypoventilation	$\uparrow HCO_3^-$ (renal)	HCO_3^- increases 1 mEq/L for each 10 mm Hg P_{CO_2}
Chronic (days)	$\uparrow P_{CO_2}$	BPD, cystic fibrosis	$\uparrow HCO_3^-$ (renal)	HCO_3^- increases 3–3.5 mEq/L for 10 mmHg of P_{CO_2}
Alkalosis				
Acute (hr)	$\downarrow P_{CO_2}$	Mechanical ventilation for $\uparrow$ intracranial pressure, hysteria	$\downarrow HCO_3^-$ (renal)	HCO_3^- falls 2.5 mEq/L for 10 mmHg of P_{CO_2}
Chronic (days)	$\downarrow P_{CO_2}$	Persistent mechanical ventilation	$\downarrow HCO_3^-$ (renal)	HCO_3^- falls 5 mEq/L for 10 mmHg of P_{CO_2}

BPD = bronchopulmonary dysplasia.
(Data from Narins R: In Maxwell M, Kleeman C, Narins R: Clinical Disorders of Fluid and Electrolyte Metabolism. 4th ed. New York, McGraw-Hill, 1987; and DuBose T: Med Clin North Am 67:799, 1983.)

Table 16–10. Etiology of Metabolic Alkalosis

Initiation	Maintenance	Maintenance Mechanism	Urine Chloride	Example
Loss of Acid				
GI tract	(1) Volume contraction	(1) ↑ tubular HCO_3^- reabsorption	<10 mEq/L	Pyloric stenosis
	(2) Decreased GFR	(2) ↑ fractional HCO_3^- reabsorption		Congenital chloride diarrhea
	(3) Chloride depletion	(3) ↓ GFR, ↓ Cl^- causes ↑ H^+ secretion; ↑ renin		
Renal sodium delivery to tubule	K^+ depletion plus those for GI tract	↑ Aldosterone, ↑ H^+ secretion plus above	>20 mEq/L on diuretics, <10 mEq/L off therapy	Diuretics
Hyperreninemic states	As above	As above	>20 mEq/L	Bartter syndrome; primary hyperaldosteronism; Licorice ingestion
High mineral-corticoid states				Renal artery stenosis
Gain of Base				
Alkalizing salts	Volume contraction	As above plus continued source	>20 mEq/L	Milk alkali syndrome
	Continued base therapy, K^+ deficit	As above		Citrate in blood products
Posthypercapnic State				
	Volume contraction; decreased GFR; K^+ and Cl^- depletion	As above	<10 mEq/L	Slow correction of chronic respiratory acidosis

GI = gastrointestinal.

(Data from Cogan M., et al: Med Clin North Am 67:903, 1983; and Sabatin S, Kurtzman N: In Maxwell M, Kleeman C, Narins R: Clinical Disorders of Fluid and Electrolyte Metabolism. 4th ed. New York, McGraw-Hill, 1987.)

METABOLIC ACIDOSIS

Loss of bicarbonate in gastrointestinal fluid (diarrhea) or urine and either endogenous acid production (retention as in uremia) or exogenous acid administration (salicylate toxicity) are the predominant etiologies of metabolic acidosis. The **anion gap** can be useful to differentiate bicarbonate loss from net acid gain as the etiology of acidosis (Table 16–11). In the presence of acidosis, the undetermined anion above the normal range (10–15 mEq/L) is considered to be net acid gained. If the anion gap is normal, bicarbonate loss by the gastrointestinal system or kidney is the probable cause.

Lactic acidosis is a frequent cause of a net increase of endogenous acid production and is the result of multiple pathophysiologic mechanisms (Table 16–12).

The *clinical manifestations* of metabolic acidosis may include tachycardia, ventricular arrhythmias, reduced cardiac contractility, Kussmaul respiration, abdominal pain, increased serum uric acid, and hyperkalemia. The *treatment* of increased anion gap acidosis depends on the underlying disease and would include insulin for diabetic ketoacidosis; dialysis for uremia; oxygen for carbon monoxide poisoning; removal of toxins (e.g., salicylate); and provision of sodium bicarbonate when acidosis is severe or not rapidly corrected by the above measures. The dose of bicarbonate may be calculated by the following equation:

$$(\text{Normal } HCO_3^- - \text{current } HCO_3^-)$$

$$\times\ 0.3 \times \text{wt (kg)}$$

Overalkalinization should be avoided because it

Table 16–11. Acidosis and the Anion Gap*

Increased Anion Gap without Acidosis
Decreased calcium, magnesium, potassium, and other *cations*
Increased albumin, other *anions*; high-dose carbenicillin

Increased Anion Gap with Acidosis
Increased endogenous anions: lactate, sulfate, phosphate (uremia), ketones (diabetes)
Increased exogenous acids: salicylate, methanol, ethanol, paraldehyde

Normal Anion Gap with Acidosis
Bicarbonate losses; diarrhea, renal tubular acidosis, carbonic anhydrase inhibitor, ureterosigmoidostomy, dilutional acidosis, pancreatic fistula

Decreased Anion Gap without Acidosis
Increased calcium, potassium, magnesium, bromide
Decreased albumin

* Normal anion gap = $Na^+ - (Cl^- + HCO_3^-)$ = 12 mEq/L.
(Adapted from Oh W, Carroll H: N Engl J Med 297:814, 1977.)

has detrimental effects, such as hypokalemia, reduced oxygen dissociation from hemoglobin, and further stimulation of lactate production. Partial correction of the acidosis is preferable while treating the underlying cause. Most children with diabetic ketoacidosis do not require bicarbonate because ketone body metabolism in the presence of insulin regenerates bicarbonate in the Kreb cycle. Intravenous bicarbonate in these patients may produce metabolic alkalosis and complicate recovery.

RENAL TUBULAR ACIDOSIS

Renal tubular acidosis (RTA) is a condition characterized by hyperchloremic normal anion gap aci-

Table 16–12. Etiology of Lactic Acidosis

Type A	
Tissue hypoxia	Shock, asphyxia, carbon monoxide toxicity
Type B	
Systemic disorders	Diabetes mellitus, renal failure, hepatic failure, malignancy, seizures, gut flora that produce D-lactate
Drugs	Biguanides, fructose, ethanol, salicylate, methanol, ethylene glycol
Inborn errors	Type I glycogen storage disease, pyruvate carboxylase deficiency, pyruvate dehydrogenase deficiency; mitochondrial myopathy, lactic acidemias, and other mitochondrial defects

dosis, which results from impaired renal acidification. Three distinctive types of renal tubular acidosis have been established: type I is distal renal tubular acidosis, type II is proximal renal tubular acidosis, and type IV is renal tubular acidosis associated with a mineralocorticoid deficiency. A type III was proposed but is most likely a variant of type I.

Proximal RTA results from reduced proximal tubular reabsorption of bicarbonate, either as a result of a failure of hydrogen ion secretion proximally or as a result of deficient carbonic anhydrase activity. Normally 85% of the filtered bicarbonate is reabsorbed in the proximal tubule. In this condition, reabsorption is reduced to 60% or less. Distal tubular bicarbonate reabsorption cannot fully compensate for this load, and, therefore, considerable filtered bicarbonate is excreted. The serum bicarbonate falls until it reaches the new bicarbonate threshold, at which time bicarbonate wasting ceases. When the serum bicarbonate reaches this level (approximately 15–16 mmol/L), bicarbonate reabsorption now can be considered complete. The urine may become acidified, because distal hydrogen ion secretion is normal. Severe hypokalemia is often an associated finding, because potassium rather than hydrogen ion is secreted concomitantly with sodium reabsorption at distal sites. Extracellular fluid contraction stimulates increased sodium chloride reabsorption, resulting in hyperchloremia, which, in turn, results in secondary hyperaldosteronism, increasing potassium wasting.

Proximal RTA occurs as a primary disease, as a part of the *Fanconi syndrome*, and in a variety of other conditions (Table 16–13). Fanconi syndrome may be idiopathic or associated with the other causes of proximal RTA. In Fanconi syndrome, a defect exists (often reversible) in proximal tubular reabsorption of glucose, phosphate, and amino acids. This is associated with proximal RTA and a defect in vitamin D metabolism, leading to reduced levels of 1,25-$(OH)_2$ vitamin D. Primary proximal RTA tends to occur more commonly in males; patients have been noted to improve with age.

Distal RTA results from an inability of the distal nephron to secrete hydrogen ion, preventing the reabsorption of the final 15% of bicarbonate (which reaches the distal tubule) and also the final acidification of the urine. In this condition, the urinary pH cannot be reduced below 5.5–6.0, despite severe systemic acidosis. Hyperchloremia and hypokalemia accompany distal RTA, although the hypokalemia is less severe than in proximal RTA. Distal RTA may be an isolated primary defect inherited as either an autosomal dominant or an autosomal

Table 16–13. Etiology of Proximal Renal Tubular Acidosis

Idiopathic or Primary
Sporadic
Fanconi syndrome

Secondary Metabolic Diseases
Cystinosis
Tyrosinemia
Galactosemia
Hereditary fructose intolerance
Type I glycogen storage disease
Lowe syndrome
Wilson disease
Osteopetrosis (carbonic anhydrase deficiency)

Drugs and Toxins
Heavy metals (lead, cadmium, mercury)
Outdated tetracycline
Carbonic anhydrase inhibitors
Vitamin D deficiency or altered metabolism

Miscellaneous
Hyperparathyroidism
Dysproteinemic states (monoclonal gammopathy)
Interstitial nephritis (renal transplant rejection, renal vein thrombosis)
Nephrotic syndrome
Prematurity
Pregnancy

recessive trait, or it may occur in association with a variety of disorders (Table 16–14). All forms of distal RTA may be complicated by nephrocalcinosis.

Mineralocorticoid deficiency, type IV RTA, results from inadequate production of or reduced responsiveness to aldosterone. It is associated with hyperkalemic and hyperchloremic acidosis. This disorder may be primary or secondary to adrenal disease or parenchymal kidney damage. *Hyporeninemic hypoaldosteronism* is another form of type IV RTA that also may result from renal disease associated with interstitial damage.

Clinical Manifestations. Children with RTA usually present with growth failure and acidosis. If Fanconi syndrome is present, rickets, nausea, anorexia, and intermittent vomiting may also occur. Hypokalemia produces muscle weakness and polyuria. Patients with systemic acidosis and alkaline urine whose bicarbonate level is below 15 mEq/L most likely have distal RTA. In children with proximal RTA, the urine becomes acidified when the bicarbonate threshold is attained. Primary RTA must be differentiated from secondary RTA because the latter requires specific therapy of the underlying disorder. For example, removal of galac-

tose (galactosemia) or fructose (hereditary fructose intolerance) from the diet reverses acquired Fanconi syndrome.

Diagnosis. Children with mild acidosis can be tested by an *ammonium chloride loading test,* which should be performed carefully by an experienced observer because severe acidosis can result. In children who have proximal RTA, the urine will acidify, whereas those who have distal RTA maintain an alkaline urine. This test also can be used to distinguish the source of a hyperchloremic metabolic acidosis. Normal patients and those with a gastrointestinal bicarbonate loss will have a negative *urine anion gap* ($Na^+ + K^+ - Cl^-$); those with renal tubular acidosis will have a positive gap. Normal patients have no defect in urine acidification and, in response to ammonium chloride loading, will increase chloride (measured) and ammonium (undetermined), thus producing a negative number. Patients with RTA will not excrete the positive am-

Table 16–14. Etiology of Distal Renal Tubular Acidosis

Primary or Idiopathic
Sporadic
Familial

Secondary Inherited Diseases
Osteopetrosis
Sickle cell anemia
Wilson disease
Hypercalciuria

Hypercalciuria/Nephrocalcinosis
Hyperparathyroidism
Hypervitaminosis D
Hyperthyroidism
Medullary sponge kidney

Drugs and Toxins
Amphotericin B
Toluene
Amiloride
Lithium

Interstitial Renal Disease
Chronic pyelonephritis
Obstructive nephropathy
Renal transplantation rejection
Hyperoxaluria

Autoimmune and Hypergammaglobulinemic States
SLE
Chronic active hepatitis
Cryoglobulinemia
Primary biliary cirrhosis
Sjögren syndrome
Thyroiditis
Pulmonary fibrosis

monium ion, the lack of which then produces a positive urine anion gap.

Treatment.   The goal of therapy is to correct the acidosis and achieve normal childhood growth. A sodium citrate–citric acid combination (Shohl solution; Bicitra) is administered that contains 1 mEq of Na citrate/mL of solution. Potassium supplementation is also given in the form of Polycitra, which contains 1 mEq/mL of sodium citrate and 1 mEq/mL of potassium citrate. Distal RTA requires a smaller dose of alkalinizing agents, which is equal to endogenous acid production (3–5 mEq/kg/day). However, because the urine cannot be acidified, nephrocalcinosis is common. Larger doses of alkali are required in proximal RTA to correct the acidosis because of the constant bicarbonate wasting resulting from the inability to reabsorb filtered bicarbonate. Proximal RTA, however, is more likely to resolve than is distal RTA. Type IV RTA most commonly results from obstructive uropathy and resolves after the obstruction is corrected. Mineralocorticoid therapy may be needed for type IV RTA associated with aldosterone deficiency.

References

Bartter F, Schwartz W: The syndrome of inappropriate secretion of antidiuretic hormone. Am J Med 42:790, 1967.

Battle D, Hizon M, Cohen E, et al: The use of the urinary anion gap in the diagnosis of hyperchloremic metabolic acidosis. N Engl J Med 318:594, 1988.

Behrman RE (ed): Nelson Textbook of Pediatrics. 14th ed. Philadelphia, WB Saunders, 1992, Sec. 6.2–6.29.

Bidani A: Electrolyte and acid base disorders. Med Clin North Am 70:1013, 1986.

Boineau F, Lewy JE: Maintenance fluids and the management of diarrheal dehydration. Pediatr Ann 10:8, 15, 1981.

Carvana R, Buckalew V: The syndrome of distal (type 1) renal tubular acidosis. Medicine 67:84, 1988.

Gill JR Jr, Frolich JC, Bowden RE, et al: Bartter's syndrome: A disorder characterized by high urinary prostaglandins and a dependence of hyperreninemia on prostaglandin synthesis. Am J Med 61:43, 1976.

Harrington J, Cohen J: Measurement of urinary electrolyte—indications and limitations. N Engl J Med 293: 1241, 1975.

Oh M, Cavrol H: Anion gap. N Engl J Med 297:814, 1977.

Rodriguez-Soriano J, Vallo A: Renal tubular acidosis. Pediatr Nephrol 4:268, 1990.

RENAL DISEASES

Approach to the Child with Hematuria

When hematuria is a chief complaint, it generally is gross hematuria (seen with the naked eye), but microscopic hematuria may be the initial manifestation observed during routine urinalysis. Microscopic hematuria is defined as greater than 5 red blood cells per high-power field in freshly voided and centrifuged urine.

The child who presents with gross hematuria needs prompt evaluation. The child with microscopic hematuria, no proteinuria, normal blood pressure, and normal renal function should have the urinalysis repeated. If the hematuria persists, further evaluation is appropriate. The first step in evaluating the child with hematuria is taking a careful history, performing a physical examination, and examining the urine. *The presence of red urine but a negative microscopic examination* and negative dipstick for blood suggests that the red urine has been caused by a substance that has colored the urine, as might occur from the child's ingesting medications such as acetophenetidin, which has a metabolite that produces a dark wine–brown color; from toxins such as benzene or carbon tetrachloride, both of which produce a red–brown color; from food dyes (beets); or from rifampin (orange–red color). The color also might be due to the side effects of treatment, such as occurs after deferoxamine administration, or due to poisoning with heavy metals, such as lead, which produces a red–brown coloration of the urine. Urates are a common cause of an orange–red discoloration on the diaper of infants.

If the *urine tests positive for blood but no red blood cells are seen* when the urine is promptly examined, the presence of free hemoglobin or myoglobin should be suspected. **Hemoglobinuria** may be present secondary to hemoglobin excretion from acute intravascular hemolysis (e.g., glucose-6-phosphate dehydrogenase deficiency or paroxysmal nocturnal hemoglobinuria) or from intravascular coagulation (e.g., sepsis, hemolytic–uremic syndrome). It may be seen in freshwater drowning, mismatched blood transfusions, and other causes of hemolysis. Rhabdomyolysis and **myoglobinuria** (from a crush injury, burns, myositis, asphyxia) also must be considered.

If examination of the urine reveals the presence of a *significant number of red blood cells but no casts* are observed, one must consider bleeding beyond the glomerulus and renal tubules. However, it is important to remember that casts as well as red cells will hemolyze on standing, particularly in dilute urine, and they also can be missed if the urine is not examined with reduced light and shortly after voiding.

Another mechanism for localizing hematuria to the glomerulus is by examining the morphology of

Table 16–15. Differential Diagnosis of Proteinuria and Hematuria

Proteinuria	Hematuria	Edema	Etiologies
Yes	No	No	Exercise, orthostatic (intermittent or fixed) fever, dehydration; benign; reflux nephropathy; focal segmental sclerosis; SLE
Yes	Yes	No/Mild	Acute glomerulonephritis, IgA nephropathy (Berger disease), Henoch-Schönlein purpura, hemolytic uremic syndrome, endocarditis, hereditary nephritis; interstitial nephritis; SLE, severe exercise
Yes	No	Yes	Minimal lesion (change) nephrotic syndrome; focal segmental sclerosis
Yes	Yes	Yes	Acute glomerulonephritis, atypical minimal lesion nephrotic syndrome, membranoproliferative (mesangiocapillary) glomerulonephritis, membranous nephropathy
No	Yes	No	Benign hematuria, IgA nephropathy, hereditary nephritis, sickle cell anemia, tumor, trauma, interstitial nephritis, nephrolithiasis, idiopathic hypercalciuria

the red blood cells. Carefully examining the urine by phase-contrast microscopy frequently documents altered red cell morphology in glomerular hematuria, whereas morphology characteristically is unaltered when nonglomerular causes are present. However, the absence of casts or the absence of alterations in red blood cell morphology by no means excludes a glomerular etiology.

The presence of *red cells in the absence of casts* is seen in some patients with hematuria associated with sickle cell trait or disease, in some children following marked exercise, or in patients after renal trauma. The presence of a coagulopathy (acute or inherited) may be associated with hematuria, although bleeding from the urinary tract in the absence of bleeding into other organ systems (e.g., skin or joints) is unusual. A family history of hematuria, renal failure, or deafness or the finding of hematuria on a urinalysis performed on siblings or parents suggests the possibility of a familial nephritis. Hypercalciuria is an important cause of isolated hematuria in children; 25–30% of children with isolated hematuria have calcium excretion rates greater than 4 mg/kg/24 hr and/or urinary calcium-to-creatinine ratios greater than 0.2:1.

Urolithiasis is an uncommon cause of hematuria, although it may be seen in children who have idiopathic hypercalciuria, in children who have been immobilized for long periods of time, and in those with urinary tract malformations and recurrent infections. Idiopathic nephrolithiasis does occur with uric acid, calcium oxalate, and ammonium acid urate stones, but it is uncommon. Nephrocalcinosis also may be seen in distal RTA, cystinuria, hyperoxaluria, the milk alkali syndrome, and other uncommon conditions.

A benign (hemangioma, hamartoma) or malignant (Wilms) *tumor must be excluded in patients with*

hematuria. Urinary tract infection *may be associated with hematuria;* therefore, a urine culture is an important part of evaluating a child with hematuria. The differential diagnosis of hematuria and its association with proteinuria and edema is noted in Table 16–15. The minimal screening evaluation is noted in Table 16–16.

Congenital obstructions of the kidney, cystic disease, infiltrative processes (e.g., leukemia), and severe reflux each may be exhibited in association with hematuria. Nephrosonography or IVP is an important part of evaluating the child with hematuria to assess these possibilities. *Interstitial nephritis,* which may be drug induced or idiopathic, also may be associated with hematuria, eosinophilia, and urinary eosinophils without casts.

If the urinalysis reveals the presence of *hematuria and casts,* one of a variety of glomerular diseases should be considered. Glomerular injury may be the result of immunologic injury (e.g., acute poststreptococcal glomerulonephritis), inherited disease (e.g., Alport syndrome), or vascular injury (e.g., acute tubular or cortical necrosis).

Table 16–16. Basic Work-up of the Child with Hematuria

1. *History:* Present, past, family
2. *Physical Examination:* Height, weight, blood pressure, optic fundi, presence or absence of abdominal mass, skin appearance, genitalia, edema, complete physical examination
3. *Laboratory:* Urinalysis, urine culture, CBC, smear, platelets, serum BUN, creatinine, calcium, streptozyme, serum complement (C3 as screen), quantitative urinary protein, calcium and creatinine, intravenous pyelogram and/or nephrosonogram

BUN = blood urea nitrogen; CBC = complete blood count.

MICROSCOPIC HEMATURIA WITH CASTS OR ALTERED RED CELL MORPHOLOGY BUT LITTLE OR NO PROTEINURIA

Immunoglobulin A Nephropathy (Berger Disease)

Microscopic hematuria or recurrent gross hematuria (the more usual of the two) shortly following an upper respiratory infection (1–2 days) and not associated with the signs and symptoms of an acute nephritic syndrome (edema, hypertension, renal insufficiency) suggests the possibility of immunoglobulin (Ig) A nephropathy or "benign" recurrent familial or nonfamilial idiopathic hematuria (see below). The cause of Berger disease is not known, but a consistent finding on renal biopsy is the presence of mesangial proliferation accompanied by mesangial deposits of IgA and variable deposition of IgG and IgM. The course generally is benign in children but may be associated with recurrent bouts of hematuria following or during respiratory infections. Berger disease is not inherited, is more common in males than in females, and is characteristically associated with normal renal function and normal serum levels of C3. Although the prognosis is good in children, progressive disease has been demonstrated to develop in about 20% of adults. No therapy currently is known that alters the course of the disease. The presence of IgA in a skin biopsy suggests a possible relationship of this condition to Henoch-Schönlein purpura with nephritis.

Idiopathic Hematuria

Idiopathic hematuria may be familial or nonfamilial. Benign familial hematuria is a common nonprogressive, autosomal dominant disorder, demonstrating thinning of the glomerular basement membrane on electron microscopy. Renal biopsy in patients with the nonfamilial form may be normal or reveal only mild mesangial hypercellularity. Patients who have **Alport syndrome** often present with microscopic hematuria. This familial disorder is associated with progressive bilateral neurosensory deafness (high tones) after age 6 yr and progressive renal failure during adolescence and young adulthood, particularly in males. Ocular findings include cataracts, keratoconus, and spherophakia. Electron microscopy of the renal biopsy reveals characteristic splitting and layering of the basement membrane of the glomerulus. The prognosis for patients with nonfamilial or the non-

Alport form of idiopathic familial hematuria is excellent, but long-term follow-up is required to exclude the progressive forms of familial hematuria.

HEMATURIA WITH CASTS AND MILD TO MODERATE PROTEINURIA

Children who have hematuria associated with casts and less than 1 g of proteinuria/m^2/day usually have nephritis.

Acute Poststreptococcal Glomerulonephritis

This disorder is the prototype of the acute nephritic syndrome. Acute glomerulonephritis (AGN) is associated with a sudden onset of gross hematuria in approximately two thirds of children, edema in three fourths, and hypertension in one half and with variable degrees of renal insufficiency.

Etiology and Pathophysiology. AGN characteristically follows streptococcal pharyngitis or impetigo–pyoderma by 7–21 days. Only certain strains of group A beta-hemolytic streptococci are nephritogenic. Acute poststreptococcal glomerulonephritis is immunologically mediated by activation of the complement system, which initiates a glomerular proliferative and inflammatory response. Streptococcal antigen and its antibody induce an antigen–antibody complex that deposits in the glomerular basement membrane, producing complement activation. Edema is formed as a result of reduced GFR and hence decreased filtration plus enhanced distal Na$^+$ reabsorption. Plasma volume is elevated and plasma renin is suppressed.

Clinical Manifestations. Signs and symptoms may be delayed for 5 days to 3 wk (10-day average) after streptococcal infections. Children may have asymptomatic hematuria. Edema and tea- or cola-colored urine are the most common initial signs. Oliguria, edema, and hypertension may induce complications, such as heart failure or encephalopathy.

Diagnosis. The diagnosis is based on the typical findings of edema, hematuria, and hypertension. Oliguria may occur, and pulmonary vascular congestion may be apparent on chest roentgenogram. Encephalopathy is infrequent. In addition to hematuria, urinalysis reveals mild to moderate proteinuria, concentrated urine, and the presence of many casts, including coarse and fine granular and red cell casts. Previous streptococcal infection should be documented by the streptozyme test.

Confirmation of activation of the complement system is determined by low C3 levels. Renal biopsy usually is not indicated in children with typical AGN; it reveals electron-dense deposits in the subepithelial space. The C3 returns to normal in 1–6 wk. Renal failure, if present, usually resolves in 2–3 wk, as do hypertension and gross hematuria.

Treatment.   Specific therapy includes diuretics for hypertension, heart failure, pulmonary edema, and oliguria; hydralazine or nifedipine for hypertension alone; or nifedipine, diazoxide, or nitroprusside for severe hypertension or hypertensive encephalopathy. Proteinuria and edema characteristically decline fairly rapidly (5–10 days), but microscopic hematuria may persist for months or occasionally years, a circumstance that does not alter the generally excellent *prognosis* of this disease, from which greater than 95% of children recover completely.

The absence of evidence for a poststreptococcal glomerulonephritis does not exclude the diagnosis of *acute postinfectious glomerulonephritis*, because multiple etiologies (*Pneumococcus, Staphylococcus*) have been implicated. Hypocomplementemia persisting beyond 8 wk of the illness, however, suggests the diagnosis of mesangiocapillary glomerulonephritis.

Mesangiocapillary (Membranoproliferative) Glomerulonephritis

This disorder may present in a manner similar to that of acute poststreptococcal glomerulonephritis, but, characteristically, persistent hypocomplementemia is present. This membranoproliferative disease frequently appears as a nephrotic syndrome, which is present in less than 10% of patients with AGN (see Nephrotic Syndrome).

Hemolytic–Uremic Syndrome

Hemolytic–uremic syndrome (HUS) is characterized by a microangiopathic hemolytic anemia, renal cortical injury (sometimes progressing to renal cortical necrosis), and thrombocytopenia. HUS is a major cause of acute renal failure in children.

Etiology and Epidemiology.   HUS may be sporadic, epidemic, and, in some countries (e.g., Argentina), endemic. The disease occurs between the ages of 4 mo and 4 yr. The etiology is unknown. Circulating toxins have been implicated, especially if HUS follows *Escherichia coli* or *Shigella* enteritis. HUS following hemorrhagic colitis has been associated with a verotoxin-producing *E. coli* 0157:H7. Verotoxin is similar to shiga-toxin (*Shigella*) and binds to a specific receptor on endothelial cells, producing endothelial swelling. Familial disease may be due to an alteration in the thromboxane–prostacyclin relationship, which favors endothelial platelet activation.

In most cases, the primary event appears to be endothelial cell injury and subsequent localized clotting and platelet activation. Evidence for disseminated intravascular coagulation rarely is present. Microangiopathic hemolytic anemia results from mechanical damage to red cells as they pass through the damaged vascular endothelium. Thrombocytopenia results from platelet adhesion.

Clinical Manifestations and Diagnosis.   The onset usually appears as a gastroenteritis, with or without intestinal bleeding, followed in 7–10 days by weakness, lethargy, irritability, and oliguria. Physical examination reveals pallor, edema, petechiae, hepatosplenomegaly, and irritability. The diagnosis is supported by finding microangiopathic hemolytic anemia, thrombocytopenia, and acute renal failure. Seizures may indicate CNS involvement. A smear of peripheral red blood cells reveals schistocytes, helmet and burr cells, and fragmented erythrocytes. The reticulocyte count is elevated, and plasma haptoglobin levels are diminished. A Coombs test is negative. Leukocytosis is common. Urinalysis reveals microscopic hematuria, proteinuria, and casts. Other causes of microangiopathic hemolytic anemia should be excluded.

Treatment.   Acute renal failure requires immediate therapy. Many patients (60–80%) require early intervention with dialysis. Most children survive the acute phase and recover normal renal function. Steroids and plasmapheresis are not helpful; heparinization, platelet inhibitors, and streptokinase remain of unproven benefit. Although careful medical management with early-onset dialysis frequently is associated with recovery, children nevertheless should be observed for the late development of hypertension or chronic renal failure. Epidemic disease has the best *prognosis*, whereas familial cases, disease in older patients, HUS without diarrhea, and sporadic HUS have a poorer outcome.

Rapidly Progressive Glomerulonephritis

Rapidly progressive glomerulonephritis (RPGN) is a clinical syndrome of rapidly progressing nephritis accompanied by renal failure, the pathologic hallmark of which is epithelial cell proliferation and *crescent* formation. One histologic pattern is that of linear immunoglobulin and complement deposition (idiopathic, Goodpasture syndrome). The more common type is the appearance of immune complexes in a "lumpy" pattern in the basement membrane (SLE, poststreptococcal AGN, polyarteritis, Henoch-Schönlein purpura, mesangiocapillary or idiopathic glomerulonephritis). RPGN is more common in late childhood, when patients present with edema, gross hematuria, hypertension, and renal failure. Some children with rapidly progressive lupus nephritis respond to pulse prednisone or cyclophosphamide therapy, whereas other children with poststreptococcal glomerulonephritis recover spontaneously. The prognosis for recovery of renal function is poor for the remaining types of RPGN. Fortunately, transplantation benefits most children having end-stage renal disease associated with the "lumpy" immune complex pattern of RPGN, but not in conditions associated with antiglomerular basement membrane antibodies, such as Goodpasture syndrome.

References

Behrman RE (ed): Nelson Textbook of Pediatrics. 14th ed. Philadelphia, WB Saunders, 1992, Sec. 18.3–18.23.

Boineau FG, Lewy JE: Evaluation of hematuria in children and adolescents. Pediatr Rev 11:101, 1989.

Editorial: Unravelling HUS. Lancet 1:1437, 1987.

Lieu TA, Grasmeder HM, Kaplan BS: An approach to the evaluation and treatment of microscopic hematuria. Pediatr Clin North Am 38:579, 1991.

Makker SP, Kher KK: IGA nephropathy in children. Semin Nephrol 9:112, 1989.

Stapleton FB, Roy S III, Noe HN, et al: Hypercalciuria in children with hematuria. N Engl J Med 310:1345, 1984.

Trompeter R, Schwartz R, Chantler C, et al: Haemolytic-uremic syndrome: An analysis of prognostic features. Arch Dis Child 58:101, 1983.

HEMATURIA WITH CASTS AND MARKED PROTEINURIA

Children who present with hematuria and marked proteinuria (greater than 1 g/m²/day) may have a nephrotic syndrome (see Table 16–15).

Approach to the Child with Proteinuria
(Table 16–17)

A small amount of protein is found in the urine of healthy children. The normal amount of urine protein is less than 4 mg/m²/hr or less than 100 mg/

Table 16–17. Evaluation of a Child with Proteinuria*

1. Complete history and physical examination
2. Confirmation of presence of proteinuria by repeat urinalysis
3. Twenty-four–hour urine collection to quantitate proteinuria; if quantitatively increased, proteinuria is present
4. Orthostatic test; if orthostatic test reveals persistent proteinuria, continue with tests listed in steps 5–7
5. Serum BUN, creatinine (calculate creatinine clearance), total protein, albumin, cholesterol, electrolytes
6. Streptozyme, C3', ANA
7. Renal ultrasound or intravenous pyelogram

* If steps 4–7 are abnormal; or there is a family history of renal disease, hematuria, hypertension, edema; or other manifestations of renal or systemic disease is present, biopsy may be needed.
ANA = antinuclear antibody; BUN = blood urea nitrogen.

m²/24 hr. *Nephrotic proteinuria* is defined as greater than 40 mg/m²/hr or greater than 1 g/m²/24 hr. The intermediary amounts are abnormal but not within the nephrotic range. Qualitative proteinuria of 1+ or greater on at least two to three random urine specimens suggest proteinuria that should be confirmed quantitatively. A semiquantitative evaluation of proteinuria is possible by measuring the urine protein-to-creatinine ratio on a single voided urine. The normal ratio generally is less than 0.2:1 when measured in the first morning specimen. The nephrotic urine protein-to-creatinine ratio is generally >3.5:1.

Initially, one must determine whether the proteinuria is transient or persistent. If persistent, one must assess its severity (see Glomerular Proteinuria, below). *Transient proteinuria* is seen following vigorous exercise and occasionally in children with fevers exceeding 38.5° C (101.3° F). The proteinuria usually is mild, transient, and reproducible.

A third type of transient proteinuria is *postural (orthostatic) proteinuria*. Children with this condition excrete normal amounts of protein while recumbent but have significant, although moderate, proteinuria when in the upright position. Hematuria is absent and renal function, complement levels, and renal ultrasound or IVP are entirely normal. This transient proteinuria is best evaluated by collecting a timed urine specimen while the patient is recumbent (usually overnight), followed by a timed urine collection during a normally active day. The presence of significant moderate proteinuria during the active period and a decrease in the proteinuria to normal or nearly normal levels during recumbency confirm the diagnosis of orthostatic proteinuria. It is important to remember that "fixed" proteinuria associated with renal disease also will have orthostatic accentuation during activity. Orthostatic proteinuria generally is thought to be benign. If proteinuria is *persistent* ("fixed"), renal disease should be considered (see Table 16–15).

TUBULAR PROTEINURIA

Normal children filter low-molecular-weight proteins, which are reabsorbed in the proximal tubule. Proximal tubular injury results in diminished reabsorptive ability (e.g., Fanconi syndrome) that produces mild to moderate proteinuria characteristically unassociated with edema.

GLOMERULAR PROTEINURIA

Glomerular proteinuria is classified by its degree. Intermittent or *mild proteinuria* (less than 0.5 g/m^2/day) is seen in pyelonephritis, cystic diseases, obstructive uropathies (congenital obstructions and reflux nephropathy), and mild glomerulonephritis. *Moderate proteinuria* (0.5–1 g/m^2/day) is seen in acute poststreptococcal glomerulonephritis, mild Henoch-Schönlein nephritis, severe pyelonephritis, chronic glomerulonephritis, and HUS. *Severe proteinuria* (>1 g/m^2/day) characteristically is associated with the nephrotic syndrome.

Nephrotic Syndrome

The nephrotic syndrome is an accumulation of symptoms and signs and is characterized by *proteinuria* (mainly albuminuria) greater than 1 g/m^2/24 hr, by *hypoproteinemia* (mainly albumin) with a total protein less than 5.5 g/dL and serum albumin less than 2.5 g/dL, by *hypercholesterolemia* (>250 mg/dL), and by *edema*. The primary disorder is an increase in glomerular permeability to proteins, most likely caused by a loss of the sialoproteins, which, in turn, results in the loss of the negative charge on the basement membrane. This increase in glomerular permeability causes massive proteinuria accompanied by secondary hypoproteinemia. Plasma oncotic pressure is diminished, resulting in a shift of fluid from the vascular to the interstitial compartment and a contraction in plasma volume. Renal blood flow and GFR are not usually diminished, and in some instances GFR may be above normal. With profound hypoalbuminemia, GFR is diminished. In addition to hypoproteinemic reduction of plasma oncotic pressure, formation of edema is enhanced by a reduction in effective blood volume and by an increase in tubular sodium chloride reabsorption produced by the activation of the renin–angiotensin–aldosterone system. Most serum lipids (including cholesterol and triglycerides) and levels of lipoprotein are elevated because hypoproteinemia stimulates hepatic lipoprotein synthesis; lipid metabolism is diminished.

MINIMAL CHANGE NEPHROTIC SYNDROME OF CHILDHOOD

Minimal change nephrotic syndrome (MCNS) is the most common form of the nephrotic syndrome (80% of cases). There is a male preponderance of 2:1. Hematuria sometimes is present (10–20% of cases) but transient. Hypertension is infrequent. Serum complement characteristically is normal. Serum cholesterol usually is elevated and often markedly so (>400 mg/dL). Of all childhood patients having MCNS, children 1–7 yr old are very likely to have steroid-responsive MCNS (87%) and, therefore, corticosteroid therapy may be initiated without performing renal biopsy if the presentation is typical. Children 7–16 yr of age still have a 50% chance of having MCNS on the basis of age alone, and if the children in this age group have a "typical" nephrotic syndrome, a trial of steroid therapy is indicated, because prednisone responsiveness increases the chance of MCNS to 86%. Typical nephrotic syndrome is defined as absence of severe or persistent hematuria, renal insufficiency, hypertension, and hypocomplementemia. Dependent pitting edema (pretibial, pedal, sacral, scrotal, labial, periorbital) with weight gain or ascites is the most common presentation of nephrotic syndrome. Diarrhea (intestinal edema) or respiratory distress (pulmonary edema, pleural effusion) also may be present.

Management.   If a child has the typical nephrotic syndrome, treatment consists of efforts to reduce edema and specific therapy with prednisone. The child who has a newly developed nephrotic syndrome usually requires hospitalization for diagnostic and therapeutic purposes.

The *edema* of the nephrotic syndrome is treated by restricting salt and water intake, and by occasionally optimizing the excretion of these elements by administering diuretics and, if the patient is refractory to diuretics alone, increasing plasma volume. Sodium chloride intake should be reduced to at least a "no-added-salt" diet, usually to a 2-g sodium diet. This salt restriction may be relaxed when the edema has resolved. Fluid intake should be moderately restricted. Diuretics may be required but should be given carefully because their overzealous use may further diminish plasma volume, resulting in hypotension and a fall in GFR.

Potassium supplementation may have to be provided if GFR is normal, because considerable urine potassium can be lost as a result of a combination of secondary hyperaldosteronism and diuretic therapy. Hydrochlorothiazide often is effective in treating edema of the nephrotic syndrome unless the serum albumin is quite low or the GFR is impaired. If the GFR is normal, spironolactone may be added to minimize potassium losses. Furosemide generally is effective in inducing diuresis and natriuresis despite moderately decreased GFR and hypoalbuminemia. The administration of furosemide should be started with relatively small doses (1–2 mg/kg), and the patient should be monitored closely for volume depletion and electrolyte disturbances; occasionally even furosemide may be relatively ineffective in alleviating severe hypoalbuminemia in children. In these children, cautious volume expansion with salt-poor albumin (0.5 g/kg IV over 2 hr) followed by furosemide at 1–2 mg/kg intravenously usually results in diuresis. This therapy may be repeated once or twice as needed. The infused albumin will be excreted quantitatively over 48–72 hr by patients with the nephrotic syndrome. Once adequate volume expansion has been achieved, further therapy with furosemide alone may suffice. Albumin should be given only in the presence of volume contraction, and the patient should be monitored closely for excessive volume expansion, which could lead to congestive cardiac failure.

Specific therapy is the administration of prednisone in a dosage of 2 mg/kg/day (60 mg/m^2/24 hr) divided into three to four doses per day. Approximately 10% of patients respond (urine protein becoming negative or reduced to trace levels) by the end of 1 wk, 70% by the end of 2 wk, 85% by the end of 3 wk, and 92% by the end of 4 wk of therapy. Prednisone is continued at this dosage until the urine protein is qualitatively negative or reduced to trace levels for 5 consecutive days or for a maximum of 4 wk. Five days after the urine is free of protein or at the maximum of 4 wk, the dosage is changed to 1.5 mg/kg/day (40 mg/m^2/24 hr) taken every other day as a single dose with breakfast. This alternate-day regimen is continued for an additional 6 wk. In the steroid-responsive patient following completion of 6 wk of alternate-day therapy, the prednisone is tapered over a 2-wk period and then discontinued.

If a child does not respond to daily prednisone therapy, a renal biopsy is indicated, because steroid resistance greatly increases the chance that the

Table 16–18. Complications of Nephrotic Syndrome

Acute renal failure
Hypertension
Hypercoagulable state (renal vein thrombosis, pulmonary embolism)
Spontaneous bacterial peritonitis
Malnutrition
Exacerbation by immunization
Steroid-related toxicity
Antimetabolite-related toxicity

underlying pathology is other than MCNS. In these circumstances, the diagnosis most likely will be focal segmental glomerulosclerosis or mesangiocapillary (membranoproliferative) glomerulonephritis.

The treatment of each relapse of the nephrotic syndrome is similar to that given during the initial therapy. A relapse is defined either as persistent proteinuria for 7 days in the absence of a respiratory infection or other intercurrent infection, or as the recurrence of edema. The definition is not simply the recurrence of proteinuria, because during an upper respiratory infection many children with the nephrotic syndrome will have transient proteinuria that resolves spontaneously. Frequent relapses or steroid resistance may require immunosuppressant therapy (cyclophosphamide, chlorambucil).

Complications. (Table 16–18). Infection is a major complication in children with the nephrotic syndrome. Peritonitis, particularly with *Streptococcus pneumoniae* or *E. coli*, may occur. Fever and signs of peritonitis may be masked by providing corticosteroid therapy. Therefore, a high index of suspicion and prompt evaluation is indicated. Side effects of steroids are most common in initial nonresponders and frequently relapsing patients.

FOCAL SEGMENTAL GLOMERULOSCLEROSIS

The presentation of focal segmental glomerulosclerosis (FSGS) may be identical to that of MCNS. In some cases, FSGS is thought to progress from MCNS, but in most circumstances it appears to be a separate entity. FSGS accounts for approximately 10% of children with the nephrotic syndrome. More than 80% of these patients are *steroid resistant*, and even those who initially respond frequently become steroid resistant subsequently. No clearly effective therapy for FSGS exists, although treatment with chlorambucil may produce remission in some patients and alleviate edema in others. Unfortunately, a considerable number of these patients progress to end-stage renal disease within 2–5 yr. Children with FSGS who have progressed to end-stage renal disease and who have received kidney transplants also are more likely to have a recurrence in the transplanted kidney.

MEMBRANOUS NEPHROPATHY

Membranous nephropathy is an infrequent cause of the nephrotic syndrome in childhood. Approximately 1% of children with the nephrotic syndrome have this lesion. It is seen most commonly in adolescents and in children who have potentially curable systemic diseases such as hepatitis B, syphilis, malaria, and toxoplasmosis and as a result of drug therapy (gold salts, penicillamine). These patients may present with the nephrotic syndrome or with proteinuria only. Hematuria is common. The presence of proteinuria in a patient with one of the predisposing diseases indicates a renal biopsy.

OTHER TYPES OF NEPHROTIC SYNDROME

The nephrotic syndrome has been diagnosed in patients during therapy with penicillamine, gold, mercury compounds, and other drugs. It also has been described in association with several extrarenal neoplasms, such as lymphomas (particularly Hodgkin disease).

The *congenital nephrotic syndrome* appears in two forms during the first 6 mo of life. The Finnish type is an autosomal recessive disorder most common in persons of Scandinavian descent. Prenatal diagnosis may be possible by detecting elevated amniotic fluid alpha-fetoprotein; the placenta is enlarged. Proteinuria characteristically is present at birth and the nephrotic syndrome becomes apparent within the first 3 mo. Unfortunately, most of these children have died as a result of infection or renal failure by the age of 5 yr. Renal transplantation may be of value. The other type of congenital nephrotic syndrome is a heterogeneous group of abnormalities mostly associated with drugs or infections, such as syphilis and toxoplasmosis.

References

Arbus GS, Poucell S, Bacheyie GS, et al: Focal segmental glomerulosclerosis with idiopathic nephrotic syndrome: Three types of clinical response. J Pediatr 101:40, 1982.

Behrman RE (ed): Nelson Textbook of Pediatrics. 14th ed. Philadelphia, WB Saunders, 1992, Sec. 18.24–18.33.

Brodehl J: The treatment of minimal change nephrotic syndrome. Eur J Pediatr 150:380, 1991.

Cameron JS: Membraneous nephropathy in childhood and its treatment. Pediatr Nephrol 4:193, 1990.

Hoyer JR, Anderson CE: Congenital nephrotic syndrome. Clin Perinatol 8:333, 1981.

International Study of Kidney Diseases in Children: Minimal change nephrotic syndrome in children: Deaths during the first 5–15 years of observation. Pediatrics 73:497, 1984.

Melvin T, Bennett W: Management of nephrotic syndrome in childhood. Drugs 42:30, 1991.

Norio R, Rapola J: Congenital and infantile nephrotic syndrome. Prog Clin Biol Res 305:179, 1989.

ACUTE RENAL FAILURE

A significant decrease in GFR or in tubular function is designated as acute renal failure, which generally is associated with a GFR that is reduced sufficiently so that waste products cannot be excreted and body fluid homeostasis is altered. Early recognition and management are critical.

Etiology and Pathophysiology.   The major causes of acute renal insufficiency are listed in Table 16–19. *Prerenal renal failure* characteristically occurs when the circulating blood volume decreases, hypotension is present, or the effective blood volume decreases. Under these conditions dehydration produced by vomiting, diarrhea, or a markedly increased insensible water loss can lead to hypovolemia. However, if the underlying cause of inadequate renal perfusion is reversed, renal function usually returns to normal. If the inadequate circulation persists, intrinsic renal damage supervenes.

Postrenal renal failure characteristically is obstructive in nature. Correcting or temporarily bypassing the obstruction will restore renal function unless renal parenchymal damage also has occurred. *Intrinsic renal failure* may be caused by vascular, immunologic, inflammatory, or toxic injury to the kidney.

Acute Tubular Necrosis.   Two principal mechanisms have been suggested to explain the renal failure exhibited in acute tubular necrosis. One hypothesis suggests that tubular injury caused by one of the conditions listed in Table 16–19 results in decreased reabsorption of solutes and water. Thus, increased delivery of salt and water to the distal nephron is present, which stimulates the intrinsic renin–angiotensin system and tubuloglomerular feedback. The release of vasoactive substances produces increased cortical vascular resistance, which decreases cortical blood flow and produces further tubular injury. In addition, the release of vasoactive substances results in a diminished GFR, and,

Table 16–19. Causes of Acute Renal Failure

Prerenal/Hypovolemia/Hypotension
Dehydration
    Vomiting
    Diarrhea
    Febrile illness
    Massive reduction in colloid oncotic pressure (pro-
        tein-losing enteropathy, nephrotic syndrome)
Septic shock
Heart failure
Hemorrhage
Burns
Peritonitis, ascites, cirrhosis

Postrenal (Obstruction)
Urethral obstruction
    Stricture
    Posterior urethral valves
    Diverticulum
    Phimosis
Ureteral obstruction
    Calculi
    Crystals (drugs, urate)
    Papillary necrosis
    Clotted blood
    Tumor
Ureterocele
Solitary renal unit with ureterovesical or ureteropelvic
    junction obstruction
Extrinsic tumor compressing bladder outlet
Extrinsic urinary tract tumors
Neurogenic bladder

Intrinsic
Acute tubular necrosis
    Prolonged hypotension secondary to
        Vomiting
        Diarrhea
        Shock
    Nephrotoxins
    ↓ Organ perfusion
Glomerulonephritis
    Primary (poststreptococcal)
    Secondary (SLE, endocarditis)
Interstitial nephritis
    Primary
    Secondary
        Drugs (allergic)
        Toxins
Vascular
    Renal vein thrombosis
    Arterial thromboemboli (umbilical artery catheter)
    Acute tubular necrosis
    Acute cortical necrosis
    Disseminated intravascular coagulation
    Immune-mediated (scleroderma)
Pigmenturia
    Hemoglobinuria
    Myoglobinuria

when severe, acute renal failure. A second hypothesis suggests that tubular injury results in tubular cell necrosis. Necrotic materials produce intratubular obstruction, raising intratubular resistance and thereby diminishing net glomerular filtration and tubular flow, which results in acute renal failure. In addition, the cellular necrosis results in loss of integrity of the renal tubule, with backleak of solute and fluid leading to reabsorption of most of the glomerular ultrafiltrate. Evidence exists for each of these theories, and probably both play a role in the pathophysiology of acute renal failure.

Severe vascular compromise may lead to arterial or venous thrombosis or to *acute cortical necrosis.* Whereas acute tubular necrosis commonly is reversible, acute cortical necrosis results in eventual scarring of the damaged glomeruli and permanent loss of renal function.

Diagnosis. History, physical examination, and laboratory data are helpful in evaluating the child with acute renal failure (Table 16–20).

The child with a *prerenal* cause for renal failure frequently has evidence of a precipitating illness associated with vomiting and diarrhea or an inadequate oral intake, or has a history of one of the predisposing factors (Table 16–19). The physical examination may show signs of dehydration accompanied by decreased weight, decreased skin turgor, and perhaps tachycardia and hypotension. Mucous membranes of the mouth may be dry, and CNS signs of poor perfusion, such as irritability or lethargy, may be present. Urine volume characteristically is decreased. Oliguric renal failure in adults is defined as less than 500 mL/day, whereas in children less than 1–2 mL/kg/hr is considered oliguria. Nonoliguric renal failure may occur and often is complicated by fluid and electrolyte disturbances in addition to azotemia. Urinary osmolality is significantly greater than serum osmolality. Measurement of urinary sodium usually reveals a sodium concentration less than 20 mEq/L. Urinalysis reveals a high specific gravity and, frequently, the absence or rare finding of cellular elements.

Postrenal renal failure often is found in early infancy and is associated with an obstructive lesion. Physical findings of dehydration are absent. Urinary output may be decreased, normal, or increased. Urinary osmolality frequently is similar to that of plasma, and urinary sodium concentration often is greater than 50 mEq/L. Urinalysis reveals no sediment abnormalities. Renal ultrasonography, voiding cystourethrogram, or a radionuclide scan are useful tests in assessing the possibility of postrenal failure.

Table 16–20. Laboratory Differential Diagnosis of Renal Insufficiency

	Prerenal		Renal		
	Child	*Neonate*	*Child*	*Neonate*	**Postrenal**
Urine Na$^+$ (mEq/L)	<20	<20–30	>40	>40	Variable, may be >40
FE$_{Na}$* (%)	<1	<2–5	>2	>2–5	Variable, may be >2
Urine osmolality (mOsm/L)	>500	>300–500	~300	~300	Variable, may be <300
RFI† (%)	<1	<2–5	>2	>2–5	Variable
Serum BUN/creatinine	>20	≥10	~10	≥10	Variable, may be >20
Response to volume	Diuresis		No change		No change
Response to furosemide	Diuresis		No change		No change/diuresis
Urinalysis	Normal		RBC, WBC, casts, proteinuria		Variable/normal
Comments	Hx: diarrhea, vomiting, hemorrhage, diuretics		Hx: hypotension, anoxia, exposure to nephrotoxins		Hx: poor urine stream/output
	Px: volume depletion		Px: hypertension, edema		Px: Flank mass, distended bladder

* FE$_{Na}$ = fractional excretion of sodium (%) = (urine sodium/plasma sodium ÷ urine creatinine/plasma creatinine) × 100.
† RFI = renal failure index = (urine sodium ÷ urine creatinine/plasma creatinine) × 100.
BUN = blood urea nitrogen; Hx = history; Px = physical signs; RBC = red blood cells; WBC = white blood cells.

The child with *intrinsic renal failure* may have a history compatible with one of the predisposing conditions. Physical examination may show signs of adequate, increased, or decreased fluid balance. Papilledema, hypertension, cardiac enlargement, or a gallop rhythm may be present that suggests vascular overload. Signs of systemic involvement resulting from underlying disease may be noted (e.g., in SLE, Henoch-Schönlein purpura, HUS). Urine output characteristically is decreased. Urinary osmolality may be isotonic, hypotonic, or hypertonic. Urinary sodium concentration generally is increased and frequently is greater than 40 mEq/L. Urinalysis usually will contain red cell and granular casts. Usually hematuria and proteinuria and, sometimes, leukocyturia are exhibited. C3 complement may be depressed in acute poststreptococcal glomerulonephritis, SLE, or membranoproliferative (mesangiocapillary) glomerulonephritis. Evidence of an earlier infection may be present, which can be demonstrated by the presence of a positive streptozyme or hepatitis B surface antigen. Anemia and thrombocytopenia may be present in conditions such as SLE or HUS. A chest roentgenogram may reveal evidence of pulmonary edema and cardiomegaly, suggesting vascular overload.

Treatment. Treatment depends upon the cause of acute renal insufficiency, although certain modalities commonly are used for many children with acute renal failure. The first step is to develop a plan of comprehensive monitoring. The patient should be weighed at least at 12-hr intervals to determine fluid balance, because acute weight changes reflect water loss or gain. Initial fluid and electrolyte therapy and a plan for frequent re-evaluation should be established. Urine output and electrolyte composition should be determined frequently during the acute phase.

Reversible conditions that can be treated should be given prompt attention. Obstructions of the urinary tract should be corrected or bypassed. Infection and/or shock should be treated. Hypovolemia should be corrected promptly. Dopamine may improve renal blood flow in low doses and is effective in various states of poor cardiac output. In addition, dobutamine may improve renal perfusion by enhancing myocardial contractility. If the presence of severe, intrinsic renal failure is in question, a catheter may be placed into the bladder to assess whether urine is present and to remove the urine promptly. If acute renal failure is present, there is no advantage in monitoring small volumes of urinary output.

Fluid Requirements. The degree of dehydration should be estimated. If hypovolemia is apparent, intravascular volume should be expanded by intravenously administering physiologic saline (0.9% sodium chloride), giving 20 mL/kg intravenously over 30–60 min. Once volume depletion has been corrected, giving an intravenous dose of furosemide, 2 mg/kg, in the presence of anuria is reasonable. If urinary output is not increased, a second dose of furosemide may be given. If no response occurs, further infusion generally is not helpful and increases the risk of ototoxicity.

If the patient shows evidence of excessive weight gain or fluid overload, fluid intake should be reduced to insensible water loss, plus urinary and stool output, plus any fluid drainage (nasogastric tube), minus a planned weight loss. Patients who have acute renal failure are catabolic and lose approximately 1% of body weight/day in the form of tissue losses and not as fluid losses. When the patient maintains weight in the presence of acute renal failure, this generally indicates fluid retention. Diuretics should be used as initial therapy to mobilize retained fluids. Severe fluid overload in the presence of marked oliguria or anuria is one indication for dialysis.

Hyperkalemia. This condition frequently is found in patients with acute renal failure resulting from the absence of potassium excretion and catabolism. High-potassium–containing foods, fluids, and medications should be restricted until renal function is re-established. Lead II of the electrocardiogram is useful for assessing hyperkalemia (see Disturbances of Electrolytes, Acid–Base Balance, and Fluids).

Acidosis. This is common in renal failure as a consequence of catabolism and the inability of the failed kidney to secrete hydrogen ion. When severe, intravenous $NaHCO_3$ should be administered as noted above, but should be given cautiously in order to avoid fluid overload, hypernatremia, and hypertension.

Hypocalcemia. This is seen commonly in acute renal failure in association with hyperphosphatemia. Treatment primarily involves efforts to lower the serum phosphorus. Milk and other high-phosphorus foods are severely limited, and oral calcium carbonate is given to bind phosphorus. Aluminum hydroxide gels previously used to treat hyperphosphatemia have been associated with aluminum intoxication (dementia, rickets). If the patient shows evidence of tetany, an intravenous infusion of 10% calcium gluconate (0.5 mL/kg) may be given slowly.

Caloric Needs. It is important to maintain an adequate caloric intake in patients with acute renal failure in order to minimize catabolism. At least 70% of the regular daily allowance of calories and 0.5–1.0 g of high-quality protein/kg/day should be provided.

Dialysis. In children with renal insufficiency, dialysis is indicated in order to treat (1) hyperkalemia unresponsive to medical therapy, (2) acidosis unresponsive to medical therapy, (3) hyperkalemia or acidosis in the presence of hypernatremia, (4) fluid overload unresponsive to fluid restriction or to diuretics, or (5) symptoms and signs of "uremia." The method used may be peritoneal dialysis, hemodialysis, or modifications of hemodialysis, such as hemoperfusion.

Complications. The most serious potential complications of acute renal failure are infections, vascular overload, and hyperkalemia. Other potential complications are uremic encephalopathy, seizures, pericardial effusion, hypertension, peptic ulceration, platelet dysfunction, and anemia. In addition, carefully monitoring blood levels of drugs excreted by the kidney and appropriately adjusting either the total dose or the dosing interval are necessary to avoid toxicity (e.g., acyclovir, aminoglycosides, penicillins, cephalosporins, vancomycin, cimetidine, digoxin). The recovery phase of obstructive renal failure and acute tubular necrosis may be complicated by a polyuric phase associated with poor concentrating ability and hypo- or hyperkalemia. The plan of management that minimizes the use of urinary catheters, avoids fluid overload and electrolyte excess, and effectively treats hyperkalemia generally is rewarded by the patient's recovery.

Prognosis. Recovery depends on the etiology of acute renal failure. Prerenal failure, postrenal failure, and intrinsic renal failure are reversible in most types of renal disease. In patients with acute tubular necrosis, the period of anuria/oliguria usually lasts 7–10 days and is followed by 2–7 days of polyuria. With good supportive care and steady monitoring, all patients should recover from acute tubular necrosis. Lack of improvement suggests acute cortical necrosis or some other etiology. Renal failure associated with RPGN, renal vascular thrombosis, and cortical necrosis may not be reversible and may require chronic dialysis and eventual renal transplantation.

References

Behrman RE (ed): Nelson Textbook of Pediatrics. 14th ed. Philadelphia, WB Saunders, 1992, Sec. 18.35.

Corwin H, Bonventre J: Acute renal failure. Med Clin North Am 70:1037, 1986.

Gaudio KM, Siegal NJ: Pathogenesis and treatment of acute renal failure. Pediatr Clin North Am 34:771, 1987.

CHRONIC RENAL FAILURE

Etiology. The cause of chronic renal failure in childhood is closely related to the age of the child at the time that renal failure occurs. Between birth and 5 yr of age, congenital and obstructive abnormalities are the most common causes. After age 5, acquired diseases, such as focal segmental glomerulosclerosis, chronic glomerulonephritis, reflux nephropathy, HUS, and progressive hereditary disorders (Alport syndrome, cystic disease), are likely causes of chronic renal failure. In each category, renal function progressively deteriorates and is accompanied by the contraction of the renal parenchyma with subsequent end-stage renal failure. The progression to end-stage renal failure is variable and depends on features such as hyperfiltration, ongoing immunologic injury, proteinuria, hypertension, secondary hyperparathyroidism, and infection.

Clinical Manifestations. *Growth failure* in children with chronic renal failure is prominent. The factors associated with growth retardation include undernutrition, osteodystrophy, hormonal abnormalities, medications (e.g., steroids), and acidosis. Growth failure generally does not occur until GFR is less than 25 mL/min/1.73 m². Increased calorie intake leads to a slight increase in growth, but considerably more calories are needed than are necessary to achieve comparable growth in children with normal renal function. Children with chronic renal failure also have progressive anemia, frequently are hypertensive, are at increased risk for infection or CNS disturbances, and demonstrate severe osteodystrophy.

Treatment. The management of children with chronic renal failure and their complex problems requires a team of pediatric nephrologists, clinical nursing specialists, nutritionists, social workers, psychiatrists, psychologists, recreational and occupational therapists, and various other professionals.

Diet. Children with chronic renal insufficiency have diminished growth velocity and progressive retardation of bone age prior to puberty. They should be provided with more than 70% of the recommended dietary allowance of calories. Infants often require greater than 125% of the recommended daily allowance in order to achieve moderate growth. Protein should be provided at a level of 1.5 g/kg/24 hr or greater and should consist of high-biologic-value proteins. Milk must be restricted because of its high phosphate content. In infants, a high-quality protein formula, such as PM60/40 (Ross Laboratories), used in conjunction with calcium carbonate as a phosphate binder, may be indicated. Supplemental calcium usually is necessary because the child must avoid milk products. Children with renal insufficiency also need vitamin supplementation, because they become deficient in water-soluble vitamins.

In order to keep the serum bicarbonate in the 19–20 mEq/L range, acidosis should be treated by providing appropriate doses of sodium bicarbonate or sodium citrate (Bicitra). Water balance usually is maintained reasonably well until dialysis is required, and, therefore, water restriction rarely is necessary. A "no-added-salt" diet will provide adequate but not excessive sodium intake, although, as a consequence of obstructive uropathies, some children with renal insufficiency may be salt wasters and require increased salt intake. Patients with intrinsic renal disease usually have hypertension, for which salt restriction is needed. High-potassium foods should be avoided once renal failure is established.

Renal Osteodystrophy. Renal osteodystrophy (most commonly osteitis fibrosa) is a nearly constant accompaniment of chronic renal failure and is associated with hyperphosphatemia, high serum alkaline phosphatase activity, and secondary hyperparathyroidism. The initial therapy is to restrict phosphate in the diet, most commonly by restricting milk. In addition, calcium carbonate may be used to bind phosphate in the gastrointestinal tract. The phosphate level should be kept in the 5–6 mg/dL range to minimize secondary hyperparathyroidism while providing enough phosphate for new bone formation. Milk restriction leads to inadequate calcium intake, so a child should receive approximately 1 g of elemental calcium from all sources per day. Because that is not provided in the diet, calcium gluconate supplements should be given.

Chronic renal failure is associated with an inability of the kidney to convert 25-hydroxycholecalciferol to 1,25-dihydroxycholecalciferol. Therapy with either synthetic vitamin D (dihydrotachysterol) or 1,25-dihydroxycholecalciferol usually is necessary.

Anemia. Anemia is a common finding in chronic renal failure in children. There is an ongoing debate as to whether the anemia results primarily from toxic depression of erythropoiesis by abnormal or retained metabolites or from a failure of the kidney to produce erythropoietin in response to anemia. Reduced serum iron and elevated iron-binding capacity are common but do not indicate iron deficiency because the anemia is normochromic and normocytic and the ferritin levels are normal or elevated. Transfusions should be restricted to symptomatic children to avoid hemosiderosis and hepatitis or to prepare them for transplantation. They rarely are needed if recombinant-produced erythropoietin is administered. Children on continuous ambulatory peritoneal dialysis (CAPD) or continuous cycling peritoneal dialysis (CCPD) usually have higher hematocrits than those on hemodialysis.

Growth. Therapy with recombinant-produced growth hormone continue to be studied in children with chronic renal failure. Results are promising, although cost and availability limit its use at present.

Treating End-Stage Renal Failure. The principal treatment of end-stage renal failure is *renal transplantation.* Cadaver donors and living related donors have been used extensively for renal transplantation. Children with progressive renal failure should be referred to a center specializing in renal transplantation for children for evaluation when the serum creatinine reaches 5–6 mg/dL. Thoroughly evaluating the cause of chronic renal failure, listing potential donors, and beginning to prepare the family and child for dialysis and transplantation should be begun before the threat of end-stage renal failure becomes immediate. *Dialysis* is effective for sustaining the patient who is awaiting renal transplantation or in whom renal transplantation is not possible. Few children are given hemodialysis as the preferential mode of dialysis. The development of CAPD and CCPD has made chronic dialysis an effective and well-tolerated technique during the necessary time prior to transplantation. The principal complication of peritoneal dialysis is peritoneal infection (*S. epidermidis*). Because of improved techniques used in dialysis and immunosuppressive drugs used for transplantation (e.g., cyclosporine), the outlook for children with end-stage renal disease is encouraging. Patient and graft survival are highest in pediatric patients beyond infancy.

References

Baum M, Powell D, Calvin S, et al.: Continuous ambulatory peritoneal dialysis in children. N Engl J Med 307:1537, 1982.

Behrman RE (ed): Nelson Textbook of Pediatrics. 14th ed. Philadelphia, WB Saunders, 1992, Sec. 18.36.

Fine R, Salusky I, Ettenger R: The therapeutic approach to the infant, children and adolescent with end-stage renal disease. Pediatr Clin North Am 34:789, 1987.

Fine RN, Pyke-Grim K, Nelson PA, et al: Recombinant human growth hormone treatment of children with chronic renal failure: Long term (1–3 year) outcome. Pediatr Nephrol 5:477, 1991.

HYPERTENSION

Systolic and diastolic blood pressure values increase gradually between birth and 18 yr of age. During this period and adulthood, most patients "track" in a constant percentile around the mean. The younger the hypertensive patient, the greater the chance the hypertension will be secondary to another disease rather than being essential.

Etiology. Hypertension in children may be due to renal (Table 16–21), endocrine (Table 16–22), vascular (Table 16–23), and neurologic (Table 16–24) disorders and to miscellaneous disorders,

Table 16–21. Renal Causes of Hypertension

Congenital Anomalies
Dysplastic kidney
Polycystic disease
Obstructive uropathy

Acquired Lesions
Wilms tumor
Acute glomerulonephritis
Hemolytic–uremic syndrome
Henoch-Schönlein purpura
Systemic lupus erythematosus
Familial nephritis (Alport syndrome)
Reflux nephropathy
Segmental hypoplasia (Ask-Upmark kidney)
Drugs, toxins (cyclosporine, steroids, lead)

Table 16–22. Endocrine Causes of Hypertension

Neuroblastoma
Pheochromocytoma
Adrenal genital syndrome (11-hydroxylase deficiency)
Cushing syndrome
Hyperparathyroidism
Hyperaldosteronism
Hyperthyroidism
Diabetic nephropathy

Table 16–23. Vascular Causes of Hypertension

Coarctation of aorta
Postcoarctation repair
Renal artery embolism (neonate with umbilical artery
    catheter)
Renal vein thrombosis
Endocarditis
Renal artery stenosis
Fibromuscular dysplasia
Neurofibromatosis
Arteritis (Takayasu, periarteritis nodosa)
Sarcoidosis

such as essential hypertension, drugs or foods (steroids, licorice), or prolonged immobilization.

Clinical Manifestations. The signs and symptoms of hypertension include heart failure, stroke, seizures, headache, coma, polyuria, oliguria, and blurred vision. However, many patients are asymptomatic, which emphasizes the importance of obtaining a blood pressure reading from every infant and child at each physician visit. In young infants, blood pressure may be measured with the Dynamap machine, whereas in older patients, standard sphygmomanometry and auscultation are sufficient. Additional physical findings include papilledema, abdominal bruits (renovascular), arm blood pressure greater than leg pressure (aortic coarctation), café-au-lait spots (neurofibromatosis), flank masses (hydronephrosis, renal dysplasia, neuroblastoma, Wilms tumor), ataxia, opsoclonus (neuroblastoma), tachycardia, flushing, diaphoresis (pheochromocytoma), tetany, weakness, polydipsia (primary aldosteronism), and truncal obesity, acne, striae, and buffalo hump (Cushing syndrome).

Diagnosis. The diagnostic evaluation of patients with hypertension includes urinalysis, blood urea nitrogen, creatinine, electrolytes, acid–base balance, chest roentgenogram, and renal ultrasound. Clues from the history, physical examination, mode of presentation, initial laboratory data, and age should determine the next sequence of tests.

Table 16–24. Neurologic Causes of Hypertension

Neurofibromatosis
Guillain-Barré syndrome
Subdural hemorrhage
Dysautonomia (Riley-Day syndrome)
Increased intracranial pressure (with bradycardia)
Poliomyelitis
Quadriplegia
Encephalitis
Stress, anxiety

A renal scan and the determination of plasma hormone levels (catecholamines, thyroxine, cortisol, renin) and urine hormone levels (vanillylmandelic acid, homovanillic acid, dopamine, steroid hormones) are more specific and noninvasive methods. Finally, renal arteriography and renal biopsy are invasive tests that may provide definitive diagnosis.

Treatment. Before treatment is initiated, it is important to determine whether the hypertension is persistent or intermittent; whether the measurements are accurate (appropriate-size blood pressure cuff); and that the hypertension is not compensatory, as occurs with increased intracranial pressure or as a result of a coarctation of the aorta. For mild hypertension resulting from volume overload, a diuretic is indicated (e.g., chlorothiazide, furosemide); for moderate hypertension, the administration of a vasodilator such as nifedipine is useful. Alternately, a beta-blocker and a diuretic may be used. If severe, a vasodilator (e.g., nifedipine), and a diuretic may be effective, or an angiotensin-converting enzyme inhibitor (e.g., captopril, enalapril) may be used. Renovascular hypertension may be approached with renal artery angioplasty or reconstruction of the vessel with autotransplantation of the kidney. Primary diseases, such as SLE, thyrotoxicosis, and coarctation of the aorta, require specific therapy.

Prognosis. The prognosis depends on the primary disorder. Essential hypertension, when present in adolescents and not associated with morbidity at presentation, contributes to the cardiovascular, CNS, and renal morbidity associated with hypertension in older patients.

References

Behrman RE (ed): Nelson Textbook of Pediatrics. 14th ed.
    Philadelphia, WB Saunders, 1992, Sec. 15.80.
Editorial: Screening for hypertension in childhood. Lancet
    1:918, 1988.
Feld LG, Springate JE: Hypertension in children. Curr Probl
    Pediatr 18:317, 1988.
Ingelfinger J: Pediatric Hypertension. Phildelphia, WB
    Saunders, 1982.

GENITAL DISORDERS

Anomalies of the Penis

HYPOSPADIAS

In *hypospadias*, which occurs in approximately 1:500 newborn infants, the urethral meatus is located below and proximal to its normal position, an abnormality resulting from a failure of the urethral folds to fuse completely over the urethral groove. The ventral foreskin also is lacking, while the dorsal portion gives the appearance of a hood. *Chordee* is a term for a ventral curvature of the penile shaft. The meatus may be on the glans or at any point along the penis to the penile–scrotal junction. Rarely, the urethra opens onto the perineum. In this circumstance, the chordee is extreme, and the scrotum is biphid and sometimes extends to the dorsal base of the penis. Testes are undescended in 10% of boys with hypospadias, and inguinal hernias are common. The differential diagnosis of severe hypospadias with undescended testes must include the various causes of ambiguous genitalia (e.g., congenital adrenal hyperplasia, masculinization of females). The frequency of other anomalies of the urinary tract in males with hypospadias is relatively low, except in those whose urethral opening is very close to the penile–scrotal junction.

Males with hypospadias should not be circumcised because the foreskin often is necessary for later repair. The ideal age of repair remains controversial, although most pediatric urologists tend to operate before the patient is 18 mo of age, most frequently when the patient is 13–15 mo of age.

PHIMOSIS

In 90% of uncircumsized males, the prepuce becomes retractable by the age of 3 yr, but after this age, the inability to retract the prepuce is termed phimosis. The condition may be congenital or a sequel to inflammation. Severe phimosis usually requires surgical enlargement of the opening or circumcision. Accumulation of smegma is not pathologic and does not require surgical treatment. *Paraphimosis* occurs when the prepuce is retracted behind the coronal sulcus and cannot be returned to its normal position, which usually is due to venous stasis and edema and leads to severe pain. Occasionally, when discovered early, reduction of the foreskin is possible with lubrication. In some cases, circumcision is needed.

Disorders and Abnormalities of the Scrotum and its Contents

UNDESCENDED TESTES (CRYPTORCHIDISM)

Undescended testes are found in 0.7% of children after 1 yr of age. The frequency is higher in full-term newborn infants (3.4%) than in older children. In cases discovered at birth, the percentage increases with prematurity (17% in infants with birth weights between 2000 and 2500 g and 100% in infants weighing less than 900 g). Although spontaneous testicular descent does not occur beyond the age of 1 yr, failure to find one or both testes in the scrotum does not necessarily indicate undescended testicles. *Retractile testes*, absent testes, and ectopic testes also may be the cause. The true undescended testis is found along the path of normal descent, usually with a patent processus vaginalis. The undescended testis commonly is associated with an *inguinal hernia*; it also is subject to *torsion*. A higher incidence of infertility in adulthood, a risk of development of tumor in the undescended testis, and untoward psychologic effects in adolescence and adulthood are associated with the condition. Cryptorchidism is bilateral in up to 30% of reported cases. Infertility is uniform in adults with untreated bilateral cryptorchidism. Because infertility also is common in adults with a history of unilateral undescended testicle, the contralateral descended testis may also be abnormal.

The undescended testis usually is histologically normal at birth, but atrophy and poor development are found by the end of 1 yr. Although still a subject of controversy, reports indicate that surgical correction at an early age results in a greater probability of fertility in adulthood. The development of a malignant tumor in the cryptorchid testis has been reported to occur 20–44% of the time, usually in the third or four decade of life. The greatest risk seems to be in those who underwent surgical correction during or after puberty.

Indirect inguinal hernias accompany undescended testes and also are seen frequently with ectopic testes. Torsion, with or without infarction, may occur and probably is related to excessive mobility of these testes. *Orchidopexy* usually is undertaken in the 2nd yr of life. Most testes that are extraabdominal can be brought into the scrotum when the associated hernia is corrected. If the testis is not palpable, ultrasonography will determine its location. The closer the testis is to the internal inguinal ring, the better the chance of successful orchidopexy.

RETRACTILE TESTES

Retractile testes are normal testes that have retracted into the inguinal canal as a result of an exaggeration of the cremasteric reflex. The diagnosis of retractile testes is likely if testes are palpable in the newborn examination but not at a later examination. Retractile testes frequently can be identified and brought into the scrotum by palpation when the child is warm and relaxed, and they characteristically remain in the scrotum permanently with puberty. The retractile testis does not develop the complications commonly associated with a true undescended testis.

TORSION OF THE TESTIS

This condition is an emergency that requires prompt diagnosis and treatment. It accounts for approximately 40% of cases of acute scrotal pain and swelling at all ages and is the major cause in patients under the age of 6 yr. It usually is caused by an abnormal fixation of the testis to the scrotum. If the tunica vaginalis covers both the testis and the epididymis as well as the distal spermatic cord, the testis can rotate freely and torsion is facilitated. Testicular torsion produces severe acute pain and swelling of the scrotum. On examination, the swelling is apparent, tenderness is severe, and the cremasteric reflex is absent.

The *differential diagnosis* includes an incarcerated hernia and torsion of the testicular epididymal appendices. Torsion of the appendices is associated with point tenderness over the lesion and minimal swelling. In adolescence, the differential diagnosis must include **epididymitis**. Epididymitis is the most common cause of acute scrotal pain and swelling in older adolescents. The differential diagnosis frequently is helped by an antecedent history of sexual activity (infection with *Chlamydia, gonococcus*) or urinary tract infection (infection with *E. coli*). Testicular torsion must be considered as the principal diagnosis when severe acute testicular pain is present.

If radiologic studies are in doubt, prompt surgical exploration should be performed. If the testis is explored within 6 hr of torsion, the gonads will survive (in up to 90% of cases). The procedure is detorsion and fixation of the testis to the scrotum. The contralateral testis usually is fixed to the scrotum to prevent future torsion. If torsion of the appendices is found at the time of exploration, removal of the necrotic tissue is indicated.

References

Behrman RE (ed): Nelson Textbook of Pediatrics. 14th ed. Philadelphia, WB Saunders, 1992, Sec. 18.45–18.46.
Burbige K, Hensle T: Posterior urethral valves in the newborn: Treatment and functional results. J Pediatr Surg 22: 165, 1987.
Colodny AH: Undescended testes—is surgery necessary? N Engl J Med 314:510, 1986.
Fallon B, Welton M, Hawtrey C: Congenital anomalies associated with cryptorchidism. J Urol 127:91, 1987.

URINARY TRACT INFECTIONS

Urinary tract infections (UTIs) are the most common genitourinary disease of childhood.

Clinical Manifestations. The symptoms and signs of UTI vary markedly with age. *Neonates* commonly present with failure to thrive, feeding problems, diarrhea, vomiting, fever, and hyperbilirubinemia. The *1 mo–2 yr old* infant with a UTI usually has nonurinary tract manifestations, such as feeding problems, failure to thrive, diarrhea, and unexplained fever. This age group also presents with a UTI masquerading as gastrointestinal illness, such as "colic," irritability, and screaming periods. In the 1st mo of life, a male preponderance is seen in patients with UTI. The sex ratio of UTI has a female preponderance from the 2nd mo of life to adulthood. The *2–6 yr old* child may have gastrointestinal symptoms, but in this age group the classic signs of urinary tract infection, such as urgency, dysuria, frequency, and abdominal pain, begin to appear. The *6–18 yr old* most commonly will have urgency, frequency, dysuria, and abdominal or flank pain. Urinary tract infections occur in 1–2% of school-age females. In all children, *unexplained fevers* and sustained abdominal symptoms without explanation are indicators to examine the urine and perform a urine culture.

Congenital genitourinary tract abnormalities predispose patients to UTI, and UTI should be suspected when unexplained fevers or other symptoms are found in a child with these problems.

Diagnosis. The diagnosis of UTI is made by finding a *positive culture of bacteria* in the urine. The finding of any bacteria in urine obtained by bladder catheterization or by suprapubic bladder puncture indicates infection. A properly collected voided urine, promptly plated, that grows more than 100,000 colonies/mL of a single organism on quantitative bacterial culture has a 95% positive correlation with suprapubic aspiration. A count of less than 10^5 bacterial colonies on a voided specimen has diminished value. The presence of *leukocytes* in the urine suggests that infection may be present in the symptomatic child, but inflammatory diseases such as acute poststreptococcal glomerulonephritis also are associated with leukocyturia. *Blood* in the urine may be present in UTI, particularly in adolescent females, but the presence of blood or leukocytes in the urine is not diagnostic. The presence of numerous motile bacteria in a freshly voided and examined urine (uncentrifuged urine) specimen from symptomatic infants and children has a 94% correlation with a positive culture of a suprapubic aspiration. The presence of even scant bacteria has an 82% correlation with a positive suprapubic aspiration. A delay of 1–2 hr in the examination of a voided specimen frequently will lead to bacterial multiplication and, hence, to a false impression of infection.

The most common cause of bacteriuria in the absence of a UTI is contamination of the urine by periurethral and anterior urethral flora. Colony counts will be low, however, if the urine is plated for culture promptly. In a few cases, bacterial colony counts of less than 100,000 on a voided specimen occur when a UTI is present. This may happen in the very well-hydrated child who is voiding frequently and has a dilute urine. It also may occur if the child has received recent antimicrobial therapy or if bacterial inhibitors are present. Less than 10^5 bacterial colonies also may be seen when UTI is caused by fastidious organisms (e.g., tuberculosis).

Localization of a UTI is important because infection of the upper urinary tract is associated more frequently with anatomic abnormalities than is infection of the lower urinary tract. Unfortunately, the clinical presentation is of limited help in determining the site of infection in neonates, infants, and toddlers. Fever and abdominal pain can occur with either lower or upper UTI, although high fevers favor upper tract involvement. Direct methods of investigation, such as bladder washout specimens, usually are contraindicated because of their invasiveness. Indirect methods, including examining the urine for glitter cell and white cell casts (which, if present, indicate upper tract infection), finding evidence of an inability to maximally concentrate the urine, finding antibody-coated bacteria measured by immunofluorescence, beta$_2$-microglobulin excretion in 24-hr urine collections, and performing lactic dehydrogenase differential excretion all have been suggested as possible but limited ways to differentiate upper from lower UTIs. A high erythrocyte sedimentation rate, leukocytosis, and bacteremia are noted in pyelonephritis.

Predisposing Factors.   The short urethra in girls predisposes them to UTI. Uncircumsized males are also at risk for UTI. The *E. coli* serotypes from bowel flora frequently are found in UTI. Furthermore, certain strains of bacteria have increased adherence to uroepithelial cells, which correlates with the presence of bacterial pili. A hydronephrotic kidney, vesicoureteral reflux, a poorly emptying bladder, congenital malformations, nephrolithiasis, and other factors leading to *urinary stasis* predispose the patient to UTI. The specific role of vesicoureteral reflux in the pathogenesis of UTI is unclear. A high incidence of vesicoureteral reflux is reported in association with UTI, but its pathogenic significance remains unclear. However, the presence of vesicoureteral reflux and infection is a predisposing factor for chronic UTI and renal scarring.

The most common bacteria isolated from symptomatic or asymptomatic children experiencing their first UTI, occurring at any age and in both boys and girls, is *E. coli*. Other organisms, such as *Klebsiella*, *Proteus*, enterococci, and *Staphylococci saprophyticus*, appear more frequently in the presence of obstruction or abnormalities of the urinary tract.

Treatment.   UTI should be treated promptly. Neonates require 10–14 days of parenteral antibiotic therapy because UTI is often associated with bacteremia. Older children with *acute cystitis* should receive a 5–7 day course of oral antibiotic therapy. The most common therapy is with amoxicillin or trimethoprim–sulfamethoxazole. In children with high fevers, white cell casts, or other symptoms or signs of *acute pyelonephritis*, the initial use of broad-spectrum parenteral antibiotics is indicated. In children with pyelonephritis who do not have toxic symptoms, treatment includes parenteral antibiotics such as ampicillin or a cephalosporin. Patients who show evidence of toxicity (chills, high fever) often are treated with ampicillin and gentamicin (or another aminoglycoside) or a third-generation cephalosporin alone. Once systemic toxicity has resolved and the patient is afebrile, oral therapy with an agent to which the cultured organism is sensitive should be administered to complete at least 14 days of therapy. It is important to repeat the urine culture 4–7 days after the therapy is discontinued because many relapses are asymptomatic. UTI has a tendency to recur, even without predisposing factors. Follow-up urine cultures also should be obtained after recurrent cystitis or pyelonephritis, first at 1-mo intervals and subsequently at 3-mo intervals for at least 1 yr.

Follow-Up Evaluation of the Urinary Tract.   The decision as to whether a work-up is indicated following UTI depends on the likelihood that complicating abnormalities are present. A history of treatment failure, the presence of unusual organisms, growth disturbances, and frequent recurrences suggest a more complex problem. The indications for radiologic evaluation include (1) UTI in a male, (2) UTI in the 1st yr of life, (3) UTI in a female who shows evidence of pyelonephritis or who does not respond to treatment, and (4) recurrent UTI in a female. The timing of evaluation is important. If the patient has toxic symptoms, responds slowly or poorly to therapy, or has a mass or bladder distention, prompt nephrosonography and ultrasound of the bladder are indicated. If the symptoms are those of lower UTI and response is rapid, it is best to wait approximately 3 wk before carrying out the evaluation, because infection-induced reflux may not be persistent at this time. An experienced nephrosonographer can provide most of the important anatomic information by using renal ultrasound. However, small scars and slight calyceal dilations may be missed. Therefore, some prefer a renal scan or an IVP. A voiding cystourethrogram is essential to assess reflux, bladder wall thickness, and bladder emptying.

Reference

Behrman RE (ed): Nelson Textbook of Pediatrics. 14th ed. Philadelphia, WB Saunders, 1992, Sec. 18.39–18.40.

Endocrine Disorders

17

Dennis M. Styne
Mark A. Sperling
Steven P. Chernausek

Endocrine disorders generally manifest in one of four ways: (1) by an excess of hormone (in thyrotoxicosis, of thyroid hormone; in Cushing syndrome, of cortisol); (2) by a deficiency of hormone (in diabetes mellitus, of insulin; in hypothyroidism, of thyroid hormone); (3) by an abnormal response of target tissues to hormone (in testicular feminization syndrome, by resistance to male sex hormones); and (4) by simple gland enlargement (in nonfunctioning pituitary adenoma, by neurologic signs and symptoms). Because hormones are circulating chemical messengers, the location of action often is distant from the specialized organ (gland) of origin. Consequently, signs and symptoms of an endocrine disorder usually are related to the peripheral tissue's response to the hormone excess or deficiency. Indeed, functioning endocrine tumors frequently produce profound physiologic changes that reveal the pathologic process long before the appearance of signs and symptoms related to tumor mass.

Peptide hormones act through specific cell membrane receptors (Fig. 17–1). *Steroid hormones* work by attachment to intracellular receptors, which then translocate the hormone to the nucleus where they interact with DNA (hormone response elements upstream to the specific gene), causing appropriate effects (Fig. 17–2). Hormones generally are involved in a feedback loop so that the production of a substance is regulated by its effect; corticotropin-releasing factor (CRF) stimulates adrenocorticotropic hormone (ACTH) to produce cortisol, which in turn feeds back to suppress CRF and ACTH production so that an equilibrium is reached. The equilibrium's set point may change with development; in prepuberty small amounts of sex steroids completely suppress gonadotropin secretion, but during pubertal development the sensitivity of this feedback decreases and increased sex steroid production is allowed before gonadotropin secretion is inhibited.

Receptor number and avidity may be regulated by hormones as well; excessive continuous exposure to gonadotropin-releasing hormone (GnRH) down-regulates receptor numbers on pituitary gonadotropes for GnRH. Some hormones exert their effects locally on the cell of origin or a neighboring cell (Fig. 17–3).

The interpretation of serum endocrine hormone levels must be related to their controlling factors; a given value of parathyroid hormone may be normal in a eucalcemic patient but may be inadequate in a hypocalcemic patient and excessive in a hypercalcemic patient.

The *hypothalamus* controls many endocrine systems. Hypothalamic releasing factors travel down the pituitary portal system to stimulate the anterior pituitary gland to release the related hormones specific for the releasing factor (Fig. 17–4). These pituitary hormones then circulate and reach their target glands to exert their effect and create other hormones that then feed back to suppress hypothalamic and pituitary secretion. Prolactin is the only pituitary hormone that is suppressed by a hypothalamic factor, prolactin inhibitory factor (dopamine). Hypothalamic deficiency will lead to a decrease in most pituitary hormone secretion but may lead to an increase in prolactin secretion.

In childhood, increased *pituitary* secretion of various hormones as a result of an adenoma is rare, although cases of pituitary gigantism (growth hormone excess) are described. Destructive lesions of the pituitary gland or hypothalamus are more common in childhood. A craniopharyngioma, a tumor of Rathke pouch, may descend into the sella turcica, causing erosion and calcification and destroying pituitary and hypothalamic tissue as it enlarges. Hypopituitarism in this case will be due to lack of functioning pituitary and or hypothalamic cells. Acquired hypopituitarism also may result from pituitary infections, from infiltration such as with histiocytosis X, lymphoma, and sarcoidosis, or following radiation therapy and trauma. Congenital hypopituitarism usually is due to absence of hypothalamic releasing factors, even though the pituitary gland can be stimulated by exogenous hy-

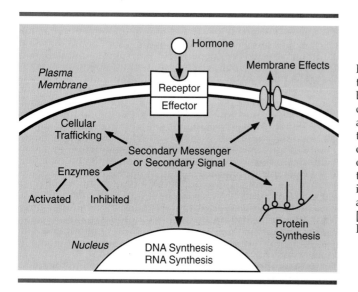

Figure 17–1. A general model for the action of peptide hormones, catecholamines, and other membrane-active hormones. The hormone in the extracellular fluid interacts with the receptor and activates an associated effector system. This activation results in generation of an intracellular signal or second messenger that produces the final effects of the hormone on metabolic enzyme activity, protein synthesis, membrane transport, cellular trafficking, DNA and RNA synthesis, and cellular growth and differentiation. (From Wilson JD, Foster DW [eds]: Williams Textbook of Endocrinology. 8th ed. Philadelphia, WB Saunders, 1990, p 92.)

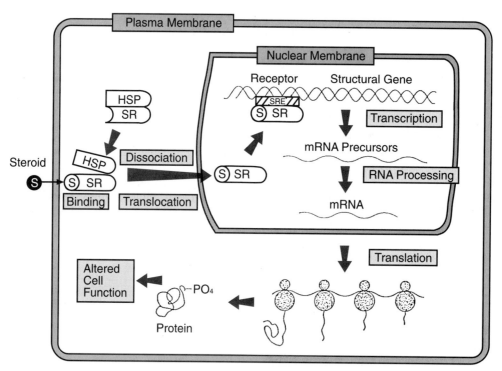

Figure 17–2. Proposed mechanism of action of steroids (glucocorticoids, estrogens, progesterone) in activation of specific gene transcription. The steroid (S) readily diffuses across the plasma membrane and binds to a cytosolic receptor (SR). In the absence of steroid, the receptor resides in the cytoplasm as an inactive complex with heat shock protein (HSP). When the steroid binds to the receptor, the HSP dissociates from it. The steroid–receptor complex is translocated to the nucleus, where it binds to a chromatin receptor consisting of the steroid receptor response DNA element (SRE), thereby activating the transcription of specific genes involved in steroid hormone action. RNA transcripts are translated into proteins that mediate changes in cell function. Some evidence suggests an alternative model in which the steroid receptor resides in the nucleus and not in the cytoplasm. In this model, presumably, steroid diffuses through the cytoplasm into the nucleoplasm, where it binds to the receptor before gene activation occurs. (Adapted from Chan L, O'Malley BW: Mechanism of action of the sex steroid hormones. N Engl J Med 294:1322, 1976; reprinted by permission.)

Figure 17–3. Schematic representation of modalities by which hormones and growth factors reach target tissues. Whereas traditional hormones are formed in glands of internal secretion and are transported to distant sites of action through the bloodstream (endocrine modality), peptide growth factors more often are produced locally by the target cells themselves (autocrine modality) or by neighboring cells (paracrine modality). (From Wilson JD, Foster DW [eds]: Williams Textbook of Endocrinology. 8th ed. Philadelphia, WB Saunders, 1990, p 1087.)

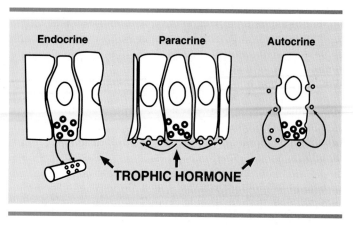

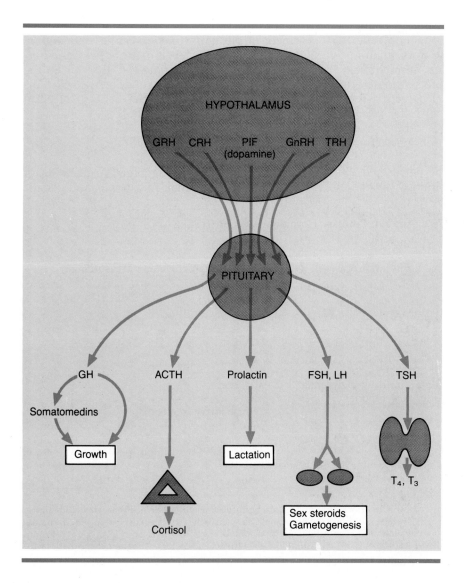

Figure 17–4. Hormones and regulation of the anterior pituitary. CRH = corticotropin-releasing hormone; FSH = follicle-stimulating hormone; GH = growth hormone; GRH = growth hormone–releasing hormone; LH = luteinizing hormone; PIF = prolactin-inhibiting factor, T_3 = triiodothyronine; T_4 = thyroxine; TRH = thyrotropin-releasing hormone, TSH = thyrotropin.

Table 17–1. Diagnostic Evaluation of Hypopituitarism

Manifestation	Cause(s)	Tests*
Growth failure	GH deficiency and/or TRH/TSH deficiency	Provocative GH tests, T$_4$, bone age, IGF-1, IGF BP3
Hypoglycemia	GH deficiency and/or ACTH/cortisol insufficiency	Provocative GH tests, test of cortisol secretion
Micropenis, pubertal delay/arrest	Hypogonadotrophic hypogonadism	Sex steroids (E$_2$, testosterone), LH, FSH after GnRH administration
Polyuria, polydipsia	ADH deficiency	Urine analysis (sp. gr.), serum electrolytes, water deprivation test

* Each patient with documented, acquired hypopituitarism should have a head computerized tomography scan or magnetic resonance imaging as part of evaluation to determine the etiology of the condition.

ADH = antidiuretic hormone; E$_2$ = estradiol; FSH = follicle-stimulating hormone; GH = growth hormone; LH = luteinizing hormone; sp. gr. = specific gravity; T$_4$ = thyroxine; TRH = thyrotropin-releasing hormone; TSH = thyroid-stimulating hormone; IGF-1 = insulin like growth factor; IGF BP3 = insulin like growth factor binding protein 3.

pothalamic releasing factors. Congenital hypopituitarism rarely indicates a tumor. Congenital defects of pituitary secretion may result from anatomic malformations of the hypothalamus, from pituitary hypoplasia or aplasia, or from more subtle defects of hormone secretion. Congenital defects associated with panhypopituitarism include *holoprosencephaly* (cyclopia, cebocephaly, orbital hypotelorism) and *septo-optic dysplasia* (optic nerve hypoplasia, absent septum pellucidum).

Pituitary function testing can be performed directly by measuring the specific pituitary hormone in the basal state or after stimulation. Indirect assessment of pituitary function can be obtained by measuring circulating levels of the target gland hormones. The most appropriate test depends on the specific hormone in question and the type of information sought (Table 17–1). Several tests of pituitary function are listed in Table 17–2.

GROWTH

Normal growth is the aggregate expression of hormonal, environmental, nutritional, and genetic

Table 17–2. Anterior Pituitary Hormone Function Testing

Random Hormone Measurements	Provocative Stimulation Test	Target Hormone Measurement
GH	Arginine* L-dopa* Insulin-induced hypoglycemia* Clonidine* GRH Sleep (Stage IV) 12–24 hr integrated GH levels	IGF-1, IGF BP3
ACTH	Cortisol after insulin-induced hypoglycemia* 11-desoxycortisol after metyrapone* CRH	A.M. cortisol 24-hr urinary free cortisol
TSH†	TRH	FT$_4$*
LH, FSH†	GnRH	Testosterone* Estradiol*
Prolactin*	TRH	None

* These tests, in general, are the most useful in pediatric practice.

† Random measurement is not useful for assessing anterior pituitary function but is very useful for detecting target gland failure.

CRH = corticotropin-releasing hormone; FSH = follicle-stimulating hormone; GH = growth hormone; GRH = growth hormone-releasing hormone; L-dopa = L-dihydroxyphenylalanine, LH = luteinizing hormone; FT$_4$ = free thyroxine; TRH = thyrotropin-releasing hormone; TSH = thyroid-stimulating hormone; IGF-1 = insulin like growth factor; IGF BP3 = insulin like growth factor binding protein 3.

Table 17–3. Hormonal Effects on Growth

Hormone	Bone Age	Growth Rate	Adult Height*
Androgen excess	Advanced greatly	Increased	Diminished
deficiency	Normal or delayed (late)	Normal or decreased	Increased slightly or normal
Thyroxine excess	Advanced slightly	Increased slightly	Normal
deficiency	Retarded slightly	Decreased	Diminished
Growth hormone excess	Normal	Increased	Excessive
deficiency	Retarded	Decreased	Diminished
Cortisol excess	Retarded	Decreased	Diminished
deficiency	Normal	Normal	Normal

* Effect in most patients with treatment.

(Adapted from Underwood LE, Van Wyk JJ: Normal and aberrant growth. *In* Wilson JD, Foster DW [eds]: Textbook of Endocrinology. p 1083. 8th ed. Philadelphia, WB Saunders, 1992.)

factors (see Chapter 1). Consequently, the range of pathology that alters growth is quite large, but maintenance of a normal linear growth pattern is good evidence of overall health. The effects of certain hormones on growth and ultimate height are listed in Table 17–3. It is important to recognize that stature influences psychologic, social, and, potentially, economic well-being. Frequently, it is parental concern about the psychosocial penalty of abnormal stature that causes a family to seek medical attention.

Measurement of Growth

Periodic, accurate measurements of height and weight should be plotted on appropriate growth charts for the timely and efficient diagnosis of growth disorders (see Chapter 1). The correct method of measuring an infant requires two adults, one to hold the baby's head still and the other to extend the feet with the soles perpendicular to the lower leg. A calipers-like device, such as an infantometer or the moveable plates on a baby scale are slid until one rests at the top of the baby's head and the other at the bottom of the baby's feet perpendicular to a ruler so that the exact distance between the two plates can be determined.

After 2–3 yr of age the measurement of a child may be performed standing. A roughly 1.25-cm decrease in height measurements may occur on taking the measurement in the standing position as compared to the lying position, and many referrals are made incorrectly for a child who appears "not to be growing" when in fact the position and the device of measurement are all that have changed. Children in the standing position should be measured barefoot against a hard surface where they can place their backs with legs straight, bare feet together, and all aspects of the body pressed as far

back as possible against the upright surface. Barrettes or hair buns must be removed.

Arm span is a useful measurement of the distance between the tips of the fingers when the patient holds a horizontally outstretched arm position while standing against a solid surface. Measurement of arm span is essential when the diagnosis of Klinefelter syndrome, short-limbed dwarfism, or other dysmorphic conditions are considered. The upper-to-lower segment ratio is the result of the division of the measurement from the symphysis pubis to the floor (lower segment) subtracted from the total height by the lower segment; this ratio changes with age. A normal term baby has an upper/lower ratio of 1.7:1, a 1 yr old has a ratio of 1.4:1, and a 10 yr old has a ratio of 1:1. Conditions of hypogonadism lead to much-decreased upper-to-lower ratio whereas hypothyroidism leads to a very high upper-to-lower ratio.

Endocrine Factors Affecting Growth

Growth hormone (GH), or somatotropin, is a 191–amino acid peptide secreted by the pituitary gland under the stimulatory control of hypothalamic growth hormone–releasing factor (GRF) and the inhibitory control of growth hormone–releasing inhibitory factor (somatostatin or SRIF) (Fig. 17–4). GH secretion is enhanced by alpha-adrenergic stimulation, hypoglycemia, starvation, exercise, and stress. GH secretion is inhibited by beta-adrenergic stimulation, hyperglycemia, and GH treatment. GH has direct effects (diabetogenic activity) and indirect effects mediated by the insulin-like growth factors (IGFs). Serum concentrations of GH are low throughout most of the day but several peaks occur within a 24-hr period, most notably during electroencephalographic stage III or IV sleep. The determination of a random GH concentration is of little value, unless the sample is obtained during an episode of secretion. GH deficiency or the inability to release GH cannot be determined by a single GH determination; a stimulated sample is necessary to measure peak GH secretion (Table 17–2).

Most of GH's growth effects are due to GH stimulated production of *insulin like growth factors.* Serum IGF-I usually is related directly to GH secretion, rising in GH excess and decreasing in GH deficiency. IGF-II decreases in GH deficiency but does not rise in GH excess. IGF-I is considered to function as a paracrine, autocrine, or endocrine agent (Fig. 17–3). IGF-I is the agent most closely associated with linear growth.

Thyroid hormone is essential in normal postnatal growth, although a GH- or thyroid hormone–deficient fetus will achieve a normal birth length. Thyroid hormone is necessary in sufficient quantities to allow the secretion of GH, and hypothyroid patients may falsely appear to be GH deficient. The effects of other hormones on growth are noted in Table 17–3.

Abnormalities of Growth

Short Stature of Nonendocrine Causes (Tables 17–4 and 17–5)

Short stature is defined as subnormal height relative to other children of the same sex, age, and ethnic background. Usually, the 3rd or 5th percentile of the growth curve is selected for demarcation. *Growth failure,* however, is a slow growth rate irrespective of stature. Plotted on a growth chart, growth failure appears as a curve that crosses percentiles (Fig. 17–5). The distinction is critically important because it is the presence of growth failure that signifies persistent pathology requiring a diagnostic evaluation (Table 17–6).

Nutrition is the most important factor affecting growth (see Chapter 2). Infants may develop *failure to thrive* as a result of maternal deprivation (nutritional, psychosocial) or, less often, of organic illness (anorexia, increased metabolism, or nutrient losses). Chronic disease can affect growth either through persistent inflammation (rheumatoid arthritis) or because of the disease's effect on nutrition (anorexia, nutrient losses, hypermetabolism). Psychologic difficulties can affect growth, as in *psychosocial dwarfism.* In this situation the child is psychologically abused and develops functional GH deficiency and poor growth.

The common condition **constitutional delay in**

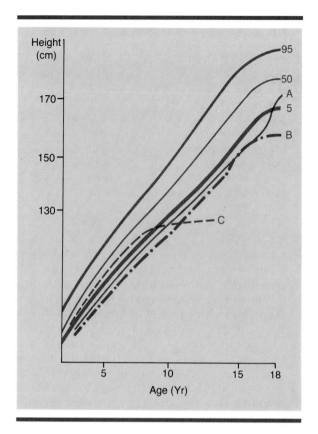

Figure 17–5. Patterns of linear growth. Normal growth percentiles (5th, 50th, 95th) are shown along with typical growth curves for constitutional delay of growth and adolescence *(A),* familial short stature *(B),* and acquired pathologic growth failure *(C)* (e.g., acquired primary hypothyroidism).

growth is a variation of normal growth (Fig. 17–5, Table 17–5). There usually is a family history of a close relative who has grown poorly during childhood but achieves a relatively normal final height. The bone age is delayed, but the growth is appropriate for bone age. The combination of constitutional growth delay and *genetic short stature* leads to exceptional short stature and brings the child to medical attention sooner than usual. Constitutional delay in growth usually leads to constitutional delay in puberty, so that secondary sexual development is delayed. **Genetic familial short stature** (Fig. 17–5, Table 17–5) refers to a child born to a family with short parents. These children would be expected to reach a lower than average height.

Recognizable physical syndromes of short stature often include obesity and decreased height (Table 17–4). The *Prader-Willi syndrome* includes

Table 17–4. Causes of Short Stature

Variations of Normal
Constitutional (delayed bone age)
Genetic (short familial heights)

Endocrine Disorders
GH deficiency
  Congenital
    Isolated GH deficiency
    With other pituitary hormone deficiencies
    With midline defects
    Pituitary agenesis
    With IgG deficiency
  Acquired
    Hypothalamic/pituitary tumors
    Histiocytosis X
    CNS infections and granulomas
    Head trauma (birth and later)
    Hypothalamic/pituitary radiation
    CNS vascular accidents
    Hydrocephalus
    Autoimmune
    Psychosocial dwarfism (functional GH deficiency)
    Amphetamine treatment for hyperactivity(?)
Laron dwarfism (increased GH and decreased IGF-I)
Pygmies (normal GH and IGF-II but decreased IGF-I at
    puberty)
Hypothyroidism
Glucocorticoid excess
  Endogenous
  Exogenous
Diabetes mellitus under poor control
Diabetes insipidus (untreated)
Hypophosphatemic vitamin D–resistant rickets
Virilizing congenital adrenal hyperplasia (tall child,
    short adult)
P-450$_{c21}$, P-450$_{c11}$ deficiencies

Skeletal Dysplasias
Osteogenesis imperfecta
Osteochondroplasias

Lysosomal Storage Diseases
Mucopolysaccharidoses
Mucolipidoses

Syndromes of Short Stature
Turner syndrome (syndrome of gonadal dysgenesis)
Noonan syndrome (pseudo–Turner syndrome)
Autosomal trisomy 13, 18, 21
Prader-Willi syndrome
Laurence-Moon-Biedl syndrome
Autosomal abnormalities
Dysmorphic syndromes (Russell-Silver, Cornelia de
    Lange)
Pseudohypoparathyroidism

Chronic Disease
Cardiac disorders
  Left-to-right shunt
  Congestive heart failure
Pulmonary disorders
  Cystic fibrosis
  Asthma
GI disorders
  Malabsorption (e.g. celiac disease)
  Disorders of swallowing
  Inflammatory bowel disease
Hepatic disorders
Hematologic disorders
  Sickle cell anemia
  Thalassemia
Renal disorders
  Renal tubular acidosis
  Chronic uremia
Immunologic disorders
  Connective tissue disease
  Juvenile rheumatoid arthritis
  Chronic infection
  AIDS
Hereditary fructose intolerance

Malnutrition
Kwashiorkor, marasmus
Iron deficiency
Zinc deficiency
Anorexia due to chemotherapy of neoplasms

AIDS = acquired immunodeficiency syndrome; CNS = central nervous system; GI = gastrointestinal; IGF = insulin-like growth factor.
  (Modified from Styne DM: Growth disorder. *In* Fitzgerald PA [ed], Handbook of Clinical Endocrinology. Norwalk, CT, Appleton & Lange, 1992, pp. 73–99.)

fetal and infantile hypotonia, small hands and feet (acromicria), postnatal acquired obesity and insatiable appetite, developmental delay, hypogonadism, almond-shaped eyes, and abnormalities of the 15th chromosome. *Laurence-Moon-Bardet-Biedl syndrome* includes various combinations of short stature, obesity, retinitis pigmentosum, and hypogonadism in an autosomally inherited pattern.

SHORT STATURE CAUSED BY GROWTH HORMONE DEFICIENCY (Tables 17–4 and 17–5)

Classic severe GH deficiency occurs in 1:4000–10,000 children. Congenital GH deficiency may be associated with congenital anomalies (midline facial defects, microphallus). Acquired GH de-

Table 17–5. Differential Diagnosis

	Hypopituitarism Including Gonadotropin Deficiency (Possibly with ACTH or TRF Deficiency)	Constitutional Delay	Familial Short Stature
Family history	Rare	Frequent	Always
Phenotypic sex	Both	Males > females	Both
Facies	Immature or with midline defect (e.g., cleft palate or optic hypoplasia)	Normal	Normal
Sexual development	Delayed	Delayed	Normal
Bone age	Delayed	Delayed	Normal
Dentition	Delayed	Slight delay	Normal
Hypoglycemia	Variable	No	No
Karyotype	Normal	Normal	Normal
Free T_4	Low or normal	Normal	Normal
Stimulated growth hormone	Low	Normal	Normal
Insulin-Like Growth Factor I	Low	Normal for bone age	Normal
Therapy	Replace deficiencies	Reassurance; sex steroids to initiate secondary sexual development in selected patients	None; GH therapy controversial

T_4 = thyroxine; TRF = thyrotropin-releasing factor.

ficiency suggests a serious etiology (e.g., tumor). Idiopathic GH deficiency is a hypothalamic disease because GRF is either not present or does not exert an effect; the pituitary gland manufactures GH but does not secrete it. Less often, GH deficiency is due to anatomic defects of the pituitary gland. In other cases portions of the GH gene are missing. Classic GH deficiency indicates virtually no secretion of GH, but intermediate forms of decreased GH secretion, referred to as partial GH deficiency or neurosecretory disorder, are described.

Clinical Manifestations. Infants with congenital GH deficiency achieve a normal birth length and weight but soon the growth rate slows and they become chubby and short. Observation in the 1st yr of life may indicate the diagnosis, although most patients are not diagnosed until several years have passed. A classic GH-deficiency patient has the appearance of a cherub (a chubby angelic appearance), with a high-pitched voice resulting from an immature larynx but with intellectually age-appropriate speech. Male neonates with isolated GH deficiency with or without gonadotropin deficiency may have a **microphallus,** which is defined as a stretched penile length of less than 2.5 cm. Severe fasting hypoglycemia leading to seizures in the newborn occurs because of decreased gluconeogenesis. Patients who lack ACTH in addition to GH may have more profound hypoglycemia, because cortisol is another factor in gluconeogenesis.

Dysraphism (midline defects) of the head may be associated with hypothalamic deficiency leading to hypopituitarism; 7% of patients with cleft palate are GH deficient. Patients with pendular nystagmus (sign of poor vision as a result of optic hypoplasia) and absence of the septum pellucidum (septo-optic dysplasia) frequently have anterior and posterior pituitary hormone deficiencies.

and Therapy of Short Stature

Deprivational Dwarfism	Turner Syndrome	Hypothyroidism	Chronic Disease
No	No	Variable	Variable
Both	Female	Both	Both
Normal	Turner facies or normal	Coarse, cretin	Normal
Delayed	Prepubertal	Usually delayed, may be precocious if severe	Delayed
Usually delayed; growth arrest lines	Delayed	Delayed	Delayed
Variable	Normal	Delayed	Normal
No	No	No	No
Normal	45,X or partial deletion of X chromosome or mosaic	Normal	Normal
Normal or low	Normal: hypothyroidism may be acquired	Low	Normal
Possibly high	Usually normal	Low	Variable
Low	Normal	Low	Low or normal (depending on nutritional status)
Change or improve environment	Sex hormone replacement, GH; oxandrolone appears useful	T₄	Treat malnutrition, organ failure (e.g., dialysis, transplant, cardiotonic drugs, insulin)

Diagnosis (Table 17–5). Classic GH-deficient patients are unable to increase their GH levels after stimulation by various secretagogues. There are patients who can release GH in response to secretagogues but cannot spontaneously release GH during the day. An operational definition of GH deficiency might be that patients who require GH will grow more when administered a normal dose of GH. GH testing should be offered to a patient who is short (well below the 5th percentile), usually more than 3.5 standard deviations below the mean, who is growing poorly (less than the 5th percentile growth rate for age), and/or who is below the 5th percentile for height when corrected for family heights. After eliminating chronic disease and routine laboratory testing (Table 17–6), two GH stimulatory tests are performed (Table 17–2).

Treatment. Classic GH deficiency is treated by administering biosynthetic recombinant DNA–derived GH. The dose is given subcutaneously 6 times per week or daily. GH also is administered to patients with partial GH deficiency, but its use in patients who have normal GH responsiveness is controversial. Human cadaver pituitary GH is no longer used because of the risk of contamination with the neurodegenerative infectious *Jakob-Creutzfeldt agent*.

GH is effective in increasing growth rate and final height in Turner syndrome and, possibly, in chronic renal failure. GH treatment carries the risk of a small but increased incidence of slipped capital femoral epiphysis and leukemia.

Psychologic support of children with severe short stature is important. School-age children are aware of their height, and the shortest children may be ridiculed by their peers. Marital status, satisfaction with life, and vocational achievement may be decreased in children of short stature who are not given supportive measures.

Table 17–6. Growth Failure: Screening Test

Test	Rationale
CBC	*Anemia:* nutritional, chronic disease, malignancy *Leukocytosis:* inflammation, infection *Leukopenia:* bone marrow failure syndromes *Thrombocytopenia:* malignancy, infection
ESR & CRP	Inflammation of infection, inflammatory diseases, malignancy
SMA 20 (electrolytes, liver enzymes, BUN)	Signs of acute or chronic hepatic, renal, adrenal dysfunction; hydration and acid–base status
Carotene and prothrombin time	Assess malabsorption of vitamin A and K
Urinalysis	Signs of renal dysfunction, hydration, water and salt homeostasis; renal tubular acidosis
Karyotype	Determines Turner (XO) or other chromosomal syndromes
Cranial imaging (MR, CT)	Assesses hypothalamic–pituitary tumors (craniopharyngioma, glioma, germinoma) or congenital midline defects
Bone age	Compare with height age, and eventual height potential
IGF-I, IGF BP3	Reflects GH status
Free thyroxine	Detects panhypopituitarism or isolated hypothyroidism
Prolactin	Elevated in hypothalamic dysfunction or destruction

BUN = blood urea nitrogen; CBC = complete blood count; CRP = C-reactive protein; CT = computerized tomography; ESR = erythrocyte sedimentation rate; MR = magnetic resonance; IGF BP3 = insulin like growth factor binding protein 3.

TALL STATURE (Table 17–7)

Constitutional tall stature indicates an advancement of bone age and physical development leading to tall stature during childhood but an ultimate normal adult height. Moderate obesity may lead to this situation by advancing the bone age and leading to taller than average stature. *Genetic tall stature* occurs when parents are tall.

Cerebral gigantism or *Soto syndrome* manifests in infancy by increased growth rate, prominent forehead, sharp chin, high arched palate, hypertelorism, and, frequently, developmental delay. There are no known chemical abnormalities in cerebral gigantism, and by mid-childhood the growth rate normalizes.

Marfan syndrome combines tall stature with arm span exceeding height, a very low upper-to-lower segment ratio, long thin fingers (arachnodactyly) and toes, hyperextensibility of the joints, aortic dilation, and superior subluxations of the lens. Homocystinuria may present with a phenotype similar to that of Marfan syndrome. Mental retardation is characteristic and there is increased urinary secretion of the homocysteine. The lens subluxation in this condition may be inferior.

Endocrine Etiologies of Tall Stature

Pituitary gigantism caused by excess GH secretion is quite rare.

Clinical Manifestations. If a GH-secreting adenoma occurs after puberty, a patient will have acromegaly, but in infancy the child will grow remarkably because the epiphyses are not closed. Height velocity is increased; leonine faces and acromegalic facial features may occur. Organomegaly may be noted and glucose intolerance or diabetes mellitus may result. Elevated fasting GH or IGF-1 concentrations will confirm the diagnosis.

Diagnosis. The initial evaluation should include an estimation of the patient's genetic height poten-

Table 17–7. Causes of Tall Stature

Variations of Normal	Nonendocrine Disorders
Constitutional	Marfan's syndrome
Genetic	Klinefelter's syndrome
Exogenous obesity	XYY syndrome
	Cerebral gigantism
Endocrine Disorders	(Sotos syndrome)
Pituitary gigantism	Homocystinuria
Sexual precocity	Weaver Smith syndrome
Thyrotoxicosis	
Beckwith-Wiedemann syndrome	

(Modified from Styne DM: Growth disorder. *In* Fitzgerald PA [ed], Handbook of Clinical Endocrinology. Norwalk, CT, Appleton & Lange, 1992, pp 73–99.)

tial. The corrected mid-parental height is obtained by determining the average height of the parents and adding 6.5 cm if the patient is male or subtracting 6.5 cm if the patient is female. By plotting this number ±8 cm on the mature end of the growth chart, the range of expected adult heights for the patient can be estimated. If the patient's current height-for-age is within the expected parental range, the patient probably has familial tall stature and no further studies are needed. (Assessing the genetic potential for height in this way also is helpful in evaluating children with short stature.) If familial tall stature is not a possibility or if other signs are present, laboratory tests specific for the diagnosis of pituitary gigantism (GH, IGF-I levels, magnetic resonance imaging, chromosomes) should be performed.

Treatment.   A request for treatment most often occurs with girls who are going to be taller than 5'10". Estrogen therapy, if the bone age has not reached 10 yr, may reduce the final height in girls who are predicted to be more than 5'10". Such therapy achieves a more rapid pubertal progression, leading to earlier epiphyseal fusion.

References

Behrman RE (ed): Nelson Textbook of Pediatrics. 14th ed. Philadelphia, WB Saunders, 1992, Sec. 19.1–19.5.

Bramswig JH, Fasse M, Holthoff M-L, et al: Adult height in boys and girls with untreated short stature and constitutional delay of growth and puberty: Accuracy of five different methods of height prediction. J Pediatr 117: 886, 1990.

Cara J, Johanson A: Growth hormone for short stature not due to classic growth hormone deficiency. Pediatr Clin North Am 37:1229, 1990.

Grunt JA, Schwartz ID: Growth, short stature, and the use of growth hormone: Considerations for the practicing pediatrician. Curr Prob Pediatr 22:390, 1992.

LaFranchi S, Hanna CE, Mandel SH: Constitutional delay of growth: Expected versus final adult height. Pediatrics 87:82, 1991.

PUBERTY AND ITS DISORDERS
(see Chapters 1 and 7)

The staging of pubertal changes and the sequence of events are discussed in Chapter 7 (Figs. 7–1 through 7–4; Tables 7–1 through 7–3). Control of the onset of puberty involves adrenal, hypothalamic, pituitary, and gonadal maturation.

Table 17–8.   Classification of Delayed Puberty and Sexual Infantilism

Constitutional Delay in Growth and Puberty (Delayed Activation of Hypothalamic GnRH Pulse Generator)

Hypogonadotropic Hypogonadism
Central nervous system disorders
   Tumors (craniopharyngioma, germinoma, glioma)
   Congenital malformations
   Radiation therapy
   Other causes
Isolated gonadotropin deficiency
   Kallmann syndrome (anosmia–hyosmia)
   Other disorders
Idiopathic and genetic forms of multiple pituitary hormone deficiencies
Miscellaneous disorders
   Prader-Willi syndrome
   Laurence-Moon-Biedl syndrome
   Functional gonadotropin deficiency
      Chronic systemic disease and malnutrition
      Hypothyroidism
      Cushing disease
      Diabetes mellitus
      Hyperprolactinemia
      Anorexia nervosa
      Psychogenic amenorrhea
      Impaired puberty and delayed menarche in female athletes and ballet dancers (exercise amenorrhea)

Hypergonadotropic Hypogonadism
Klinefelter syndrome (syndrome of seminiferous tubular dysgenesis) and its variants
Other forms of primary testicular failure
Anorchia and cryptorchidism
Syndrome of gonadal dysgenesis and its variants (Turner syndrome)
Other forms of primary ovarian failure
XX and XY gonadal dysgenesis
   Familial and sporadic XX gonadal dysgenesis and its variants
   Familial and sporadic XY gonadal dysgenesis and its variants
Pseudo-Turner syndrome
Galactosemia

(Modified from Wilson JD, Foster DW [eds]: Williams Textbook of Endocrinology. 8th ed. Philadelphia, WB Saunders, 1990, p 170.)

Delayed Puberty (Table 17–8)

Puberty is delayed when there is no sign of pubertal development by age 13 yr in girls and 14 yr in boys.

CONSTITUTIONAL DELAY IN GROWTH AND ADOLESCENCE (see Table 17–5 and Abnormalities of Growth)

Patients who have a delayed bone age but who always have grown at the normal rate for their bone age would be expected to have a delayed onset of pubertal development. This is a variation of normal and often is familial. Puberty usually begins by the time the bone age reaches 12 yr of age in boys and 11 yr in girls. Such patients usually begin pubertal development by 18 yr of age.

HYPOGONADOTROPIC HYPOGONADISM (Tables 17–8 and 17–9)

Patients with hypogonadotropic hypogonadism have eunuchoid proportions because their long bones grow for a longer than normal period of time, producing an upper-to-lower ratio below 0.9. If the patient has concurrent GH deficiency, stature will be exceptionally short.

Isolated Gonadotropin Deficiency.   If there is an inability to release gonadotropins, but no other pituitary abnormality, the patient has isolated gonadotropin deficiency. Patients grow normally until the time of the pubertal growth spurt, when they do not accelerate growth. Patients may have associated midline facial defects, such as cleft palate or optic hypoplasia.

Kallmann syndrome combines isolated gonadotropin deficiency with abnormal olfaction. There is genetic heterogeneity; some patients have a decreased sense of smell, others have abnormal reproduction, and some have both.

Abnormalities of the Central Nervous System.   Central nervous system (CNS) tumors are a serious cause of gonadotropin deficiency. Craniopharyngiomas have a peak incidence in the teenage years and may lead to any type of anterior or posterior hormone deficiency. Craniopharyngiomas calcify, erode the sella turcica, and may impinge on the optic chiasm, leading to bitemporal hemianopsia as well as optic atrophy. Germinomas are noncalcifying hypothalamic tumors that frequently produce human chorionic gonadotropin (hCG) and headaches.

Table 17–9. Differential Diagnostic Features of Delayed Puberty and Sexual Infantilism

	Stature	Plasma Gonadotropins	GnRH Test: LH Response	Plasma Gonadal Steroids	Plasma DHAS	Karyotype	Olfaction
Constitutional Delay in Growth and Adolescence	Short for chronologic age, usually appropriate for bone age	Prepubertal, later pubertal	Prepubertal, later pubertal	Low, later normal	Low for chronologic age, appropriate for bone age	Normal	Normal
Hypogonadotropic Hypogonadism							
Isolated gonadotropin deficiency	Normal, absent pubertal growth spurt	Low	Prepubertal or no response	Low	Appropriate for chronologic age	Normal	Normal
Kallmann syndrome	Normal, absent pubertal growth spurt	Low	Prepubertal or no response	Low	Appropriate for chronologic age	Normal	Anosmia or hyposmia
Idiopathic multiple pituitary hormone deficiencies	Short stature and poor growth since early childhood	Low	Prepubertal or no response	Low	Usually low	Normal	Normal
Hypothalamo-pituitary tumors	Decrease in growth velocity of late onset	Low	Prepubertal or no response	Low	Normal or low for chronologic age	Normal	Normal
Primary Gonadal Failure							
Syndrome of gonadal dysgenesis and variants	Short stature since early childhood	High	Hyper-response for age	Low	Normal for chronologic age	XO or variant	Normal
Klinefelter syndrome and variants	Normal to tall	High	Hyper-response at puberty	Low or normal	Normal for chronologic age	XXY or variant	Normal
Familial XX or XY gonadal dysgenesis	Normal	High	Hyper-response for age	Low	Normal for chronologic age	XX or XY	Normal

DHAS = dehydroepiandrosterone sulfate; LH = luteinizing hormone.
(From Wilson JD, Foster DW [eds]: Williams Textbook of Endocrinology. 8th ed. Philadelphia, WB Saunders, 1990, p 1183.)

Idiopathic Hypopituitarism. Congenital absence of various combinations of pituitary hormones may produce idiopathic hypopituitarism. Inheritance may be X-linked or autosomal recessive; sporadic types of congenital idiopathic hypopituitarism are more common.

Congenital hypopituitarism may manifest in a male with GH deficiency and/or associated gonadotropin deficiency with a microphallus (stretched neonatal penile length less than 2.5 cm). The concurrent absence of GH and ACTH may lead to hypoglycemia from decreased gluconeogenesis.

Syndromes of Hypogonadism. Weight loss resulting from voluntary dieting, malnutrition, or chronic disease will lead to decrease gonadotropin function when weight falls below 80% of ideal weight. *Anorexia nervosa* is characterized by striking weight loss (see Chapters 2 and 3). Primary or secondary amenorrhea frequently is found in affected girls, and pubertal development is absent or minimal, depending on the level of weight loss. Regaining weight reverses the condition. Increased physical activity even without weight loss can lead to decreased menstrual frequency and gonadotropin deficiency. When physical activity is interrupted, menstrual function may return. *Hypothyroidism* will inhibit the onset of puberty and delay menstrual periods. Severe hypothyroidism may also lead to precocious puberty.

HYPERGONADOTROPIC HYPOGONADISM

Hypergonadotropic hypogonadism is characterized by elevated gonadotropins resulting from primary gonadal failure.

Ovarian Failure. Turner syndrome is a common cause of ovarian failure. The incidence of Turner syndrome is 1:2000–5000 births (see Chapter 4). Patients with variants of Turner syndrome, gonadal dysgenesis, galactosemia, or following radiation therapy also may have ovarian failure (Table 17–8).

Testicular Failure. Klinefelter syndrome (seminiferous tubular dysgenesis) is the most common cause of testicular failure. The incidence is approximately 1:1000 males. Testosterone levels may be close to normal because Leydig cell function may be spared, but seminiferous tubular function characteristically is lost, causing infertility. The age of onset of puberty usually is normal but secondary sexual changes may not progress because of inadequate Leydig cell function (see Chapter 4).

DIFFERENTIAL DIAGNOSIS OF DELAYED PUBERTY

Once it is determined that no secondary sexual development is present after the upper age limits of normal pubertal development, gonadotropin determinations should be obtained to determine whether the patient has hypogonadotropic or hypergonadotropic hypogonadism (Table 17–9). Differentiation between constitutional delay in growth and hypogonadotropic hypogonadism is difficult if no family history for the former or no CNS abnormalities for the latter are identified. Sometimes a period of observation for months or years is necessary before the diagnosis is confirmed.

TREATMENT OF DELAYED PUBERTY

If a permanent condition is apparent, replacement with sex steroids is indicated. Girls are given ethinyl estradiol in daily doses until breakthrough bleeding occurs, at which time cycling is started with a dose being given on the first 21 days of the month; on days 12–21, a progestational agent such as medroxyprogesterone acetate is added to mimic a normal menstrual period. In boys, testosterone enanthate given once every 4 wk may be started. This regimen is appropriate for patients with hypo- or hypergonadotropic hypogonadism. Boys with hypogonadotropic hypogonadism may receive better virilization if hCG is added to their androgen dose. Patients with hypogonadotropic hypogonadism may be able to achieve fertility by the administration of gonadotropin therapy or hypothalamic-releasing hormone therapy.

Estrogen replacement in Turner syndrome may be offered at the normal age of puberty in low doses to ensure feminization and improve psychologic function as well as to attempt to decrease the likelihood of osteoporosis. Several patients with Turner syndrome have received in vitro fertilization with a donor ovum.

Precocious Puberty
(Tables 17–10 and 17–11)

Precocious puberty is secondary sexual development occurring before the age of 9 yr in boys or 8 yr in girls. There is usually early gonadal maturation, and development is *isosexual* (same sex). Precocious puberty should be distinguished from feminization or virilization in which there is no gonadal development leading to gametogenesis. The condition is true precocious puberty or central precocious puberty if it emanates from premature reacti-

Table 17–10. Classification of Sexual Precocity

True Precocious Puberty or Complete Isosexual Precocity (Premature Reactivation of the Hypothalamic GnRH Pulse Generator)
Idiopathic true precocious puberty
CNS tumors
  Hamartomas (ectopic GnRH pulse generator)
  Other tumors
Other CNS disorders
True precocious puberty after late treatment of congenital virilizing adrenal hyperplasia

Incomplete Isosexual Precocity (GnRH-Independent Sexual Precocity)
Males
  Chorionic gonadotropin–secreting tumors (hCG-dependent sexual precocity)
    CNS tumors (e.g., germinoma, chorionepithelioma, and teratoma)
    Tumors in locations outside the CNS (hepatoblastoma)
    LH-secreting pituitary adenoma
  Increased androgen secretion by adrenal or testis
    Congenital adrenal hyperplasia (21-OH deficiency, 11-OH deficiency)
    Virilizing adrenal neoplasm
    Leydig cell adenoma
    Familial testotoxicosis (familial pituitary gonadotropin–independent sexual precocity)
Females
  Estrogen-secreting ovarian or adrenal neoplasms
  Ovarian cysts
Males and females
  McCune-Albright syndrome
  Primary hypothyroidism
  Peutz-Jeghers syndrome

Iatrogenic Sexual Precocity

Variations of Pubertal Development
Premature thelarche
Premature menarche
Premature adrenarche
Adolescent gynecomastia

Contrasexual Precocity
Feminization in males
  Adrenal neoplasm
  Increased extraglandular conversion of circulating steroids to estrogen
Virilization in females
  Congenital adrenal hyperplasia
    21-OH deficiency
    11-OH deficiency
    3β-ol deficiency
  Virilizing adrenal neoplasms
  Virilizing ovarian neoplasms (e.g., arrhenoblastomas)

LH = luteinizing hormone; OH = hydroxylase.
(From Wilson JD, Foster DW [eds]: Williams Textbook of Endocrinology. 8th ed. Philadelphia, WB Saunders, 1990, p 1186.)

vation of the hypothalamic–pituitary–gonadal axis (GnRH dependent), or incomplete precocious puberty if the hypothalamic–pituitary–gonadal axis is not involved in the process (GnRH independent). A boy may have incomplete precocious puberty as a result of autonomous production of testosterone or other androgens, or of a tumor that produces hCG, stimulating the production of androgens. A girl might have precocious puberty as a result of autonomous production of estrogens from the ovaries or adrenal glands. Members of some families enter puberty prior to the lower limits of normal (*constitutional or familial precocious puberty*). In these cases, every aspect of pubertal development is normal but early.

Idiopathic Precocious Puberty. Although the endocrine changes of puberty, such as increased pulsatile gonadotropin secretion or increased response of luteinizing hormone (LH) to GnRH, are the same as in normal puberty, the clinical course may be waxing and waning. Idiopathic precocious puberty occurs approximately 9 times more often in girls than boys. Boys have a higher incidence of CNS disorders such as tumors or hamartomas (precipitating the precocious puberty. Hamartomas of the cinereum have characteristic appearance on computerized tomography (CT) or magnetic resonance imaging (MRI) and do not need biopsy for diagnosis. The resulting precocious puberty is very amenable to medical therapy. Optic or hypothalamic gliomas (with or without neurofibromatosis), astrocytomas, and ependymomas also can cause precocious puberty by exerting mass effects on those areas of the CNS that characteristically inhibit pubertal development. Almost any condition that affects the CNS, including hydrocephalus, meningitis, encephalitis, suprasellar cysts, head trauma, and irradiation, has been reported to precipitate central precocious puberty. Children with epilepsy and mental retardation have an increased incidence of precocious puberty.

Incomplete GnRH-Independent or Pseudoprecocious Puberty (Tables 17–10 and 17–11). Because of an abnormality in the G-protein system, several endocrine organs may autonomously function, creating the **McCune-Albright syndrome.** Characteristically these patients have irregular café-au-lait spots, polyostotic fibrous dysplasia of the long bones, and precocious puberty. Other patients may have hyperthyroidism, hyperadrenalism, or acromegaly in addition.

Evaluation of Sexual Precocity (Table 17–11). On physical examination, it should be noted whether changes characteristic of normal puberty

Table 17–11. Differential Diagnosis of Sexual Precocity

	Serum Gonadotropin Concentration	LH Response to GnRH	Serum Sex Steroid Concentrations	Gonadal Size	Miscellaneous
True Precocious Puberty (Premature Reactivation of Hypothalamic GnRH Pulse Generator)	Prominent LH pulses, initially during sleep	Pubertal	Pubertal values of testosterone or estradiol	Normal pubertal testicular enlargement or ovarian and uterine enlargement (by sonography)	CT scan of brain to rule out CNS tumor or other abnormality; skeletal survey for McCune-Albright syndrome
Incomplete Sexual Precocity (Pituitary Gonadotropin Independent)					
Males					
Chorionic gonadotropin– secreting tumor in males	High hCG	Prepubertal	Pubertal values of testosterone	Slight to moderate uniform enlargement of testes	Hepatomegaly suggests hepatoblastoma; CT scan of brain if chorionic gonadotropin–secreting CNS tumor suspected
Leydig cell tumor in males	Prepubertal	Prepubertal	Very high testosterone	Irregular asymmetric enlargement of testes	
Familial testotoxicosis	Prepubertal	Prepubertal	Pubertal values of testosterone	Testes symmetric and larger than 2.5 cm but smaller than expected for pubertal development; spermatogenesis occurs	Familial; probably sex-limited, autosomal dominant trait
Premature adrenarche	Prepubertal	Prepubertal	Prepubertal testosterone; DHAS or urinary 17-ketosteroid values appropriate for pubic hair stage 2	Testes prepubertal	Onset usually after 6 yr of age; more frequent in brain-injured children
Females					
Granulosa cell tumor (follicular cysts may present similarly)	Low	Prepubertal	Very high estradiol	Ovarian enlargement on physical examination, MRI, CT, or sonography	Tumor often palpable on abdominal examination
Follicular cyst	Low	Prepubertal	Prepubertal to very high estradiol values	Ovarian enlargement on physical examination, MRI, CT, or sonography	Single or repetitive episodes; exclude McCune-Albright syndrome (skeletal survey)
Feminizing adrenal tumor	Low	Prepubertal	High estradiol and DHAS values	Ovaries prepubertal	Unilateral adrenal mass
Premature thelarche	Prepubertal	Prepubertal	Prepubertal or early pubertal estradiol	Ovaries prepubertal	Onset usually before 3 yr of age
Premature adrenarche	Prepubertal	Prepubertal	Prepubertal estradiol; DHAS or urinary 17-ketosteroid values appropriate for pubic hair stage 2	Ovaries prepubertal	Onset usually after 6 yr of age; more frequent in brain-injured children

CT = computerized tomography; DHAS = dehydroepiandrosterone sulfate; LH = luteinizing hormone; GnRH = gonadotropin-releasing factor; hCG = human chorionic gonadotropin.
(Modified from Wilson JD, Foster DW [eds]: Williams Textbook of Endocrinology. 8th ed. Philadelphia, WB Saunders, 1990, p 1205.)

are apparent (see Chapter 7). In boys it is important to note whether the testes are enlarged over 2.5 cm, which suggests ectopic production of hCG or central (GnRH-dependent) precocious puberty. If the testes are not enlarged but virilization is progressing, the source of the androgens may be the adrenal glands.

Laboratory examinations include sex steroid and gonadotropin levels, usually in the GnRH-stimulated state (Table 17–11). Thyroid hormone determination is useful. If there is a possibility of a CNS anomaly or a tumor (CNS, hepatic, adrenal, ovarian, testis), a CT scan or MRI of the appropriate location is indicated.

Table 17–12. Pharmacologic Therapy of Sexual Precocity

Disorder	Treatment	Action and Rationale
GnRH dependent true or central precocious puberty	GnRH agonists	Desensitization of gonadotropes; blocks action of endogenous GnRH
GnRH independent incomplete sexual precocity		
Girls		
Autonomous ovarian cysts	Medroxyprogesterone acetate	Inhibition of ovarian steroidogenesis; regression of cyst (inhibition of FSH release)
McCune-Albright syndrome	Medroxyprogesterone acetate*	Inhibition of ovarian steroidogenesis; regression of cyst (inhibition of FSH release)
	Testolactone* or fadrozole	Inhibition of P-450 aromatase; blocks estrogen synthesis
Boys		
Familial testotoxicosis	Ketoconazole*	Inhibition of P-450$_{c17}$ (mainly 17,20-lyase activity)
	Spironolactone* or flutamide *and* testolactone or fadrozole	Antiandrogen Inhibition of aromatase; blocks estrogen synthesis
	Medroxyprogesterone acetate*	Inhibition of testicular steroidogenesis

* If true precocious puberty develops, a GnRH agonist can be added.
FSH = follicle-stimulating hormone; GnRH = gonadotropin–releasing hormone.
(Modified from Grumbach MM, Kaplan SL: Recent advances in the diagnosis and management of sexual precocity. Acta Paediatr Jpn 30(Suppl):155, 1988.)

Treatment of Sexual Precocity (Table 17–12). Long-acting analogues of GnRH are the treatment of choice for central precocious puberty as they suppress gonadotropin secretion. The early sexual development and height of the patient with precocious puberty requires psychologic counseling for the children and families. In many cases of incompletely precocious puberty, the removal of the hormone-secreting tumor will be curative. Boys with GnRH-independent premature Leydig cell and germinal cell maturation cannot be treated with GnRH analogues but require treatment with ketoconazole, spironolactone, or testolactone (all inhibitors of testosterone synthesis or effect).

Variations in Pubertal Development

INAPPROPRIATE BREAST DEVELOPMENT

Benign premature thelarche is the term used to describe the isolated appearance of unilateral or bilateral breast tissue in girls ages 6 mo to 3 yr. There are no other signs of puberty and no evidence of excessive estrogen effect (e.g., thickening of the vaginal secretions or bone age acceleration). Ingestion or application of estrogen-containing compounds must be excluded as etiology. Vaginal bleeding is absent and no acceleration in growth velocity is noted. Laboratory investigations usually are not necessary, but a pelvic ultrasound study may be performed to exclude ovarian pathology. Girls with this condition should be re-evaluated at intervals of 6–12 mo to ensure that premature thelarche is not the beginning of isosexual precocious puberty. The prognosis is excellent, and no treatment other than reassurance is necessary.

In boys, the appearance of breast tissue is referred to as *gynecomastia*, which is discussed in Chapter 7.

ISOLATED PREMATURE ADRENARCHE (PUBARCHE)

In girls, the appearance of pubic hair before the age of 8 yr is relatively common. The critical issue is whether the pubic hair is associated with any other features of virilization, such as clitoral enlargement, advanced bone age, or other signs of virilization, such as acne, rapid growth, and voice change. With rapid progression of pubic hair, a detailed investigation for virilizing cause must be undertaken. In such cases, measurements of hormones, such as testosterone, 17-hydroxyprogesterone (17-OHP), and dehydroepiandrosterone (DHEA), are indicated. An ultrasound study may reveal a virilizing adrenal or ovarian tumor, whereas the presence of excessive 17-OHP or DHEA will indicate an enzyme defect consistent with congenital adrenal hyperplasia. Most cases of isolated pubic hair, however, do not have these abnormal signs of progressive virilization and reflect a poorly defined condition known as *benign premature pubarche*. Premature activation of DHEA-S secretion from the adrenal gland (adrenarche) by an undefined mechanism is postulated. Bone age may be slightly advanced, but testosterone levels are normal, whereas DHEA-S levels usually are consistent with Tanner stages II to III (see Figs. 7–1 and 7–4).

References

Behrman RE (ed): Nelson Textbook of Pediatrics. 14th ed. Philadelphia, WB Saunders, 1992, Sec. 3.9, 10.14, 10.18, 19.6–19.9, 19.23, 19.32, 19.37.

Conn PM, Crowley WF Jr: Gonadotropin-releasing hormone and its analogues. N Engl J Med 324:93, 1991.

Englund AT, Geffner ME, Nagel RA, et al: Pediatric germ cell and human chorionic gonadotropin-producing tumors. Am J Dis Child 145:1294, 1991.

Lee P, O'Dea L: Primary and secondary testicular insufficiency. Pediatr Clin North Am 37:1359, 1990.

Pescovitz OH, Barnes KM, Cutler GB Jr: Effect of deslorelin dose in the treatment of central precocious puberty. J Clin Endocrinol Metab 72:60, 1991.

Wheeler M, Styne D: Diagnosis and management of precocious puberty. Pediatr Clin North Am 37:1255, 1990.

THYROID

Disorders of thyroid function are among the most common endocrine problems in pediatrics. Interpretation of thyroid function is based on recognizing the interrelationships within the hypothalamic–pituitary–thyroid axis (Fig. 17–6).

Thyroid Physiology and Development

Thyrotropin-releasing hormone (TRH), a tripeptide synthesized in the hypothalamus, governs the pituitary's release of thyroid-stimulating hormone (TSH). TRH cannot be measured in peripheral serum but can be administered for diagnostic tests. Pituitary TSH is a glycopolypeptide that stimulates the synthesis and release of thyroid hormones by the thyroid gland. Normal plasma concentrations of TSH are less than 10 μU/mL.

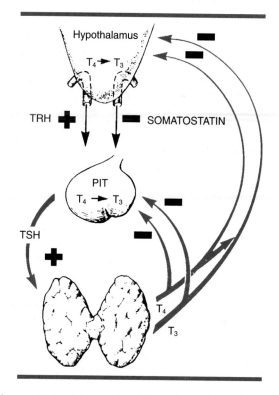

Figure 17–6. Interrelationships of the hypothalamic–pituitary–thyroid axis. Thyroid-stimulating hormone (TSH) from the pituitary (PIT) stimulates the secretion of both thyroxine (T_4) and tri-iodothyronine (T_3). These act at the pituitary level to control secretion of TSH by a negative feedback mechanism. In addition, T_4 is degraded to the much more potent T_3 within the pituitary by a monoiodinase. Secretion of TSH is stimulated by thyrotropin-releasing hormone (TRH) from the hypothalamus and inhibited by somatostatin and, to a lesser extent, by dopamine. Hypothalamic factors thus interact at the pituitary level to determine the secretion rate. Thyroid hormone acts at the hypothalamus to stimulate secretion of somatostatin (somatostatin acts as a negative signal to the pituitary secretion of TSH). The effect of thyroid hormones on secretion of TRH has not been determined precisely. Finally, within the hypothalamus, T_4 also is degraded to T_3, and this degradation may play a role in feedback control. (From Wilson JD, Foster DW [eds]: Williams Textbook of Endocrinology. 8th ed. Philadelphia, WB Saunders, 1990, p 169.)

Thyroid function develops in three stages: (1) embryogenesis occurs from the floor of the primitive oral cavity, and the gland descends to its definitive position in the anterior lower neck by the end of the 1st trimester; (2) the hypothalamic–pituitary–thyroid axis matures in the 2nd trimester; and (3) peripheral metabolism of thyroid hormones matures in the 3rd trimester. This final process extends into the newborn period. The fetal thyroid gland is autonomous; thyroxine (T_4), tri-iodothyronine (T_3), and TSH do not cross the placenta from mother to fetus, so the concentration in fetal serum reflects fetal secretion and metabolism. However, antithyroid antibodies, thyroid-stimulating immunoglobulins (TSIs), and drugs, such as iodides (including radioactive iodides), propylthiouracil, and methimazole, do cross the placenta and affect fetal thyroid function in the same way that they affect maternal thyroid function.

The thyroid gland efficiently concentrates and organifies iodine into tyrosine; with subsequent coupling of two tyrosines, T_4 or T_3 is synthesized, representing the major thyroid hormones. Mole for mole, T_3 is about four times as potent as T_4. The major fraction of circulating T_3 (approximately two thirds) is derived from peripheral conversion of T_4 to T_3. Both hormones are carried by a specific serum carrier protein, thyroxine-binding globulin (TBG). Only the fraction of T_4 and T_3 (~2%) not bound to this or to other serum carriers (i.e., the free T_4 and free T_3) is biologically active and exerts a negative feedback on TSH release. The conversion of T_4 to T_3 requires the removal of one iodine from the outer ring; removing an iodine from the inner ring results in reverse T_3 (rT_3), which has little biologic effect. Conversion of T_4 to T_3 or rT_3 is not a random event; preferential conversion to rT_3 occurs in utero and in all forms of severe illness, including respiratory distress syndrome, fevers, anorexia, cachexia, and starvation. In contrast, conversion from T_4 to T_3 occurs preferentially immediately after birth and with excessive caloric intake.

At birth, there are several dramatic changes in thyroid function (Table 17–13). Appropriate interpretation of thyroid function tests must take into account the influence of TBG as assessed directly or indirectly via the T_3 resin uptake test (Fig. 17–7) and the age-related changes in circulating thyroid hormone concentrations (Table 17–13). When TBG concentrations are normal, the T_3 resin uptake is increased in hyperthyroidism and decreased hypothyroidism (Fig. 17–7), reflecting the change in number of unoccupied binding sites; that is, the thyroid hormone level and T_3 resin uptake test results vary in the same direction. In contrast, with altered TBG capacity, the T_4 level and T_3 resin uptake lead in opposite directions; there is an elevated T_4 level with reduced T_3 resin uptake when there is TBG excess and a low T_4 level with high T_3 resin uptake when there is TBG deficiency. Certain drugs appear to alter TBG capacity and, hence, may affect thyroid function tests. Factors increasing TBG capacity (and total but not free T_4) are estrogens, oral contraceptives, pregnancy, genetic increased TBG, acute hepatitis, maturity (neonates), narcotic abuse, and acute intermittent porphyria; factors decreasing TBG capacity (and total but not free T_4) are competing drugs (phenytoin, salicylates), congenital TBG deficiency, nephrotic syndrome, glucocorticoids, severe nonthyroid illness, androgens, and severe liver failure with cirrhosis. Total T_4 measurements are commonly performed but because free T_4 is physiologically the most important hormone, the direct measurement of free T_4 is available in many laboratories.

A summary of laboratory test results in various types of thyroid abnormalities is illustrated in Table

Table 17–13. Normal Serum Thyroid Hormone, T_3 Uptake, and TSH Concentrations in Childhood

Age	T_4 (μg/dL)	TSH (μU/mL)	T_3 Uptake (% Normal Serum)	T_3 (ng/dL)
Cord blood	10.9* (6.6–18.1)	9.0 (<2–40)		50 (15–85)
2–5 days	15.1 (8.5–22)	<20	1.0 (0.88–1.12)	185 (115–285)
3–12 mo	11.0 (7.6–16.0)	<10	1.0 (0.88–1.12)	176 (110–275)
1–5 yr	10.5 (7.3–15.0)	<10	1.0 (0.88–1.12)	168 (105–269)
6–10 yr	9.3 (6.4–13.3)	<10	1.0 (0.88–1.12)	150 (94–241)
11–16 yr	8.1 (5.6–11.7)	<10	1.0 (0.88–1.12)	133 (8.3–213)

* Mean value, usual range in parentheses.

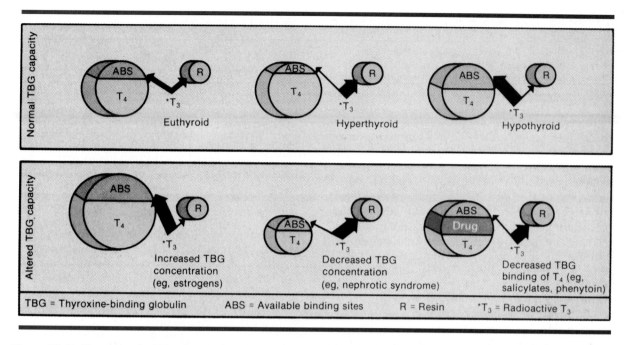

Figure 17–7. Note that the T_3 resin uptake test measures available binding sites not occupied by endogenous thyroid hormones, principally T_4. Thickness of arrows indicates direction of T_3 uptake relative to the normal state (euthyroid). Effects of thyroid disease with normal TBG and of alterations in TBG on results of T_4 and T_3 resin uptake are illustrated. (From Sperling MA: How to recognize and treat thyroid disease in children. Drug Ther, Nov. 1982, p. 79.)

17–14. Thyroid scans rarely are indicated in pediatric thyroid disease. A thyroid scan performed with short-lived ^{123}I will indicate the size, shape, and location of the thyroid gland. Agenesis or ectopic glands and hyperfunctioning "hot" nodules or nonfunctioning "cold" nodules may be detected.

Thyroid Disorders

HYPOTHYROIDISM

Hypothyroidism is considered to be congenital or acquired and, in each instance, as goitrous or nongoitrous.

Congenital Hypothyroidism

This condition occurs in approximately 1:4000 live births. The female-to-male ratio is 2:1. Over 90% of these patients have a dysgenetic (agenesis, aplasia, ectopia) malformation of the thyroid gland. Thyroid tissue usually is not palpable (i.e., nongoitrous), although a radionucleotide scan may reveal some thyroid tissue in an ectopic location. The T_4 concentration is low, whereas circulating TSH is elevated, documenting primary hypothyroidism (see Table 17–13 for normal levels). Such infants are identified through routine neonatal screening programs. Typically, T_4 is measured in neonates at 2–3 days of life, and a subsequent T_4 and TSH

Table 17–14. Laboratory Test Results in Various Types of Thyroid Function Abnormalities in Children*

	Serum Total T_4	Free T_4	Serum TSH	Serum T_3 Resin Uptake	Serum TBG
Primary hypothyroidism	↓	↓	↑	↓	N
Hypothalamic (TRH) hypothyroidism	↓	↓	N	↓	N
Pituitary (TSH) hypothyroidism	↓	↓	N	↓	N
TBG deficiency	↓	N	N	↑	↓
excess	↑	N	N	↓	↑

* N = normal; ↓ = decreased; ↑ = increased.

measurement is made if the original T_4 value is low, although primary TSH screening is more frequently favored.

Congenital TBG deficiency occurs in about 1:10,000 live births and will be associated with a low T_4 and a normal TSH value. Secondary (pituitary) or tertiary (hypothalamic) hypothyroidism can be distinguished from TBG deficiency by determining the free T_4 and TBG concentrations or by determining the T_3 resin uptake, which is elevated in TBG deficiency and normal or low in hypothyroidism. Secondary or tertiary hypothyroidism is rare, occurring in 1:100,000 live births. When tertiary or secondary hypothyroid is detected, structural abnormalities of the CNS should be suspected, and investigation of pituitary–hypothalamic anatomy via CT or MRI may be indicated, along with assessment of other pituitary hormones.

Goitrous congenital hypothyroidism is unusual, occurring in less than 5% of cases. The existence of a goiter indicates an inborn error of metabolism in the pathway of iodide incorporation and thyroid hormone synthesis or reflects the transplacental passage of antithyroid drugs. Inborn errors require lifelong thyroxine treatment.

Clinical manifestations of congenital hypothyroidism include gestation greater than 42 wk (50%), birth weight greater than 4 kg (25%), hypothermia (33%), acrocyanosis (33%), respiratory distress (22%), larger posterior fontanel (33%), abdominal distention (50%), lethargy and poor feeding (40%), jaundice more than 3 days after birth (75%), edema (70%), umbilical hernia (60%), mottled skin (50%), constipation (45%), large tongue (45%), dry skin (45%), hoarse cry (40%), and congenital anomalies (2–4%). In the immediate newborn period the symptoms and signs usually are subtle but become more evident weeks or months after birth. Thyroid hormones are crucially important for maturation and differentiation of tissues, such as bone (bone age is often delayed) and brain. Hence, the importance of newborn screening to make an early diagnosis and initiate thyroid replacement therapy.

When *treatment* is initiated within 1–4 mo of birth, the overall prognosis for normal intellectual development is excellent, although subtle defects in intellect or coordination may become apparent. However, if the diagnosis is missed and therapy instituted after 6 mo or more, when the signs of hypothyroid cretinism are present, the likelihood of normal intellectual function is markedly decreased, despite improved growth associated with ~id replacement.

Acquired Hypothyroidism

The *etiologies* of acquired hypothyroidism are listed in Table 17–15 and the *clinical manifestations* are summarized in Table 17–16. The signs and symptoms may be subtle, and hypothyroidism should be suspected in any child who has a decline in growth velocity, especially if not associated with weight loss. The most common cause in older children is autoimmune thyroiditis (Hashimoto thyroiditis). The failure of the thyroid gland may be heralded by a rise of TSH before T_4 levels fall.

Hashimoto Thyroiditis

Also known as autoimmune or lymphocytic thyroiditis, Hashimoto thyroiditis is a common cause of goiter and acquired thyroid disease in older children and adolescents. A genetic predisposition may be present, because a family history of thyroid disease is present in 25–35% of patients. The *etiology* is an autoimmune process targeted against the thyroid gland with lymphocytic infiltration, anti-

Table 17–15. Causes of Hypothyroidism in Infancy and Childhood

Age	Manifestation	Cause
Newborn	No goiter	Thyroid gland dysgenesis*
	Goiter	Inborn defect in hormone synthesis or effect
		Maternal goitrogen ingestion, including propylthiouracil, methimazole, iodides
		Severe iodide deficiency (endemic)
1–10 yr	No goiter	Thyroid gland dysgenesis
		Cystinosis
		Hypothalamic–pituitary insufficiency
	Goiter	Inborn defect in hormone synthesis or effect
		Hashimoto thyroiditis: chronic lymphocytic thyroiditis*
		Goitrogenic drugs
10–18 yr	Goiter	Hashimoto thyroiditis*
		Inborn defect in hormone synthesis or effect
		Goitrogenic drugs
		Surgical after thyrotoxicosis or thyroglossal duct cysts

* Most common for age group indicated.

Table 17–16. Symptoms and Signs of
Hypothyroidism*

Ectodermal	Poor growth
	Dull facies—thick pale lips, large tongue, depressed nasal bridge, periorbital edema
	Dry scaly skin
	Sparse brittle hair
	Diminished sweating
	Carotenemia
	Vitiligo
Circulatory	Sinus bradycardia/heart block
	Cold extremities
	Cold intolerance
	Pallor
	ECG changes—low-voltage QRS complex
Neuromuscular	Muscle weakness
	Hypotonia—constipation, potbelly
	Myxedema coma (CO_2 narcosis, hypothermia)
	Pseudohypertrophy of muscles
	Myalgia
	Physical and mental lethargy
	Delayed relaxation of reflexes
	Paresthesias (nerve entrapment: carpal tunnel syndrome)
	Umbilical hernia
	Cerebellar ataxia
Metabolic	Myxedema
	Serous effusions (pleural, pericardial, ascites)
	Hoarse voice (cry)
	Weight gain (in adolescent)
	Menstrual irregularity
	Arthralgia
	Elevated CPK
	Macrocytosis (anemia)

* Other features in infants and children: delayed bone maturation; long bone growth delay and epiphyseal dysgenesis; delayed dentition; elevated cholesterol; elevated prolactin; and, occasionally, "precocious puberty."
CPK = creatine phosphokinase; ECG = electrocardiogram.

microsomal or antithyroglobulin antibodies, and lymphoid follicle and germinal center formation preceding fibrosis and atrophy.

Clinical manifestations include firm, nontender euthyroid, hypothyroid or, rarely, hyperthyroid (Hashitoxicosis) diffuse goiter and an insidious onset after 6 yr of age (the incidence peaks in adolescence, with a female predominance); a pea-sized Delphian lymph node above the thyroid isthmus; and later hypothyroidism. Associated autoimmune diseases include diabetes mellitus, adrenal insufficiency (Schmidt syndrome), and hypoparathy-roidism; trisomy 21 or Turner syndrome may predispose to autoimmune thyroiditis.

The *diagnosis* may be confirmed by biopsy; this is rarely indicated. Serum antimicrosomal, antithyroglobulin, anti-TSH receptor or antithyroid nuclei antibodies may be present.

Treatment is indicated for biochemical and clinical signs of hypothyroidism. Patients without manifestation of hypothyroidism require periodic thyroid function testing (TSH, T_4); some patients undergo spontaneous remission.

HYPERTHYROIDISM

Most children with hyperthyroidism have **Graves disease,** which is produced by a variety of autoantibodies (thyroid-stimulating antibodies; TSIs) which stimulate thyroid gland activity, simulating the effects of TSH. The resulting excessive synthesis, release, and peripheral metabolism of thyroid hormones produce the clinical features. Antimicrosomal and antithyroglobulin antibodies may be present; exceptionally high titers may indicate coexistent Hashimoto thyroiditis with the eventual risk of delayed hypothyroidism. In Graves disease, T_4 and/or T_3 are elevated while TSH is suppressed. Rare causes of hyperthyroidism include McCune-Albright syndrome, thyroid neoplasm, TSH hypersecretion, and iodine or thyroid hormone ingestion.

The *clinical manifestations* of fully expressed Graves disease consist of hyperthyroidism (Table 17–17), exophthalmos, ophthalmopathy, dermopathy, myopathy, and acropachy (clubbing). In children, Graves disease is about 5 times more common in females than in males, with a peak incidence in adolescence. However, most children do not exhibit all of these clinical features. Personality changes, mood instability, and poor school performance are common presenting problems. The tremor, anxiety, inability to concentrate, and weight loss may be insidious and confused with a psychologic disorder until thyroid function tests reveal the elevated T_4 level. Rarely, T_4 is near normal while T_3 is selectively elevated (T_3 toxicosis), a situation more common in patients with adenomas or autonomous "toxic" nodules. Goiter usually is present, but may not readily be perceived because of its insidious nature. Many patients complain of neck fullness and, in older subjects, a change in the size of their shirt collars. Thyroid gland enlargement is best visualized with the neck extended and with the examiner lateral to the patient; palpation of the thyroid gland is best performed with the examiner's hands around the neck

Table 17–17. Clinical Manifestations of Hyperthyroidism

Increased catecholamine effects	Nervousness Palpitations Tachycardia Atrial arrhythmias Systolic hypertension Tremor Brisk reflexes
Hypermetabolism	Increased sweating Shiny, smooth skin Heat intolerance Fatigue Weight loss—increased appetite Increased bowel movement (hyperdefecation)
Myopathy	Weakness Periodic paralysis Cardiac failure—dyspnea
Miscellaneous	Proptosis, stare, exophthalmos, lid lag Hair loss Inability to concentrate Personality change (emotional lability) Goiter Thyroid bruit Onycholysis Acute thyroid storm (hyperpyrexia, tachycardia, coma, high-output heart failure, shock)

and having the patient swallow so the examiner can feel the size, consistency, nodularity, and motion of the gland.

For Graves disease, three *treatment* choices are available: medical, surgical, and radioactive iodine. Medical therapy consists of propranolol to reduce excessive beta-adrenergic cardiac manifestations and propylthiouracil, 5–10 mg/kg/24 hr t.i.d., to block thyroid hormone synthesis. The propranolol is tapered after 1–2 mo when the pulse rate is reduced to less than 100 beats/min. Propylthiouracil usually is continued for 1–2 yr, with a remission rate of approximately 30–40%. In patients adhering to the treatment regimen, the 2-yr course of treatment can be repeated. Propylthiouracil should suppress all thyroid function, hence thyroid hormone replacement is needed. Complications of propylthiouracil include lupus-like syndrome, rash, granulocytopenia, and jaundice. Methimazole is an alternate agent. Partial thyroidectomy or radioiodine therapeutic doses may be used. Surgery is effec-

tive and its results immediate, but it entails some risks in anesthesia and in the possibility that the thyroid removal will be excessive, causing hypothyroidism, or will be inadequate, resulting in persistent hyperthyroidism; risks also include keloid formation, recurrent laryngeal nerve palsy, and hypoparathyroidism. Radioiodine (^{131}I) has none of the acute surgical complications but is slower in its therapeutic effects, may require repeated dosing, may cause hypothyroidism, and may be associated with possible long-term sequelae. Whatever the choice of treatment, continued evaluation is mandatory, especially in anticipating the development of hypothyroidism.

Thyroid storm (Table 17–7) is a rare medical emergency that requires reducing the hyperthermia with a cooling blanket, and administering propranolol to control tachycardia. Iodine, a blocker of thyroid hormone release, may be given after propylthiouracil blocks hormone synthesis. Cortisol may be indicated for suspected relative adrenal insufficiency, and therapy for heart failure may include diuretics and digoxin.

Congenital hyperthyroidism results from transplacental passage of material TSIs. The clinical features in the neonate may be masked for several days until the short-lived effects of transplacental maternal antithyroid medication wear off, at which time the effects of TSIs are observed. Irritability, tachycardia (often with signs of cardiac failure simulating "cardiomyopathy"), polycythemia, craniosynostosis, poor feeding, and failure to thrive are the clinical hallmarks. Biochemically, T_4 and T_3 are higher than the levels of the normal neonate. These features may be anticipated if the mother is known to be thyrotoxic in pregnancy. However, the mother may have been cured of her hyperthyroidism before pregnancy by surgery or radioiodine treatment, which limits or curtails T_4 production but not the underlying immune disturbance producing TSIs. Treatment for the neonate includes oral propranolol at 2–3 mg/kg/24 hr in divided doses and propylthiouracil approximately 5 mg/kg/24 hr PO in three divided doses. Because the half-life of immunoglobulin is several weeks, spontaneous resolution of neonatal thyrotoxicosis resulting from transplacental passage of TSIs usually occurs by 2–3 mo of life.

Tumors of the Thyroid

Carcinoma of the thyroid is rare in children; papillary and follicular carcinoma can occur and represent 90% of thyroid cancers. A history of low-dose (<500 rads) therapeutic head or neck irradiation may be related by the patient. Girls are more commonly affected than boys, and the mean age is 9 yr. Carcinoma usually presents as a firm to hard, painless, nonfunctional solitary nodule and occasionally is spread to adjacent lymph nodes. Rapid growth, hoarseness (recurrent laryngeal nerve involvement), and lung metastasis may be present. If the nodule is solid on ultrasound, "cold" on radioiodine scanning, and feels hard, the likelihood of a carcinoid is high. Fine-needle aspiration biopsy may alleviate the need for surgery if demonstrating that the cytology is compatible with a benign thyroid nodule, thyroiditis, or multinodular goiter. **Medullary carcinoma** of the thyroid may be asymptomatic and usually can be detected by the presence of elevated calcitonin levels, either in the basal state or following pentagastrin stimulation. This tumor may occur with multiple endocrine neoplasia (possibly with pheochromocytoma) or alone.

References

Behrman RE (ed): Nelson Textbook of Pediatrics. 14th ed. Philadelphia, WB Saunders, 1992, Sec. 19.10–19.16.

Garcia CJ, Daneman A, Thorner P, et al: Sonography of multinodular thyroid gland in children and adolescents. Am J Dis Child 146:811, 1992.

Geffner DL, Hershman JM: β-adrenergic blockade for the treatment of hyperthyroidism. Am J Med 93:61, 1992.

Grant DB, Smith I, Fuggle PW, et al: Congenital hypothyroidism detected by neonatal screening: Relationship between biochemical severity and early clinical features. Arch Dis Child 67:87, 1992.

Hashizume K, Ichikawa K, Sakurai A, et al: Administration of thyroxine in treated Graves' disease: Effects on the level of antibodies to thyroid-stimulating hormone receptors and on the risk of recurrence of hyperthyroidism. N Engl J Med 324:947, 1991.

Tonglet R, Bourdoux P, Minga T, et al: Efficacy of low oral doses of iodized oil in the control of iodine deficiency in Zaire. N Engl J Med 326:236, 1992.

Zimmerman D, Gan-Gaisano M: Hyperthyroidism in children and adolescents. Pediatr Clin North Am 37:1273, 1990.

DISORDERS OF SEXUAL DIFFERENTIATION

Normal Sexual Development

Maleness or femaleness can be delineated by karyotype (genotypic or chromosomal sex), by morphology of internal organs and gonads (gonadal sex), by the appearance of the external genitalia and the form of secondary sex characteristics (phenotypic sex), by the self-perception of the individual (gender identity), and by the perception of others (gender role). In most children these features blend and conform, but in some patients one or more features may be aberrant. The biochemical bases of many of the defects in sexual development are now known. Consequently, specific diagnoses can be made in many instances.

Ambiguous genitalia in a newborn must be considered an endocrine emergency. Insensitive handling of the situation may lead to a lifelong pattern of gender uncertainty in both parents and patient. Before a sex is assigned or a name is given to the child, various laboratory evaluations are required that may take days or weeks to be completed.

Diagnosis and management of disorders of sex differentiation are understood easily when the embryology and hormonal control of normal sex differentiation is known. The internal and external genitalia are completely formed by the 13th wk of gestation. Every fetus, regardless of karyotype, has the capacity to become a normally formed individual of either sex. Development is programmed to proceed toward the female phenotype unless a specific "male" influence alters development. The male or female phenotype develops internally from bipotential gonads and internal ducts, and externally from bipotential anlaga (Fig. 17–8). In the presence of a testes-determining gene on the Y chromosome, the primitive fetal gonad differentiates into a testes (Fig. 17–9). The testes secretes testosterone, which has direct effects (stimulation of development of the wolffian ducts). Testosterone is locally converted into dihydrotestosterone (DHT) by 5-alpha-reduction; DHT causes enlargement, rugation, and fusion of the labia majora into a scrotum, fusion of the ventral surface of the penis to enclose a penile urethra, and enlargement of the phallus with ultimate development of male external genitalia (Figs. 17–8 and 17–9). Testicular production and secretion of müllerian duct–inhibitory substance causes the regression and disappearance of the müllerian ducts so that the remaining male wolffian ducts develop. In the presence of testosterone, the wolffian ducts develop into the vas deferens, seminiferous tubules, and prostate.

In the absence of testis-determining factor, an ovary spontaneously develops from the bipotential, primitive gonad. In the absence of fetal testicular secretion of müllerian-inhibitory substance, a normal uterus, fallopian tubes, and posterior third of the vagina develop out of the müllerian ducts as the wolffian ducts degenerate. In the total absence of androgens, the external genitalia appear female. In the absence of adequate virilization because of abnormal development of the testes, biosynthetic

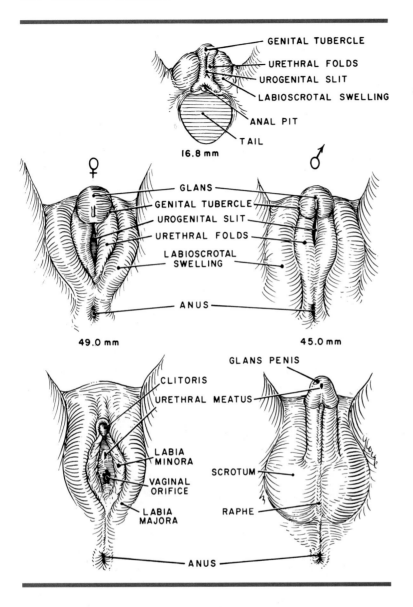

Figure 17–8. Differentiation of male and female external genitalia as proceeding from a common anlage. (From Grumbach MM, Conte FA: Disorders of sexual differentiation. *In* Wilson JD, Foster DW [eds]: Textbook of Endocrinology. 8th ed. Philadelphia, WB Saunders, 1990, p 873. Adapted from Spaulding MH: The development of the external genitalia in the human embryo. Contrib Embryol Carnegie Instit 1921;13:69–88.)

defects of testosterone or DHT, or androgen receptor defects, any phenotype between female and male may develop; the patient has ambiguous genitalia or an intersex condition.

Abnormal Sexual Development

VIRILIZATION OF THE GENOTYPIC XX FEMALE (FEMALE PSEUDOHERMAPHRODITISM)

Masculinization of the external genitalia of genotypic females always is due to the presence of excessive androgens during the critical period of development (8–13 wk gestation) (Table 17–18). The magnitude of the changes will reflect the quantity and duration of exposure to androgens. The degree of virilization can range from mild clitoral enlargement to that of a "male" phallus with a penile urethra and fused scrotum with raphe. Ambiguous genitalia in females is most commonly the result of an enzyme deficiency that impairs adrenal cortisol synthesis but does not affect testosterone production (see Adrenal Gland). Under these conditions, ACTH stimulates hyperplasia of the adrenal cortex and excessive adrenal production of testosterone.

INADEQUATE MASCULINIZATION OF THE GENOTYPIC XY MALE (MALE PSEUDOHERMAPHRODITISM)

Underdevelopment of the male external genitalia occurs because of a relative deficiency of testosterone production or action (Table 17–19). The penis is small, with various degrees of hypospadias (penile or perineal) and associated chordee; unilateral, but more often bilateral, cryptorchidism may be present. The testis (gonad) should be carefully sought in the inguinal canal or labioscrotal folds. Very rarely, a palpable gonad in the inguinal canal or labioscrotal fold represents a herniated ovary or an ovotestis in a hermaphrodite. The latter patients have both ovarian and testicular tissue, usually an XX genotype (80%), and ambiguous external genitalia. Production of testosterone by a gonad in utero implies that testicular tissue is present and that some cells carry Y chromosomal DNA.

Testosterone production can be reduced by specific deficiencies of the enzymes needed for androgen biosynthesis or by dysplasia of the gonads. In the latter, if müllerian-inhibiting substance production also is reduced, a rudimentary uterus and fallopian tubes will be present. Enzyme defects in testosterone biosynthesis, which also block cortisol production, produce adrenal hyperplasia. Hypopituitarism with LH deficiency does not result in ambiguous genitalia because placental hCG present in the fetal circulation stimulates gonadal testosterone synthesis. Congenital gonadotropin deficiency

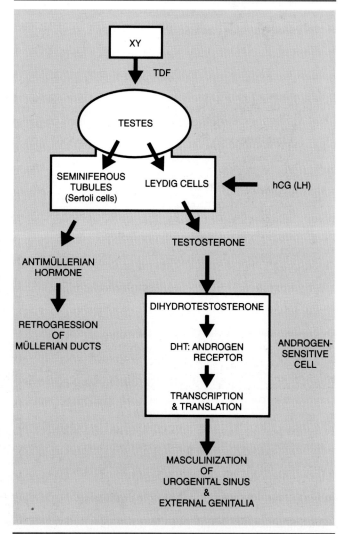

Figure 17–9. A diagrammatic scheme of male sex determination and differentiation. DHT = dihydrotestosterone; TDF = testis determining factor. (From Wilson JD, Foster DW [eds]: Williams Textbook of Endocrinology. 8th ed. Philadelphia, WB Saunders, 1990, p 918.)

Table 17–18. Causes of Virilization in the Female

Condition	Additional Features
P-450 C_{21} deficiency	Salt loss in some
3β-Hydroxysteroid dehydrogenase deficiency	Salt loss
P-450 C_{11} deficiency	Salt retention/hypertension
Androgenic drug exposure (e.g., progestins)	Exposure by 12th wk gestation
Mixed gonadal dysgenesis*	Karyotype = 45, X/46, XY
True hermaphrodite	Testicular and ovarian tissue present
Maternal virilizing adrenal or ovarian tumor	Rare, positive history

* Or mosaic Turner syndrome.

Table 17–19. Causes of Inadequate Masculinization in the Male

Condition	Additional Features
P-450$_{scc}$ deficiency	Salt loss
3β-Hydroxysteroid dehydrogenase deficiency	Salt loss
P-450$_{c17}$ deficiency	Salt retention/hypertension
17,20-Desmolase deficiency	Adrenal function normal
17β-Hydroxysteroid oxidoreductase deficiency	Adrenal function normal
Dysgenetic testes	Possible abnormal karyotype
Leydig cell hypoplasia	Rare
Testicular feminization syndrome (complete)*	Female external genitalia, absence of müllerian structures
Testicular feminization syndrome (partial)*	As above with ambiguous external genitalia
Partial androgen insensitivity syndromes	Family history frequently positive
5α-Reductase deficiency	Autosomal recessive, virilization at puberty

* Or androgen insensitivity.

may produce a microphallus and often is combined with deficiencies of growth hormone and ACTH, causing neonatal hypoglycemia.

The complete form of *testicular feminization syndrome* is the most dramatic example of androgen insensitivity. Absolute resistance of target tissues to the actions of the androgens in some patients occurs because the androgen receptor cannot bind DHT. In others, a postreceptor defect is presumed. Affected patients have a 46,XY karyotype, normally formed testes usually located in the inguinal canal or labia majora, and feminine-appearing external genitalia with a short vagina and no internal müllerian structures. At the time of puberty, testosterone concentrations rise to the normal male range. Because some of the testosterone is converted to estradiol in peripheral tissues, breast development ensues without growth of sex hair or the occurrence of menstruation.

Approach to the Infant with Genital Ambiguity

The major goals of caring for these infants are to quickly determine the correct sex of rearing and to identify any accompanying disorders important to the baby's biologic function (e.g., salt loss). Sex assignment is based on the prognosis of the underlying hormonal defect and the feasibility of genital reconstruction rather than on karyotype or gonadal histology. For example, it would be inappropriate to raise a female infant virilized from adrenal hyperplasia as a male, even if a virtually normal phallus and penile urethra existed. To do so would complicate the hormonal therapy as well as deny the patient the potential for future fertility. Likewise, a karyotypic male with an extremely small phallus that cannot be increased in size with androgen therapy probably should be raised female because surgical construction of a fully functional phallus is very difficult. For many reasons, it is wise to assign sex as rapidly as possible; however, premature speculation with parents about sex assignment must be avoided. The naming of the infant can be delayed until the correct choice is clear.

The first step toward *diagnosis* is to determine if the disorder represents virilization of a female (androgen excess) or underdevelopment of a male (androgen deficiency) (Fig. 17–9). Inguinal gonads that are evident on palpation nearly always are testes and indicate that incomplete development of a male has occurred. Similarly, absence of female internal genitalia (detected by ultrasound) implies that müllerian-inhibiting substance was secreted by fetal testes.

Most virilized females have adrenal hyperplasia, and 90% have 21-hydroxylase deficiency. The diagnosis is established by measuring the plasma concentration of 17-OHP (see Adrenal Gland), which typically is 10–100 times above the normal range. Other enzymatic defects also can be diagnosed by quantifying the circulating levels of the steroid that serves as the defective enzyme's substrate.

Accurate diagnoses are more difficult to obtain in underdeveloped males. When adrenal hyperplasia coexists, excessive ACTH secretion will elevate levels of specific adrenal steroid precursors substantially. If the defect is restricted to testosterone biosynthesis, the measurement of testosterone and its precursors after stimulation by hCG may be required. Patients with normal levels of testosterone either have persistent androgen resistance or had an interruption of normal morphogenesis at a critical time. Abnormalities of the sex chromosomes suggest dysgenetic gonads, as does persistence of müllerian structures.

Treatment consists of replacing deficient hormones (e.g., cortisol in adrenal hyperplasia and testosterone at the time of puberty in androgen biosynthetic defects); surgical restoration; and psychologic support of the whole family. Gonads and internal organs discordant for the sex of rearing are removed. Reconstructive surgery should be started by 2 yr of age so that genital structure will reflect sex of rearing during the time when gender identity is acquired. Dysgenetic gonads should be removed because gonadoblastomas or dysgerminomas may develop in the future.

References

Behrman RE (ed): Nelson Textbook of Pediatrics. 14th ed. Philadelphia, WB Saunders, 1992, Sec. 19.29–19.43.
Editorial: The secret of sex? Lancet 336:348, 1990.
Griffin JE: Androgen resistance—the clinical and molecular spectrum. N Engl J Med 326:611, 1992.
McCauley E: Disorders of sexual differentiation and development: Psychological aspects. Pediatr Clin North Am 37:1405, 1990.
Pagon RA: Diagnostic approach to the newborn with ambiguous genitalia. Pediatr Clin North Am 34:1019, 1987.

ADRENAL GLAND

The adrenal gland consists of an outer cortex, responsible for the synthesis of steroids, and an inner medulla derived from neuroectodermal tissue, which synthesizes catecholamines. The **adrenal cortex** consists of three zones: an outer glomerulosa whose end product is the mineralocorticoid aldosterone, which regulates sodium balance; a middle zone, the fasciculata, whose end product is cortisol; and an inner reticularis that synthesizes sex steroids. The general scheme of these synthetic steps is shown in Figure 17–10.

The hypothalamic–pituitary–adrenal axis comprises a classic negative feedback system. A hypothalamic corticotropin-releasing hormone (CRH) stimulates the release of pituitary ACTH, derived by selective processing from pro-opiomelanocortin. The sequence of melanocyte-stimulating hormone (MSH) is contained within the ACTH molecule. ACTH governs the synthesis and release of cortisol and adrenal androgens. Cortisol deficiency from any defect in the adrenal results in an oversecretion of ACTH; cortisol deficiency also may occur from CRH or ACTH deficiency causing low serum ACTH concentrations. Endogenous glucocorticoids feed back to inhibit ACTH and CRH secretion. Exogenous cortisol or equivalent glucocorticoids also suppress ACTH. The renin–angiotensin system, as well as potassium, regulates aldosterone secretion.

Steroids that are free (i.e., not bound to cortisol-binding protein [transcortin]) may cross the placenta from mother to fetus. Because the fetal CRF–ACTH–adrenal axis is operational in utero, deficiencies in cortisol synthesis lead to excessive ACTH secretion and adrenal hyperplasia in some cases. The normal ranges for serum cortisol concentration are not appropriate for the neonate; cortisol's diurnal variation may not be established until the end of the 1st yr of life.

Adrenal Insufficiency

The *clinical manifestations* of inadequate adrenal function result from the inadequate secretion or action of glucocorticoids, mineralocorticoids, or both (Table 17–20). In addition, in the case of enzyme defects that commonly affect the gonad as well as the adrenal gland, overproduction or underproduction of potent androgens can occur, depending on the site of blockade (Fig. 17–10). Thus, there may be progressive virilization of the external genitalia in females and males or incomplete virilization in males. Ambiguity of the external genitalia is therefore a common manifestation of disordered fetal adrenal function. Precise *diagnosis* is essential for the prescription of appropriate therapy, long-term outlook, and genetic counseling. Table 17–21 presents a diagnostic classification of adrenal insufficiency in infancy and childhood.

The dominant clinical features of adrenal insufficiency in infancy are related to mineralocorticoid

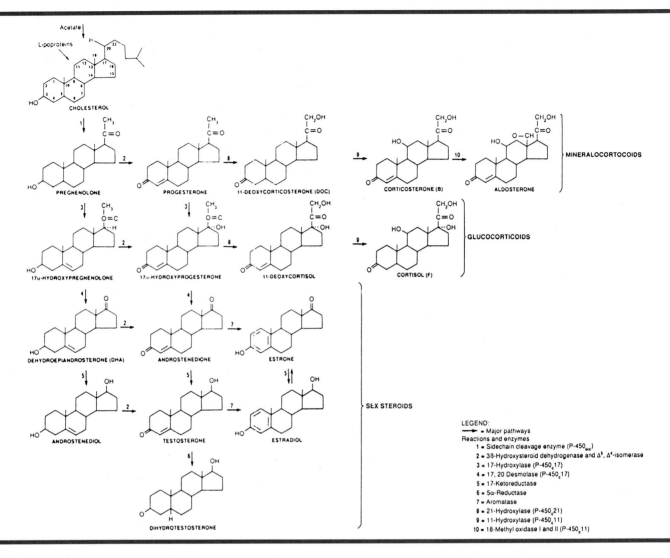

Figure 17–10. Steroid hormone biosynthetic pathways. (From Styne DM: Sexual differentiation. In Fitzgerald PA [ed], Handbook of Clinical Endocrinology. Norwalk, CT, Appleton & Lange, 1900, pp. 73–99.)

deficiency. Vomiting begins several days after birth and may lead to severe dehydration. Serum electrolyte measurement reveals hyponatremia, hyperkalemia, and acidosis. In females, ambiguous genitalia resulting from excessive androgen secretion is often a major clue. In males, the diagnosis of adrenal insufficiency may be overlooked or confused with pyloric stenosis. However, in pyloric stenosis, the vomiting of HCl results in hypochloremia; serum potassium is normal or low and alkalosis is present. This distinction may be lifesaving in preventing unnecessary investigations, inappropriate therapy, or surgery. Scrotal pigmentation suggests excess ACTH (MSH) secretion.

In congenital adrenal hypoplasia or in adrenal hemorrhage, the secretion of all adrenal steroids will be low. In contrast, congenital adrenal hyperplasia (adrenogenital syndrome), as a result of one of the enzyme defects listed in Figure 17–10, leads to a diagnostic steroid pattern in blood and urine. Deficiency of 21-hydroxylase is most common (95%) and serves as a paradigm for these disorders.

21-HYDROXYLASE DEFICIENCY

Deficient 21-hydroxylase activity results in the decreased conversion of 17-OHP to 11-desoxycortisol and of progesterone to desoxycorticosterone

Table 17–20. Clinical Manifestations of Adrenal Insufficiency

Cortisol Deficiency
Hypoglycemia
Inability to withstand stress
Vasomotor collapse
Hyperpigmentation (primary adrenal insufficiency with ACTH excess)
Apneic spells
Hypoglycemic seizure
Muscle weakness, fatigue

Aldosterone Deficiency
Vomiting
Hyponatremia
Urinary sodium wasting
Salt craving
Hyperkalemia
Acidosis
Failure to thrive
Volume depletion
Hypotension
Dehydration
Shock
Diarrhea
Muscle weakness

Androgen Excess or Deficiency (Caused by Enzyme Defect)
Ambiguous genitalia

(Fig. 17–10). The obligatory decreased production of cortisol stimulates hypersecretion of ACTH, which, in turn, stimulates the synthesis of steroids immediately proximal to the block and causes shunting of precursors to the androgen pathway, leading to the overproduction of testosterone. The latter results in many of the *clinical manifestations.* Virilization of the external genitalia of the female occurs in utero; the development of the ovaries, fallopian tubes, and uterus is unaffected. The degree of virilization in the external genitalia of the female is variable, ranging from mild clitoromegaly to complete fusion of labioscrotal folds, simulating a phallus (see Disorders of Sexual Differentiation). A male infant with this defect appears normal at birth, although penile enlargement may be apparent. The deficiency in aldosterone found in about 75% of patients causes salt wasting with shock and dehydration unless appropriate treatment is given.

Inadequately treated, or milder forms, demonstrate postnatal virilization, causing excessive growth, early appearance of pubic hair, progressive penile or clitoral enlargement, and progressive advancement in the bone age that is accompanied by early epiphyseal fusion, ultimately yielding

short stature. Normal puberty is impossible in untreated girls, whereas males have adequate penile size but subnormal testes and azoospermia.

Biochemical diagnostic studies demonstrate decreased urinary excretion of cortisol (17-hydroxycorticosteroids) and aldosterone, whereas 17-ketosteroids, representing the excretion products of the androgen pathway, are increased. In serum, cortisol and aldosterone are low whereas testosterone is elevated, as is the major substrate of 21-hydroxylase, 17-OHP. The major urinary metabolite of this compound is pregnanetriol, leading to an excretion rate in affected subjects that exceeds the normal value of 2 mg/24 hr.

There may be variable allelic forms of this disorder or other individual factors that result in variable

Table 17–21. Causes of Adrenal Insufficiency in Infancy and Childhood

Congenital Adrenal Hypoplasia
Secondary to ACTH deficiency
Autosomal recessive
X-linked

Adrenal Hemorrhage

Congenital Adrenal Hyperplasia
$P-450_{scc}$ (Cholesterol side chain cleavage) deficiency
3β-Hydroxysteroid dehydrogenase deficiency
$P-450 \; C_{21}$ (21-Hydroxylase) deficiency
$P-450 \; C_{11}$ (11β-Hydroxylase) deficiency
$P-450 \; C_{17}$ (17-Hydroxylase) deficiency

Isolated Deficiency of Aldosterone Synthesis
$P-450_{c11}$ (18-Hydroxylase) deficiency
$P-450_{c11}$ (18-Hydroxysteroid dehydrogenase) deficiency

Pseudohypoaldosteronism—End-Organ Unresponsiveness to Aldosterone

Congenital Adrenal Unresponsiveness to ACTH

Addison Disease
Autoimmune
Infections of the adrenal gland
   Tuberculosis
   Histoplasmosis
   Meningococcosis
Infiltration of the adrenal gland
   Sarcoidosis
   Hemochromatosis
   Amyloidosis
   Metastatic cancer
Adrenoleukodystrophy

Drugs (Suppress Adrenal Steroidogenesis)
Withdrawal of steroid therapy given for more than 7–10 days
Metyrapone
Ketoconazole

expression of the defect, in terms of salt wasting and age at presentation. This genetic and clinical heterogeneity has given rise to terms such as classic, nonclassic, salt-wasting, simple virilizing, and late-onset forms to define a group of fundamentally similar disorders. The incidence of classical 21-hydroxylase deficiency is about 1:12,000 among various Caucasian populations. Two genes on chromosome 6 code for 21-hydroxylase; 1 of 5 common deletions or mutations accounts for most cases, permitting prenatal diagnosis.

Chronic *treatment* consists of providing glucocorticoid at a dose of approximately 15–20 mg/m^2/24 hr of hydrocortisone or its equivalent. Various other glucocorticoid regimens and dose schedules have been recommended in an attempt to ensure adequate suppression of excessive ACTH, and hence of adrenal by-products, without inducing cushingoid features and growth failure that develop from administering excessive glucocorticoids. For those who are salt losers, mineralocorticoid therapy, usually 9-alpha-fludrocortisone (Florinef) at a dose of approximately 0.1–0.2 mg/24 hr, is used along with sodium chloride supplementation, which is especially recommended for infants in the 1st yr of life. Surgical correction of ambiguous external genitalia begins by 1 yr of life to permit normal development of gender identity. The adequacy of glucocorticoid replacement therapy is monitored by determining blood concentrations of 17-OHP or testosterone and by assessing linear growth and skeletal age. Higher doses of glucocorticoids are given during stressful states such as febrile illnesses to avoid adrenal insufficiency. Prenatal treatment with dexamethasone to suppress fetal ACTH-induced androgen production has been reported as successful if begun at approximately the 7th wk of gestation.

OTHER ENZYME DEFECTS

In these disorders, an elevation in the precursor steroid is present immediately above the block, a deficiency of steroids is present below the block, and an overflow drains into whichever pathway is available (Fig. 17–10). The excessive secretion and excretion of precursor steroids are suppressed by administering glucocorticoid; the suppressive response confirms the diagnosis. The incidence of the other enzyme defects is rare in comparison to that of 21-OH deficiency; 11-OH deficiency is the next most common.

In *11-OH deficiency*, virilization occurs but salt wasting with hyponatremia and hyperkalemia do not, as a result of the build-up of desoxycorticosterone (Fig. 17–10), a potent mineralocorticoid. Hypertension may develop in these patients along with hypokalemia, mimicking excessive aldosterone production

A summary of the clinical and biochemical features of adrenal insufficiency in infancy is listed in Table 17–22.

Table 17–22. Clinical and Biochemical Features in Newborn Adrenal Insufficiency

| | | Ambiguous Genitalia | | Serum | | | | | Urine | | |
	Electrolyte Disturbance	Virilized Female	Incomplete Male	Cortisol	Aldosterone	17-OHP	DHEA	17-OHCS	17-KS	Pregnanetriol
Hypoplasia	Severe	No	No	Decrease	Decrease	Decrease	Decrease	Decrease	Decrease	Decrease
Hemorrhage	Moderate–severe	No	No	Decrease	Decrease	Decrease	Decrease	Decrease	Decrease	Decrease
P-450$_{scc}$ deficiency	Severe	No	Yes	Decrease	Decrease	Decrease	Decrease	Decrease	Decrease	Decrease
3β-HSD	Severe	Yes	Yes	Decrease	Decrease	Decrease	Increase	Decrease	Increase	Decrease
P-450$_{c21}$ deficiency	Absent–severe	Yes	No	Decrease	Decrease	Increase	Increase	Decrease	Increase	Increase
Aldosterone synthesis block	Severe	No	No	Normal	Decrease	Normal	Normal	Normal	Normal	Normal
Pseudohypoaldosteronism	Severe	No	No	Normal	Increase	Normal	Normal	Normal	Normal	Normal
P-450 C$_{11}$ deficiency	None	Yes	No	Decrease	Decrease	Normal–sl. Increase	Normal	Increase	Increase	Normal–sl. Increase
P-450 C$_{17}$ deficiency	None	No	Yes	Decrease	Normal–decrease	Decrease	Decrease	Decrease	Decrease	Decrease
Unresponsiveness to ACTH	None	No	No	Decrease	Normal–low	Normal–low	Normal–low	Decrease	Decrease	Normal–low

HSD = hydroxysteroid dehydrogenase; 17-KS = 17-ketosteroid; 17-OHCS = 17-hydroxycorticosteroid; sl. = slight.

ADDISON DISEASE

This rare disorder of childhood usually is associated with autoimmune destruction of the adrenal cortex. *Clinical manifestations* are hyperpigmentation, salt craving, postural hypotension, fasting hypoglycemia, and episodes of shock during severe illness. Baseline and ACTH-stimulated cortisol values are subnormal, thereby confirming the *diagnosis*. Replacement *treatment* with glucocorticoids at 15–20 mg/m^2/24 hr of hydrocortisone is indicated, with supplementation during stress at 3 times the normal maintenance dosage. Mineralocorticoid replacement with Florinef also may be required. Associated autoimmune disorders include diabetes mellitus, hypothyroidism, oophoritis, pernicious anemia, malabsorption, chronic hepatitis, vitiligo, alopecia, and mucocutaneous candidiasis.

CUSHING SYNDROME

Classic *clinical manifestations* of Cushing syndrome in children include progressive central obesity, marked failure of longitudinal growth, hirsutism, weakness, a nuchal fat pat (buffalo hump), acne, striae, hypertension and hyperpigmentation only if secondary to an ACTH-secreting pituitary adenoma (Cushing disease). Most affected children have adrenal adenoma, carcinoma, or, occasionally, nodular hyperplasia. Increased in glucocorticoids as well as sex steroids in plasma and urine, which are usually nonsuppressible by standard doses of exogenous dexamethasone. The high-dose dexamethasone suppression test (2 mg every 6 hr for 48 hr) will suppress glucocorticoid secretion in Cushing disease. Excessive excretion of urinary free cortisol (normal levels are less than 100 µg/day) helps establish the *diagnosis* of Cushing syndrome but precise localization may require MRI or CT. Parenteral glucocorticoids are necessary during and immediately after surgical removal of the etiology of the syndrome to avoid a crisis of adrenal insufficiency.

Spontaneous Cushing syndrome is rare in childhood, but iatrogenic Cushing syndrome is far more common and produces similar features; the latter may be induced by the use of potent glucocorticoids for chronic inflammatory, neoplastic, and collagen vascular disorders, and suppression of the immune response. Depending on the potency of glucocorticoid used and its duration of use, both adrenal gland size and secretory ability and pituitary ACTH are suppressed. Recovery of pituitary ACTH secretion precedes that of adrenal gland function. Hence, glucocorticoids should be withdrawn gradually over a number of weeks. During this tapering process, any needed emergency glucocorticoid therapy at triple the physiologic dose should be provided in the form of short-acting hydrocortisone, the effects of which wear off within hours. The ability of the adrenal to respond to ACTH with a doubling of plasma cortisol to levels of at least 15–20 µg/dL indicates recovery of pituitary–adrenal function.

Treatment of Cushing syndrome includes excision of autonomous adrenal, pituitary, or ectopic ACTH-secreting tumors. Rarely, adrenalectomy or adrenal ablative agents (mitotane-*o,p'*-DDD) are needed to control hyperglucocorticoid symptoms.

References

Behrman RE (ed): Nelson Textbook of Pediatrics. 14th ed. Philadelphia, WB Saunders, 1992, Sec. 19.21–19.28.

Cutler GB Jr, Laue L: Congenital adrenal hyperplasia due to 21-hydroxylase deficiency. N Engl J Med 323:1806, 1990.

Miller WL, Levine LS: Molecular and clinical advances in congenital adrenal hyperplasia. J Pediatr 111:1, 1987.

Pang S, Pollack MS, Marshall RN, et al: Prenatal treatment of congenital adrenal hyperplasia due to 21-hydroxylase deficiency. N Engl J Med 322:111, 1990.

Speiser PW, Agdere L, Ueshiba H, et al: Aldosterone synthesis in salt-wasting congenital adrenal hyperplasia with complete absence of adrenal 21-hydroxylase. N Engl J Med 324:145, 1992.

Young MC, Hughes IA: Response to treatment of congenital adrenal hyperplasia in infancy. Arch Dis Child 65:441, 1990.

BONE/MINERAL ENDOCRINOLOGY

Parathyroid Hormone and Vitamin D (see Chapter 2)

The two most important circulating regulators of calcium and phosphate metabolism are parathyroid hormone (PTH) and vitamin D. The function of PTH is to maintain the plasma ionized calcium level in the normal range. PTH is secreted in response to a decrease serum ionized calcium level and then acts via adenylate cyclase to mobilize calcium from bone and to enhance fractional reabsorption of calcium while inducing phosphate excretion by the kidney; these combined events raise the serum calcium concentration. Because PTH increases renal 1-hydroxylase activity, it also acts indirectly to elevate serum calcium concentration by stimulating the production of 1,25-dihydroxyvitamin D.

Vitamin D enhances calcium absorption from the

gut, resulting in increased bone mineralization. Circulating vitamin D (from sun exposure or food) must be sequentially modified first to 25-hydroxyvitamin D in the liver and then to the metabolically active form, 1,25-dihydroxyvitamin D, in the kidney. However, the serum concentration of 25-hydroxyvitamin D is ordinarily the best measurement of vitamin D sufficiency.

Hypocalcemia

Regardless of etiology, the predominant *clinical manifestations* of hypocalcemia (ionized calcium < 4.5 mg/dL; total calcium < 8.5 mg/dL) reflect increased neuromuscular irritability and include muscle cramps, carpopedal spasm (tetany), weakness, paresthesia, laryngospasm, or seizures. Latent tetany can be detected by producing facial spasms by lightly tapping over the facial nerve (Chvostek sign) or by demonstrating carpal spasms when arterial blood flow to the hand is occluded for 3 min with a blood pressure cuff inflated to 15 mmHg above systolic blood pressure (Trousseau sign). Total calcium concentration commonly is measured even though serum ionized calcium (approximately half of the total) is the biologically active form. Albumin is the major reservoir of protein-bound calcium, and the fraction of ionized calcium is inversely related to plasma pH. Therefore, disorders that alter plasma pH or serum albumin concentration must be considered when assessing circulating calcium concentrations.

Hypocalcemia can be caused by defects in PTH secretion or action. In **primary hypoparathyroidism,** the gland itself malfunctions because of congenital malformation (e.g., DiGeorge syndrome) or postnatal destruction (e.g., associated with thyroidectomy or resulting from autoimmunity). Hypoparathyroidism does not cause rickets.

In **pseudohypoparathyroidism,** circulating PTH is secreted normally and is biologically active, but the patient is unresponsive to the hormone because he or she is unable to generate cyclic adenosine monophosphate or respond to it. Patients with pseudohypoparathyroidism frequently are diagnosed in mid-childhood, even though the condition is inherited (X-linked dominant) and may become manifest at birth. Other clinical features of pseudohypoparathyroidism include short stature, short 4th and 5th metacarpals, calcification of the basal ganglia, and often mental retardation. Some of these manifestations likely reflect the inherited symptom complex, whereas others presumably result from chronic hypocalcemia and hyperphosphatemia.

Hypocalcemia caused by attenuated PTH release is found in infants of mothers with hyperparathyroidism and hypercalcemia; the latter suppresses fetal PTH release, thereby causing **transient hypoparathyroidism** in the neonatal period. During the first 3 days of life, calcium concentrations normally decline in response to withdrawal of the maternal calcium supply so that sluggish PTH response in the neonate results in a transient hypocalcemia.

Normal serum magnesium concentrations also are required for normal parathyroid gland function and action. Thus, **hypomagnesemia** may cause a secondary hypoparathyroidism that will respond poorly to therapies other than magnesium replacement.

Neonatal tetany resulting from excessive phosphate consumption classically occurs in the week-old infant fed cow's milk. The resultant hyperphosphatemia drives down the serum calcium, causing symptomatic hypocalcemia (see Chapter 6).

The etiologies of hypocalcemia usually can be discerned by combining features of the clinical presentation with determinations of serum total or ionized calcium, albumin, magnesium, phosphate, creatinine, and alkaline phosphatase and with roentgenograms of the hands or wrists and knees. The most important diagnostic test is quantitating the serum PTH at a time when the calcium is low. If the PTH concentration is not elevated appropriately, hypoparathyroidism (transient, primary, caused by hypomagnesemia) is present. Vitamin D stores can be estimated by measuring serum 25-hydroxyvitamin D and renal function assessed with a serum creatinine measurement (Table 17–23).

Treatment of severe tetany or seizures resulting from hypocalcemia consists of intravenous calcium gluconate (2 mL/kg of 10% solution) given slowly over 10 min while monitoring cardiac status for bradycardia. Chronic treatment of hypoparathyroidism involves administering vitamin D and calcium. Therapy is adjusted to keep the serum calcium in the lower half of the normal range to avoid episodes of hypercalcemia that might produce nephrocalcinosis and pancreatitis.

Rickets

Rickets occurs when growing bone is inadequately mineralized and the proportion of osteoid (the organic portion of the bone) becomes excessive. As a result, the bone becomes soft and the metaphyses widen. Poor linear growth, bowing of the legs on weight bearing, thickening at the wrists and knees, and prominence of the costochondral

Table 17–23. Important Physiologic Changes in Bone/Mineral Diseases

Condition	Calcium	Phosphate	PTH	25(OH)D
Primary hypoparathyroidism	↓	↑	↓	Nl
Pseudohypoparathyroidism	↓	↑	↑	Nl
Vitamin D deficiency	Nl (↓)	↓	↑	↓
Familial hypophosphatemic rickets	Nl	↓	Nl (Sl ↑)	Nl
Hyperparathyroidism	↑	↓	↑	Nl
Immobilization	↑	↑	↓	Nl

Nl = normal; ↑ = high; ↓ = low; Sl = slightly; 25(OH)D = 25-hydroxyvitamin D.

junctions (rachitic rosary) develop. At this stage, the roentgenographic findings are unmistakable.

Rickets develops because of an imbalance in bone mineral metabolism. In *nutritional vitamin D deficiency*, calcium is not adequately absorbed from the intestine (see Chapter 2). Poor vitamin D intake (food fads or poor maternal diet, both affecting breast milk vitamin D) or avoidance of sunlight also may contribute to the development of rickets. Fat malabsorption resulting from hepatobiliary disease (biliary atresia, neonatal hepatisis) or other causes also may produce vitamin D deficiency, because vitamin D is a fat-soluble vitamin. Defects in vitamin D metabolism by the kidney (renal failure, autosomal recessive deficiency of 1-alpha-hydroxylation, **vitamin D–dependent rickets**) or liver also can cause rickets. Very-low–birth weight infants have an increased incidence of rickets of prematurity (see Chapter 6).

In *familial hypophosphatemic rickets*, the major defect in mineral metabolism is failure of the kidney to resorb filtered phosphate adequately. This X-linked disease usually is diagnosed within the first few years of life and typically is more severe in males, although it can occur in females.

The etiology of rickets usually can be determined by assessing the mineral and vitamin D (25-hydroxyvitamin D < 8 ng/mL suggests nutritional vitamin D deficiency) status as outlined and analyzing the results in accordance with the clinical presentation and expected laboratory features of the different disorders (Table 17–23). Further testing of mineral balance or measuring of other vitamin D metabolites may be required in more difficult cases.

Several chemical forms of vitamin D can be used for *treatment* of the different rachitic conditions, but their potencies vary widely and required dosages depend on the condition being treated (see Chapters 2 and 16). In hypophosphatemic rickets, phosphate supplementation must accompany vitamin D therapy, which is given to suppress secondary hyperparathyroidism. Adequate therapy restores normal skeletal growth and produces resolution of the roentgenographic signs of rickets. Vitamin D–dependent rickets is treated with 1,25-hydroxyvitamin D.

Hypercalcemia

Hypercalcemia is rare in children. It is due to hyperparathyroidism, immobilization (body casts), hypervitaminosis D (food faddism or incorrectly prepared commercial formula), fat necrosis, maternal hypoparathyroidism with subsequent fetal hypocalcemia, autosomal dominant–familial hypocalciuric hypercalcemia, William syndrome, and malignancy. The overt symptoms are nonspecific (mental disturbances, anorexia, constipation, lethargy, vomiting, weakness, and polyuria) and relate to the degree of hypercalcemia. With time, chronic hypercalcemia usually will produce pancreatitis or nephrolithiasis and/or renal insufficiency.

References

Behrman RE (ed): Nelson Textbook of Pediatrics. 14th ed. Philadelphia, WB Saunders, 1992, Sec. 4.29, 19.17–19.20, 24.60–24.66.

Glorieux FH: Rickets, the continuing challenge. N Engl J Med 325:1875, 1991.

Jacobus CH, Holick MF, Shao Q, et al: Hypervitaminosis D associated with drinking milk. N Engl J Med 326:1173, 1992.

McMurtry CT, Schranck FW, Walkenhorst DA, et al: Significant developmental elevation in serum parathyroid hormone levels in a large kindred with familial benign (hypocalciuric) hypercalcemia. Am J Med 93:247, 1992.

Ratcliff WA, Hutchesson ACJ, Bundred NJ, et al: Role of assays for parathyroid-hormone-related protein in investigation of hypercalcaemia. Lancet 339:164, 1992.

DIABETES MELLITUS

Diabetes mellitus is the most common childhood endocrine disorder and is a chronic metabolic dis-

Table 17–24. Classification of Diabetes Mellitus in Children and Adolescents

Classification	Criteria
Diabetes mellitus Insulin-dependent (Type 1)	Typical symptoms Glycosuria, ketonuria, random PG >200 mg/dL
Noninsulin-dependent (Type II)	Fasting PG >140 mg/dL with 2 hr value >200 mg/dL on OGTT* more than once and in absence of precipitating factors
Other types	Type I or II criteria with genetic syndromes (Turner syndome, Down syndome, Prader-Willi syndrome), drug treatment (steroids, L-asparaginase); pancreatic disease (cystic fibrosis, hemochromatosis), or other known causes or associations
Impaired glucose tolerance	FPG <140 mg/dL with 2 hr >140 mg/dL on OGTT*
Gestational diabetes	2 or more abnormal of: FPG >105 1 hr >190 2 hr >165 3 hr >145 mg/dL on OGTT*
Statistical risk Previous abnormal glucose tolerance	Normal OGTT* following an abnormal one, spontaneous hyperglycermia or gestational diabetes
Potential abnormal glucose tolerance	Genetic predisposition (identical twin of affected sib); islet cell antibodies

* Oral glucose tolerance testing—1.75 g/kg body weight to a maximum of 75 g.
FPG = fasting plasma glucose; PG = plasma glucose.
(Data from Rosenbloom AL, Kohrman A, Sperling MA: J Pediatr 98:320, 1981; National Diabetes Data Group: Diabetes 28: 1039, 1979.)

order caused by the absolute or relative deficiency of insulin. The overall prevalence is approximately 1:500 children 18 yr of age and younger. The annual incidence rate is approximately 12 new cases per 100,000 population aged less than 20 yr, a rate equal to all forms of childhood cancer. The incidence rates vary from as high as 30:100,000 in northern Scandinavia to less than 1:100,000 in Japan. The rate in American blacks is approximately one quarter of that of Caucasians. Peak ages of presentation are 6–7 yr and around puberty.

Insulin deficiency affects the metabolism of carbohydrate, protein, and fat, but its hallmark is hyperglycemia with resultant osmotic diuresis (polyuria), compensatory excessive drinking (polydipsia), and weight loss. Although several types of diabetes mellitus are known, the predominant form affecting children is Type I or insulin-dependent diabetes mellitus (Table 17–24). Other forms of diabetes mellitus are uncommon in childhood and usually are accompanied by obesity, pancreatic disease (e.g., cystic fibrosis), and rare but distinct syndromes.

Type I Insulin-Dependent Diabetes Mellitus

Etiology and Epidemiology.   Type I diabetes mellitus is an autoimmune disorder. Islet cell antibodies (ICAs) directed against cell surface (possibly cross-reacting with an epitope of cow's milk–derived bovine serum albumin) or cytoplasmic (possibly glutamic acid decarboxylase) components of islets are present at clinical onset in close to 90% of patients. Patients also may have spontaneous antiinsulin autoantibodies (IAAs) at diagnosis (i.e., before they receive exogenous insulin), suggesting an immune response to altered endogenous insulin. Abnormalities in cellular immunity exhibited by the ratio of T helper to T suppressor cells have been shown, as have alterations in mediators of inflammation, such as the interleukins. A lymphocytic infiltrate around islets has been observed in autopsy specimens within months of diagnosis. ICAs disappear within 5 yr of established disease but may reappear after successful transplantation of the pancreas between identical twins, suggesting reactivation of the immune response by fresh antigen. Type I diabetes is associated with other autoimmune diseases such as Hashimoto thyroiditis, Graves disease, Addison disease, celiac disease, and juvenile rheumatoid arthritis.

The D antigens are part of the class II antigens of the major histocompatability complex (MHC). Over 90% of patients with type I diabetes possess either human leukocyte antigen (HLA)-DR3 or HLA-DR4, or both. Possession of DR3 or DR4 increases the relative risk of diabetes by 3- to 4-fold, whereas possession of both DR3 and DR4 increases

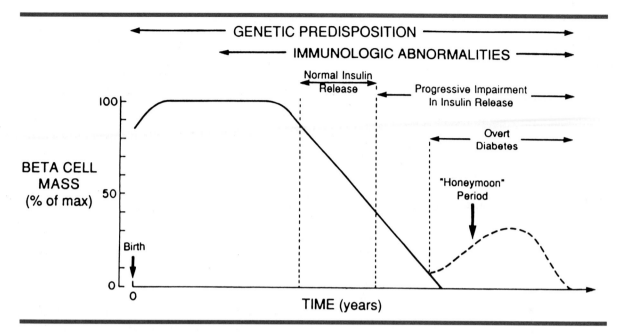

Figure 17–11. Schematic representation of the autoimmune evolution of diabetes in genetically predisposed individuals. See text for details.

the relative risk 10-fold. Siblings who are HLA identical have a 20-fold greater risk of being affected by diabetes. However, even in identical twins, the concordance rate for type I diabetes is only 50%. These observations indicate that genetic factors alone are not responsible for the disease; the genetic factors appear to predispose the patient to an autoimmune process. The practical implications are that the risk to siblings is at worst 50% in the case of identical twins and empirically 5% in siblings or offspring, unless HLA typing demonstrates identity.

The current concepts of the etiology of Type I diabetes are summarized in Figure 17–11. Genetic predisposition is inherited via the HLA-D complex. At some unknown point in time, a trigger, possibly a viral illness or other environmental factor, initiates an autoimmune response. Evidence of autoimmunity in the form of ICAs or IAAs may be present for months to years before the clinical appearance of disease. During this time, there is progressive destruction of insulin-secreting tissue and, eventually, progressive impairment in insulin release. The clinical manifestations of overt diabetes, such as polyuria, polydipsia, polyphagia, and weight loss, become manifest only when the insulin secretory reserve is reduced to 10–20% of normal. The decompensation phase may be hastened by an intercurrent viral infection or by the stress of evolving

dehydration. Resolution of these stress factors may permit the resumption of spontaneous insulin secretion, exhibited as the "honeymoon period," but the primary immune disturbance continues and results in eventual total destruction of insulin-secreting cells.

Pathophysiology. Feeding and the high-insulin state are associated with anabolism (glucose uptake, protein synthesis) and the curtailment of catabolic processes; conversely, fasting and the low-insulin state are associated with the curtailment of anabolic processes and activation of catabolism (glycogenolysis, gluconeogenesis, ketogenesis, proteolysis). In this way, the basal blood glucose concentration of approximately 80 mg/dL rarely exceeds 120 mg/dL after meals. The gradual impairment of insulin secretion (Figure 17–11) results in a permanent low-insulin state in which catabolic processes predominate over those of anabolic processes. Thus, glucose production by glycogenolysis and/or by gluconeogenesis proceeds, but its peripheral utilization is limited, resulting in hyperglycemia. When the renal threshold of approximately 180 mg/dL is exceeded, glucosuria accompanied by resultant polyuria, polydipsia, and weight loss ensue. Breakdown of protein and fat stores to provide the substrate for gluconeogenesis and ketone body production also proceeds. Thus, the production of organic acids, such as beta-hydroxybutyric and acetoacetic acids, exceeds their capacity for utilization and buffering, ultimately leading to the clinical picture of diabetic ketoacidosis.

Clinical Manifestations. Most patients present with the typical symptoms of polyuria, polydipsia, polyphagia, and weight loss of several weeks' duration. Hyperglycemia must be documented to exclude a renal tubular defect producing glucosuria. About 10% of patients present with diabetic ketoacidosis (dehydration, Kussmaul respiration, cerebral obtundation). Vaginal infection with candida may be the presenting feature in pubertal females.

Diabetic ketoacidosis (DKA) is considered to be present when there is hyperglycemia (blood glucose >300 mg/dL), acidosis with pH less than 7.25 and bicarbonate less than 15 mEq/L, and ketonemia, accompanied by total ketones in serum exceeding 3 mmol/L or positive at 1:2 dilution in serum or in undiluted urine as detected by the sodium nitroprusside reaction (Acutest, Ketostix, Chemstrips UGK). Glycosuria produces an obligate renal fluid and electrolyte loss, whereas the anionic ketones require the excretion of additional cations (Na^+, K^+) during ketonuria. The presence of severe lactic acidosis or ketoacidosis in the absence of hyperglycemia should arouse suspicion of an inborn error of metabolism or of an ingestion (salicylates).

The cause of DKA is an absolute or relative deficiency of insulin. Insulin deficiency is absolute in a newly presenting patient with diabetes or in one who has deliberately or inadvertently omitted a scheduled insulin injection. Insulin deficiency may be relative if the stress of an intercurrent illness has stimulated the excessive secretion of counter-regulatory hormones (catecholamines, growth hormone, cortisol), which antagonize the effects of insulin. Such stresses include infections, trauma, and emotional stress. Therefore, a precipitating event, including deliberate omission of insulin, should be sought carefully.

In the absence of insulin, excessive amounts of free fatty acids are released from adipose tissue and transported to the liver but are no longer re-esterified. Rather, they enter mitochondria and are partially oxidized to ketones. The generation of beta-hydroxybutyrate and acetoacetate exceeds their capacity for peripheral utilization and contributes to the acidosis, low bicarbonate, and developing anion gap. An element of lactic acidosis also is present as a result of dehydration and poor tissue perfusion.

The evolution of DKA may take hours to days;

polyuria, polydipsia, nausea, vomiting, and anorexia are usually the major presenting manifestations. Abdominal pain (paralytic ileus, gastric distention) that may mimic an acute abdominal condition is common in children but often resolves with intravenous fluid therapy; persistence of abdominal pain suggests the possibility of the presence of an intra-abdominal process, such as acute appendicitis, which triggered the DKA. Dehydration, Kussmaul respiration, the fruity odor of acetone on the breath, and an altered mental status ranging from disorientation to coma are the major signs. The altered mental status correlates best with the degree of elevation in serum osmolality.

Blood glucose concentration may range from 200 to greater than 1000 mg/dL. The degree of ketoacidosis usually is underestimated because the common tests used to measure "ketone bodies" react with acetoacetate but not with beta-hydroxybutyrate. In addition, beta-hydroxybutyrate may be converted to acetoacetate during treatment of DKA, giving the false impression that ketosis is worsening, whereas acidosis as judged by pH and bicarbonate actually is improving. Additional laboratory tests reveal hypertriglyceridemia, azotemia (dehydration), elevated amylase (not from acute pancreatitis), and leukocytosis (not from infection). Pseudohyponatremia may be present and is due to high glucose (there is a decrease of 1.6 mEq Na^+ per 100 mg/dL rise of glucose) and triglycerides. Hyperkalemia may be due to a transcellular shift of potassium from the cell to plasma during acidosis or to dehydration-induced renal insufficiency. Hyperosmolality may be due to hyperglycemia and the elevated blood urea nitrogen (BUN) from prerenal azotemia caused by intravascular contraction from dehydration (see Chapter 16). **Hyperosmolar nonketotic coma** is associated with high blood glucose levels (900–2000 mg/dL), minimal ketosis, and disturbances of cerebral function.

Treatment of DKA. In the course of evolving, DKA is associated with fluid and electrolyte losses (see Chapter 16). Fluid management is critical to the management of DKA. Current fluid replacement regimens call for acute fluid resuscitation (normal saline) to correct shock, poor tissue perfusion (re-establishes renal blood flow), and dehydration of approximately 5–10%. Normal saline (20 mL/kg; maximum 1 L) given in the 1st hr usually is sufficient to improve the circulation. In the subsequent 2–4 hr, normal saline is given according to weight: less than 10 kg, at 7 mL/kg/hr; 10–20 kg, at 6 mL/kg/hr; 20–40 kg, at 5 mL/kg/hr; and greater than 40 kg, at 4.5 mL/kg/hr (maximum 250 mL/hr).

This modified fluid protocol may reduce the incidence of hyperchloremic acidosis and cerebral edema, yet replaces deficit and ongoing fluid losses. After 4 hr, 0.5 normal saline or 0.5 normal saline in 5% glucose can be substituted at the same rate.

Blood glucose levels fall during the initial normal saline resuscitation. Insulin therapy by continuous intravenous infusion (0.1 U/kg priming dose followed by 0.1 U/kg/hr regular insulin) begins in the 1st hr of management of DKA. All patients should be managed with a diabetic flow sheet to carefully monitor laboratory data. Patients should be managed in an intensive care unit.

Children with DKA are *hyperosmolar* because of the contribution of hyperglycemia to osmolality. Because too-rapid correction of hyperglycemia and osmolality by hypotonic intravenous fluid therapy may result in rapid shifts of water from the extracellular to the intracellular compartment, predisposing the patient to cerebral edema, it generally is recommended that rehydration take place over at least 36 hr. For the same reason, blood glucose concentration should be maintained at 200–300 mg/dL, if necessary by the inclusion of 5–10% glucose in the infusate. Failure of the serum sodium level to increase above 130 mEq/L during fluid therapy is a risk factor for cerebral edema.

Total body potassium stores usually are depleted even though serum potassium may appear to be normal or elevated because of the combined effects of acidosis, catabolism, and dehydration. With provision of fluids and insulin and correction of acidosis, plasma potassium concentrations may fall and predispose the patient to arrhythmias. Therefore, potassium should be added to the intravenous fluids at a concentration of 20–40 mEq/L, beginning with the 2nd hr of therapy, after serum electrolytes and the status of renal function are known and urine flow is established.

Total body *phosphate depletion* may also occur, and the repletion of phosphate by potassium phosphate infusion has theoretical benefit. In addition, providing potassium phosphate limits the excessive provision of chloride. Calcium levels should be monitored to avoid phosphate-induced hypocalcemia.

Blood glucose concentration invariably falls more quickly than the acidosis can be corrected. It is therefore imperative to infuse 5–10% glucose to prevent hypoglycemia and to continue administering insulin (at the usual or possibly half the usual rate) until acidosis has almost been corrected (i.e., bicarbonate is greater than 15 mEq/L and pH greater than 7.3).

Bicarbonate therapy is not necessary in most cases. Providing fluids and insulin will correct acidosis, and bicarbonate therapy should be used only when the pH is less than 7.1. Bicarbonate should be given as an infusion and not as a bolus. The acidosis during DKA may be a high-anion-gap acidosis resulting from accumulation of ketones or lactate or the hemoconcentration of plasma protein anions. Accumulation of ketone bodies during DKA most commonly is noted when significant volume depletion reduces renal blood flow (high BUN) and, hence, reduces renal excretion of ketones. Insulin therapy will convert ketones to bicarbonate by improving ketone oxidation in the Krebs cycle, whereas fluid resuscitation will enhance renal blood flow. Alternately, a hyperchloremic metabolic acidosis may be present and is due to normal saline infusion plus persistent renal losses of ketones (bicarbonate) in those patients with preserved renal blood flow (normal BUN) and urine output.

Bicarbonate therapy for DKA is controversial because of potential adverse side effects. Rapid infusion of bicarbonate may shift the oxygen–hemoglobin dissociation curve to the left and reduce tissue oxygen delivery. Furthermore, once bicarbonate neutralizes circulating acid, CO_2, which is produced in the systemic circulation, may diffuse readily across the blood–brain barrier and result in a paradoxical CNS acidosis and altered CNS function. In addition, rapidly correcting the acidosis will shift potassium into cells and contribute to hypokalemia. Bicarbonate therapy may improve cardiac output and may improve recovery from the hypercholoremic acidosis resulting from loss of bicarbonate in the urine. The latter type of acidosis usually corrects more slowly than the high-anion-gap acidosis because of the relative paucity of bicarbonate-generating circulating ketone bodies. Bicarbonate also will be helpful in those patients who have significant hyperkalemia and poor cardiac output.

Each of the complications of treating DKA usually can be avoided by careful monitoring of physical findings, electrolytes, glucose, and acid–base status. Assessment at hourly intervals for the first 4 hr and 2–4 hr intervals thereafter until acidosis resolves is recommended. *Cerebral edema* is a rare but feared complication that occurs during treatment of DKA in children. Its etiology remains unknown; too-rapid correction of metabolic disturbances has not been consistently implicated. Cerebral edema may manifest as a headache, confusion, lethargy, seizures, papilledema, or brain stem herniation.

Transition Management. When the acidosis is corrected and the patient rehydrated, clear fluids should be introduced until the patient can tolerate full meals. The customary insulin dose for a known diabetic should be introduced before discontinuing the intravenous insulin infusion. In newly diagnosed patients, regular insulin (fast acting, soluble) should be used at a dose of 0.1–0.25 units/kg at 4–6 hr intervals to maintain blood glucose concentration within the range of 80–180 mg/dL. Alternately, the amount of insulin given in the previous 24-hr continuous infusion may be converted to the subsequent 24-hr requirement. Subcutaneous regular human insulin is administered in proportions of the total daily dose: one third at breakfast, one fourth at lunch, one third at dinner, one twelfth at bedtime. A sliding scale modifies these doses according to the fingerstick blood glucose that is measured at these times. If the blood glucose is less than 60 mg/dL, no insulin is administered. At a blood glucose between 60 and 80 mg/dL, the expected insulin dose is decreased 10%; between 120 and 180 mg/dL the dose is increased 10%; between 180 and 240 mg/dL the dose is increased 15%; between 240 and 300 mg/dL the dose is increased 20%, and at greater than 300 mg/dL the dose is increased 30% and a test for ketones is performed.

Over 1–2 days, as success with subcutaneous regular insulin is achieved, a split dose of regular- and intermediate-acting insulin, such as NPH, is added. Two thirds of the morning, lunchtime, and evening insulin requirements are administered as NPH; the remaining morning, noontime, dinner, and bedtime doses are administered as regular insulin. The sliding scale adjusts the regular dose in this b.i.d. schema, while changes in NPH occur after several days of observation as the dose of regular insulin becomes established.

Routine Management

Importance of Metabolic Control. In general, management of insulin-dependent diabetes in children is governed by the increasing evidence that normal growth and development, both physical and emotional, can be achieved, and that the risks of long-term microvascular complications can be minimized by maintaining metabolic control, usually equated with glycemic control. Micro- or macrovascular complications rarely become manifest in children. Also, evidence has been found that instituting strict metabolic control can restore normal retinal, neural, and renal function in those patients with early functional impairment but cannot reverse anatomic changes. The biochemical bases of certain complications are related directly to hyperglycemia.

Principles. The principles of management involve appropriately using and adjusting insulin; providing nutrition consistent with the requirements of a growing child, appropriately geared to insulin administration and exercise; educating and involving the patient and family unit in the minimal goal of obtaining a level of knowledge that may enable the patient to live independently outside of the hospital; and providing short- and long-term monitoring by physical examination and appropriate laboratory tests. For newly diagnosed patients, these initial steps toward stabilization are accomplished best in an inpatient setting that considers individual learning skills and recognizes the influence of fear, anger, denial, grief, mourning, and guilt as feelings that affect initial adjustment. The ultimate level of metabolic control must be mutually acceptable to the physician and family and must lie within their emotional, educational, and financial resources. Furthermore, it should be recognized that the benefits of strict metabolic control are putative and long-term, whereas the consequences of severe hypoglycemia are all too readily apparent. At a minimum, patients and their families should be capable of adjusting their daily routine with respect to insulin treatment, meal planning, home blood glucose monitoring, and recognition of the signs and symptoms of hyperglycemia and hypoglycemia and their precipitating events. They also should be able to take the elementary steps to adjust insulin, food intake, and exercise to avoid or treat these problems as they emerge. Phone contact after discharge and during crisis is helpful.

Insulin. Some commonly available insulins are listed in Table 17–25. All available insulins in the United States are now highly purified, and human

Table 17–25. Insulin Preparations

Type	Onset	Peak Action	Duration
Short-Acting Insulin			
Regular	½–2 hr	2–4 hr	6–12 hr
Semilente			
Intermediate Insulin			
NPH	1–4 hr	4–12 hr	16–28 hr
Lente			
Long-Acting Insulin			
Protamine zinc	4–6 hr	8–20 hr	24–36 hr
Ultralene			

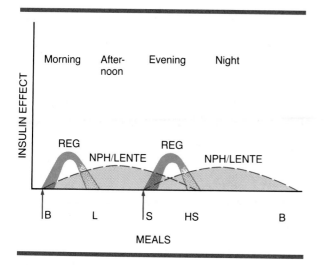

Figure 17–12. Representative profile of insulin effect using a twice-daily injection regimen that combines an intermediate-acting insulin (NPH or Lente) with regular (short-acting) insulin. (Reprinted with permission from Schade DS, Santiago JV, Sykler JS: Intensive Insulin Therapy. Excerpta Medica, 1983.)

insulin is available. No insulin regimen currently available can mimic the precision of endogenously secreted insulin delivered into the portal vein in precisely the right amounts at the right time. Therefore, all insulin treatment regimens represent a compromise. The most common compromise is to give two daily injections, combining intermediate-acting and short-acting insulins as outlined in Figure 17–12. The ratio should be approximately 2:1 or 3:1 of the intermediate-acting insulin to the short-acting insulin, with about two thirds of the total daily dose given in the morning before breakfast and about one third of the total dose given in the evening before supper. Individual adjustments are made according to individual responses. At the outset of the disease, when endogenous insulin secretion is still present, the total daily dose may vary between 0.2 and 0.7 U/kg/24 hr. After about 1 yr of established disease, the dose of insulin tends to be 1–2 U/kg/24 hr, although this is variable and requires individual adjustment. A predictable increase in insulin requirement of about 40–50% occurs with the adolescent growth spurt. Although not invariable, those who exceed 1 U/kg/24 hr in the 1st yr after diagnosis or those taking more than 2 U/kg/24 hr may be subject to problems of instability, such as the Somogyi phenomenon. In contrast, those whose daily insulin requirement is less than 0.5 U/kg/24 hr after more than 1 yr of diabetes

should be suspected of not receiving enough insulin.

The **Somogyi phenomenon** is the term given to the hyperglycemic surge that occurs in the early morning hours as a result of counter-regulatory hormones that increase glucose production in response to nocturnal hypoglycemia. Hypoglycemia may cause morning headache, night terrors, and diaphoresis; the resultant rebound hyperglycemia becomes manifest by excessive glycosuria. Measurement of glucose at 3 A.M. identifies hypoglycemia; moving NPH administration from dinner to bedtime may avoid this problem. The **dawn phenomenon** is the term given to significant early morning hyperglycemia in the absence of antecedent hypoglycemia. The distinction between these two phenomena is important, because the former requires a reduction or modification of the time of the evening dose, whereas the latter requires an increase in the evening dose. Therefore, management demands that hypoglycemia or hyperglycemia be documented in the early hours of the morning by appropriately monitored blood glucose determinations at home.

Nutrition. The nutritional requirements of diabetic children are similar to those of healthy children of similar age, sex, weight, and activity who are eating the foods of their own cultural, social, and ethnic background. The calories should consist of approximately 55% carbohydrate, 30% fat, and 15% protein. It is recommended that approximately 70% of the carbohydrate content be derived from complex carbohydrates, such as starch, whereas highly refined sugars be avoided or limited. Diets with high fiber content are useful in improving control of blood glucose in patients with diabetes by delaying the absorption of food and, hence, eliminating wide swings in blood glucose concentrations. The cholesterol intake should be reduced, and the polyunsaturated-to-saturated ratio of fat ideally is increased to 1.2:1. The regularity of the eating pattern for the chosen dose of insulin is paramount. The total daily caloric intake may be divided so as to provide 20% at breakfast, 20% at lunch, and 30% at dinner, leaving 10% each for a mid-morning, mid-afternoon, and evening snack. In older children, the mid-morning snack may be omitted and the extra 10% of balanced calories taken with lunch or spread out to dinner and the evening snack. Special adjustments in meal planning and insulin dose must be made to meet the needs of each individual patient, and flexibility rather than rigidity is of the essence in managing children with diabetes.

Exercise. Special adjustments in meal planning and insulin dose must be made during anticipated vigorous exercise to avoid hypoglycemia. A regular exercise program is highly beneficial, and no form of exercise should be prohibited to children with diabetes.

Monitoring. The use of home blood glucose monitoring is an integral component of diabetes management and is encouraged for all patients. Blood is obtained by a spring-loaded device. A drop of blood is placed on a chemically impregnated plastic strip that undergoes a color change in proportion to the glucose concentration. This color change can be visually matched against a chart or used in a calibrated reflectance meter. Parents (patients) should record all blood glucose levels; some devices have memories that can be used to check the patient's compliance. This method has good agreement with standard laboratory measurements of glucose. Target blood glucose concentrations should be 80–180 mg/dL. Values consistently less than 60 mg/dL or greater than 180–240 mg/dL at certain times of the day require adjustment of the appropriate insulin type and dose, as well as continued monitoring. Initially, monitoring should take place before breakfast, lunch, dinner, and the evening snack. Once a stable pattern of insulin dosage and glucose profile is established, monitoring can be performed twice a day at the time of the two insulin doses. A third determination at noon, bedtime, or 3 A.M. may be indicated and depends on the degree of control and suspicion of nocturnal hypoglycemia (3 A.M.). Parents can be advised to alter insulin type and/or dose as well as nutrition depending on the observed response, providing the reported measurements are accurate and honest.

Glycosylated hemoglobin measurement should be performed 4 times/yr and reflects the time-averaged integral of the prevailing blood glucose concentration over the preceding 6–8 wk. Total glycosylated hemoglobin and hemoglobin A_{1c} are not completely synonymous, and the former is generally 1–2 percentage points higher. Table 17–26 summarizes the correlation between clinical and biochemical indices of glycemic control. Clinical judgment remains paramount, however, because certain hemoglobinopathies interfere with the commonly used glycohemoglobin tests. Thus, with sickle cell trait, glycohemoglobin values may be spuriously low. In contrast, with syndromes of persistent fetal hemoglobin production (e.g., thalassemia major), glycohemoglobin values may be spuriously high.

Table 17–26. Correlation between Clinical and Biochemical Indices of Glycemic Control

Minimal Control
HbA_{1c} 11.0–13.0% and GHb 13.0–15.0%
Many SMBG values of 300 mg/dL or greater
Intermittent spontaneous ketonuria

Average Control
HbA_{1c} 8.0–9.0% and GHb 10.0–11.0%
Premeal SMBG 160–200 mg/dL
Intermittent positive urine glucose
Rare ketonuria

Intensive Control
HbA_{1c} 6.0–7.0% and GHb 7.0–8.0%
Premeal SMBG 70–120 mg/dL; postmeal SMBG <180 mg/dL
Essentially no positive urine glucose or ketones

GHb = glycohemoglobin; HbA_{1c} = hemoglobin A_{1c}; SMBG = self-monitored blood glucose.

Observation for abnormalities in linear growth, weight gain, and pubertal development and for the appearance of other autoimmune conditions, especially Hashimoto thyroiditis, is an integral component of long-term monitoring. Limited joint mobility, often associated with thick, tight, shiny, waxy, scleroderma-like skin, should be sought at routine physical examination; it can be documented easily by observing the gap between the fingers when the hands are held in the "prayer" position at a right angle to the wrist. Limited joint mobility is strikingly associated with certain microvascular complications, such as retinopathy and nephropathy. If it is present, the fundi should be examined carefully for evidence of retinopathy, and the urine should be collected for an assessment of macroalbuminuria (>200 μg/min) or microalbuminuria (>20 to <200 μg/min) as an index of early renal dysfunction. Progression of microalbuminuria to more severe renal disease may be attenuated by angiotensin-converting enzyme inhibitors.

Prognosis: Long-Term Microvascular and Macrovascular Complications. Diabetes is the leading cause of blindness, with approximately 5000 new cases of blindness per year. Diabetic nephropathy is responsible for about one third of all new cases of end-stage renal failure. Diabetic neuropathy, including autonomic neuropathy, can be disabling. Macrovascular disease leading to premature myocardial infarction and lower extremity amputations is increased greatly in patients with diabetes. These complications usually appear after 10–20 yr of diabetes but infrequently may be seen before puberty. Hence, diabetes in children may be viewed as deceptively benign. The possible relationship between control and complications forms the basis of attempts to intensity metabolic control and mimic normal metabolism as closely as possible.

Attempts to arrest diabetes at clinical presentation and preserve residual insulin secretory capacity via drugs that suppress the immune response (cyclosporine) presently are experimental and do not have a role in routine management. Transplantation of the pancreas also is an experimental procedure usually reserved for those requiring simultaneous renal transplantation.

References

Adrogue HJ, Barrero J, Eknoyan G: Salutary effects of modest fluid replacement in the treatment of adults with diabetic ketoacidosis. JAMA 262:2108, 1989.

Amiel S: "Brittle" diabetes: Usually settles down. BMJ 303:260, 1991.

Behrman RE (ed): Nelson Textbook of Pediatrics. 14th ed. Philadelphia, WB Saunders, 1992, Sec. 8.52–8.58.

Daugirdas JT, Kronfol NO, Tzamaloukas AH, et al: Hyperosmolar coma: Cellular dehydration and the serum sodium concentration. Ann Intern Med 110:855, 1989.

DCCT Research Group: Epidemiology of severe hypoglycemia in the diabetes control and complications trial. Am J Med 90:450, 1991.

Drash A, Arslanian S: Can insulin dependent diabetes mellitus be cured or prevented? A status report on immunomodulatory strategies and pancreas transplantation. Pediatr Clin North Am 37:1467, 1990.

Dunger DB: Diabetes in puberty. Arch Dis Child 67:569, 1992.

Hammond P, Wallis S: Cerebral oedema in diabetic ketoacidosis: Still puzzling—and often fatal. BMJ 305:203, 1992.

Krane E: Diabetic ketoacidosis: Biochemistry, physiology, treatment and prevention. Pediatr Clin North Am 34:935, 1987.

Morris L, Murphy M, Kitabichi A: Bicarbonate therapy in severe diabetic ketoacidosis. Ann Intern Med 105:836, 1986.

Orchard TJ, Dorman JS, Maser RE, et al: Prevalence of complications in IDDM by sex and duration: Pittsburgh epidemiology of diabetes complications study II. Diabetes 39:1116, 1990.

Shah SC, Malone JI, Simpson NE: A randomized trial of intensive insulin therapy in newly diagnosed insulin-dependent diabetes mellitus. N Engl J Med 320:550, 1989.

Sperling MA: Outpatient management of diabetes mellitus. Pediatr Clin North Am 34:917, 1987.

Tarn A, Smith C, Spencer K, et al: Type I (insulin-dependent) diabetes: A disease of slow clinical onset? BMJ 294:342, 1987.

Watkins P: Long-term complications of diabetes. Endocrinol Metab Clin 15:715, 1986.

HYPOGLYCEMIA

Hypoglycemia reflects a failure to maintain normal glucose homeostasis because of a defect in either available substrate (gluconeogenesis, glycogenolysis, alternate fuels), enzymes, or hormones. Hypoglycemia of infants and children may conveniently be classified as occurring at two times:

1. Hypoglycemia in the neonatal period, discussed in Chapter 6.
2. In infancy and childhood. Hypoglycemia is less common in these age groups and usually is due to an acquired lesion of the endocrine system, to environmental insults, and, occasionally, to persistence of congenital or developmental abnormalities.

Definition. After 48 hr of life, serum glucose values less than 45 mg/dL are abnormal and require treatment. Hypoglycemic symptoms may be present at higher blood glucose levels and, if they are due to hypoglycemia, the symptoms will respond to glucose administration. This response is particularly relevant among diabetics, when a sudden decline of hyperglycemia to the low-euglycemic range may produce symptoms. *Whipple triad* refers to low blood glucose levels, symptoms compatible with hypoglycemia, and a response to glucose administration in which symptoms and signs are alleviated.

Clinical Manifestations. Symptoms and signs of hypoglycemia in older children are listed in Table 17–27. In infants, these features may be subtle and include cyanotic episodes, apnea, refusal to feed, weak spells, myoclonic jerks, somnolence, subnormal temperatures, and convulsions. Because these symptoms are nonspecific and may occur in other

Table 17–27. Symptoms and Signs of Hypoglycemia

Features Associated with Epinephrine Release*	Features Associated with Cerebral Glucopenia
Perspiration	Headache
Palpitation (tachycardia)	Mental confusion
Pallor	Somnolence
Paresthesia	Dysarthria
Trembling	Personality changes
Anxiety	Inability to concentrate
Weakness	Staring
Nausea	Hunger
Vomiting	Convulsions
	Ataxia
	Coma
	Diplopia
	Stroke

* These features may be blunted if the patient is receiving beta-blocking agents.

conditions, such as sepsis, asphyxia, intraventricular hemorrhage, and congenital heart disease, or as side effects of drugs, it is important to demonstrate that the blood glucose level is low at the time of the manifestations and that they disappear when parenteral glucose is given in amounts adequate to elevate blood glucose concentrations.

Significance and Classification of Hypoglycemia. The major impetus for recognizing and treating neonatal hypoglycemia is to permit normal brain development; the long-term sequelae of severe, symptomatic neonatal hypoglycemia are retarded brain development and epileptic seizures. The younger the infant and the more severe or prolonged the hypoglycemia, the greater the risk for permanent neurologic damage. Similar concerns about the morbidity form hypoglycemia are relevant for the older infant and child. A general classification of hypoglycemia is presented in Table 17–28 (see also Table 6–26).

Diagnosis. An approach to the diagnosis of hypoglycemia in children and in infants beyond the

---

Table 17–28. Classification of Hypoglycemia in Infants and Children

Neonatal—Transient Hypoglycemia
Associated with inadequate substrate or enzyme function
  Prematurity
  Small for gestational age
  Smaller of twins
  Infant with severe respiratory distress
  Infant of toxemic mother
Associated with hyperinsulinemia
  Infant of diabetic mother
  Infant with erythroblastosis fetalis

Neonatal—Infantile or Childhood-Persistent Hypoglycemia
Hyperinsulinemic states
  Nesidioblastosis
  Beta cell hyperplasia
  Beta cell adenoma
  Beckwith-Wiedemann syndrome
  Leucine sensitivity
  Falciparum malaria
Hormone deficiency
  Panhypopituitarism
  Isolated growth hormone deficiency
  ACTH deficiency
  Addison disease
  Glucagon deficiency
  Epinephrine deficiency
Substrate limited
  Ketotic hypoglycemia
  Branched-chain ketonuria (maple syrup urine disease)
Glycogen storage disease
  Glucose-6-phosphatase deficiency
  Amylo-1,6-glucosidase deficiency
  Liver phosphorylase deficiency
  Glycogen synthetase deficiency
Disorders of gluconeogenesis
  Acute alcohol intoxication
  Hyperglycinemia, carnitine deficiency
  Salicylate intoxication
  Fructose-1,6-diphosphatase deficiency
  Pyruvate carboxylase deficiency
  Phosphoenolpyruvate carboxykinase (PEPCK) deficiency

Other enzyme defects
  Galactosemia: galactose-1-phosphate uridyltransferase deficiency
  Fructose intolerance: frustose-1-phosphate aldolase deficiency
Disorders of fat (alternate fuel) metabolism
  Primary carnitine deficiency
  Secondary carnitine deficiency
  Carnitine palmitoyltransferase deficiency
  Long–medium–short chain fatty acid acyl-CoA dehydrogenase deficiency
Poisoning–drugs
  Salicylate
  Alcohol
  Oral hypoglycemic agents
  Insulin
  Propranolol
  Pentamidine
  Quinine
  Ackee fruit (unripe)–hypoglycin
Liver disease
  Reye syndrome
  Hepatitis
  Cirrhosis
  Hepatoma
Amino acid and organic acid disorders
  Maple syrup urine disease
  Propionicacidemia
  Methylmalonicacidemia
  Tyrosinosis
  Glutaricaciduria
  3-Hydroxy-3-methylglutaricaciduria
Systemic disorders
  Sepsis
  Carcinoma/sarcoma
  Heart failure
  Malnutrition
  Malabsorption
  Anti-insulin receptor antibodies
  Neonatal hyperviscosity

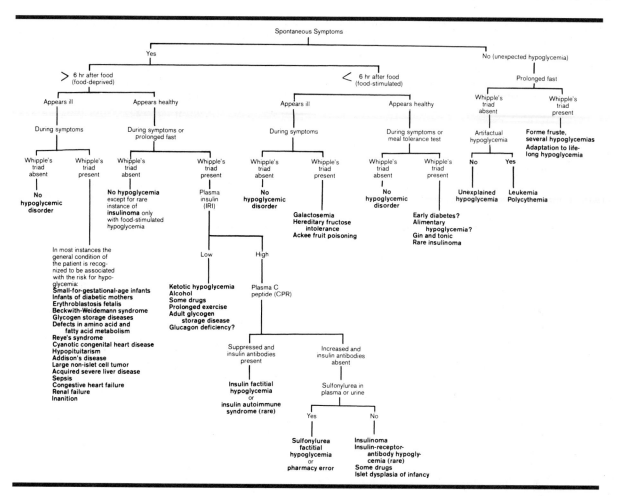

Figure 17–13. Evaluation of the hypoglycemic disorders. (From Service FJ: Hypoglycemic disorders. *In* Wyngaarden JB, Smith LH Jr [eds]: Cecil Textbook of Medicine. 17th ed. Philadelphia, WB Saunders, 1985, p. 1343.)

immediate newborn period is outlined in Figure 17–13.

Neonatal Persistent Hypoglycemia. When hypoglycemia and symptoms persist or recur despite increasing the rates of glucose infusion from 6–8 mg/kg/min to 12–16 mg/kg/min, hormone excess (hyperinsulinemia) is most likely. Hormone deficiency (cortisol, GH) or an inborn error of glycogen degradation or gluconeogenesis is less likely. Rates of glucose infusion of up to 20–25 mg/kg/min may be necessary to maintain euglycemia. Clinical clues to the existence of one of these syndromes are often present: large size (macrosomia) in those with hyperinsulinemia; microphallus or mid-line facial defects in hypopituitarism; and hepatomegaly in glycogen storage disease.

At the time of the onset of hypoglycemic manifestations, the critical step in diagnosis is to obtain a blood sample before glucose administration. Analysis of the blood sample should include determination of glucose, insulin, ketones, free fatty acids (FFAs) lactate, pyruvate, GH, cortisol, and, if appropriate, a blood gas and anion gap. Occasionally hypoglycemia may need to be induced by a planned fast. While these samples are being analyzed for substrates and hormones, therapy is begun with increasing rates of glucose infusion (up to 15–20 mg/kg/min by central vein). If hyperinsulinemia is suspected, diazoxide (10–20 mg/kg/24 hr PO, t.i.d.) is begun. If diazoxide is ineffective, long-acting somatostatin analogues are indicated. Both diazoxide and somatostatin suppress insulin release.

Hyperinsulinemic States. If the infant is macrosomic, the ketones are absent or low, and the FFAs are low, hyperinsulinemia is most likely. An insulin level greater than 10 μU/mL at a time when glucose is less than 30 mg/dL confirms this diagnosis. Confirmation of whether the infant has islet cell hyperplasia, adenoma, or nesidioblastosis can be made only by histologic examination of pancreatic tissue; some infants have all three components in a spectrum of islet cell dysplasia. Therefore, subtotal (80%) or near-total (95%) pancreatectomy often is indicated when the diagnosis of hyperinsulinemia is confirmed and hypoglycemia persists despite intravenous glucose in excess of 10 mg/kg/min, in addition to treatment with glucocorticoids, somatostatin, and diazoxide. This group of patients is most likely to suffer permanent neurologic deficits if definitive treatment by surgery is delayed. Hyperinsulinemia and hypoglycemia also occur in approximately 50% of infants with the **Beckwith-Wiedemann syndrome,** which is characterized by gigantism, omphalocele, macroglossia, visceromegaly, and distinctive earlobe fissure.

Hormone Deficiency. Severe neonatal hypoglycemia occurs with panhypopituitarism resulting from to congenital hypoplasia, aplasia of the pituitary gland, or functional separation of the hypothalamus and its releasing factors from the anterior pituitary gland. Despite deficient GH, these infants are of normal size at birth. In males, the presence of a microphallus and undescended testes provides a strong clue to the existence of gonadotropin deficiency in utero; jaundice and hepatomegaly frequently are associated with this syndrome, which may be familial. An anterior midline facial defect also may occur in some patients.

The critical blood sample at the time of hypoglycemia will reveal low insulin levels (less than 10 μU/mL) in association with low cortisol and low GH; low T_4 and low TSH also may be present. The level of GH must be interpreted with the knowledge that normal newborns have basal concentrations of 20–40 ng/mL in the initial days of life. Ketones, FFAs, and uric acid will be normal. Infants with this condition respond dramatically to replacement with glucocorticoid and GH. Rarely, isolated GH deficiency or isolated ACTH–cortisol deficiency may be responsible for neonatal hypoglycemia. Diagnosis is established on the screening blood sample. Replacement therapy with the hormone ameliorates the symptoms.

Metabolic Defects. Metabolic defects that cause hypoglycemia in the immediate newborn include type I glycogen storage disease, galactosemia, and maple syrup urine disease (see Chapter 5). Affected infants have metabolic acidosis, hepatomegaly, elevated uric and lactic acid concentrations, ketonemia, ketonuria, high triglycerides, and elevated FFAs. They also may have a reducing sugar (galactose) in the urine. Plasma levels of hormones are normal, but the glycemic increment after glucagon is markedly diminished or absent.

Profound neonatal hypoglycemia may be present in infants with type I glycogen storage disease (glucose-6-phosphatase deficiency), because both glycogen breakdown and gluconeogenesis are reduced by the deficiency of this enzyme at the final critical step for hepatic release of glucose. Galactosemia also should be considered in an infant with jaundice, hepatomegaly, and a reducing sugar that is not glucose in the urine; hypoglycemia, however, is not consistently present. Individuals with inborn errors of metabolism may present later in infancy rather than in the immediate newborn period.

Infancy and Childhood. Hypoglycemia in infants and children is uncommon and usually signifies an altered response to fasting, a milder form of hyperinsulinemia, hormone deficiency, or inborn metabolic error. An inability to maintain euglycemia during fasting and an acquired deficiency of hormones predominate during late infancy and childhood. A common time for presentation of milder hyperinsulinemia and defects in gluconeogenesis is 3–6 mo of life, when infants sleep through the night for progressively longer periods so that feedings are no longer given at 3–4 hr intervals.

Clinical manifestations of hypoglycemia may be dramatic and include seizure activity and coma, or may be mild and include irritability, motor incoordination, or wilting spells. A blood sample at the time of the appearance of symptoms or signs can document hypoglycemia and can be used for measuring substrates or hormones to establish the diagnosis. In any infant presenting with seizures for the first time, hypoglycemia should be excluded. Hyperinsulinemic infants and toddlers have a big appetite and become obese. If the critical blood sample is not obtained at the time of symptoms but hypoglycemia is clinically suspected, the child should be admitted to the hospital for a 10–20 hr fast under observation.

Hyperinsulinemia. The findings from the initial blood sample at the time of symptoms are similar to those for neonatal hyperinsulinemia. Treatment of the 3–6 mo infant differs from that of the neonate, however, in that a more prolonged trial of oral diazoxide, at a dose of 5–15 mg/kg/24 hr in three divided doses, is warranted. Frequently, diazoxide at these doses can maintain euglycemia in these patients and can be continued for months to years. However, if hypoglycemia recurs despite adequate doses of diazoxide, or if side effects such as hirsutism, edema, hypotension, or hyperuricemia become intolerable, partial pancreatectomy is indicated.

Factitious Hyperinsulinemia. Deliberate injections of insulin (as a form of child abuse) may mimic spontaneous hypoglycemia resulting from endogenous hyperinsulinemia and result in repeated episodes of symptomatic hypoglycemia. Suspicion may be raised by the presence of inappropriately high insulin levels (greater than 100 μU/mL), which then require measurement of C peptide concentration in the same sample. Because the C peptide concentration reflects endogenous insulin secretion, it will be low, whereas insulin levels are high in factitious hypoglycemia.

Ketotic Hypoglycemia. This is a common cause of hypoglycemia in infants and children age 6 mo to 6 yr. Its cause appears to be the inability to adapt to fasting; however, the specific mechanisms are not understood. Hypoglycemia, occasionally with severe symptoms such as seizures, occurs after limited oral intake during intercurrent infection or gastrointestinal disturbances combined with a relatively long fast. In the critical blood sample, glucose and insulin are low whereas ketones are high, and ketonuria may be present. A subnormal glycemic increment is noted with glucagon challenge, and the syndrome may be reproduced by a fast of 14–24 hr. Because the syndrome may be produced by hormone deficiency, the levels of GH and cortisol always should be measured.

Typically, hormone deficiency is not present, and treatment consists of a high-carbohydrate, high-protein diet with frequent feedings. During intercurrent illness, high-glucose–containing drinks are encouraged and the urine is checked for ketones. The appearance of ketonuria despite high-carbohydrate feeding or high-carbohydrate–containing liquids warrants hospital admission for temporary intravenous glucose at a rate of 6–8 mg/kg/min to avoid a serious hypoglycemic reaction. Most patients respond well to the high-carbohydrate, high-protein feeding regimen and spontaneously resolve the tendency to hypoglycemia by 7–8 yr of age.

Hormone Deficiency. Deficiency of GH or cortisol, rarely, can cause hypoglycemia after the 1st mo of life, and this hypoglycemia is likely to occur only during prolonged fasting, when glucose declines while FFAs and ketones increase, thereby

simulating ketotic hypoglycemia. Clinical clues may be present in older children, such as short stature, poor growth velocity, or symptoms associated with a space-occupying intracranial lesion indicative of pituitary pathology; there also may be hyperpigmentation, salt craving, hyponatremia, and hyperkalemia in progressive adrenal failure, such as occurs in Addison disease.

Carnitine Deficiency. See Chapter 5.

Enzyme Deficiencies. See Chapter 5.

Alcohol and Other Drugs. An important cause of hypoglycemia in infants and children is alcohol ingestion, which causes an acute interruption of gluconeogenesis. The metabolism of alcohol to acetaldehyde requires cofactors also essential for gluconeogenesis. Hepatic alcohol metabolism, however, seems to take preference, thereby depleting the cofactors essential for gluconeogenesis. Consequently, alcohol-induced hypoglycemia occurs only when liver glycogen stores are depleted after some 6–8 hr of fasting. The response to intravenous glucose is dramatic. No laboratory investigations for an isolated episode of hypoglycemia is necessary if a history of alcohol ingestion is elicited. Counseling is indicated.

Reactive Hypoglycemia. This form of postprandial hypoglycemia frequently is suspected in children and adolescents but actually is uncommon. Diagnosis requires demonstrating blood glucose levels less than 50 mg/dL and precipitation of symptoms between the 3rd and 5th hours of an oral glucose tolerance test (i.e., 1.75 g/kg, with a maximum of 75 g after 3 days of normal carbohydrate intake).

References

Baker L, Thornton PS, Stanley CA: Management of hyperinsulinism in infants. J Pediatr 119:755, 1991.

Behrman RE (ed): Nelson Textbook of Pediatrics. 14th ed. Philadelphia, WB Saunders, 1992, Sec. 8.59, 9.57.

Cornblath M, Schwartz R, Aynsley-Green A, et al: Hypoglycemia in infancy: The need for a rational definition. Pediatrics 85:834, 1990.

Dodek AB, Sadeghi-Nejad AB: Value of selective pancreatic angiography in the evaluation of hyperinsulinemic hypoglycemia in infancy. Pediatrics 90:636, 1992.

Haymond MW: Hypoglycemia in infants and children. Endocrinol Metab Clin North Am 18:211, 1989.

Lucas A, Morley R, Cole TJ: Adverse neurodevelopment outcome of moderate neonatal hypoglycaemia. BMJ 397:1304, 1988.

Woolf DA, Leonard JV, Trembath RC, et al: Nesidioblastosis: Evidence for autosomal recessive inheritance. Arch Dis Child 66:529, 1991.

Neurology

Michael J. Painter
Ira Bergman

Neurologic disorders include diseases of the central nervous system (CNS), of the peripheral nervous system, of muscle, and of the special senses. These diseases may be localized to one site of the nervous system or may be part of a generalized multisystem disorder (acquired immunodeficiency syndrome-dementia, systemic lupus erythematosus-psychosis, lead poisoning). The pathogenesis of neurologic disorders includes trauma; infections; inborn errors of metabolism and storage diseases; congenital anomalies; metabolic and toxic disturbances; anoxic, ischemic, embolic, and thrombotic complications; primary or metastatic neoplasms; and autoimmunity.

Neurologic diseases become manifest within a narrow range of symptoms and signs, which include pain (headache, paresthesia); altered mental function (encephalopathy, encephalitis, intoxication–poisoning, hypoxia–ischemia, degenerative disorders); altered motor function (cortical, cerebellar, spinal, anterior horn cell, peripheral nerve, neuromuscular junction, or muscle lesion); and/or seizures. These disorders may be congenital or acquired, acute or chronic, progressive or static, and reversible or irreversible.

DEVELOPMENT OF THE CENTRAL NERVOUS SYSTEM

The precursor of the nervous system is the embryonic ectodermal neural plate, which is present at 18 days of gestation. The neural plate gives rise to the neural tube, which forms the CNS (brain, spinal cord), and the neural crest cells, which give rise to the peripheral nervous system (e.g., the cranial, spinal, and autonomic nerves and ganglia). Neural crest cells thus constitute the cardiac, celiac, mesenteric, and Meissner plexuses, as well as the chromaffin cells, melanocytes, meninges, and adrenal medulla cells.

The neural tube begins to form on the 22nd day of gestation. The fusion of the neural tube proceeds in a cranial and caudal direction, thus leaving temporary rostral and caudal openings, which close on the 25th and the 27th days of gestation, respectively. The rostral end forms the brain, and the caudal region forms the spinal cord; the lumen of the neural tube forms the ventricles of the brain and the central canal of the spinal cord.

Congenital Anomalies of the Nervous System

Defective closure of the caudal neuropore at the end of the 4th wk of gestation produces defects of the vertebral arches known as *spina bifida* (divided spine). Nonfusion of spinal arches may be isolated to vertebral defects (L5, S1) (**spina bifida occulta**) and is noted in 10% of people, who usually are asymptomatic. A small dimple or tuft of hair may be present over the affected vertebra. **Spina bifida cystica** occurs in 1:1000 births and is a sac-like lesion that has multiple unfused vertebrae and an associated *meningocele* or *meningomyelocele* if the meninges or meninges and spinal cord, respectively, form the sac. Spina bifida with *myeloschisis* is noted when the lesion is an open neural tube without an overlying sac. Spina bifida cystica and myeloschisis produce severe neurologic deficits that correlate to the level of the neural tube defect. Loss of sensation, paralysis, and loss of bowel and bladder control are common and depend on the level of the lesion. Thoracic lesions are associated with the poorest neurologic outcome and vertebral instability. Most patients with any of these lesions have bowel and bladder dysfunction. The bladder dysfunction results in repeated episodes of urinary tract infections, reflux nephropathy, and renal insufficiency. Meningomyelocele usually is accompanied by hydrocephalus that is due to an **Arnold-Chiari malformation**, producing downward displacement of the medulla and cerebellum accompanied by obstruction of the 4th ventricle.

MENINGOMYELOCELE

Treatment of infants with this malformation includes operative skin closure of an open or thin-walled spinal defect, ventricular–peritoneal shunting of hydrocephalus, bracing of the lower extremities to permit ambulation of low vertebral lesions, intermittent bladder catheterization to avoid urinary stasis, and physical therapy. Most children have a normal IQ. *In utero detection* is possible by screening for a high maternal serum alpha-fetoprotein level followed by performing fetal ultrasonography and amniocentesis to confirm elevated amniotic fluid alpha-fetoprotein and acetylcholinesterase levels. *Prevention* may be possible by providing supplements of vitamins and folate early in pregnancy, before neural tube development.

DIASTEMATOMYELIA

In this malformation, the spinal cord is split by bone spicules or by a fibrous band. This split condition and a lipomatous tumor (lipomeningocele) produce the **tethered cord syndrome**, with resultant abnormalities of distal sensation, gait, and bladder or bowel function. The *treatment* is surgery.

CRANIAL DEFECTS

These defects may produce anterior or posterior encephaloceles containing either meninges or meninges and brain. Severe malformations resulting from failure of rostral neuropore closure produce exencephaly (exposed brain) or anencephaly. The latter is noted in 1:1000 births in the United States and is uniformly lethal.

Neonates with **anencephaly** have a rudimentary brain stem or midbrain but no cortex or cranium. *Prenatal diagnosis* is possible by detecting elevated maternal serum alpha-fetoprotein levels and by performing fetal ultrasonography. The recurrence risk in subsequent pregnancies for either cranial or spinal neural tube defects is 10%. Within a family, an anencephalic birth may be followed by the birth of a second child affected with a lumbar–sacral meningomyelocele. The inheritance of neural tube defects is polygenic.

References

Behrman RE (ed): Nelson Textbook of Pediatrics. 14th ed. Philadelphia, WB Saunders, 1992, Sec. 3.2, 20.2–20.16.

McCarthy G: Treating children with spina bifida. BMJ 302: 65, 1991.

Volpe J: Neurology of the Newborn. 2nd ed. Philadelphia, WB Saunders, 1987.

Werler MM, Shapiro S, Mitchell AA: Periconceptional folic acid exposure and risk of occurrent neural tube defects. JAMA 269:1257, 1993.

NEUROLOGIC EVALUATION

The results and evaluation of the neurologic examination of children vary with chronologic age. The examination of the newborn is unique, whereas examination of the older child approximates that of the adult. Examining the young child is a challenging process, because the patient often is uncooperative and has limited ability to assist.

The neurologic evaluation includes a history of the evolution of the illness, its character, and the presence of the illness in similarly affected family members. One attempts to establish the abnormalities as "progressive," "intermittent," "static," or "saltatory." *Static* abnormalities noted in the first few months of life suggest congenital abnormalities or brain injury sustained during the neonatal period. *Progressive* disorders suggest degenerative CNS disease, whereas abnormalities that are *intermittent* with return to normal neurologic function indicate paroxysmal disorders. *Saltatory* disorders, characterized by exacerbation and partial recovery, are seen with demyelinating and vascular diseases.

Findings on the general examination often are clues to diagnosis. Abnormalities of hair, skin, teeth, and nails, all of neuroectodermal origin, may reflect nervous system lesions. Neurocutaneous lesions, such as café-au-lait spots, neurofibroma, or adenoma sebaceum occur in several disorders (Table 18–1). The occipital frontal head circumference reflects underlying brain growth and/or the presence of anomalies. The *head circumference* is measured using paper disposable tape and plotted against appropriate standard growth curves (see Figs. 1–4 and 1–10). A measurement of 3 standard deviations above or below the mean is abnormal

Table 18–1. Differential Diagnosis of Café-au-Lait Spots

—Neurofibromatosis
—Tuberous sclerosis
— Bloom syndrome
—McCune-Albright syndrome
—Fanconi anemia
—Gaucher disease
—Russel-Silver dwarf
—Ataxia–telangiectasia
—Epidermal nevi

and reflects either macrocephaly or microcephaly. Measurements plotted over time may show an accelerating or decelerating pattern of growth indicating hydrocephalus or growth impairment or destruction of brain, respectively.

During infancy, the anterior fontanel is slightly depressed and pulsatile when the infant is placed in the sitting position. When the fontanel is tense or bulging, this bulging is an indication of increased intracranial pressure. An unusual shape of the head may indicate premature closure of one or more of the sutures (**craniosynostosis**). Abnormal shape, location, and condition of the ears are found in a number of syndromes (e.g., whether the ears are low set and/or posteriorly rotated). An examination of the eyes should include searching for epicanthal folds, coloboma, conjunctival telangiectasias, or cataracts. Examining the optic fundus with a direct ophthalmoscope helps assess the status of the optic discs and macula. A complete examination of the retina requires dilating the pupil and using an indirect ophthalmoscope. Examining the hands and feet reveals the presence of abnormal creases, polydactyly, or syndactyly (see Chapter 19). An examination of the neck and spine should include searching for *midline defects*, which may be obvious, such as spina bifida with myelomeningocele, or subtle, such as cutaneous dimples, small openings or sinus tracts, or tufts of hair or subcutaneous lipomas, suggesting the possiblity of vertebral or spinal cord abnormalities. Kyphosis and scoliosis are important features to note in abnormalities of the central and peripheral nervous systems.

Neonatal Examination

Because the brain is immature, an examination of the neonate is used mainly to assess the function of the subcortical structures.

REFLEXES

A number of primitive reflexes noted at birth (Table 18–2) indicate the functional integrity of the brain stem. As a group, they are symmetric and disappear at 4–6 mo of age, indicating the normal maturation of descending inhibitory cerebral influences. The *Landau* and *parachute* reflexes become apparent after the newborn period, indicating proper maturation of appropriate brain structures. The *grasp* and *rooting* reflexes are inhibited by maturation of frontal lobe structures and may reappear later in life with frontal lobe lesions. Asymmetry

of the primitive reflexes often indicates focal brain or peripheral nerve lesions.

POSTURE

Posture is defined as the position that the infant naturally assumes when placed supine. An infant at 28 wk of gestation will demonstrate total extension, whereas at 32 wk a slight increase in tone of the lower extremities is noted. At 34 wk, the lower extremities are flexed and the upper extremities extended. At term, the infant flexes both lower and upper extremities. Recoil is defined as a liveliness with which an extremity springs back to its original position after passive stretching and release. Recoil is essentially absent in the small premature infant but very brisk at term.

MOVEMENT/TONE

As gestational age increases, spontaneous movements of the infant change from extensive, generalized, and athetoid to those that are localized and brief. Spontaneous movements of the small premature infant normally are slow, whereas those of the term infant are rapid and jerk-like.

The popliteal angle, heel-to-ear maneuver, scarf maneuver, and head control are utilized in assessing muscle tone and estimating gestational age (see Chapter 6 and Fig. 6–4).

Interpretation

Persistence of the primitive reflexes beyond 4–6 mo of age indicates dysfunction of brain structures responsible for their inhibition. Increased resistance to such maneuvers as the elicitation of the scarf reflex or the popliteal angle in the premature infant may be a manifestation of rigidity or of spasticity, whereas decreased resistance in the performance of these maneuvers in the term infant may be a manifestation of hypotonia. Because CNS maturation is incomplete, one must be cautious in establishing a prognosis based on the newborn neurologic examination alone.

Cranial Nerve Evaluation

The evaluation of cranial nerve function depends on the stage of maturation of the child's brain and on the ability of the child to cooperate.

EVALUATION OF CRANIAL NERVE I

The child's sense of smell is difficult to assess. Beginning at the age of 2–3 yr, one can discern

Table 18–2. CNS Reflexes of Infancy

Reflex	Description	Age of Appearance	Age of Disappearance	Origin in CNS
Moro	Sudden head extension causes extension followed by flexion of the arms and legs	Birth	4–6 mo	Brain stem vestibular nuclei
Grasp	Placing a finger in palm results in flexing of the infant's hand, accompanied by flexion at elbow and shoulder	Birth	4–6 mo	Brain stem vestibular nuclei
Rooting	Tactile stimulus about the mouth results in the infant's mouth pursuing the stimulus	Birth	4–6 mo	Brain stem trigeminal system
Trunk incurvation	Infant withdraws from stroking stimulus along the ventral margin	Birth	9–6 mo	Spinal cord
Placing	Infant places foot on examining surface when dorsum of foot is brought into contact with the edge of the surface	Birth	4–6 mo	Cerebral cortex
Crossed extension	One leg held firmly in extension and the dorsum and sole of the foot stimulated results in a sequence of flexion, extension, and adduction, followed by toe fanning of the opposite leg	Birth	4–6 mo	Spinal cord
Tonic neck	With the infant supine, turning of the head results in ipsilateral extension of the arm and leg in a "fencing" posture	Birth	4–6 mo	Brain stem vestibular nuclei
Parachute	With the infant sitting, tilting to either side results in extension of the ipsilateral arm in a protective fashion	6–8 mo	Never	Brain stem vestibular nuclei
Landau	With the infant held about the waist and suspended, extension of the neck produces extension of the arms and legs	6–8 mo	15 mo–2 yr	Brain stem

whether or not the child can smell. Aromatic substances, such as perfumes and ground coffee, should be utilized, not volatile substances such as ammonia that irritate the nasal mucosa and do not test smell. Once the child has established speech, it often is possible to assess the ability to perceive and name an odor. Anosmia may be due to head trauma, fractures, meningitis, diseases of the nose, or brain tumors.

EVALUATION OF CRANIAL NERVE II

Vision can be assessed grossly in the neonate by noting a blinking response to bright light. The visual acuity at birth is approximately 20/400. Utilizing visual evoked responses, the visual acuity has been found to be 20/20 by 6 mo of age. An indication of peripheral vision can be obtained by noting the infant's detection of objects brought into the visual field from behind. The ability of the child to visually locate and track small objects estimates visual acuity in the infant, whereas in older children standard visual acuity charts and confrontational testing of peripheral vision are utilized. Lesions of the anterior visual pathways, including the optic nerves, chiasm, and tract, are expressed by a reduced pupillary reaction to light, which may be bilateral or unilateral (afferent pupillary defect). Lesions of the posterior visual pathway, involving the occipital cortex, lateral geniculate, and optic radiations, are expressed by loss of visual fields and normal pupillary reactions.

EVALUATION OF CRANIAL NERVES III, IV, AND VI

Extraocular movements may be assessed in the neonate by observing eye movements in response to visual stimuli and by noting extraocular movements when stimulating vestibular reflexes by gently spinning the infant. Beyond the newborn period, extraocular movements are observed as the infant follows objects. The pupillary reflex is assessed using a focused bright light. The pupil reacts to light by 30 wk of gestation. Cranial nerve III innervates the levator palpebrae superioris, the medial, superior and inferior recti, and the inferior oblique muscles. Cranial nerve IV innervates the superior oblique muscle, which adjusts the globe in the adducted position, and cranial nerve VI innervates the lateral rectus muscle. Because cranial nerve VI has a long intracranial route, VIth cranial palsies may be nonspecific signs of increased intracranial pressure. Cavernous sinus infection affects cranial nerves III, IV, V, and VI. Abnormalities of cranial nerves III, IV, and VI may cause diplopia.

Clinical syndromes may affect cranial nerve III and produce *miosis* or *mydriasis*. A constricted pupil (miosis) may be associated with a **Horner syndrome** (miosis, ptosis, anhidrosis) resulting from a unilateral sympathetic nervous lesion. Additional causes of miosis include the **Argyll Robinson pupil**, drugs (opiates, cholinergic agents), and pontine lesions (sympathetic paralysis). Mydriasis (dilated pupil) is seen with drugs (anticholinergic, sympathomimetic), botulism, IIIrd nerve compression, and thyrotoxicosis.

EVALUATION OF CRANIAL NERVE V

In newborns and small infants, the muscles of mastication can be assessed while watching the infant suck and swallow. The masseter muscles may be directly palpated. In later childhood, as coopera-

tion improves, pterygoid function may be assessed by voluntary jaw deviation. The *corneal reflex* can be tested (cranial nerves V and VII) at any age. Facial sensation of light touch and pain can be determined with cotton gauze and pinprick.

EVALUATION OF CRANIAL NERVE VII

The assessment of facial symmetry at rest and during sucking activity can be utilized in assessing the small infant. Beyond infancy, the muscles of facial expression are assessed on a voluntary basis. Complete facial weakness suggests a peripheral lower motor neuron lesion, whereas lower facial weakness suggests an upper motor neuron lesion. Taste to the anterior two thirds of the tongue is difficult to assess, but the ability to discriminate between salt and sugar can be assessed in a cooperative child once language is acquired.

EVALUATION OF CRANIAL NERVE VIII

The neonate will demonstrate eye blinking in response to loud noises. At approximately 4 mo of age, an infant will turn to the sound stimulus. The use of spoken words whispered at 2 feet is a more reliable technique and may be used once the child has acquired speech. Conductive versus sensorineural hearing loss can be differentiated by the fact that air conduction of a turning fork sound should last twice as long as bone conduction. Symptoms of lesions of cranial nerve VIII include deafness, tinnitus, and vertigo.

Lesions of the vestibular component of the acoustic nerve may produce manifestations such as vertigo, nausea, vomiting, diaphoresis, and nystagmus. Lesions in cranial nerve VIII, the cerebellopontine angle, or the junction of the pons and medulla all may produce these problems. The differential diagnosis of vertigo is noted in Table 18–3. Testing of the labyrinth system can be performed by irrigating the ear canal with warm or cold water. Warm calorics stimulate nystagmus toward the irrigated side, whereas cold produces nystagmus to the opposite direction. Nystagmus is defined by the direction of the quick component.

EVALUATION OF CRANIAL NERVES IX AND X

The gag reflex is brisk at all ages except in the very immature neonate. Uvula deviation toward the stronger unaffected side suggests unilateral palsy of cranial nerves IX and/or X. Nasal speech

Table 18–3. Differential Diagnosis of Vertigo*

Peripheral Causes
Benign positional vertigo
Acute vestibulopathy (labyrinthitis)
Ménière syndrome
Toxic labyrinthopathy
Motion sickness

Central Causes
Multiple sclerosis
Cerebrovascular disease
Cerebellopontine tumors (acoustic neuroma)
Migraine

* Peripheral vertigo has no other auditory (except Ménière syndrome) or neurologic deficts. Often, an intense sense of severe spinning with nausea, vomiting, a positive Romberg test, past pointing, and rotatory or horizontal nystagmus are present. Vertical nystagmus is due to brain stem lesions.

and vocal cord paralysis (recurrent laryngeal nerve) are additional signs of lesions of cranial nerve X.

EVALUATION OF CRANIAL NERVE XI

The functions of the trapezius and sternocleidomastoid muscles are assessed by observing the infant's posture and spontaneous activity. Head tilt and drooping of the shoulder are suggestive of lesions involving cranial nerve XI. In later childhood, direct examination of these muscles is possible.

EVALUATION OF CRANIAL NERVE XII

Examination of the tongue for atrophy and fasciculation is accomplished at any age. By 1 yr of age, specific tongue movements can be assessed by having the child follow a lollypop with the tongue, and, by 3–4 years of age, tongue movement to command is possible. The tongue deviates toward the weak side in unilateral lesions.

Motor Examination

In the neonate and the small infant, this examination utilizes the observation of spontaneous activity, primitive reflexes, and muscle tone previously described. When the infant begins to walk, gait is assessed. In early infancy, the gait is broad based and unsteady. The base narrows with age, so that by the 6th year a child is able to tandem walk. *Pyramidal track* dysfunction will result in a stiff, shuffling gait caused by spasticity, whereas a similar gait is noted in *extrapyramidal* motor dysfunction on the basis of rigidity. Abnormalities of the anterior horn cell, peripheral nerve, neuromuscular junction, and muscle (lower motor neuron)

result in a wide-based, unsteady gait caused by weakness. Cerebellar dysfunction results in a broad-based, unsteady gait accompanied by difficulty in executing turns. The ability of the child to stand from the supine posture evaluates strength of the back, hip, and proximal leg muscles. The ability of the child to walk on the heels tests the anterior tibial muscles. Toe walking assesses strength of the gastrocnemius and soleus muscles. Dexterity of movements of the upper extremities are assessed in the small infant by having the child reach for objects and, in the older child, by demonstrating the ability to perform finger-to-finger and finger-to-nose maneuvers.

In the toddler, muscle strength is assessed by observation. Arm and shoulder muscle strength is tested by observing the child's ability to raise the arms above the head and the resistance the examiner feels when lifting the child by placing his or her hands in the infant's axillae. Muscle weakness of pyramidal origin is spastic, extrapyramidal weakness is rigid, and weakness of lower motor neuron origin is flaccid. Muscle fasciculations suggest denervation.

ASSESSMENT OF MUSCLE BULK AND TONE

Although atrophy eventually is seen in both pyramidal and extrapyramidal lesions, it is most striking in lesions involving the lower motor neuron. Bulk is assessed by observation, palpation, and comparison to contralateral extremities. Excessive muscle bulk is seen in myotonia congenita and pseudohypertrophic muscular dystrophy. Muscle tone is assessed by measuring the extremity's resistance to passive motion. In extrapyramidal disease, an increase in resistance is present throughout passive movement of a joint (*rigidity*). In pyramidal disease, increased resistance to passive movement that suddenly gives way at a critical point (*clasped knife response*) is noted. In lower motor neuron disease, decreased resistance to passive movement is present.

EVALUATION OF DEEP TENDON REFLEXES

Myotactic reflexes (triceps, biceps, knee, ankle) are elicited by sudden tendon stretch and can be obtained at any age. The Babinski response is not helpful in the neonate, because the plantar response may be extensor or flexor. The plantar response is consistently flexor (downward) after 2 yr of age.

INVOLUNTARY MOVEMENTS

See Movement Disorders.

Sensory Examination

Evaluation of the sensory system includes an assessment of pain, touch, hot and cold temperature, and joint position senses. The sensory examination of the newborn and infant is limited to observing the perception of a pinprick by watching for crying, eye closure, facial grimace, or sucking response while feeding. Normal newborns will interrupt their continuous sucking activity as they perceive a light pin stimulus. Simple withdrawal of the involved body part may be all that can be observed in the small infant, and without simultaneous facial changes, withdrawal may indicate a spinal cord reflex. In the cooperative child, once language has been achieved, touch, hot and cold, and position sense can be evaluated. Cortical sensation (two-point discrimination, stereognosis, and others) can be assessed reliably only in older children. Properly demarcating a sensory level can help localize a lesion.

Mental Status Evaluation

The assessment of mental status is a critical aspect of the examination. *Alertness* is assessed in the newborn and small infant by observing spontaneous activities, feeding behavior, and the ability of the infant to visually fix and follow the movement of objects. The child's response to tactile, visual, and auditory stimuli is noted. Does the child localize sound, follow objects visually, and verbalize to noxious stimuli? In circumstances of altered consciousness, the response to painful stimuli is noted. Does the child simply withdraw from pain, or is vigorous withdrawal accompanied by vocalization?

Language function is both expressive (involving speech and the use of gestures such as pointing or shaking the head) and receptive (understanding speech or gesture). Abnormalities of language resulting from disorders of the cerebral hemispheres are referred to as aphasias. Anterior, expressive, or **Broca aphasia** is characterized by sparse, nonfluent language. Posterior, receptive, or **Wernicke aphasia** is characterized by an inability to understand language. Speech is fluent but nonsensical. **Global aphasia** is the term applied to impaired expressive and receptive language.

The use of a Denver Developmental Standard Screening Test is an efficient means of relating the child's behavior to appropriate age norms (see Chapter 1). Older children should have short-term and long-term *memory* tested with current events and other factors. Orientation to person, place, and time should be assessed, as well as cognitive activities such as mental solution of mathematical problems (e.g., serial subtraction of 7 from 100).

Special Diagnostic Procedures

ELECTROENCEPHALOGRAPHY

The (EEG) records electrical activity generated by the cerebral cortex. EEG rhythms mature throughout childhood. The EEG of the premature infant is discontinuous and accompanied by a predominance of slower frequencies (2–4 Hz) until 36 wk of gestation, when the waking portion of the record is continuous. Sleep is characterized by a discontinuous pattern (trace alternans). In later childhood, the occipital portion of the EEG is characterized by 8–12 Hz activity (alpha), whereas faster rhythms (13–30 Hz) (beta) are seen anteriorly. Theta rhythms (4–7 Hz) are intermixed. Fixed slow-wave foci (1–3 Hz) delta rhythms suggest an underlying structural abnormality. When delta activity is seen diffusely, increased intracranial pressure or other encephalopathy is suspected. Spikes, polyspikes, and spike-and-wave abnormalities indicate an underlying seizure tendency.

EVOKED RESPONSES

Evoked responses are computer-analyzed CNS responses to afferent stimuli. The stimulus (a click for auditory testing, a flash or pattern stimulus for visual testing, and a vibratory stimulus for somatosensory testing) is applied and the CNS response monitored over the scalp. Repetitive stimuli are computer averaged and a response pattern is obtained. Abnormalities of the components of the response pattern can be localized to specific areas of the CNS. Somatosensory responses are of value in assessing peripheral nerve, spinal cord, and cerebral hemispheric function, whereas visual and auditory responses are of value in assessing hearing, central auditory function, and abnormalities of visual acuity and the visual pathways. Auditory evoked responses also are known as brain stem evoked responses, because they assess auditory pathways at the level of the brain stem. Evoked responses are of particular value in small infants and in patients with altered consciousness.

ELECTROMYOGRAPHY

This procedure is used primarily to assess abnormalities of the lower motor neuron and muscles. Needles inserted into muscles frequently will reveal denervation patterns when anterior horn or peripheral nerve disease is present. Normal muscle is electrically silent at rest, and the presence of spontaneous discharge of motor units (fibrillations) or muscle fasciculus (fasciculation) is indicative of denervation. Abnormalities of the motor pattern on muscle contraction are seen in denervation and primary muscle disease. Repetitive nerve stimulation may demonstrate excessive fatigue in *myasthenia gravis*.

Electromyography (EMG) in conjunction with muscle biopsy in which tissue is examined histochemically and with electron microscopy frequently is necessary to establish specific diagnoses in neuromuscular disease.

NEURORADIOLOGY

Imaging the brain and spinal cord is accomplished utilizing computerized tomography (CT), myelography, cerebral angiography, and magnetic resonance imaging (MRI).

References

Behrman RE (ed): Nelson Textbook of Pediatrics. 14th ed. Philadelphia, WB Saunders, 1992, Sec. 3.3, 20.1.

DISORDERS OF CONSCIOUSNESS

Consciousness is a process by which a person is aware of self and environment. Coma is defined as being unresponsive to stimuli and differs from sleep in that the person in a coma cannot be aroused. Arousal is impaired either by small lesions involving the reticular activating system (RAS), extensive bilateral cerebral lesions, or unilateral cerebral lesions that distort the upper brain stem (i.e., herniation syndromes). The RAS is a network of neurons located in the core of the brain stem extending from the mid-pons through the midbrain and hypothalamus to the thalamus. The RAS projects widely to the cerebral cortex and serves a general arousing function.

Depression of consciousness may be acute, chronic, transitory, or recurring.

Acute Disorders of Consciousness
(See also Chapter 3)

Approach. Acute changes in consciousness vary in degree from mild lethargy and confusion to deep coma. The differential diagnosis of altered consciousness is presented in Table 18–4. An initial approach to the comatose patient is discussed in Chapter 3. In childhood the most common causes of coma include infections, hypoxia-ischemia (after cardiac arrest, drowning), intoxications, head trauma, and the postictal state.

Metabolic derangements may require adjustments of certain blood chemistries (glucose, calcium, sodium, bicarbonate, blood urea nitrogen, ammonia) by intravenous infusions or dialysis. Toxic ingestions may necessitate gastric lavage, charcoal administration, forced diuresis, dialysis, or specific antidotes (see Chapter 3). Infections are treated with antibiotics or antiviral agents (see Chapter 10). Structural brain lesions may require surgical excision or medical treatment of raised intracranial pressure (see Chapter 3).

Clinical Manifestations. A detailed history and physical examination usually will provide sufficient clues to differentiate among the three major diagnostic categories producing coma: metabolic/toxic, infectious, and structural. Fever, petechiae, chills, and sweats suggest infection. Pain on neck flexion, photophobia, and pain on movement of the eyes are symptoms of meningeal irritation. Associated symptoms of abdominal pain, diarrhea, sore throat, conjunctivitis, cough, or rash point to viral encephalitis or a parainfectious syndrome. Neck motion should be avoided in patients with suspected trauma or drowning until the cervical spine films rule out vertebral fracture or subluxation. Headache and severe vomiting can be caused by raised intracranial pressure. A very abrupt loss of consciousness suggests a stroke: stupor progressing to deep, unarousable "sleep" over hours suggests drug intoxication; and a chronic gradual fading of alertness over weeks suggests a growing intracranial mass. Chronic medical conditions or their treatment (e.g., diabetes mellitus, insulin administration, leukemia), head trauma, use of "street drugs," social and emotional difficulties, exposure to sick animals, or travel to areas with known endemic diseases (e.g., Rocky Mountain spotted fever, Lyme disease) all provide specific clues.

Neurologic examination begins with observation. Breathing patterns, posture, and spontaneous actions often provide important clues to the depth, localization, and etiology of the depressed consciousness. Important recognizable respiratory patterns include **Cheyne-Stokes respirations**, central neurogenic hyperventilation, and gasping respirations. In Cheyne-Stokes respirations, a period of

Table 18–4. Diagnostic Approach to Coma

Cause	Diagnostic Approach
Metabolic Derangements	Na^+, K^+, Cl^-, CO_2, BUN, creatinine, SGOT, SGPT, PT, PTT, blood gas, ammonia, lead level, pyruvate, lactate, urinalysis, and urine amino and organic acids
Hypoglycemia	
Hyponatremia	
Hypernatremia	
Hyperosmolarity	
Hypercapnia	
Uremia	
Hyperammonemia	
Hepatic failure	
Reye syndrome	
Urea cycle enzyme deficiency	
Fatty acid–acyl-coenzyme A dehydrogenase deficiency	
Methylmalonicaciduria	
Proprionicaciduria	
Mitochondrial Diseases	
Diabetes mellitus	
Lead intoxication	
Causes with CSF Abnormalities	CSF analysis, CT, MRI, angiogram
Bloody CSF	
Subarachnoid hemorrhage	
Subdural hemorrhage	
Intraparenchymal hemorrhage (trauma, arteriovenous malformations, coagulopathy)	
Excess WBCs	
Meningitis	
Encephalitis	
Parainfectious syndrome	
Vasculitis	
Carcinomatosis	
Subacute bacterial endocarditis	
Causes with CT or MRI Abnormalities	CT, MRI
Infarction	
Global (anoxia)	
Multifocal	
Unilateral, large	
Focal midbrain, hypothalamus or thalamus	
Mass lesion	
Tumor	
Hemorrhage	
Hydrocephalus	
Abscess	
Inflammatory mass	
Cyst	
Causes with Normal CT and CSF	Blood and urine analyses for toxic substances, EEG
Drug intoxication or withdrawal	
Epilepsy	
Concussion	
Hypoxic–ischemic injury	

BUN = blood urea nitrogen; CSF = cerebrospinal fluid; PT = prothrombin time; PTT = partial thromboplastin time; SGOT = serum glutamic oxaloacetic transaminase; SGPT = serum glutamic pyruvic transaminase; WBCs = white blood cells.

hyperventilation with a crescendo–decrescendo pattern alternates with a shorter period of apnea. Cerebral, thalamic, or hypothalamic modulation of respirations has been lost but brain stem control is intact. This pattern also can be observed in patients with heart failure or primary respiratory disease. Midbrain disease yields **central neurogenic hyperventilation**, which consists of sustained rapid deep breathing. Gasping respirations are irregularly irregular. They indicate dysfunction of the low brain stem–medulla and usually will be followed by terminal apnea.

Body posture can indicate the degree of depression of consciousness. Mild depression is manifested by a comfortable "sleeping" posture with limbs slightly flexed, body tilted to one side, and eyes fully closed. Frequent readjustments of position, yawns, and sighs are observed. Deep coma is exhibited by patients who lie in a flat, extended, unvarying position with eyes half-open. An asymmetric posture suggests motor dysfunction of one side.

Observation will reveal focal and generalized seizures, tremors, myoclonus, asterixis, choreoathetosis, dystonia, and ballismus. Focal seizures imply focal brain disease but also may be noted in children with meningitis or hypoglycemia. Generalized tremors, myoclonus, and asterixis are seen with metabolic–toxic diseases. Choreoathetosis, dystonia, and ballismus imply basal ganglia dysfunction.

Hallucinations can involve any sensory modality. Typically, olfactory and gustatory hallucinations indicate structural brain disease; visual and tactile hallucinations indicate metabolic–toxic disease, and auditory hallucinations indicate psychiatric illness.

Formal assessment of the degree of unconsciousness is performed utilizing the **Glasgow Coma Scale** (Table 18–5). Unresponsive patients are stimulated with noise, light touch, and pain. Words used to describe lack of full consciousness and their usual meaning are listed in Table 18–6. However, a full description of what is observed should be noted.

The detailed neurologic examination of the comatose patient focuses on the eyes, patterns of motor movement, tone, and reflexes. Eye movements are observed and then elicited with the **doll's head maneuver** (oculocephalic response) and cold caloric stimulation (oculovestibular response) (Fig. 18–1). Doll's head movement should not be performed until the cervical spine has been cleared of fracture or subluxation. Persons who are awake always can move their eyes whenever and

Table 18–5. Glasgow Coma Scale

Best motor response	1. Nil (flaccid)
	2. Extensor response
	3. Abnormal flexion
	4. Withdrawal
	5. Localization of pain
	6. Obeys
Best verbal response	1. Nil
	2. Incomprehensible sounds
	3. Inappropriate words
	4. Confused conversation
	5. Oriented, fluent speech
Best eye opening response	1. Nil
	2. To pain
	3. To speech
	4. Spontaneous

wherever they wish, either by making a quick jumping (i.e., saccadic) eye movement or by slowly following (i.e., pursuing) a target. **Uninhibited eye movements** are seen with an intact brain stem but a poorly functioning cerebrum; the normal oculomotor brain stem reflexes are not controlled or inhibited by the aware brain. There may be no spontaneous eye movements, or the eyes may spontaneously rove slowly side to side. In the doll's head maneuver, the eyes move opposite to the direction of head movement at exactly the same pace, as if they were freely floating "ball bearings" within the orbits. To cold caloric stimulation, the eyes deviate fully and conjugately toward the ear that has been stimulated. Nystagmus is not observed. **Incomplete eye movements** are observed when the brain stem, peripheral oculomotor nerves, neuromuscular junctions, or eye muscles are not functioning properly. With complete loss of oculomotor function, the eyes will remain in the center of the orbit, as if they are "painted on," regardless of any

Table 18–6. Stages of Depressed Consciousness

Stage	Manifestations
Lethargy–irritability	Sleepy, poor attention, fully arousable
Confusion	Poor orientation
Delirium	Agitated confusion, hallucinations, autonomic abnormalities (e.g., excess sweating, tachycardia, hypertension)
Obtundation	Arousable only to severe stimuli
Stupor	Unarousable, localizes pain
Coma	Unarousable, does not localize pain

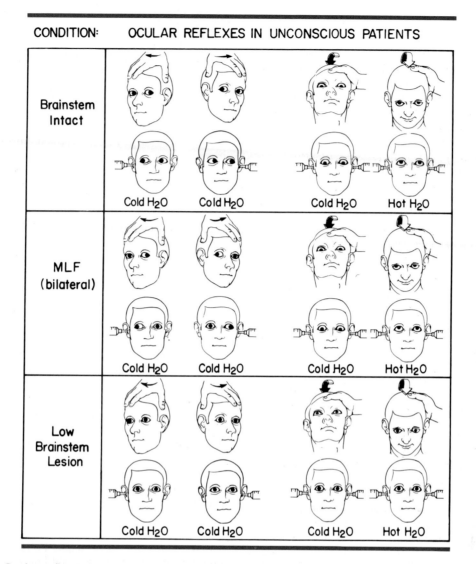

CONDITION: OCULAR REFLEXES IN UNCONSCIOUS PATIENTS

Brainstem Intact	Cold H₂O	Cold H₂O	Cold H₂O	Hot H₂O
MLF (bilateral)	Cold H₂O	Cold H₂O	Cold H₂O	Hot H₂O
Low Brainstem Lesion	Cold H₂O	Cold H₂O	Cold H₂O	Hot H₂O

Figure 18–1. Ocular reflexes in unconscious patients. The upper section illustrates the oculocephalic (above) and oculovestibular (below) reflexes in an unconscious patient whose brain stem ocular pathways are intact. Horizontal eye movements are illustrated on the left and vertical eye movements on the right: lateral conjugate eye movements (upper left) to head turning are full and opposite in direction to the movement of the face. A stronger stimulus to lateral deviation is achieved by douching cold water against the tympanic membrane(s). There is tonic conjugate deviation of both eyes toward the stimulus; the eyes usually remain tonically deviated for 1 min or more before slowly returning to the midline. Because the patient is unconscious, there is no nystagmus. Extension of the neck in a patient with an intact brain stem produces conjugate deviation of the eyes in the downward direction, and flexion of the neck produces deviation of the eyes upward. Bilateral cold water against the tympanic membrane likewise produces conjugate downward deviation of the eyes, whereas hot water (no warmer than 44°C [111.2°F]) causes conjugate upward deviation of the eyes.

In the middle portion of the drawing, the effects of bilateral medial longitudinal fasciculus (MLF) lesions on oculocephalic and oculovestibular reflexes are shown. The left portion of the drawing illustrates that oculocephalic and oculovestibular stimulation deviates the appropriate eye laterally and brings the eye, which normally would deviate medially, only to the midline, because the medial longitudinal fasciculus, with its connections between the abducens and oculomotor nuclei, is interrupted. Vertical eye movements often remain intact.

The lower portion of the drawing illustrates the effects of a low brain stem lesion. On the left, neither oculovestibular nor oculocephalic movements cause lateral deviation of the eyes because the pathways are interrupted between the vestibular nucleus and the abducens area. Likewise, in the right portion of the drawing, neither oculovestibular nor oculocephalic stimulation causes vertical deviation of the eyes. On rare occasions, particularly with low lateral brain stem lesions, oculocephalic responses may be intact even when oculovestibular reflexes are abolished. (From Plum F, Posner J: The Diagnosis of Stupor and Coma. 3rd ed. Philadelphia, FA Davis, 1980, p 55.)

stimulation. With partial loss, only the affected portion will be nonfunctioning regardless of stimulation.

Abnormal positioning of the eyes or pupils and failure of specific extraocular movements can localize the site of neurologic dysfunction.

Certain characteristic postures and tone can define the level or locus of neurologic disability. **Decorticate posturing** consists of rigid extension of the legs and feet, flexion and supination of the arms, and fisting of the hands. It occurs when the midbrain and red nucleus control body posture without inhibition by diencephalon, basal ganglia, and cortical structures. **Decerebrate posturing** consists of rigid extension of legs, arms, trunk, and head with hyperpronation of lower arms. It indicates pontine and vestibular nucleus control of posture without inhibition from more rostral structures. These postures may be exhibited unilaterally or bilaterally, indicating equal or unequal dysfunction of the two sides of the brain. Sometimes stereotyped rigid postures are exhibited that do not fall easily into the category of decerebrate or decorticate positions. These postures also indicate lack of cerebral and diencephalic control of upper brain stem motor reflexes.

Metabolic causes of acute coma are suggested by spontaneous fluctuations in the level of consciousness; tremors, myoclonus, and asterixis; visual and tactile hallucinations; and deep coma with preservation of pupillary light reflexes. Acute metabolic or toxic disorders also usually produce a hypotonic limp state, but hypertonia, rigidity, and decorticate and decerebrate posturing sometimes are observed in coma caused by hypoglycemia, hepatic encephalopathy, and short-acting barbiturates. Focal abnormalities on the neurologic examination (i.e., hemiparesis, cortical blindness, choreoathetosis, ataxia) suggest *structural brain disease*.

Intracranial Pressure Elevation. Papilledema or cranial nerve III palsies in patients with depressed consciousness are strong evidence of elevated intracranial pressure (ICP), which is a medical emergency. More commonly, progressive loss of consciousness accompanied by a characteristic progression of motor, oculomotor, pupillary, and respiratory signs, as detailed in Table 18–7, warns of incipient transtentorial herniation. Uncal herniation is another sign of severe increased ICP with early unilateral IIIrd nerve palsy and contralateral hemiparesis. Medical therapy must be instituted and emergency cranial CT performed. The initial study is done without contrast material to clearly identify blood and calcifications. If the patient's condition permits, a study with contrast material follows, to identify inflammatory and neoplastic lesions. Some metabolic derangements give rise to severe elevations of ICP without producing recognizable CT abnormalities. These derangements include hepatic encephalopathy, Reye syndrome, hyponatremia, lead encephalopathy, trauma, treatment of diabetic ketoacidosis, and global or multifocal hypoxic–ischemic injury.

Lumbar puncture increases the risk of transtentorial herniation in patients with raised ICP pressure and should be avoided.

Differential Diagnosis. See Table 18–4.

Toxic or Metabolic Abnormalities. Metabolic imbalances associated with depression of consciousness are most severe when the metabolic derangement has developed acutely and rapidly. The neurologic deficits associated with uremia and hypercapnia without hypoxia usually are fully reversible. The other metabolic disorders, however, may produce permanent neurologic disability if they are not treated at an early stage. Pathologic examination of brain tissue has revealed neuronal loss in the presence of hypoglycemia; vascular damage and parenchymal hemorrhages with hypernatremia; cerebral edema with hyponatremia, hepatic failure, Reye syndrome, and lead encephalopathy; and astrocytosis with hepatic failure. Focal deficits are uncommon in metabolic encephalopathy. The presence of asterixis signals hepatic or uremic encephalopathy or hypercapnia. Reye syndrome pro-

Table 18–7. Progression of Stages and Anatomic Levels of Transtentorial Central Herniation

Signs	Thalamus ⟶	Midbrain ⟶	Medulla*
Consciousness	Confusion; stupor	Coma	
Respirations	Sighs; Cheyne-Stokes type	Central neurogenic hyperventilation	Gasping; absent
Pupils	Small, reactive	3–5 mm, fixed	
Extraocular movements	Roving; uninhibited	Incomplete, dysconjugate	Absent
Motor response	Spastic; decorticate	Decerebrate	Flaccid

* Uncal herniation with unilateral oculomotor nerve palsy and/or hemiplegia is another sign of severe increased ICP.

Table 18–8. Effect of Coma-Producing Toxins on Pupillary Size

Pupils Small
Narcotics (except meperidine)
Sedatives
   Barbiturates
   Alcohol
Major tranquilizers
Phenothiazines
Cholinergic agonists
   Organophosphate insecticides
   Nicotine
   Certain plants and mushrooms

Pupils Large
Anticholinergics
   Antihistamines
   Tricyclic antidepressants
   Phenothiazines
Glutethimide

Pupils Normal
Salicylates
Acetaminophen

duces an easily recognizable clinical picture consisting of pernicious vomiting, lethargy accompanied by belligerence, hyperventilation, and large pupils.

Systemic acidosis and alkalosis do not significantly depress consciousness but are characteristic features of a number of diseases that produce encephalopathy. Consciousness often is reduced in patients with diabetic ketoacidosis, but the severity of unresponsiveness correlates with the degree of hyperosmolarity, not with the degree of acidosis. Proper treatment results in rapid return of full consciousness (see Chapter 17). Rare diabetic patients will lapse into stupor hours after treatment is begun because of the development of brain swelling and central herniation; mortality is high. Medical therapy to reduce cerebral swelling may be very effective if instituted when consciousness first wanes (see Chapter 3).

The *common drugs and toxins* that cause stupor and coma and their effects on pupillary size are listed in Table 18–8. Delirium can be produced by amphetamines, cocaine, psychedelics, anticholinergics, and withdrawal from alcohol or barbiturates. The clinical profile of depressant drug overdose consists of lethargy, ataxia, dysarthria, and nystagmus, followed by coma in a flaccid state, with diminished stretch reflexes, incomplete extraocular muscle responses, and small reactive pupils.

Cerebrospinal Fluid Abnormalities. Red blood cells in the cerebrospinal fluid (CSF) indicate primary subarachnoid hemorrhage or parenchymal hemorrhage that has ruptured into the CSF. The former usually is caused by rupture of a **saccular "berry" aneurysm** of one of the major cerebral arteries in the circle of Willis. These aneurysms are presumed to result from localized developmental defects in the arterial walls. Rupture is rare in childhood, but the usual manifestations are the sudden onset of intense headache followed by collapse and loss of consciousness. Focal neurologic deficits are variable, but nuchal rigidity almost invariably is present. Retinal or subhyloid hemorrhages are common. The patient is treated in an ICU with bed rest, sedation, and therapy to eliminate vascular spasm until surgical approach to the aneurysm is feasible.

Spontaneous parenchymal hemorrhages in children are usually caused by **arteriovenous malformations** (AVMs). These are developmental anomalies consisting of tangled or dilated vessels that form a communication between the arterial and venous systems. The entire complex may enlarge slowly with age. Clinical presentation most commonly occurs between 10 and 40 yr of age with intraparenchymal and subarachnoid hemorrhages, seizures, headaches, or slowly progressive neurologic deficits. The rare AVM that produces a very enlarged "vein of Galen aneurysm" can cause heart failure in infancy as a result of large-volume blood flow through the shunt. In early childhood, these AVMs also can cause hydrocephalus as a result of compression of the aqueduct by the enlarged vein of Galen. A loud cranial bruit, if present, suggests an AVM. Management of AVMs consists of performing surgical ligation of the entire lesion, if possible. Intravascular resins or embolization with particulate matter also has been utilized to halt flow.

Other etiologies of parenchymal hemorrhages include cerebral trauma, disorders of hemostasis, hypertension, tumors, or hemorrhagic infarctions.

White blood cells in the CSF usually denote infectious meningitis or meningoencephalitis but also may be associated with subacute bacterial endocarditis, vasculitis, carcinomatous meningitis, or a parainfectious syndrome.

Parainfectious syndromes closely resemble episodes of viral meningoencephalitis but are the consequence of acute multifocal, immunologically mediated demyelination rather than of direct viral invasion of the brain. Fever, stiff neck, depression of consciousness, and focal neurologic deficits occur a few days following a benign systemic viral syndrome. The course is variable, but most children recover without sequelae within a few days to weeks. Systemic viral infection appears to trigger the syndrome by an unknown mechanism. These syndromes were first described following measles, mumps, rubella, and chickenpox and also after vaccination against smallpox and rabies.

CT Abnormalities. Cerebral CT of a child with an acute consciousness disorder may disclose either a space-occupying or a destructive lesion. To depress consciousness, unilateral cerebral lesions must either directly compress and distort the diencephalon and brain stem, increase intracranial pressure by their bulk and associated edema, or block CSF pathways and produce hydrocephalus with increased ICP. Focal midbrain and diencephalic lesions that impair the RAS also can depress consciousness. Space-occupying lesions include tumors, abscesses, hemorrhages, cysts, and inflammatory masses.

Destructive lesions include infarcts and demyelinating plaques. When visible by CT, both appear as low-density areas but the latter are confined to the white matter. Cerebral infarctions can impair consciousness when the lesions are global, multifocal, located in the midbrain, or unilateral and large. The latter create brain swelling and elevations of ICP, which then depress consciousness. Hypoxic–ischemic injury is the major cause of infarcts in children. Cerebral MRI provides a clearer image of both small infarctions and small demyelinating plaques than does CT. The major diseases that produce demyelinative plaques are multiple sclerosis and parainfectious syndromes. The former chronic condition rarely presents in an acute disseminated manner to produce coma. Parainfectious syndromes, in contrast, occur acutely and frequently give rise to multifocal lesions that impair consciousness.

Hypoxic–ischemic Injury (see also Chapter 6). Deprivation of oxygen to the brain, caused by either deficient oxygen in the blood (hypoxemia) or deficient delivery of blood to the brain (ischemia), impairs consciousness (Table 18–9). Severe ischemia will produce loss of consciousness within seconds and permanent brain damage within a few minutes. Sometimes progressive deterioration in functioning takes place for several hours after a severe hypoxic–ischemic insult. Some irreversibly damaged cells may continue to function for a brief period of time and then die. Release of metabolites from dead and dying cells may initiate a chemical cascade leading to loss of membrane stability in adjacent cells, intracellular influx of calcium ions, and cell death. In addition, the initial injury may be compounded by the development of circulatory failure from anoxic cardiac injury, disseminated intravascular coagulation or cerebral edema.

Rarely, patients undergo delayed *postanoxic encephalopathy*, which becomes manifest by an initial hypoxic–ischemic event that causes stupor or coma. The patients awaken in 24–48 hr, but several days to weeks later become irritable, apathetic, and confused, and then develop a spastic quadriplegia accompanied by pseudobulbar palsy. Pathologic and radiologic studies reveal severe bilateral leukoencephalopathy. The pathogenesis is unknown. Patients may die, recover completely, or remain in a spastic state.

The *prognosis* of cerebral hypoxic–ischemic injury is extremely variable in children. In general, short duration of coma (hours to 1–2 days) and presence of intact brain stem function on admission to the hospital imply a good prognosis. The most common permanent neurologic sequelae are ataxia, choreoathetosis, parkinsonian syndrome, intention or action myoclonus, memory loss, visual agnosia, and impairments of learning and attention. Improvement can occur for several months to 1 yr following the insult. *Treatment* involves physical therapy, occupational therapy, rehabilitative services, and education.

Occult Etiologies. Some causes of coma remain unclear after the entire diagnostic work-up is completed. The most common occult etiologies are drug or toxin exposure, cranial trauma, seizures, and hypoxic–ischemic injury. Sometimes a diagnosis is verified only as the natural history of the illness unfolds and the results of repeated examinations and testing are known.

Table 18–9. Causes of Hypoxia and Ischemia

Hypoxemia
PO_2 decreased
  Pulmonary disease
  Cardiac disease; right-to-left shunt
  Hypoventilation
    Exogenous (e.g., drowning, choking, suffocation)
    Neuromuscular disease
    Central respiratory drive decreased
PO_2 normal; decreased O_2 content
  Severe anemia
  Carbon monoxide poisoning
  Methemoglobinemia

Ischemia
Cardiac disease (decreased cardiac output)
  Myocardial infarction
  Arrhythmia
  Valvular disease
  Pericarditis
Pulmonary embolism
Hypotension, shock
Hanging, strangulation
Extensive cerebrovascular disease

Table 18–10. Guidelines for Determination of Brain Death*

No spontaneous movements, communication, or interaction with the environment

No superspinal response to externally applied stimuli (pain, touch, light, sound)

Absence of brain stem reflexes (including pupillary light, oculocephalic, oculovestibular, corneal, oropharyngeal–gag, and tracheal–cough)

Apnea

Electrocerebral silence on an EEG

* All of the criteria listed should be present on multiple examinations at least 6–24 hr after the onset of coma and apnea. There must be documented absence of drug intoxication (including sedatives and neuromuscular blocking agents), hypothermia, and cardiovascular shock. A cause of coma sufficient to account for the loss of brain function should be established.

Prognosis. The outcome of coma relates to many variables, including the etiology (intoxication has a good prognosis, hypoxia has a bad prognosis), the duration of coma, the age (children have a better outcome than adults), and the Glasgow coma score on admission. Complete recovery from traumatic coma of several days' duration is possible in children. Long-term outcomes of survivors of severe coma include persistent vegetative state and serious neuropsychiatric disability.

Brain Death. Death of the whole brain (cortex and brain stem) generally is accepted as death of the person. Brain death means irreversible cessation of all functions. Table 18–10 lists the usual guidelines. In addition, total absence of cerebral blood flow on four-vessel intracranial angiography is definitive confirmation of brain death. Application of the criteria of brain death can be very difficult, particularly in newborns.

Transient Recurrent Depression of Consciousness

Seizures may cause transient recurrent depression of consciousness.

Basilar artery migraine attacks last hours and may consist of confusion accompanied by agitation, ataxia, cortical blindness, vertigo, or cranial nerve palsies; headache may precede or follow the neurologic signs. Ischemia of the tissues supplied by the basilar artery also can produce amnesia and, infrequently, total loss of consciousness.

Cardiac arrhythmias or an obstructive cardiomyopathy (e.g., septal hypertrophy, left atrial myxoma, critical aortic stenosis) can cause recurrent episodes of syncope. Children with syncope require a cardiac examination, an electrocardiogram, and a tilt test.

Hypoglycemia can give rise to recurrent episodes of lethargy, confusion, seizures, or coma. Attacks often are heralded by anxiety, excess sweating, tremulousness, and hunger. A typical spell usually can be aborted by feeding the child orange juice or other sugar-containing solutions.

Several metabolic disorders cause recurrent bouts of hyperammonemia (see Table 18–4). Symptoms include nausea, vomiting, lethargy, confusion, ataxia, hyperventilation, and coma. Unlike episodes of hypoglycemia, which evolve over minutes, these spells worsen over hours. They often are precipitated by high-protein dietary intake or systemic viral infections. Early intravenous therapy is required to prevent permanent brain damage or death.

References

Bannister R: Brain's Clinical Neurology. 6th ed. Cambridge, England, Oxford University Press, 1985.

Behrman RE (ed): Nelson Textbook of Pediatrics. 14th ed. Philadelphia, WB Saunders, 1992, Sec. 2.6, 3.59, 6.33–6.35, 20.55–20.56.

Levy D, Bates D, Caronna J: Prognosis in nontraumatic coma. Ann Intern Med 94:293, 1981.

Plum F, Posner JB: The Diagnosis of Stupor and Coma. Philadelphia, FA Davis, 1980.

Task Force for the Determination of Brain Death in Children: Guidelines for the determination of brain death in children. Ann Neurol 21:616, 1987.

CRANIOCEREBRAL TRAUMA

Children with head trauma either may have depression of consciousness and neurologic deficits or may be alert without neurologic deficits. The former require neurosurgical management, and the latter requires neurologic observation. Most serious trauma results from motor vehicle accidents, sports, recreation-related injuries, and violence.

Patients with Neurologic Deficits

Patients in this category may have awakened following the injury (lucid interval) and then relapsed into coma or may have remained abnormal from the time of injury. Some patients are stable; others progressively deteriorate, develop acute irreversible loss of brain function, and require immediate neurosurgical care. The circulation must be supported, bleeding controlled, all systemic problems identified, proper IV fluids maintained, the neck

Table 18–11. Syndromes of Post-traumatic Intracranial Hemorrhage

Syndrome	Clinical and Radiologic Characteristics	Treatment
Epidural	Onset over minutes to hours Uncal herniation with IIIrd nerve palsy and contralateral hemiparesis Lens-shaped extracerebral hemorrhage compressing brain	Surgical evacuation or observation Prognosis good
Acute subdural	Onset over hours Uncal herniation Focal neurologic deficits Crescentic extracranial hemorrhage compressing brain	Surgical evacuation Prognosis guarded
Chronic subdural	Onset over weeks to months Anemia, macrocephaly Seizures, vomiting Crescentric low-density mass on CT	Subdural taps as necessary Prognosis good
Intraparenchymal	Depressed consciousness Focal neurologic deficits Additional multiple contusions	Supportive care Prognosis guarded
Subarachnoid	Stiff neck Late hydrocephalus	Supportive care Prognosis variable
Contusion	Focal neurologic deficits Brain swelling with transtentorial herniation CT: Mutifocal low-density areas with punctate hemorrages	Medical treatment of elevated intracranial pressure Prognosis guarded

carefully immobilized in a neutral position, and the cerebral lesions managed immediately. A baseline neurologic evaluation should be followed by intubation, ventilation if indicated, and pharmacologic paralysis or sedation. If consciousness and the neurologic deficits are stable, other life-threatening problems (e.g., an acute abdomen) may take precedence over immediate neurosurgical evaluation or treatment. Skull and cervical spine roentgenograms and cranial CT are obtained as soon as possible. Syndromes of post-traumatic hemorrhage are summarized in Table 18–11).

If surgery is not required, children should be taken to an intensive care unit and followed (see Chapter 3). If the child's neurologic condition worsens or the child already is comatose, ICP monitoring may be indicated.

Children with cerebral contusion who survive the acute cerebral swelling may improve rapidly or slowly, or remain vegetative. Those who show daily improvement starting within days of the injury usually will recover completely. Maximal recovery may take weeks, months, or even a year in some patients. Caution must be used in providing families with a prognosis. Coma lasting for weeks following head trauma still is compatible with an ultimately good outcome, although the risk of late sequelae is increased. Patients who remain in a vegetative state for months following head injury without any clear evidence of improvement are unlikely to improve.

Awake, Alert Children without Neurologic Deficits Who Have Headaches, Sleepiness, or Vomiting

Although the vast majority of children in this category will recover fully and uneventfully, a few develop early or late complications that must be recognized and treated.

CONCUSSION

Concussion is a brief (lasting seconds or minutes) period of unconsciousness occurring immediately after head trauma, followed by normal arousal. Retrograde and antegrade amnesia often follow concussion. *Retrograde amnesia* is the inability to remember events immediately prior to the trauma and may extend backward in time for minutes, hours, days, or weeks. Usually, retrograde memory gradually is regained and permanent amnesia is only for the few minutes immediately prior to the blow. *Antegrade amnesia* is the inability to form new memories and becomes manifest by the patient incessantly repeating the same questions shortly after they have been answered (e.g., "Where am I?," "Why am I here?"). This state often persists for hours. The period of amnesia, both retrograde and antegrade, usually correlates with the severity of the trauma.

The pathophysiology of concussion is thought to be a shearing lesion of white matter as the brain is shaken within the cranium, resulting in a temporary failure of axon conduction. If loss of consciousness is maintained for longer than an hour or if recovery of consciousness is slow and accompanied by focal neurologic deficits, the pathophysiology is likely to include contusion and laceration, which may lead to focal or generalized *brain swelling*.

HEMORRHAGE

See Table 18–11.

MALIGNANT POST-TRAUMATIC CEREBRAL SWELLING

Occasionally, epidural hemorrhage, other intracranial hemorrhage, or a rapid life-threatening increase in ICP develops unexpectedly in children who appear stable for hours following head trauma. Diagnosis and management proceed as detailed in Table 18–11; a significant number of epidural hemorrhages can be observed and treated supportively.

SYNCOPE

Some patients faint a few minutes after head trauma or on awakening from their initial concussion. These patients complain of "dizzy" lightheadedness and loss of vision and slowly slump to the ground in a sleep-like state. Spontaneous arousal to full orientation occurs within a couple of minutes. Presumably, the psychic trauma produces a vagal discharge resulting in bradycardia and hypotension. Treatment consists of maintaining the recumbent position until the patient is fully aroused, well perfused, and reassured that all is well.

TRANSIENT NEUROLOGIC DISTURBANCE

These conditions sometimes develop in a few minutes following minor or severe head trauma and last for minutes to hours before clearing. The most common symptoms are occipital blindness and a confusional state, but hemiparesis, ataxia, or any other neurologic deficit may appear. These symptoms may represent migraine precipitated by trauma in susceptible children.

POST-TRAUMATIC SEIZURES

See Seizure Disorders.

DROWSINESS, HEADACHE, AND VOMITING

These manifestations are common following head trauma and are not by themselves of concern if consciousness is preserved and the neurologic examination is normal. Children are especially susceptible to severe sleepiness following head trauma but should be easily arousable to alert wakefulness. If these symptoms persist unabated for more than 1–2 days, CT or MRI is indicated.

SKULL FRACTURES

These fractures may be linear, diastatic (spreading the suture), depressed (an edge displaced inferiorly), or compound (bone fragments breaking the skin surface). Compound fractures or penetrating injuries require surgical débridement but not prophylactic antibiotic therapy. Tetanus prophylaxis must be assured. The risk of local brain contusion and early seizures is high. Linear and diastatic fractures require no treatment but indicate severe trauma capable of producing an underlying hematoma. Small depressed fractures have the same significance as linear fractures, but if the depression is more than 0.5–1 cm, surgical elevation of bone fragments and repair of associated dural tears is recommended. Clinical indicators of skull fracture include localized bogginess and pain; subcutaneous bleeding over the mastoid process (*Battle sign*) or around the orbit (*raccoon eyes*); blood behind the tympanic membrane (*hemotympanum*); or CSF leak from nose (*rhinorrhea*) or ear (*otorrhea*). Rarely, following linear skull fractures, a soft pulsatile scalp mass is palpable within a few weeks to months. Radiographically, the fracture edges are separated by a soft tissue mass that consists of fibrotic and accumulated brain and meningeal tissue and perhaps a leptomeningeal cyst. Surgical excision of abnormal tissue and dural repair is recommended.

CEREBROSPINAL FLUID LEAK

This condition occurs when a skull fracture tears adjacent dura, creating communications between the subarachnoid space and the nose, paranasal sinuses, mastoid air cells, or middle or external ear. Clear fluid leaking from the nose or ear following head trauma is presumed to be CSF. The presence of air within the subdural, subarachnoid, or ventricular space also indicates a dural tear and open communication between the nose or paranasal sinuses and brain. In most cases the dura heals spontaneously when the patient's head is kept elevated. If the leak persists or recurs, or if meningitis supervenes, the fracture site is identified and the dura surgically repaired.

CRANIAL NERVE PALSIES

Palsies following laceration or contusion from skull fracture may be transitory or permanent. Longitudinal fractures of the petrous bone produce conductive hearing loss and facial palsy, which begins hours after the injury and usually resolves spontaneously. Transverse petrous fractures produce sensorineural hearing loss and immediate facial palsy, with a poor prognosis for spontaneous recovery. Disruption of the ossicular chain is a cause of hearing loss and can be cured with proper surgery. Permanent loss of olfaction following head injury is due to a vibrational rupture of the thin olfactory nerves within the cribriform plate. Disruption of cranial nerve III, IV, or VI produces ophthalmoplegia, diplopia, and head tilt.

CERVICAL SPINE INJURIES

These injuries should be suspected in any unconscious child, especially if bruises are present on the back. In conscious children, findings of neck or back pain, burning or stabbing pains radiating to the arms, paraplegia, or asymmetric motor or sensory responses of arms or legs are indications of spinal cord injury. Cervical spine injury also may result in complete transection with spinal shock, loss of sensation, and flaccid paralysis. A contused cord may be exhibited in a similar manner, but complete recovery occurs by 24 hr. Any patient with a clinical or radiologic abnormality of the spine requires immediate stabilization and neurosurgical consultation.

SUBDURAL FLUID

The presence of subdural fluid can be caused either by active accumulation of fluid or by atrophy of adjacent brain tissue. The former process usually begins with a subdural hemorrhage. Vascular membranes arising from dura surround the hemorrhage and leakage of proteinaceous exudate or small hemorrhages from these membranes may enlarge the subdural collection. Symptoms consist of slowly evolving focal neurologic deficits, focal seizures, or evidence of raised ICP. Treatment may

require repeated subdural taps or a subdural-peritoneal shunt.

POST–HEAD TRAUMA SYNDROME

Some children experiencing uncomplicated concussion will complain for days or weeks of headaches, dizziness, forgetfulness, inability to concentrate, slowing of response time, mood swings, irritability, and other subtle aberrations of cerebral function. These deficits almost always resolve spontaneously. Children may require brief periods of special schooling, home tutoring, and reassurance. Persistent severe headaches often respond to prophylactic therapy with propranolol, 1 mg/kg/day.

Management

Children who have been unconscious from a head injury or who have amnesia after the event, even if loss of consciousness is not documented, should be observed in an emergency room for several hours following the injury, even if they initially appear to be entirely well. High-risk patients include those with persistent depressed level of consciousness, focal neurologic signs, decreasing level of consciousness, and penetrating skull injury or depressed skull fractures. These patients warrant CT or MRI examination.

The period of observation should increase with the severity of the injury, and there should be no hesitation to admit children without neurologic deficits to the hospital for observation for 1–2 days. If the child appears well after several hours and is discharged home, parents should be instructed to call their physician for any change in alertness, orientation, or neurologic functioning, or increase in headache or vomiting. They should be taught how to test consciousness, orientation, extraocular motions, pupillary reactions, and gait and told to check these functions every 2–4 hr for 1 day following the injury. If conditions at home preclude this type of detailed observation, the child should be admitted to the hospital.

Damage to the brain from the trauma occurs immediately and is not treatable. The goal is to prevent secondary brain injury from hemorrhage, cerebral edema, and hypoxia–ischemia.

Prognosis

Children suffering from concussion without subsequent neurologic deficits do well; late sequelae are rare. Children with contusions are likely to make surprisingly good recoveries, even in the face of relatively persistent neurologic signs that continue for weeks; subtle deficits may persist. Poor memory and slowing of motor skills are most common, but a generalized decrease in cognitive skills, behavioral alterations, and attention deficits also occurs. Language function, especially in the young child, frequently makes a good recovery. Rehabilitation consists of physical therapy, behavior management, and appropriate education. *Poor prognostic features* include a Glasgow coma score of 3–4 on admission without improvement in 24 hr, absent pupillary light reflexes, and persistent plantar reflex. Extracranial trauma also contributes to the morbidity of these patients (e.g., adult respiratory distress syndrome, sepsis, emboli).

References

Behrman RE (ed): Nelson Textbook of Pediatrics. 14th ed. Philadelphia, WB Saunders, 1992, Sec. 6.32–6.33, 20.57, 20.77.

Duhaime AC, Alario AJ, Lewander WJ, et al: Head injury in very young children: Mechanisms, injury types, and ophthalmologic findings in 100 hospitalized patients younger than 2 years of age. Pediatrics 90:179, 1992.

Harris JH Jr, Edeiken-Monroe B, Kopaniky DR: A practical classification of acute cervical spine injuries. Orthop Clin North Am 17:15, 1986.

Lieh-Lai MW, Theodorou AA, Sarnaik AP, et al: Limitations of the Glasgow Coma Scale in predicting outcome in children with traumatic brain injury. J Pediatr 120:195, 1992.

White RJ, Likavec MJ: The diagnosis and initial management of head injury. N Engl J Med 327:1507, 1992.

INCREASED INTRACRANIAL PRESSURE

Normal ICP measurements vary depending on the site of determination and the position of the child. In the lateral recumbent position, ICP should be below 170 mm of CSF and is equal in the ventricle, cisterna magna, and lumbar subarachnoid space. Lumbar subarachnoid pressure rises and ventricle pressure falls in the sitting position, and the opposite occurs in the head-down position.

The diagnosis and treatment of the child with increased ICP is a medical emergency. Treatment should be initiated before ICP rises to a level that significantly compromises *cerebral perfusion pressure* (CPP). CPP equals the mean arterial blood pressure minus the ICP. Increased ICP also may result in movement of the brain from normal compartments of the skull across dural structures that divide these compartments (*herniation*). The direction of herniation is dictated by movements from regions of high pressure to regions of lower pressure. Herniation distorts the cortex and brain stem and their vascular supply, resulting in injury and, if not reversed, death.

In infancy, partial compensation for raised ICP is accomplished by spreading the cranial sutures and distending the anterior fontanel. Suture diastasis also may occur in chronically increased ICP and may be detected as late as 10 yr of age. After the sutures close, the intracranial volume is constant, consisting of the volume of the brain tissue, CSF, and blood. Any normal or abnormal (e.g., brain tumor, extravascular blood, inflammation) increase in one component is accompanied by a simultaneous decrease in one or more of the other components. Normally, the brain accounts for 80–85% of the volume, CSF 10–15%, and blood 5–10%. CSF is displaced readily from the intracranial compartment to the lumbar subarachnoid space and is the first mechanism of normalizing ICP when acute increases occur. Pathologic processes that block the flow of CSF deprive the patient of this compensatory maneuver.

Clinical Manifestations. The clinical presentation of increased ICP varies with age (Table 18–12). Hypertension, bradycardia, and irregular respirations (Cushing triad) also signify increased ICP. The abducens nerve (cranial nerve VI) has the longest intracranial course and is most susceptible to increased ICP. Therefore, VIth nerve paresis is a false localizing sign when ICP is elevated. Swelling of the optic nerve head (**papilledema**) is one of the most reliable signs of increased ICP. It frequently

Table 18–12. Frequent Signs and Symptoms of Increased Intracranial Pressure

Infants	Older Children
Symptoms	
Irritability	Irritability
Lethargy	Lethargy
Vomiting (initially, in the morning)	Vomiting (initially morning)
	Headache
	Visual obscurations
	Diplopia
Signs	
Tense or bulging fontanel	Papilledema
Distended scalp veins	VIth nerve paralysis
Head enlargement	Altered mental status
VIth nerve paralysis	Signs of herniation
Altered mental status	
Signs of herniation	

Table 18–13. Herniation Syndromes

Location	Description	Clinical Findings
Transtentorial		
Central	Caudal displacement of cerebral hemispheres, resulting in downward displacement of diencephalon and midbrain	Altered mental status Cheyne-Stokes to central neurogenic hyperventilation Decorticate to decerebrate posturing Loss of oculovestibular reflexes Death
Uncal	Temporal lobe displacement into the tentorial opening Third nerve, posterior cerebral artery, and midbrain compression	Unilateral pupillary dilation followed by oculomotor paralysis Hemiplegia Death
Cerebellar		
Downward	Cerebellar tonsils displaced through the foramen magnum Compression of medulla, posterior inferior cerebellar artery	Neck stiffness Respiratory, cardiac arrest Lower cranial nerve dysfunction Death
Upward	Cerebellar tissue displaced through tentorial opening Compression of midbrain and superior cerebellar arteries	Paralysis of upgaze Pupillary dilation Central hyperventilation Death
Transfalcial		
(cingulate)	Unilateral cerebral lesions result in displacement of the cingulate gyrus beneath the falx cerebri, compromising the gyrus and the callosal pericallosal arteries	Cingulate gyrus necrosis and ischemia lead to edema and central transtentorial herniation

is absent in infants, but its absence at any age does not exclude the diagnosis of ICP. Swelling of the optic nerve head also may be due to processes other than elevated ICP (e.g., papillitis, optic neuropathy).

Herniation of brain tissue from one compartment of the skull to another is a common cause of death in elevated ICP. Herniation of cerebral or cerebellar tissue results in necrosis of the herniated tissue and compression of vital CNS structures. The common herniation syndromes and their clinical characteristics are noted in Table 18–13 (see also Table 18–7).

Etiology. The most common causes of raised ICP in childhood are cerebral edema, hydrocephalus, pseudotumor cerebri, trauma, infection, and tumors.

Cerebral edema is the abnormal accumulation of fluid within brain tissue, resulting in volumetric expansion. Edema is of two varieties, vasogenic and cytotoxic. *Vasogenic edema* is due to alterations in the vasculature resulting in increased vessel permeability and fluid escape (e.g., edema surrounding tumors, abscesses, hematomas, or infarcts). *Cytotoxic edema* is due to abnormal cellular function resulting in fluid accumulation, which is primarily intracellular (e.g., edema seen in anoxia, water intoxication, encephalitis, and Reye syndrome). Cytotoxic edema does not respond to steroids but does respond to osmotic agents, whereas the vasogenic edema responds to both.

The common causes of cerebral edema in childhood are listed in Table 18–14. Anoxic cerebral

Table 18–14. Common Causes of Cerebral Edema in Childhood

Vasogenic Edema	Cytotoxic Edema
Tumor	Anoxia
Abscess	Heavy metal poisoning (Pb, Hg, As)
Hemorrhage	
Infarct	Infection: bacterial and viral meningoencephalitis
Infection: bacterial and viral meningoencephalitis	Pseudotumor cerebri
	Metabolic disorders
	Methylmalonicacidemia
	Propionicacidemia
	Acyl-coenzyme A dehydrogenase deficiency
	Urea cycle deficiency
	Reye syndrome
	Hepatic coma
	Hypertensive encephalopathy

Table 18–15. Abnormalities Associated with Pseudotumor Cerebri

Endocrine Considerations	Medication Related
Obesity	Vitamin A excess
Menarche	Vitamin A
Addison disease	deficiency
Adrenal hyperplasia	Tetracycline
Pregnancy	(infancy)
Hypoparathyroidism	Steroid therapy
Catch-up growth following	(usually during
malnutrition	tapering of
	therapy)
Other Disorders	Nalidixic acid
Iron-deficiency anemia	Oral contraceptives
Galactosemia	
Polycythemia	
Middle ear disease	

edema is seen following neonatal asphyxia and asphyxia with smoke inhalation, near-drowning, and cardiac arrest. Infectious processes can produce a combination of vasogenic and cytotoxic cerebral edema. In brain abscess, the degree of surrounding edema usually is severe. The degree of edema in viral meningoencephalitis is variable. In enteroviral infection and mumps, it usually is mild, but, with herpes simplex meningoencephalitis, edema frequently is severe and may lead to herniation.

Pseudotumor cerebri (benign intracranial hypertension) is a disorder characterized by markedly elevated ICP without focal neurologic signs or altered mental status. The underlying pathogenesis and the degree to which cerebral edema and/or subarachnoid fluid accumulation is responsible for the process are unknown. Benign intracranial hypertension is associated with a variety of conditions, among which endocrine abnormalities are prominent (Table 18–15). Loss of vision as a result of papilledema may develop.

Tumors of the brain are a common cause of raised ICP (see Chapter 15).

Diagnosis of Increased ICP. Symptoms of brief duration associated with an altered state of consciousness are ominous. Fever suggests an infectious process. The risk associated with *lumbar puncture* must be weighed against the benefits of obtaining CSF from the lumbar region. Herniation of tissue will occur during lumbar puncture if obstruction of flow within the CSF pathways exists and if the flow of CSF through the lumbar puncture needle and/or subarachnoid space is faster than at any level in the subarachnoid pathways. If meningitis is suspected, but signs of increased ICP are present (other than a bulging fontanel), alternative

sources of isolating organisms should be sought. Institution of broad-spectrum antibiotics and therapy for elevated ICP before lumbar puncture should be considered, as well as the safety and feasibility of obtaining ventricular fluid. Lumbar puncture is contraindicated in patients with brain abscess. *CT scan and MRI* studies are indicated to assess the degree of cerebral edema present.

Laboratory studies of blood and urine are essential in establishing toxic causes of cerebral edema. Blood ammonia is elevated and partial thromboplastin and prothrombin times are prolonged in Reye syndrome. Urine samples for amino and organic acids establish the diagnosis of brain edema secondary to propionicaciduria and methylmalonicaciduria as well as to acyl-coenzyme A dehydrogenase deficiency and to certain amino acidopathies. A measurement of blood ammonia and plasma amino acids will elucidate disorders of the urea cycle. The EEG usually is diffusely slow in toxic and metabolic cerebral edema irrespective of cause.

Treatment. The management of any child with increased ICP should encompass basic mechanisms by which ICP is increased. Hypoxia and hypercapnia increase brain blood flow, brain blood volume, and, thus, ICP. Protection of the airway and proper ventilation is therefore essential. *Hyperventilation* is an effective measure to reduce ICP acutely. The patient should be placed in the head-up position flexed approximately 45 degrees at the waist; constriction of the neck should be avoided to facilitate venous return from the brain. Screaming, thrashing, and seizure activity aggravate increased ICP.

The advantage of *ICP monitoring* is that it provides continuous objective information as a basis for adjusting therapy. The disadvantage is that, in the encephalopathic patient, neuromuscular paralysis must be used to obtain satisfactory ICP monitoring and most of the signs and symptoms that must be observed in the neurologic examination are therefore lost. ICP monitoring can be performed by either intraventricular, subarachnoid, epidural, or intraparenchymal routes, and, in neonates, measurements can be obtained from the anterior fontanel (see Chapters 3 and 6).

Systemic hypotension resulting from *intravascular volume depletion*, phenobarbital induced myocardial depression, or low peripheral vasomotor tone should be corrected with either crystalloid volume expansion or dopamine to improve CPP. Fluid overload contributes to cerebral edema and should be avoided. Vasodilator therapy should be avoided or used very cautiously in the treatment of systemic hypertension because decreases in mean arterial pressure without concomitant decreases in ICP jeopardize cerebral perfusion. Fluid and electrolyte management should limit the availability of free water, which diffuses rapidly to the brain, adding to cerebral edema. Deficient antidiuretic hormone (ADH) may follow injuries to the hypothalamus or the pituitary tract. Inappropriate ADH secretion may occur in tumor, infection, or trauma or, initially, following neurosurgical procedures. Fluid restriction for inappropriate ADH secretion, and vasopressin therapy in diabetes insipidus, may be indicated.

Control of Intracranial Volume. Normalization of ICP is attempted by correcting the volume–pressure relationships within the cranial cavity. This may be accomplished by hyperventilation; the administration of steroids, osmolar and loop diuretics; removal of CSF; and giving agents to decrease CSF production.

CSF production may be transiently decreased by administering dexamethasone or acetazolamide. Steroids decrease CSF production by inhibiting the sodium-potassium pump–activated ATP pathways in the choroid plexus, whereas acetazolamide decreases production by inhibiting carbonic anhydrase. In the presence of hydrocephalus or a tumor, a direct surgical approach is appropriate. Steroid therapy is appropriate as an initial measure to reduce peritumor edema.

Osmotic therapy requires an intact blood–brain barrier. The administration of an osmotic agent results in free water shifts from brain to the intravascular space. Subsequent renal clearance of free water from the general circulation results in clinically significant reduction of brain edema. Clearance of the osmotic agent from the circulation may result in reversal of the osmotic gradient and rebound intracranial hypertension, especially if a significant leak of the osmotic agent into the extracellular space of the brain has occurred. Mannitol (0.25–1.0 g/kg infused over 10–30 min) is the most commonly employed osmotic agent. Glycerol has the advantages of being effective by the oral route, being metabolized by the liver, and not requiring renal function for elimination. However, it may produce intravascular hemolysis.

Serum osmolality should be kept below 320 mOsm/L. Levels of 350 mOsm/L may result in progressive renal failure and osmolality over 375 mOsm/L may result in intracellular dehydration severe enough to produce systemic acidosis. Chronic serum hyperosmolality also may result in neuronal production of intracellular fixed osmoles, which lead to the development of neuronal swelling and damage.

The *treatment of pseudotumor cerebri* includes steroids, repeated lumbar punctures, or, if severe, shunting of CSF.

References

Behrman RE (ed): Nelson Textbook of Pediatrics. 14th ed. Philadelphia, WB Saunders, 1992, Sec. 6.34–6.35, 9.23, 20.55, 20.57.

Miller D: Intracranial pressure monitoring. Arch Neurol 42: 1191, 1986.

Schulte FJ: Intracranial tumors in childhood: Concepts of treatment and prognosis. Neuropediatrics 15:3, 1984.

HEADACHES AND MIGRAINE

The evaluation of children with *headaches* is straightforward. If the neurologic examination reveals any abnormalities, cranial CT or MRI is obtained. If neurologic and general physical examinations are negative, the likely diagnoses are either migraine or tension headaches. Most headaches are of extracerebral origin and are due to dilation of extracranial vessels (vascular headache) or to contraction of the scalp or neck muscles (tension headache).

Any *space-occupying lesion* within the cranium can cause headache, either by pressure (inflammation, stretching, distortion) on adjacent pain-sensitive structures or by obstruction of CSF circulation and the production of hydrocephalus. Lesions within the posterior fossa usually produce occipital pain, whereas supratentorial lesions produce frontal, temporal, or vertex pain. *Hydrocephalus* usually causes early morning frontal headache that may awaken the child, and often is associated with vomiting with or without nausea. *Aneurysms* almost always appear as an acute subarachnoid hemorrhage and are characterized by severe headache, change in consciousness, and stiff neck. *Pseudotumor cerebri* presents with severe daily headaches, as well as with signs of raised ICP.

Acute headache also may be caused by hypertension (intermittent), trauma, lumbar puncture, fever, and infection. It is a common symptom in meningitis, encephalitis, sinusitis, pharyngitis, and systemic viral illness. Headache also is associated with a variety of disorders involving the eyes, ears, nose, teeth, and neck.

Many patients with headache visit a doctor only

for reassurance that there is no serious underlying disease and thereafter are content to treat the headache symptomatically. An unremarkable history and physical examination is sufficient to provide this reassurance. Sometimes the neurologic examination yields equivocal findings or the history is so compelling for serious intracranial pathology that CT or MRI is required despite a normal examination. Worrisome headaches are those that are most severe on awakening, awaken the patient in the middle of the night, are severely exacerbated by coughing or bending, are acute without a previous history of headache, are present daily and getting progressively more severe in a crescendo pattern, and are accompanied by vomiting with or without nausea.

Migraine and *tension headaches* are the most common chronic recurrent headaches in both children and adults (Table 18–16). Migraine is thought to be due to a hereditary paroxysmal vasoregulatory instability, with release of inflammatory mediators, characterized by a phase of intracerebral arterial constriction followed by a phase of extracranial, and sometimes intracranial, arterial dilation. Migraine frequently begins in childhood; infants and toddlers who are unable to verbalize the source of their discomfort may present with spells of irritability, sleepiness, pallor, and vomiting. Young children with migraine frequently lack many of the typical features. Periodic headaches in children accompanied by nausea or vomiting and relieved by rest are likely to be migraine. Sometimes even the periodic nature of the headache is not appreciated because the children will have frequent mild to moderate headaches between major attacks of severe headaches. The name "common migraine" sometimes is attached to these moderate atypical headaches without other neurologic manifestations or an aura.

There are several migraine syndromes called "complicated migraine" that produce longer lasting neurologic dysfunction than that experienced with the usual aura. The diagnosis is suggested by the distinctive headaches, visual losses, confusion, previous attacks of classic migraine, or strong family history of migraine: structural CNS lesions must be considered. The distinction between complicated migraine and epileptic seizures occasionally is difficult (see later). Hemiplegic migraine is another variant that may rarely produce permanent hemiplegia. *Amaurosis fugax* (acute reversible monocular blindness) is another variant.

Treatments for migraine include prophylactic medications taken daily to reduce the frequency and severity of attacks and symptomatic medications taken during attacks to reduce their intensity and duration (Table 18–17). The first step in migraine prophylaxis is to identify precipitating agents and eliminate as many as possible. Prophylactic medications are utilized when headaches are occurring frequently (more than one per month) and interfering with activities of daily life. Symptomatic therapy requires early administration of analgesic and sedative medication, immediate rest, and sleep in a quiet, dark room. Unfortunately, administration of oral medication often is impossible because of severe nausea and vomiting.

Headache frequently is caused by psychologic stresses and diseases. These *tension headaches* have a different clinical profile than that of migraine (see Table 18–16). These headaches can be acute and related to environmental stresses or can be chronic and a symptom of underlying psychiatric illness, such as anxiety neurosis, hysterical neurosis, or depression. Treatment consists of psychologic support or counseling, biofeedback, mild analgesics, mild tranquilizers, antidepressants, or psychiatric intervention.

Table 18–16. Features of Classic Migraine Versus Tension Headache

Migraine	Tension
Aura	
Flashes of light	
Wavy or zigzag lines	
Enlarging scotoma surrounded by luminous changes	
Unilateral numbness	
Duration of 10–30 min	
Unilateral	Daily
Throbbing	Present all day with worsening in afternoon
Nausea/vomiting	
Photophobia, audiophobia	Moderate band-like or boring pain
Relief by rest	
Periodic attacks (lasting hours)	Multiple somatic complaints (e.g., shortness of breath, abdominal pain, dizziness)
Precipitating factors	
Psychologic stresses	
Lack of food or sleep	
Menses	
Exertion	
Foods or drugs	
Monosodium glutamate	
Cheeses	
Chocolate	
Oral contraceptive pills	
Family history	

Table 18–17. Treatment for Migraine

Nonmedical Treatment	Serotonin Agonists
Eliminate precipitating factors	Sumatriptan
Reassurance	
Biofeedback	
Psychotherapy	
Analgesics	**Prophylactic Agents**
Aspirin	Propranolol
Acetaminophen	Phenytoin
Propoxyphene	Cyproheptadine
Codeine	Methysergide
Oxycodone	
Meperidine	*NSAID*
	Naproxen
Ergotamine (PO, PR, Sublingual, Inhaler, Subcutaneous)	*Calcium Channel Blockers*
	Nimodipine
Minor Tranquilizers	Verapamil
Barbiturates	
Benzodiazepines	*Tricyclic Antidepressants*
Chloral hydrate	Amitriptyline
Hydroxyzine	Imipramine
Major Tranquilizers	**Combinations of Medications**
Nonsteroidal Anti-inflammatory Drugs (NSAIDs)	Aspirin, caffeine, barbiturate
Ibuprofen	Ergotamine, belladonna, barbiturate
Fenoprofen	
Sulindac	

References

Bateman D: Sumatriptan. Lancet 341:221, 1993.

Behrman RE (ed): Nelson Textbook of Pediatrics. 14th ed. Philadelphia, WB Saunders, 1992, Sec. 20.35–20.38.

Rossi L, Cortinouis I, Bellettini G, et al: Diagnostic criteria for migraine and psychogenic headache in children. Devel Med Child Neurol 34:516, 1992.

PAROXYSMAL DISORDERS

Paroxysmal disorders of the nervous system are characterized by the abrupt onset of a clinical episode that tends to be stereotyped and repetitive, lasts seconds to minutes (rarely hours), and ends abruptly. Depending on the etiology of the episode, there may be a warning before or a state of altered awareness afterward, but the child usually recovers quickly. Although seizures are the most commonly encountered paroxysmal disorder, vascular, vestibular, and other causes should be considered. The EEG is of distinct value in distinguishing seizure from nonseizure paroxysmal disorders.

However, on occasion normal children have epileptiform EEG patterns, and children with seizures may have normal interictal EEGs. The differential diagnosis of paroxysmal disorders is listed in Table 18–18.

Seizure Disorders

A classification of individual seizures and some of the more frequently seen epileptic syndromes is presented in Table 18–19. The clinical seizure classification describes individual events, whereas epileptic syndromes consider age of onset, etiology, and association of seizure types.

GENERALIZED TONIC, CLONIC, AND TONIC–CLONIC SEIZURES

These seizures (occurring alone or in combination with other seizure types) are the most common childhood type. Typically, the attack begins abruptly, occasionally preceded by a prodrome of myoclonic jerks. The presence of an aura indicates a focal origin of the attack. Consciousness and control of posture are lost, followed by tonic stiffening and upward deviation of the eyes. Pooling of secretions, pupillary dilation, diaphoresis, hypertension, and piloerection are common. Clonic jerks follow the tonic phase, and then the child is briefly tonic again. Thereafter, the child remains flaccid and urinary incontinence may occur. As the child awakens, irritability and headache are common. Children, particularly young children, often are unaware of an aura or focal onset of their seizure, and caretakers frequently witness only the generalized aspects of the event. During an attack, the EEG demonstrates repetitive synchronous bursts of spike activity followed by periodic paroxysmal discharges. Approximately 10% of children with generalized clonic seizures have abnormalities on brain

Table 18–18. Paroxysmal Disorders of Childhood

Seizure disorders
Syncope
Breath-holding spells
Migraine
Narcolepsy, cataplexy
Apnea
Neonatal clonus
Paroxysmal torticollis
Paroxysmal vertigo (benign)
Paroxysmal dystonia
Paroxysmal choreoathetosis
Night terrors

Table 18–19. Classification of Epileptic Seizures and Some Epileptic Syndromes

Clinical Seizure Types	Epileptic Syndrome
Partial Seizures	Benign focal epilepsy
Simple partial	Juvenile myoclonic
(consciousness not	epilepsy
impaired)	West syndrome
Motor signs	Lennox-Gastaut
Special sensory (visual,	syndrome
auditory, olfactory,	Acquired epileptic
gustatory, vertiginous,	aphasia
or somatosensory)	Benign neonatal
Autonomic	convulsions
Psychic (déjà vu, fear, and	
others)	
Complex partial	
(consciousness impaired)	
Impaired consciousness at	
onset	
Development of impaired	
consciousness	
Generalized Seizures	
Absence	
Typical	
Atypical	
Tonic–clonic	
Atonic	
Myoclonic	
Tonic	
Clonic	
Unclassified	
Neonatal	

imaging; the incidence rises to 25% when only children with an abnormal neurologic examination are considered. *Febrile* and *post-traumatic seizures* fall into the category of primarily generalized tonic–clonic seizures.

Brief seizures of any type are not believed to produce brain damage directly. However, generalized tonic–clonic activity of 30 min or longer is defined as *status epilepticus* and carries inherent risks for brain damage. Although the majority of children with exclusively primary generalized tonic–clonic seizures have idiopathic epilepsy, a significant minority have an identifiable etiology (Table 18–20). Consideration of hypocalcemia frequently is overlooked, and the manifestations of hypoparathyroidism may mimic a degenerative neurologic disease. It is important to distinguish primary generalized tonic and/or clonic seizures from *partial seizures* exhibiting generalized spread. The latter are symptomatic of a focal cerebral lesion.

Treatment is outlined in Table 18–21.

Post-traumatic Seizures

Seizures following head trauma are a common problem. Approximately 5% of children have seizures in the 1st wk following head trauma (early post-traumatic seizures or epilepsy), and another 5% have seizures after the 1st wk (late post-traumatic seizures or epilepsy). The treatment and significance of early seizures are controversial. However, a generalized seizure occurring within seconds of the injury, the so-called *impact seizure*, is benign and not associated with an increased risk of epilepsy.

Early post-traumatic seizures indicate that a severe head injury has occurred; about 25% of these children have underlying skull fractures. Approximately 10% of children with depressed skull fractures and 25% of those with intracranial hematomas have early post-traumatic seizures. If the child has focal neurologic signs following injury, the risk of early post-traumatic seizures is 15%. In children, in contrast to adults, the occurrence of early post-traumatic seizures does not predict the development of late post-traumatic seizures.

Table 18–20. Etiology of Seizures

Perinatal Conditions	**Poisoning**
Cerebral malformation	Lead
Intrauterine infection	Drugs (see Chapter 3)
Hypoxic-ischemic*	Drug withdrawal
Trauma	
Hemorrhage*	**Neurocutaneous**
	Syndromes
Infections	Tuberous sclerosis
Encephalitis*	Neurofibromatosis
Meningitis*	Sturge-Weber syndrome
Brain abscess	Klippel-Trenaunay-
	Weber syndrome
Metabolic Conditions	Linear sebaceous nevus
Hypoglycemia*	Incontinentia pigmenti
Hypocalcemia	
Hypomagnesemia	**Systemic Disorders**
Hyponatremia	Vasculitis (CNS or
Hypernatremia	systemic)
Storage diseases	SLE
Reye syndrome	Hypertensive
Degenerative disorders	encephalopathy
Porphyria	Renal failure
Pyridoxine dependency	Hepatic encephalopathy
(deficiency)	
	Other
	Trauma*
	Tumor
	Febrile*
	Idiopathic*
	Familial

* Common.
SLE = systemic lupus erythematosus.

Table 18–21. Treatment of Seizure Disorders

Seizure Type	Drug(s)*	Therapeutic Serum Levels (μg/mL)	Drug Complications
Tonic–clonic	Carbamazepine	6–12	Drowsiness, agranulocytosis, hyponatremia; aplastic anemia
	or		
	Phenytoin	10–20	Gingival hyperplasia, hirsutism, nystagmus, pseudolymphoma; Stevens-Johnson syndrome, SLE, rickets
	or		
	Phenobarbital	15–35	Sedation, reduced cognition; Stevens-Johnson syndrome; hyperactivity
	or		
	Valproate	50–100	Drowsiness, pancreatitis, fatal liver failure (Reye-like syndrome) if under 2 yr old
Partial	Carbamazepine		
	or		
	Phenytoin		
	or		
	Valproate		
Absence	Ethosuximide	40–100	Nausea, lethargy, hiccups, SLE, Stevens-Johnson syndrome; blood dyscrasia
	or		
	Valproate		
	Clonazepam as alternate	0.013–0.072	Ataxia, lethargy, blood dyscrasia
Atonic, myoclonic	Valproate		
	Clonazepam as alternate		
Infantile spasms	ACTH		Immunosuppression, hypertension, infection
	or		
	Corticosteroids		Adrenal suppression, cataracts, osteoporosis, hypertension, immunosuppression, infection
	Clonazepam, valproate as alternates		

SLE = systemic lupus erythematosus.
*See appendix for dosages.
(Modified from Med Lett 28:91, 1986.)

Abnormal EEGs are more common in patients who develop late post-traumatic seizures than in those who do not, but this relationship has no predictive value for the individual patient.

The treatment of post-traumatic seizures does not differ from that for other seizure types (see Table 18–21). Phenytoin is preferred because its use does not alter mental status.

Febrile Seizures

Seizures with fever may be due to infection of the nervous system, underlying epilepsy triggered by fever, or *simple febrile convulsions*. The latter represent a genetic predisposition to seizures in infancy that are precipitated by a rapid rise in body temperature issuing from any cause and that are seen in 2–4% of children between the ages of 6 mo and 7 yr; half occur between 1 and 2 yr.

The simple febrile seizure occurs within hours of the onset of fever, is brief (less than 15 min), is single, does not have focal features, and does not occur more than once in a 24-hr period. The risk of recurrence of febrile seizures is approximately 30%. Half of children with onset in the 1st yr and 28% of children with onset after 1 yr have a recurrence. Recurrence decreases to 10% with onset after 3 yr.

If focal, prolonged, or multiple, the seizure is referred to as a *complex febrile seizure*. These seizures do not predict further complicated febrile seizures but may (in association with a family history) predict future nonfebrile seizures or epilepsy. Three quarters of complex febrile seizures occur as the 1st seizure, and only 8% of children have subsequent complex attacks. About 10% of children with febrile seizures have three or more recurrences. The risk of multiple recurrences is greater in infants with onset in the 1st year.

Children with febrile seizures, including those

with recurrences, are at no greater risk for intellectual or growth abnormalities than their peers. The risk of subsequent afebrile epilepsy is 3-fold higher (9.6%) in children with a prior abnormal neurologic or developmental status, complex febrile seizures, and a family history of afebrile seizures than in children without these complications.

Recurrence of simple febrile seizures can be reduced markedly with chronic administration of phenobarbital or valproic acid. However, the risk of adverse effects from valproic acid contraindicates its use for febrile seizures. Phenobarbital may be indicated after many recurrences but has serious behavioral side effects in toddlers. Phenobarbital is ineffective if given with the onset of a febrile illness because a therapeutic level cannot be reached quickly; thus, it must be given for the period of risk (next 2 yr). Rectal or oral valium given at the onset of a febrile illness can reduce the incidence of recurrent febrile seizures and is effective in terminating febrile seizures.

Status Epilepticus

Status epilepticus is a seizure of sufficient duration or frequency to create a fixed epileptic condition. The duration of seizure activity necessary to reach status epilepticus varies, but after 20–30 min of convulsive status, reductions in cortical partial pressure of oxygen occur in experimental animals, indicating a risk of irreversible brain injury. The mortality rate of status epilepticus is less than 10%.

In children under the age of 15 yr who had a seizure or a series of seizures without regaining consciousness for 1 hr or more, generalized tonic–clonic activity will occur in 43%, unilateral clonic seizures in 39%, and generalized tonic seizures in 8%. A single seizure of prolonged duration is seen much more frequently than repetitive seizures accompanied by regained consciousness.

About 25% of children presenting in status epilepticus will have an acute brain injury, such as purulent or aseptic meningitis, encephalitis, electrolyte disorders, or acute anoxia. Twenty percent are children with a history of previous brain injury or congenital malformation. Half of the cases of status epilepticus have no definable etiology, but, in 50% of this group, status is associated with fever. Sudden cessation of anticonvulsant medication is another frequent cause.

Treatment of Status Epilepticus.   The first priority is to ensure an adequate airway and to assess the cardiovascular status (see Chapter 3). The child's mouth and throat should be cleared, the oral pharynx suctioned, and a plastic oral airway placed. If any doubt is present concerning the adequacy of the airway, the child should be intubated. Oxygen is administered. The child should be examined for focal neurologic signs and evidence of meningeal irritation. A history is obtained with specific reference to previous seizures and anticonvulsant treatment. An intravenous infusion should be begun and blood obtained for a complete blood count, glucose, calcium, blood urea nitrogen, and electrolytes. When indicated by history, a toxicology screen and plasma anticonvulsant levels should be obtained. In the event that muscle activity endangers ventilation, muscle paralysis and artificial ventilation are undertaken. Underlying disorders should be treated.

The International Symposium on Status Epilepticus recommends the simultaneous administration of diazepam, 0.2–0.4 mg/kg (up to 10 mg) given intravenously at a rate of 1 mg/min, and phenytoin, 20 mg/kg (up to 1.0–1.5 g), at a rate of 1 mg/kg/min. Diazepam distributes rapidly to the brain but has a short duration of action, whereas phenytoin distributes more slowly but has a longer duration. An alternative, equally efficacious approach is to give lorazepam 0.1 mg/kg intravenously. If diazepam and phenytoin are ineffective, a loading dose of 10 mg/kg of phenobarbital is given, which may be repeated in 10 min. If this approach is ineffective, preparations for general anesthesia are undertaken. While waiting for anesthesia, continuously infused diazepam or pentobarbital is recommended. Once status epilepticus stops, maintenance therapy is initiated with the appropriate anticonvulsant.

Pseudoseizures

Children with hysteria occasionally may present with seizures, and children with seizure disorders may consciously or subconsciously exhibit activity that simulates their own seizures. Pseudoseizures differ from real seizures in that tremulousness or thrashing rather than true tonic-clonic activity is noted. Verbalization and pelvic thrusting are more commonly seen in pseudoseizures, and pseudoseizures are more likely to be initiated or terminated by suggestion. An EEG performed during pseudoseizure activity does not demonstrate typical epileptiform patterns.

Absence Seizures

Approximately 6–20% of epileptic children have typical absence seizures. The clinical hallmark of absence seizures is brief loss of environmental awareness accompanied by eye fluttering, but 90%

of children will have other associated manifestations, such as automatisms, changes in postural tone, turning of the head and/or eyes, autonomic changes, or vocalizations, such as humming. Less than 25% of children with absence seizures have focal neurologic abnormalities, and these are mild and nonprogressive. No more than 10% have abnormalities on CT scan, indicating a very low incidence of underlying structural brain disease. The absence seizure is uncommon before age 4 or after age 25. There is a 75% concordance rate in monozygotic twins, suggesting an autosomal mode of inheritance. The characteristic EEG patterns consist of synchronous 3-Hz spike-and-wave activity with frontal accentuation. The clinical seizure invariably is accompanied by the electrical discharge, and both are provoked by hyperventilation or light stimulation. Approximately 40–50% of children with absence seizures will have associated generalized seizures; 60% will occur before and 40% after the onset of absence seizures.

Differentiating absence from partial complex seizures can be difficult; both seizure types include automatisms, staring spells, and vocalizations. Partial complex seizures, however, often are followed by postictal confusion, whereas absence seizures are not. Absence seizures are provoked by hyperventilation and usually last a few seconds, whereas partial complex seizures are not thus provoked and usually last several minutes. Treatment is outlined in Table 18–21.

Myoclonic, Tonic, Atonic and Atypical Absence Seizures

Approximately 10–15% of childhood epilepsies consist of a group of seizure types that are frequently, but not invariably, associated with underlying structural brain disease and are difficult to treat and classify. These seizures often occur in combination with each other and with generalized tonic–clonic seizures.

Atypical Absence Seizures

These seizures appear as episodes of impaired consciousness with automatisms, autonomic phenomena, and/or motor manifestations, such as eye opening, eye deviation, and body stiffening. The EEG does not show the typical absence pattern but is composed instead of several frequencies of epileptiform discharges superimposed on an abnormal background. In children with chronic brain syndromes, the interictal record is abnormal, and, during seizure activity, the spike wave discharge is usually of slower than 3 Hz frequency, not necessarily symmetric, and often associated with other varieties of epileptiform activity.

MYOCLONUS

Myoclonus is a brief flexion contraction that may be epileptic or nonepileptic. The latter occurs as a normal phenomenon in physiologic sleep jerks as well as in numerous disease states (e.g., spinal cord lesions and disorders of the basal ganglia). Myoclonic seizures almost always are associated with other seizure forms, and the reveals seizure discharges. Progressive myoclonic epilepsy syndromes should be distinguished from more benign forms of myoclonic epilepsy.

Myoclonic absence refers to the body jerks that commonly accompany absence seizures and atypical absence seizures. Bilateral massive epileptic myoclonus is symmetric and varies in intensity. It may involve only facial muscles or also limbs in single or repetitive muscle contractions; both types are serious. The peak age of occurrence is within the 1st yr (37%), and status epilepticus is the first ictal manifestation in 77% of patients.

Astatic–akinetic or atonic seizures have their onset between 1 and 3 yr of age, although they may occur later. The seizures last 1–4 sec and are characterized by a loss of body tone, with falling to the ground, dropping of the head, or pitching forward or backward. A tonic component usually is associated. These seizures frequently result in repetitive head injury if the child is not protected (e.g., with a hockey or football helmet). They are most frequent on awakening and on falling to sleep; 50 or more daily seizures is usual. Children with astatic–akinetic seizures usually are retarded and have underlying brain damage. Those children without underlying brain damage tend to have later onset of seizures, normal intelligence, and better response to therapy.

Infantile spasms (West syndrome) are characterized by a brief contraction of the neck, trunk, and arm muscles, followed by a phase of sustained muscle contraction lasting from 2 to 10 sec. The initial phase consists of flexion and extension in various combinations such that the head may be thrown either backward or forward. The arms and legs may be either flexed or extended. As with most seizures, spasms occur most frequently when the child is awakening or falling asleep. Smiling or crying commonly is associated with an attack. The episodes of flexion or extension are followed by relaxation and repetition of the seizure such that these seizures occur in clusters of unpredictable and variable duration. Hundreds of these seizures occur daily. The peak age of onset is 3–8 mo, and 86% of infants will experience the onset of seizures before age 1 yr. In circumstances in which flexion of the thighs and crying are prominent, this syndrome often is mistaken for colic.

Mental retardation may accompany or follow the onset of infantile spasms. Approximately 41% of children have no apparent etiology to their seizures (cryptogenic) and respond promptly to treatment; some of this group have a normal outcome. The other 59% have a known etiology (symptomatic) and poor response to therapy, and more than 90% of this group will be developmentally impaired. The etiologies of infantile spasms are outlined in Table 18–22.

The EEG during the waking state, **hypsarrhythmia**, is dramatically abnormal, consisting of high-voltage slow waves, spikes, and polyspikes accompanied by background disorganization. Commonly, burst suppression patterns are seen during sleep. Hypsarrhythmia is seen in half of the infants with infantile spasms and sometimes is present in infants who do not have spasms. CT scanning is abnormal in 58–75% of infants, most frequently demonstrating intracranial calcifications, congenital anomalies, and atrophy. The most common anomaly is agenesis of the corpus callosum. Regardless of the seizure response to therapy, infants with abnormal CT scans have a poor prognosis, whereas those with normal CT scans, prompt response to therapy, and normal development prior to the onset of their spasms have a good chance for normal outcome.

Therapy of infantile spasms includes adrenocorticotropic hormone (ACTH), oral steroids, benzodiazepines, and valproic acid. Hypertension, glycosuria, and severe infections are complications to be anticipated with steroid therapy. Valproic acid and clonazepam may be of value in the treatment of infantile spasms refractory to ACTH.

PARTIAL SEIZURES

These seizures comprise between 40 and 60% of the classifiable epilepsies of childhood. *Simple partial seizures* arise from a specific anatomic focus, and clinical symptomatology may include motor, sensory, psychic, and/or autonomic abnormalities. Location and direction of spread of the seizure focus determines clinical symptomatology. *Complex partial seizures* have the same array of clinical abnormalities but differ from simple partial seizures in that consciousness is impaired.

The clinical manifestations in partial seizures may involve disturbances of olfaction (uncinate seizures), usually characterized by the perception of an unpleasant odor; emotional abnormalities, such as uncontrolled laughing (gelastic epilepsy); the appearance of shivering (pilomotor epilepsy); autonomic phenomena, such as tachycardia, increased gastrointestinal motility, or fever; anterior temporal lobe discharges, resulting in lip smacking; posterior temporal foci, causing episodes of vertigo, macropsia, micropsia, and/or altered depth perception; limbic discharges, resulting in dreamlike states (déjà vu); simple visual phenomena, like flashing lights and spots; and bizarre combinations of sensory, motor, and psychic abnormalities. Partial seizures may secondarily generalize and young children may not report sensory experiences.

Fifty to 80% of children with partial seizures have abnormalities on CT scan, and approximately 80% of the abnormalities are focal. The lesions of greatest concern are cerebral hemisphere tumors and arteriovenous malformations. Agenesis of the corpus callosum, focal atrophy, medial temporal sclerosis, cortical dysplasia, and hamartomas are addi-

Table 18–22. Etiologies of Infantile Spasms

Metabolic
Phenylketonuria
Biotinidase deficiency
Maple syrup urine disease
Isovalericacidemia
Ornithine accumulation
Nonketotic hyperglycinemia
Pyridoxine dependency
Hypoglycemia
Lipidosis

Developmental Malformations
Polymicrogyria
Lissencephaly
Schizencephaly
Down syndrome and other chromosomal disorders
Aicardi syndrome
Organoid nevus syndrome

Neurocutaneous Syndrome
Tuberous sclerosis
Sturge-Weber syndrome

Congenital Infections
Toxoplasmosis
Cytomegalovirus
Syphilis

Encephalopathies
Postasphyxia
Posthemorrhagic
Trauma
Postimmunization (pertussis)

tional prominent lesions associated with partial seizures. Children with refractory partial seizures who have normal intelligence, normal neurologic examinations, and a persistence of focally slow EEGs are more likely to harbor a tumor than children with partial seizures who are intellectually impaired, have focal abnormalities on examination, diffusely abnormal EEGs, and known risk factors for seizures. MRI is superior to CT scanning in detecting gliomas in children with partial complex seizures. Although a high incidence of underlying structural brain disease as the cause of partial seizures has been noted, genetic factors also play a role. Treatment is outlined in Table 18–21.

BENIGN FOCAL EPILEPSY

This epileptic syndrome, also known as **rolandic epilepsy,** usually begins between the ages of 5 and 10 (rarely before 2 yr). The incidence may be as high as 21:100,000, comprising 16% of all afebrile seizures below the age of 15 yr. The seizures usually are focal motor with generalized spread. In approximately half of the children affected, seizures occur only during sleep or on awakening. When the seizure occurs in the awake state, symptomatology is motor or sensory, involving the tongue, mouth, and face. Speech and swallowing commonly are impaired. A family history is found in 13% of patients. This disorder disappears in adolescence to early adulthood, intelligence is normal, and no associated neurologic or CT scan abnormalities are present.

JUVENILE MYOCLONIC EPILEPSY (JANZ)

This occurs in adolescence and is an autosomal dominant disorder with variable penetrance. Myoclonus, predominantly in the morning, with or without generalized seizures characterizes the disorder. Seizures respond only to valproic acid and treatment is life long.

LENNOX-GASTAUT SYNDROME

This is an epileptic syndrome with variable age of onset, but most children present before age 5 yr. The disorder is characterized by multiple seizure types, including atonic–astatic, partial, atypical absence, and generalized tonic, clonic, or tonic–clonic varieties. Many children have underlying brain injury or malformations (etiologies similar to infantile spasms), but a minority have no demonstrable etiology. These seizures as a rule respond poorly to treatment, although a significant minority respond well to valproic acid.

ACQUIRED EPILEPTIC APHASIA (LANDAU-KLEFFNER)

This seizure syndrome is characterized by language disability related to partial seizures. It appears that the seizures are an epiphenomenon related to underlying acquired brain injury.

BENIGN NEONATAL CONVULSIONS

This is an autosomal dominant syndrome located on chromosome 22 and characterized by generalized clonic seizures occurring toward the end of the 1st wk of life. Response to treatment is variable, but the outlook generally is favorable.

PRINCIPLES OF SEIZURE THERAPY

Therapy is not considered for benign febrile seizures unless more than three recurrences have occurred. Absence seizures, infantile spasms, atypical absence seizures, and astatic–akinetic seizures are universally recurrent at the time of diagnosis, and therapy is indicated. If the seizure is symptomatic of acute neurologic illness, 23% of patients can be expected to have a recurrence during the illness, and treatment is limited to the acute illness. The overall risk of recurrence for children whose first seizure is generalized tonic–clonic is approximately 50%, and it seems reasonable to wait for recurrence before therapy is instituted.

When treatment is initiated, the goal is to achieve optimal function. Medication risks should be weighed against the risk of seizure type. Initially, a single agent should be chosen, because this reduces cost, improves compliance, and avoids toxicity. Approximately 50% of children will obtain satisfactory seizure control with one drug. A second agent is considered only when therapeutic anticonvulsant levels are obtained with the first drug. Anticonvulsant levels are helpful in adjusting medication but should be interpreted in light of the patient's clinical state. Because of phenobarbital's very long half-life, phenobarbital plasma levels can be determined anytime throughout the day; levels of carbamazepine and phenytoin may vary significantly between peak and trough as a result of their shorter half-lives. In disease states in which drug binding is likely to be altered (i.e., hepatic or renal disease), free and bound anticonvulsant determinations can be helpful. Hazardous physical activities are best avoided, and many advise against direct contact sports such as football. Although children with epilepsy have a greater risk of submersion accidents, if anticonvulsant drug levels are maintained in the therapeutic range and the child is afforded appropriate supervision, accidents should be avoidable.

Discontinuation of Therapy

Children with generalized tonic, clonic, and tonic–clonic seizures, absence seizures, and certain partial seizures may not require therapy beyond 4 yr. The risk of recurrence is higher when partial seizures occur. When prophylaxis is used for febrile seizures, the duration need not be longer than 2 yr. Children with myoclonic seizures, progressive myoclonic epilepsy, atypical absence seizures, and the Lennox-Gastaut syndrome will require treatment for life. As a rule, children who are neurologically abnormal, have seizures that were initially difficult to control, and have persistently paroxysmal EEGs are at highest risk for recurrence when therapy is discontinued.

References

Annegers J, Hauser W, Shirts S, et al: Factors prognostic of unprovoked seizures after febrile seizures. N Engl J Med 316:493, 1987.
Behrman RE (ed): Nelson Textbook of Pediatrics. 14th ed. Philadelphia, WB Saunders, 1992, Sec. 20.17–20.34.
Berkovic S, Andermann F, Carpenter S, et al: Progressive myoclonus epilepsies: Specific causes and diagnosis. N Engl J Med 315:296, 1986.
Callaghan N, Garrett A, Goggin T: Withdrawal of anticonvulsant drugs in patients free of seizures for two years. A prospective study. N Engl J Med 318:942, 1988.
Camfield C, Camfield P, Gordon K, et al: Outcome of childhood epilepsy: A population-based study with a simple predictive scoring system for those treated with medication. J Pediatr 122:861, 1993.
Holmes GL: Use of EEG in childhood epilepsy. Int Pediatr 7:223, 1992.
Holmes GL: Severe seizures in infancy and early childhood. Int Pediatr 7:237, 1992.
Rosman NP, Colton T, Labazzo J, et al: A controlled trial of diazepam administered during febrile illnesses to prevent recurrence of febrile seizures. N Eng J Med 329: 79, 1993.

ATAXIA

Ataxia is an abnormality of coordination resulting in an impairment of direction, rate, and strength of voluntary movement. A broad-based unsteady gait is termed ataxic, whereas *dysmetria* and *dysdiadochokinesis* refer to ataxic abnormalities of coordination in the extremities. Ataxia may have its origin in lesions of the peripheral nerves, spinal cord, brain stem, cerebellum, thalamus, or cerebral hemispheres. Ataxia may appear suddenly (acute ataxia) or manifest gradually (chronic ataxia). In either circumstance, the condition may be static or progressive.

Acute Ataxia

Infectious/postinfectious and toxic etiologies are encountered most commonly when ataxia begins abruptly. The former include varicella, Epstein-Barr virus, and encephalitis viruses. Accidental ingestion is most common between the ages of 1 and 4 yr, and the causative agents include barbiturates, other soporifics, alcohol, and antihistamines. Later in childhood, drug ingestion of the same agents as a suicide gesture is encountered. Overdose of phenytoin should be considered in children with epilepsy. Children with ataxia secondary to drug ingestion usually have an altered sensorium. Treatment is based on the specific offending agent.

As a group, the metabolic causes of ataxia tend to be episodic; aggravated by intercurrent infections or other stresses, resulting in a catabolic state; and slowly progessive (saltatory progression).

The vascular disorders include migraine, vasculitis (systemic lupus erythematosus), or vasculopathy involving the cerebellum or its pathways. Spontaneous cerebellar hemorrhage seen in coagulopathies and AVMs presents with acute ataxia, nystagmus, and gaze paresis and may be accompanied by an altered sensorium. The hemorrhage is detected readily on CT scan, and therapy consists of clot evacuation and correction of coagulopathy.

Posterior fossa tumors, primarily involving the cerebellum or the brain stem, produce ataxia that may be acute or gradual in onset, but, once present, it follows a progressive course. The ataxia, dysmetria, and titubation (inability to maintain a steady sitting posture) may result from the primary cerebellar lesion and/or from obstruction of the CSF pathways and resultant hydrocephalus. Hydrocephalus causes ataxia by exertion of pressure on the corticopontocerebellar pathways as they sweep over the lateral ventricles.

Chronic Ataxia

A number of congenital malformations of the brain result in chronic static or slowly progressive ataxia. Despite the embryologic origin of these conditions, the age of presentation is frequently in in-

Table 18–23. Congenital Causes of Chronic Ataxia

Disorder	Age of Presentation	Clinical Manifestations	Mechanism of Ataxia, Diagnoses, and Treatment
Cerebellar hypoplasia	Early infancy (occasionally delayed)	Developmental delay, hypotonia, athetosis, chorea, delayed walking, ataxic gait	Absent cerebellar granular cells; CT shows small cerebellum
Vermal aplasia Dandy-Walker malformation	Early infancy	Macrocephaly, enlarged occipital region; ataxia	Hydrocephalus and cystic dilation of the fourth ventricle; treatment is by shunting of hydrocephalus and/or the posterior fossa cyst
Joubert syndrome	Early infancy	Neonatal episodic hyperpnea and apnea; hypotonia, nystagmus	MRI and CT demonstrate agenesis of the superior cerebellar vermis
Arnold-Chiari malformation	Variable	Headache, neck pain, lower cranial nerve dysfunction, nystagmus, ataxia; this variety does not have associated myelomeningocele	MRI and CT demonstrate a caudal fourth ventricle; distortion of the brain stem; treatment is by posterior fossa decompression
Hydrocephalus	Variable	Macrocephaly, vomiting, ataxia	CT and MRI demonstrate enlarged lateral ventricles; in aqueductal stenosis, the third ventricle is particularly large, whereas the fourth ventricle is normal or small

fancy or later in childhood (Table 18–23). The hereditary and familial metabolic causes are genetic in origin and have varying ages of presentation (Table 18–24). Children with chronic ataxia may have episodes of worsening of their disease, resulting in a process exhibiting an apparently static baseline but with superimposed periods of exacerbation. Some of the causes of acute ataxia also may cause chronic ataxia (brain tumors, toxins, migraine).

References

Barbeau A: The hereditary ataxias: Pathogenesis and treatment. Neurol Neurosurg 37:2, 1979.
Stumpf D: Acute ataxia. Pediatr Rev 8:303, 1987.

PSYCHOMOTOR RETARDATION
(see also Chapter 1)

Nonprogressive Psychomotor Retardation

In many children with severe mental retardation (MR), the history and general physical examination are unremarkable. No focal neurologic deficits are present and laboratory evaluation is unrevealing. Most children with this idiopathic condition probably have microscopic aberrations of CNS development involving the structure of neurons or neuronal organelles, aggregation of neurons, myelinization of white matter, synapse formation, or interneuronal connections. Although the management of MR includes educational programs, such as infant stimulation, no treatment program can increase inherent learning capacity.

CONGENITAL MALFORMATIONS OF THE BRAIN

Most brain malformations can be produced by a variety of injuries occurring during a vulnerable period of gestation. These precipitating factors include chromosomal, genetic and metabolic abnormalities (see Chapters 4 and 5); infections (cytomegalovirus, TORCH; see Chapters 6 and 10); and exposure to X-radiation, certain drugs, and maternal illness during pregnancy.

In all types of *congenital hydrocephalus*, the degree of ventricular enlargement correlates roughly with outcome, but examples of neonates with severe hydrocephalus who receive ventriculoperitoneal shunts and then have normal development are well known. There often are associated defects in the closure of the neural tube.

Hydranencephaly consists of virtual absence of the cerebrum with an intact skull. The thalamus, brain stem, and some occipital cortex are present. Children who are affected may have a normal outward appearance but do not achieve developmental milestones.

Holoprosencephaly represents varying degrees of failure of the primary cerebral vesicle to divide and expand laterally and often is associated with midline facial defects (e.g., hypotelorism, cleft lip and cleft palate). This anomaly may occur in an isolated fashion, can be associated with a chromosomal or genetic disorder, and may be mild or severe. The outlook for infants with alobar holoprosencephaly is uniformly poor; that for infants with the semilobar form is somewhat better. Cognitively normal

Table 18–24. Hereditary Causes of Ataxia

Disorder	Usual Age of Onset	Hereditary Pattern	Clinical Characteristics	Etiology and Treatment
Friedreich ataxia	2–16 yr	Recessive	Ataxia, scoliosis, pes cavus, posterior column sensory loss, areflexia, cardiomyopathy	Supportive
Ataxia–telangiectasia	Early infancy (1–2 yr)	Recessive	Ataxia, oculomotor apraxia, sinopulmonary infections, telangiectasia of conjunctiva and skin	B and T cell dysfunction; cellular immunity is impaired; supportive
Machado-Joseph disease	12–15 yr	Dominant	Cerebellar, pyramidal, extrapyramidal degeneration; anterior horn cell disease; Portuguese ancestry	Supportive
Metachromatic leukodystrophy	(see Psychomotor Retardation)			
Refsum disease	4–7 yr	Recessive	Ataxia, neuropathy, retinitis pigmentosa, ichthyosis	Phytanic acid hydroxylase deficiency; phytol-free diet
Leigh disease	Infancy to adolescence	Recessive	Ataxia, lactic acidosis, hypotonia, abnormalities of respiration	Some Leigh disorders of pyruvate metabolism; supportive
Wilson disease	Infancy to adulthood	Recessive	Hepatic disease, tremor, dystonic, athetosis, chorea	Ceruloplasmin deficiency; penicillamine
Abetalipoproteinemia	5–15 yr	Recessive	Ataxia, dysmetria, fat malabsorption, acanthocytosis, retinitis pigmentosa, sensory loss	Low fat diet, Vitamin E and A supplementation
Juvenile gangliosidosis	3–5 yr	Recessive GM_1 or GM_2 forms	Ataxia, spasticity, rigidity, dementia	None available
Ramsay Hunt syndrome	7–10 yr	Sporadic	Ataxia, tremor, myoclonus, dementia	Supportive
Marinesco-Sjögren syndrome	Infancy to 5 yr	Recessive	Cataracts, ataxia, growth failure, mental retardation	Supportive
Juvenile sulfate lipidosis (juvenile MLD)	Infancy to 5 yr	Recessive	Dementia, ataxia, spasticity, aryl sulfidase A deficiency	Supportive

MLD = metachromatic leukodystrophy.

individuals with lobar holoprosencephaly occasionally are seen.

A number of malformations result from the failure of the normal migration of neurons from the germinal matrix zone at 1–5 mo of gestation. Often, multiple malformations exist in the same patient. *Schizencephaly* is characterized by symmetric clefts within the cerebral hemispheres that extend from the cortical surface to the ventricular cavity; the neurologic deficit is severe in the open lip variety but may be mild in the closed lip form. *Lissencephaly* indicates smooth brain with absence of sulcation. The normal six-layered cortex does not develop, and affected children present with seizures and severe developmental delay. This anomaly most commonly is part of a genetic or chromosomal disorder. In *macrogyria*, the gyri are few in number and too broad, whereas in *microgyria* the gyri are too many and too small. *Gray matter heterotopias* are abnormal islands of neurons within the central cerebral white matter that never completed the migration to the cerebral surface. *Agenesis of the corpus callosum* may be partial or complete and may occur in an isolated fashion or in association with other anomalies of cellular migration. Neurologic development with all of these anomalies is variable and depends on the extent of the malformations.

Megalencephaly, or large brain, is diagnosed by finding a large head with radiographically normal-appearing intracranial contents. Most often, this is a familial trait of no clinical significance. Sometimes, it is associated with disorders of neuronal migration and a clinical syndrome of developmental retardation. *Neurofibromatosis* and *Soto syndrome* (cerebral gigantism) are two genetic syndromes associated with megalencephaly and sometimes with MR. Megalencephaly is also a feature of a number of metabolic diseases that produce a progressive degenerative encephalopathy.

Microcephaly usually is produced by failure of normal brain growth. Any injury to the brain, intrauterine or postnatal, can retard subsequent brain growth. Autosomal recessive genetic illnesses resulting in microcephaly and MR have been described. Brain malformations often are associated with microcephaly. In general, children with head circumferences more than three standard deviations below the mean, regardless of the cause, will exhibit retarded intellect.

CHROMOSOMAL DISORDERS

Chromosomal trisomies (trisomy 21, XXY, XXX) are associated with retardation. A common chromosomal cause of MR in males is the fragile X syn-

Table 18–25. Laboratory Evaluation for Degenerative Neurologic Metabolic Diseases

CBC (leukocyte vacuolations)	**Urine**
	Ketones
Blood gas determination	Screen for inborn errors
Ammonia	Organic acids
Na$^+$, K$^+$, Cl$^-$, CO$_2$ (anion gap), CPK, uric acid, fasting blood glucose, cholesterol, triglycerides	24-hr amino acids
	24-hr mucopolysaccharides
	Carnitine: free, esterified, total
	Sialyloligosaccharides
Lactate, pyruvate	
Amino acids	**Imaging**
Long-chain fatty acids	Skull
Biotinidase level	Vertebrae
	Long bones
Lysosomal Enzymes	CNS, MRI
WBC	
Serum fibroblasts	**Biopsy**
	Skin
DNA Probes	Bone marrow
Many disorders	Muscle
	Nerve

CBC = complete blood count; CPK = creatine phosphokinase; WBC = white blood cells; CNS = central nervous system; MRI = magnetic resonance imaging.

drome (Chapter 4). These children are severely affected and present with autistic behavior, large ears, macro-orchidism, and an elongated narrow face. Females may be affected but usually not as severely as males.

Progressive Mental Retardation

A complete laboratory evaluation is listed in Table 18–25. Degenerative hereditary/metabolic diseases usually are symmetric in their manifestations and slowly progressive over weeks, months, and years. However, some acquired diseases can simulate this clinical picture and must be excluded because they are more likely to be treatable than the degenerative conditions.

ACQUIRED ILLNESSES MIMICKING DEGENERATIVE DISEASES

Some children with epilepsy experience *seizures* so frequently that they are continuously in either an ictal or postictal state and appear stuporous. A treatment program employing high doses of multiple anticonvulsants may compound this problem. The children's decline in alertness arouses suspicion of a progressive illness, but readjustment of medications and amelioration of the seizure disorder return the children to previous levels of functioning.

Chronic drug overdose with sedatives, tranquilizers, and anticholinergics as well as anticonvulsants can bring about progressive mental confusion, lethargy, and ataxia. *Lead poisoning* may become manifest as a chronic cause of MR or as irritability, listlessness, anorexia, and pallor leading to fulminant encephalopathy. Deficiencies of the *vitamins* thiamine, niacin, B_{12}, and E can produce encephalopathy as well as peripheral neuropathy. Both congenital and acquired *hypothyroidism* impair intelligence and retard movement; congenital disease produces irreversible damage if it is not treated immediately after birth. *Structural brain diseases* also may mimic dementia.

Certain *indolent brain infections* cause mental and neurologic deterioration over months and years (e.g., syphilitic and fungal infections), but usually many associated clinical manifestations are present. Rubeola (measles), rubella (German measles), and human immunodeficiency virus (HIV) also can cause chronic infection of the CNS, which subsequently results in MR. Measles produces subacute sclerosing panencephalitis, a dementing illness that has a course that can vary from weeks to years. Rubella virus produces a similar panencephalitis accompanied by prominent motor abnormalities usually in children who have the congenital rubella syndrome. Congenital HIV brings about both failure of normal developmental gains and regression of acquired skills.

Severe *psychosocial deprivation* in infancy can give rise to apathy and failure to attain developmental milestones. *Depression* in older children can lead to blunting of affect, social withdrawal, and poor school performance that raise the question of encephalopathy and dementia.

HEREDITARY/METABOLIC DEGENERATIVE DISEASES

Degenerative diseases may affect white matter, gray matter, or focal regions of the brain. Many of the white and gray matter degenerative illnesses represent specific enzymatic deficiencies in the metabolism of one category of brain lipids, the sphingolipids. Gray matter is rich in gangliosides, whereas the myelin of white matter is rich in proteolipid protein and galactolipids.

Degenerative Diseases with Focal Manifestations

Although certain enzyme deficiencies usually are expressed in classic patterns of disease, such as Niemann-Pick disease, Gaucher disease, and Tay-Sachs disease, the same enzyme deficiencies sometimes produce unusual clinical syndromes that vary widely in age of onset, rate of progression, and neurologic signs. Therefore any patient with a degenerative neurologic condition of unknown cause should have leukocytes or skin fibroblasts submitted for measurement of a standard battery of lysosomal enzymes (see Chapter 5).

Friedreich ataxia is a relentlessly progressive autosomal recessive disorder that becomes manifest in the early teenage years with ataxia, dysmetria, dysarthria, pes cavus, hammer toes, diminished proprioception and vibration sensation, diminished or absent reflexes, upgoing toes, kyphoscoliosis, nystagmus, and a hypertrophic cardiomyopathy.

Lesch-Nyhan syndrome is a sex-linked recessive disorder caused by deficiency of hypoxanthine–guanine phosphoriboyltransferase, leading to the formation of excess uric acid. Infants appear normal until late in the 1st yr of life, when they develop psychomotor retardation, choreoathetosis, spasticity and severe self-mutilation. Gouty arthritis and renal calculi with renal failure also develop. The hyperuricemia and renal complications are treated with allopurinol, a xanthine oxidase inhibitor, but no effective treatment for the neurologic disease is available.

Wilson disease is an example of a treatable degenerative condition that exhibits signs of both cerebellar and basal ganglia dysfunction. It is an autosomal recessively inherited inborn error of copper metabolism. Serum copper and ceruloplasmin are low, and abnormal copper deposition is found in the liver, producing cirrhosis; in the peripheral cornea, producing a characteristic green–brown (Kayser-Fleischer) ring; and in the CNS, producing neuronal degeneration and protoplasmic astrocytosis. Neurologic symptoms characteristically begin in the early teenage years with dysarthria, dysphasia, drooling, fixed smile, tremor, dystonia, and emotional lability. Treatment is with a copper-chelating agent such as oral penicillamine.

Subacute necrotizing encephalomyelopathy, or *Leigh disease*, is a degenerative inherited CNS disease primarily involving the periaqueductal region of the brain stem, caudate, and putamen. Symptoms usually begin prior to 2 yr of age and consist of hypotonia, feeding difficulties, respiratory irregularity, weakness of extraocular movements, and ataxia. Blood pyruvate and lactate are elevated. Decreased pyruvate carboxylase or pyruvate dehydrogenase activity, biotinidase deficiency, and cytochrome c oxidase deficiency have been identified as causative in some cases.

Degenerative Diseases of the White Matter

The prominent signs of diseases affecting primarily white matter are spasticity, ataxia, optic atrophy, and peripheral neuropathy. Seizures and dementia are late manifestations. In general, life expectancy ranges from months to a few years. *Metachromatic leukodystrophy* is an autosomal recessive lipidosis caused by deficiency of the enzyme aryl-sulfatase. Demyelination of the central and peripheral nervous systems occurs, and children present between 1 and 2 yr of age with stiffening and ataxia of gait, spasticity, optic atrophy, intellectual deterioration, absent reflexes, upgoing toes, raised CSF protein, and slowing of motor nerve conduction velocities. *Krabbe disease* (globoid cell leukodystrophy) presents a similar clinical picture that begins at 6 mo of age and includes irritability, macrocephaly, hyperacusis, and seizures. The same combination of upper and lower motor neuron signs is noted as a result of demyelination of both the central and peripheral nervous systems. Krabbe disease is also an autosomal recessive lipidosis and is caused by a deficiency of the enzyme galactocerebrosidase.

Adrenal leukodystrophy is a sex-linked, recessively inherited disorder associated with progressive central demyelination and adrenal cortical insufficiency. It is caused by an impaired capacity of a subcellular organelle, the *peroxisome*, to degrade saturated unbranched very-long-chain fatty acids, particularly hexacosanoate (C26:0). The diagnosis is achieved by finding an elevated hexacosanoate level in plasma lipids of the serum and a typical CT scan. The disease most commonly is exhibited in males in the early school years, with subtle behavior changes and intellectual deterioration followed by cortical visual and auditory deficits and stiff gait. Later, spastic quadriparesis, coma, and seizures supervene. Symptomatic adrenocortical insufficiency with fatigue, vomiting, and hypotension develop in 20–40% of patients, usually at the same time as the neurologic illness.

Degenerative Diseases of the Gray Matter with Visceromegaly (Chapter 5)

The prominent signs of gray matter encephalopathy are dementia and seizures. To aid diagnosis, these diseases are divided into those with and without hepatosplenomegaly. All the illnesses discussed below, except for Rett syndrome, are genetic disorders. All are autosomal recessive traits except for Hunter syndrome, which is sex-linked recessive, and the mitochondrial encephalopathies, in which the disease may be transmitted through either nuclear or mitochondrial DNA defects.

In the *mucopolysaccharidoses*, degradation of mucopolysaccharides (MPS) is defective because of the absence of a variety of lysosomal hydrolases. MPS, important matrix constituents of connective tissue, skin cartilage, bone, and cornea, accumulate within lysosomes and abnormally large amounts are excreted in the urine. The clinical manifestations of these disorders are dwarfism, kyphoscoliosis, coarse facies, hepatosplenomegaly, cardiovascular abnormalities, and corneal clouding. Neurologic involvement is seen in MPS types 1H (Hurler syndrome), II (Hunter syndrome), III (Sanfilippo syndrome), and VII. Children with Hurler syndrome, the most severe of these illnesses, appear normal during the first 6 mo of life and then develop the characteristic skeletal and neurologic features. Mental deficiency, spasticity, deafness, and optic atrophy are progressive. Hydrocephalus frequently develops because of obstruction to CSF flow by thickened leptomeninges.

Mucolipidosis II (I-cell disease), mucolipidosis III, GM$_1$ gangliosidosis, fucosidosis, and mannosidosis resemble Hurler syndrome clinically but do not exhibit excess excretion of MPS and involve different disorders in lysosomal hydrolases. Diagnosis is achieved by analysis of enzymes in white blood cells, serum, and skin fibroblasts.

Classic *Niemann-Pick disease* is caused by a deficiency of the enzyme sphingomyelinase. Sphingomyelin accumulates in foam cells of the reticuloendothelial system of the liver, spleen, lungs, and bone marrow; it also distends neurons of the brain. Intellectual retardation and regression, myoclonic seizures, hypotonia, hepatosplenomegaly, jaundice, and, sometimes, retinal cherry-red spots are noted within the 1st yr of life. The diagnosis is confirmed by finding foam cells in the bone marrow and sphingomyelinase deficiency in leukocytes and skin fibroblasts.

Although the most common form of *Gaucher disease* is an indolent illness of adults, there is a rapidly fatal infantile form featuring severe neurologic involvement caused by the same enzyme deficiency of glucocerebrosidase. Glucoceramide accumulates in the liver, spleen, and bone marrow. The characteristic neurologic signs are neck retraction, extraocular movement palsies, trismus, difficulty swallowing, apathy, and spasticity. Gaucher cells are found in bone marrow, and serum acid phosphatase is increased.

Degenerative Disease of the Gray Matter without Visceromegaly

Tay-Sachs disease occurs most commonly in Jewish children of eastern European background. The disease is confined to the CNS. It is caused by deficiency of hexosaminidase A and the accumulation of GM_2 ganglioside in cerebral gray matter and cerebellum. Infants are normal until 6 mo of age, when they develop listlessness, irritability, hyperacusis, intellectual retardation, and a **retinal cherry-red spot**. The ganglion cells of the retina and macula are distended when ganglioside is present and appear as a large area of white surrounding a small red fovea that is not covered by ganglion cells. Within months, blindness, convulsions, spasticity, and opisthotonos develop.

Rett syndrome is a recently described but common neurodegenerative disorder affecting only females, with onset at about 1 yr of age. It is characterized by the loss of purposeful hand movements and communication skills; social withdrawal; gait apraxia; stereotypic repetitive hand movements that resemble washing, wringing, or clapping of the hands; and acquired microcephaly. The illness then plateaus for many years before seizures, spasticity, and kyphoscoliosis develop. The etiology, genetic basis, and neurobiologic pathogenesis of the disease are unknown.

Several syndromes of *mitochondrial myopathy* and *progressive encephalopathy* have been described. Skeletal muscle biopsy reveals ragged red fibers representing proliferating abnormal mitochondrial elements. Neurologic signs have included seizures, focal deficits, and dementia in the **MELAS** (*mitochondrial myopathy, encephalopathy, lactic acidosis, and stroke-like episodes*) **syndrome**, and seizures, dementia, hearing loss, optic nerve atrophy, ataxia, and loss of deep sensation in the **MERRF** (*myoclonus, epilepsy, and ragged red fibers*) **syndrome**. Elevation of creatine phosphokinase, lactic acidosis, and calcification of the basal ganglia suggest this class of disorders. Onset is usually between 5 and 10 yr of age and progression occurs over years.

Many degenerative encephalopathies defy diagnosis despite extensive laboratory analysis. The diagnosis of leukodystrophy usually can be made confidently on the basis of extensive cerebral white matter changes on CT or MRI in the absence of cortical abnormalities. The diagnosis of hereditary/metabolic gray matter encephalopathy without histologic or biochemical confirmation is much less secure. Acquired lesions (infectious, inflammatory, vascular, toxic) are difficult to exclude completely.

Unless roentgenographic lesions are demonstrated, brain biopsy is not likely to be helpful.

References

Al-Mateen M, Philippart M, Shields D: Rett syndrome. A commonly overlooked progressive encephalopathy in girls. Am J Dis Child 140:761, 1986.

Behrman RE (ed): Nelson Textbook of Pediatrics. 14th ed. Philadelphia, WB Saunders, 1992, Sec. 3.58, 8.7–8.35, 8.43–8.44, 20.58–20.69.

Kalter H, Warkany J: Congenital malformations. Etiological factors and their role in prevention. N Engl J Med 308: 424, 1983.

Opitz J: Mental retardation. Biologic aspects of concern to pediatricians. Pediatr Rev 2:41, 1980.

Smith DW: Recognizable Patterns of Human Malformation. Genetic Embryological and Clinical Aspects. Philadelphia, WB Saunders, 1988.

Taft L: Cerebral palsy. Pediatr Ann 15:176, 1986.

MACROCEPHALY AND MICROCEPHALY

Abnormalities of head size are among the most common problems encountered by pediatricians. Head circumference varies with race and sex, but measurements greater than 3 standard deviations above the mean constitute **macrocephaly**. Macrocephaly may be due to *macrocrania*, increased skull thickness; *hydrocephalus*, enlargement of the ventricles; or *megalencephaly*, enlargement of the brain. Head circumference measurements more than 3 standard deviations below the mean are termed **microcephaly**. In most circumstances, microcephaly reflects *micrencephaly*, a small brain. With *craniosynostosis* (premature closure of one or more skull sutures), compensatory growth in the vertical or horizontal dimension will result in an altered head circumference measurement, which inaccurately reflects intracranial volume. If brain volume is reduced above the cranial base, as in *microcephaly vera*, in which intracranial content is decreased as a result of deficiency of the frontal lobes, the occipital frontal head circumference may not completely reflect the deficiency. Definitions of microcephaly do not apply to dwarfism, in which head circumference is proportional to body size and intellectual development is normal. As a general rule, macrocephaly and microcephaly raise a concern about cognitive ability, but head circumference alone should never be used to establish a prognosis for intellectual development.

Macrocephaly

HYDROCEPHALUS

This important cause of macrocephaly is due to increased production, a block in the flow, or impaired absorption of CSF. CSF is an ultrafiltrate of plasma continuously produced by the choroid plexus of the lateral, 3rd, and 4th ventricles. The normal volume of CSF is approximately 50 mL in neonates and reaches the adult volume of 150 mL by late childhood or early adolescence. CSF normally flows from the lateral ventricles through the intraventricular foramen of Monro to the 3rd ventricle. From the 3rd ventricle, it passes through the cerebral aqueduct to the 4th ventricle. CSF exits the 4th ventricle from the single midline foramen of Magendie and the two lateral foramina of Luschka. Subarachnoid flow occurs superiorly to the cisterns of the brain and inferiorly to the spinal subarachnoid space. Absorption of CSF is accomplished by the arachnoid villi, which are microtubular invaginations into the large dural sinuses and are most concentrated along the superior sagittal sinus, and by transependymal absorption. Increased ICP neither effectively facilitates CSF absorption nor inhibits CSF formation.

The etiology of hydrocephalus is obstruction of CSF flow anywhere along its course (Table 18–26). **Obstructive or internal hydrocephalus** is due to a block before CSF reaches the subarachnoid space. Impairment of CSF flow within the subarachnoid space or impairment of absorption is known by the misnomer **communicating hydrocephalus** (actu-

Table 18–26. Causes of Hydrocephalus

Obstruction Region	Clinical Characteristics	Etiology
Intraventricular foramina	Acutely or slowly evolving, unilateral ventricular dilation; can be exhibited at any age	Congenital, parasellar mass, intraventricular tumors
Aqueduct of Sylvius (cerebral aqueduct)	May be exhibited in utero or in adults; usually noted in infancy; slowly evolves	Neurofibromatosis, intrauterine toxoplasmosis; post-mumps meningoencephalitis; periaqueductal mass lesions: tumors, vein of Galen malformations; congenital dysplasia; hereditary, sex-linked
Impaired flow from the fourth ventricle		
Dandy-Walker malformation	Enlarged occipital shelf; slowly evolving; marked transillumination of the posterior fossa; usually is exhibited in infancy but may be delayed until adult life	Referred to as atresia of the foramina of Luschka and Magendie but actually due to agenesis of the cerebellar vermis, resulting in cystic dilation of the fourth ventricle and aqueductal compression
Arnold-Chiari malformation	May or may not be associated with myelomeningocele; may be exhibited in later life with cranial nerve dysfunction, with or without hydrocephalus	Congenital malformation resulting in a small posterior fossa, caudal displacement of the fourth ventricle and cerebellum, and distortion of the brain stem
Congenital bone lesions of the cranial base	Slowly evolving hydrocephalus, stiff neck; lower cranial nerve dysfunction	Achondroplasia, rickets, basilar impression; these lesions compress the posterior fossa, preventing CSF flow and distorting the brain stem
Extraventricular obstruction (communicating)	Acutely or slowly evolving; is exhibited at any age	Congenital, due to hypoplasia of the arachnoid villi; following infection or hemorrhage due to destruction of arachnoid villi or subarachnoid fibrosis, causing obstruction to CSF flow (following superior sagittal sinus occlusion, preventing absorption of CSF)

ally extraventricular obstructive hydrocephalus) or **external hydrocephalus**. Hydrocephalus caused by overproduction of CSF without true obstruction is seen in choroid plexus papillomas, which account for 2–4% of childhood intracranial tumors and are exhibited in early infancy.

The *clinical manifestations* of hydrocephalus are caused by ventricular distention and increased intracranial pressure. Dilation of the lateral ventricles results in stretching of the corticopontocerebellar and corticospinal pathways, which sweep around the lateral margins of these ventricles to reach the cerebral peduncles. This stretching results in ataxia and spasticity that initially is most marked in the lower extremities. Distention of the 3rd ventricle may compress the hypothalamic regions and result in endocrine dysfunction. The optic nerves, chiasm, and tracts also are in close proximity to the anterior 3rd ventricle, and visual dysfunction results when these structures are compressed. Dilation of the cerebral aqueduct compresses the surrounding periaqueductal gray matter, a vertical gaze center, causing paresis of upward gaze. Manifestations of increased ICP may evolve slowly in obstructive hydrocephalus when there is time for transependymal absorption of CSF to compensate partially for the obstruction, or they may evolve acutely when compensation is absent. Acute manifestations consist of headache, vomiting, cranial nerve dysfunction, herniation, and coma in rapid sequence. They usually follow acute complete obstruction to CSF flow resulting from tumors, infection, or hemorrhage. Gradually evolving hydrocephalus results in macrocephaly, scalp vein distention caused by obstruction of flow from the bridging veins of the scalp to the sagittal sinus, impairment in upward gaze eventually causing the "sunsetting sign," ataxia, spasticity, papilledema or optic atrophy, and endocrine dysfunction, which most commonly is exhibited as growth failure.

The *treatment* of hydrocephalus is both medical and surgical. Following subarachnoid hemorrhage or meningitis, the flow or absorption of CSF may be transiently impaired. In this circumstance, the use of agents such as acetazolamide, which transiently decreases CSF production, may be of benefit. Surgical treatment consists of removing the obstructive lesion (tumor, cyst, or aneurysm) or placing a shunt. A shunt consists of polyethylene tubing, with or without a valve, that bypasses the obstruction and diverts CSF to other sites for absorption. The cranial end usually is placed in the lateral ventricles. In the instance of Dandy-Walker malformation, the cranial end may be placed in the posterior fossa cyst. The distal end usually is placed in the peritoneal cavity. Shunts carry the hazards of infection (*Staphylococcus epidermidis, Corynebacterium*) or sudden occlusion with signs and symptoms of acute hydrocephalus.

MEGALENCEPHALY

This may be due to an embryologic proliferative abnormality of the brain and is associated with several rare syndromes (Sotos syndrome, Riley-Smith syndrome, Alexander and Canavan diseases). Megalencephalic brains may be two to three times as large as normal brains. Megalencephaly also may be due to chronic brain edema (i.e., pseudotumor cerebri); tumors (ganglioneuromas, neurocutaneous syndrome); and the accumulation of abnormal metabolic substances. Megalencephaly is seen in achondrodysplasia.

MACROCRANIA

Macrocrania refers to a number of processes that directly (abnormalities of bone metabolism) or indirectly (hemolytic processes) result in thickening of the calvaria.

Microcephaly

Microcephaly is a sign of many heterogeneous disorders. Brain growth is rapid during the perinatal period, and any insult (e.g., infectious, metabolic, toxic, or vascular disorder) sustained during this period or early infancy is likely to impair brain growth and result in microcephaly. In children who have microcephaly vera, endochondral bone formation at the base of the skull is normal but severely deficient membranous bone formation of the calvaria is present secondary to hypoplasia of the frontal regions of the brain. This results in a normal-sized face but a markedly small calvaria that sharply recedes in the frontal regions. Children affected with this condition are free of associated malformations but are severely impaired intellectually. A myriad of syndromic and metabolic disorders are associated with microcephaly, some of which are hereditary (Table 18–27). Although premature closure of all the skull sutures, sometimes associated with hyperthyroidism, is a treatable cause of microcephaly, once a brain insult has resulted in microcephaly, subsequent brain growth is severely limited.

Table 18–27. Microcephaly

Etiology	Comment
Recognized Chromosomal Disorders	
Partial deletion, trisomy, or ring abnormalities; deletion of the short arm of 5 (cri du chat syndrome)	
Genetic Disorders	
Microcephaly vera	
Microcephaly with lissencephaly, schizencephaly, pachygyria, micropolygyria	Some are autosomal recessive
Agenesis of the corpus callosum	
Male microcephaly	Sex-linked recessive, autosomal dominant
Microcephaly with normal intelligence and minor malformations	
Microcephaly with Syndromes	
Prader-Willi syndrome	Hypotonia, cryptorchidism, obesity
Smith-Lemli-Opitz syndrome	Cryptorchidism, hypospadias, vomiting, seizures
Cornelia de Lange syndrome	Anteverted nostrils, low birth weight, carp mouth, micromelia, synophrys
Seckel dwarf syndrome	Bony defects, joint dislocations
Cockayne syndrome	Retinal degeneration, cataracts, brain calcifications
Leprechaunism	Sunken eyes, low-set ears, absent subcutaneous fat, hypoglycemia
Rubinstein-Taybi syndrome	Broad thumbs and toes, narrow nose, maxillary hypoplasia
Lowe syndrome	Cataracts, hypotonia, glaucoma, aminoaciduria, X-linked
Zellweger syndrome	Hypotonia, high forehead, seizures, absent DTRs, recessive inheritance, paroxysmal disorder
Hallermann-Streiff syndrome	Microphthalmia, small nose
Infections	
Congenital rubella	
CMV	
Herpes simplex	
Toxoplasmosis	
Syphilis	
Toxic Causes	
Maternal radiation	
Maternal alcohol and aminopterin ingestion	
Maternal PKU	
Vascular Causes	
Intrauterine or neonatal hypoxia–ischemia	

CMV = cytomegalovirus; DTRs = deep tendon reflexes; PKU = phenylketonuria.

References

Behrman RE (ed): Nelson Textbook of Pediatrics. 14th ed. Philadelphia, WB Saunders, 1992, Sec. 3.5, 3.10, 20.14–20.16.

DeMyer W: Megalencephaly in children. Neurology 22: 634, 1972.

Warkany J, Lemire R, Cohen M: Mental Retardation and Congenital Malformations of the Central Nervous System. Chicago, Year Book Medical Publishers, 1981.

WEAKNESS

Introduction and Neuroanatomy

Voluntary movement is directed by a conscious "will," utilizing a large number of subconscious motor mechanisms. Maintenance of proper tone and coordination of agonist, antagonist, synergistic, and fixating muscle groups involve motor nuclei of the spinal cord, cerebellum, brain stem, thalamus, basal ganglia, and motor cortex of cerebrum.

The corticospinal tract and its neurons that subserve voluntary motor activity are known as the *upper motor neuron*. The *lower motor neuron* includes the anterior horn cells in addition to their motor roots and peripheral motor nerves, the neuromuscular junctions, and the muscles. Destruction of the upper motor neuron causes loss of voluntary control but not total loss of movement. Motor nuclei of the basal ganglia, thalamus, and brain stem have their own tracts that innervate anterior horn cells and produce simple or complex stereotyped patterns of movement. Destruction of the spinal cord leaves intact simple stereotyped reflex movements coordinated by local spinal reflexes below the level of the lesion. Destruction of the lower motor neuron leads to total absence of movement because it is the final common pathway producing muscle activity.

Weakness caused by disease of the lower motor unit is different in quality from weakness produced by central, corticospinal tract lesions. The latter often is not so much an inability to move the limb as a loss of dexterous movements. The corticospinal tract permits fine motor activity, and its function is best tested by asking the patient to perform rapid alternating movements of the distal extremities. Mild dysfunction produces slowed, stiff motions. More severe dysfunction produces stiff, abnormal postures that do not respond to voluntary command. Characteristically, the posture in corticospinal tract disease consists of the forearm being flexed at the elbow and wrist and adducted close to the chest, with the leg extended and adducted. Disease of the lower motor unit produces progressive loss of strength with hypotonia and no abnormality of posture. Function is best tested by measuring the strength of individual muscle groups or, in the young child, by observing the ability to perform tasks requiring particular muscle groups (e.g., walk up or down stairs, arise from the ground, walk on toes or heels, raise the hands above the head, squeeze a ball). Table 18–28 characterizes the

Table 18–28. Corticospinal (Upper) Versus Neuromuscular (Lower) Loss of Motor Function

Clinical Sign	Neuromuscular	Corticospinal
Posture	Flaccid	Arm flexed, leg extended
Tone	Decreased	Increased
Reflexes	Decreased	Increased
Babinski reflex	Absent	Present
Atrophy	Possible	Absent
Fasciculations	Possible	Absent

findings in weakness of upper and lower motor neuron type.

Disease of the Upper Motor Neuron

Stroke is the most common cause of damage to the corticospinal tract. Tumors, trauma, infections, demyelinating syndromes, and metabolic and degenerative diseases also injure the corticospinal tract.

STROKE IN CHILDHOOD

Obstruction of blood flow may occur in arteries or veins and may be caused by local thrombosis or embolization from distant sites. Cerebral embolization characteristically occurs without warning, produces its full deficit within seconds, and may be associated with focal seizures, headache, and hemorrhagic infarction. The most common sources of cerebral emboli are the heart and the carotid artery in the neck. Cerebral thrombosis may be preceded by transient ischemic attacks that resolve completely. The deficits themselves evolve over hours in a stepwise or stuttering progression. The sudden emergence of neurologic deficits implies cerebral vascular disease, and the site of occlusion is suggested by the neurologic deficits. If clinical assessment does not reveal the cause of the stroke, a complete laboratory investigation should be undertaken.

Clinical assessment will uncover the most common sources of childhood stroke, which are congenital heart disease, sickle cell anemia (SS), meningitis, and acute and congenital hemiplegias of childhood. Less common causes include hypoxic–ischemic encephalopathy, emboli from the placenta or a dead twin fetus, infections (especially sepsis), disseminated intravascular coagulopathy, collagen vascular or related inflammatory disease, cerebral vasculitis, accidental air or fat emboli, polycythemia, drugs (amphetamines, birth control pills, cocaine), atlantoaxial dislocation, the syndrome of antiphospholipid–anticardiolipin antibodies associated with systemic lupus erythematosus, and rare complications of migraine and metabolic disorders (homocystinuria, mitochondrial myopathy with lactic acidosis).

Heart disease and its complications may give rise to thromboses in cerebral arteries or veins or emboli to cerebral arteries. Cerebral venous and arterial thromboses occur in 1–2% of infants with cyanotic congenital heart disease and probably are related to local congestion of blood flow. Predisposing factors include acute episodes of severe cyanosis, febrile illnesses, dehydration, polycythemia, hyperventilation, and iron-deficiency anemia. Sources of emboli include mural thrombi from dilated poorly contracting cardiac chambers, bacterial endocarditis, nonbacterial endocarditis, valvular disease, atrial myxoma, cardiac catheterization, and cardiac surgery. Septic emboli producing cerebral infarcts occur in 10–20% of patients who develop bacterial endocarditis.

Often, a thorough evaluation of the child with a stroke does not reveal the etiology and angiography may disclose the site of vascular occlusion, but the pathogenetic mechanism remains unknown. This condition has been labeled as *acute hemiplegia of childhood*. Children with this condition suffer a single acute episode, are not at risk for further recurrences, and do not require special treatment.

A similar problem in defining etiology pertains to children with *congenital hemiplegia*. Affected infants typically present at 6–9 mo of age with decreased use of one side of the body. CT reveals an area of encephalomalacia in the contralateral cerebral hemisphere. The details of the child's intrauterine, labor, delivery, and postnatal history often are unremarkable. Some neonates manifest focal seizures. The timing of the injury is unknown.

Completed strokes do not benefit from medical treatment. Strokes in evolution, transient ischemic attacks, or ongoing cerebral embolization may be treated with anticoagulants (intravenous heparin and oral warfarin [Coumadin]), platelet antiaggregants (aspirin and dipyridamole), or surgery to enlarge stenosed channels, excise sources of emboli, or provide alternative sources of intracerebral blood flow.

Disease of the Lower Motor Unit

Each motor neuron in the spinal cord and brain stem gives rise to a single myelinated axon that extends to muscle. After numerous branchings, each axon twig terminates in a synapse with a single muscle fiber. The presynaptic axon terminal releases acetylcholine, which traverses the synaptic cleft, binds to receptors on the muscle membrane, initiates muscle contraction, and is inactivated by acetylcholinesterase. The lower motor unit consists of all of these components.

Neuromuscular disease is illness of any component of the motor unit. The distribution of muscle weakness can point toward specific diseases (Table 18–29). Diseases affecting each component of the motor unit are lised in Table 18–30 and briefly summarized below.

Table 18–29. "Topography" of Neuromuscular Diseases

Proximal Muscle Weakness
Dystrophy
 Duchenne
 Limb girdle
Dermatomyositis; polymyositis
Kugelberg-Welander disease (late-onset spinal muscular atrophy)

Distal Limb Weakness
Polyneuropathy
 HMSN I
 HMSN II
Myotonic dystrophy
Distal myopathy

Ophthalmoplegia and Limb Weakness
Myasthenia gravis
Botulism
Myotonic dystrophy
Congenital structural myopathy

Facial and Bulbar Weakness
Myasthenia gravis
Botulism
Myotonic dystrophy
Congenital structural myopathy
Facioscapulohumeral dystrophy

HMSN = hereditary motor sensory neuropathy.

DISEASE OF THE SPINAL CORD

Acute spinal cord disease may produce a flaccid, areflexic paralysis that simulates neuromuscular disease. A child who presents with an acute or subacute flaccid paraparesis is most likely to have either an acute cord syndrome, such as transverse myelitis, a cord tumor, or the Guillain-Barré syndrome. The hallmarks of spinal cord disease are a sensory level, a motor level, disturbance of bowel and bladder function, and local spinal pain or tenderness.

DISEASES OF THE ANTERIOR HORN CELL

Werdnig-Hoffmann Disease or Spinal Muscular Atrophy

Progressive degeneration of anterior horn cells is the sole manifestation of this genetic illness, which may begin in intrauterine life or anytime thereafter and may progress at a rapid or slow pace. In general, the earlier in life that the process starts, the more rapid is the progression. Infants who already are affected at birth or who become weak within the first several months of life usually progress to flaccid quadriplegia with bulbar palsy, respiratory

Table 18–30. Diseases of the Lower Motor Unit in Infants and Children

Anterior Horn Cell	**Muscle**
Spinal muscular atrophy*	Dystrophy
Poliomyelitis	Duchenne
	Becker
Peripheral Nerve	Limb girdle
Guillain-Barré syndrome	Facioscapulohumeral
Tick paralysis	Myotonic*
Hereditary*	Congenital*
Vitamin E, B$_{12}$, and B deficiencies	Myositis
Toxins	Congenital structural myopathy
Lead	Central core
Organophosphates	Nemaline rod
Diphtheria	Centronuclear
Collagen vascular disease	Congenital fiber type of dysproportion
Paraneoplastic	Congenital muscular dystrophy
	Miscellaneous types
Neuromuscular Junction	
Myasthenia gravis	**Metabolic, Endocrine, and Mineral**
Acquired	Glycogen storage disease II (Pompe disease)
Neonatal transitory*	Carnitine metabolism abnormalities
Congenital*	Mitochondrial abnormalities
Botulism*	Thyroid excess or deficiency
	Cortisol excess or deficiency
	Hyperparathyroidism; calcium excess
	Potassium excess or deficiency

* Infants.

failure, and death within the 1st yr of life. This early fulminant form of the illness is called Werdnig-Hoffmann disease. A mild form of the illness, *Kugelberg-Welander syndrome*, begins in late childhood with proximal weakness of the legs and progresses slowly over decades. Between these extremes the illness may be unpredictable: it may begin between 6 mo and 6 yr of age and may progress rapidly, slowly, or rapidly initially and then seemingly plateau. The inheritance of all of these forms is autosomal recessive. It seems highly probable that acute and chronic spinal muscular atrophy generally are due to mutations at the same gene locus, which has been mapped by linkage studies to chromosome 5q.

The *clinical manifestations* usually are similar in all affected siblings within a single family. Infants present with progressive weakness, especially proximally; decreased spontaneous movement; and floppiness. Atrophy may be marked. Head control is lost. With time, the legs stop moving altogether and the children play only with toys placed in their hands. The range of facial expression diminishes, and drooling and gurgling increase. The eyes remain bright, open, mobile and engaging. Weakness is flaccid, with early loss of reflexes. Fasciculations sometimes can be seen in the tongue and are searched for best when the child is asleep. The infants have normal mental, social, and language skills and sensation. Breathing becomes rapid, shallow, and predominantly abdominal. In the very weak child, respiratory infections lead to atelectasis, pulmonary infection, and death. Creatine phosphokinase may be mildly elevated. The EMG shows fasciculations, fibrillations, positive sharp waves, and high-amplitude, long-duration motor units.

No *treatment* for the condition exists. Symptomatic therapy is directed toward minimizing contractures, preventing scoliosis, aiding oxygenation, preventing aspiration, and maximizing social, language, and intellectual skills. Respiratory infections are managed early and aggressively with pulmonary toilet, chest physical therapy, oxygen, and antibiotics. The use or nonuse of artificial ventilation must be individualized for each patient in each stage of the illness.

Poliomyelitis

See Chapter 10.

PERIPHERAL NEUROPATHY

The principal peripheral nerve diseases in childhood are Guillain-Barré syndrome, hereditary motor sensory neuropathy, and tick paralysis. Peripheral neuropathy produced by diabetes mellitus, alcoholism, chronic renal failure, amyloid, exposure to industrial or metal toxins, vasculitis, or the remote effects of neoplasms is a common cause of weakness and sensory loss in adults but is rare in infants and children.

Guillain-Barré Syndrome

This condition is an idiopathic peripheral neuropathy that often occurs following a respiratory or gastrointestinal infection; it is exhibited most characteristically by areflexia, flaccidity, and relatively symmetric weakness beginning in the legs and ascending to involve the arms, trunk, throat and face. Progression can occur rapidly, in hours or days, or more indolently, over weeks. Typically, the children complain of numbness or paresthesia in hands and feet and then develop a heavy weak feeling in the legs, followed by the inability to walk. The examination often reveals complete absence of reflexes even when strength is good. Objective signs of sensory loss usually are minor compared with the dramatic weakness. Meningeal signs frequently are noted. Progression to bulbar and respiratory insufficiency may occur rapidly, and close monitoring of respiratory function is necessary. The loss of arm reflexes, the absence of a sensory level, lack of spinal tenderness, and, usually, normal bowel and bladder function serve to distinguish neuropathy from a spinal cord syndrome. Dysfunction of autonomic nerves can lead to hypertension, hypotension, orthostatic hypotension, tachycardia and other arrhythmias, urinary retention or incontinence, stool retention, or episodes of abnormal sweating, flushing, or peripheral vasoconstriction. A cranial nerve variant (Miller-Fisher) may be isolated or simultaneous with peripheral nerve involvement.

Porphyria and tick paralysis may simulate Guillain-Barré syndrome. Other causes of peripheral neuropathy include vasculitis, heredity, nutritional deficiency (vitamins B_1, B_{12}, and E), endocrine disorders, infections (diphtheria, Lyme disease) and toxins (organophosphate, lead).

CSF often is normal in the 1st wk of the illness and then shows elevated protein levels without pleocytosis. Nerve conduction velocity EMG also may be normal early in the disease but then shows delay in motor nerve conduction velocity and decreased amplitude and temporal dispersion of the evoked compound motor action potential.

This illness resolves spontaneously and 75% of patients recover normal function within 1–12 mo. Twenty percent of patients are left with mild to moderate residual weakness in the feet and lower legs. The mortality rate is 5%, and death is caused by respiratory failure or complications of mechanical ventilation, cardiovascular collapse, or pulmonary embolism.

Children with moderate or severe weakness or rapidly progressive weakness should receive *treatment* in a pediatric intensive care unit. Endotracheal intubation should be performed electively in patients who exhibit either early signs of hypoventilation, accumulation of bronchial secretions, or obtunded pharyngeal or laryngeal reflexes. Prior to mechanical ventilation, respiratory sufficiency is monitored by frequent spirometric studies, including vital capacity and maximum inspiratory force. Therapy is symptomatic and rehabilitative and directed at hypertension, hypotension, and cardiac arrhythmias; pulmonary embolism; nutrition, fluids, and electrolytes; pain; skin, cornea, and joints; bowel and bladder; infection; psychologic support; and communication. Controlled studies have not supported the efficacy of ACTH or steroids but suggest that plasma exchange and intravenous immunoglobulin may be beneficial in rapidly progressive disease.

Hereditary Motor Sensory Neuropathy Charcot-Marie-Tooth Disease

Hereditary motor sensory neuropathy (HMSN), commonly called Charcot-Marie-Tooth disease, is a chronic, genetically determined polyneuropathy characterized by weakness and wasting of distal limb muscles and foot deformity. Most often, complaints begin in the preschool years with *pes cavus deformity of feet* and weakness of the ankles with frequent tripping. Examination reveals high-arched feet, bilateral weakness of foot dorsiflexors, and normal sensation despite occasional complaints of paresthesia. Progression is slow, extending over years and decades. Eventually, patients develop weakness and atrophy of the entire lower legs and hands and mild to moderate sensory loss in the hands and feet. Some patients with HMSN never develop more than mild deformity of their feet, loss of ankle reflexes, and electrophysiologic abnormalities, whereas others in the same family may be confined to a wheelchair and have difficulties performing everyday tasks with their hands in early adult life.

HMSN is a demyelinating illness with severely decreased nerve conduction velocity and hypertrophic changes on nerve biopsy. HMSN-α is a neuronal form with normal or mildly decreased nerve conduction velocity and no hypertrophic changes. Both are inherited as autosomal dominants with variable expressivity. HMSN often is caused by a large DNA duplication within chromosome 17p11.2.

Specific treatment is not available, but braces such as those that maintain the feet in dorsiflexion can improve function measurably. Early surgery is contraindicated because the progression of the disease destabilizes even good repair.

NEUROMUSCULAR JUNCTION

Acquired Myasthenia Gravis

Classic myasthenia gravis may begin in the teenage years with the acute onset of ptosis; diplopia; and ophthalmoplegia, with or without weakness; and fatigability of extremities, neck, face, and jaw. *Clinical manifestations* are least prominent on awakening in the morning and worsen as the day progresses or with exercise. In some children the disease never advances beyond ophthalmoplegia and ptosis, but others develop a progressive and potentially life-threatening illness involving all musculature, including that of respiration and swallowing.

Edrophonium chloride (Tensilon) intravenously but not saline control usually will improve strength and decrease fatigability significantly. Antiacetylcholine receptor antibodies usually can be detected in the serum, and EMG reveals a decremental response to repetitive nerve stimulation.

Treatment includes an acetylcholine esterase inhibitor such as pyridostigmine (Mestinon), thymectomy, prednisone, plasmapheresis, and immunosuppressive agents. When respirations are compromised, immediate intubation and admission to an intensive care unit are indicated.

Neonatal Transitory Myasthenia Gravis

Ten to 20% of neonates born to mothers with myasthenia gravis develop a transitory myasthenic syndrome that persists for 1–10 wk (mean = 3 wk). Almost all infants born to mothers with myasthenia will demonstrate antiacetylcholine receptor antibody, and neither antibody titer nor extent of disease in the mother predicts which neonates will display clinical disease. Symptoms and signs include ptosis, ophthalmoplegia, weak facial movements, poor sucking and feeding, hypotonia, and variable extremity weakness. Diagnosis is made by demonstrating clinical improvement lasting approximately 45 min following IM administration of neostigmine methylsulfate, 0.1 mg. Treatment with oral pyridostigmine (Mestinon) or neostig-

mine 30 min prior to feeding is continued until spontaneous resolution occurs.

Muscle Disease

DUCHENNE DYSTROPHY

Muscular dystrophy is a common sex-linked recessive trait appearing in 20–30:100,000 boys. Boys present at about 3 yr of age with inability to run properly or keep up athletically with their peers. Some have an antecedent history of mild slowness in attaining motor milestones (walking, climbing stairs). Examination reveals calf hypertrophy and mild to moderate proximal leg weakness exhibited by a hyperlordotic and waddling gait and inability to arise from the ground easily. The child typically arises from sitting by climbing up on his legs and body, the Gower sign. Weakness progresses such that arm weakness is evident by 6 yr of age, and most boys are confined to a wheelchair by 12 yr of age. By 16 yr, little mobility of arms remains and respiratory difficulties increase. Death is due to pneumonia or congestive heart failure resulting from myocardial involvement. Patients may develop obesity and mild mental retardation.

Serum creatine phosphokinase always is markedly elevated. Muscle biopsy reveals evidence of muscle fiber degeneration and regeneration accompanied by increased intrafascicular connective tissue. This disease results from absence of a large protein called dystrophin. Becker muscular dystrophy arises from an abnormality in the same gene locus that results in the presence of dystrophin that is abnormal in either amount or molecular structure. Prenatal diagnosis is possible by restriction fragment length polymorphism. Approximately one third of cases represent new mutations.

Treatment is supportive, with physical therapy, bracing, proper wheelchairs, and prevention of scoliosis. A multidisciplinary approach is recommended.

BECKER DYSTROPHY

This sex-linked muscular dystrophy is indistinguishable from Duchenne dystrophy except that onset is later and progression is slower.

LIMB GIRDLE DYSTROPHY

This is usually an autosomal recessive disease presenting with proximal leg and arm weakness. The clinical manifestations are similar to those of

Duchenne dystrophy but are seen in an older child or teenager and progress slowly over years. By mid-adult life most patients are wheelchair bound and incapacitated.

FASCIOSCAPULOHUMERAL DYSTROPHY

This condition is usually an autosomal dominant disease presenting in teenagers with facial and proximal arm weakness. Children have mild ptosis, a decrease in facial expression, inability to pucker the lips or whistle, neck weakness, difficulty in fully elevating the arms, diminished scapular muscle width, and thinness of upper arm musculature. Progression is slow, and most patients retain excellent functional capabilities for decades.

MYOTONIC DYSTROPHY

Myotonic dystrophy is exhibited either at birth with severe generalized weakness or in adolescence with slowly progressive facial and distal extremity weakness and myotonia. The adolescent type is the classic illness and is associated with cardiac arrhythmias, cataracts, male pattern baldness, and infertility in males (hypogonadism). The facial appearance is characteristic, with hollowing of muscles around temples, jaw, and neck; ptosis; facial weakness; and drooping of the lower lip. The voice is nasal and mildly dysarthric.

Some mothers with myotonic dystrophy give birth to children with the disease who are immobile and hypotonic, with expressionless faces, tented upper lips, ptosis, absence of sucking and Moro reflexes, and poor swallowing and respiration. Often, weakness and atony of uterine smooth muscle during labor leads to associated hypoxic–ischemic encephalopathy and its sequelae. The presence of congenital contractures, clubfoot, or a history of poor fetal movements indicates intrauterine neuromuscular disease.

Myotonic dystrophy is an autosomal dominant genetic disease caused by progressive expansion of a triplet repeat, GCT, on chromosome 19q13.2–13.3 in a gene designated myotonin protein kinase (MP-PK). (See Chapter 4).

CONGENITAL STRUCTURAL MYOPATHIES

These disorders are a group of congenital, often genetic, either nonprogressive or slowly progressive myopathies of uncertain etiology characterized by abnormal appearance of the muscle biopsy (see Table 18–30). The typical clinical manifestations consist of a hypotonic infant with moderately diffuse weakness involving limbs and face, often accompanied by congenitally dislocated hips, high-arched palate, clubfoot, and contractures at hips, knees, ankles or elbows secondary to intrauterine weakness. The attainment of motor milestones is moderately to severely delayed and the illness is either static or slowly progressive. Progressive kyphoscoliosis represents a significant problem in some children. Reflexes are diminished, creatine phosphokinase may be mildly elevated, EMG shows a nonspecific myopathic pattern or is normal, and muscle biopsy demonstrates characteristic changes for each entity.

METABOLIC MYOPATHIES

Glycogen storage disease type II (Pompe disease) and *muscle carnitine deficiency* are discussed in Chapter 5.

Mitochondrial myopathies are characterized by muscle biopsies that sometimes reveal ragged red fibers, representing collections of abnormal mitochondria. Many of these illnesses involve abnormalities of reactions along the respiratory chain. These syndromes have clinical manifestations that are typical of congenital structural myopathies; the course is generally progressive. Some have both CNS and neuromuscular manifestations, such as the MELAS syndrome. Important clues to this class of disorders are elevations of serum lactate and, in those with cerebral involvement, calcification of the basal ganglia.

Endocrine myopathies (hyperthyroidism, hypothyroidism, hyperparathyroidism, and Cushing syndrome), either endogenous or produced by exogenous corticosteroid administration, all are associated with proximal muscle weakness (see Chapter 17).

Hypokalemia and hyperkalemia produce weakness and loss of tendon jerks but do so in the context of a larger clinical picture that usually is easily recognizable (e.g., gastroenteritis, family history, renal failure). This encompassing picture should be specifically treated.

LABORATORY EVALUATION OF NEUROMUSCULAR DISEASES

Laboratory evaluation is required in patients who have a neuromuscular disease but in whom a careful history and physical examination have not revealed a specific diagnosis (Table 18–31). EMG nerve conduction velocity testing is moderately painful, and muscle biopsy usually requires general anesthesia.

Table 18–31. Evaluation of Neuromuscular Disease

Examine parents
Complete blood count, differential, ESR, electrolytes, BUN, creatinine, glucose, Ca^{2+}, PO_4^- alkaline phosphatase, Mg^{2+}, bilirubin, blood gases, CPK, lactate, pyruvate
Chest roentgenogram, ECG
Stool: botulism culture and toxin
Tensilon test, neostigmine test
EMG-NCV
Muscle biopsy

BUN = blood urea nitrogen; CPK = creatine phosphokinase; ECG = electrocardiogram; ESR = erythrocyte sedimentation rate; NCV = nerve conduction velocity.

Patients with Duchenne muscular dystrophy, central core myopathy, and other myopathies are susceptible to the life-threatening syndrome of **malignant hyperthermia** during administration of anesthesia comprised of succinylcholine or of potent inhalation agents such as halothane. Often, a family history of unexplained death during operations is noted. Many patients who develop malignant hyperpyrexia appear normal but have mild ptosis or facial muscle wasting and thus may have subclinical myopathies. Other patients at risk include those with kyphoscoliosis, foot deformity, dislocated hips, hypermobile hips, dislocated patella, and other musculoskeletal anomalies. Children without apparent muscle disease inherit malignant hyperpyrexia as an autosomal dominant trait. Malignant hyperpyrexia is exhibited as a rapid rise of body temperature and pCO_2, muscle rigidity, cyanosis, hypotension, arrhythmias, and convulsions. *Treatment* with IV dantrolene, sodium bicarbonate, and cooling is helpful. *Diagnosis* of the patient and family is possible with the in vitro muscle contraction test. Excessive tonic contracture on exposure to halothane and caffeine in vitro indicates susceptibility.

SEQUELAE OF NEUROMUSCULAR DISEASE

The major complications of neuromuscular illness are the development of contractures, scoliosis, and pneumonia. Prophylaxis and treatment of contractures with active range of motion exercises and bracing are important because contractures can be painful or inhibit function even when strength is adequate. Surgery to release contractures or to realign tendons is most helpful in nonprogressive or in very slowly progressive conditions. Kyphoscoliosis produces loss of function, disfigurement, and life-threatening decrease of ventilatory reserve. Vigorous prophylaxis and treatment are achieved by maintaining ambulation for as long as possible, with the provision of a properly fitted wheelchair, bracing, and, eventually, stabilizing surgery. Pneumonia in the weak patient may produce heavy secretions that are difficult to clear, progressive atelectasis, and respiratory failure. Anticipatory treatment with antibiotics, hospitalization, chest physical therapy, oxygen, and ventilatory support helps in most cases.

Neonatal and Infantile Hypotonia

Neonatal and infantile hypotonia pose certain distinctive diagnostic dilemmas. First, some neuromuscular diseases are exhibited at this age, whereas others rarely or never appear. Second, the distinction between neuromuscular paralysis and cerebral depression using the criterion of lack of movement is much more difficult in neonates than in older children who, when awake and aware, can communicate. Finally, some infants develop a unique syndrome of hypotonia, "floppiness," and hypomotility accompanied by only a small loss of observable strength. This syndrome carries a differential diagnosis quite different from that of the definitely weak infant (Table 18–32).

NEONATAL IMMOBILITY

The first step in evaluating an infant who does not move spontaneously or in response to stimulation is to determine whether *awareness* is intact. If the child is bright-eyed, and able to follow objects with the eyes, and tries to smile but unable to move, cortical activity is intact. If the face and eyes are immobile and the eyelids ptotic, the problem is more difficult. Other responses include response to light, tactile stimulation, or a bell; eye movement if the eyelids are lifted (fix on the examiner); the presence of the gag and corneal reflexes; and extremities in a posture that suggests cerebral or neuromuscular disease. If the arm and hand are positioned above the face and dropped, does the hand strike the face as it would in deep coma or paralysis? Are reflexes increased as in cerebral disease, or are they absent? If clinical examination does not settle the question, an EEG will be helpful; cerebral disease sufficient to suppress all movement will produce severe slowing of the EEG. If the EEG is normal or near normal and the infant is paralyzed, a disease of the neuromuscular unit or spinal cord is present.

If the cause of the child's immobility is depression of consciousness, the differential diagnosis is very broad (see Table 18–4). The most common

Table 18–32. Approach to Differential Diagnosis of the Floppy Infant

Weakness		No Weakness
Awareness Intact	Cerebral Depression (Flaccid Encephalopathy)	
Neuromuscular disease	Severe brain illness	Acute systemic illness
Spinal cord disease	Structural	Mental retardation
Trauma	Infectious	Specific syndromes
Tumor	Metabolic (e.g., anoxia)	Down syndrome
Vascular compromise		Cerebrohepatorenal (Zellweger peroxisomal
Malformation	Intoxication through mother	disorder)
Spina bifida	Magnesium sulfate	Oculocerebrorenal (Lowe syndrome)
Syringomyelia	Barbiturates	Kinky hair disease (Menkes
	Narcotics	syndrome—copper metabolism disorder)
	Benzodiazepines	Neonatal adrenal leukodystrophy
	General anesthesia	
		Prader-Willi syndrome
	Metabolic abnormality	
	Hypoglycemia	Connective tissue disorder
	Kernicterus	Ehlers-Danlos syndrome
		Marfan syndrome
		Congenital laxity of ligaments
		Nutritional–metabolic disease
		Rickets
		Renal tubular acidosis
		Celiac disease
		Biliary atresia
		Congenital heart disease
		Benign congenital hypotonia

causes of neonatal immobility are severe hypoxic–ischemic encephalopathy (HIE) or endogenous or exogenous intoxication. Severe HIE can result acutely in a flaccid, areflexic infant with complete ptosis, ophthalmoplegia, absent corneal and gag reflexes, and pupillary reactions that may be absent or preserved.

Mothers who, during labor, receive drugs that are cerebral depressants, such as magnesium sulfate, barbiturates, narcotics, benzodiazepines, and inhalation anesthetics, can give birth to children who are transiently floppy, apneic, and unresponsive. Rarely, infants whose mothers received magnesium sulfate and who are themselves treated with an aminoglycoside for suspected sepsis develop neuromuscular weakness because these antibiotics inhibit acetylcholine release at the neuromuscular junction. Finally, infants who are themselves treated with drugs that are cerebral depressants, who develop severe hyperbilirubinemia accompanied by kernicterus, or who develop hypoglycemia can present with a flaccid encephalopathy. Seizures may occur when the metabolic encephalopathies and HIE are present, but are unusual with drug intoxication.

HYPOTONIA WITHOUT MAJOR WEAKNESS

Some infants who appear to move well when supine in their cribs clearly are "floppy" when handled or moved. They often are first perceived as having a problem when gross motor milestones, such as rolling over, sitting, and walking, are delayed. When placed on their backs, most of these children are bright-eyed, have expressive faces, and can lift their arms and legs without apparent difficulty. However, when they are lifted, their heads flop, they "slip through" at the shoulders, do not stand upright on their legs, and form an "inverted U" in prone suspension. When placed prone as neonates, they may lay flat instead of having their arms tucked underneath them and their rumps up in the air. Passive tone is decreased, but reflexes are normal.

When this syndrome is present in the severe form in an infant who appears mentally alert but is having severe feeding problems leading to failure to thrive, the probable diagnosis is the *Prader-Willi syndrome*. Paradoxically, these children will develop severe hyperphagia and obesity in early childhood. The presence of a small penis, small testicles, or cryptorchidism in the male is a useful clue to diagnosis; small hands and feet may be seen in either sex. Approximately 60–70% of affected individuals have an interstitial deletion of chromosome 15q11q13, the origin of which is consistently paternal. Clinical manifestations similar to those of Prader-Willi syndrome, with or without feeding difficulties, occur in Down syndrome and in some infants who will later prove to have nonspecific *mental retardation*. Infants in whom the combination of severe floppiness with mental dullness or cerebral depression is seen may have one of several syndromes (Table 18–32).

Children who have a *connective tissue disorder*, such as Ehlers-Danlos syndrome, Marfan syndrome, or familial laxity of the ligaments, may exhibit marked passive hypotonia, "double jointedness," and increased skin elasticity but have normal strength and mentation. They usually achieve motor milestones normally and present to the orthopedist with peculiar postures of their feet or an unusual gait.

Finally, there are children who have *benign congenital hypotonia*. Typically, the child has been well, with an uneventful history, and appears robust except that motor milestones are delayed. The child usually presents at 9–12 mo unable to sit well or achieve a sitting position alone and unable to crawl up on hands and knees but with good verbal, social, and manipulative skills and an intelligent appearance. The head may lag a bit when the child is lifted, the child slips through slightly at the shoulders, and the extremities are floppy when shaken but the child briskly kicks arms and legs when sitting in the mother's lap and can easily bring the toes to the mouth. Parents may remember that the infant has seemed floppy from birth. This diagnosis represents a miscellaneous category of unknown causes. Some children may have mild congenital myopathies, and others mild cerebellar immaturity or dysfunction, but extensive laboratory investigation will be unrevealing and is not warranted. Most catch up to their peers and appear normal by 3 yr of age. Often, other family members have exhibited a similar developmental pattern.

References

Behrman RE (ed): Nelson Textbook of Pediatrics. 14th ed. Philadelphia, WB Saunders, 1992, Sec. 21.21–21.51.

Buist NRM, Powell BR: Approaches to the evaluation of muscle diseases. Int Pediatr 7:320, 1992.

Dubowitz V: Evaluation and differential diagnosis of the hypotonic infant. Pediatr Rev 6:237, 1985.

Gold A, Carter S: Acute hemiplegia of infancy and childhood. Pediatr Clin North Am 23:413, 1976.

Jansen PW, Perkin RM, Ashwal S: Guillain-Barré syndrome in childhood: Natural course and efficacy of plasmapheresis. Pediatr Neurol 9:16, 1993.

Miller G, Wessel HB: Diagnosis of dystrophinopathies: Review for the clinician. Pediatr Neurol 9:3, 1993.

Tulinius MH, Holme E, Kristiansson B, et al: Mitochondrial encephalomyopathies in childhood. 11. Clinical manifestations and syndromes. J Pediatr 199:251, 1991.

Tulinius MH, Holme E, Kristiansson B, et al: Mitochondrial encephalomyopathies in childhood 1. Biochemical and morphologic investigations. J Pediatr 119:242, 1991.

van der Meché FGA, Schmitz PIM, the Dutch Guillain-Barré Study Group: A randomized trial comparing intravenous immune globulin and plasma exchange in Guillain-Barré syndrome. N Engl J Med 326:1123, 1992.

NEUROCUTANEOUS DISORDERS

The skin, teeth, hair, and nails have the same embryologic origin from neuroectoderm as the brain, and abnormalities of these structures frequently are clues to neurologic disorders. Neurocutaneous disorders are dysplastic in nature, with varying neoplastic tendencies that share CNS lesions with visceral and cutaneous abnormalities. The term *phakomatosis* refers to tuberous sclerosis and neurofibromatosis, and designates the cutaneous lesions as "mother spots" or "birthmarks." Not all of the so-called neurocutaneous disorders, however, have characteristic cutaneous lesions, and not all are of neuroectodermal origin. Von Hippel–Lindau disease does not have characteristic cutaneous lesions, and both von Hippel–Lindau disease and Sturge-Weber disease are of mesenchymal rather than ectodermal origin. Over 40 conditions are referred to as neurocutaneous syndrome, but neurofibromatosis, tuberous sclerosis, Sturge-Weber disease, von Hippel–Lindau disease, and ataxia–telangiectasia are the major disorders.

Neurofibromatosis

This complex and heterogenous autosomal dominant disorder presents in two distinct fashions, neurofibromatosis (NF) I and NF II. Its frequency is approximately 1:3000. The gene for NF I is located on chromosome 17 and the gene for NF II is located on chromosome 22.

The major clinical features of NF I are the characteristic pigmented skin lesion referred to the café-au-lait spot (see Table 18–1), pigmented hamartomas of the iris called Lisch nodules, and neurofibromas of the skin.

Café-au-lait spots eventually are present in over 90% of patients who have NF I, but they may take a year to appear. More than five café-au-lait spots larger than 5 mm should suggest the possibility of NF I. In addition, freckling commonly is seen in the axillae or other intertriginous areas in NF I. The margins of café-au-lait spots may be smooth or irregular.

Lisch nodules also increase in frequency with age and eventually are present in over 90% of adults who have NF I. Approximately 25% of children will exhibit these iris nodules.

Neurofibromas may be discrete or diffuse and are composed of various combinations of Schwann cells, fibroblasts, neurons, and vascular elements. Although benign histologically and almost always involving skin, they may invade and compromise viscera, the spinal cord, or blood vessels, occasionally producing life-threatening airway, neurologic, or vascular compromise. Other manifestations include optic glioma, pheochromocytoma, skeletal dysplasias, macrocephaly, and renovascular hypertension.

Once present, as a rule, the lesions are progressive. Surgical removal of significant approachable tumors is a mainstay of *treatment*. Orthopedic management of scoliosis and pseudoarthrosis is indicated. The response of seizures to anticonvulsants and of attention deficit disorders to medication is unpredictable. Concern for the psychologic burdens of this disorder and attention to genetic counseling should be emphasized.

NF II, or central neurofibromatosis, is not associated with café-au-lait spots, Lisch nodules, or other peripheral manifestations. These children have associated brain tumors. Bilateral acoustic neuromas are diagnostic; other children have other tumors such as meningiomas or neoplasms of glial origin.

Tuberous Sclerosis

Tuberous sclerosis is an autosomal dominant disorder characterized by adenoma sebaceum, MR, and seizures. Like neurofibromatosis, developmental abnormalities of ectoderm result in disorders of segmentation and migration of cells of the brain that frequently are associated with seizures, brain tumor, and/or intellectual impairment. Tuberous sclerosis is a frequent etiology of infantile spasms.

The manifestations of tuberous sclerosis are quite different when the disorder is encountered in infancy compared with childhood or adolescence. The clinical characteristics of tuberous sclerosis that occurs in infancy include abnormal hair pigmentation, hypopigmented skin (Ash leaf) macules, seizures, rhabdomyoma of the heart, MR, and retinal hamartomas. The lesions of *adenoma sebaceum*, which actually are vascular angiokeratomas (angiofibromas) surrounding sweat glands, usually are not encountered until 2–5 yr of age. These skin lesions predominate in the malar regions and appear as pink or red macules. *Seizures*, particularly mixed astatic–akinetic and generalized tonic–clonic seizures, are prevalent in early childhood as well. In later childhood, *angioleiomyomas* involving the kidney result in hypertension and abdominal masses. *Shagreen patches*, elevated rough plaques of skin with a predilection for the lumbar and gluteal regions, develop in late childhood to early adolescence. Nodules of tissue beneath the nails (*subungual keratomas*) also become evident at this age.

Intracranial calcifications typically are subependymal in location, with a predilection for the regions around the intraventricular foramina of Monro. Subependymal lesions have a propensity to enlarge, resulting in significant intracranial masses or obstructive hydrocephalus.

Sturge-Weber Disease

This disorder is characterized by a unilateral pink–purple vascular nevus (hemangiomata) over the face ("port-wine nevus") and a similar angiomatous malformation involving the meninges over the ipsilateral side of the brain. The *facial nevus* always involves the region between the forehead and eye (the distribution of the first division of the trigeminal nerve) when the meninges are involved but also may involve the face in the distribution of the second and third divisions of the trigeminal nerve in varying combinations. The disease is not hereditary.

The *meningeal nevus* is a slow-flow angioma resulting in hypoxia and encephalomalacia of the developing underlying cortex and is most marked over the occipital and posterior parietal regions of the brain. The vascular lesion and accompanying brain encephalomalacia (cortical atrophy) result in seizures, progressive mental retardation, and contralateral hemiparesis. The seizures as well as the hemiparesis and behavioral abnormalities progress as the child becomes older. Calcium becomes detectable in the gyri of the brain underlying the angioma, and, as the intervening sulci are spared, the radiologic picture of "tram track" or "railroad track" calcifications is seen in about 60% of cases.

The *treatment* of Sturge-Weber disease is controversial. Children treated with successful early surgical resection appear to develop more normally and have better seizure control than those treated with anticonvulsants alone. The degree of hemiparesis also is significantly less in those managed surgically, but significant morbidity and mortality as a result of the hemispherectomy are noted.

The vascular nevus involves the canal of Schlemm in about 25% of children (those with lesions above and below the orbit) and results in obstructive glaucoma. Ophthalmologic evaluations and treatment therefore are mandatory in these children. Laser treatment may improve the cutaneous lesion.

References

Behrman RE (ed): Nelson Textbook of Pediatrics. 14th ed. Philadelphia, WB Saunders, 1992, Sec. 20.39–20.44.

Chalhub EG: Neurocutaneous syndromes in children. Pediatr Clin North Am 23:499, 1976.

Korf BR: Diagnostic outcome in children with multiple café au lait spots. Pediatrics 90:924, 1992.

Riccardi VM: Type 1 neurofibromatosis and the pediatric patient. Curr Probl Pediatr 22:66, 1992.

MOVEMENT DISORDERS

Movement disorders are due to abnormalities of the extrapyramidal system, which is composed of the basal ganglia and its connections. Disorders of movement may be *bradykinetic*, slowness of movement; *hypokinetic*, paucity of movement; or *hyperkinetic*, excessive involuntary movements. Bradykinesia and hypokinesia describe the agonizingly slow gait, halting speech patterns, apparent inactivity, and paucity of facial expression seen in children with extrapyramidal disorders. The hyperkinetic disorders are associated with many disease states and, as a group, are activated by stress and fatigue but disappear in sleep. *Segmental myoclonic* abnormalities refer to activity in isolated muscle groups (e.g., the palatal myoclonus) that does not disappear in sleep.

Chorea

Chorea is a hyperkinetic, rapid, unsustained, irregular, purposeless, nonpatterned movement. Muscle tone is decreased. Choreiform movement abnormalities may be congenital, familial, metabolic, vascular, toxic, infectious, or neoplastic in origin. The movements may occur alone or as part of a more extensive neurologic disorder (e.g., Sydenham chorea, Huntington chorea, cerebral palsy, Wilson disease, toxins, drugs). Fidgety behavior, inability to sit still, clumsiness, dysarthria, and an awkward gait may occur. The exact site of dysfunction within the extrapyramidal system is unknown.

Athetosis

Athetosis is a hyperkinetic, slow, coarse, writhing movement that is more pronounced in distal muscles. Muscle tone is increased. Athetosis frequently is seen in combination with chorea (choreoathetosis) and usually is present in conjunction with other neurologic signs. It may be seen in virtually all the disorders mentioned for chorea, but the most prominent cause is encephalopathy. Athetosis is a prominent feature of Hallervorden-Spatz disease, Wilson disease, and Pelizaeus-Merzbacher dystrophy.

Dystonia

Dystonia is a hyperkinetic, sustained, slow, twisting motion (torsion spasm) that may progress to a fixed posture and can be activated by repetitive movement (i.e., action dystonia). It usually begins in the legs when appendicular muscles are involved, and in the neck or trunk when axial muscles are involved. Dystonia is a movement disorder with many causes and associated neurologic signs. *Tardive dyskinesia* usually is associated with antipsychotic drug use; darting tongue movements, incessant flexion and extension of the distal muscles, standing and marching in place, and a perception of restlessness are common.

Tremor

Tremor is a hyperkinetic, rhythmic, oscillatory movement caused by simultaneous contractions of antagonistic muscles. The amplitude and frequency are regular. In children, tremor is usually of physiologic, familial, or cerebellar origin, but may be seen in association with other disease processes (thyrotoxicosis, hypoglycemia, Wilson disease) or drugs (bronchodilators, amphetamines, or tricyclic antidepressants).

Myoclonus

Myoclonus is a hyperkinetic, brief flexion contraction of a muscle group, resulting in a sudden jerk. Myoclonus may be epileptic or nonepileptic. Nonepileptic myoclonus is distinguished from tremor in that it is a simple contraction of an agonist muscle, whereas tremor is a simultaneous contraction of agonist and antagonist muscles. Myoclonus is seen as a manifestation of various epilepsies as well as of infectious, toxic, and metabolic encephalopathies.

Tic

Tic movements are similar to myoclonus but are much more stereotyped and involve the face, shoulder, and arm. Motor tics in association with vocal tics are characteristic of Tourette syndrome.

Tourette syndrome consists of a chronic tic disorder that begins in early childhood. The severity and form of the tics vary over months and years; vocal tics are common. The pathophysiology underlying the tics is unknown, but a family history of tics is elicited in more than 50% of cases. Treatment consists of psychologic support and pharmacologic therapy.

References

Appel S: Movement disorders. Neurol Clin 2:1, 1981.
Behrman RE (ed): Nelson Textbook of Pediatrics. 14th ed. Philadelphia, WB Saunders, 1992, Sec. 20.45–20.48.

Common Orthopaedic Problems of Children

19

George H. Thompson

GENERAL CONSIDERATIONS

Multiple mechanisms produce orthopaedic problems that are specific to childhood; other pathologic mechanisms are common to all age groups (Table 19–1). Most pediatric orthopaedic problems involve the spine and lower extremities, especially the hips and feet. Upper extremity abnormalities, other than trauma, occur less frequently. It is important to have a basic understanding of the various pediatric musculoskeletal system disorders, including diagnosis and nonoperative management. In addition to the challenge of identifying pathologic processes, the necessity for clearly discerning ongoing physiologic, developmental, or maturational changes from abnormal events confronts the pediatrician. What may be normal at one age may be pathologic at another.

In Utero Positioning

In the neonate, the imprint of intrauterine posture may be evident. Posture, which reflects the position in utero, produces joint and muscle contractures and affects torsional alignment and bowing of long bones, especially of the lower extremities (Fig. 19–1). All normal full-term newborns have 20–30 degree hip and knee flexion contractures. These decrease to neutral by 4–6 mo of age. The newborn hip externally rotates in extension 80–90 degrees and has limited internal rotation to 0–10 degrees. The normal newborn foot also may reflect the in utero position. Most commonly, in utero feet are in the tucked-under position, which can be observed after birth. On inspection, the forefoot appears adducted or deviated inwardly with respect to the hindfoot, the heel may be inclined medialward, and the foot tends to be pointed down at the ankle. If the foot can be positioned so that the lateral border is straight, the heel inclined slightly toward the lateral aspect, and the foot dorsiflexed to above a right angle, the clinical diagnosis of normal in utero posturing is validated.

The face also may be distorted, whereas the spine and upper extremities are less affected by in utero positioning. The effects of in utero position therefore are physiologic in origin but produce parental concern. The child may be 3–4 yr of age before the intrauterine effects resolve.

Developmental Milestones/Neurologic Maturation

Neural maturation, marked by the passage of motor milestones at the regular intervals, is important for normal musculoskeletal development (see Chapter 1). A trophic relationship exists between skeletal form and gross motor development. The concept of normal neurologic development, therefore, must be included in the definition of a normal musculoskeletal system. Any process that produces a neurologic abnormality may secondarily cause an aberration of normal skeletal growth. Some of the neurologic influence on skeletal growth is mediated by normal muscle function, and, thus, diseases that primarily affect skeletal muscle also may produce aberrations of growth and development.

Gait

Disturbances of gait, including limp, are common manifestations of pediatric orthopaedic disorders (Tables 19–2 and 19–3). Understanding the normal development aspects of gait is helpful in distinguishing maturational from pathologic processes. Normal gait (walking on level ground) is composed of a stance phase and a swing phase. The gait cycle is the interval between stance phases on the same limb. The stance phase (60%) is performed when the foot, which bears all weight, contacts the ground; it begins with the heel strike and ends with the toeoff. In the swing phase (40%), the foot is off the ground. The early child's or toddler's (12–18 mo) gait is very hesitant and inconsistent. The gait is broad based and characterized by forefoot, flatfoot, or heel-type initial ground contact, not accompanied by the reciprocal arm swing.

Table 19–1. Mechanisms of Common Pediatric Orthopaedic Problems

Category	Mechanism	Example
Congenital		
Malformation	Teratogenesis prior to 12th wk of gestation	Spina bifida
Disruption	Amniotic band constriction Fetal varicella infection	Extremity amputation Limb scar/atrophy
Deformation	Leg compression Neck compression	Developmental hip dislocation Torticollis
Dysplasia	Abnormal cell growth or metabolism	Osteogenesis imperfecta Skeletal dysplasias
Acquired		
Infection	Pyogenic—hematogenous spread	Osteomyelitis, septic arthritis
Inflammation	Antigen–antibody reaction Immune mediated	Juvenile rheumatoid arthritis Systemic lupus erythematosus
Trauma	Mechanical forces, overuse	Child abuse, sports injuries, accidents, fractures, dislocations, tendonitis
Tumor	Primary bone tumor Metastasis to bone from other site Bone marrow tumor	Osteosarcoma Neuroblastoma Leukemia, lymphoma

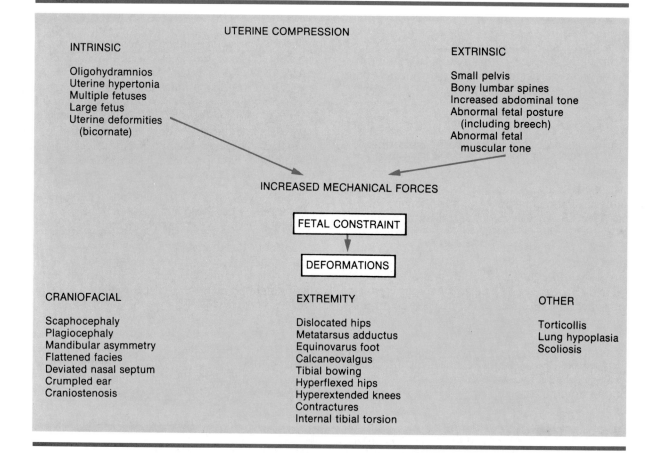

Figure 19–1. Deformation abnormalities resulting from uterine compression.

Table 19–2. Differential Diagnosis of Gait Disturbances (Limping)

Early Walker (1–3 yr)
Painful Limp
    Septic arthritis/osteomyelitis
    Transient monoarticular synovitis
    Occult trauma ("toddler's fracture")
    Intervertebral discitis

Painless Limp
    Developmental dysplasia of the hip (DDH)
    Neuromuscular disorder
        Cerebral palsy
    Lower extremity length inequality

Child (3–10 yr)
Painful limp
    Septic arthritis/osteomyelitis
    Transient monoarticular synovitis
    Trauma
    Rheumatologic disorders
        Juvenile rheumatoid arthritis
    Intervertebral discitis
    Legg-Calvé-Perthes disease (LCPD)—acute

Painless Limp
    DDH
    LCPD—chronic
    Lower extremity length inequality
    Neuromuscular disorder
        Cerebral palsy
        Muscular dystrophy (Duchenne)

Adolescent (11 yr–maturity)
Painful Limp
    Septic arthritis/osteomyelitis
    Trauma
    Rheumatologic disorder
    Slipped capital femoral epiphysis (SCFE)—acute

Painless limp
    SCFE—chronic
    DDH—acetabular dysplasia
    Lower extremity length inequality
    Neuromuscular disorder

. *Limping* is either painless or painful (Table 19–2). A painful limp is characterized by acute onset and usually is due to trauma, infection (including sepsis), or acquired disorders producing noninfectious, inflammatory disease (Table 19–3). Stance phase and stride length are shortened in an attempt to spend as little time as possible on the involved limb. Trunk shift to the opposite side also decreases stress while maintaining balance. This is referred to as an **antalgic gait.** A painless limp is characterized by normal stance phase but with a persistent trunk sway. This type of gait is called a **Trendelenburg gait.** Painless limping (Table 19–2) may be associated with neuromuscular disorders produc-

ing muscle weakness about the hip, especially in the gluteus medius muscle, the major hip abductor. This muscle stabilizes the pelvis during stance phase and prevents a pelvic drop to the opposite side. Trauma and then weakness of this muscle or inflammatory hip disorders are the most common causes of limping. Disorders that have bilateral involvement produce a **waddling gait.**

Knee pathology, usually from trauma, can produce a limp by limiting knee flexion and causing the child to circumduct the leg and elevate the pelvis during swing phase. It also produces a short-

Table 19–3. Mechanisms of Gait Disturbances and Extremity Pain

Mechanical
Trauma, fracture, sprain
Sports injury; overuse injury
Child abuse
Dysplastic lesions

Osseous
Legg-Calvé-Perthes disease
Slipped capital epiphysis
Osteomyelitis
Discitis
Osteoid osteoma

Articular
Septic arthritis
Toxic synovitis
Rheumatic disease (JRA, SLE)
Hemophilia

Neurologic
Guillain-Barré syndrome (other peripheral neuropathies)
Intoxication
Cerebellar ataxia
Brain tumor
Lesion occupying spinal cord space
Myopathy
Hemiplegia
Sympathetic reflex dystrophy

Hematologic
Sickle cell pain crisis
Leukemia
Metastatic tumor
Bone tumor
Histiocytosis

Other
Kawasaki disease
Conversion reaction
Gaucher disease
Scurvy
Rickets

JRA = juvenile rheumatoid arthritis; SLE = systemic lupus erythematosus.

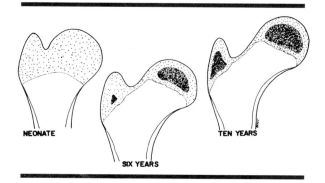

Figure 19–2. Lightly stippled areas represent cartilage composition, whereas heavily darkened areas are zones of ossification. (From Tachdjian MO: Congenital Dislocation of the Hip. New York, Churchill Livingstone, 1982, p 104.)

ened stance phase. Poor dorsiflexion of the foot resulting from weakness (peroneal nerve injury or peripheral neuropathy) or trauma causes increased knee flexion for toe clearance during the swing phase, resulting in a **steppage gait.** Toe-walking, which is common in early walkers, may be due to habit, leg length discrepancy, underlying neuromuscular disorder (cerebral palsy), or a congenital contracture of the gastrocnemius and soleus muscles (tendo Achillis or heel cord).

Growth and Development

During the growing years, the ends of long bone contain a much greater proportion of cartilage than after maturity (Fig. 19–2). The high cartilage content (articular and growth plate or physeal) leads to a unique vulnerability from trauma and metaphyseal infections of the physis and joint space.

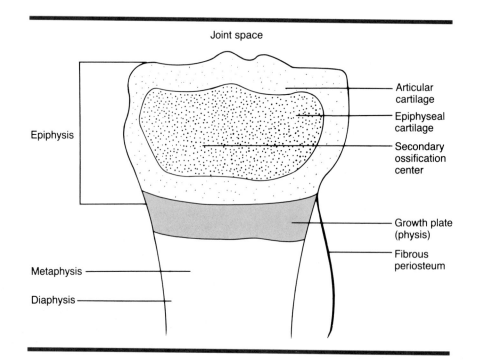

Figure 19–3. Schematic of long bone structure. The shaft, or *diaphysis,* is distal to the *metaphysis,* which is the closest extension of endochondral bone. The epiphyseal growth plate *(physis)* is the avascular cartilage between the articular surface and the metaphyseal bone. The growth plate is the region of longitudinal bone growth. The contribution to eventual bone length varies: 80% for the proximal humerus, 20% for the distal humerus, 75% for the distal radius, 80% for the distal ulna, 70% for the distal femur, 57% for the proximal tibia, and 60% for the proximal fibula. When growth is complete, the epiphyseal growth plate is ossified or closed. The cartilaginous epiphyseal plate is supported by internal interdigitation with the metaphyseal bone and externally by the insertion of the fibrous periosteum. (Modified from Shapiro F: Epiphyseal disorders. N Engl J Med 317:1702, 1987.)

Table 19–4. Glossary of Orthopaedic Terminology

Abduction	Movement away from the midline
Adduction	Movement toward and possibly across the midline
Anteversion	Increased angulation of the femoral head and neck with respect to the knee in the frontal plane
Apophysis	Bone growth center that is not a growth plate and that has a strong muscle insertion (e.g., greater trochanter of femur)
Arthroplasty	Surgical reconstruction of a joint
Arthrotomy	Surgical incision into a joint
Calcaneus	Dorsiflexion of hindfoot
Cavovarus	High longitudinal or medial arch of foot with plantar-flexed supinated forefoot and hindfoot varus
Cavus	High longitudinal arch of the foot (usually plantar-flexed forefoot)
Dislocation	Complete loss of contact between two joint surfaces
Equinus	Plantar flexion of the forefoot, hindfoot, or entire foot
Extension	Means to straighten, and is the reverse of flexion
External or lateral rotation	Lateral rotation away from the midline
Flexion	Means to bend
Internal or medial rotation	Inward rotation, toward the midline
Subluxation	Incomplete loss of contact between two joint surfaces
Valgum	Angulation of a bone or joint in which the apex is toward the midline; genu valgum results in knock-knee, because the angulation of the knee is midline
Varum	Angulation of a bone or joint away from the midline; genu varum results in bowleg because the angulation is away from the midline

Special anatomic features within the child's skeletal system stimulate and support the various kinds of skeletal growth that continuously occur in the immature skeletal (Fig. 19–3). The epiphyseal growth plate, also called the physis, provides for longitudinal growth of the bones. Articular cartilage provides for enlargement of the bone ends and also for growth of some of the small bones largely covered by articular cartilage, such as the carpals and tarsals. The perichondrium and the perios-

teum provide apositional growth or circumferential growth of the cartilaginous and bony skeletal, respectively. Trauma, infection, nutritional deficiency (rickets), regional soft tissue processes, inborn errors of macromolecular metabolism (mucopolysaccharidosis, mucolipidosis, Gaucher disease, and disorders of collagen or cartilage synthesis), and other metabolic processes (oxalosis, renal tubular acidosis, uremia, and endocrine excess or deficiencies) may affect each of these processes, producing a distinct aberration in the particular growth function.

Orthopaedic Terminology

The terminology used in orthopedics to describe position, motion, and function can be confusing. Some of the common orthopaedic terminology is summarized in Table 19–4.

References

Behrman RE (ed): Nelson Textbook of Pediatrics. 14th ed. Philadelphia, WB Saunders, 1992, Sec. 24.1.

Scoles PV (ed): Pediatric Orthopaedics in Clinical Practice. 2nd ed. Chicago, Year Book Medical Publishers, 1988.

Todd FN, Lamoreaux LW, Skinner SR, et al: Variations in the gait of normal children. A graph applicable to the documentation of abnormalities. J Bone Joint Surg 71-A:196, 1989.

THE HIP

The hip is a ball (femoral head) and socket (acetabulum) design that provides the skeleton with structural balance and stability. The femoral head and acetabulum have a trophic relationship and are interdependent for normal growth and development (Fig. 19–4). When this trophic relationship is interrupted, abnormal hip development follows. Additionally, muscle balance and activity related to appropriate gross motor development are essential to normal development of the hip. The blood supply to the capital femoral epiphysis (femoral head) is quite unique. The capital femoral epiphysis and femoral neck lie intracapsularly but the blood supply is extraosseous, lying on the surface of the femoral neck and entering the epiphysis peripherally. This makes the blood supply to the femoral head vulnerable to damage from septic arthritis, trauma, and other vascular insults. *Avascular necrosis* or *osteonecrosis*, either as an idiopathic process or secondary to other disorders, is a common problem in children.

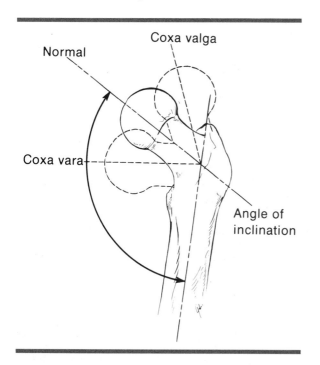

Figure 19–4. Coxa vara and coxa valga. The neck shaft angle or α angle is measured on an anteroposterior roentgenogram. This angle is formed by a line drawn through the femoral shaft center and one bisecting the head and neck. Normally, the value of this angle decreases with age. A reasonably accurate neck–shaft angle measurement may be made on an anteroposterior pelvic roentgenogram by placing the patient's hips in maximum internal rotation. Otherwise, because of the illusion caused by anteversion or external rotation on a one-plane roentgenogram, the measured neck–shaft angle value may be considerably larger than the true value. Internal femur rotation has a negligible effect on the neck–shaft angle. (From Chung SMK: Hip Disorders in Infants and Children. Philadelphia, Lea & Febiger, 1981, p 85.)

Developmental Dysplasia of the Hip

This disorder represents abnormal development or dislocation of the hip; the hips at birth usually are not dislocated but rather "dislocatable." Dislocations tend to occur following delivery. Because dislocations are not truly congenital in origin, the term development dysplasia of the hip (DDH) is suggested rather than congenital dysplasia or dislocation. DDH is classified into two major groups: *typical*, in a neurologically normal infant, and *teratologic*, when there is an underlying neuromuscular disorder (myelodysplasia or arthrogryposis multiplex congenita) or syndrome complex. This latter type of dislocation occurs in utero. Typical DDH is the most common form and is discussed below.

Etiology. The etiology of DDH is multifactorial. Physiologic factors include: positive family history (20%), generalized ligamentous laxity, maternal estrogen and other hormones associated with pelvic relaxation, and female predominance (9:1). Mechanical factors include primigravida (first born), breech presentation, and postnatal posturing. The positive family history and the generalized ligamentous laxity are related factors. Maternal estrogens and other hormones associated with pelvic relaxation also result in further, although temporary, relaxation of the newborn hip joint.

Approximately 60% of children with typical DDH are first born and 30–50% are breech. In this presentation, the fetal pelvis is positioned in the maternal pelvis, resulting in extreme hip flexion and limitation of hip motion. Increased hip flexion results in stretching of the already lax capsule and ligament teres. It also produces posterior uncoverage of the femoral head. This position, as well as decreased hip motion, alters the normal trophic relationship of the hip, resulting in abnormal development of the cartilaginous acetabulum. The sex ratio of infants with DDH who developed in a breech presentation declines to 2:1 female to male. This decline substantiates the importance of the mechanical factors of the breech position in the development of DDH. There is also an association of congenital muscular torticollis (14–20%) and metatarsus adductus (1–10%) with DDH. The presence of either of these two conditions requires a careful examination of the hips.

Postnatal factors also are important determinants in the development of DDH. Maintaining the hips in the position of adduction and extension is a major factor leading to dislocation. Placing the extremities in this position puts the unstable hip under pressure as a result of the normally present hip flexion and abduction contractures. The femoral head, as a consequence, can be displaced from the acetabulum over several days, weeks, or perhaps months.

Clinical Manifestations. Common physical findings in infants with DDH include positive Barlow test (unstable or dislocatable hip), positive Ortolani test (dislocated hip), limitation of hip abduction, asymmetric thigh skinfolds, uneven knee levels (Galeazzi sign), and the absence of normal knee flexion contracture.

The *Barlow test* is the most important maneuver in examining the newborn hip. This is a provocative test that attempts to dislocate the unstable hip. This test is performed by stabilizing the pelvis with one hand and then flexing and adducting the oppo-

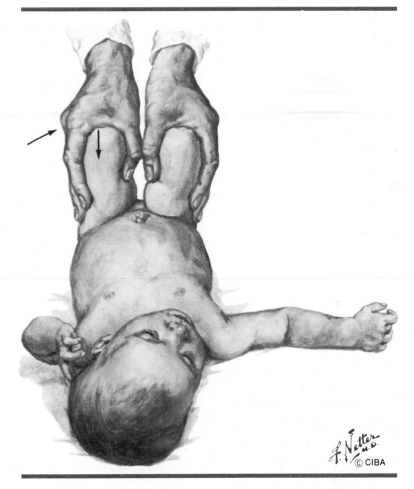

Figure 19–5. Barlow (dislocation) test. Reverse of Ortolani test. If the femoral head is in the actabulum at the time of examination, the Barlow test is performed to discover any hip instability. The baby's thigh is grasped as above and adducted with gentle downward pressure. Dislocation is palpable as the femoral head slips out of the acetabulum. Diagnosis is confirmed with the Ortolani test. (From Robert N, Hensinger MD: Congenital dislocation of the hip. Clin Symp 31[1]:5, 1979. Copyright 1978. CIBA-GEIGY Corporation. Reproduced with permission from Clinical Symposia by Frank H. Netter, M.D. All rights reserved.)

site hip and applying a posterior force (Fig. 19–5). If the hip is dislocatable, this usually is felt readily. Following release of the posterior pressure, the hip usually will spontaneously relocate. It has been estimated that only 1:100 newborns has clinically unstable hips (subluxation or dislocation) and only 1:800–1000 infants eventually develops a true dislocation. The *Ortolani test* is a maneuver to reduce a recently dislocated hip. It is most likely to be positive in infants that are 1–2 mo of age because adequate time must have passed for the true dislocation to have occurred. In performing this test, the thigh is flexed and abducted and the femoral head is lifted anteriorly into the acetabulum (Fig. 19–6). If reduction is possible, the relocation will be felt as a "clunk," not a "click." After 2 mo of age, manual reduction of a dislocated hip usually is not possible because of the development of soft tissue contractures. Limitation of hip abduction is indicative of soft tissue contractures and may indicate DDH (Fig. 19–7). Conversely, hip abduction contractures

may indicate dysplasia of the contralateral hip. An asymmetric number of thigh skinfolds and apparent shortening of an extremity when the supine infant's feet are placed together on the examining table with the hips and knees flexed is suspicious for DDH because these findings suggest proximal displacement of the femoral head. In older or walking children, complaints of limping, waddling (bilateral DDH), increased lumbar lordosis (swayback), toe-walking, and in-toeing may be associated with an unrecognized DDH.

A common concern regarding an unstable hip is the presence of a hip "click." These usually are not pathologic and are secondary to breaking the surface tension across the hip joint, snapping of gluteal tendons, patellofemoral motion, or femorotibial (knee) rotation.

Roentgenographic Evaluation. Ultrasonography is a popular method for initial evaluation and following the results of conservative treatment in

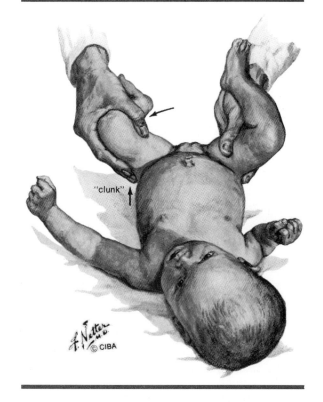

"clunk"

Figure 19–6. Ortolani (reduction) test. With the baby relaxed and content on a firm surface, the hips and knees are flexed to 90 degrees. The hips are examined one at a time. The examiner grasps the baby's thigh with the middle finger over the greater trochaner, and lifts the thigh to bring the femoral head from its dislocated posterior position to opposite the acetabulum. Simultaneously, the thigh is gently abducted, reducing the femoral head into the acetabulum. In a positive finding, the examiner senses reduction by a palpable, nearly audible "clunk." (From Robert N, Hensinger MD: Congenital dislocation of the hip. Clin Symp 31[1]:5, 1979. Copyright 1979. CIBA-GEIGY Corporation. Reproduced with permission from Clinical Symposia by Frank H. Netter, M.D. All rights reserved.)

newborns and infants (<3 mo) with DDH. Hip stability as well as acetabular development can be assessed accurately by an experienced ultrasonographer, and this avoids the use of ionizing radiation.

Roentgenographic evaluation is useful in older infants (>3 mo) and includes an anteroposterior (AP) and Lauenstein (frog) lateral roentgenographs of the pelvis. The ossific nucleus does not appear until 4–6 mo of age and may be further delayed in DDH. Line measurements usually are made in order to determine the relationship of the femoral head to the acetabulum. Arthrography, computer-ized tomography (CT) scans, and magnetic resonance imaging (MRI) may be beneficial in select or difficult cases.

Treatment.   The treatment of DDH is individualized and depends on the child's age at diagnosis. The goal is a concentric and stable reduction that results in normal growth and development of the hip. When an unstable hip is recognized at birth, maintenance of the hip in the position of flexion and abduction ("human" position) for 1–2 mo usually is sufficient. This position maintains reduction of the femoral head and allows for tightening of the ligamentous structures as well as for stimulation of normal growth and development of the femoral head and acetabulum. Usually double or triple diapers are sufficient. Treatment usually is continued until there is clinical stability of the hip and the radiographic or ultrasonography measurements are within normal limits. Between 1 and 6 mo of age the Pavlik harness is indicated. It places the hips in the human position by flexing the hips more than 90 degrees (preferably 100–110 degrees) and providing gentle abduction. This redirects the femoral head toward the acetabulum. Usually, spontaneous relocation of the femoral head occurs within 3–4 wk. The Pavlik harness is approximately 95% successful in dysplastic or subluxated hips and 80% in true DDH. If a reduction does not occur, a surgical closed reduction is attempted. This consists of preliminary skin traction for 1–3 wk to stretch the soft tissue contractures, percutaneous adductor tenotomy, closed reduction, and application of a hip spica cast in the "human" position. In the older infant (6–18 mo), surgical closed reduction is the major method of treatment. If, at the time of closed reduction, the hip shows significant residual instability, an open reduction may be indicated. Beyond 18 mo of age, the dysplastic changes are so advanced that open reduction followed by pelvic or femoral osteotomy, or both, is necessary.

Complications.   The most important and severe complication of DDH is avascular necrosis (osteonecrosis) of the femoral head or capital femoral epiphysis (CFE). This is an iatrogenic complication. Reduction of the femoral head under pressure produces cartilaginous compression, and this can result in occlusion of the intra-articular, extraosseous epiphyseal vessels and produce partial or total CFE infarction. Revascularization follows, but abnormal growth and development may occur, especially if the growth plate is severely damaged. The hip is most vulnerable to this complication prior to the development of the ossific nucleus (4–6 mo).

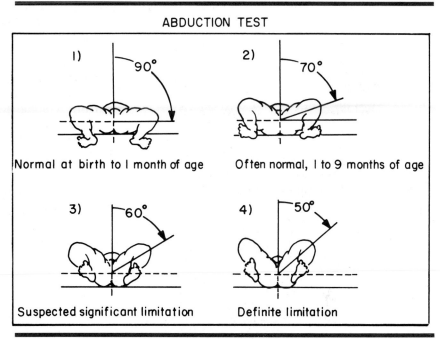

Figure 19–7. Hip abduction test. Place the child supine, flex the hips 90 degrees, and fully abduct. While the normal abduction range is quite broad, one can suspect hip disease in any patient who lacks more than 35–45 degrees of abduction. (From Chung SMK: Hip Disorders in Infants and Children. Philadelphia, Lea & Febiger, 1981, p 69.)

Septic Arthritis and Osteomyelitis

See Chapter 10.

Transient Monoarticular Synovitis

Transient synovitis of the hip is a common cause of limping and is characterized by acute onset of pain, limp, and mild restriction of hip motion, especially abduction and internal rotation. This is a diagnosis of exclusion because septic arthritis of the hip must be excluded. The etiology of transient synovitis remains uncertain. Possible etiologies have included active or recent infection, especially viral syndromes; trauma; and hypersensitivity. Approximately 70% of involved children have a nonspecific viral upper respiratory infection 7–14 days prior to the onset of hip symptoms. Biopsy specimens from the hip joint of patients with transient synovitis have demonstrated synovial hypertrophy secondary to nonspecific inflammatory reaction. Hip joint aspirations, if necessary, will be negative, although a small synovial effusion is common.

Clinical Manifestations. The mean age of onset is 6 yr, with most patients being 3–8 yr of age. The acute onset of pain is felt in the groin, anterior thigh, or knee. It must be remembered that any child with nontraumatic anterior thigh or knee pain must be evaluated carefully for hip pathology because this is the site of referred pain. Patients usu-

ally are ambulatory and the hip is not held in the flexed, abducted, and laterally rotated position typical of septic arthritis unless a significant effusion is present. Children usually are afebrile and limp. The white blood cell count and erythrocyte sedimentation rate usually are normal or slightly elevated.

Roentgenographic Evaluation. AP and frog lateral roentgenographs of the pelvis usually will be normal. Occasionally, ultrasound of the hip may be useful in demonstrating the hip joint effusion. Bone scans help differentiate a septic process.

Treatment. Bed rest (~7 days) and non–weight bearing until the pain resolves, followed by limited activities (1–2 wk) thereafter, are the treatments of choice. This sometimes is difficult because children want to return to normal activities when their symptoms resolve. If the child returns to normal activities too early, exacerbation of symptoms can occur. Nonsteroidal anti-inflammatory agents may be helpful.

Legg-Calvé-Perthes Disease

Legg-Calvé-Perthes disease (LCPD) is idiopathic avascular necrosis (osteonecrosis) of the CFE and the associated complications in a growing child. This disorder is caused by an interruption of the

CFE blood supply. It is more common in males (4–5:1) and is bilateral in approximately 20% of patients. Children with LCPD have delayed bone ages, disproportionate growth, and mild short stature.

Clinical Manifestations. The clinical onset occurs between the ages of 2 and 12 yr (mean age of 7 yr). There is mild or intermittent pain in the anterior thigh, limp, or both. The classic presentation has been described as a "painless" limp. The pertinent early physical findings include antalgic gait; muscle spasm and mild restriction of motion, especially abduction and internal rotation; proximal thigh atrophy; and mild shortness of stature.

Roentgenographic Evaluation. Roentgenographic assessment is necessary to determine the disease progression, sphericity of the femoral head, possibility of CFE collapse and extrusion, and the response to treatment. AP and frog lateral pelvic roentgenographs usually are adequate, but occasionally additional procedures such as arthrography, bone scans, and MRI may be useful. Bone scans and MRI are helpful in recognizing early LCPD but are of limited value in assessing the extent of CFE involvement or following the disease progression.

Prognosis. The short-term prognosis concerns femoral head deformity at the completion of the healing stage. The long-term prognosis involves the potential for osteoarthritis of the hip in adulthood. The six prognostic factors for the short-term prognosis are sex, age at clinical onset, extent of CFE involvement, femoral head containment, hip range of motion, and premature CFE closure. The prognostic factors for the development of late degenerative arthritis include femoral head deformity and age at clinical onset. Older children with significant residual femoral head deformity are at risk for the development of degenerative arthritis. The incidence is essentially 100% in children who are 10 yr of age or older at onset. This is compared to a negligible risk in children 5 yr or less and 38% when onset occurs between 6 and 9 yr.

Treatment. LCPD is a local, self-healing disorder. Prevention of femoral head deformity and secondary osteoarthritis are the only justifications for treatment. There are four basic treatment goals: elimination of hip irritability; restoration and maintenance of a good range of hip motion; prevention of CFE collapse, extrusion, or subluxation; and attainment of a spherical femoral head at healing. Treatment utilizes the concept of containment; the femoral head is contained within the acetabulum so the latter acts as a mold for the reossifying CFE. This is accomplished by nonsurgical containment using abduction casts and orthoses or by surgical containment with proximal femoral varus osteotomy, with or without derotation, and pelvic osteotomies to redirect the acetabulum and thereby contain the femoral head in the position of weight bearing. The long-term results of containment treatment, orthotic or surgical, are 75–90% satisfactory (round or oval femoral head).

Slipped Capital Femoral Epiphysis

Slippage of the capital femoral epiphysis (SCFE) is the most common adolescent hip disorder.

Etiology. The etiology of SCFE is unknown. An endocrine basis has been suggested because SCFE frequently occurs in adolescents who are either obese and have delayed skeletal maturation or tall and thin, following a recent growth spurt. In obese children, a low level of sex hormones has been postulated, whereas in tall, thin children an overabundance of growth hormone is implicated. It is known that both sex hormones and growth hormones alter the rate of proliferation of the cartilage cells in the growth plate (physis) and the rate of skeletal growth. SCFE also can occur as a complication of an underlying endocrine disorder, such as hypothyroidism, pituitary disorders, pseudohypoparathyroidism, and treatment with recombinant growth hormone. When a SCFE occurs prior to puberty, a hormonal abnormality or systemic disorder should be suspected. Nonetheless, the histopathology of SCFE indicates mechanical factors as the ultimate cause of slippage. Obesity produces high shear forces across the weakened and obliquely oriented growth plate.

Roentgenographic Evaluation. AP and frog lateral roentgenographs of the pelvis are used for assessment of the hips. The earliest sign of SCFE is widening of the growth plate without slippage. This is considered a preslip condition. As slippage occurs, the CFE stays in the acetabulum and the femoral neck rotates anteriorly and occasionally superiorly, resulting in a varus, retroverted femoral head and neck (Fig. 19–8). The degree of slippage between the CFE and the femoral neck can be classified into mild (0–33%), moderate (34–50%), and severe (>50%) by roentgenographic measurement techniques. Slippage resulting in a valgus deformity is rare except in metabolic disorders such as renal osteodystrophy and Marfan syndrome, and as a sequela to irradiation therapy.

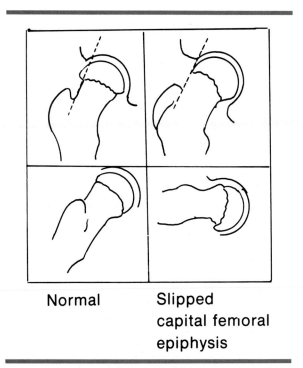

Normal   Slipped capital femoral epiphysis

Figure 19–8. Klein line extends along the lateral femur neck and normally passes through a small part of the lateral femoral head. In slipped capital femoral epiphysis (SCFE), the line does not pass through the head, but just touches its lateral margin. A frog-leg lateral, rather than an anteroposterior, projection gives the clearest view of SCFE. (From Chung SMK: Hip Disorders in Infants and Children. Philadelphia. Lea & Febiger, 1981, p 85.)

Classification. SCFE is classified into four distinct clinical groups.

Preslip. The growth plate is wide but slippage has not occurred. There may be mild discomfort but the physical examination usually is normal. Preslips frequently are seen in the opposite hip of an adolescent with a previous SCFE.

Acute SCFE. In acute SCFE there usually are no or only mild antecedent symptoms, such as pain or limp for less than 3 wk. Slippage occurs suddenly, with or without significant trauma; the pain is so severe that the child usually is unable to stand or bear weight.

Acute-on-Chronic SCFE. In acute-on-chronic SCFE, the epiphysis slips acutely on an existing chronic slip. These adolescents have had previous symptoms (pain, limp, out-toed gait) for several months. Trauma is a potential underlying factor that results in the sudden slippage.

Chronic SCFE. This is the most common type. There is usually a several-month history of the previously described symptoms. The symptoms typically worsen as the slip progresses. However, because there is continuity between the femoral neck and CFE, the symptoms are not severe and the child is able to walk, albeit with a mildly antalgic, externally rotated gait.

Clinical Manifestations. The physical findings in SCFE depend on the degree of slippage and the classification. In acute or acute-on-chronic slip, the physical examination is limited by pain with any attempted hip motion. In chronic SCFE, the patient will have an antalgic gait and the affected extremity is externally rotated. Hip range of motion will demonstrate a lack of medial rotation and increased lateral rotation. Also, as the hip is flexed it will become progressively laterally rotated. Limitation of flexion and abduction also may be present as a result of a varus deformity of the proximal femur. Adolescents, especially those who are obese, with nontraumatic knee pain (referred pain) should be evaluated carefully for SCFE.

Treatment. The goals of treatment for SCFE are to prevent further slippage and minimize complications. This is accomplished by performing an epiphysiodesis of the CFE. The technique selected depends on the classification and the severity of the slippage. The current methods include: in situ internal fixation with pins or screws (single or multiple); open bone graft epiphysiodesis; closed bone graft epiphysiodesis; osteotomies of the femoral neck or subtrochanteric regions to realign the proximal femur; and hip spica cast immobilization.

Complications. The two serious complications in SCFE are osteonecrosis and chondrolysis. Osteonecrosis occurs as a result of injury to the retinacular vessels. This can be due to forced manipulation of an acute slip, compression from intracapsular hematoma, or direct injury during surgery. Partial forms of osteonecrosis also may occur following internal fixation as a result of disruption of the intraepiphyseal blood vessels. Chondrolysis occurs when there is destruction of the articular cartilage of the hip joint. The etiology of this complication is unclear but has been demonstrated to be associated with more severe slips, black race, pins or screws protruding out of the femoral head, and female gender.

References

Behrman RE (ed): Nelson Textbook of Pediatrics. 14th ed. Philadelphia, WB Saunders, 1992, Sec. 24.7–24.11.

Carney BT, Weinstein SL, Noble J: Long-term follow-up of slipped capital femoral epiphysis. J Bone Joint Surg 73-A:667, 1991.

Crawford AH: Current concepts review. Slipped capital femoral epiphysis. J Bone Joint Surg 70-A:1422, 1988.

Gabuzda GM, Renshaw TS: Current concepts review. Reduction of congenital dislocation of the hip. J Bone Joint Surg 74-A:624, 1992.

Harcke HT: Imaging in congenital dislocation of the hip. Clin Orthop 281:22, 1992.

Hauseisen DC, Weiner DS, Weiner SD: The characterization of "transient synovitis of the hip" in children. J Pediatr Orthop 6:11, 1986.

Wenger DR, Ward TW, Herring JA: Current concepts review. Legg-Calvé-Perthes disease. J Bone Joint Surg 73-A:778, 1991.

THE LOWER EXTREMITIES

Torsional (in-toeing and out-toeing) and angular (physiologic bowlegs and knock-knees) variations of the lower extremities are common reasons parents seek orthopedic attention for a child. Most of these complaints do not require active treatment because they will resolve with normal growth. It is important to understand the natural history, however, in order to reassure a concerned family.

Angular Variations

There are both physiologic (variations) and pathologic (deformities) reasons for angular deformities. The physiologic or angular variations, fortunately, are the most common and occur predominantly in the tibia. The femur is much less frequently involved.

PHYSIOLOGIC BOWLEGS (GENU VARUM)

The lower extremities of newborns and infants (<1 yr of age) commonly have mild to moderate bowing and internal rotation (Fig. 19–9). This is due to in utero positioning in which the hips are flexed, abducted, and externally rotated; the knees flexed and lower legs internally rotated; and the feet in slight equinus, supination, and contact with the posterolateral aspect of the opposite thigh. This position produces hip flexion, abduction, and external rotation contractures; knee flexion contractures and internal tibial torsion; and mild supination of the feet. The bowed appearance is actually a torsional combination from the external rotation of the hip (tight posterior capsule) and the internal tibial torsion. With the onset of standing and independent walking, the bowing sponta-

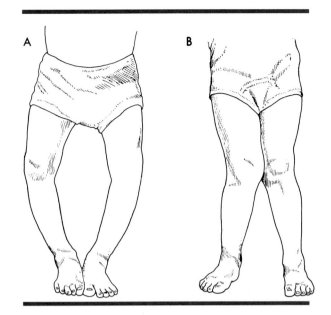

Figure 19–9. *A,* Bowleg deformity. Bowlegs are referred to as varus angulation (genu varum) because the legs distal to the knees are tilted toward the midline of the body. *B,* Knock-knee or valgus deformity of the knees. The extremity distal to the knee is tilted away from the midline. (From Scoles P: Pediatric Orthopedics in Clinical Practice. 2nd ed. Chicago, Year Book Medical Publishers, 1988, p 91. Reproduced with permission.)

neously corrects over a 6–12 mo period. Significant improvement will not occur during the 1st yr of life. The typical infant has 15 degrees of genu varum or bowleg configuration. This decreases to approximately 10 degrees by 1 yr of age. By 2 yr of age, the majority of children have straight or neutrally aligned lower extremities. Treatment is indicated for children older than 2 yr in whom there has been no documented improvement with growth.

PHYSIOLOGIC KNOCK-KNEES (GENU VALGUM)

As the spontaneous correction of physiologic bowlegs continues, there is typically an overcorrection, of variable degree, into mild genu valgum or knock-knee (Fig. 19–9). This physiologic angular variation commonly is seen between 3 and 4 yr of age but resolves spontaneously between 5 and 8 yr. As with physiologic bowlegs, treatment rarely is indicated.

Torsional Variations

The common causes for in-toeing and out-toeing are delineated in Table 19–5.

Table 19–5. Common Causes of In-Toeing and Out-Toeing

In-Toeing	Out-Toeing
Internal femoral torsion	External femoral torsion
Internal tibial torsion	External tibial torsion
Metatarsus adductus	Calcaneovalgus feet
Talipes equinovarus (clubfoot)	Hypermobile pes planus (flatfoot)

IN-TOEING

Internal Femoral Torsion

Internal or medial femoral torsion is the most common cause of in-toeing in children 2 yr of age or older. It occurs more commonly in girls than boys (2:1). Most children with this condition have generalized ligamentous laxity. The etiology of femoral torsion is controversial; it may be congenital (persistent infantile femoral anteversion) or acquired secondary to abnormal sitting habits.

Clinical Manifestations. The primary clinical feature of internal femoral torsion is an in-toed gait. While watching the undressed child walk, the entire lower leg is noted to be internally rotated. There is 80–90 degrees of internal rotation of the hip in the extended position; external rotation, as a consequence, is limited to 0–10 degrees. Generalized ligamentous laxity, including elbow and finger hyperextension, knee recurvatum, and hypermobile flatfeet (pes planus), are present. These children sit almost exclusively in the "television" or "W" position. This position may allow the lower leg to act as a lever, thereby producing the torsional change in the "biologically plastic" femur. Although this condition was called femoral anteversion, implying an abnormality of the proximal femur, it is actually a torsional abnormality throughout the femoral shaft that results in a change in the normal alignment between the hip and knee.

Roentgenographic Evaluation. Roentgenography for internal femoral torsion is not routinely necessary. Clinical measurements usually are quite accurate. CT of the hip and knee can be used to measure the degree of torsion roentgenographically.

Treatment This is primarily observation. It was previously believed that internal femoral torsion was associated with bunions, back pain, degenerative osteoarthritis of the hip and knee, and diffi-

culty with athletic ability. However, this is no longer accepted. Correction of abnormal sitting habits usually will allow this torsional variation to resolve with normal growth and development. However, it can take 1–3 yr for complete correction to occur. Children over 10 yr of age and young adolescents may not have enough remaining musculoskeletal growth for spontaneous correction to occur. After these children have been followed for 1–2 yr without improvement, and if there is significant cosmetic or functional disability, surgical correction my be necessary.

Internal Tibial Torsion

Internal or medial tibial torsion is the most common cause of in-toeing in children less than 2 yr of age and is secondary to in utero positioning. This condition may be associated with metatarsus adductus. It also is the major component of physiologic bowlegs.

Clinical Manifestations. The degree of tibial torsion can be measured by the supine or prone thigh–foot angle. In both tests, the knee is flexed to 90 degrees to neutralize the normal tibiofemoral rotation and the foot is placed in a neutral or simulated weight-bearing position. The long axis of the foot is compared to the long axis of the thigh (prone test) or tibia (supine test). An inwardly rotated foot is assigned a negative value and represents internal tibial torsion. It is important that the measurements be recorded on each visit to document improvement. Roentgenographic measurements usually are of no value in assessment of medial tibial torsion.

Treatment. This is a physiologic condition, and spontaneous resolution with normal growth and development can be anticipated. If there has been no documented improvement by 2 yr of age, a nighttime orthosis, such as a Denis-Browne splint, may be considered. Rarely, persistent internal tibial torsion in an older child or adolescent may require surgical derotation.

OUT-TOEING

External Tibial Torsion

External tibial torsion is common and always is associated with a calcaneovalgus foot (see The Foot). External tibial torsion is due to a variation in normal in utero position. When these two conditions are combined with the normally externally rotated hip (tight posterior hip capsule), it produces a very externally rotated or out-toed appearance. Fortunately, both conditions will undergo spontaneous resolution, following a clinical course similar to that of internal tibial torsion.

Pathologic Genu Varum

TIBIA VARA (BLOUNT DISEASE)

Idiopathic tibia vara, or Blount disease, is the most common pathologic disorder producing a progressive genu varium deformity. It is characterized by abnormal growth of the medial aspect of the proximal tibial epiphysis, resulting in a progressive varus angulation beneath the knee. Tibia vara can occur at any age in a growing child. It is classified based on the age at clinical onset: infantile (1–3 yr), juvenile (4–10 yr), and adolescent (11 yr or older). The infantile group is the most common; the juvenile and adolescent forms are combined as late-onset tibia vara and occur less frequently. Although the exact etiology of tibia vara remains unknown, it appears to be secondary to growth suppression from increased compressive forces across the medial aspect of the knee.

Clinical Manifestations. The characteristics of infantile tibia vara include predominance of black race and female gender, marked obesity, approximately 80% bilateral involvement, a prominent medial metaphyseal beak, internal tibial torsion, and lower extremity length inequality. Characteristics of the juvenile and adolescent (late-onset) form include black race, predominance of males, marked obesity, normal or above-normal height, approximately 50% bilateral involvement, slow progressive genu varum deformity, pain rather than deformity as the primary initial complaint, no palpable proximal medial metaphyseal beak, minimal internal tibial torsion, mild medial collateral ligament laxity, and mild lower extremity length inequality.

Roentgenographic Evaluation. Standing AP and lateral roentgenographs of the lower extremities are necessary to assess pathologic genu varum deformities. Roentgenographically, fragmentation with a protuberant step deformity and beaking of the proximal medial tibial metaphysis are considered the major features of infantile tibia vara. The changes of the proximal medial tibia are less conspicuous in the late-onset forms and are characterized by wedging of the medial portion of the epiphysis, a mild posteromedial articular depression, a serpiginous cephalad curved physis of variable width, and mild or no fragmentation or beaking of

the proximal medial metaphysis. The differences between the three tibia vara groups appear to be due primarily to the age at clinical onset, the amount of remaining growth, and the magnitude of the medial compression forces on the involved side. Thus, the infantile-onset group has the potential for the greatest deformity and the adolescent-onset group, the least.

The major deformity that must be differentiated from infantile tibia vara is the physiologic genu varum deformity. It is difficult to differentiate roentgenographically between these two disorders prior to 2 yr of age.

Treatment. Once the roentgenographic findings confirm the diagnosis, treatment should begin immediately. Orthotic management may be considered for children 3 yr of age or younger with a mild deformity. Approximately 50% of children with this criterion may achieve adequate correction using orthoses. Conservative management in the late-onset forms of tibia vara is contraindicated. The children are too large, compliance is poor, and the remaining growth too small to allow for adequate correction.

The indications for surgical treatment in infantile tibia vara include 4 yr of age or older, failure of orthotic management, and moderate to severe deformity. Proximal tibial valgus osteotomy and associated fibular diaphyseal osteotomy is the procedure of choice.

Lower Extremity Length Discrepancies

Length discrepancies in the femur, tibia, or both are common problems. The differential diagnosis is extensive, and some of the common causes are presented in Table 19–6.

Table 19–6. Common Causes of Lower Extremity Length Inequality

Congenital	Infectious
Proximal femoral focal deficiency	Pyogenic osteomyelitis with growth plate damage
Coxa vara	
Hemiatrophy/ hemihypertrophy (anisomelia)	**Trauma**
Congenital dislocation of the hip	Growth plate injury with premature closure
	Overgrowth
Developmental	Malunion (shortening)
Legg-Calvé-Perthes disease	**Tumor**
	Growth plate destruction
Neuromuscular	Radiation-induced growth
Polio	Plate injury
Cerebral palsy (hemiplegia)	Overgrowth

NORMAL GROWTH AND DEVELOPMENT

Approximately 65% of the growth of the entire lower extremity comes from the distal femoral (38%) and proximal tibial (27%) physeal plates. Thus, growth disturbances about the knee can have the most adverse effect on lower extremity length depending on the amount of remaining growth.

METHODS OF LIMB LENGTH MEASUREMENT

Clinical Measurements. The available clinical methods are less accurate than the roentgenographic techniques. The most common clinical measurement is from the anterior superior iliac spine to the medial malleolus. This minimizes measurement error secondary to pelvic obliquity. It also is possible to measure limb length by leveling the pelvis. Blocks of various thickness may be placed beneath the foot on the involved side until the iliac crests are level. The thickness indicates the amount of discrepancy.

Roentgenographic Measurements. Roentgenographic evaluations are the most accurate method of assessment of leg length. The *teleoroentgenogram* is a single exposure of both lower extremities. Its primary indication is for young children, usually under 5 yr of age. There is a small amount of magnification error present but it has the advantage of showing angular deformities. The *orthoroentgenogram* consists of three separate, slightly overlapping exposures of the hips, knees, and ankles on a long cassette. Bone length is measured directly on the roentgenograph. There is less magnification present, and angular deformities are demonstrated. It has the disadvantage of being bulky and difficult to handle. The *scanogram* is the most accurate method and consists of three narrow exposures of the hips, knees, and ankles on a standard cassette with a roentgenographic ruler next to the extremity. Minimal magnification is present and accurate measurements can be made. However, angular deformities cannot be visualized fully, which may lead to errors in interpretation. Currently, *CT scanogram* techniques are being utilized with the best accuracy.

The measured discrepancy is followed with the Moseley or Green-Anderson graph. An AP roentgenograph of the left hand and wrist for bone age determination is necessary to assess maturation.

TREATMENT

Issues in management include etiology of the discrepancy, skeletal age, ultimate discrepancy, anticipated adult height, neuromuscular status of the extremities, joint involvement, and psychologic aspects of the child and parents. Discrepancies of greater than 2 cm at maturity usually require treatment. Equalization can be achieved by nonsurgical and surgical methods. The nonsurgical methods include orthotic and prosthetic devices, whereas the surgical methods include shortening of the longer extremity, lengthening of the shorter extremity, or a combination of both. Discrepancies 2–5 cm are treated by epiphyseodesis of the affected side and discrepancies greater than 5 cm by lengthening.

References

Behrman RE (ed): Nelson Textbook of Pediatrics. 14th ed. Philadelphia, WB Saunders, 1992, Sec. 24.3–24.5.

Kling TF, Jr: Angular deformities of the lower limbs in children. Orthop Clin North Am 18:513, 1987.

Moseley CF: Leg length discrepancy. Orthop Clin North Am 18:529, 1987.

Paley D: Current techniques of limb lengthening. J Pediatr Orthop 8:73, 1988.

Staheli LT: Rotational problems of the lower extremities. Orthop Clin North Am 18:503, 1987.

Thompson GH, Carter JR: Late-onset tibia vara (Blount's disease): Current concepts. Clin Orthop 255:24, 1990.

THE KNEE

The knee joint is unique because the movement of the tibiofemoral articulation is constrained only by soft tissues rather than by the usual geometric fit between the ends of articulating bone (Fig. 19–10). Paramount among these constraints are the medial and lateral collateral ligaments, the anterior and posterior cruciate ligaments, and the medial and lateral menisci. Weight is transmitted by load path that includes both the points of articular cartilage and the menisci. A second clinically important area, the patellofemoral joint, is part of the knee and a common site of problems, especially in adolescents.

Accumulation of fluid (effusion) in the knee is common during childhood and adolescence. When fluid accumulates rapidly following an injury, blood usually is in the joint (hemarthrosis); this may indicate a serious injury to one of the ligaments or menisci. If there has been repeated trauma, an accumulation of synovial fluid may indicate a chronic internal derangement, usually a tear of a meniscus. Unexplained accumulation of fluid may occur with arthritis (septic, viral, postinfectious, juvenile rheumatoid arthritis, systemic lupus erythematosus), in associated with ligamen-

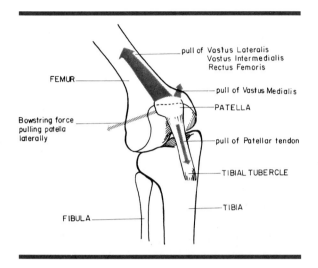

Figure 19–10. Diagram of the knee extensor mechanism. The major force exerted by the quadriceps muscle tends to pull the patella laterally out of the intercondylar sulcus. The vastus medialis muscle pulls medially to keep the patella centralized. (From Smith JB: Knee problems in children. Pediatr Clin North Am 33:1443, 1986.)

tous laxity (hypermobile joint syndrome), and with overactivity. In addition to the evaluation of other systemic manifestations and the clinical history (e.g., fever, hemophilia, rash, trauma), an analysis of an aspiration of fluid from the joint generally is indicated and expedites precise diagnosis (see Chapter 10).

Discoid Lateral Meniscus

Each meniscus is semilunar in shape, but occasionally the lateral meniscus persists as a solid disk of fibrocartilage, an entity referred to as *discoid lateral meniscus*. A normal meniscus is attached about its periphery and glides anteriorly and posteriorly with knee motion, but a discoid meniscus is less mobile and may become torn. Occasionally, there will be no peripheral attachment about is posterolateral aspect, resulting in knee flexion in which the entire discoid meniscus may suddenly displace anteriorly to produce a loud click or clunk. Most commonly the patient comes to clinical attention during the late childhood years and early adolescence (11–15 yr). AP roentgenographs often will show widening of the lateral aspect of the knee joint. Arthroscopy, arthrography, and MRI are diagnostic. Treatment in most cases is to excise tears and reshape the meniscus arthroscopically. Peripheral reattachment also is performed when necessary.

Popliteal Cyst

A popliteal cyst ("Baker cyst") commonly is seen during the middle childhood years (Fig. 19–11). The cause is distention of the gastrocnemius and semimembranosus bursa along the posteromedial aspect of the knee by synovial fluid from the tendon sheaths. In childhood, the cysts usually are benign and resolve with time, even though several years may be required. Knee roentgenographs are normal; the diagnosis is confirmed by ultrasound or aspiration. Management should be directed at reassurance because surgery usually is not indicated.

Osteochondritis Dissecans

Osteochondritis dissecans commonly involves the knee and occurs when an area of bone adjacent to the articular cartilage becomes necrotic and separates from the underlying bone. In the older child or young adolescent, this condition usually affects the lateral portion of the medial femoral condyle. AP, lateral, and "tunnel" roentgenographs of the

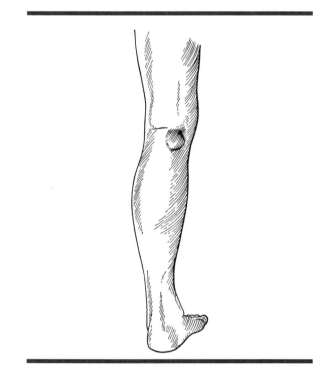

Figure 19–11. Diagram of popliteal cyst location—medial posterior aspect of knee, inferior to knee crease. (From Ferguson A: Orthopedic Surgery in Infancy and Childhood. 5th ed. Baltimore, Williams & Wilkins, 1981, p 261.)

knee are diagnostic and are used to follow the course of the disease. In the young patient, the overlying articular cartilage usually remains intact and the necrosis revascularizes and heals spontaneously. With increasing age, the risk increases for fracture of the articular cartilage and separation of the bony fragment. MRI is helpful in determining the integrity of the articular cartilage. In the young adolescent, a judgment must be made about whether to follow the lesion expectantly or to attempt to stimulate healing surgically. Once cartilage fracture takes place, surgical treatment is necessary. This may consist of arthroscopic excision, drilling of the lesion to promote revascularization and healing, and possible internal fixation.

Osgood-Schlatter Disease

The portion of the patellar ligament inserted into the tibial tubercle is vulnerable to fibrocartilage microfracture during late childhood and early adolescence. This condition, Osgood-Schlatter disease, is more common in males. The natural history almost always is benign, with activity-related pain persisting until 6 mo to 1 yr after skeletal maturity. Frequently, bony enlargement of the tibial tubercle will be a residual manifestation of the proliferative healing response. Rest, restriction of activities, and occasionally a knee immobilizer may be necessary, combined with an isometric exercise program. Anti-inflammatory medications are not beneficial.

Patellofemoral Disorders

The patellofemoral joint depends on a subtle balance among restraining ligaments, muscle forces, alignment, and articular anatomy for normal function (Fig. 19–10). On its deep surface, the patella has a V-bottom shape; it moves through a matching groove in the distal femur called the trochlea. The force of the muscle pulling through the quadriceps tendon and the patellar ligament does not act in a straight line because the patellar ligament inclines in a slightly lateral direction with respect to the line of the quadriceps tendon. This lateral movement, coupled with the movement of the restraining ligaments, tends to move the patella in a lateral direction. The vastus medialis muscle functions to counteract the laterally acting forces. An abnormality of any one or a group of these factors makes the patellofemoral joint function abnormally; the usual clinical manifestations is knee pain.

Because of the biomechanical malfunction, the articular surface of the patella is damaged and becomes tender, producing chondromalacia of the patella, a condition easily assessed by directly palpating the extended knee and also by compressing the patellofemoral joint. To elicit the latter sign, one merely exerts manual pressure against the patella as the knee is extended. Running and climbing stairs elicit pain when the knee is flexed. With early articular damage, pain usually is perceived maximally as the knee comes to within 15–20 degrees of full extension (crepitance also may be felt by the examiner). Although it may be reasonable to treat recent or mild cases empirically with anti-inflammatory medication and an exercise program aimed at developing strength and bulk in the vastus medialis muscle, persistent or refractory cases should be referred to a specialist. Patellofemoral pain is particularly prevalent among young athletes (participating in running, basketball, soccer) and in adolescent women.

Recurrent *patella subluxation and dislocation* resulting from similar muscle imbalance also can occur in late childhood and early adolescence. There are several other predisposing factors, including generalized ligamentous laxity, internal femoral torsion, genu valgum, and lateral femoral condyle hypoplasia. Acute traumatic dislocations also occur in a normal knee. Initial treatment is nonoperative, with a vigorous physical therapy program to strengthen predominantly the quadriceps muscles. If this fails, surgical correction is necessary.

References

Behrman RE (ed): Nelson Textbook of Pediatrics, 14th ed. Philadelphia, WB Saunders, 1992, Sec. 24.6.

Bentley G, Dowd G: Current concepts of etiology and treatment of chondromalacia patellae. Clin Orthop 189:209, 1984.

Dickhaut SC, Delee JC: The discoid lateral meniscus syndrome. J Bone Joint Surg 64-A:1068, 1982.

Dinham JM: Popliteal cysts in children: The case against surgery. J Bone Joint Surg 57-B:69, 1975.

Krause BL, Williams JPR, Catterall A: Natural history of Osgood-Schlatter disease. J Pediatr Orthop 10:65, 1990.

THE FOOT

In the newborn and prewalking age range, it is helpful to remember the difference between posturing and deformity. Posturing is the habitual position in which the infant holds the foot but still allows a normal range of motion, so that the examiner can position the foot in a normal shape. Deformity produces an appearance similar to posturing, but the deformed foot cannot be manually repositioned to a normal shape. Most pediatric foot disor-

Table 19–7. Differential Diagnosis of Foot Pain by Age

0–6 yr	6–12 yr	12–20 yr
Poor-fitting shoes	Poor-fitting shoes	Poor-fitting shoes
Foreign body	Sever disease	Stress fracture
Fracture	Enthesopathy (JRA)	Foreign body
Osteomyelitis	Foreign body	Ingrown toenail
Juvenile rheumatoid arthritis (JRA)	Accessory navicular	Metatarsalgia
Leukemia	Tarsal coalition	Plantar fasciitis
Puncture wound	Ewing sarcoma	Avascular necrosis of metatarsal (Freiberg infarction) or navicular bone (Köhler disease)
Drawing of blood	Hypermobile flatfoot	Sever disease
	Trauma (sprains)	Achilles tendinitis
	Puncture wound	Trauma (sprains)
		Plantar warts

ders are painless. However, foot pain does occur. The differential diagnosis of foot pain in children is presented in Table 19–7.

Metatarsus Adductus

Congenital metatarsus adductus is a common problem of infants and young children. It also is known as metatarsus varus if the forefoot is supinated as well as adducted. It occurs equally in males and females and is bilateral in 50% of patients. Metatarsus adductus has hereditary tendencies and is more common in firstborn than in later children because of the molding effect from the primigravida uterus and abdominal wall. Approximately 10% of children with metatarsus adductus will have DDH. Thus, careful examination of the hips is necessary.

Clinical Manifestations. The forefoot is adducted and occasionally supinated. The hindfoot and midfoot are normal. The lateral border of the foot is convex and the base of the fifth metatarsal appears prominent. The medial border of the foot is concave. There is usually an increased interval between the first and second toes, with the great toe being held in a greater varus position. Ankle dorsiflexion and plantar flexion are normal. Forefoot flexibility can vary from flexible to rigid. This is assessed by stabilizing the hind and midfoot in a neutral position and applying pressure over the first metatarsal head. In the walking child with an uncorrected metatarsus adductus deformity an intoed gait is noted. Abnormal shoe wear also commonly is seen.

Roentgenographic Evaluation. Routine roentgenographs of the foot usually are not necessary for metatarsus adductus. AP weight-bearing roentgenographs will demonstrate adduction of the met-

atarsals at the tarsometatarsal articulation and an increased intermetatarsal angle between the first and second metatarsals.

Treatment. The feet may be classified into three groups depending on forefoot flexibility. Type I deformities are flexible feet that can be placed into the overcorrected (abducted) position. Voluntary correction usually can be elicited by stimulating the peroneal musculature by stroking the lateral border of the foot. These feet usually require no treatment. Type II deformities are feet that correct to the neutral position both passively and actively. These feet may benefit from a trial of corrective shoes, such as straight or reversed last shoes. These shoes are worn full time (22 hr/day) and the child is re-evaluated in 4–6 wk. If the condition has improved, treatment can be continued. If no improvement occurs, serial plaster casts are necessary. Type III deformities are rigid and do not correct. These feet are treated with serial casts that are changed at 1–2 wk intervals. Usually, complete correction can be obtained in 4–6 wk depending on the age of the child and the severity of deformity. The best results are obtained when casting is initiated before 8 mo of age.

Metatarsus adductus deformities persisting or presenting after 4 yr of age usually require surgical intervention. Children 4–6 yr of age with a fixed deformity usually are considered for soft tissue release. Children 7 yr of age or older usually do not benefit from the soft tissue release and require metatarsal osteotomies.

Calcaneovalgus Feet

The calcaneovalgus foot is a relatively common finding in the newborn and appears to be secondary to in utero positioning. This condition is manifested by a hyperdorsiflexed foot with forefoot abduction and heel valgus and usually is associated with external tibial torsion. These variations usually are unilateral but may be bilateral. In utero, the plantar surface of the foot was against the wall of the uterus, forcing it into a hyperdorsiflexed, abducted, and laterally rotated position. When calcanevovlagus feet and external tibial torsion are combined with the normal newborn external rotation of the hip (tight posterior capsule), it results in an excessively externally rotated lower extremity.

Clinical Manifestations. The infant typically presents with an externally rotated extremity. The dorsum of the foot can be brought into contact with the anterior aspect of the tibia and the forefoot will have an abducted appearance.

The most common condition that must be distinguished from the calcaneovalgus foot is a vertical talus. The differentiation usually can be made clinically because a congenital vertical talus is a rigid deformity.

Roentgenographic Evaluation. Simulated weight-bearing AP and lateral roentgenographs of the feet may be necessary to differentiate between the calcaneovalgus foot and a congenital vertical talus. In a calcaneovalgus foot, the roentgenographs either are normal or show a slight increase in hindfoot valgus. In congenital vertical talus, the hindfoot is in equinus and the midfoot dorsally displaced (*rocker bottom*).

Treatment. The typical calcaneovalgus foot require no treatment. The hyperdorsiflexion of the foot will resolve during the first 3–6 mo of life. The external tibial torsion, however, will persist and follow the same natural history as internal tibial torsion. Spontaneous improvement will not occur until the child begins to pull to stand and walk independently. The majority of involved infants will have normally aligned feet and lower extremities by 2 yr of age.

Talipes Equinovarus (Clubfoot)

A clubfoot represents a deformity of not only the foot but the entire lower leg. It can be congenital, teratologic, or positional. The congenital clubfoot is usually an isolated abnormality, whereas the teratologic form is associated with neuromuscular disorders such as myelodysplasia, arthrogryposis multiplex congenita, or a syndrome complex. Positional clubfoot is a normal foot that has been held in a deformed position in utero.

Etiology. The etiology of clubfoot is unknown. There are inheritance factors that may be multifac-

torial with a major influence from a single autosomal dominant gene. Recent biopsy studies of the extrinsic muscles of the calf have suggested a probable nonprogressive neuromuscular etiology.

Clinical Manifestations. The congenital form of clubfoot, which constitutes 75% of cases, is characterized by the absence of other congenital abnormalities; variable rigidity of the foot; mild calf atrophy; and mild hypoplasia of the tibia, fibula, and bones of the foot. It occurs more commonly in males (2:1) and is bilateral in 50% of cases. The probability for the deformity to occur at random is approximately 0.1%, but within involved families the probability is approximately 3% for subsequent siblings and 20–30% for offspring of involved parents.

Examination of the infant clubfoot demonstrates hindfoot equinus, hindfoot varus, forefoot adduction, and variable rigidity. All are secondary to the medial dislocation of the talonavicular joint. In the older child, the calf and foot atrophy are more obvious than in the infant regardless of how well corrected or functional the foot. These findings are due to the neuromuscular etiology of clubfoot.

Roentgenographic Evaluation. AP and lateral standing or simulated weight-bearing roentgenographs are used in the assessment of clubfeet. Useful measurements in assessing clubfeet include the AP talocalcaneal angle, the lateral talocalcaneal angle, and the talocalcaneal overlap (Fig. 19–12). The navicular, which is the primary site of deformity, does not ossify until 3 yr in the female and 4 yr in the male. Thus, line measurements are necessary in order to determine the position of the unossified navicular.

Treatment
Conservative Management. Conservative methods of treatment include taping, malleable splints, and serial plaster casts. Taping and malleable splints are particularly useful in premature infants until they obtain an appropriate size for casting. Serial plaster casts are the major method of treatment. Failure to achieve clinical and radiographic correction by 3 mo of age is an indication for surgical treatment. Further attempts at conservative management may result in articular damage and a midfoot breech (rocker-bottom deformity).

Surgical Management. The most common method of initial surgical treatment is a complete soft tissue release simultaneously correcting all components of the clubfoot deformity. Satisfactory long-term results can be expected in 75–90% of

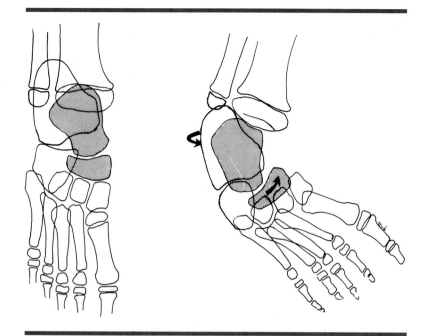

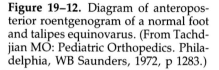

Figure 19–12. Diagram of anteroposterior roentgenogram of a normal foot and talipes equinovarus. (From Tachdjian MO: Pediatric Orthopedics. Philadelphia, WB Saunders, 1972, p 1283.)

these cases. Those feet with unsatisfactory results requiring additional treatment usually are secondary to extrinsic muscle imbalance (neuromuscular etiology) rather than incomplete correction.

Hypermobile Pes Planus (Flexible Flatfeet)

Hypermobile (flexible flatfeet) or pronated feet are common sources of parental concern. These children usually are asymptomatic and have no limitations of activities. Flexible flatfeet are common in neonates and toddlers as a result of associated ligamentous laxity and fat in the area of the medial longitudinal arch; significant improvement is noted by 6 yr of age. In the older child, flexible flatfeet usually are secondary to generalized ligamentous laxity.

Clinical Manifestations. In the non–weight-bearing position in the older child with a flexible flatfoot, the normal medial longitudinal arch is present, but in the weight-bearing position, the foot becomes pronated with varying degrees of pes planus and heel valgus. Subtalar motion will be normal or slightly increased. Loss of subtalar motion may indicate a rigid flatfoot. Common causes of rigid flatfeet include tight tendo Achillis (heel cord), tarsal coalitions, and neuromuscular abnormalities (cerebral palsy). Rigid flatfeet also may be a familial trait.

Roentgenographic Evaluation. Roentgenograms of asymptomatic flexible flatfeet usually are not indicated.

Treatment. The treatment of flexible flatfeet is conservative; the diagnosis is not possible until after 6 yr of age. Treatment is indicated only for persistent symptoms not attributable to other causes or abnormal shoe wear. Feet that are symptomatic with vigorous physical activities usually respond readily to the use of a commercially available medial longitudinal arch support.

Peroneal Spastic Flatfoot

Peroneal spastic flatfoot is a common disorder characterized by a painful, rigid valgus deformity of the mid and hindfoot (flatfoot) and peroneal (lateral calf) muscle spasm but without true spasticity. Peroneal spastic flatfoot usually is synonymous with tarsal coalition, a congenital fusion or failure of segmentation between two or more tarsal bones. Any condition that alters the normal gliding and rotatory motion of the subtalar joint may produce the appearance of a peroneal spastic flatfoot. Thus, congenital malformations, arthritis or inflammatory disorders, infection, neoplasms, and trauma can be potential, although uncommon, etiologies.

The most common tarsal coalitions occur at the medial talocalcaneal (subtalar) facet and between the calcaneus and navicular tarsal bones. Coalitions can be either fibrous, cartilaginous, or osseous. Peroneal spastic flatfoot will be bilateral in approximately 50% of involved children.

Clinical Manifestations. The onset of symptoms usually occurs during the 2nd decade of life. Although mild limitation of subtalar motion and a valgus deformity are present since early childhood, the onset of symptoms varies with the age at which the fibrous or cartilaginous bar begins to ossify and further decrease motion. The talonavicular coalitions ossify between 3 and 5 yr, the calcaneonavicular coalitions between 8 and 12 yr, and the middle-facet talocalcaneal coalitions between 12 and 16 yr of age. The pain typically is felt laterally in the hindfoot and radiates proximally along the lateral malleolus and distal fibula (peroneal muscle spasm). Symptoms frequently are aggravated by sports or walking on uneven ground. The foot is pronated both in the weight-bearing and non–weight-bearing positions. Subtalar or mid-tarsal joint motion is diminished or absent, and attempts at motion produce pain.

Roentgenographic Evaluation. The diagnosis of tarsal coalition is confirmed roentgenographically by AP oblique, and lateral weight-bearing roentgenographs of the foot. Beaking of the anterior aspect of the talus on the lateral view is suspicious for a tarsal coalition. Axial views through the posterior and middle talocalcaneal joints can be useful in the diagnosis of the middle-facet talocalcaneal coalition. However, CT is the procedure of choice in the evaluation of tarsal coalitions, especially those involving the middle facet.

Treatment. The treatment of symptomatic tarsal coalition varies according to the type of coalition, the age of the patient, the extent of the coalition, the presence or absence of degenerative osteoarthritis, and the degree of disability. Nonoperative treatment consists of cast immobilization, shoe inserts, or orthotics. When this fails, excision of the coalition and soft tissue interposition to prevent hematoma formation and reossification of the coalition is very effective in relieving pain, improving subtalar motion, and allowing resumption of normal activities.

Cavus Feet

Cavovarus foot, an exaggerated medial longitudinal arch associated with an inward cant of the heel, often appears during the middle childhood years (Fig. 19–13). Both idiopathic and neuromuscular types may be seen; in either instance, cavovarus is a progressive deformity leading to considerable compromise of foot function. In hypermobile pes planus, the foot rotates externally, but, in high arch or cavovarus posture, the foot rotates internally. The cavovarus foot also tends to be rigid. Aggressive treatment is warranted and usually involves reconstructive surgery. Special shoes and shoe modifications are not helpful from a therapeutic standpoint, but sometimes may be warranted for various types of symptomatic treatment. Because a neuromuscular etiology is possible whenever such a deformity of the foot exists, carefully assessing the patient's neurologic function is mandatory. Spinal cord pathology poliomyelitis and peripheral neuropathy (Charcot-Marie-Tooth disease) always are to be considered.

Osteochondroses

Both the tarsal navicular (Köhler disease) and the head of the second metatarsal (Frieberg disease)

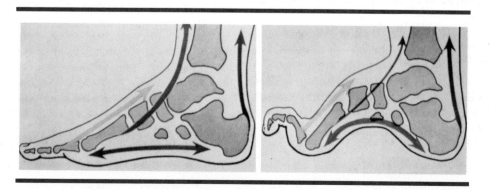

Figure 19–13. The normal muscular balance of the foot is demonstrated on the left. A right triangle of muscle forces is generated by the gastrocnemius–soleus group posteriorly, the plantar muscles distally, and the tibialis anticus anteriorly. Weakness, as demonstrated in the diagram on the right, causes imbalance in the foot with resultant pes cavus. (Redrawn from Chuinard E, Baskin M: Clawfoot deformity. J Bone Joint Surg 55-A:351, 1973.)

may undergo idiopathic avascular necrosis. These conditions are relatively uncommon, and both produce pain in the affected site on activity or weight bearing. The pathologic process involves infarction and subsequent revascularization, resorption, and replacement of the affected bone. Symptomatic treatment based on the severity of the child's complaints is appropriate.

As the child enters the pubescent growth spurt, the fibrocartilaginous insertion of major muscle groups to bone is vulnerable to microfracture through the fibrocartilage, resulting in inflammatory and healing responses. The usual site of microfracture in the foot is at the attachment of the triceps surae to the os calcis, producing *Sever disease.* Symptoms wax and wane, depending on the level of activity, until skeletal maturity is achieved. The usual residual manifestation, if any, is some bony enlargement at the tendon insertion site when the cartilage, which proliferated as part of the healing response, undergoes its normal maturation to become bone. Involvement at multiple sites is common. Treatment is symptomatic and includes the use of anti-inflammatory agents.

Toe Deformities

Extra toes **(polydactyly)** usually are recognized at birth, and it is appropriate to decide on a management strategy at that time. When the extra toe is attached to the foot by only a tag of skin and soft tissue, as commonly occurs adjacent to the 5th toe, simple amputation or ligation through the stalk is effective. When the abnormality involves the great toe or the intercalary toes, or has some rudiment of cartilage or bone connecting it with the foot proper, delayed surgical treatment targeted at the specific abnormality is indicated. Malformation syndromes may be associated with polydactyly (Table 19–8).

Fusing of the toes, or syndactyly, usually is a benign cosmetic problem that does not warrant treatment. Syndromes also may be associated with syndactyly (Table 19–9).

Puncture Wounds

Puncture wounds of the foot are common and generally trivial. For the major of these injuries,

Table 19–8. Syndromes Associated with Polydactyly

Carpenter syndrome
Ellis–van Creveld syndrome
Meckel-Gruber syndrome
Polysyndactyly
Trisomy 13
Orofaciodigital syndrome
Rubinstein-Taybi syndrome

Table 19–9. Syndromes Associated with Syndactyly

Apert syndrome
Carpenter syndrome
de Lange syndrome
Holt-Oram syndrome
Orofaciodigital syndrome
Polysyndactyly
Trisomy 21
Fetal hydantoin syndrome
Laurence-Moon-Biedl syndrome
Fanconi pancytopenia
Trisomy 13
Trisomy 18

cleansing the wound, ensuring prophylaxis for tetanus, and administering broad-spectrum oral antibiotic prophylaxis are all that is needed. When infection occurs despite these measures, *Pseudomonas aeruginosa* and *S. aureus* are the offending organisms in most cases of osteomyelitis, supposedly because these organisms normally colonize the skin surface of the foot as a result of the moist environment in a shoe. Treatment of these infections includes débriding the wound to remove necrotic tissue, which invariably is present, and administering parenteral antibiotic treatment, initially with methicillin and gentamicin. Subsequent antibiotic treatment should be based on culture and sensitivity studies. Following surgery, parenteral antimicrobial therapy is required for 10–14 days.

References

Behrman TE (ed): Nelson Textbook of Pediatrics, 14th ed. Philadelphia, WB Saunders, 1992, Sec. 24.2.

Bunnel W, Shook J: Orthopaedics in the pediatric office. Curr Prob Pediatr 22:13, 1992.

Crawford AH, Gabriel KR: Foot and ankle problems. Orthop Clin North Am 18:649, 1987.

McClusky WP, Lovell WW, Cummings RJ: The cavovarus foot deformity: Etiology and management. Clin Orthop 247:27, 1989.

Swiontkowski MF, Scranton PE, Hansen S: Tarsal coalitions: Long-term results of surgical treatment. J Pediatr Orthop 3:287, 1983.

Thompson GH, Simons GW III: Congenital talipes equinovarus (clubfeet) and metatarsus adductus. In Drennan JC (ed): The Child's Foot and Ankle. New York, Raven Press, 1992, pp 97–133.

Wenger DR, Mauldin D, Speck G, et al: Corrective shoes and inserts as treatment for flexible flatfeet in infants and children. J Bone Joint Surg 71-A:800, 1989.

THE SPINE

A simplified classification of the common spinal abnormalities is presented in Table 19–10.

Table 19–10. Classification of Spinal Deformities

Scoliosis

Idiopathic
  Infantile
  Juvenile
  Adolescent

Congenital
  Failure of formation
    Wedge vertebrae
    Hemivertebrae
  Failure of segmentation
    Unilateral bar
    Bilateral bar
  Mixed

Neuromuscular
  Neuropathic diseases
    Upper motor neuron
      Cerebral palsy
      Spinocerebellar degeneration
        Friedreich ataxia
        Charcot-Marie-Tooth disease
      Syringomyelia
      Spinal cord tumor
      Spinal cord trauma
    Lower motor neuron
      Poliomyelitis
      Spinal Muscular Atrophy
  Myopathic diseases
    Duchenne muscular dystrophy
    Arthrogryposis
    Other muscular dystrophies

Syndromes
  Neurofibromatosis
  Marfan syndrome

Compensatory
  Leg length discrepancy

Kyphosis
Postural roundback
Scheuermann disease
Congenital kyphosis

(Adapted from the Terminology Committee of the Scoliosis Research Society.)

Clinical Examination

A complete physical examination is necessary for any child or adolescent with a spinal deformity because it may indicate an underlying disease process. The back is examined with the patient in the standing position and viewed from behind (Fig. 19–14). The levelness of the pelvis is assessed first. Leg length inequality results in pelvic obliquity and can produce the appearance of scoliosis. When the pelvis is level or has been leveled with wood blocks placed under the foot, the spine is examined for symmetry. The back is observed for areas of defor-

mity, spinal curvature, and areas of tenderness. Next, the patient is asked to bend forward with the hands directed between the feet. A tangential view of the spine while standing behind (thoracic area) and in front (lumbar area) allows the observer to determine the symmetry of the back. The presence of a hump is the hallmark of a scoliotic deformity. The corresponding area opposite the hump typically is depressed. The reason for these "humps and valleys" is **spinal rotation**. Scoliosis represents a rotational malalignment of one vertebra on another. This results in rib rotation when the curve is in the thoracic area and paravertebral muscle rotation when the curve is in the lumbar region. When the trunk is viewed from the side with the patient still in the forward flexed position, the degree of roundback can be ascertained. A sharp, abrupt forward angulation in the thoracic or thoracolumbar region is indicative of a kyphotic deformity.

In a scoliosis patient other areas of the body also must be examined, including the skin (hairy patches, nevi, and lipomas for spinal dysraphism); café-au-lait spots (for neurofibromatosis), the extremities (skeletal dysplasia), the heart (murmurs for Marfan syndrome), and the neurologic system, to determine whether the scoliosis is truly idiopathic or possibly secondary to an underlying neuromuscular disorder.

Roentgenographic Evaluation

Initial roentgenograms of the spine include a posteroanterior (PA) and lateral standing roentgenogram of the entire spine. This allows assessment for scoliosis, kyphosis, lordosis, congenital malformations, and, if the iliac crests are visible, the skeletal maturity of the patient. The degree of curvature is measured from the most tilted or end vertebra of the curve superiorly and inferiorly using the Cobb method (Fig. 19–15).

Scoliosis

Alterations in normal spinal alignment that occur in the AP or frontal plane are termed scoliosis. Most scoliotic deformities are idiopathic (unknown causation). Others, however, can be congenital, secondary to an underlying neuromuscular disorder, or compensatory from a leg length inequality.

IDIOPATHIC SCOLIOSIS

The most common form of scoliosis occurs in healthy, neurologically normal children, its etiology is unknown. The incidence is only slightly

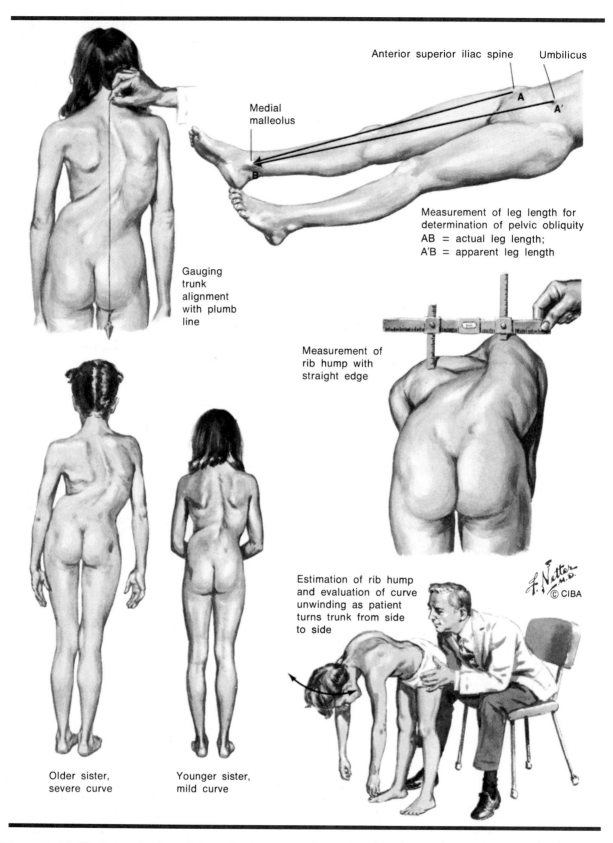

Anterior superior iliac spine

Umbilicus

Medial malleolus

A

A'

Measurement of leg length for determination of pelvic obliquity
AB = actual leg length;
A'B = apparent leg length

Gauging trunk alignment with plumb line

Measurement of rib hump with straight edge

Estimation of rib hump and evaluation of curve unwinding as patient turns trunk from side to side

Older sister, severe curve

Younger sister, mild curve

Figure 19–14. Clinical evaluation of the scoliosis patient. (From Hugo A, Keim MD: Scoliosis. Clin Symp 30[1]:16, 1978. Copyright 1978. CIBA-GEIGY Corporation. Reproduced with permission from Clinical Symposia by Frank H. Netter, M.D. All rights reserved.)

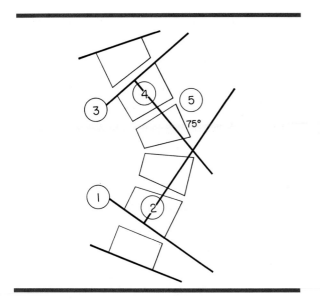

75°

Figure 19–15. Scoliosis; measurement of a curve by the Cobb (roentgenographic) method. *1,* Bottom vertebra: lowest one whose bottom tilts to concavity of curve. *2,* Erect perpendicular from bottom of bottom vertebra. *3,* Top vertebra: highest one whose top tilts to concavity of curve. *4,* Drop perpendicular from top of top vertebra. *5,* Measure intersecting angle. This is the accepted method of measurement of a curve according to the Scoliosis Research Society. Curves of 0–20 degrees are mild, 20–40 degrees are moderate, and above 40 degrees are severe. (From Ferguson A: Orthopaedic Surgery in Infancy and Childhood. 5th ed. Baltimore, Williams & Wilkins, 1981, p 856.)

higher in females, but they are more likely to progress and require treatment. Hereditary tendencies occur; approximately 20% have other family members with the same condition.

Idiopathic scoliosis is classified into three age groups: infantile (birth to 3 yr), juvenile (4–10 yr), and adolescent (11 yr and older). Idiopathic adolescent scoliosis (80% of cases) is the most common cause of spinal deformity. The right thoracic curve is the most common pattern. Infantile scoliosis is very rare in the United States but is common in England. Juvenile scoliosis is not common, but many children with the diagnosis of adolescent scoliosis actually had juvenile onset but were not diagnosed until later.

Clinical Manifestations. Idiopathic scoliosis is a painless disorder. Any child with scoliosis and back pain requires a careful neurologic examination. Left thoracic curves and back pain have an increased incidence of intraspinal pathology, such

as a tumor. These children should be evaluated by MRI.

Treatment. Treatment of idiopathic scoliosis is based on whether the curve is progressive or nonprogressive. No treatment is necessary for nonprogressive deformities. The possibility for progression varies with several factors: sex, skeletal age, curve location, and curve magnitude. The risk for progression is much higher for females (5:1). The younger the child the higher the risk for progression. The treatment of progressive idiopathic adolescent scoliosis is by orthosis (braces) or surgery; exercises alone are ineffective. Typically, progressive curves between 25 and 45 degrees in a skeletally immature patient are managed by orthoses. Curves greater than 45 degrees generally require surgery.

CONGENITAL SCOLIOSIS

Abnormalities of vertebral formation during the 1st trimester result in structural deformities of the spine that are evident at birth or become obvious in early childhood. Congenital scoliosis can be classified as partial or complete failure of vertebral formation (wedge vertebrae or hemivertebrae), partial or complete failure of segmentation (unsegmented bars), or mixed. It may occur as a single anomaly or in combination with other bone, neural, or soft tissue abnormalities of the axial or appendicular skeleton (Fig. 19–16). Congenital genitourinary malformations occur in 20% of children with congenital scoliosis. Unilateral renal agenesis is the most common abnormality, but 6% may have a silent, obstructive uropathy. Renal ultrasound is performed in all patients to assess for possible genitourinary problems. Congenital heart disease may be found in 10–15%. Spinal dysraphism occurs in approximately 20% of patients with congenital scoliosis. These include tethered spinal cord, intradural lipomas, and diastematomyelia. These abnormalities frequently are associated with cutaneous lesions of the back, such as hairy patches, skin dimples, and hemangiomas, and abnormalities of the feet and lower extremities, such as cavus feet, calf atrophy, asymmetric foot size, and neurologic changes. MRI is the procedure of choice for evaluation of possible *spinal dysraphism.* Congenital scoliosis also occurs in association with syndromes such as Klippel-Feil and VATER and spinal dysraphism disorders such as myelodysplasia.

The risk for progression of spinal deformity in a child with congenital scoliosis is variable depending on the growth potential of the malformed vertebra. Defects such as a block vertebra have little

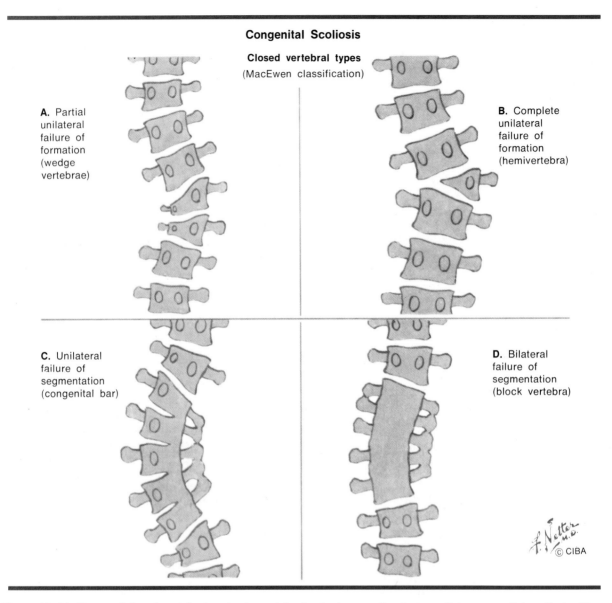

Congenital Scoliosis

Closed vertebral types
(MacEwen classification)

A. Partial unilateral failure of formation (wedge vertebrae)

B. Complete unilateral failure of formation (hemivertebra)

C. Unilateral failure of segmentation (congenital bar)

D. Bilateral failure of segmentation (block vertebra)

Figure 19–16. Types of closed vertebral and extravertebral spinal anomalies that result in congenital scoliosis. (From Hugo A, Keim MD: Scoliosis. Clin Symp 30[1]:16, 1978. Copyright 1978. CIBA-GEIGY Corporation. Reproduced with permission from Clinical Symposia by Frank H. Netter, M.D. All rights reserved.)

growth potential, whereas unilateral unsegmented bars produce progressive deformities. Seventy-five percent of involved patients will demonstrate some progression that continues until skeletal growth stops; approximately 50% will require treatment. Rapid progression can be expected during periods of rapid growth, before 2 and after 10 year of age. Early diagnosis and prompt treatment of progressive curves are essential elements in the care of congenital spinal deformity. Orthotic treatment is of limited value because these curves tend to be rigid. A posterior spinal fusion without instrumentation is the most common procedure.

NEUROMUSCULAR SCOLIOSIS

Progressive spinal deformity is a common and potentially serious abnormality associated with many neuromuscular disorders, such as cerebral palsy, Duchenne muscular dystrophy, spinal muscular atrophy, and myelodysplasia. Progression usually is continuous once scoliosis begins. The magnitude of the deformity depends on the severity and pattern of weakness and whether the disease process is progressive. In nonambulatory patients, the curves tend to be long and sweeping, produce pelvic obliquity, involve the cervical spine, and alter pulmonary function, producing restrictive lung disease. As these curve progress, sitting balance can be lost and the affected individuals must use their arms to support an upright position. Spinal alignment must be part of the routine examination of a child with a neuromuscular disorder. Ambulatory patients have a much lower incidence of spinal deformity than nonambulatory or more severely involved patients. The standing or sitting forward bending test can be used in assessing the symmetry of spinal alignment. Any asymmetry is an indication for roentgenographic evaluation, which should include a PA and lateral standing or sitting radiograph of the entire spine. If the child or adolescent cannot sit unsupported, a supine AP radiograph may be necessary.

The goal of treatment of neuromuscular scoliosis is to prevent progression and loss of function. Nonambulatory patients usually are most comfortable, more independent, and have better respiratory function when they are able to sit erect without external support. Orthotic management or bracing usually is not effective in neuromuscular scoliosis; surgery will be necessary in most cases. The current instrumentation systems are sufficiently strong and distribute the corrective forces such that postoperative immobilization usually is not necessary.

COMPENSATORY SCOLIOSIS

Adolescents with leg length inequality may have a positive screening examination for scoliosis. With a pelvic obliquity, the patient will stand erect and curve the spine in the opposite direction. The magnitude of the leg length discrepancy can be measured radiographically by a scanogram of the lower extremities. It is important to distinguish between a structural and a compensatory spinal deformity.

Kyphosis

The term "kyphosis" refers to a roundback deformity or to an increased angulation in the thoracic or thoracolumbar spine in the sagittal plane. Roundback deformities can be either postural or structural. The latter is termed *Scheuermann's kyphosis.* Kyphosis also can be congenital in origin.

POSTURAL ROUNDBACK

Postural kyphosis is secondary to bad posture and is a common concern of parents. Postural kyphosis is voluntarily corrected in both the standing and prone position. Radiographically, no vertebral abnormalities are present. There may be some increase in the normal kyphosis of the thoracic region, but a supine hyperextension film will show complete correction. The child is responsible for correcting posture. Active treatment is not indicated.

SCHEUERMANN DISEASE

Scheuermann disease is common and second only to idiopathic scoliosis as a cause of spinal deformity. It occurs equally among male and female adolescents. Its etiology is unknown; hereditary factors are present but with no definite pattern of inheritance. The differentiation between postural kyphosis and Scheuermann disease is determined by clinical and roentgenographic evaluation.

Clinical Manifestations.   A patient with Scheuermann disease cannot correct the kyphosis either in the standing position or in the prone, hyperextended position. When viewed from the side in the forward flexed position, patients with Scheuermann disease usually will show an abrupt angulation in the mid to lower thoracic region (Fig. 19–17). A patient with a postural roundback shows a smooth symmetric contour. In both conditions there is reversal of the normal lumbar lordosis. Approximately 50% of patients with Scheuermann

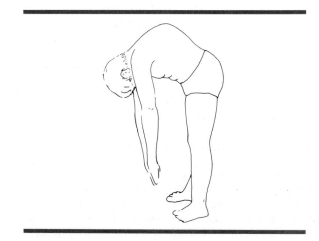

Figure 19–17. Note the sharp break in the contour in the child with kyphosis. (From Behrman RE [ed]: Nelson Textbook of Pediatrics. 14th ed. Philadelphia, WB Saunders, 1992, p 1715.)

disease will have apical back pain, especially with thoracolumbar kyphosis.

The classic roentgenographic findings of Scheuermann kyphosis include narrowing of disc space; loss of the normal anterior height of the involved vertebra, producing wedging of 5 degrees or more in three or more vertebrae; irregularities of the endplates; and Schmorl nodes.

Treatment. Treatment for Scheuermann kyphosis is similar to that for scoliosis and is dependent on the skeletal age of the patient, the degree of deformity, and the presence or absence of pain in the apical region. Nonoperative treatment consists of either corrective plaster casts or an orthosis. Permanent correction of the kyphotic deformity can be achieved with nonoperative management. Surgical treatment in Scheuermann disease rarely is necessary and is indicated for those patients who have completed growth, who have a significant deformity, or who have chronic pain in the apical region.

CONGENITAL KYPHOSIS

Congenital kyphosis includes congenital failure of formation of all or part of the vertebral body but with preservation of the posterior elements, and failure of anterior segmentation of the spine (anterior unsegmented bar). The more severe deformities usually are recognized at birth and rapidly progress thereafter. The less obvious deformities may not appear until years later. Once the progression begins, it does not cease until the end of growth. The most important factor regarding congenital kyphosis is that a progressive deformity in the thoracic spine can result in paraplegia. This usually is associated with the failure of vertebral body formation. Treatment of congenital kyphosis, when necessary, is operative. Orthotic management is ineffective.

Spondylolysis/Spondylolisthesis

Spondylolysis is a defect in the pars interarticularis without forward slippage of one vertebra on another. *Spondylolisthesis* refers to the forward slippage or displacement of one vertebra in relation to another. The lesions are not present at birth but occur in 5% of children by 6 yr of age. Children involved in certain sports, such as gymnastics, have an even higher incidence of spondylolysis. This has been attributed to repetitive hyperextension stresses.

Spondylolisthesis is classified according to the degree of slippage of one vertebra on the other: grade 1, less than 25%; grade 2, 25–50%; grade 3,

50–75%; grade 4, 75–100%; and grade 5, complete displacement. The most common location for spondylolisthesis is the fifth lumbar vertebra on the sacrum (first sacral vertebra).

Clinical Manifestations. Physical examination for spondylolysis or spondylolisthesis is similar to that for any disorder of the spine. A palpable "step-off" at the lumbosacral area and a vertically oriented sacrum indicate severe spondylolisthesis. A neurologic examination must be performed because nerve root involvement can occur, especially with severe displacement.

Roentgenographic Evaluation. Roentgenographic evaluation should include standing PA and lateral views of the entire spine with an oblique radiograph of the lumbar spine. Myelography and MRI may be required in patients with neurologic findings.

Treatment. Children and adolescents with asymptomatic spondylolysis require periodic evaluation during growth to assess for possible slippage; treatment rarely is required. Painful spondylolysis may benefit from orthotic management. If this does not relieve pain, surgical intervention with an in situ posterior spinal fusion may be required.

Adolescents with spondylolisthesis may require treatment, which depends on age, type of defect, degree of the slippage, and associated malalignment in the involved area. Grade I spondylolisthesis usually does not require treatment unless there is chronic pain. Conservative management may be tried initially and, if this fails, surgical intervention may be necessary. Grade 2 usually requires a spinal fusion because of the high risk for further progression. Grade 3 and grade 4 spondylolisthesis usually require fusion to prevent further deformity.

Disc Space Infection

This disease usually is regarded as an osteomyelitis of the vertebral endplates that secondarily invades the disc without producing an acute osteomyelitis of the vertebral body. The most common organism is *S. aureus*. The infection can occur at any age. Children may present with back pain, but also may present with abdominal or pelvic pain or irritability and refusal to walk.

Clinical Manifestations. The child typically maintains the spine in a straight, stiff, or splinted position and will refuse to flex the lumbar spine. The normal lumbar lordosis is reversed and there may be paravertebral muscle spasms. However, in comparison with other forms of osteomyelitis, there are few systemic symptoms such as fever or an elevated white blood cell count. The sedimentation rate typically is elevated.

Roentgenographic Evaluation. The roentgenographic features will vary according to the interval between the onset of symptoms and delay in diagnosis. AP, lateral, and oblique radiographs of the lumbar spine or thoracic spine, depending on the location of symptoms, usually are necessary to make the diagnosis. There is narrowing of the disc space with irregularity of the adjacent vertebral body endplates. In very early cases, bone scan or MRI may be helpful because they may be positive before routine roentgenographic changes are present.

Treatment. The treatment of disc space infection usually is antibiotic therapy. Blood cultures may be helpful in establishing a precise organism. Aspiration needle biopsy of the disc space is reserved for children who do not respond to initial treatment with antistaphylococcal antibiotics. Immobilization of the spine may be used on a symptomatic basis. However, most children will have their symptoms rapidly resolve with intravenous antibiotics. Intravenous antibiotics are continued for 1–2 wk and followed by oral antibiotics for an additional 4 wk.

Torticollis

The definition of torticollis is twisted neck, but the functional definition is shortening of the sternocleidomastoid muscle that pulls the mastoid process toward the ipsilateral sternoclavicular joint. Shortening and secondary contractures can be a primary abnormality of the sternocleidomastoid muscle (muscular torticollis) or secondary to central nervous system or upper cervical spine abnormalities.

Patients with muscular torticollis present with the ear pulled down toward the clavicle on the ipsilateral side. Their face looks upward toward the contralateral side. Early in childhood, a "tumor" is palpated in the midportion of the sternocleidomastoid muscle. This represents swelling or fibrosis of the central portion of the muscle and often is a precursor of the subsequent contracture.

Etiology. In infants, in utero malposition, birth trauma, sternocleidomastoid muscle compartment syndrome, and heredity have been implicated as etiologies. In acquired torticollis in children, central nervous system mass lesions, abnormalities of the cervical spine, and infection are more likely. Psychiatric causes may occur during adolescence.

Diagnosis. A thorough neurologic examination should be performed and AP and lateral radiographs of the cervical spine obtained. A CT scan or MRI of the head and neck is necessary for any patient with persistent neck pain or other neurologic signs and symptoms.

Treatment. Treatment goals in torticollis include ruling out an underlying disorder, increasing range of motion of the neck, and correcting the cosmetic disability. Some patients with muscular torticollis will respond to nonoperative measures, which include range of motion exercises of the head and neck, stretching the restrictive muscles several times daily. General indications for nonoperative management include age less than 1 yr, positive response to stretching exercise over several weeks, and no underlying cervical abnormalities or central nervous system findings.

Principles of surgical management of patients with muscular torticollis include identifying and releasing all restricting bands involving the sternocleidomastoid muscle and other neck structures, moving the head through a full range of motion prior to completion of the surgery, and resuming physical therapy within 2 wk of operation to prevent recurrent contracture.

Back Pain in Children

Back pain in children is unusual and should be viewed with concern. In contrast to adults, in whom back pain frequently is mechanical or psychologic in origin, back pain in children usually is due to organic causes, especially in the preadolescent. Back pain lasting more than a few days requires careful investigation. Approximately 85% of children with back pain of more than 2 mo have a specific lesion: 33% post-traumatic (occult fracture, spondylolysis), 33% developmental (kyphosis, scoliosis), and 18% infection or tumor. In the remaining 15% the diagnosis will be undetermined.

Clinical Manifestations. The history should include the onset and duration of symptoms; antecedent factors; general health; family history; location, character and radiation of pain; and neurologic symptoms such as muscle weakness, sensory changes, and bowel or bladder dysfunction. Physical examination should include a complete musculoskeletal and neurologic evaluation. Spinal alignment, mobility, muscle spasm, and areas of tenderness should be evaluated and

Table 19–11. Differential Diagnosis of Back Plain

Inflammatory Diseases
Discitis (common before 6 yr)
Vertebral osteomyelitis (pyogenic, tuberculous)
Spinal epidural abscess
Pyelonephritis
Pancreatitis
Rheumatologic Diseases
Pauciarticular juvenile rheumatoid arthritis
Reiter syndrome
Ankylosing spondylitis
Psoriatic arthritis
Developmental Diseases
Spondylolysis (common in adolescents)
Spondylolisthesis (common in adolescents)
Scheuermann syndrome (common in adolescents)
Scoliosis (especially left thoracic)
Mechanical Trauma and Abnormalities
Hip/pelvic anomalies
Herniated disc
Overuse syndromes (common with athletic training
    and in gymnasts and dancers)
Vertebral stress fractures
Upper cervical spine instability
Neoplastic Diseases
Primary vertebral tumors (e.g., osteogenic sarcoma)
Metastatic tumor (e.g., neuroblastoma)
Primary spinal tumor (e.g., neuroblastoma, lipoma)
Malignancy of bone marrow (e.g. ALL, lymphoma)
Benign tumors (e.g., eosinophilic granuloma, osteoid
    osteoma)
Other
After lumbar puncture
Conversion reaction
Juvenile osteoporosis

ALL = acute lymphocytic leukemia.

recorded. Muscle strength, sensory assessment such as pain and light touch, deep tendon reflexes, and pathologic reflexes such as the Babinski sign are tested. The danger signs in childhood back pain include persistent or increasing pain; systemic symptoms such as fever, malaise, or weight loss; neurologic findings; bowel or bladder dysfunction; young age, especially under 4 yr (suspect tumor); and painful left thoracic spinal curvatures.

Roentgenographic Evaluation   The first diagnostic procedure is PA and lateral standing films of the entire spine with right and left oblique views of the involved area. Other roentgenographs may be necessary depending on the location of the pain and the differential diagnoses. These include bone scans, CT scan, laminograms, myelography, and MRI. The latter is especially useful when intraspinal pathology is suspected.

Laboratory Evaluation.   Laboratory studies such as complete blood count, erythrocyte sedimenta-

tion rate, and tests for the juvenile forms of arthritis (juvenile rheumatoid arthritis and ankylosing spondylitis) may be necessary. Cerebrospinal fluid should be evaluated if myelography is performed.

Differential Diagnosis.   The differential diagnosis in pediatric back pain is extensive, and is presented in Table 19–11.

Treatment.   The treatment of back pain is based on an accurate diagnosis.

References

Behrman RE (ed): Nelson Textbook of Pediatrics, 14th ed. Philadelphia, WB Saunders, 1992, Sec. 24.12–24.22.

Galasko GSB, Delaney C, Morris P: Spinal stabilization in Duchenne muscular dystrophy. J Bone Joint Surg 74-B: 210, 1992.

Hensinger RN: Back pain in children. In Brandord DS, Hensinger RN (eds): The Pediatric Spine. New York, Theime Inc, 1985, pp 41–60.

Hensinger R: Current concepts review: Spondylolysis and spondylolisthesis in children and adolescents. J Bone Joint Surg 71-A:1098, 1989.

Lonstein JE, Carlson JM: The prediction of curve progression in untreated idiopathic scoliosis during growth. J Bone Joint Surg 66-A:1061, 1984.

Lonstein JE: Adolescent idiopathic scoliosis: Screening and diagnosis. In Instr Course Lect 38:105, 1989.

Lowe TG: Current concepts review: Scheurmann disease. J Bone Joint Surg 72-A:940, 1990.

McMaster MJ, Ohtsuka K: The natural history of congenital scoliosis: A study of 251 patients. J Bone Joint Surg 68-B:588, 1986.

Morrison DL, MacEwen GD: Congenital muscular torticollis: Observations regarding clinical findings, associated conditions, and results of treatment. J Pediatr Orthop 2: 500, 1982.

Scoles PV, Quinn TP: Intervertebral discitis in children and adolescents. Clin Orthop 162:31, 1982.

Thompson GH: Back pain in children. J Bone Joint Surg 75A:928, 1993.

THE SHOULDER

The shoulder joint has minimal geometric stability because of the relatively small glenoid fossa that articulates with a proportionately large hemispheric humeral head. A large range of motion is gained at the expense of intrinsic stability; consequently, the musculature about the shoulder, particularly the muscles of the rotator cuff, must function with normal glenohumeral contact. Scapulothoracic movement greatly expands the range of motion possible at the shoulder area, and the scapula, just as is the case with the glenohumeral joint, requires strong coordinated musculature to function with stability.

Sprengel Deformity

Failure of the upper extremity to descend to its normal location is Sprengel deformity, which occurs with varying degrees of severity. The scapula is located abnormally high with respect to the child's neck and thorax. Webbing of the skin and a low posterior hair line may be associated findings. In the severe form, a bone (omovertebral) may connect the scapula with the cervical spine and virtually no scapulothoracic movement may be possible; often, associated muscle anomalies are present as well that further limit strength and stability of the shoulder girdle. In the mild form, the scapula is slightly high riding, with less than normal motion. Association with congenital cervical vertebral anomalies, particularly the **Klippel-Feil anomaly,** occur and suggest the possibility of significant problems in other organ systems. The best outcome in severe Sprengel deformities is achieved in early childhood by surgically repositioning and occasionally partially resecting the scapula.

Brachial Plexus (Obstetric) Palsy
See Chapter 6.

Dislocation of the Shoulder

Dislocation of the shoulder is uncommon in childhood but becomes more frequent in adolescence. The younger the individual at the time of the initial dislocation, the more likely he or she is to develop recurrent dislocation. The chances of redislocation are so high that many orthopedic surgeons now favor early reconstruction rather than instituting conservative treatment and awaiting further dislocations.

Epiphysiolysis of the Proximal Humeral Epiphysis

The youngster who engages regularly in a throwing sport is at risk for traumatic epiphysiolysis of the proximal humeral physis. This disorder is a fatigue fracture through the physis; it heals with rest and avoidance of repetitive throwing. Pain about the shoulder is the usual presenting complaint.

Overuse Syndromes

Overuse syndromes, inflammatory responses in tendons and bursae subjected to repetitive mild trauma, are uncommon in childhood but may be seen in the adolescent. Subacromial bursitis, for example, occurs in tennis players and swimmers. Bicipital tendinitis is uncommon in the young but may produce a sensation of something snapping in the shoulder or shoulder pain when the bicipital groove is shallow and the tendon can sublux from it. In these types of inflammatory responses, direct tenderness over the involved anatomic structure is diagnostic.

References

Behrman RE (ed): Nelson Textbook of Pediatrics. 14th ed. Philadelphia, WB Saunders, 1992, Sec. 24.23.
Wagner KT, Lyne ED: Adolescent traumatic dislocations of the shoulder with open epiphyses. J Pediatr Orthop 3: 61, 1983.

THE ELBOW

The elbow joint consists of three articulations: the ulna and the humerus, the radius and the humerus, and the proximal radius and the ulna. Collectively, they provide for a hinge-type joint that allows for a palm-up (supination) and a palm-down (pronation) positioning of the wrist and hand. The elbow has great geometric stability, and the musculature moving the joint primarily motors flexion and extension at the elbow joint, but there are smaller muscles that primarily serve to rotate the radius about its long axis.

Nursemaid's Elbow

The radial head is not as bulbous in the infant as in older children. During infancy, the circular ligament that passes around its base can partially slip off the head with traction across the elbow. When the ligament slips, the entity is known as nursemaid's elbow or subluxation of the annular ligament (Fig. 19–18). The subluxation is initiated by a jerk on the arm when a child falls with the hand being held or when a child is forcefully lifted by the hand. When the subluxation occurs, the hand typically is held in a palm-down position, and the child may refuse to use the hand or may cry when the elbow is moved. Moving the hand to a palm-up position with pressure over the radial head usually reduces the ligament subluxation and restores full normal use of the extremity. The parents should be educated about the mechanism of injury and encouraged to avoid picking the child up by holding the hand or forearm. Once subluxa-

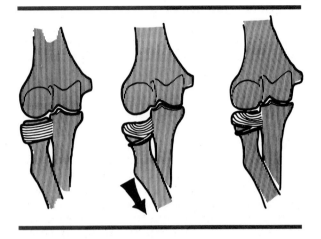

Figure 19–18. The pathology of pulled elbow. The annular ligament is torn when the arm is pulled. The radial head moves distally and, when traction is discontinued, the ligament is carried into the joint. (From Rang M: Children's Fractures. 2nd ed. Philadelphia, JB Lippincott, 1983, p 193.)

tion has occurred, there is a propensity for subsequent episodes. Generally, the problem resolves with maturation.

Panner Disease

This is an osteochondrosis that involves the ossific nucleus of the capitellum, the lateral portion of the distal humeral epiphysis. It is most common in adolescents, especially those involved in throwing activities. They complain of pain and may have crepitation and loss of motion. AP, lateral, and oblique roentgenographs, tomograms, or CT may be helpful. In the absence of a loose osteocartilaginous body, the treatment is conservative; if such a body is present, surgery is indicated.

Throwing Injuries

The elbow is especially vulnerable to throwing injuries in the skeletally immature child. The most common pathology results from abnormal compressive forces acting across the radial side of the joint. In addition to Panner disease, the ossific nucleus of the radial head may become asymmetric as compared with the opposite side, or may be fragmented. Some irregularity in shape of the cartilaginous radial head is present. Additionally, there may be irregularity of the ossific nucleus of the capitellum or compressions in the normally rounded articular cartilage of the capitellum. Rarely, cartilage flecks from the capitellum or radial head may

shed into the joint, producing loose bodies. Before the problem becomes established or severe, the child complains of an aching pain about the elbow, which generally is worse after throwing than during the time spent at the throwing activity. On physical examination, an early loss of supination (the palm-up position of the hand) can be detected. Children who develop these lesions generally have a high emotional investment in their particular sport, most commonly baseball, and nonparticipation is a difficult option for them to accept. Avoidance of pitching until the elbow is normal on physical examination and follow-up roentgenogram is the best solution. Often, switching the baseball player to another position allows the child to avoid pitching. Behind such highly motivated youngsters is usually an overzealous parent or coach in need of appropriate counseling.

References

Behrman RE (ed): Nelson Textbook of Pediatrics. 14th ed. Philadelphia, WB Saunders, 1992, Sec. 24.24, 24.26.
Bora FW: The Pediatric Upper Extremity: Diagnosis and Management. Philadelphia, WB Saunders, 1986.

THE HAND

Multiple small joints, a delicately balanced intrinsic muscle system, a powerful extrinsic muscle system, dense sensory innervation, and specialized skin combined to make the hand a highly mobile, sensitive, delicate yet powerful anatomic part.

The extrinsic muscles, those whose muscle origin is in the forearm and that motor the hand via tendons that pass to it, provide great power, whereas the intrinsic muscles, those that are located in the hand itself, modulate the effects of the powerful extrinsic musculature and provide for delicate coordinated movement. Simply asking the patient to open the hand, extending and spreading the fingers and thumb, and, subsequently, clenching the hand to a fist yields much insight, because these maneuvers require coordinated function of both the intrinsic and extrinsic musculature as well as full range of motion in the small joints of the hand. Following this maneuver, simply having the individual squeeze the examiner's fingers gives further information about the strength of the hand.

Finger Abnormalities

Extra digits **(polydactyly)** occur both as simple and complex varieties (see Table 19–8). Those skin tags and digit remnants typically seen near the metacarpophalangeal joint of the small finger or of the thumb that do not have palpable bone in their base or possess voluntary movement may simply be excised while the child is still in the nursery. Varieties of polydactyly more complex than this should be referred for amputation.

Syndactyly also occurs in both simple and complex patterns (see Table 19–9). There always is concern about the sharing of common important structures between the digits and about the tethering effect of the syndactyly on the growth of the affected digits. Referral for delineation of the specific pathology and development of a treatment strategy is indicated when the condition is recognized.

Ganglion

A synovial fluid-filled cyst about the wrist, a *ganglion*, is common in childhood. The usual site is the dorsum of the wrist near the radiocarpal joint, and a secondary site is over the volar radial aspect of the wrist. The essential pathology is a defect in one of the joint capsules; with wrist use, synovial fluid is pumped into the soft tissue, where it becomes walled off by reactive fibrous tissue. Often, in the skeletally immature child, the process is benign and tends to disappear with the passage of time. In the event that a ganglion is sufficiently large to cause pain or interfere with normal tendon function, aspiration and injection of the cyst is sometimes helpful; in refractory cases, surgical excision of the cyst accompanied by removal of the tract that extends into the joint is curative.

References

Behrman RE (ed): Nelson Textbook of Pediatrics. 14th ed. Philadelphia, WB Saunders, 1992, Sec. 24.24.
Bora FW Jr: The Pediatric Upper Extremity: Diagnosis and Management. Philadelphia, WB Saunders, 1986.
Satku K, Ganesh B: Ganglia in children. J Pediatr Orthop 5:513, 1985.

MUSCULOSKELETAL TRAUMA

Fractures in children have been estimated to account for 10–15% of all childhood injuries. Children are not small adults; their skeletal systems have anatomic, biomechanical, and physiologic differences from those of adults. These result in different fracture patterns, including epiphyseal injuries, problems of diagnosis, and variation in management techniques.

The anatomic differences in the pediatric skeleton include the presence of preosseous cartilage, growth plate (physes), and thicker, stronger periosteum that produces callus more rapidly and in greater amounts. Biomechanically, the pediatric skeletal system can absorb more energy prior to deformation and fracture than adult bone. This has been attributed to lower ash content and the greater porosity of young bone. As maturation occurs, the porosity deceases and the cortical bone becomes thicker and stronger. The thick periosteum of a child is a major determinant in whether a fracture becomes displaced. The thick periosteum also can act as an impediment to closed reduction because of the hinging phenomena. Conversely, it can help stabilize a fracture following reduction.

Unusual Features

FRACTURE REMODELING

Remodeling occurs by a combination of periosteal resorption and new bone formation. Thus, anatomic alignment in certain pediatric fractures is not always necessary. The major factors affecting fracture remodeling include: the child's age, the proximity of the fracture to a joint, and the relationship of the fracture to the plane of joint axis or motion. The amount of remaining musculoskeletal growth provides the basis for remodeling—the younger the child the greater the remodeling potential. Certain physes also have a relatively greater growth potential than others. Fractures adjacent to a physis undergo the greatest amount of remodeling, provided the residual deformity is in the plane of motion of that joint. Fracture remodeling will not be effective in: displaced intra-articular fractures, diaphyseal fractures, malrotation, and fracture displacement or deformity not in the plane of joint axis. The amount of remodeling will be significantly diminished as a child approaches skeletal maturity.

Overgrowth

Overgrowth, especially in long bones such as the femur, is due to the hyperemia associated with fracture healing. Femoral fractures in children under 10 yr of age frequently overgrow 1–3 cm. This accounts for the concept of bayonet apposition to compensate for the overgrowth that may occur over the next 1–2 yr. After 10 yr of age, overgrowth is less of a problem and end-on-alignment is recommended.

PROGRESSIVE DEFORMITY

Injuries to a physis can result in complete or partial closure. As a consequence, angular deformity, shortening, or both can occur. The magnitude depends on the bone involved and the amount of remaining growth. Growth arrest most commonly occurs in the distal femur, distal tibia, and proximal tibia.

HEALING RATE

Children heal fractures faster than adults. This is due to their growth potential and thicker, more metabolically active periosteum. As the older child and adolescent matures, the rate of healing slows and approaches that of an adult.

Pediatric Fracture Patterns

NONEPIPHYSEAL FRACTURES

Complete.   Complete fractures occur when both sides of the bone are fractured. This is the most common fracture type. These fractures may be classified as spiral, transverse, oblique, or comminuted depending on the direction of the fracture line.

Buckle or Torus Fracture.   Compression of bone produce a buckle or torus fracture. These fractures typically occur in the metaphyseal areas in young children, especially the distal radius. They are inherently stable and usually heal in 2–3 wk with simple immobilization.

Greenstick.   When a bone is angulated beyond the limits of plastic deformation, a greenstick fracture may occur. This represents bone failure on the tension side and compression or bend deformity on the opposite side. The energy was insufficient to result in a complete fracture.

Bowing or Bend Fractures.   Traumatic bowing or bend deformities are due to plastic deformation of bone. The bone was angulated beyond its limit of plastic deformation but did not fracture. Thus, no fracture line is visible roentgenographically.

EPIPHYSEAL FRACTURES

Fractures involving the physes are common and comprise 15–20% of all children's fractures. There is a male-to-female ratio of 2:1 and the upper extremity is involved twice as frequently as the lower. The peak incidence in males is 13–14 yr and in females 11–12 yr. The distal radius is the most common site, followed by the distal tibia.

Ligaments frequently insert into epiphyses. As a consequence, traumatic forces supplied to an extremity may be transmitted to the growth plate (physis). The strength of the physes is enhanced by their shape and perichondrial ring. However, the physis still is not as strong biomechanically as the metaphyseal or diaphyseal bone. The physis is most resistant to traction and least resistant to torsional or angular forces.

Salter and Harris have classified epiphyseal injuries into five groups: type I, epiphyseal separation through the physis; type II, fracture through a portion of the physis but exiting across the metaphysis, type III, fracture through the physis but exiting across the epiphysis into the joint, type IV, a fracture line extending across the metaphysis, physis, and epiphysis; and type V, a crush injury to the physis (Fig. 19–19). This classification allows gen-

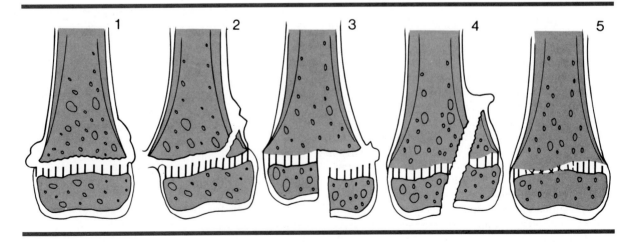

Figure 19–19.   The types of growth plate injury as classified by Salter and Harris. (From Salter RB, Harris WR: Injuries involving the epiphyseal plate. J Bone Joint Surg 45-A:587, 1963.)

eralized prognostic information regarding the risk for premature physeal closure and the indications for treatment. A type VI injury also has been suggested, which is an injury to the perichondral ring that often results in a peripheral bony bridge and rapid angular deformities.

Types I and II fractures usually can be managed by closed reduction techniques and do not require perfect alignment. A major exception are type II fractures of the distal femur. Fractures in this location have a poor prognosis unless almost anatomic alignment is obtained by either closed or open methods. Types III and IV epiphyseal fractures require anatomic alignment because of displacement of the physis and the articular surfaces. Type V fractures usually are recognized in retrospect and invariably result in premature growth plate closure.

Treatment

CLOSED TREATMENT.

The majority of pediatric fractures can be managed by closed methods.

OPERATIVE TREATMENT

Certain pediatric fractures have been demonstrated to have better prognosis if the fractures are reduced, by either open or closed techniques, and then internally fixed. Approximately 3–4% of pediatric fractures require internal fixation. The common indications for internal fixations in children and adolescents with open growth plates include: displaced epiphyseal fractures, displaced intra-articular fractures, unstable fractures, fractures in the multiply injured child, and open fractures.

In children, the goals of surgery and type of internal fixation device used are different. The goals of surgery are not rigid internal fixation but rather attainment and maintenance of anatomic alignment. Thus, simple fixation with the use of Steinmann pins, Kirschner wires, and small cortical screws is indicated. Fractures subsequently are protected with external immobilization, usually a plaster cast, until satisfactory healing has occurred. All internal fixation devices are removed following fracture healing to prevent incorporation into the callus formation and bone and to prevent physeal damage if a physis has been transgressed by a smooth wire or pin.

External fixation also has been demonstrated to be very successful in certain pediatric fractures.

The major indications have been pelvic and open extremity fractures, especially those with extensive soft tissue loss, burns, or vascular and nerve repairs.

Special Problems

NEUROVASCULAR INJURIES

The most common sites for neural or vascular injuries are the distal humerus, in which supracondylar fractures occur, and the knee, in which distal physeal fractures or dislocations occur. Careful neurovascular examination is necessary in all fractures and should be documented in the patient's medical record.

COMPARTMENT SYNDROMES

Hemorrhage and soft tissue swelling within tight fascial compartments may result in muscle ischemia and neurovascular compromise unless relieved surgically. This condition is called compartment syndrome. The forearms and lower legs are the major sites, and these syndromes tend to occur following supracondylar fractures at the distal humerus and tibial shaft fractures. The common findings are tense compartments, severe pain, decreased sensation in the nerves that transverse the involved compartment, and pain with passive stretch (fingers or toes) of involved muscles. In addition, once an injured extremity is placed in a cast, it is possible that a cast-induced compartment syndrome may develop. It is the responsibility of the treating physician to ensure that parents understand the signs of ischemia and appreciate that it is an emergency. They must contact the physician or return to the hospital immediately.

TODDLER'S FRACTURE

An oblique fracture of the distal one third of the tibia without a fibula fracture can occur with minimal trauma in children 1–3 yr of age and occasionally up to 6 yr of age. Limping or inability to bear weight is a common complaint. These fractures may not be visible roentgenographically but occasionally oblique roentgenographs may be helpful. A physical examination may show minimal soft tissue swelling, pain, and slight warmth.

CHILD ABUSE

Fractures attributable to child abuse are a special issue that constantly must be considered when assessing trauma in the infant and younger child, especially those 3 yr of age or less (see Chapter 1). Multiple fractures that are visible roentgenographically at different stages of healing are a classic sign. If a child has been shaken, frequently there will be areas adjacent to the epiphysis on the metaphyseal side that will fracture, produce the appearance of metaphyseal "corner" fractures. Long bone fractures, especially spiral fractures of the humeral, tibial, or femoral shaft, suggest that someone has forcefully twisted the extremity. When there is any suspicion of abuse, the child should be admitted to the hospital for full assessment. Roentgenographs of a specific area are appropriate, but a bone scan may be more helpful in identifying other fractures, old and new. A thorough physical examination focusing on soft tissues, the skeletal system, and the cranium, along with a careful examination of the retina for hemorrhage or detachment, is very important.

References

Behrman RE (ed): Nelson Textbook of Pediatrics. 14th ed. Philadelphia, WB Saunders, 1992, Sec. 24.25–24.28.

King J, Kiefendorf D, Apthorp J, et al: Analysis of 429 fractures in 189 battered children. J Pediatr Orthop 8:585, 1988.

Peterson HA: Partial growth plate arrest and its treatment. J Pediatr Orthop 4:246, 1984.

Rockwood CA Jr, Wilkens KE, King RE: In Fractures in Children. 3rd ed. Philadelphia, JB Lippincott, 1991, pp 000–000.

Tenenbien M, Reed MH, Block GB: The toddler's fracture revisited. Am J Emerg Med 8:208, 1990.

Thompson GH, Wilber JH, Marcus RE: Internal Fixation of fractures in children and adolescents: A comparative analysis. Clin Orthop 188:10, 1984.

Table 19–12. Benign Bone Tumors and Cysts

Disease	Characteristics	Roentgenography	Treatment	Prognosis
Osteochondroma (osteocartilaginous exostosis)	Common; distal metaphysis of femur, proximal humerus, proximal tibia; painless, hard, nontender mass	Bony outgrowth, sessile or pedunculated	Excision, if symptomatic	Excellent; malignant transformation rare
Multiple hereditary exostoses	Osteochondroma of long bones; bone growth disturbances	As above	As above	Recurrences
Osteoid ostoma	Point tenderness; pain relieved by aspirin; femur and tibia; predominantly found in boys	Osteosclerosis surrounds small radiolucent nidus, 1 cm	As above	Excellent
Giant osteoid osteoma (osteoblastoma)	As above, but more destructive	Osteolytic component; size greater than 1 cm	As above	Excellent
Enchondroma	Tubular bones of hands and feet; pathologic fractures, swollen bone; Ollier disease if multiple lesions are present	Radiolucent diaphyseal or metaphyseal lesion; may calcify	Excision or curettage	Excellent; malignant transformation rare
Nonossifying fibroma	Silent; rare pathologic fracture; late childhood adolescence	Incidental roentgenographic finding; thin sclerotic border, radiolucent lesion	None or curettage with fractures	Excellent; heals spontaneously
Eosinophilic granuloma	Age 5–10 yr; skull, jaw, long bones; pathologic fracture; pain	Small, radiolucent without reactive bone; punched out lytic lesion	Biopsy, excision rare; irradiation	Excellent; may heal spontaneously
Brodie abscess	Insidious local pain; limp; suspected as malignancy	Circumscribed metaphyseal osteomyelitis; lytic leions with sclerotic rim	Biopsy; antibiotics	Excellent
Unicameral bone cyst (simple bone cyst)	Metaphysis of long bone (femur, humerus); pain, pathologic fracture	Cyst in medullary canal, expands cortex; fluid-filled unilocular or multilocular cavity	Curettage; steroid injection into lesion	Excellent; some heal spontaneously
Aneurysmal bone cyst	As above; contains blood, fibrous tissue	Expands beyond metaphyseal cartilage	Curettage, bone graft	Excellent

METABOLIC BONE DISEASE

Metabolic bone disease may occur from disorders that primarily affect bone, cartilage, and collagen or that indirectly affect bone mineralization. Primary bone disorders often occur in the fetus or young infant, such as the skeletal dysplasias—dwarf-like syndromes (e.g., achondroplasia, Kneist dysplasia, osteogenesis imperfecta).

Patients with metabolic disorders that produce indirect effects may appear normal at birth and later develop signs of bone disease. The signs of bone disease may occur after or concomitant with the manifestations produced by the underlying metabolic disorder (e.g., homocystinuria, Marfan syndrome, Gaucher disease, renal rickets). The treatment of primary disorders of bone is limited, and therapy of inborn errors of metabolism must be tailored to the specific disease (see Chapter 5).

BONE TUMORS AND CYSTIC LESIONS

Bone tumors and cystic lesions are common in childhood. Some represent fibrous dysplasia and others are benign tumors, whereas subacute osteomyelitis (Brodie abscess) or eosinophilic granuloma represent lesions unrelated to abnormal osseous or cartilage growth (Table 19–12). Many of these lesions produce pain, pathologic fractures, or limp; others may be incidental findings on roentgenographic examination. The prognosis usually is excellent. Treatment is summarized in Table 19–12. Malignant bone tumors are discussed in Chapter 15.

Reference

Behrman RE (ed): Nelson Textbook of Pediatrics. 14th ed. Philadelphia. WB Saunders, 1992, Sec. 17.17–17.19, 24.29–24.74.

Appendices

Table AP–1. Drug Doses* (Drugs Listed Alphabetically by Generic Name)

KEY:

NB	newborn (birth to end of 1st mo)	†	available as generic preparation
IN	infant (1–12 mo)	‡	available also under other brand name(s)
CH	child (1–12 yr)		
AD	adult	g	gram
caps	capsules	mg	milligram = 10^{-3} g
div	divided	μg	microgram = 10^{-6} g
DW	dextrose in water		(sometimes abbreviated "mcg")
IM	intramuscular	ng	nanogram = 10^{-9} g
inj	injection	kg	kilogram = 10^3 g
IV	intravenous	mL	milliliter = 10^{-3} liter $\simeq$ cm^3 = cc (cubic
LO	linguo-occlusal		centimeter)
ointm	ointment	℞	Prescription
PO	per os, oral		
PR	per rectum		
SC	subcutaneous		
SL	sublingual		
sol	solution		
susp	suspension		
tabl	tablets		

I. Antibiotics

Acyclovir; antiviral agent against herpes simplex and varicella-zoster virus by selective inhibition of viral DNA synthesis

℞ in clinical herpes simplex infection in neonates: NB = IV (over 60 min): 10 mg/kg/dose every 8 hr, for 14–21 days. Dosing interval should be increased to 24 hr if renal function is less than 25% of normal

℞ in immunocompromised individuals with herpes simplex or varicella-zoster virus infection: CH = IV (over 60 min): 250 mg/m²/dose every 8 hr; AD = IV (over 60 min): 5 mg/kg/dose every 8 hr

℞ in severe first episode of herpes genitalis: CH, AD = LO: 5% ointm

ZOVIRAX: inj, ointm

Amikacin sulfate; antimicrobial aminoglycoside effective primarily against gram-negative micro-organisms

NB <7 days or <28 wk = IM, IV (over 20–30 min): 7.5 mg/kg once daily; 28–34 wk, 7.5 mg/kg every 18 hr; >34 wk, 7.5 mg/kg every 12 hr; NB >7 days <28 wk, 7.5 mg/kg every 18 hr; 28–34 wk, 7.5 mg/kg every 12 hr; >34 wk, 7.5 mg/kg every 8 hr

IN, CH = 15–20 mg/kg/24 hr, div, every 8 hr

Serum concentrations should be monitored; therapeutic peak concentration 25–35 mg/L, trough concentration <10 mg/L

AMIKIN: inj

---

* No attempt has been made to reproduce a comprehensive list of adverse side effects or of formulations available for the drugs listed. For these, the reader again is referred to standard textbooks of pharmacology, to the package inserts accompanying the commercial preparations of each drug, and to Physicians' Desk Reference, distributed annually in the United States by Physicians' Desk Reference, Box 210, Westwood, NJ 07675.

Dosages listed in the table are not specifically intended for premature and newborn infants unless so indicated.

All doses are average doses and are approximate. Variability of individual response may require alteration of dosage upward or downward. Doses based on different criteria (e.g., body weight, surface area) frequently do not correspond. Surface area may be calculated from Figure AP–1.

Doses generally are expressed as grams or milligrams per kilogram of body weight per 24 hours (g or mg/kg/24 hr), even for drugs ordinarily administered on a prn (as needed or indicated) basis.

For teratogenic effects of drugs, see Chapter 6, package inserts, and Physicians' Desk Reference.

Because of the multiplicity of proprietary names and formulations of the drugs listed, only a few representative examples have been given of the many proprietary preparations available in most instances. We have intended no bias in selecting the proprietary names used, and make due apology to any manufacturers and distributors whose products may appear to have been slighted.

See KEY to abbreviations, above; for further information about drugs, see package inserts.

Table AP–1. Drug Doses* (Drugs Listed Alphabetically by Generic Name) *Continued*

Amoxicillin; acid-resistant ampicillin congener

IN, CH = PO: 20–40 mg/kg/24 hr, div, every 8 hr

†, AMOXIL, LAROTID, ‡: caps, oral susp, pediatric drops

Amoxicillin + clavulanic acid; combination of a β-lactam antibiotic with a β-lactamase (penicillinase) inhibitor.

℞ for otitis media, sinusitis, lower respiratory tract, skin, soft fissue, and urinary tract infections: CH = PO: amoxicillin 20–40 mg/kg/24 hr + clavulanic acid 5–10 mg/kg/24 hr, div, every 8 hr

Note: May cause diarrhea, abdominal pain, urticaria and other rashes, possibly due to clavulanic acid alone.

Amoxicillin is available as single component.

AUGMENTIN: tabl of 2 strengths: 250 mg amoxicillin + 125 mg clavulanic acid, and 500 mg amoxicillin + 125 mg clavulanic acid; oral susp with amoxicillin 125 mg + clavulanic acid 31.25 mg/5 mL, or amoxicillin 250 mg + clavulanic acid 62.5 mg/5 mL

Ampicillin; acid-resistant penicillin congener

NB (≤7 days old) = IV (over 15–30 min), IM: 50 mg/kg/24 hr, div, every 12 hr

℞ for meningitis: IV: 100 mg/kg/24 hr, div, every 4 hr

NB (>7 days old) = IV (over 15–30 min), IM: 75 mg/kg/24 hr, div, every 8 hr

℞ for meningitis: IV: 200 mg/kg/24 hr, div, every 4 hr

IN, CH = PO: 50–100 mg/kg/24 hr, div, every 6 hr

℞ for septicemia: IV (over 15–30 min), IM: 100–200 mg/kg/24 hr, div, every 4 hr (IV) or every 6 hr (IM)

℞ for meningitis: IV (over 15–30 min): 400 mg/kg/24 hr, div, every 4 hr

ampicillin sodium, for injection, OMNIPEN-N, PEN-BRITIN-S, ‡: inj

ampicillin trihydrate, †, OMNIPEN, PENBRITIN, ‡: caps, oral susp, pediatric drops

Carbenicillin disodium; semisynthetic penicillin susceptible to destruction by penicillinase

℞ for systemic use: NB = IV (over 15–30 min), IM: initial dose 100 mg/kg, followed by maintenance therapy according to the following criteria:

≤2000 g + ≤7 days old: 225 mg/kg/24 hr, div, every 8 hr

≤2000 g + >7 days old: 400 mg/kg/24 hr, div, every 6 hr

>2000 g + ≤7 days old: 300 mg/kg/24 hr, div, every 6 hr

>2000 g + >7 days old: 400 mg/kg/24 hr, div, every 6 hr

IN, CH = IV (over 15–30 min), IM: 400–600 mg/kg/24 hr, div, every 4 hr (IV) or every 6 hr (IM)

GEOPEN: inj; 1 g carbenicillin disodium contains 6.5 mEq Na⁺

℞ for treatment of urinary tract infection only: CH = PO: 10–30 mg/kg/24 hr, div, every 6 hr

carbenicillin indanyl sodium; GEOCILLIN: tabl

Cephalosporins, semisynthetic derivatives of 7-aminocephalosporanic acid, structurally related to penicillins

a. **First-generation cephalosporins:** active against most gram-positive cocci (excluding enterococci and methicillin-resistant *Staphylococcus aureus*), some strains of *Escherichia coli, Klebsiella pneumoniae,* and *Proteus mirabilis*

Note: First-generation drugs do not cross the blood–brain barrier and therefore are ineffective for treatment of infections within the central nervous system.

Cefadroxil: relatively resistant against β-lactamases; absorption appears unaffected by food intake; minimal inhibitory concentrations for *E. coli, P. mirabilis, Klebsiella* species may be maintained in urine for about 20 hr after single dose

℞ CH = PO: 30 mg/kg/24 hr, div, every 12 hr

DURICEF, ULTRACEF: caps, powder for oral susp

Cefazolin sodium: NB = IV (over 15–30 min), IM: 40 mg/kg/24 hr, div, every 12 hr; IN, CH = IV (over 15–30 min), IM: 50–100 mg/kg/24, div, every 6 hr

ANCEF, KEFZOL: inj

Cephalothin: NB = IV (over 15–30 min), IM: ≤7 days old: 40 mg/kg/24 hr, div, every 12 hr; >7 days old: 60 mg/kg/24 hr, div, every 8 hr; IN, CH = IV: 80–160 mg/kg/24 hr, div, every 4 hr

KEFLIN; inj

ANSPOR, VELOSEF; caps, oral susp, inj

b. **Second-generation cephalosporins:** more active against gram-negative bacteria such as *Haemophilus influenzae* type b, *Neisseria gonorrhoeae,* and enteric gram-negative bacilli

Cefaclor: effective against some β-lactamase–producing, ampicillin-resistant strains of *H. influenzae;* absorption not affected by food intake

℞ for treatment of otitis media and infections of the upper and lower respiratory tracts, urinary tract, skin, and soft tissues with susceptible organisms: IN, CH = PO: 20–40 mg/kg/24 hr, div, every 8 hr

CECLOR: powder for oral susp, caps

Cefoxitin: IN (>3 mo old), CH = IV, IM: 80–160 mg/kg/24 hr, div, every 4–6 hr

Note: May cause renal impairment and cross-reaction with penicillin.

MEFOXIN: vials, infusion bottles, inj

c. **Third-generation cephalosporins:** less active against gram-positive cocci than older cephalosporins but more active against most strains of enteric gram-negative bacilli, moderately active against *Pseudomonas aeruginosa,* highly active against *H. influenaze* and *N. gonorrhocae.*

Ceftriaxone sodium: biliary and renal excretion

℞ misc. infection 50–75 mg/kg/24 hr (not to exceed 2 g) divided q 12 hr; meningitis 100 mg/kg/24 hr (not to exceed 4 g) divided q 12 hr

Cefotaxime: IN, CH = IV, IM: 50–150 mg/kg/24 hr, div, every 4–6 hr

See KEY to abbreviations, p. 747; for further information about drugs, see package inserts.

Table AP–1. Drug Doses* (Drugs Listed Alphabetically by Generic Name) *Continued*

℞ in neonatal meningitis: NB = IV 150–200 mg/kg/ 24 hr, div, every 4–6 hr

Note: May cause hypersensitivity reactions in penicillin-sensitive patients. Adjust dose with renal failure. Nephrotoxicity may develop with combined use of a cephalosporin and an aminoglycoside.

CLAFORAN: vials, inj

Ceftazidime: possesses antipseudomonal activity

NB = IV, IM: <7 days <2000 g, 100 mg/kg/24 hr, div, every 12 hr; >2000 g, 100 mg/kg/24 hr, div, every 8 hr; >7 days, 100–150 mg/kg/24 hr, div, every 8 hr

IN, CH = IV, IM: 100–150 mg/kg/24 hr, div, every 8 hr (meningitis, 150 mg/kg/24 hr, div, every 8 hr)

FORTAZ, TAZIDIME: inj

Chloramphenicol: derivative of dichloracetic acid combined to a structure containing a nitrobenzene ring

NB = IV (over 15–30 min), (PO):

≤14 days old, irrespective of weight: 25 mg/kg/24 hr, div, every 4 hr

15–30 days old and ≤2000 g: 25 mg/kg/24 hr, div, every 4 hr

15–30 days old and >2000 g: 50 mg/kg/24 hr, div, every 4 hr

IN, CH = PO: 50–100 mg/kg/24 hr, div, every 6 hr; IV (over 15–30 min): 100 mg/kg/24 hr, div, every 4 hr

Caution: Newborn infants susceptible to development of high blood levels and gray-baby syndrome on usual doses; therefore, careful monitoring (of blood levels, if available) mandatory. Dose-duration–related suppression of erythrocyte production universal; weekly hematocrit or hemoglobin and reticulocyte count mandatory. Idiosyncratic aplastic anemia occasionally occurs without warning and may be lethal. **Use only when specifically indicated.**

CHLOROMYCETIN: caps

chloramphenicol palmitate, CHLOROMYCETIN palmitate: oral susp

chloramphenicol sodium succinate, CHLOROMYCETIN sodium succinate: inj

Chloroquine, a 4-aminoquinoline antimalarial agent; drug of choice for the treatment of attacks of malaria caused by *Plasmodium vivax, P. ovale, P. malariae,* and susceptible strains of *P. falciparum.* Not advised for use in treatment of juvenile rheumatoid arthritis.

℞ oral treatment of uncomplicated attacks (excluding those caused by chloroquine-resistant *P. falciparum*):

Chloroquine diphosphate: CH = PO:

first day: 25 mg/kg/first 24 hr (equivalent to base: 15 mg/kg/first 24 hr), div in initial dose of 16.5 mg/ kg (equivalent to base 10 mg/kg) and subsequent dose of 8.5 mg/kg (equivalent to base 5 mg/kg) 6 hr later;

second and third day: 8.5 mg/kg/24 hr (equivalent to base 5 mg/kg/24 hr), as single daily dose

℞ intramuscular treatment of severe illness (excluding malaria caused by chloroquine-resistant *P. falciparum*):

Chloroquine dihydrochloride: CH = IM: 6 mg/kg/dose (equivalent to base 5 mg/kg/dose), every 12 hr, until clinical response is obtained and treatment can be completed by the oral route

℞ clinical prophylaxis of malaria (prevention of clinical manifestations from infection with any of the *Plasmodium* species):

Chloroquine diphosphate: CH = PO: 8.5 mg/kg/dose (equivalent to base 5 mg/kg/dose) once every 7 days, beginning 2 wk before entering the malarious area and continuing for 8 wk after return. For eradication of *P. vivax* and *P. ovale,* treatment for 14 days with primaquine should be considered on leaving malarious area.

Chloroquine diphosphte, ARALEN diphosphate, (RESOCHIN) diphosphate: tabl

chloroquine dihydrochloride, ARALEN dihydrochloride: inj

(1 mg chloroquine base is equivalent to 1.65 mg chloroquine diphosphate or 1.2 mg chloroquine dihydrochloride)

Caution: Irreversible retinal damage may occur with prolonged use; frequent ophthalmologic examination necessary to detect early changes. *Note:* Chloroquine does not cause hemolysis in individuals with G-6-PD deliciency

Chlortetracycline: see Tetracyclines

Clindamycin: semisynthetic derivative of lincomycin

NB <7 days <2000 g, 10 mg/kg/24 hr, div, every 12 hr; >7 days <2000 g, 15 mg/kg/24 hr, div, every 8 hr; <7 days >2000 g, 15 mg/kg/24 hr, div, every 8 hr; >7 days >2000 g, 20 mg/kg/24 hr, div, every 6 hr

IN, CH: 20–45 mg/kg/24 hr, div, every 6–8 hr

Note: Therapy may be associated with the development of pseudomembranous colitis.

clindamycin hydrochloride, CLEOCIN hydrochloride: caps

clindamycin palmitate hydrochloride, CLEOCIN pediatric: oral susp

clindamycin phosphate, CLEOCIN phosphate: inj

Cloxacillin sodium monohydrate; penicillinase-resistant penicillin

IN, CH = PO: 50–100 mg/kg/24 hr, div, every 6 hr (expressed in terms of the base)

TEGOPEN: caps, oral susp

Demeclocycline; see Tetracyclines

Dicloxacillin sodium monohydrate; penicillinase-resistant penicillin

IN, CH = PO: 12.5–25 mg/kg/24 hr, div, every 6 hr

DYNAPEN: caps, oral susp

Doxycycline; see Tetracyclines

See KEY to abbreviations, p. 747; for further information about drugs, see package inserts.

Table AP-1. Drug Doses* (Drugs Listed Alphabetically by Generic Name) *Continued*

Erythromycin; macrolide antimicrobial agent

IN, CH = PO: 30–50 mg/kg/24 hr, div, every 6 hr; IV: 15–20 mg/kg/24 hr, div, every 6 hr

erythromycin, †, ILOTYCIN, ‡: tabl

erythromycin estolate, ILOSONE: tabl, oral susp

erythromycin ethylsuccinate, PEDIAMYCIN, ‡: tabl, oral susp drops

erythromycin gluceptate, ILOTYCIN gluceptate IV: inj

erythromycin lactobionate, ERYTHROCIN lactobionate IV: inj

erythromycin stearate, ERYTHROCIN stearate, ‡: tabl

Ethambutol hydrochloride; antituberculous agent used concomitantly with isoniazid

℞ in the treatment of tuberculosis as part of multiple drug regimen. Conditions for safe use in children not firmly established. In adults: 15–25 mg/kg/24 hr, as single daily dose, for course of treatment or retreatment. *Because of rare side effects of optic neuritis and decreased visual acuity,* eye examinations are indicated before inception of treatment and at monthly intervals thereafter.

MYAMBUTOL: tabl

Fluconazole; synthetic broad-spectrum *bis*-triazole antifungal drug. Selective inhibitor of fungal cytochrome P_{450} sterol C-14 α-demethylation; limited data in pediatrics available.

℞ for the treatment of fungal infections; CH = PO, IV: 3–6 mg/kg/24 hr, div, every 12–24 hr

DIFLUCAN: tabl, inj

Gentamicin sulfate; antimicrobial aminoglycoside

NB = IV (30–60 min), IM: <7 days <34 week <1500 g, 3 mg/kg every 24 hr; <34 wk >1500 g, 2.5 mg/kg every 18 hr; >34 wk >1500 g, 2.5 mg/kg every 12 hr; >7 days and term NB, 5 mg/kg/24 hr, div, every 12 hr

IN, CH = IM, IV (30–60 min): 5–7.5 mg/kg/24 hr, div, every 6–8 hr

Serum concentrations should be monitored, therapeutic peak concentration 5–10 mg/L, trough <2 mg/L. Dosage and interval may require modification for treatment of patients with cystic fibrosis

GARAMYCIN: inj

Caution: Ototoxic, nephrotoxic

Griseofulvin; antifungal agent

℞ against deep-seated mycotic infections (skin, hair, nails) with organisms of the species *Microsporum, Trichophyton, Epidermophyton:* CH = PO (microcrystalline): 10 mg/kg/24 hr for 4–6 wk (4–6 mo for fingernails, 6–12 mo for toenails)

Note: "Ultramicrosize" form is an ultramicrocrystalline suspension for which 125 mg is biologically equivalent to 250 mg of a "microsize" preparation. The daily dose of an ultramicrosize preparation is reduced to 5 mg/kg/24 hr and offers comparable efficacy without additional advantages.

griseofulvin, microcrystalline, †, FULVICIN-U/F, GRIFULVIN V, ‡: tabl, oral susp

griseofulvin, ultramicrocrystalline, GRIS-PEG: tabl

Isoniazid (INH), isonicotinic acid hydrazide; tuberculostatic agent

℞ in the treatment of active tuberculosis, in combination with other antituberculous drugs: IN, CH = PO, IM: 10–20 mg/kg/24 hr, div, every 8–12 hr; maximum daily dose: 500 mg/24 hr. AD = PO, IM: 5–10 mg/kg/24, div, every 8–12 hr; maximum daily dose: 300 mg/24 hr

℞ for prophylaxis of complications in recent conversion to positive tuberculin reaction (primary tuberculosis), or after suspected exposure: IN, CH = PO: 5–10 mg/kg/24 hr, as single dose, or div, every 12 hr; maximum daily dose: 300 mg/24

Note: "Slow" acetylators (homozygous) need only about 0.20–0.50 of this dose to reach therapeutically effective plasma concentrations achieved by "rapid" acetylators (homozygous and heterozygous). Higher than necessary plasma concentrations of unmetabolized isoniazid seem not to be associated with risk of isoniazid hepatotoxicity.

†, INH: tabl, syrup, inj

Caution: Formation of toxic metabolite in some patients may lead to hepatic necrosis with usual doses (rare under 20 yr of age).

Kanamycin sulfate; antimicrobial aminoglycoside

NB = IM, IV (over 20–30 min):

≤2000 g and ≤7 days old: 15 mg/kg/24 hr, div, every 12 hr

≤2000 g and >7 days old: 20 mg/kg/24 hr, div, every 12 hr

>2000 g and ≤7 days old: 20 mg/kg/24 hr, div, every 12 hr

>2000 g and >7 days old: 30 mg/kg/24 hr, div, every 8 hr

IN, CH = IM, IV (over 20–30 min): 6–15 mg/kg/24 hr, div, every 8–12 hr. Usual duration therapy: 7–10 days; not indicated in long-term therapy because of ototoxic hazard.

Caution: Ototoxic, nephrotoxic

KANTREX: inj

Mebendazole; antihelmintic agent that blocks glucose uptake by the susceptible parasites and interferes with their survival

℞ against pinworms (*Enterobius vermicularis*; cure rate 90–100%): CH = PO: 100 mg/dose, as single dose; against whipworms (*Trichuris trichiura*; cure rate 61–75%), roundworms (*Ascaris lumbricoides*; cure rate 91–100%), and hookworms (*Ancylostoma duodenale, Necator americanus*; cure rate 96%); alternative method = PO: 200 mg/24 hr, div, every 12 hr, for 3 consecutive days. If patient is not free of parasites 3 wk after treatment, a 2nd course is indicated.

Note: Not extensively studied in children under 2 yr of age.

VERMOX: chewable tabl

See KEY to abbreviations, p. 747; for further information about drugs, see package inserts.

Table AP–1. Drug Doses* (Drugs Listed Alphabetically by Generic Name) *Continued*

Methicillin sodium; semisynthetic penicillinase-resistant penicillin

NB = IM, IV (over 15–30 min):

≤2000 g and ≤14 days old: 50 mg/kg/24 hr, div, every 12 hr

≤2000 g and 15–30 days old: 75 mg/kg/24 hr, div, every 8 hr

>2000 g and ≤14 days old: 75 mg/kg/24 hr, div, every 8 hr

>2000 g and 15–30 days old: 100 mg/kg/24 hr, div, every 6 hr

IN, CH = IV (over 15–30 min), IM: 200–400 mg/kg/24 hr, div, every 4 hr (IV) or every 6 hr (IM)

CELBENIN, STAPHCILLIN: inj

Metronidazole hydrochloride; synthetic antibacterial agent highly active against most obligate anaerobes, including *Bacteroides* species such as *B. fragilis,* and *Clostridium* and *Peptostreptococcus* species. The drug also is effective in the treatment of amebiasis, *Giardia,* and *Trichomonas.*

℞ for amebiasis: CH = PO: 35–50 mg/kg/24 hr, div, every 8 hr

℞ for the treatment of anaerobic infections: IV

NB <2000 g, 15 mg/kg/24 hr, div, every 12 hr

NB >2000 g, <7 days: 15 mg/kg/24 hr, div, every 8 hr

NB >2000 g, >7 days: 30 mg/kg/24 hr, div, every 8 hr

℞ for giardiasis: CH = PO: 15 mg/kg/day, div, every 8 hr

℞ for trichomonas vaginitis: CH = PO: 15 mg/kg/24 hr, div, every 8 hr, for 7 days.

Topical therapy: Apply and rub in thin film twice daily to affected area. May be administered as vaginal suppositories.

Caution: Patient should not ingest alcohol for 24 hr after receiving a dose of this drug (disulfiram-type reaction). Drug interactions possible; may prolong anticoagulant effect of warfarin-type anticoagulants

†, FLAGYL: tabls, inj

Miconazole; synthetic antifungal imidazole derivative effective against systemic infections with *Coccidioides immitis, Candida albicans, Cryptococcus neoformans, Paracoccidioides brasiliensis.* IV infusion alone is inadequate for the treatment of fungal meningitis and urinary bladder infection; intrathecal administration and bladder instillation also must be carried out.

℞ for treatment of proved coccidioidomycosis, candidosis, cryptococcosis, or paracoccidioidomycosis: CH = IV (after dilution with isotonic saline or 5% D/W and over 30–60 min): 20–40 mg/kg/24 hr, div, every 8 hr, until clinical and laboratory tests no longer indicate activity of fungal infection. Dose may vary with type of fungus involved; MONISTAT IV; ampules for IV inj

Minocycline; see Tetracyclines

Nafcillin sodium; semisynthetic penicillinase-resistant penicillin

NB = IM, IV (over 15–30 min); ≤7 days old: 40 mg/kg/24 hr, div, every 12 hr; >7 days old: 60 mg/kg/24 hr, div, every 8 hr

IN, CH = PO: 50–100 mg/kg/24 hr, div, every 6 hr; IM, IV (over 15–30 min): 100–200 mg/kg/24 hr, div, every 6 hr (IM) or every 4 hr (IV)

UNIPEN: caps, tabl, oral susp, inj

Nystatin; antifungal agent; 1 mg = 2000 units; seems to be active by altering permeability of cell membrane of yeasts

℞ for topical treatment of candidosis of the buccal cavity (thrush) and the gastrointestinal tract. Very poorly absorbed. In oral candidosis, spread nystatin suspension into recesses of mouth:

NB (<2000 g) = PO: 200,000–400,000 units/24 hr, div, every 4–6 hr

NB (>2000 g), IN = PO: 400,000–800,000 units/24 hr, div, every 4–6 hr

CH = PO: 800,000–2,000,000 units/24 hr, div, every 4–6 hr

†, MYCOSTATIN, NILSTAT: oral susp, tabl

Oxacillin sodium; semisynthetic penicillinase-resistant penicillin

NB = IV (over 15–30 min), IM: for dosage same criteria apply as for methicillin in newborns; *see* Methicillin sodium

IN, CH = PO: 50–100 mg/kg/24 hr, div, every 6 hr; IV (over 15–30 min), IM: 100–200 mg/kg/24 hr, div, every 4 hr (IV) or every 6 hr (IM)

BACTOCILL, PROSTAPHLIN: caps, oral susp, inj

Penicillin G, benzylpenicillin; potassium penicillin G (1 mg = 1595 units); sodium penicillin G (1 mg = 1667 units). One million units of these salts of penicillin contain either 1.68 mEq K^+ or Na^+; in other terms, 1 g contains either 2.7 mEq K^+ or 2.8 mEq Na^+.

NB = IV (over 15–30 min), IM:

<2000 g: 50,000 units/kg/24 hr, div, every 12 hr

℞ for meningitis: 100,000 units/kg/24 hr, div, every 12 hr

>2000 g: 75,000 units/kg/24 hr, div, every 8 hr

℞ for meningitis: 150,000–200,000 units/kg/24 hr, div, every 8 hr

IN, CH = PO, IM, IV (15–30 min): 100,000–250,000 units/kg/24 hr, div, every 4–6 hr

℞ for meningitis: 200,000–300,000 units/kg/24 hr, div, every 4 hr

(The higher doses should be chosen for meningitis caused by group B streptococci.)

IN, CH = PO, IM, IV (over 15–30 min) (minor infections): 25,000–50,000 units/kg/24 hr, equivalent to 15.5–31 mg/kg/24 hr, div, every 4–6 hr; if given PO, administer penicillin G 0.5 hr before or 2 hr after the meal.

℞ for prophylaxis of rheumatic fever; PO: 200,000 units/dose, equivalent to 125 mg/dose, twice daily, spaced from meals

See KEY to abbreviations, p. 747; for further information about drugs, see package inserts.

Table AP–1. Drug Doses* (Drugs Listed Alphabetically by Generic Name) *Continued*

Penicillin G benzathine, for injection; combination of 1 mole of dibenzylethylenediamine with 2 moles of penicillin G; 1 mg = 1211 units

℞ for prophylaxis of rheumatic fever: CH = IM: 600,000–1,200,000 units, equivalent to 500–1000 mg penicillin G, once a month

†, BICILLIN L-A, PERMAPEN, ‡: susp for inj

†, PENTIDS, PFIZERPEN G, ‡: tabl, caps, oral susp, inj (IV)

Penicillin G procaine, for injection; combination of penicillin G with procaine, mole for mole (1 mg = 1009 units)

NB = IM: 50,000 units/kg/24 hr, equivalent to 50 mg/kg/24 hr, in single daily dose

IN, CH = IM: 25,000–50,000 units/kg/24 hr, equivalent to 25–50 mg/kg/24 hr, in single daily dose

†, CRYSTICILLIN, DURACILLIN A.S., ‡: susp for IM inj

Penicillin V, phenoxymethyl penicillin; acid-resistant penicillin; 1 mg = 1695 units

IN, CH = PO: 25,000–50,000 units/kg/24 hr, equivalent to 15–30 mg/kg/24 hr, div, every 6–8 hr. *Note:* 400,000 units = 250 mg (approx.).

†, PEN-VEE K, VEETIDS, ‡: tabl, oral susp, drops

Primaquine; 8-aminoquinoline antimalarial agent, used for prophylaxis against *Plasmodium vivax*, *P. ovale*, and *P. malariae* and for "radical" cure for *P. vivax* and *P. ovale*.

IN, CH = PO: 0.55 mg/kg/24 hr (equivalent to 0.3 mg/kg/24 hr of base), as single daily dose, for 14 days

Note: Degree of intravascular hemolysis in individuals with G-6-PD deficiency is related to dosage and particular variant of the deficiency

PRIMAQUINE DIPHOSPHATE: tabl

Pyrantel pamoate; antihelmintic agent effective by means of neuromuscular paralysis of the parasite

℞ against pinworms (*Enterobius vermicularis*), *Ascaris lumbricoides*, and hookworms (*Necator americanus*, *Ancylostoma duodenale*): pyrantel pamoate has not been extensively studied in infants and children below 2 yr of age, hence particular attention should be given to children of this age group during treatment of parasitic infestation with pyrantel. CH = PO: 11 mg/kg/dose, as single dose and without regard to food intake or time of day; purging not necessary prior to, during, or after therapy

Note: In pinworm infestation, in which possibility of reinfection with eggs from the host exists, a 2nd treatment 2–3 wk after the 1st might be indicated.

ANTIMINTH: oral susp

Pyrimethamine; inhibitor of dihydrofolate reductase, antimalarial agent; for use in treatment of toxoplasmosis

℞ for clinical prophylaxis of malaria, especially effective against *Plasmodium falciparum*: IN, CH = PO: 0.5–0.75 mg/kg/dose, once every 7 days. Begin prophylaxis 2 wk before entering malarious area and continue for 8 wk after leaving. To eradicate *P. vivax* and *P. ovale* infections, treatment for 14 days with primaquine should be considered immediately on leaving malarious area while pyrimethamine prophylaxis is still in effect.

Note: Hematologic abnormalities (anemia, thrombocytopenia, leukopenia) secondary to folic and folinic acid depletion can be prevented or reversed by IM administration of folinic acid (leucovorin) without affecting the efficacy of pyrimethamine.

DARAPRIM: tabl

Quinacrine hydrochloride, mepacrine hydrochloride; acridine derivative formerly used as antimalarial agent and against infestation with tapeworms, presently regarded as drug of choice against giardiasis

℞ against *Giardia lamblia*: CH = PO: 6 mg/kg/24 hr, div, every 8 hr, for 5 consecutive days; maximum daily dose: 300 mg/24 hr

ATABRINE: tabl

Ribavirin; synthetic nucleoside antiviral drug, Ribavirin possesses antiviral inhibitory activity in vitro against respiratory syncytial virus (RSV), influenza virus, and herpes simplex virus. Various protocols exist for the use of this compound; the drug usually is reserved for use in the treatment of severe lower respiratory tract infections due to RSV. Ribavirin is administered by the aerosol route as a continuous aerosolization for 12–18 hr daily for 3–7 days. Aerosol solution usually is prepared in sterile water, without preservatives, to a final concentration of 20 mg/ml.

VIRAZOLE: aerosol

Rifampin; macrocytic antimicrobial and antimycobacterial agent, interfering with RNA-polymerase of infecting organisms

℞ in treatment of tuberculosis, in conjunction with at least 1 other antituberculous agent (isoniazid) and

℞ in carriers of *Neisseria meningitidis* resistant to sulfonamide; treatment course of 4 consecutive days (possibility of rapid emergence of resistance); IN, CH = PO: 10–20 mg/kg/24 hr, in single daily dose (1 hr before or 2 hr after meal): maximum daily dose: 600 mg (= adult dose)

RIFADIN, RIMACTANE: caps

Sulfonamides; analogues of *para*-aminobenzoic acid, interfering with the synthesis of tetrahydrofolic acid in sensitive bacteria

Sulfadiazine, sulfisoxazole, and trisulfapyrimidines: IN, CH = PO: initial dose 75 mg/kg/1st dose, followed by 120–150 mg/kg/24 hr, div, every 4–6 hr; IV (over 30 min), SC: 100–110 mg/kg/24 hr, div, every 4–6 hr

Sulfadiazine, †: tabl

sulfadiazine sodium, †: inj

sulfisoxazole, †, GANTRISIN: tabl

sulfisoxazole acetyl, GANTRISIN acetyl: oral susp, syrup

See KEY to abbreviations, p. 747; for further information about drugs, see package inserts.

Table AP–1. Drug Doses* (Drugs Listed Alphabetically by Generic Name) *Continued*

sulfisoxazole diolamine, GANTRISIN diolamine: inj
trisulfapyrimidines (equal parts of sulfadiazine, sulfamerazine, and sulfamethazine), †, ‡: tabl, oral susp
Sulfamethoxazole: IN, CH = PO: initial dose 50–60 mg/kg/1st dose, followed by 50–60 mg/kg/24 hr, div, every 12 hr GANTANOL: oral susp, tabl
Trimethoprim–sulfamethoxazole (combination of TMP + SMX): IN (>2 mo old), CH = PO: 6–12 mg TMP + 30–60 mg SMX/kg/24 hr, div, every 12 hr
℞ in severe urinary tract or *Shigella* infection: CH = PO, IV: 8–10 mg TMP + 40–60 mg SMX/kg/24 hr, fiv, every 6–8 hr
℞ against *Pneumocystis carinii:* CH = PO, IV: 15–20 mg TMP + 75–100 mg SMX/kg/24 hr, div, every 6–8 hr
Caution: Do not use in infants less than 2 mo old. Reduce dose in severe renal insufficiency. May cause bone marrow depression.
BACTRIM, SEPTRA: susp: 40 mg TMP + 200 mg SMX/5 mL; tabl: 80 mg TMP + 400 mg SMX/tabl or 160 mg TMP + 800 mg SMX/tabl; ampule: 80 mg TMP + 400 mg SMX/5 mL

Tetracyclines; a group of derivatives of polycyclic naphthacenccarboxamide
Chlortetracycline hydrochloride: CH = PO: 25–50 mg/kg/24 hr, div. every 6 hr
AUREOMYCIN: caps, inj (IV)
Demeclocycline and *demeclocycline hydrochloride:* CH = PO: 7–13 mg/kg/24 hr, div, every 6–12 hr
DECLOMYCIN: pediatric drops, syrup
DECLOMYCIN hydrochloride: caps, tabl
Doxycycline monohydrate and *doxycycline hyclate:* CH = PO: 5 mg/kg/24 hr, div, every 12 hr
†, VIBRAMYCIN monohydrate: oral susp
†, VIBRAMYCIN hyclate: caps, inj (IV)
Methacycline hydrochloride: CH = PO: 7–13 mg/kg/24 hr, div, every 6–12 hr
RONDOMYCIN: caps, syrup
Minocycline hydrochloride: CH = PO, IV: initial dose 4 mg/kg, followed by 4 mg/kg/24 hr, div, every 12 hr
MINOCIN, VECTRIN: caps, syrup, inj (IV)
Oxytetracycline, oxytetracycline hydrochloride, oxytetracycline calcium: same dosage as tetracycline hydrochloride, below TERRAMYCIN: tabl, inj (IM)
TERRAMYCIN hydrochloride, †: caps, inj (IV, IM)
TERRAMYCIN calcium: pediatric drops, syrup
Tetracycline hydrochloride: CH = PO: 25–50 mg/kg/24 hr, div, every 8 hr; IM (often very painful): 15–25 mg/kg/24 hr, div, every 8–12 hr; IV: 10–20 mg/kg/24 hr, div, every 12 hr
†, ACHROMYCIN V, PANMYCIN, ‡: caps, inj (IV, IM); sol for IM inj contains local anesthetic. Pediatric drops, oral susp, and syrup prepared with tetracycline base
Note: Tetracyclines have limited indications in infancy and childhood because of their accumulation in bone and teeth and their potential to interfere with growth. Their use should be avoided insofar as pos-

sible until formation of dental enamel is complete in most permanent teeth (at about 8 yr), to avoid unsightly discolored, pitted teeth. Tetracyclines may cause increased intracranial pressure in infants (pseudotumor cerebri).

Ticarcillin disodium; semisynthetic penicillin susceptible to penicillinase; each gram of drug contains 5.2 mEq of sodium.
NB = IV (over 20–30 min), IM: <7 days <2000 g; 150 mg/kg/24 hr, div, every 12 hr; >2000 g: 225 mg/kg/24 hr, div, every 8 hr; >7 days <2000 g: 225 mg/kg/24 hr, div, every 8 hr; >7 days >2000 g: 300 mg/kg/24 hr, div, every 8 hr
IN, CH = IV (over 20–30 min), IM: 200–300 mg/kg/24 hr, div, every 4–6 hr. IM injection is painful.
TICAR: IV and IM inj

Ticarcillin + clavulanic acid; combination of a β-lactam antibiotic (ticarcillin) with a β-lactamase (penicillinase) inhibitor (clavulanic acid). The addition of clavulanic acid extends the activity of ticarcillin to include β-lactamase–producing strains of *Haemophilus influenzae,* and other drug-resistant pathogens. Doses administered as either IM or IV are the same as those for ticarcillin noted above.

Tobramycin sulfate; antimicrobial aminoglycoside
NB = IV (30–60 min), IM: <7 days <34 wk <1500 g: 3 mg/kg every 24 hr; <34 wk >1500 g: 2.5 mg/kg every 18 hr; >34 wk >1500 g: 2.5 mg/kg every 12 hr; >7 days and term NB; 5 mg/kg/24 hr, div, every 12 hr
IN, CH = IV (30–60 min), IM: 5–7.5 mg/kg/24 hr, div, every 6–8 hr. Serum concentration should be monitored; therapeutic peak concentration 5–10 mg/L, trough <2 mg/L. Dosage and interval may require modification for the treatment of patients with cystic fibrosis.
Caution: Ototoxic, nephrotoxic
†, NEBCIN: inj

Vancomycin; complex glycopeptide that inhibits synthesis of cell wall in gram-positive bacteria and is effective against methicillin-resistant staphylococci; in oral application effective in pseudomembranous colitis caused by toxin-producing bacteria such as *Clostridium difficile* and *Staphylococcus aureus;* excreted mainly by kidneys
NB = IV: 20–30 mg/kg/24 hr div, every 12 hr if ≤1 wk old, every 8 hr if >1 wk old
CH = IV (<500 mg/30 min): 40 mg/kg/24 hr, div, every 6 hr (maximum 2 g/24 hr)
Note: Reduce dosage in renal insufficiency. May cause ototoxicity and renal impairment, skin rashes, peripheral neuropathy
VANCOCIN: vials

Vidarabine; antiviral agent used for treatment of neonatal herpes simplex infections
IN = IV: 15–30 mg/kg infused over 12 hr q 24 hr for 14–21 days

See KEY to abbreviations, p. 747; for further information about drugs, see package inserts.

Note: May rarely cause hepatic and hematologic toxicity.

VIRA-A: 200-mg/mL vial inj

II. DRUGS OTHER THAN ANTIBIOTICS

Acetaminophen, paracetamol, APAP, NAPAP

℞ antipyretic, analgesic: IN, CH = PO: 60 mg/kg/24 hr, div, every 4–6 hr, prn

†, LIQUIPRIN, TYLENOL, ‡: tabl, liquid preparations

Caution: Massive overdose may cause hepatic necrosis through formation of a toxic metabolite. Lesser overdoses frequently cause reversible jaundice.

Acetylcysteine; mucolytic agent; detoxifying agent in acetaminophen overdose

℞ to loosen tenacious bronchial secretions by local application to the bronchial tree with nebulizer: 3–5 mL 20% sol diluted with equal volume of sterile water or saline, or 6–10 mL of 10% sol, every 6–8 hr; or by direct instillation: 1–2 mL of 10% or 20% sol every 1–4 hr

℞ in acetaminophen overdose: CH, AD = PO: 140 mg/kg/1st dose, followed by 70 mg/kg/dose every 4 hr for a total of 72 hr

MUCOMYST: vials 10% (100 mg/mL) or 20% (20 mg/mL)

Acetylsalicylic acid, ASA

℞ antipyretic, analgesic, anti-inflammatory: IN, CH = PO: 30–65 mg/kg/24 hr, div, every 4–6 hr, prn. This dosage corresponds to 27–58 mg salicylate sodium/kg/24 hr, or 20–50 mg salicylic acid/kg/24 hr

℞ antirheumatic: CH = PO: 65–130 mg/kg/24 hr, div, every 4–6 hr

†, ASPIRIN, BUFFERIN, ‡: tabl; also contained in many combination products

Caution: Acute or chronic overdose may cause life-threatening poisoning syndrome.

Activated charcoal; adsorbent for treatment of oral drug overdose PO: 10 times (by weight) estimated quantity of drug ingested or 1 g/kg orally; may repeat every 4 hr when necessary

Adenosine; endogenous nucleoside, treatment of choice to terminate supraventricular tachycardia; causes acute transient AV nodal conduction block

NB, IN, CH = IV; 0.05 mg/kg/dose rapid injection (1–2 sec), increase to 0.10 mg/kg/dose, then 0.15 mg/kg/dose, then 0.20 mg/kg/dose if prior doses were ineffective (in 1–2 min)

Albuterol; catecholamine analogue; β-adrenergic receptor agonist with preferential effect on β₂-adrenergic receptors

℞ bronchodilator: CH = PO: 0.1 mg/kg, div, every 8 hr; 6–12 yr; 2 mg 3–4 times/24 hr; nebulization: 0.01–0.03 mL/kg of 5 mg/mL solution.

VENTOLIN, PROVENTIL: tab, liquid, inhalation

Atropine sulfate, *dl*-hyoscyamine; anticholinergic agent used mainly in premedication for anesthesia, as anti-

arrhythmic agent, and as antiispasmodic. Dosage varies according to indications and sensitivity of patients. On the average for IN, CH = SC, PO (IV): 0.01 mg/kg/dose, to be repeated prn after 2 hr until desired effect is obtained or adverse effects preclude further increase; for continued ℞: PO: 0.04 mg/kg/24 hr, div, every 6 hr, preferably with meals

†: inj, tabl

Beclomethasone dipropionate; chlorinated synthetic corticosteroid

℞ topical treatment to the bronchial tissues in long-term steroid-dependent asthma. Delivered from metered-dose aerosol unit, releasing approximately 50 μg beclomethasone by activation of the dispenser unit: CH (6–12 yr): 1–2 inhalations every 6–8 hr. Effect usually apparent within 1–4 wk after beginning of steroid inhalations

Caution: On transfer from systemic steroid therapy for asthma to inhalation therapy, adrenocortical competency of the patient must be watched and supported, if indicated, because inhalation therapy does not contribute to systemic corticosteroid supply.

VANCERIL: inhaler

Captopril; competitive inhibitor of angiotensin I–converting enzyme, antihypertensive agent, congestive heart failure

℞ for cardiovascular response: NB = PO: 0.1–0.4 mg/kg/dose administered every 6–24 hr; IN = PO: 0.5–0.6 mg/kg/24 hr, div, every 6–12 hr; CH = PO: 0.15 mg/kg every 4–8 hr. Dose may be increased slowly to desired effect.

Note: May cause renal impairment, neutropenia, rashes, and disturbances of taste. Adjust dose with renal failure. Limited experience in children.

CAPOTEN: tabl

Carbamazepine; anticonvulsant agent; structurally related to tricyclic antidepressants

CH = PO: initially 10 mg/kg/24 hr, div, every 8–12 hr; to be increased progressively, if needed, to 20 mg/kg/24 hr, div, every 12 hr or as a single daily dose, if tolerated. On the basis of presently available information, 30 mg/kg/24 hr should not be exceeded.

TEGRETOL: tabl

Chloral hydrate; trichloro derivative of acetaldehyde; tolerance to its hypnotic effect may develop

℞ for sedation: IN, CH = PO: 25 mg/kg/24 hr, div, every 6–8 hr

℞ for sleep: IN, CH = PO, (PR): 25–75 mg/kg/dose, to be repeated prn after 12–24 hr

†, NOCTEC, SOMNOS, ‡: elixic, syrup, suppos

Chlorothiazide; saluretic, inhibiting sodium reabsorption and interfering with dilution of urine

IN, CH = PO: 20 mg/kg/24 hr, div, every 12 hr

†, DIURIL: tabl, oral susp

Table AP–1. Drug Doses* (Drugs Listed Alphabetically by Generic Name) *Continued*

Chlorpromazine; phenothiazine with aliphatic side chain

℞ for sedation: CH = PO: 2 mg/kg/24 hr, div, every 4–6 hr, prn; IM: 2 mg/kg/24 hr, div, every 6–8 hr, prn THORAZINE: suppos

chlorpromazine hydrochloride, THORAZINE hydrochloride: tabl, syrup, inj

Caution: Overdose may produce parkinsonian syndrome. Diphenhydramine may be antidotal.

Cimetidine; H$_2$-receptor antagonist inhibiting gastric acid secretion

℞ for treatment of duodenal and gastric ulcers and for relief of symptoms caused by gastroesophageal reflux; compatible with concomitant treatment with oral antacids (which should be given at frequent intervals and in adequate dosage) and/or anticholinergic antispasmodics. Clinical experience in children is extremely limited, and the benefit/risk ratio should be considered carefully: PO: 20–40 mg/kg/24 hr, div and given with every meal, have been used, as well as same dosage, IV, div, every 4 hr.

TAGAMET: tabl, inj

Clonazepam; benzodiazepine with selective anticonvulsant effect

CH = PO: start with 0.01–0.05 mg/kg/24 hr, div, every 8 hr, and progressively increase up to 0.3 mg/kg/24 hr, div, every 8 hr, if needed.

Caution: Concomitant use of clonazepam and valproate sodium may lead to petit mal status.

CLONOPIN: tabl

Codeine phosphate or sulfate; narcotic analgesic

℞ as antitussive: CH = 1–1.5 mg/kg/24 hr, div, every 4 hr prn

℞ against moderately severe pain: CH = PO: 4 mg/kg/24 hr, div, every 4–6 hr, prn; SC: 3 mg/kg/24 hr, div, every 4–6 hr, prn

†: tabl, oral susp, inj; mostly in combination with other drugs

Corticosteroids

℞ physiologic replacement; *cortisone:* PO 1 mg/kg/24 hr, div, every 8 hr; IM: 0.5 mg/kg/24 hr, every 24 hr. (*Note:* "Increased demand" under stressful situation; e.g., in children with congenital adrenogenital syndrome, receiving replacement therapy, for stressful situation in which 2 mg/kg/24 hr of cortisol may be safer)

℞ use in pharmacologic doses (leukemia, lymphoma, nephrosis, rheumatic carditis, certain types of tuberculosis, immunologic reactions, and other types of autoimmune disease): adjust dosage to the specific situation.

cortisone: PO: 10 mg/kg/24 hr, div, every 6–8 hr; IM: 3–6 mg/kg/24 hr, div, every 12 hr

prednisone: PO: 2 mg/kg/24 hr, div, every 6–8 hr (or analogue in equally effective dosage: see Table)

(For continued treatment after initial response, adjust dosage, frequency of administration, and duration of treatment according to type of disease and side effects to be avoided.)

℞ in status asthmaticus refractory to other types of treatment: methylprednisolone IV: 2–4 mg/kg/dose every 4–6 hr

Relative Potencies of Corticosteroids

Drug	Anti-inflammatory Effect (mg)	Sodium-Retaining Effect (mg)
Hydrocortisone (cortisol)	100	100
Cortisone	80	80
Prednisolone	20	100
Prednisone	20	100
Methylprednisolone	16	0
Triamcinolone	16	0
Dexamethasone	2	0
Desoxycorticosterone	0	2

dexamethasone, DECADRON, GAMMACORTEN, ‡: tabl; elixir dexamethasone sodium phosphate, DECADRON phosphate

hydrocortisone, †, CORTEF, HYDROCORTONE, ‡: tabl, oral susp; hydrocortisone sodium phosphate, †, HYDROCORTONE phosphate: inj; hydrocortisone sodium succinate, †, SOLUCORTEF: inj

methylprednisolone, MEDROL: tabl; methylprednisolone sodium succinate, SOLU-MEDROL: inj

prednison, †, DELTASONE, METICORTEN, ‡: tabl

prednisolone, †, DELTA-CORTEF, METICORTELONE, ‡: tabl

triamcinolone, ARISTOCORT, KENACORT: tabl, syrup

Caution: May inhibit clinical signs of infection.

Cromolyn sodium

℞ topical prophylaxis of bronchial asthma, allergic rhinitis: not useful in the treatment of acute asthmatic attack because it is not a bronchodilator. CH (≥5 yr) = inhalation of 20 mg every 6 hr; nebulize contents of one ampule (2 ml) every 6–8 hr; aerosol inhaler, 1–2 puffs 4 times daily.

AARANE, INTAL: inhalation with Spinhaler, sol, nasal spray

Cyproheptadine hydrochloride; piperidine; serotonin and histamine antagonist with mild anticholinergic and mild sedative effect

℞ antiallergic effect: CH = PO: 0.25 mg/kg/24 hr, div, every 6 hr

PERIACTIN: tabl, syrup

Deferoxamine; chelating agent for treatment of iron intoxication; may cause hypotension; contraindicated

See KEY to abbreviations, p. 747; for further information about drugs, see package inserts.

Table AP–1. Drug Doses* (Drugs Listed Alphabetically by Generic Name) *Continued*

in renal failure or acute anuria unless concomitant hemodialysis is used.
IV: 10–15 mg/kg/hr infusion
DESFERAL: 500 mg/vial inj

Desmopressin acetate; synthetic analogue of vasopressin indicated as replacement therapy in the management of central diabetis insipidus. Toxicities include headache, abdominal cramping, excessive water retention.
Nasal insufflation: 0.03–0.05 mL divided b.i.d. or t.i.d. dose determined by patient response.
DDAVP: 0.1 mg/mL for nasal insufflation

Dexamethasone; see Corticosteroids

Diazepam; benzodiazepine with anxiolytic and muscle-relaxant effects
℞ in status epilepticus: NB, IN, CH = IV (slowly as controlled "push" injection); 0.1–0.3 mg/kg/dose; may be repeated 2 times after intervals of 5 min; give IM if impossible to give IV (efficacy diminished)
℞ for symptomatic relief of anxiety: CH = PO: 0.1–0.3 mg/kg/24 hr, div, every 6 hr; adjust dosage according to response
VALIUM: tabl, inj
Caution: Confusion and prolonged extreme drowsiness may follow overdose or concurrent ingestion of alcohol in any form.

Digoxin; cardiac glycoside with rapid onset of action and half-life of approximately 48 hr
℞ for digitalization: 0.5 × digitalizing dose initially, 0.25 × digitalizing dose 8 and 16 hr later.
(Digitalizing dose: NB = IV, IM: 0.010–0.030 mg/kg div in fractions, or PO: 0.040 mg/kg, div in fractions. IN = IV, IM, PO: same doses as indicated for NB)
℞ for maintenance: begin maintenance dosage 24 hr after 1st fraction of digitalizing dose. NB = PO: 0.010 mg/kg/24 hr, div, every 12 hr. IN, CH = PO: 0.015 mg/kg/24 hr, div, every 12 hr
Note: Digitalizing and maintenance doses must be adjusted to the condition of the patient.
†, LANOXIN: tabl, elixir, inj
Caution: Fatal arrhythmia may follow overdose.

Diphenhydramine hydrochloride; ethanolamine; antihistamine with mild anticholinergic, sedative, antiemetic, and antitussive effects
℞ antiallergic effect; sometimes used as sedative. IN, CH = PO, IM, IV: 5 mg/kg/24 hr, div, every 6–8 hr
†, BENADRYL: caps, elixir, inj

Epinephrine, catecholamine (α- and β-adrenergic agonist)
℞ bronchodilator (β₂ stimulatory effect), in acute asthma attack: IN, CH = SC: 0.01 mg/kg/dose, repeat prn every 20 min, 2 times
Note: With epinephrine solution 1:1000 this corresponds to 0.01 mL/kg/dose.
Caution: Cardiac arrhythmia and/or acute hypertension may follow overdose.

Epinephrine racemic; inhalation treatment of acute spasmodic croup
Inhalation: 0.25–0.5 mL of 2.25% solution diluted in 3 mL of saline given via nebulizer
VAPONEPHRINE: inhalation 2.25% solution

Furosemide; saluretic with a duration of action of about 2 hr when given IV; inhibits chloride and sodium reabsorption and interferes with concentration of urine
IN, CH = PO: start with 2 mg/kg/dose; if needed, increase progressively to 3–6 mg/kg/dose, at intervals of 6–8 hr; IV: start with 1 mg/kg/dose; if needed, increase progressively to 6 mg/kg/dose, with an interval of at least 2 hr between doses
LASIX: tabl, oral sol, inj

Hydralazine hydrochloride; phthalazine derivative; causes relaxation of vascular smooth muscles, especially of arterioles
℞ as antihypertensive in long-term treatment: CH = PO: initially 0.75 mg/kg/24 hr, div, every 6 hr; increase progressively until desired response or daily maximum dose of 3.5 mg/kg/24 hr is reached
℞ for emergency reduction of hypertension: IV (immediate onset of action), IM (onset of action after 15–20 min): 0.15 mg/kg/dose; repeat prn every 30–90 min up to daily dose of 1.7–3.6 mg/kg/24 hr, switch to oral administration if conditions permit
Note: Hydralazine may produce sodium retention and usually increases plasma renin activity.
Caution: May induce lupus erythematosus–like syndrome: frequency related to dosage.
†, APRESOLINE, ‡: tabl, inj

Hydrochlorothiazide; saluretic, inhibiting sodium reabsorption and interfering with dilution of urine
IN, CH = PO: 2 mg/kg/24 hr, div, every 12 hr
†, ESIDRIX, HYDRODIURIL, ‡: tabl

Hydroxyzine hydrochloride; neuroleptic agent of the piperazine type, with sedative and antihistamine effects
℞ for sedation and/or antihistamine effect: CH = PO: 2 mg/kg/24 hr, div, every 6–8 hr, prn
ATARAX: tabl, syrup
VISTARIL I.M.: inj (IM)
hydroxyzine pamoate, VISTARIL: caps, oral susp

Ibuprofen; nonsteroidal anti-inflammatory agent of the propionic acid class that possesses analgesic and antipyretic activities. The drug's mechanism of action remains to be described but may involve prostaglandin synthetase inhibition. Pharmacologic effect appears to be equivalent to that of equipotent doses of acetaminophen or aspirin.
℞ as antipyretic or for mild analgesia: CH = PO: 10–15 mg/kg/dose at intervals of 4–6 hr
℞ for juvenile rheumatoid arthritis: CH = PO: 30–70 mg/kg/24 hr, div, every 4–6 hr
Note: complete scope of associated adverse reactions in infants and children remains to be described. Ad-

See KEY to abbreviations, p. 747; for further information about drugs, see package inserts.

Table AP–1. Drug Doses* (Drugs Listed Alphabetically by Generic Name) *Continued*

verse effects appear to be similar to those associated with aspirin administration, including gastritis, platelet dysfunction, and possible compromise in renal function. Drug should be used cautiously in patients with renal insufficiency.

†, ADVIL, MEDIPRIN, MOTRIN, NUPRIN: tabs, caps, susp

Ipecac; emetic agent used in the adjunctive management of poisoning or intoxication. Active ingredient emetidine produces local gastric irritation and central effect, resulting in emesis, which usually occurs within 15–35 min of drug administration

℞ to induce vomiting:

IN >8 mo of age, CH = PO: 15–30 ml/dose; if no effect occurs same dose may be repeated in 30 min

N <8 mo of age = PO: 1 mL/kg single dose

Note: Children usually vomit 3–5 times within 1 hr of receiving Ipecac. Ipecac should be available in all households with young infants and children but should not be administered except on the advice of a physician or a poison control center.

Iron preparations

℞ Daily maintenance iron requirement, as elemental iron: PO: 0.5–1 mg/kg/24 hr, in single dose or divided

℞ In iron deficiency anemia, as elemental iron: PO: 6 mg/kg/24 hr, div, with meals

Note: Iron supply at this dosage level ought to be continued for 2–3 mo to compensate for the deficits in erythrocytes and iron stores. Only iron in the ferrous form (Fe^{2+}) is absorbed from the gastrointestinal tract. The content of elemental iron in different preparations varies. The percentage of dry weight as elemental iron of ferrous choline citrate is 20; ferrous fumarate, 33; ferrous gluconate, 12; ferrous lactate, 19; ferrous sulfate, 20; and iron-dextran complex (ferric hydroxide), 2.

℞ Dose calculation for parenteral iron administration: elemental Fe deficit = 2.5 mg/kg × deficit of hemoglobin concentration (in g/dL) in blood. (The deficit of the hemoglobin concentration is obtained as the difference between the measured and the desirable value, expressed in g/dL.) When iron must be supplied by the parenteral route, deep IM injection is preferable to IV administration. In either case, a test dose of approximately 25 mg elemental Fe in the form of the dextran complex should precede the administration of the total dose. If the total dose is large, it should be divided in separate daily doses of which none should exceed 5 mg/kg/24 hr of elemental iron.

Note: An additional 20–30% of the calculated deficit is needed to restore the tissue iron reserves.

Caution: Acute overdose may lead to shock, CNS depression, death.

Isoproterenol hydrochloride; β-adrenergic agent

℞ to overcome atrioventricular block: IV infusion: Example: to prepare a solution containing 0.004 mg/ mL, mix 1 mg isoproterenol in 250 mL 5% D/W or appropriate electrolyte solution and infuse at rate adjusted to response in patient (beginning with approximately 0.0001–0.0002 mg/kg/min)

†, ISUPREL: inj

Lidocaine hydrochloride; anesthetic agent used systemically for its antiarrhythmic effects: delayed slow diastolic depolarization, diminished automaticity. Does not affect normal conduction but seemingly improves conduction velocity in damaged areas of myocardium. In therapeutic doses does not depress myocardial contractility or atrioventricular conduction.

℞ against ventricular tachyarrhythmia: IN, CH = IV (slowly, as 20 mg/mL sol): 1 mg/kg/dose, to be repeated prn after 20 min, or continuous IV infusion as 1 mg/mL sol: 0.020–0.050 mg/kg/min, to a maximum total dose of 5 mg/kg/24 hr

XYLOCAINE hydrochloride IV: inj

Caution: Excessive depression of cardiac conductivity may occur; ECG monitoring indicated during treatment.

Mannitol; osmotic diuretic

℞ test dose for oliguria: CH = IV: 0.2 g/kg/dose, injected within 3–5 min

℞ in cerebral edema: CH = IV: 1–2.5 g/kg/dose, injected as 15–25% sol over 30–60 min

†, OSMITROL, ‡: IV inj

Meperidine hydrochloride; synthetic narcotic analgesic agent; addictive

℞ against severe pain: CH = PO, SC, IM: 6 mg/kg/24 hr, div, prn every 4–6 hr (maximum single dose: 100 mg)

†, DEMEROL hydrochloride, ‡: tabl, elixir, inj

Caution: May produce respiratory depression, seizures, coma in some sensitive patients. Test dose advisable. Naloxone is antidote.

Metaproterenol sulfate; catecholamine analogue; β-adrenergic receptor agonist with relatively selective effect on $β_2$-adrenergic receptors

℞ bronchodilator: IN, CH (<6 yr of age) = PO: 1.3–2.6 mg/kg/24 hr div every 6–8 hr; >6 yr of age: 10–20 mg/dose administered 3–4 times daily

†, ALUPENT; METAPREL; syrup, tabl, inhalation

Methylphenidate hydrochloride; piperidine derivative structurally related to amphetamine; CNS stimulant with more prominent effects on mental than on motor activities

℞ in minimal brain dysfunction (MBD): drug treatment of MBD not recommended below the age of 3 yr or in nonstructured therapeutic situation. CH (over 3 yr) = PO: initiate treatment with 5 mg dose given at the onset of daytime activities and again 4–6 hr later; if needed, increase the dose at weekly intervals by increments of 5 mg/dose and adjust the size of the respective doses (early morning and mid-day) according to the response in the patient; daily dose

See KEY to abbreviations, p. 747; for further information about drugs, see package inserts.

Table AP–1. Drug Doses* (Drugs Listed Alphabetically by Generic Name) *Continued*

usually should not exceed 2 mg/kg/24 hr. To avoid insommia do not administer closer than 6 hr before bedtime.

Caution: Reduction of growth rate and weight gain might accompany prolonged use. Chronic abuse can lead to tolerance.

R in narcolepsy: PO: proceed for dosage adjustment as in MBD, with correction of the abnormal symptomatology as the end point.

RITALIN: tabl

Metoclopramide hydrochloride; gastrointestinal prokinetic agent that increases lower esophageal sphincter pressure and rate of gastric emptying, and augments gastrointestinal peristaltic activity. Use of this drug for the treatment of symptomatic gastroesophageal reflux in infants and children remains controversial. Drug is also used for the treatment of diabetic gastroparesis and as an adjunctive measure facilitating small bowel intubation when the tube does not pass the pylorus with conventional maneuvers. High-dose metoclopramide therapy has been shown to be an effective aid in the adjunctive management of nausea and vomiting associated with cancer chemotherapy.

R for gastroesophageal reflux or gastrointestinal dismotility: CH = PO: 0.1 mg/kg/dose administered 4 times a day

R for prevention of chemotherapy-induced emesis: 2–3 mg/kg/dose administered before and after chemotherapeutic drug; timing of dose and actual regimen are dependent on the specific chemotherapeutic agent administered.

Caution: Metoclopramide possesses dopamine receptor antagonist activity; thus, acute dystonic reactions may occur and are relatively frequent with high-dose therapy. Diphenhydramine may be used to treat metoclopramide (or phenothiazine)-induced acute dystonic reaction. It may be appropriate to co-administer diphenhydramine with high-dose metoclopramide to prevent dystonic reactions in patients receiving this therapy for nausea and vomiting associated with cancer chemotherapy.

†, REGLAN: tabs, syrup, inj

Mineral oil; indigestible liquid hydrocarbon with limited absorbability; lubricant

R mild laxative: PO: 0.5 mL/kg/dose

†, liquid petrolatum: plain liquid or emulsion

Morphine sulfate; narcotic analgesic agent; addictive

R against severe pain: CH = SC: 0.6–1.2 mg/kg/24 hr, div, prn every 4 hr, equivalent to 0.1–0.2 mg/kg/dose, to be repeated prn every 4 hr

†: inj

Caution: Overdose produces severe respiratory depression, hypothermia, coma. Naloxone antidotal.

Naloxone hydrochloride; opioid antagonist; nonaddictive

R in respiratory depression due to opioids: NB, IN, CH = IV, IM, SC: 0.01 mg/kg/dose, to be repeated prn after 2–3 min up to 3 times. After satisfactory response, the dose must be repeated every 1–2 hr, as long as opioid depression persists

NARCAN, NARCAN neonatal: inj

Nitroprusside; sodium nitrosylpentacyanoferrate Na_2-$Fe(CN)_5 \cdot NO \cdot 2H_2O$; vasodilator by direct action on smooth muscles of blood vessels; effect appears almost immediately and ends promptly, 1–10 min after stopping of administration of nitroprusside

R for emergency reduction of hypertension: IV infusion: Example: to prepare a solution of nitroprusside containing 0.1 mg/mL, dissolve 50 mg nitroprusside first in 2–3 mL 5% dextrose in water, and transfer this amount to 500 mL 5% D/W,* and start continuous infusion using a microdrip regulator or an infusion pump that allows precise measurement of flow; begin with infusion rate of 0.003 mg/kg/min (equivalent to 0.03 mL/kg/min of solution containing 0.1 mg/mL nitroprusside), and decrease or increase dosage according to response, for which there exists a wide dosage range (0.0005–0.008 mg/kg/min)

*Only 5% dextrose in water solution should be used to prepare nitroprusside solution, and no other drug should be added. To prevent decomposition of nitroprusside by exposure to light, protect infusion bottle and possibly tubing from light; for instance, by wrapping in aluminum foil.

Caution: Fall in arterial blood pressure is dose-dependent, with risk of hypotensive circulatory failure on overdosage if careful monitoring of blood pressure does not lead to prompt adjustment of infusion rate.

Note: In patients receiving concomitant antihypertensive medications, a smaller dosage of nitroprusside is required for comparable reduction of hypertension.

NIPRIDE: powder for preparation of solution prior to inj

Paraldehyde; cyclic ether compound that decomposes to acetaldehyde on exposure to light and air; rapidly acting hypnotic agent

R in status epilepticus: CH = IM (injection remote from nerves because of risk of damage): 0.15 g/kg/dose, corresponding to 0.15 mL/kg/dose of paraldehyde solution containing 1 g/mL; occasionally 1 additional dose may be given after 30 min, prn

Note: Use glass syringe, because paraldehyde reacts with plastic equipment. When given IV, injection should be slow and paraldehyde solution should be diluted with isotonic sodium chloride solution to lessen risk of thrombophlebitis. IV use is not recommended.

R to calm agitation: CH = PO, IM (PR, diluted in equal amount of olive oil): 0.15 mL/kg/dose, to be repeated prn after 4–6 hr

Caution: Before use, make sure that drug is not decomposed (acetaldehyde, acetic acid).

†, PARAL: liquid for inj, oral use (risk of gastric irritation), and rectal use.

See KEY to abbreviations, p. 747; for further information about drugs, see package inserts.

Table AP-1. Drug Doses* (Drugs Listed Alphabetically by Generic Name) *Continued*

Phenobarbital; central nervous system depressant with long duration of action; initially, hypnotic effect of 8–12 hr; tolerance to hypnotic effect may develop on continued use

℞ for sedation: IN, CH = PO, IM: 2–3 mg/kg/24 hr, div, every 8–12 hr

℞ for sleep; IN, CH = PO, IM: 2–3 mg/kg/dose, repeat prn after 12–24 hr

℞ as anticonvulsant for long-term therapy: IN, CH = PO: start with 1.5 mg/kg/24 hr, div, every 12 hr; increase according to tolerance and therapeutic effect to 4–6 mg/kg/24 hr, div, every 12 hr, or as single daily dose, preferably at bedtime in order to minimize daytime drowsiness from hypnotic effect

℞ as adjunct in treatment of status epilepticus: CH = IV: 5–7.5 mg/kg/1st dose, by slow IV injection; followed prn after interval of 5 min by 2.5–3 mg/kg/dose, to be repeated once prn. If status epilepticus has been interrupted by drugs not including a barbiturate, phenobarbital can be given IM: 5–10 mg/kg/dose, followed by PO anticonvulsant regimen

†, LUMINAL: elixir, tabl
phenobarbital sodium, †, LUMINAL sodium: inj

Phenytoin, diphenylhydantoin; anticonvulsant agent; effective also in certain types of cardiac arrhythmias; antiarrhythmic effects similar to those of lidocaine; delayed slow diastolic depolarization, diminished automaticity; may facilitate conduction in damaged myocardial areas; does not depress myocardial activity

℞ as anticonvulsant for long-term therapy: IN, CH = PO: 3–8 mg/kg/24 hr, div, every 12 hr

℞ as adjunct in the treatment of status epilepticus: CH = IV (slow infusion under monitoring of heart rate): 10–15 mg/kg/dose

℞ as adjunct in the treatment of ventricular tachyarrhythmia: CH = IV (over 5 min): 2–4 mg/kg/dose, to be repeated prn after 20 min

†, DILANTIN: oral susp
phenytoin sodium, †, DILANTIN sodium: caps, inj

Procainamide hydrochloride; antiarrhythmic agent with general cardiodepressant effects; diminished myocardial excitability (decreased threshold potential, prolonged refractory period), reduced conduction velocity, diminished automaticity; decreases myocardial contractility; effects similar to those of quinidine

℞ for ventricular tachyarrhythmia: IN, CH = IM: 20–30 mg/kg/24 hr, div, every 4–6 hr; IV loading dose 10–15 mg over 30 min followed by continuous IV maintenance infusion of 20–80 μg/kg/min; PO: 15–50 mg/kg/24 hr, div, every 3–6 hr. Serum concentration should be monitored for both procainamide and its active metabolite N-acetyl procainamide (NAPA).

†, PRONESTYL: tabl, caps, inj

Promethazine hydrochloride; phenothiazine with aliphatic side chain

℞ for sedation, prevention or treatment of motion sickness, and as antihistamine: CH = PO: 1 mg/kg/24 hr, divided into half dose at bedtime and quarter doses every 6 hr of the remaining daytime

†, PHENERGAN: syrup, tabl, suppos

Propranolol hydrochloride; β-adrenergic blocking agent (β₁ and β₂); racemic mixture of D- and L-propranolol, of which only L form has adrenergic blocking activity

℞ against selected forms of supraventricular and ventricular tachycardia: IN, CH = IV: 0.01–0. 10 mg/kg/dose given slowly; repeat every 6–8 hr prn. PO: 0.5–4 mg/kg/24 hr, div, every 6–8 hr

℞ as antihypertensive in long term therapy. CH = PO: initially 1 mg/kg/24 hr div, every 6 hr, and progressive increase of dosage, if needed up to 5 mg/kg/24 hr, div every 6 hr.

Combination with diuretic and/or hydralazine indicated, because propranolol blocks physiologic compensatory mechanisms such as adrenergic inotropic and chronotropic responses, as well as renin activity.

℞ for prevention of migraine attack in severe cases and to combat the manifestations of thyrotoxicosis: Propranolol requirements vary widely from patient to patient because of individual differences in severity of underlying disease, endogenous sympathetic neuronal activity, sensitivity of β-adrenergic receptors to blockade, degree of protein binding, hepatic blood flow. For comparable effect, oral dose 6–10 times higher than intravenous dose in spite of good absorption from the gut because of inactivation of important fraction of propranolol in liver after entrance through portal vein.

Measures in case of exaggerated response: against bradycardia, atropine, if no response, isoproterenol, *cautiously;* against cardiac failure, digitalization and diuretics; against hypotension, epinephrine; against bronchospasm, isoproterenol, theophylline (aminophylline)

INDERAL: tabl, inj

Spironolactone; aldosterone antagonist and potassium-sparing diuretic, which interferes with sodium reabsorption

℞ as diuretic in selected cases (with normal renal function), most effective in combination with a potassium-wasting diuretic: CH = PO: 1.5–3 mg/kg/24 hr, div, every 4–8 hr

Note: Monitoring of serum concentration of potassium, of potassium intake, and of renal function is indicated during treatment with spironolactone.

ALDACTONE: tabl

Terbutaline sulfate, catecholamine; β-adrenergic receptor agonist with preferential effect on β₂-adrenergic receptors

℞ bronchodilator: Dosage in pediatric age group not firmly established. PO: 0.10–0.15 mg/kg/24 hr, div, every 8 hr. β₂-selectivity is reduced with increasing dosage or on parenteral administration. SC: 0.005

See KEY to abbreviations, p. 747; for further information about drugs, see package inserts.

760 Appendices

Table AP–1. Drug Doses* (Drugs Listed Alphabetically by Generic Name) *Continued*

mg/kg/dose, to be repeated prn after 20 min, once only
BRETHINE, BRICANYL: tabl, inj

Theophylline; methylxanthine commonly used in acute and chronic management of reversible airways disease (asthma), and neonatal apnea, bronchopulmonary dysplasia, among others. Cellular mechanism of action originally believed to be a result of phosphodiesterase inhibition; however, pharmacologic effect is most likely a result of adenosine receptor antagonism.

Ŗ in neonatal apnea: IV, PO: initial loading dose 5 mg/kg followed by maintenance therapy depending on age: preterm NB (<36 wk): 1–2 mg/kg/24 hr, div, every 8–12 hr; term infants (>36 wk): 2–4 mg/kg/24 hr, div, every 8–12 hr

Ŗ in status asthmaticus: Initial loading dose IV: 4–7 mg/kg/dose, infused after dilution in equal volume of intravenous fluid over 20–30 min, followed by maintenance IV: 20 mg/kg/24 hr, div, every 4–6 hr, or by continuous IV drip; switch to PO maintenance as soon as possible. Daily theophylline dose adjustment necessary relative to patient age and hepatic and cardiac function.

Ŗ oral maintenance: PO: 20 mg/kg/24 hr, div, every 6 hr; as conditions permit, taper to lowest effective dosage, usually around 10 mg/kg/24 hr, div, every 6 hr. Time-release theophylline preparations permit extension of the dosage interval (i.e., administration every 8–12 hr).

Note the content of theophylline in the following formulations; theophylline (anhydrous), 100%; aminophylline, 85%; theophylline monoethanolamine, 75%; dihydroxypropyltheophylline, 70%; oxtriphylline, choline salt, 64%; theophylline sodium glycinate, 50%; theophylline calcium salicylate, 48%. Serum concentration should be monitored; therapeutic range for neonatal apnea, 7–13 mg/L: in the management of bronchospasm, 10–20 mg/L.

theophylline, †, ELIXOPHYLLIN elixir, ELIXICON oral susp, SLOPHYLLIN caps, oral susp, SOMOPHYLLIN caps, ‡; component of many combination products
aminophylline, †, SOMOPHYLLIN oral liquid, ‡: inj, oral preparations
Caution: Circulatory collapse, seizures, coma may result from acute or chronic overdose.

Valproate sodium, dipropylacetate sodium; anticonvulsant agent with singular mode of action (effective probably by increasing γ-aminobutyric acid in brain tissues)

Ŗ in the treatment of simple petit mal and of complex absence seizures, either alone or in combination with other drugs (see reservation below) according to the results: CH = PO: start with 15 mg/kg/24 hr, div, every 8–12 hr; if needed, dosage increased by weekly increments of 5–10 mg/kg/24 hr up to a maximum recommended dose of 30 mg/kg/24 hr, div, every 8 hr

Caution: Concomitant use of valproate sodium and clonazepam might result in petit mal status. Blood concentrations of phenobarbital and phenytoin may be affected by addition of valproate sodium to the regimen.
DEPAKENE: caps (valproic acid), syrup (valproate sodium)

Verapamil; calcium channel blocker; toxic effects include allergic reactions, urticaria, bronchospasm, hypotension, decreased cardiac output, and asystole. Cardiac monitoring should be used during administration.
IN = IV: 0.1–0.2 mg/kg infused over 2 min
CH = IV: 0.1–0.3 mg/kg infused over 2 min
Maintenance dose = 1–2 mg/kg q 8 hr
CALAN, ISOPTIN: IV 2.5 mg/mL vial inj, PO tabs: 80, 120 mg

(Modified from Behrman RE [ed]: Nelson Textbook of Pediatrics. 14th ed. Philadelphia, WB Saunders, 1992, pp 1827–1844.

See KEY to abbreviations, p. 747; for further information about drugs, see package inserts.

Table AP–2. Drug Interactions of Potential Importance in Pediatric Practice (Partial Listing)*

Interacting Drugs	Adverse Effects	Interacting Drugs	Adverse Effects
Acetaminophen		Salicylates	↓ Absorption
Alcohol	Hepatotoxicity	Tetracycline	↓ Absorption
Oral anticoagulants	↑ Anticoagulation	Theophylline	↑ Toxicity
Probenecid	↑ Acetaminophen toxicity		
Zidovudine	Granulocytopenia	*Aspirin*	
		Anticoagulants (oral)	↑ Bleeding
Acyclovir		Captopril	↓ Antihypertensive effect
Narcotics	↑ Narcotic toxicity?		
Zidovudine	Lethargy	*Barbiturates*	
		Anticoagulants (oral)	↓ Anticoagulation
Alcohol		Beta-adrenergic blockers	↓ Beta-blockade
Antidepressants (tricyclic)	↑ Toxicity	Carbamazepine	↑ Production of carbamazepine epoxide
Barbiturates	↑ CNS depression (acute)		
Benzodiazepines	↑ CNS depression	Chloramphenicol	↑ Barbiturate toxicity
Cephalosporins (not all)	Disulfiram effect	Contraceptives (oral)	↓ Contraception
Chloral hydrate	↑ CNS depression	Corticosteroids	↓ Steroid effect
Doxycycline	↓ Antibiotic effect	Influenza vaccine (viral)	↑ Barbiturate toxicity
Isoniazid	↑ Hepatotoxicity	Rifampin	↓ Barbiturate effect
Metronidazole	Disulfiram effect	Theophylline	↓ Theophylline effect
Phenothiazines	Impaired coordination	Valproate	↑ Barbiturate toxicity
Phenytoin	↑ Phenytoin toxicity		
		Bleomycin	
Allopurinol		Oxygen	↑ Pulmonary toxicity
Aluminum hydroxide	↓ Allopurinol absorption		
Ampicillin	Rash	*Captopril*	
Anticoagulants (oral)	↑ Anticoagulant effect	Allopurinol	↑ Cutaneous hypersensitivity
Azathioprine	↑ Azathioprine toxicity		
Captopril	↑ Cutaneous hypersensitivity	Aspirin	↓ Antihypertensive effect
		Cimetidine	Neuropathy
Cyclophosphamide	↑ Cyclophosphamide toxicity	Nonsteroidal anti-inflammatory agents	↓ Antihypertensive effect
Theophylline	↑ Theophylline toxicity	Potassium	Hyperkalemia
Thiazide diuretics	↑ Allopurinol toxicity	Spironolactone	Hyperkalemia
Aminoglycoside Antibiotics		*Carbamazepine*	
Amphotericin B	↑ Nephrotoxicity	Anticoagulants (oral)	↓ Anticoagulation
Bumetanide	↑ Ototoxicity	Antidepressants (tricyclic)	↑ Both toxicities
Cisplatin	↑ Nephrotoxicity	Cimetidine	↑ Carbamazepine toxicity
Cyclosporine	↑ Nephrotoxicity	Contraceptives (oral)	↓ Contraception
Furosemide	↑ Nephrotoxicity and ototoxicity	Corticosteroids	↓ Steroid effect
		Cyclosporine	↓ Cyclosporine effect
Magnesium	↑ Neuromuscular blockade	Erythromycins	↑ Carbamazepine toxicity
		Influenza vaccine (viral)	↑ Carbamazepine toxicity
Neuromuscular blocking agents	↑ Blockade	Isoniazid	↑ Both toxicities
		Phenytoin	↓ Carbamazepine effect
Vancomycin	↑ Nephrotoxicity?	Theophylline	↓ Theophylline effect
		Valproate	↓ Valproate effect
Antacids			
Beta-adrenergic blockers	↓ Absorption	*Cimetidine*	
Captopril	↓ Absorption	Alcohol	↑ Alcohol effect
Cimetidine	↓ Absorption	Antacids	↓ Cimetidine effect
Corticosteroids	↓ Absorption	Anticoagulants (oral)	↑ Anticoagulation
Digoxin	↓ Absorption	Antidepressants (tricyclic)	↑ Antidepressant toxicity
Iron	↓ Absorption	Benzodiazepines	↑ Benzodiazepine toxicity
Isoniazid	↓ Absorption	Beta-adrenergic blocking agents	↑ Beta-blockade toxicity
Ketoconazole	↓ Absorption		
Nonsteroidal anti-inflammatory agents	↓ Absorption	Captopril	Neuropathy
		Carbamazepine	↑ Carbamazepine toxicity
Phenytoin	↓ Absorption	Digoxin	↑ Digoxin toxicity

Table AP–2. Drug Interactions of Potential Importance in Pediatric Practice (Partial Listing)* *Continued*

Interacting Drugs	Adverse Effects	Interacting Drugs	Adverse Effects
Ketoconazole	↓ Ketoconazole absorption	*Isoniazid*	
		Alcohol	Hepatitis
Metoclopramide	↓ Cimetidine effect	Antacids	↓ INH absorption
Phenytoin	↑ Phenytoin toxicity	Carbamazepine	↑ Toxicity (both)
Theophylline	↑ Theophylline toxicity	Ketoconazole	↓ Ketoconazole effect
		Phenytoin	↑ Phenytoin toxicity
Contraceptives (Oral)		Rifampin	↑ Hepatotoxicity
Anticoagulants (oral)	↓ Anticoagulation	Valproate	↑ Hepatic and CNS toxicity
Antidepressants (tricyclic)	↑ Antidepressant toxicity		
Barbiturates	↓ Contraception	*Ketoconazole*	
Carbamazepine	↓ Contraception	Antacids	↓ Absorption
Griseofulvin	↓ Contraception	Anticoagulants (oral)	↑ Anticoagulation
Penicillins (ampicillin, oxacillin)	↓ Contraception?	Cimetidine	↓ Ketoconazole effect
		Cyclosporine	↑ Nephrotoxicity
Phenytoin	↓ Contraception	Isoniazid	↓ Ketoconazole effect
Rifampin	↓ Contraception	Phenytoin	Altered metabolism of both drugs
Theophylline	↑ Theophylline toxicity		
		Rifampin	↓ Effects of both drugs
Cyclosporine			
Alkylating agents	↑ Nephrotoxicity	*Methotrexate:*	
Aminoglycosides	↑ Nephrotoxicity	Blood transfusion	↑ Toxicity
Amphotericin B	↑ Nephrotoxicity	Cisplatin	↑ Methotrexate toxicity
Carbamazepine	↓ Cyclosporine effect	Etretinate	↑ Hepatotoxicity
Erythromycins	↑ Cyclosporine toxicity	Nonsteroidal anti-inflammatory agents	↑ Methotrexate toxicity
Furosemide	Gout		
Ketoconazole	↑ Nephrotoxicity	Trimethoprim–sulfamethoxazole	Megaloblastic anemia
Metoclopramide	↑ Cyclosporine toxicity		
Nafcillin	↓ Cyclosporine effect	*Metoclopramide*	
Phenytoin	↓ Cyclosporine effect	Carbamazepine	Neurotoxicity
Rifampin	↓ Cyclosporine effect	Cimetidine	↓ Cimetidine effect
		Cyclosporine	↑ Cyclosporine toxicity
Digoxin		Digoxin	↓ Absorption
Antacids	↓ Absorption	Narcotics	↑ Sedation
Anticholinergics	↑ Digoxin toxicity		
Cholestyramine	↓ Absorption	*Nifedipine*	
Cimetidine	↑ Digoxin toxicity	Beta-adrenergic blockers	Heart failure, A-V block
Diuretics (hypokalemia)	↑ Digoxin toxicity	Cyclosporine	↑ Gingival hyperplasia
Phenytoin	↓ Digoxin effect	Phenytoin	↑ Phenytoin toxicity
Quinidine	↑ Digoxin toxicity	Prazosin	Hypotension
Verapamil	↑ Digoxin toxicity	Quinidine	↓ Quinidine effect
Erythromycins		*Phenytoin*	
Anticoagulants (oral)	↑ Anticoagulation	Alcohol	↑ Toxicity (acute)
Astemizole (Hismanal)	↑ Astemizole toxicity: arrhythmias	Antacids	↓ Phenytoin effect
		Anticoagulants (oral)	↑ Phenytoin toxicity, ↑ ↓ Anticoagulation
Carbamazepine	↑ Carbamazepine toxicity		
Cyclosporine	↑ Cyclosporine toxicity	Antidepressants (tricyclic)	↑ Phenytoin toxicity
Phenytoin	↓ Phenytoin effect	Carbamazepine	↓ Carbamazepine effect
Terfenadine (Seldane)	↑ Terfenadine toxicity: arrhythmias	Chloramphenicol	↑ Toxicity (both)
		Cimetidine	↑ Phenytoin toxicity
Theophylline	↑ Theophylline toxicity	Contraceptives (oral and implant)	↓ Contraception
Fluoroquinolones		Corticosteroids	↓ Corticosteroid effect
Antacids	↓ Antibiotic effect	Cyclosporine	↓ Cyclosporine effect
Theophylline	↑ Theophylline toxicity	Digoxin	↓ Digoxin effect
		Dopamine	Hypotension
Griseofulvin		Folic acid	↓ Phenytoin effect
Anticoagulants (oral)	↓ Anticoagulation		
Contraceptive (oral)	↓ Contraception		

Table AP–2. Drug Interactions of Potential Importance in Pediatric Practice (Partial Listing)* *Continued*

Interacting Drugs	Adverse Effects	Interacting Drugs	Adverse Effects
Isoniazid	↑ Phenytoin toxicity	Quinidine	↓ Quinidine effect
Miconazole	↓ Phenytoin effect	Theophylline	↓ Theophylline effect
Neuromuscular blocking agents	↓ Blockade	Verapamil	↓ Verapamil effect
Nifedipine	↑ Phenytoin toxicity	***Theophylline***	
Quinidine	↓ Quinidine effect	Barbiturates	↓ Theophylline effect
Rifampin	↓ Phenytoin effect	Beta-adrenergic blockers	↑ Theophylline toxicity
Theophylline	↓ Effects (both)	Carbamazepine	↓ Theophylline effect
Valproate	↑ Phenytoin toxicity	Cimetidine	↑ Theophylline toxicity
		Erythromycins	↑ Theophylline toxicity
Quinidine		Fluoroquinolones	↑ Theophylline toxicity
Amiodarone	↑ Quinidine toxicity	Influenza vaccine (viral)	↑ Theophylline toxicity
Anticoagulants (oral)	↑ Anticoagulation	Interferon	↑ Toxicity?
Barbiturates	↓ Quinidine effect	Marijuana smoking	↓ Theophylline effect
Cimetidine	↑ Quinidine toxicity	Phenytoin	↓ Effect (both)
Digoxin	↑ Digoxin toxicity	Rifampin	↓ Theophylline effect
Metoclopramide	↓ Quinidine effect	Tobacco smoking	↓ Theophylline effect
Phenytoin	↓ Quinidine effect	Troleandomycin	↑ Theophylline toxicity
Procainamide	↑ Procainamide toxicity		
Rifampin	↓ Quinidine effect	***Trimethoprim–Sulfamethoxazole***	
Verapamil	Hypotension	Anticoagulants (oral)	↑ Anticoagulation
		Antidepressants (tricyclic)	Depression
Rifampin		Mercaptopurine	↓ Antileukemia effect
Anticoagulants (oral)	↓ Anticoagulation	Methotrexate	Megaloblastic anemia
Barbiturates	↓ Barbiturate effect		
Beta-adrenergic blockers	↓ Beta-blockade	***Valproate***	
Chloramphenicol	↓ Chloramphenicol effect	Barbiturates	↑ Phenobarbital toxicity
Contraception (oral)	↓ Contraception	Benzodiazepines	↑ Diazepam toxicity
Corticosteroids	↓ Corticosteroid effect	Carbamazepine	↓ Valproate effect
Cyclosporine	↓ Cyclosporine effect	Cimetidine	↑ Valproate toxicity?
Isoniazid	↑ Hepatotoxicity	Ethosuximide	↑ Ethosuximide toxicity?
Ketoconazole	↓ Effects (both)	Phenytoin	↑ Phenytoin toxicity
Phenytoin	↓ Phenytoin effect		

* When possible, an alternate drug combination should be given. If not possible, drug levels *and* signs of toxicity must be monitored.

A-V = atrioventricular; CNS = central nervous system; INH = isoniazid; ? = possible effect.

Modified from Rizack M, Hillman C: The Medical Letter Handbook of Adverse Drug Interactions. New Rochelle, The Medical Letter, 1989.)

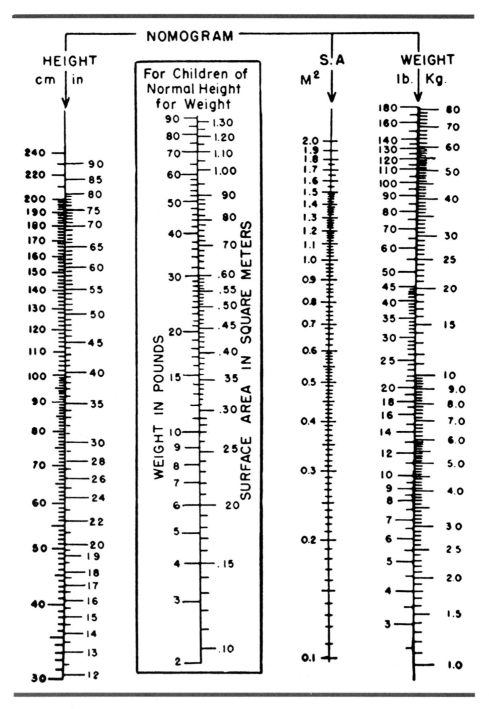

Figure AP–1. Nomogram for estimation of surface area. The surface area is indicated where a straight line that connects the height and weight levels intersects the surface area column; or the patient is roughly of average size, from the weight alone (enclosed area). (Nomogram modified from data of E. Boyd by C. D. West.)

Index

ISBN 0-7216-3775-2